Modern System of Ophthalmology (MSO) Series

Disorders of
Retina and Vitreous

Modern System of Ophthalmology (MSO) Series

Disorders of
Retina and Vitreous

Editor-in-Chief

AK Khurana MS, CTO (London)
Fellow, Moorfields Eye Hospital, London
Senior Professor and Head
Regional Institute of Ophthalmology
Pt BD Sharma Postgraduate Institute of Medical Sciences
Rohtak, Haryana

Editors

S Sood MS
Fellow, Vitreo-retina, Doheny Eye Institute, USA
Professor and Head
Vitreo-retina and Uvea Services
Department of Ophthalmology
Government Medical College, Chandigarh

Atul Kumar MD
Professor
Vitreo-retina Services
Dr RP Centre for Ophthalmic Sciences
All India Institute of Medical Sciences
New Delhi

Associate Editors

Subina Narang MS
Associate Professor, Vitreo-retina and Uvea
Department of Ophthalmology
Government Medical College and Hospital
Chandigarh

Aruj K Khurana DNB
Consultant Ophthalmologist
Cataract and Medical Retina Services
Nirmal Eye Institute
Rishikesh

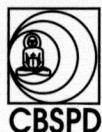

CBSPD

CBS Publishers & Distributors Pvt Ltd

New Delhi • Bengaluru • Chennai • Kochi • Kolkata • Lucknow • Mumbai
Hyderabad • Jharkhand • Nagpur • Patna • Pune • Uttarakhand

Modern System of Ophthalmology (MSO) Series

Disorders of Retina and Vitreous

ISBN: 978-81-239-2410-6

Copyright © AK Khurana

First Edition 2014
 Reprint   2019, **2025**

Published by Satish Kumar Jain and produced by Varun Jain for

CBS Publishers & Distributors Pvt Ltd

4819/XI Prahlad Street, 24 Ansari Road, Daryaganj, New Delhi 110 002, India.
Ph: 011-23266838, 23289259   Website: www.cbspd.com
                                                      e-mail: delhi@cbspd.com

Corporate Office: 204 FIE, Industrial Area, Patparganj, Delhi 110 092
Ph: 011-4934 4934   Fax: 011-4934 4935   e-mail: publishing@cbspd.com;
                                                                          publicity@cbspd.com

Branches

- **Bengaluru:** Seema House 2975, 17th Cross, KR Road, Banasankari 2nd Stage, Bengaluru 560 070, Karnataka, India
  Ph: +91-80-26771678/79   Fax: +91-80-26771680   e-mail: bangalore@cbspd.com
- **Chennai:** 7, Subbaraya Street, Shenoy Nagar, Chennai 600 030, Tamil Nadu, India
  Ph: +91-44-26680620, 26681266   Fax: +91-44-42032115   e-mail: chennai@cbspd.com
- **Kochi:** 42/1325, 1326, Power House Road, Opp KSEB, Power House, Ernakulum Kochi 682 018, Kerala, India
  Ph: +91-484-4059061-65,67   Fax: +91-484-4059065   e-mail: kochi@cbspd.com
- **Kolkata:** 147, Hind Ceramics Compound, 1st Floor, Nilgunj Road, Belghoria, Kolkata-700056, West Bengal, India
  Ph: +033-25633055, 033-25633056   e-mail: kolkata@cbspd.com
- **Lucknow:** Basement, Khushnuma Complex, 7 Meerabai Marg (Behind Jawahar Bhawan), Lucknow-226001, UP, India
  Ph: +0522-4000032   e-mail: tiwari.lucknow@cbspd.com
- **Mumbai:** PWD Shed, Gala no 25/26, Ramchandra Bhatt Marg, Next to JJ Hospital Gate no. 2, Opp. Union Bank of India, Noorbaug, Mumbai-400009, Maharashtra, India
  Ph: 022-66661880/89   e-mail: mumbai@cbspd.com

Representatives

• Hyderabad	0-9885175004	• Jharkhand	0-9811541605	• Nagpur	0-8692091830
• Patna	0-9334159340	• Pune	0-9664372571	• Uttarakhand	0-9716462459iv

Printed at   Magic International, Noida, UP, India

Foreword

It is indeed a pleasure for me to write the foreword to *Disorders of Retina and Vitreous* one of the eleven books in the series *Modern System of Ophthalmology* by Dr Ashok Khurana (Editor-in-Chief). I have known Dr Ashok Khurana as a very sharp observer in the clinics and a highly sought after author whose books in the past have been received with great enthusiasm by the students of ophthalmology. A concise and comprehensive series like this was much needed for the residents in ophthalmology.

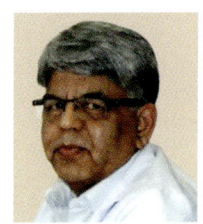

Undoubtedly highly specialized training and studies are required to manage patients with vitreo-retinal disorders. However, an advanced training in the subspeciality of vitreo-retina requires a strong foundation laid during the residency training itself. I appreciate the efforts of the editorial team in this regard for presenting a complete and up-to-date text in a very systematic manner for the trainee residents. The book comprises six sections, each covering, respectively, the relevant basic aspects, examination techniques, disorders of vitreous and retina, endophthalmitis and vitreo-retinal surgeries in detail. The book provides adequate material with recent advances in each chapter.

Dr Ashok Khurana has chosen Prof Sunandan Sood and Prof Atul Kumar, two of the most experienced teachers and eminent vitreo-retinal surgeons, to edit this volume. They have made an impressive collection of chapters. The contributors present a lucid and easy to comprehend text with the help of abundant high quality fundus photographs, angiograms, ultrasound scans and line diagrams.

I have no doubt, this volume of *Modern System of Ophthalmology*, like other volumes brought out by Prof Khurana, will serve as a highly useful resource for the residents and the general ophthalmologists alike. It will also serve as a handbook for vitreo-retinal fellows. I am quite confident that this work will be well received by the readership.

Amod Gupta
Professor and Head
Department of Ophthalmology
Advanced Eye Centre
Postgraduate Institute of
Medical Education and Research
Chandigarh, India

*M*odern System of Ophthalmology (MSO) series comprises separate volumes on different subspecialities of ophthalmology. Each volume is planned with a very specific aim to cater to the needs of postgraduate students in ophthalmology.

Salient Features of MSO Series

- Each volume is edited by different editors, yet the layout and organization has been kept similar for all the volumes.
- Editors of different volumes are masters in their subspeciality with an uncanny knack of picking up the right perspectives.
- Text matter is designed to meet the needs of residents in ophthalmology with a comprehensive coverage in a concise manner. Text is complete and up-to-date with recent advances incorporated.
- Text is organized in such a way that the students can easily understand, retain and reproduce it. Various levels of headings, subheadings, bold face and italics given in the text will be helpful for a quick revision of the subject.

Disorders of Retina and Vitreous. Disorders of retina and vitreous, most of the time need specialised services for management. However, it is imperative for each and every budding ophthalmologist to be well aware of these during their residency training. Therefore, this volume has been primarily planned to provide information on the principles and practice of disorders of vitreous and retina to residents in ophthalmology. An attempt has been made to present the subject in a more easily understood form. In a bid to simplify the text, at places the description looks more dogmatic than is warranted by the facts.

The text has been arranged in six sections. Section 1 is devoted to embryology, anatomy and physiology of retina and vitreous covering both basic and applied aspects. Section 2 is on examination and investigative techniques and covers all the available modalities. Sections 3 and 4 cover in detail various disorders of vitreous and retina. Section 5 is on endophthalmitis with a comprehensive coverage. Section 6 describes vitreo-retinal surgeries in detail.

Editors of this volume Prof S Sood, Head, Department of Ophthalmology, GMCH, Chandigarh, and Prof Atul Kumar, Vitreo-retina Services, Dr RP Center for Ophthalmic Sciences, AIIMS, New Delhi, are dedicated masters and renowned posterior segment surgeons. This volume is an outcome of their devotion and hard work. The Associate Editors, Dr Subina Narang, Associate Professor, Department of Ophthalmology, GMCH, Chandigarh, and Dr Aruj K Khurana, Consultant, Cataract and Retina Services, Nirmal Eye Institute, Rishikesh, have also contributed actively.

Compilation of this volume has been made possible due to the chapters received from many selfless contributors. My sincere thanks are due to all of them. I am grateful to Dr Amod Gupta, Professor and Head, AEC, PGIMER, Chandigarh, for providing Figs 21.5 to 21.9 and Prof MR Dogra for providing figures for the chapter on retinopathy of prematurity. I want to express my gratitude to Prof CS Dhull, Director, PGIMS, and Prof SS Sangwan, Vice-Chancellor, UHS, Rohtak, for providing an atmosphere conducive to such academic activities. I shall also like to thank Dr Atul Sachdev, Director-Principal, GMCH, Chandigarh, for providing an excellent academic atmosphere and encouraging Prof S Sood and Dr Subina Narang. My gratitude is also to Dr RV Azad, Chief of Dr RP Center for Ophthalmic Sciences, AIIMS, New Delhi, for encouraging Padma Shri Prof Atul Kumar, an eminent vitreo-retinal surgeon of India from his center.

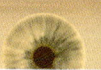

The enthusiastic cooperation received from Mr SK Jain, Managing Director, Mr YN Arjuna, Senior Director—Publishing, Editorial and Publicity, and Mrs Ritu Chawla, Manager—Production, CBS Publishers & Distributors, New Delhi, needs special acknowledgement. Mr. Sanju, graphic artist, and Mrs Jyoti Kaur, DTP operator, need special mention because of their efforts to provide considerable beauty to this volume.

In spite of the best efforts, a venture like this is unlikely to be error-free. Constructive criticism and suggestions from the readers are invited for further improvements in this volume.

AK Khurana
Editor-in-Chief

Editorial Board and Contributors

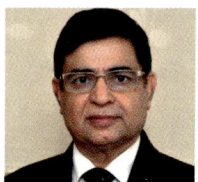
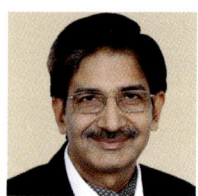
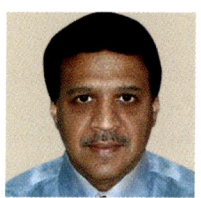
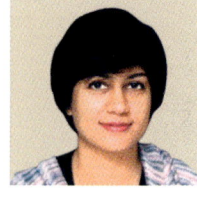
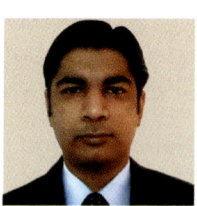

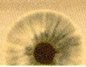

Bhawna Khurana MS DNB
Consultant Ophthalmologist
Nirmal Eye Institute, Rishikesh

G Suguneshwari MS
Ocular Oncology and Vitreo-retina
Sankara Nethralaya, Chennai

Indu Khurana MD
Senior Professor, Department of Physiology
Pt BD Sharma Postgraduate Institute of
Medical Sciences, Rohtak, Haryana (India)

Manisha Nada MS
Professor, RIO
PGIMS, Rohtak

MR Dogra MS
Professor
Advanced Eye Centre
PGIMER, Chandigarh

Michael T Trese MD
Consultant
Associated Retina Consultant
Royal Oak, MI, USA

Mohan Raj MS
SR, RPCOS
AIIMS, New Delhi

Mohit Dogra MS
SR, Department of Ophthalmology
GMCH, Chandigarh

Neha Khurana MS
SR, Department of Ophthalmology
GMCH, Chandigarh

Panchmi Gupta
JR, Department of Ophthalmology
GMCH, Chandigarh

Parul Chawla MS
SR, Department of Ophthalmology
GMCH, Chandigarh

Parul Ichhpujani MS
Assistant Professor
Department of Ophthalmology
GMCH, Chandigarh

Pradeep Venktesh MS
Associate Professor, Vitreo-retina, RPCOS
AIIMS, New Delhi

Pratik Topiwala
SR, Department of Ophthalmology
GMCH, Chandigarh

Rajiv Gupta MS
Consultant Grewal Eye Institute
Chandigarh

RK Bansal MS
Assistant Professor
Department of Ophthalmology
GMCH, Chandigarh

Reema Bansal MS
Consultant AEC
PGIMER, Chandigarh

Ritu Gera
SR, Department of Ophthalmology
GMCH, Chandigarh

Sandhya Hegde
Fellow, Ocular Oncology and Vitreo-retina
Department of Ophthalmology
Sankara Nethralaya, Chennai

Shaveta Bhayana
SR, Department of Ophthalmology
GMCH, Chandigarh

Shibal Bhartiya
Consultant, Fortis Hospital
Department of Ophthalmology
Gurgaon

Shyna Kansal Jain
SR, Department of Ophthalmology
GMCH, Chandigarh

Thirumalesh MD
SR, RPCOS, AIIMS
New Delhi

Vikas Khetan
Consultant, Ocular Oncology
and Vitreo-retina
Department of Ophthalmology
Sankara Nethralaya, Chennai

Contents

SECTION 1: DEVELOPMENT, ANATOMY AND PHYSIOLOGY OF RETINA AND VITREOUS

SECTION 2: EXAMINATION AND INVESTIGATIVE TECHNIQUES FOR RETINA AND VITREOUS

SECTION 3: DISORDERS OF VITREOUS

SECTION 4: DISORDERS OF RETINA

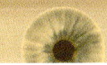

SECTION 5: ENDOPHTHALMITIS

SECTION 6: VITREORETINAL SURGERIES

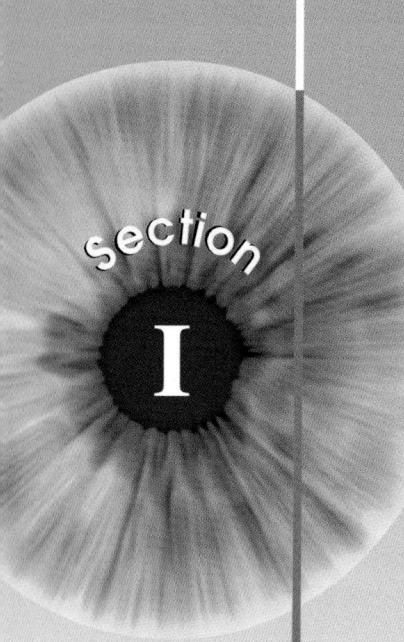

1 DEVELOPMENT AND ANATOMY OF RETINA

AK Khurana, Indu Khurana,
Aruj K Khurana, Bhawna Khurana

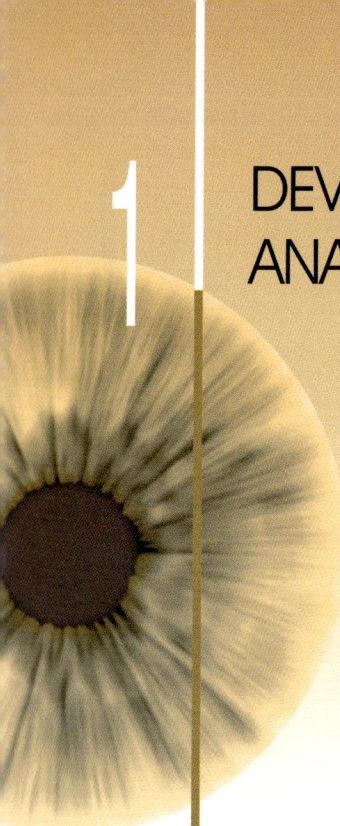

DEVELOPMENT OF RETINA

FORMATION OF OPTIC VESICLE AND OPTIC STALK

The first evidence of primitive eye formation occurs during the third week of gestation. The region of neural plate (Fig. 1.1A), which is destined to form the prosencephalon shows a linear thickened area on either side (Fig. 1.1B), which soon becomes depressed to form the optic sulcus (Fig. 1.1C). Meanwhile the neural plate becomes converted into prosencephalic vesicle. As the optic sulcus deepens, the walls of the prosencephalon overlying the sulcus bulge out to form the *optic vesicle* (Fig. 1.7D and E). The proximal part of the optic vesicle becomes constricted and elongated to form the *optic stalk* (Fig. 1.1F to H).

FORMATION OF THE OPTIC CUP

During the fourth week of gestation (embryo 7.6–7.8 mm), while the lens vesicle is forming, simultaneously the optic vesicle is converted into a double-layered *optic cup.* It appears from Fig. 1.2A to D that this has happened because the developing lens has invaginated itself into the optic vesicle. However, this is not so. The conversion of the optic vesicle to the optic cup is due to differential growth of the walls of the vesicle. The margins of optic cup grow over the upper and lateral sides of the lens to enclose it. However, such a growth does not take place over the inferior part of the lens, and therefore, walls of the cup show deficiency in this part. This deficiency extends to some distance along the inferior surface of the optic stalk and is called the *choroidal* or *fetal fissure* (Fig. 1.3). This embryonic ocular fissure closes by 6th week of gestation. When the lips of the fissure fail to fuse by 6th or 7th week, typical colobomas result. By the end of 7th week of gestation, most of the basic structures of the eye are present. Thereafter, ocular development is mainly a process of differentiation and modification, of various parts of the globe.

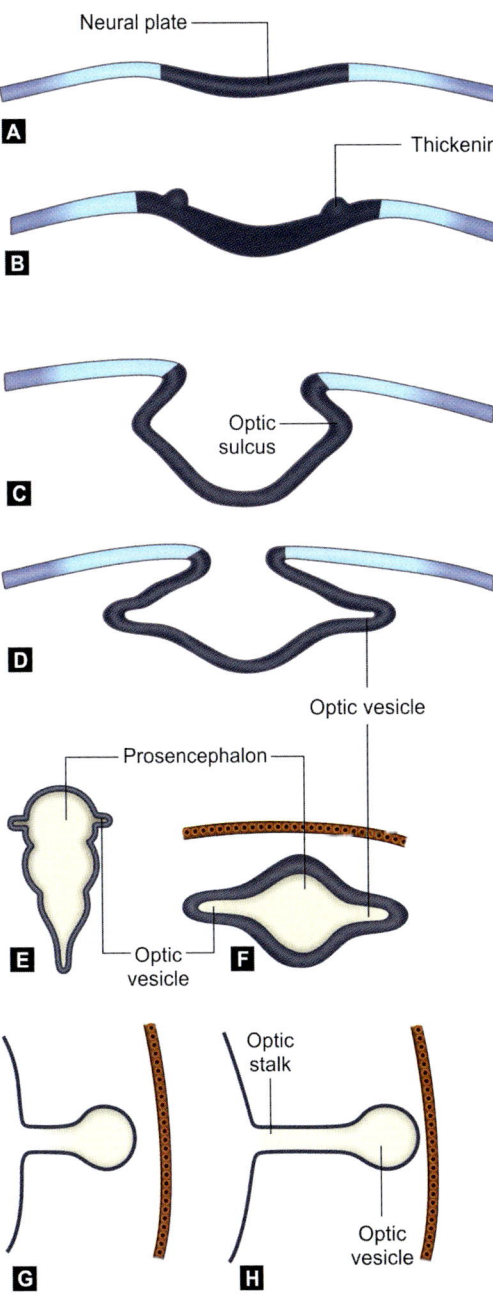

Fig. 1.1 *Formation of optic vesicle and optic stalk*

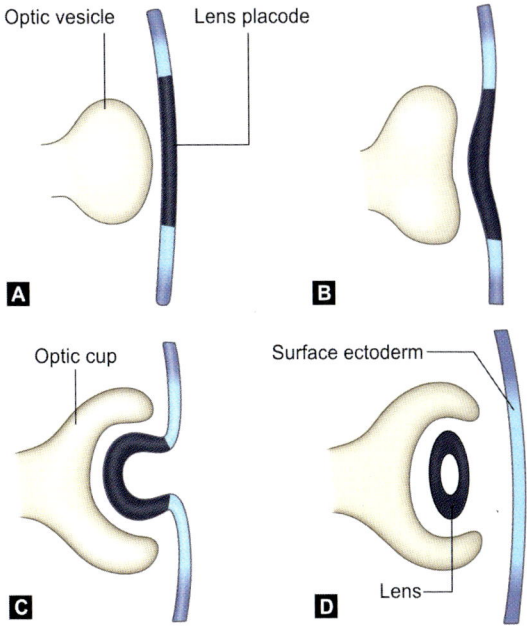

Fig. 1.2 *Formation of optic cup*

FORMATION OF RETINA

Retina is developed from the two parts of the optic cup: (a) Neurosensory retina from the inner wall and (b) Retinal pigment epithelium from the outer wall (Fig. 1.4).

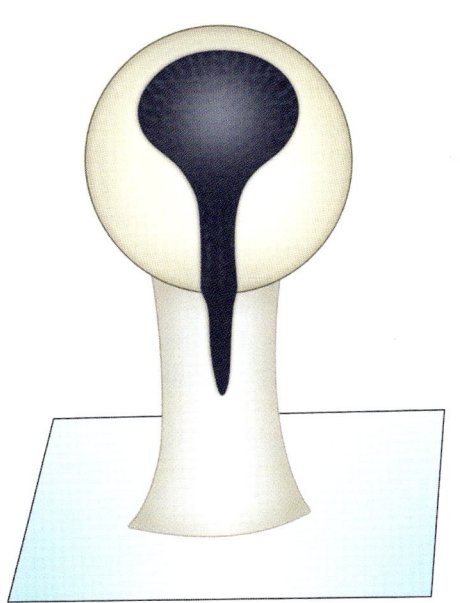

Fig. 1.3 *Optic cup and stalk seen from below to show the choroidal fissure*

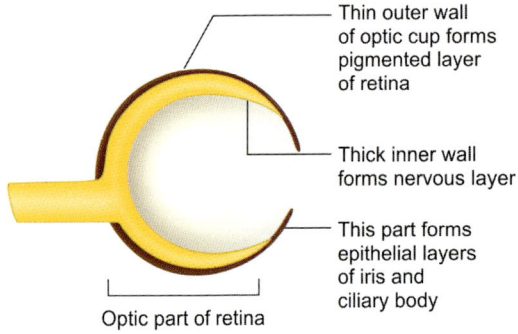

Thin outer wall of optic cup forms pigmented layer of retina

Thick inner wall forms nervous layer

This part forms epithelial layers of iris and ciliary body

Optic part of retina

Fig. 1.4 *Development of the retina*

NEUROSENSORY RETINA

Inner wall of the optic cup is a single-layered epithelium with an internal and an external basement membrane. As the development proceeds, this layer proliferates and during 4th–5th week of gestation, the primitive retina formed is arranged in two zones: an outer *primitive zone* (nuclear zone or germinal epithelium) filled with eight to nine rows of nuclei and an inner *marginal zone* (layer of HIS) devoid of nuclei (Fig. 1.5A).

The neuroepithelial cells actively divide by mitosis and by 6th to 7th week of gestation are differentiated into two layers, the *inner* and *outer neuroblastic layers.* These layers are separated by the *transient fiber layer of Chievitz*, which disappears subsequently (Fig. 1.5B).

The *inner neuroblastic layer* differentiates to form ganglion cells (the cells which develop first of all), Müller's cells and the amacrine cells.

The *outer neuroblastic layer* differentiates to form rods and cones, the bipolar cells and the horizontal cells.

The nerve fiber layer becomes identifiable on the inner aspect of the inner neuroblastic layer owing to the growth of ganglion cell axons that converge towards the optic stalk. A zone where the processes of cells from the inner neuroblastic layer intermingle (inner plexiform layer), becomes identifiable at approximately 10.5 weeks, thereby obliterating the transient layer of Chievitz (Fig. 1.5C). A new intermediate nuclear layer, the inner nuclear layer, becomes identifiable in the posterior pole retina and already contains the amacrine and Müller's cell bodies and shortly afterwards the bipolar and the horizontal cells differentiate from the outer neuroblastic layer and migrate into this new nucleated layer (Fig. 1.5C). The remaining components of the outer neuroblastic layer will form the outer nuclear layer containing the cell bodies of photoreceptors (rods and cones). The zone where fibers from this layer intermingle with those of the inner nuclear layer constitutes the new outer plexiform layer (Fig. 1.5D). The external limiting membrane (not a membrane per se) of the retina is identifiable in the early stages as rows of tight junctions between, adjacent neuroblasts. Thus the differentiation of the retinal layer starts during 6th week of gestation and by 5½ months of gestation all the layers of the adult retina are recognizable. In the macular area, the development is delayed up to 8th month of gestation. Further differentiation of the retina and specialization of the macular region continues until several months after birth.

Some important landmarks in retinal development include:
- Synaptogenesis in cone pedicles occurs at approximately 4 months and in rod spherules around 5 months.
- Photoreceptor outer segment formation commences around the 5th month.
- Horizontal cells become distinguishable around the 5th month.
- Microglia (resident tissue macrophages) invade the retina via the retinal vasculature (4 months) and peripheral subretinal space (10 weeks onwards).
- The terminal expansion of Müller's cells beneath the inner limiting membrane mature around 4.5 months, at around the same time as their processes can be identified between the rods and cones.

*A **brief summary*** of scheme of the general development of the retina and the pathway that the various cellular layers and membranes take in their formation is illustrated in Fig. 1.6.

RETINAL PIGMENT EPITHELIUM

Cells of the outer wall of the optic cup become pigmented around 6th week of gestation. Its posterior part forms the retinal pigment epithelium (RPE) of the retina and the anterior

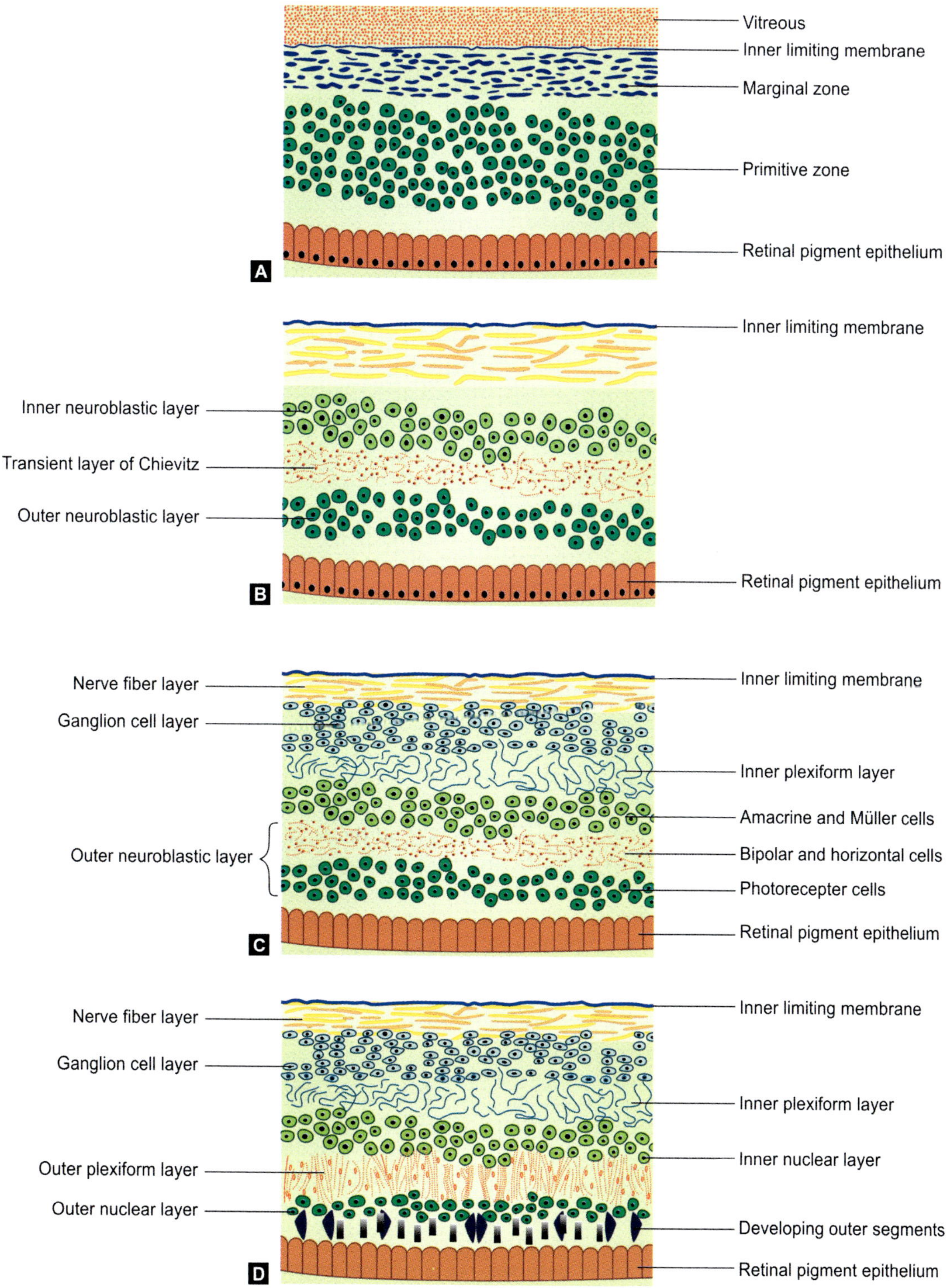

A

- Vitreous
- Inner limiting membrane
- Marginal zone
- Primitive zone
- Retinal pigment epithelium

B

- Inner limiting membrane
- Inner neuroblastic layer
- Transient layer of Chievitz
- Outer neuroblastic layer
- Retinal pigment epithelium

C

- Nerve fiber layer
- Ganglion cell layer
- Inner limiting membrane
- Inner plexiform layer
- Amacrine and Müller cells
- Outer neuroblastic layer
- Bipolar and horizontal cells
- Photorecepter cells
- Retinal pigment epithelium

D

- Nerve fiber layer
- Ganglion cell layer
- Inner limiting membrane
- Inner plexiform layer
- Inner nuclear layer
- Outer plexiform layer
- Outer nuclear layer
- Developing outer segments
- Retinal pigment epithelium

Fig. 1.5 *Zones of primitive retina during:* **(A)** *4th–5th week of gestation;* **(B)** *6th–8th week of gestation;* **(C)** *10th–12th week of gestation; and* **(D)** *4th month of gestation*

part continues forward in ciliary body and iris as their pigmented epithelium. Initially, the RPE comprises a mitotically active pseudostratified columnar ciliated epithelium. The cilia disappear as melanogenesis commences. The mitotic activity ceases by birth, thereafter growth of eye and consequently of the RPE itself is accommodated by hypertrophy or enlargement of existing cells. The mature RPE cells are hexagonal in shape, homogenous in size and in section appear as simple cuboidal epithelium.

ANATOMY OF RETINA

Retina, the innermost tunic of the eyeball, is a thin, delicate and transparent membrane. Its thickness at the posterior pole in the peripapillary region is approximately 0.56 mm, at

the equator 0.18 to 0.2 mm, and at the ora serrata approximately 0.1 mm. It is the most highly developed tissue of the eye. It appears purplish-red due to visual purple of the rods. After death of a person, the retina appears white opaque.

GROSS ANATOMY

Retina extends from the optic disc to the ora serrata and has a surface area of about 266 mm.[2] Grossly, on ophthalmoscopic examination it can be divided into three distinct regions: optic disc, macula lutea and rest of the peripheral retina (general fundus) (Fig. 1.7A and B).

OPTIC DISC

• It is a pale pink, well-defined circular area of about 1.5 mm diameter. The color of the disc is seldom uniformly pink and the tint shows considerable variations within normal limits.

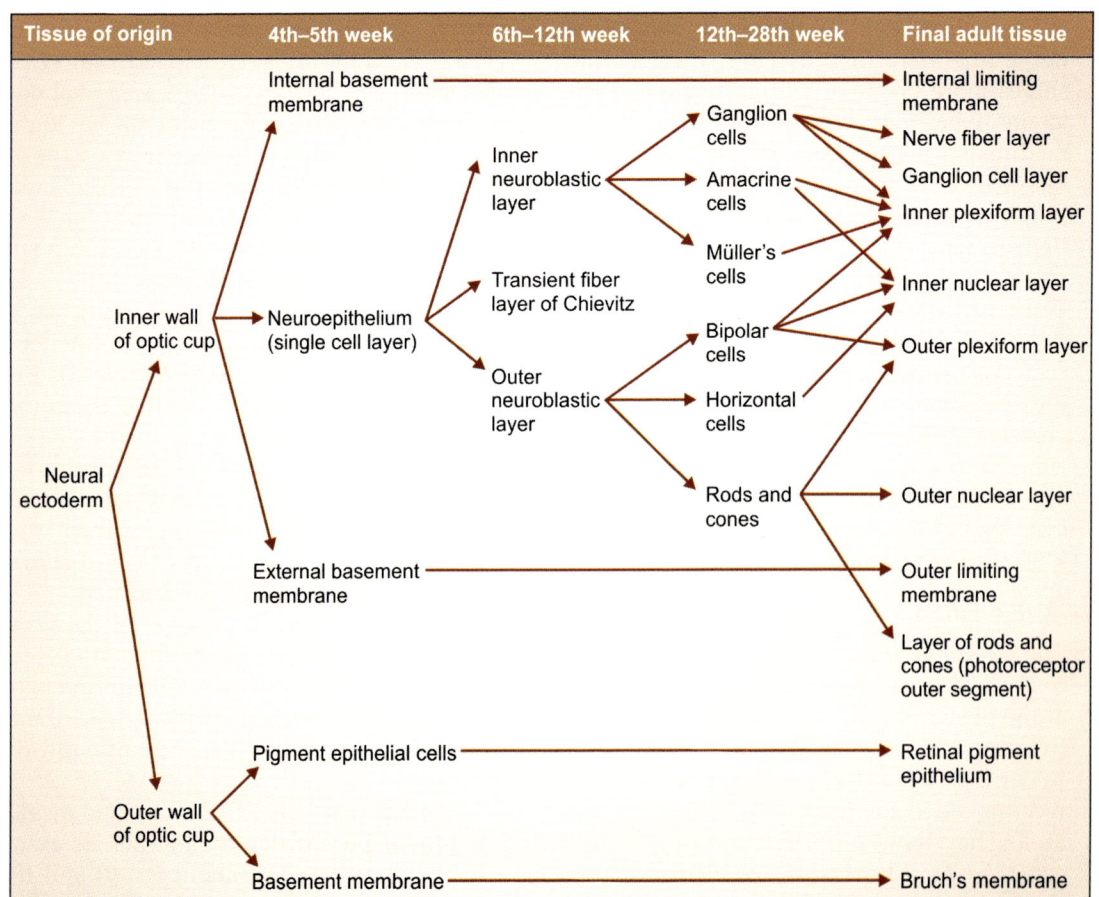

Fig. 1.6 *A schematic flowchart showing the cellular origin of various layers of the retina during embryogenesis*

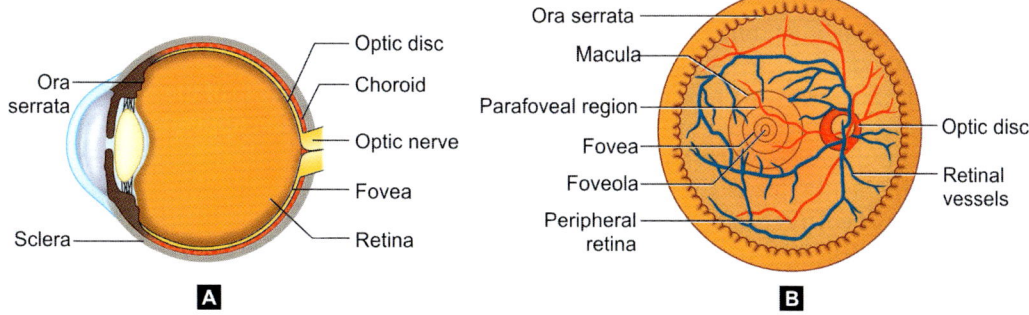

Fig. 1.7 *Gross anatomy of the retina*

- At the optic disc, all the retinal layers terminate except the nerve fibers, which pass through the lamina cribrosa (sieve-like sclera) to run into the optic nerve.
- In comparison to the rest of retina, the optic disc appears white due to lamina cribrosa and medullated nerve fibers behind it and absence of vascular choroid. In the center, where the nerve fibers are thinnest, the white lamina shines more brightly. The grey spots in the lamina, when they are seen, are due to the non-medullated nerve fibers reflecting less light than the white connective tissue fibers.
- The physiological cup of the optic disc is a depression seen in it. The central retinal vessels emerge through the centre of this cup. The cup varies in size, shape, position and depth in different eyes. Sometimes there is scarcely any physiological cup, in which case the disc is more uniformly pink and the central vessels may have already divided before they come to the surface. Increase in the size of the cup and/or difference in the size of cup of two eyes should be watched with suspicion and investigated to exclude glaucoma.

MACULA LUTEA

- The *macula lutea* (yellow spot) is a comparatively dark area 5.5 mm in diameter, situated at the posterior pole of the eyeball, temporal to the optic disc.
- Recently, Tripathi and Tripathi have recommended the term *area centralis* for this area. They have reported that in fact area *centralis* is a horizontally ellipsed area demarcated approximately by the upper and lower arcuate and temporal retinal vessels. It corresponds to approximately 15° of the visual field and that photopic vision and color vision are primarily functions of this area. Tripathi and Tripathi have also recommen-ded that the term *macula lutea* should be used for an oval zone of yellow coloration (about 3 mm in diameter, with the centre being the foveola) which can be seen with red-free light. However, they further reported that with special optical devices macular area of about 5 mm in diameter can be observed having a faint yellow color. Introduction of these different terms—the area centralis, macula lutea and macular area—has definitely caused confusion. However, the clinicians will have to bear this with the researchers.
- *Fovea centralis* is the central depressed part of the macula. It is about 1.85 mm in diameter and about 0.25 mm in thickness. It corresponds to 5° of visual field and is the most sensitive part of the retina.
  - *Foveola* (0.35 mm in diameter) forms the central floor of the fovea. It is situated about 2 disc diameter (3 mm) away from the temporal edge of the optic disc and about 1 mm below the horizontal meridian.
  - The *umbo* is a tiny depression in the very centre of the foveola which corresponds to the ophthalmoscopically visible foveolar reflex, seen in most normal eyes. Loss of the foveolar reflex may be an early sign of damage.
  - *Foveal avascular zone* (FAZ) is located inside the fovea but outside the foveola, its exact diameter is variable (about 500 μ) and its location can be determined with accuracy only by fluorescein angiography.

- Surrounding the fovea are *parafoveal* and *perifoveal* areas about 0.5 mm and 1.5 mm in diameter, respectively.

PERIPHERAL RETINA

The peripheral retina can be divided into four regions:

Near periphery. The near periphery refers to a circumscribed region of about 1.5 mm around the area centralis.

Mid periphery. The mid periphery occupies a 3 mm wide zone around the near periphery.

Far periphery. The far periphery is a region that extends from the optic disc, 9–10 mm on the temporal side and 16 mm on the nasal side in the horizontal meridian. Location of optic disc on the nasal side accounts for this asymmetry.

Ora serrata. It is the serrated peripheral margin where the retina ends and ciliary body starts. The dentate processes, consisting of tooth-like extensions of the retina on the pars plana separated by oral bays, are well marked on the nasal half of the retina. At the ora, the sensory retina is firmly attached both to the vitreous and retinal pigment epithelium. Ora serrata is 2.1 mm wide temporally and 0.7–0.8 mm wide nasally. Its distance from the limbus is 6.0 mm nasally and 7.0 mm temporally. It is located 6–8 mm away from the equator and 25 mm from the optic nerve on the nasal side.

MICROSCOPIC STRUCTURE OF THE RETINA

Retina consists of 3 types of cells and their synapses arranged (from without inward) in the following layers (Fig. 1.8):
1. Retinal pigment epithelium
2. Layer of rods and cones
3. External limiting membrane
4. Outer nuclear layer
5. Outer molecular (plexiform) layer
6. Inner nuclear layer
7. Inner molecular (plexiform) layer
8. Ganglion cell layer
9. Nerve fiber layer
10. Internal limiting membrane

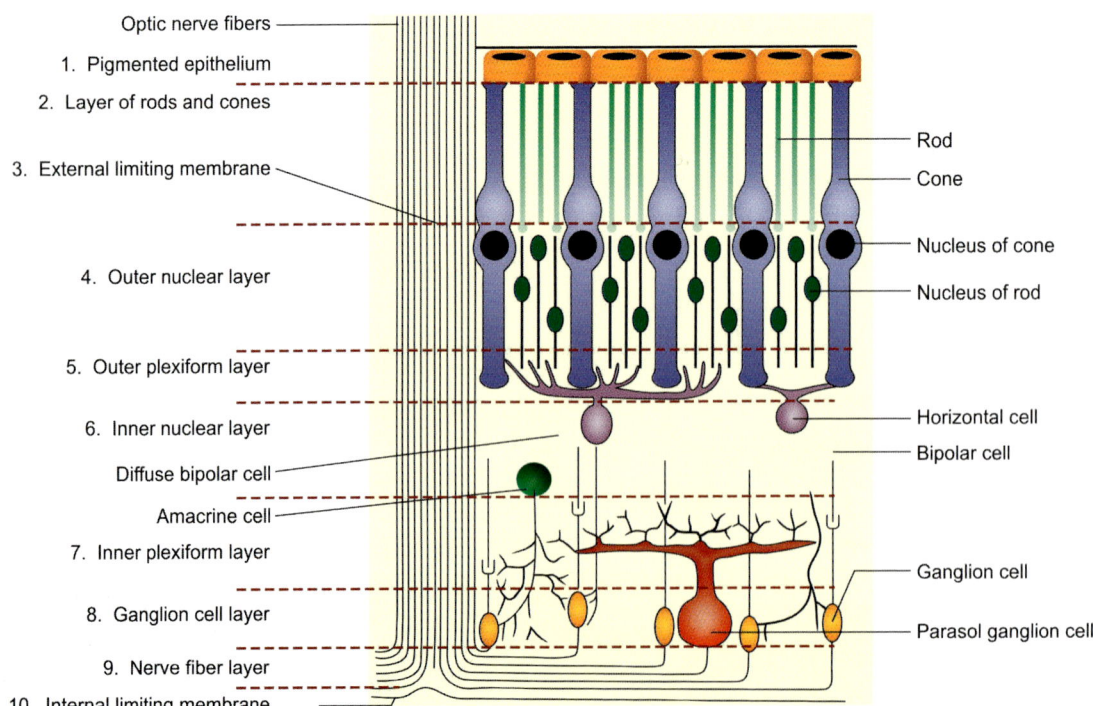

Fig. 1.8 *Microscopic structure of the retina*

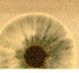

1. RETINAL PIGMENT EPITHELIUM (RPE)

It is the outermost layer of retina. It consists of a single layer of hexagonal-shaped cells containing pigment. The RPE cells show fine mottling due to unequal pigmentation of the cells and this is responsible for granular appearance of the fundus. RPE is firmly adherent to the underlying Bruch's membrane (basal lamina of the choroid) and loosely attached to the layer of rods and cones. The potential space between RPE and the sensory retina is called subretinal space. A separation of the RPE from the sensory retina is called retinal detachment, and the fluid between the two layers is called subretinal fluid (SRF).

Electron microscopy shows that adjacent RPE cells are connected with each other by tight junctions (zonulae occludens and zonulae adherens) and constitute the outer blood-retinal barrier. The RPE cells at the fovea are taller, thinner, and contain more and larger pigment granules than elsewhere in the fundus, thereby giving a dark color to this area. The optical part of RPE cells is formed by the microvilli which project between the rods and cones processes.

Functions of RPE

- Plays important role in photoreceptor renewal and recycling of vitamin A.
- Maintains integrity of subretinal space by forming outer blood-retinal barrier and actively pumping ions and water out of this (subretinal) space.
- RPE is involved with transport of nutrients and metabolites through the blood-retinal barrier and elaboration of the extracellular matrix.
- Probably RPE cells have phagocytic action.
- Provides mechanical support to the processes of photoreceptors.
- They manufacture pigment which presumably has an optical function in absorbing light.

2. LAYER OF RODS AND CONES (NEUROEPITHELIUM)

DENSITY AND DISTRIBUTION OF PHOTORECEPTORS

- Rods and cones *(photoreceptors)* are the end organs of vision which transform light energy into visual (nerve) impulse.

- Rods contain a photosensitive substance visual purple *(rhodopsin)* and subserve the peripheral vision and vision of low illumination (scotopic vision).
- Cones also contain a photosensitive substance and are primarily responsible for highly discriminatory central vision (photopic vision) and color vision.
- There are about 120 million rods and 6.5 million cones.
- The highest density of cones is at fovea with an average of 199000 cones/mm², but their number is highly variable and ranges from 100000 to 324000 cones/mm² with the highest density in an area as large as 0.032 degree. The number of cones falls off rapidly outside the fovea; being only 6000 cones/mm² 3 mm away from fovea and about 4000 cones/mm² 10 mm away. Cone density is 40–45% greater on the nasal than on the temporal aspect of human retina, and slightly lower in the superior than in the inferior retina at the mid-periphery.
- Rods are absent at the fovea in an area of 0.35 mm (rod-free zone) which corresponds to 1.25° of the visual field; but are present in a large number (160,000/mm²) in a ring-shaped zone 5–6 mm from the fovea. These are maximum below the optic disc (170,000/mm²) and their number reduces towards the periphery. The entire nasal retina has 20–25% more rods than does temporal retina, and the superior retina has 2% more than the inferior retina.

STRUCTURE OF PHOTORECEPTOR

Each *photoreceptor* consists of a cell body and nucleus (which lie in the outer nuclear layer), cell process that extends into outer plexiform layer and inner and outer segments (which form the layer of rods and cones). The long axis of the photoreceptor is oriented perpendicular to the retinal surface.

THE ROD CELL (Fig. 1.9)

- Each rod is about 40–60 μm long.
- The *outer segment* of the rod is cylindrical, highly refractile, transversly striated and contains visual purple. It is composed of numerous lipid protein lamellar discs stacked one on top of the other and surrounded by a

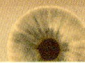

cell membrane. The number of discs varies between 600 and 1000/rod and each disc is 22.5–24.5 nm in thickness. The discs contain 90% of the visual pigment is scattered on the surface of plasmalemma. The outer segment is attached to the inner segment by a cilium with a characteristic of 9 + 0 configuration (nine doublets around the periphery with no central microtubule).

- The *inner segment* of the rod is thicker than the outer segment. It consists of two regions: ellipsoid and myoid.
  - *Ellipsoid* (the outer portion) is adjacent to the outer segment and contains abundant number of mitochondria.
  - *Myoid* (the inner portion) contains the glycogen as well as the usual organelles.
- *An outer rod fiber* arises from the inner end of rod, which passes through the external limiting membrane and swells into a densely staining nucleus—the rod granule (lies in the outer nuclear layer); and then terminates as *inner rod fiber* (lies in the outer molecular layer) which at its end has an end bulb called the rod spherule that is in contact with the cone foot.

THE CONE CELL (Fig. 1.10)

- Each cone cell is 40–80 µm long. It is largest at the fovea (80 um) and shortest at the periphery (40 µm).
- The *cone outer segment* is conical in shape, much shorter than that of rod and contains the iodopsin. The lamellar discs, which are narrower than those of the rods, maintain continuity with the surface plasma membrane. There are about 1000–1200 discs/cone.
- The *cone inner segment* and cilium are similar to the rod structures; however the cone ellipsoid is very plump and contains a large number of mitochondria.
- Unlike rod, the inner segment of the cone becomes directly continuous with its nucleus and lies in outer nuclear layer. A stout cone inner fiber runs from the nucleus which at the end is provided with lateral processes called *cone foot* or *cone pedicle* (lies in the outer plexiform layer).

The interphotoreceptor matrix (IPM) and inter-photoreceptor retinoid binding protein (IRBP)
The IPM occupies the space between the photo-receptor outer segments and the retinal pigment epithelium. It is a complex structure consisting

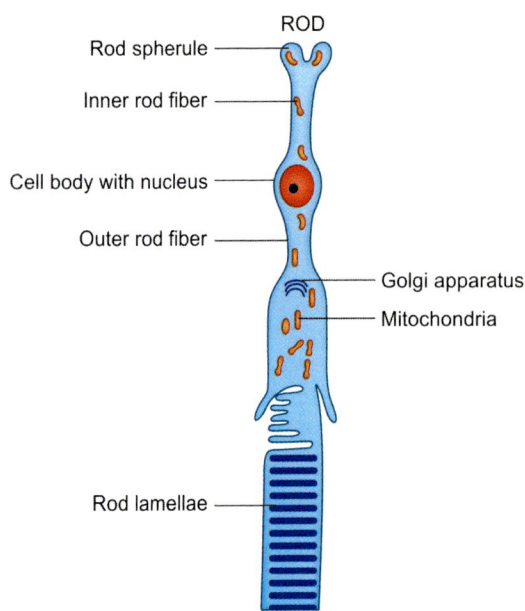

Fig. 1.9 *Microscopic structure of a rod cell*

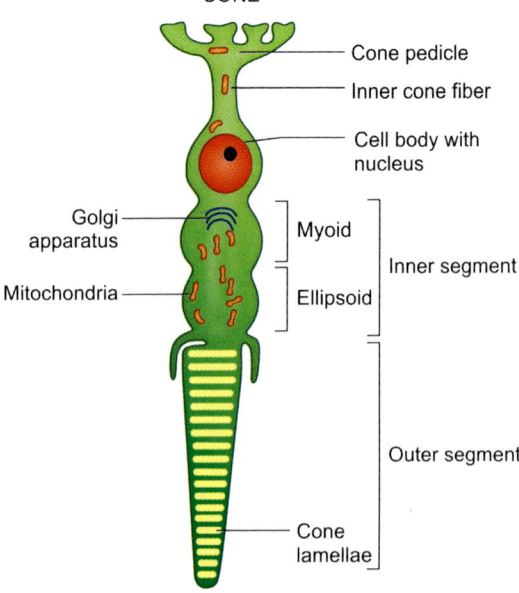

Fig. 1.10 *Microscopic structure of a cone cell*

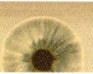

of proteins, glycoproteins, GAGs and proteo-glycans such as chondroitin sulphate. The IPM has a diverse range of functions, including retinal attachment and adhesions in molecular trafficking, facilitation of phagocytosis and probably photoreceptor outer segment alignment IRBP accounts for 70% of the soluble proteins in the IPM. In humans, it is produced by photoreceptors (mainly cones) and can bind all-*trans-retinol*, 14-*cis*-retina, α-tocopherol, retinoic acid and cholesterol. Although the primary function of IRBP is the efficient trans-port of retinoids between the photoreceptors and the retinal pigment epithelium, it may also serve to minimize fluctuations in retinoid availability, and to protect the plasma membranes from the damaging effects of high retinoid concentrations. IRBP is not the only binding protein found in the retina. Cellular retinoid binding proteins are a subgroup of the fatty acid binding proteins that orchestrate reisomerisation in the retinal pigment epithelium and may also have a role in early retinal development. Cellular fatty acid binding proteins (cellFABP) are also found in the retina. They protect retinal processes from toxic effects of fatty acids and take part in cell growth and differentiation.

3. *EXTERNAL LIMITING MEMBRANE*

In low magnification, it appears as a fenestrated membrane extending from the ora serrata to the edge of the optic disc; through which pass processes of the rods and cones. Electron microscopy studies show that the external limiting membrane is formed by the junctions (zonulae adherentes) between the cell membrane of photoreceptors and Müller's cells and thus it is not a basement membrane.

4. *OUTER NUCLEAR LAYER*

This layer is primarily formed by the nuclei of rods and cones; cone nuclei are somewhat larger (6–7 μm) than the rod nuclei (5.5 μm) and lie in a single layer next to the external limiting membrane. Rod nuclei form the bulk of this multilayered outer nuclear layer except in the cone dominated foveal region. The number of rows of nuclei and thickness of this layer varies from region to region as follows:

- Nasal to the disc—8 to 9 layers of nuclei and 45 μm thickness.
- Temporal to disc—4 rows of nuclei and 22 μm thickness.
- Foveal region—10 rows of nuclei and 50 μm thickness.
- Rest of the retina except ora serrata—one row of cone nuclei and 4 rows of rod nuclei with a thickness of 27 mm.

5. *OUTER PLEXIFORM LAYER*

This layer contains the synapses between the rods spherules and cone pedicles with the dendrites of the bipolar cells and processes of the horizontal cells (Fig. 1.11). In other words, this layer marks the junction of the end organs of vision and first-order neurons in the retina. It is thickest at the macula (51 μm) and consists predominantly of oblique fibers that have deviated from the fovea and is also known as Henle's layer.

6. *INNER NUCLEAR LAYER*

Under microscope, this layer resembles the outer nuclear layer except that it is very thin. This layer disappears at fovea and in rest of the retina consists of the following:
- Bipolar cells
- Horizontal cells
- Amacrine cells
- The soma of the Müller's cells
- Capillaries of the central retinal vessels.

I. BIPOLAR CELLS (NEURONS)

These are the neurons of first order of vision. The body of the bipolar cells consists entirely of the nucleus which lies in the inner nuclear layer. Their dendrites arborize with the rod spherules and cone pedicels in the outer plexiform (molecular) layer and their axons arborize with the dendrites of ganglion cells in the inner molecular layer. On the basis of morphology and synaptic relationship, nine types of bipolar cells are seen under light microscopy:
- Rod bipolar cells
- Invaginating midget bipolar cells
- Flat midget bipolar cells
- Invaginating diffuse bipolar cells
- Flat diffuse bipolar cells
- On-centre blue cone bipolar cells

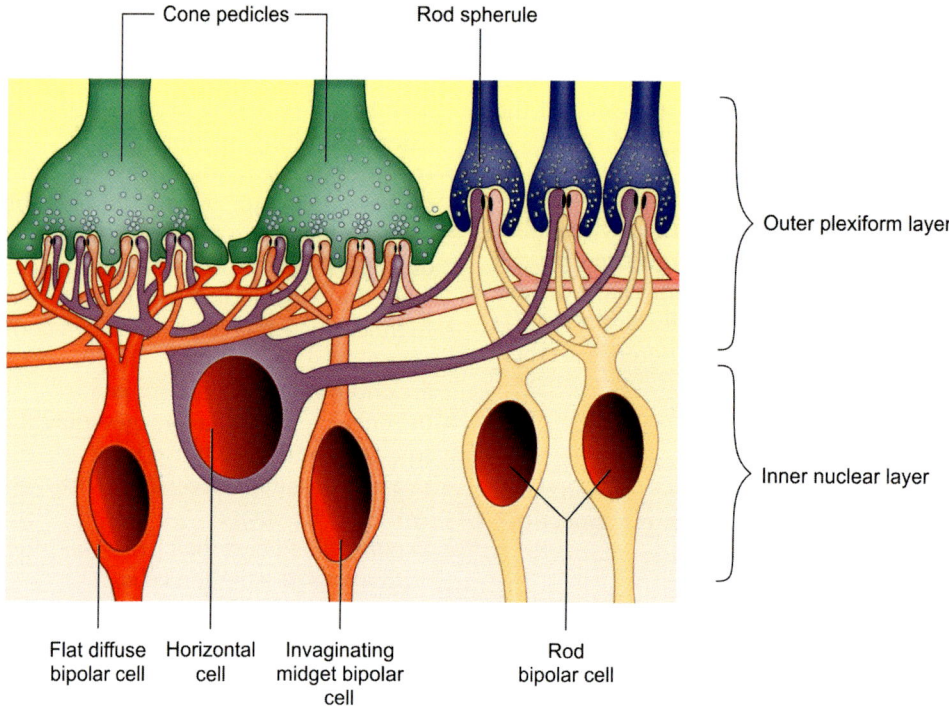

Cone pedicles   Rod spherule

Outer plexiform layer

Inner nuclear layer

Flat diffuse | Horizontal | Invaginating | Rod
bipolar cell | cell | midget bipolar | bipolar cell
| | cell |

Fig. 1.11 *Cell connections in outer plexiform layer*

- Off-centre blue cone bipolar cells
- Giant bistratified bipolar cells
- Giant diffuse invaginating bipolar cells.

Rod bipolar cells. These have large soma and profuse dendrites which arborize only with the rod spherules. Axons of these bipolar cells have synapses with the soma of up to four ganglion cells (Figs 1.11 and 1.12). These constitute about 20% of the total bipolar cells.

Midget bipolar cells. Invaginating midget cells are relatively small and make connections only in the triads of cone pedicle. Their dendrites deeply invaginate the cone pedicle. The *flat midget bipolar cells* resemble the invaginating midget bipolar cells except that they do not invaginate but make a superficial contact with the cone pedicle. Their axons synapse with a single ganglion cell (Figs 1.11 and 1.12).

Flat and invaginating diffuse bipolar cells. Their dendrites make contact with the cone pedicle only but not with their triads and their axons synapse with a number of ganglion cells of all types (Fig. 1.12).

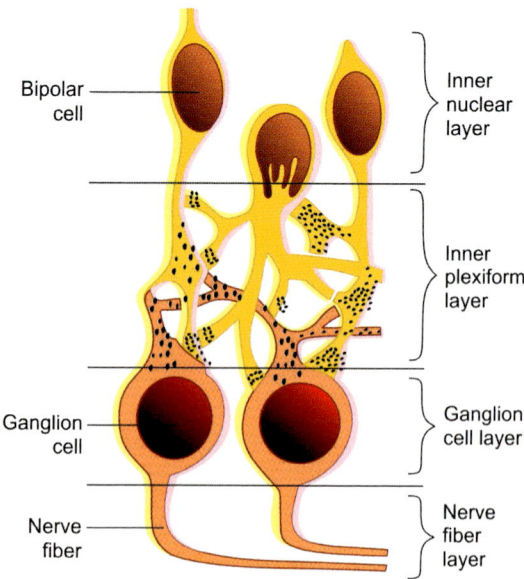

Bipolar cell

Inner nuclear layer

Inner plexiform layer

Ganglion cell

Ganglion cell layer

Nerve fiber

Nerve fiber layer

Fig. 1.12 *Cell connections in inner plexiform layer*

Blue-cone bipolar cells. There are two types of blue cone bipolar cells—the ON-centre or BBb variety and OFF-center or BBa variety. Like the

diffuse bipolar cells, blue cone bipolars innervate more than one pedicle. The axon terminal of ON-center cells arborize in stratum 5 and that of OFF-center cell arborize in stratum 1 of the inner plexiform layer.

Giant bipolar cells. These are of two types— giant bistratified and giant diffuse invaginating bipolar cells which are distinguished by the extent of their dendritic spread. Giant diffuse bipolar cells are morphologically similar to flat diffuse cells except for the difference in their dendritic fields.

II. HORIZONTAL NEURONS

- These are flat cells having numerous horizontal associative and neuronal interconnections between photoreceptors and bipolar cells in the outer plexiform layer.
- The *type A horizontal cells* have seven groups of dendrites which have contact with triad of seven cone pedicles and their single axon has contact (perhaps) with distant cone triad.
- The *type B horizontal cells'* dendrites have contact with rod receptors only and (perhaps) their axons with the distant rod cells.

III. AMACRINE CELLS

These cells are situated within the innermost part of this layer. These have a piriform body and a single process which passes inwards in the inner plexiform layer and forms connections with the axons of the bipolar cells and the dendrites and soma of the ganglion cells. Thus they perform an integrative function similar to that of the horizontal cells (Fig. 1.12).

IV. MÜLLER'S CELLS

The nucleus and cell bodies of the Müller's cells are located within the inner nuclear layer. Fibers from their outer ends extend up to the external limiting membrane and those from their inner ends reach up to the internal limiting membrane. In contrast to most other elements of the retina which possess either a photoreceptive or neural function, the Müller's cells provide structural support and contribute to the metabolism of the sensory retina. Their role in various layers is as follows:

- In external limiting membrane, junctions between the terminal parts of the fibers form the outer ends of the Müller's cells and cell membrane of the photoreceptors form the external limiting membrane.
- In outer nuclear layer, the Müller's cells provide reticulum around the cells somata.
- In outer plexiform layer, the major processes of Müller's cell produce side branches which form the horizontal extending reticulum.
- In inner nuclear layer, lie their cell bodies and secondary branches form the reticulum around the various cell somata.
- In inner plexiform layer, they play the same role as in outer plexiform layer.
- In layer of ganglion cells, provide reticulum around cell somata.
- In nerve fiber layer, their processes interweave with axons of ganglion cells.
- In internal limiting membrane, the inner fibers of the Müller's cells take part in the formation of this membrane.

V. OTHER GLIAL CELLS

In addition to Müller's cells, the retina contains other glial cells—astrocytes, microglia and (rarely) oligodendrocytes.

The astrocytes are most abundant and are located around the blood vessels.

7. *INNER PLEXIFORM LAYER*

This layer essentially consists of synapses between the axons of bipolar cells (first order neurons), dendrites of ganglion cells (second order neurons) and the processes of integrative Amacrine cells (Fig. 1.12).

Fibers from the Muller's cells courses vertically through this layer and their side branches form the horizontal extending reticulum.

This layer is absent at the foveola.

8. *GANGLION CELL LAYER*

The cell bodies and the nuclei of the ganglion cells (second order neurons of visual pathway) lie in this layer. Throughout most of the retina the ganglion cell layer is composed of a single row of cells, except in the macular region where it becomes multilayered (6–8 layers of the cells) and on temporal side of the disc where it has two

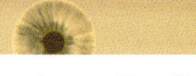

layers. Ganglion cell layer is absent in the region of foveola. Ganglion cells have been variously classified. A few of the popular classifications are as follows:

a. W, X and Y ganglion cells.
b. P (P_1 and P_2) and M ganglion cells.
c. OFF-centre and ON-centre ganglion cells.
d. Monosynaptic and polysynaptic ganglion cells.

MONOSYNAPTIC OR MIDGET GANGLION CELLS

These cells predominate in the central retina. Dendrite of each such cell synapses with the axon of the single midget bipolar cell (Fig. 1.12).

POLYSYNAPTIC GANGLION CELLS

These cells lie predominantly in peripheral retina. These cells have large dendritic fields and so synapse with multiple bipolar cells. There are complex connections between the dendrites of ganglion cells, axons of bipolar cells and amacrine neurons in the inner plexiform layer. The axons of the ganglion cells form the nerve fiber layer and then after passing through optic nerve, chiasma, and optic tracts, ultimately synapse with cells in the lateral geniculate body (third order neuron of visual pathway).

9. NERVE FIBER LAYER (STRATUM OPTICUM)

- This layer essentially consists of the unmyelinated axons of the ganglion cells which converge at the optic nerve head, pass through lamina cribrosa and become ensheathed by myelin posterior to lamina. In addition to axons of the ganglion cells (centripetal nerve fibers), this layer also contains the following:
- Centrifugal nerve fibers, which are thicker than the centripetal nerve fibers. Their exact origin and termination is not known.
- Processes of Müller's cells, which interweave with the axons of the ganglion cells.
- The neuroglial cells that are present in the nerve fiber layer are categorized as macroglia and microglia. Macroglia are constituted by two types of astrocytes (fibrous and proto-plasmic) derived from the neural crest. Microglia are small cells that are derived from the mesodermal invasion of the retina at the time of vascularization. Macroglia have a

structural role in the retina while microglial cells take the role of wandering tissue histiocytes in response to tissue injury and phagocytose debris which is carried to the vasculature for removal from the retina.
- Retinal vessels lie in the nerve fiber layer but as a rule do not project on the surface of retina. A rich bed of superficial capillary network is present in this layer (Fig. 1.17).

FEATURES OF NERVE FIBERS

The nerve fibers vary in their thickness from 0.5 to 2 µm and are non-myelinated. The cytoplasm of the axons contains microtubules, fine fibrils, mitochondria and occasional vesicles.

ARRANGEMENT OF NERVE FIBERS IN THE RETINA

In contrast to the remaining fibers of the sensory retina, which course perpendicular to the surface of the retina, the fibers within the nerve fiber layer course parallel to the surface in the following manner (Fig. 1.13):
- Fibers from the nasal half of the retina come directly to the optic disc as superior and inferior radiating fibers (srf and irf).
- Fibers from the macular region pass straight in the temporal part of the disc as papillo-macular bundle (pmb).
- Fibers from the temporal retina arch above and below the macular and papillomacular

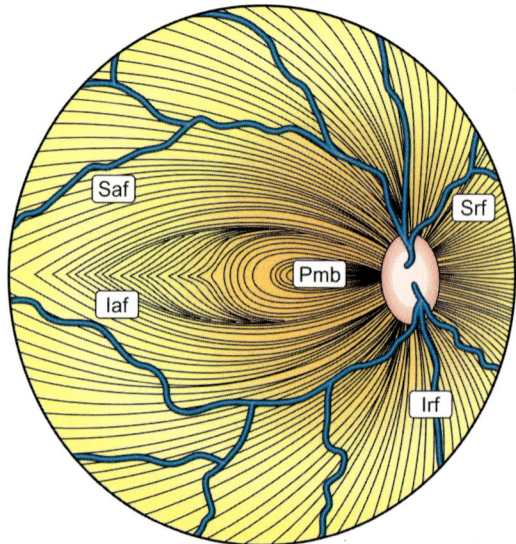

Fig. 1.13 *Arrangement of nerve fibers in the retina*

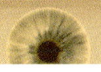

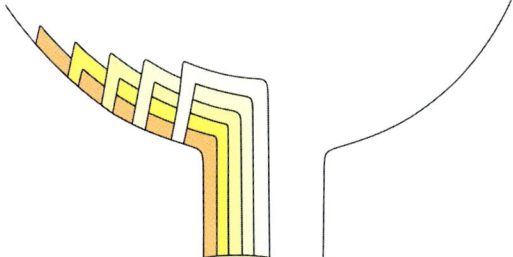

Fig. 1.14 *Arrangement of nerve fibers at the optic nerve head*

bundle as superior and inferior arcuate fibers (saf and iaf) with a horizontal raphe in between.

ARRANGEMENT OF NERVE FIBERS OF THE OPTIC NERVE HEAD

Fibers from the peripheral part of the retina lie deep in the retina but occupy the most peripheral (superficial) part of the optic disc. While the fibers originating closer to the optic nerve head lie superficially in the retina and occupy a more central (deep) portion of the disc (Fig. 1.14).

THICKNESS OF NERVE FIBER LAYER AT THE DISC

Thickness of the nerve fiber layer around the different quadrants of the optic disc margin progressively increases in the following order:
- Most lateral quadrant (thinnest)
- Upper temporal and lower temporal quadrant
- Most medial quadrant
- Upper nasal and lower nasal quadrant (thickest)

CLINICAL SIGNIFICANCE OF DISTRIBUTION AND THICKNESS OF NERVE FIBERS AT THE OPTIC DISC MARGIN

- Papilloedema appears first of all in the thickest quadrant (upper nasal and lower nasal) and last of all in the thinnest quadrant (most lateral).
- Arcuate nerve fibers which occupy the superior temporal and inferior temporal quadrants of optic nerve head are most sensitive to glaucomatous damage, accounting for an early loss in corresponding regions of visual field.
- Macular fibers occupying the lateral quadrant are most resistant to glaucomatous damage

and explain the retention of the central vision till end.

10. *INTERNAL LIMITING MEMBRANE*

It mainly consists of a PAS positive true basement membrane (unlike external limiting membrane) that forms the interface between retina and vitreous. The fibrils of the vitreous merge with the internal lamellae of this membrane. Externally, the basal foot processes of the Müller's cells abut with the membrane and probably play a role in its formation. Thus the internal limiting membrane consists of four elements:
- Collagen fibrils;
- Proteoglycans (mostly hyaluronic acid) of the vitreous;
- The basement membrane; and
- The plasma membrane of the Müller's cells and possibly other glial cells of the retina.

STRUCTURE OF FOVEA CENTRALIS

- In this area, there are no rods, cones are larger, in abundance and tightly packed, and other layers of retina are very thin (Fig. 1.15).
- Its central part (foveola) largely consists of cones and their nuclei covered by a thin internal limiting membrane. All other retinal layers are absent in the foveolar region.
- In the foveal region surrounding the foveola, the cone axons are arranged obliquely (Henle's layer) to reach the margin of the fovea.

BLOOD SUPPLY OF THE RETINA

- *Outer four layers* of the retina viz. pigment epithelium, layer of rods and cones, external limiting membrane, and outer nuclear layer get their nutrition from the choriocapillaris.
- *The six inner layers* viz. outer plexiform layer, inner nuclear layer, inner plexiform layer, layer of ganglion cells, nerve fiber layer and internal limiting membrane get their supply from the central retinal artery.
- The outer plexiform layer gets its blood supply partly from the central retinal artery and partly from the choriocapillaris by diffusion.
- The fovea is an avascular area mainly supplied by the choriocapillaris.
- *The macular region* gets its blood supply by small twigs from the superior and inferior

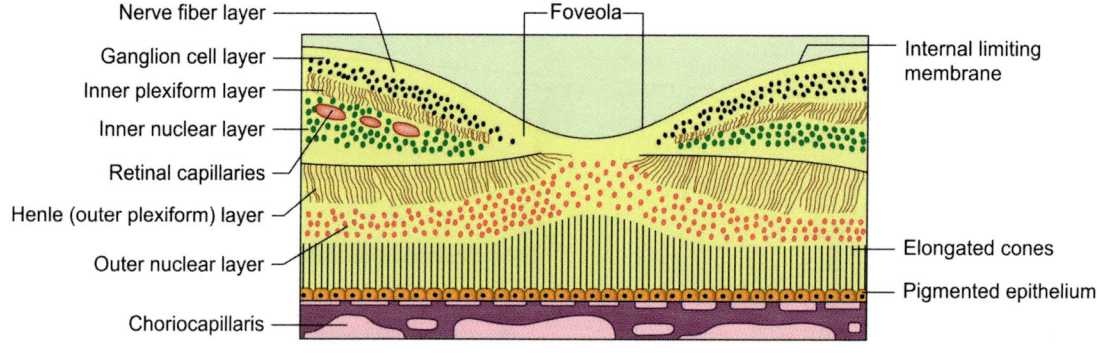

Nerve fiber layer

Ganglion cell layer

Inner plexiform layer

Inner nuclear layer

Retinal capillaries

Henle (outer plexiform) layer

Outer nuclear layer

Choriocapillaris

Foveola

Internal limiting membrane

Elongated cones

Pigmented epithelium

Fig. 1.15 *Microscopic structure of the fovea centralis*

temporal branches of central retinal artery. Sometimes, *cilioretinal artery* (a branch from the ciliary system of vessels) is seen originating in a hook-shaped manner within the temporal margin of the disc. It runs towards the macula and supplies it; thus, when present, it helps to retain the central vision in the event of occlusion of the central retinal artery.

- The retinal vessels are end arteries, i.e. they do not anastomose with each other. However, anastomosis between the retinal vessels and ciliary system of vessels does exist (in the neighbourhood of the lamina cribrosa) with the vessels which enter the optic nerve head from the arterial circle of Zinn or Haller. This arterial circle is formed by an anastomosis between 2 and 4 or more short posterior ciliary arteries and lies in the sclera around the optic nerve. From it, numerous branches pass forward to the choroid, inward to the optic nerve and backward to the pial network. Branches which pass inward, invade lamina cribrosa and also send branches to the optic nerve head and the surrounding retina.

CENTRAL RETINAL ARTERY

It arises from the ophthalmic artery near the optic foramen and courses ahead with 5–6 right angle bends as follows (Fig. 1.16):

- *Outside the optic nerve:* It runs a wavy course forward, below the optic nerve, but adherent to the dural sheath to about 10–15 mm behind the eyeball, where at a point along the inferomedial aspect of the nerve it bends

upwards to pierce the dura and arachnoid, from both of which it receive covering.

- *In the subarachnoid space:* It bends forwards and after a short course it again bends upwards at nearly right angle and invaginates the pia to reach the centre of the nerve. The entering vessel is thus clothed by the pia along with the pial vessels. It is also surrounded by a sympathetic nerve plexus (nerve of Tiedemann).
- *In the centre of optic nerve:* The artery bends forwards and then in company with the vein, which lies on its temporal side, it passes anteriorly and pierces the lamina cribrosa to appear inside the eye.
- *In the optic nerve head:* It lies superficially in the nasal part of physiology cup, covered only by that layer of glial tissue (connective tissue meniscus of Kuhnt) which closes the physiological cup. Here, it divides into two branches—a superior the an inferior, each of which subdivides into a temporal and a nasal branch at or near the margin of the optic disc.
- *In the retina:* The four terminal branches of central retina artery namely, the superior nasal, superior temporal, inferior nasal and inferior temporal, divide dichotomously as they proceed towards the ora serrata, where they end without anastomosis.

ARRANGEMENT OF RETINAL CAPILLARIES

The terminal fundus arterioles bend sharply and dip almost vertically into the retina, forming the capillary network arranged as follows:

- In most of the extramacular fundus, there are two retinal capillary networks—a superficial and a deep.

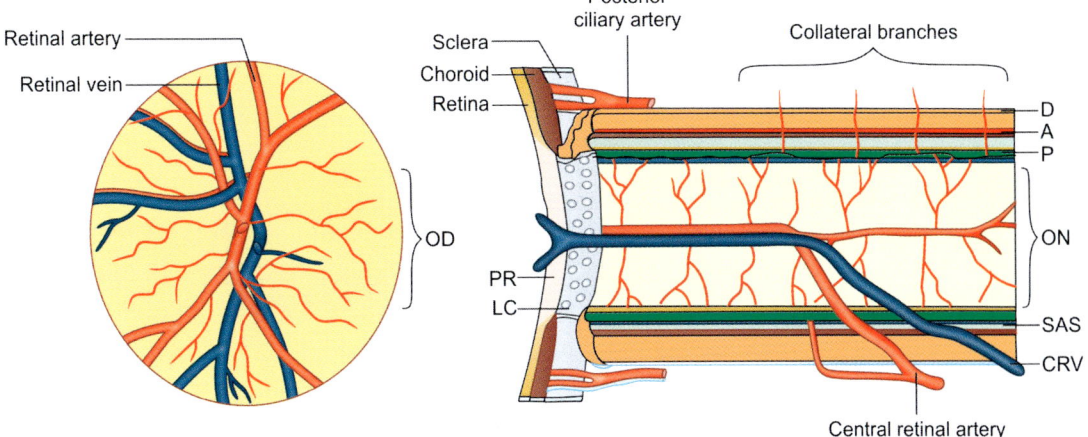

Fig. 1.16 *Course of central retinal artery. OD: optic disc, PR: prelaminar region, LC: lamina cribrosa, D: dura, A: arachnoid, P: pia, ON: optic nerve, SAS: subarachnoid space, CRV: central retinal vein*

The superficial capillary network lies at the level of the nerve fiber layer and the deep network lies between the inner nuclear layer and the outer plexiform layer (Fig. 1.17). The deep capillary network is more dense and complex than the superficial. There are anastomotic capillaries which run from one to the other. Peripherally, as the ora serrata is approached, the capillary network is reduced to a scanty single layer.

- In the parafoveal zone, the capillary network is especially well developed and is three-layered. However, there exists a capillary-free zone in the fovea, known as foveal avascular zone (FAZ) of about 500 µm in diameter.
- In the peripapillary region, the capillary network becomes four-layered to support the extremely thick nerve fiber layer characteristic of this region.

BLOOD-RETINAL BARRIER

INNER BLOOD-RETINAL BARRIER

The endothelial cells of a normal retinal capillary are closely bound together about the lumen by intercellular junctions of the zonula occludens type. These junctions normally prohibit a free flow of fluids and solutes from the vascular lumen into the retinal interstitium and thus form a blood-retinal barrier. Presence of this barrier is confirmed by absence of fluorescein leakage from these capillaries.

The endothelial cells of retinal capillaries are encircled by a basement membrane around which is present a layer of pericytes (mural cells). Pericytes are also surrounded by a layer of basement membrane. Normally, the endothelial cells and pericytes are present in a one to one ratio in young individuals. However, in certain diseases, such as diabetes mellitus, there occurs a relative decrease in the number of pericytes. On the other hand with increasing age, there occurs a gradual decrease in the number of endothelial cells.

OUTER BLOOD-RETINAL BARRIER

The adjacent retinal pigment epithelial (RPE) cells are connected with each other by tight junctions (zonulae occludens and zonulae adherens) and constitute the outer blood-retinal barrier, which maintains the integrity of subretinal space. RPE is involved with transport of nutrients and metabolites through the blood-retinal barrier and elaboration of the extracellular matrix.

APPLIED ASPECTS

- In retinal detachment the 9 layers of neurosensory retina separate from retinal pigment epithelium underneath. This can be explained by embryology and development of retina. There is potential space between RPE and neurosensory retina.

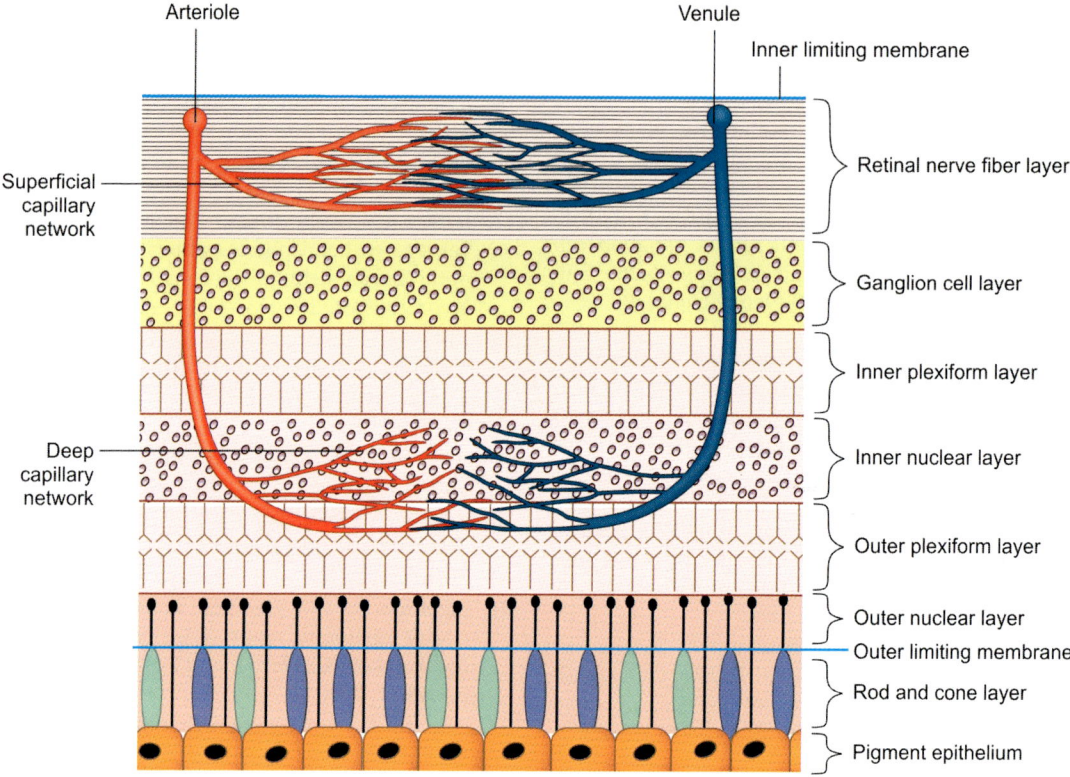

Arteriole

Venule

Inner limiting membrane

Superficial capillary network

Retinal nerve fiber layer

Ganglion cell layer

Inner plexiform layer

Deep capillary network

Inner nuclear layer

Outer plexiform layer

Outer nuclear layer

Outer limiting membrane

Rod and cone layer

Pigment epithelium

Fig. 1.17 *Arrangement of retinal capillaries*

- Optical coherence tomography (OCT) has been likened to in vivo histopathology when various layers of retina are reflected as hyporeflective and hyperreflective bands.

- In cases of central artery occlusion due to ischemic damage the cloudy swelling of retinal layers give it pale color. The cherry red spot is due to intact choroidal vasculature which shines through the thin overlying retina. In ophthalmic artery occlusion we do not see cherry red spot as the choroidal circulation is also affected.

- In central retinal vein occlusion, the anastomotic channels develop between the retinal and choroidal circulation which are seen on disc.

- In open globe injury, if the extent is beyond 5 mm of limbus (Zone III open globe injury) the prognosis becomes bad as retina may be involved by the penetrating wound.

BIBLIOGRAPHY

1. Adler R. (2000). A model of retinal cell differentiation in the chick embryo. Progress in Retinal and Eye Research, 19, 529–557.
2. Agathocleous M, & Harris WA (2009). From progenitors to differentiated cells in the vertebrate retina. Annual Reviews: Cell Developmental Biology, 25, 45–69.
3. Agathocleous M, Iordanova I, Willardsen MI, Xue XY, Vetter ML, Harris W, Badea TC, Cahill H, Ecker J, Hattar S, & Nathans J (2009).
4. B Harris, & R. Wong (Eds.), Retinal development (pp. 75–98). Cambridge: Cambridge University Press.
5. Baker GE, & Reese BE. (1993). Chiasmatic course of temporal retinal axons in the developing ferret. Journal of Comparative Neurology, 330, 95–104.
6. Baye LM, & Link BA. (2007). Interkinetic nuclear migration and the selection of neurogenic cell divisions during vertebrate retinogenesis. Journal of Neuroscience, 27, 10143–10152.

7. Blankenship AG, & Feller MB. (2010). Mechanisms underlying spontaneous patterned activity in developing neural circuits. Nature Reviews Neuroscience, 11, 18–29.

8. Curcio CA, Sloan KR, Kalina RE et al 1990. Human photoreceptor topography. J. Comp. Neural, 292, 497.

9. Fabre PJ, Shimogori T, & Charron F. (2010). Segregation of ipsilateral retinal ganglion cell axons at the optic chiasm requires the Shh receptor Boc. Journal of Neuroscience, 30, 266–275.

10. Farajian R, Raven MA, Cusato K, & Reese BE (2004). Cellular positioning and dendritic field size of cholinergic amacrine cells are impervious to early ablation of neighboring cells in the mouse retina. Visual Neuroscience, 21, 13–22.

11. Huberman AD, Murray KD, Warland DK, Feldheim DA, & Chapman, B. (2005). Ephrin-As mediate targeting of eye-specific projections to the lateral geniculate nucleus. Nature Neuroscience, 8, 1013–1021.

12. Incerti B, Cortese K, Pizzigoni A, Surace EM, Varani S, Coppola M, et al. (2000). Oa1 knock-out: New insights on the pathogenesis of ocular albinism type 1. Human Molecular Genetics, 9, 2781–2788.

13. Jacobson M. (1978). Developmental neurobiology. New York: Plenum Press. pp. 1–562.

14. Jadhav AP, Roesch K, & Cepko CL. (2009). Development and neurogenic potential of Müller glial cells in the vertebrate retina. Progress in Retinal and Eye Research, 28, 249–262.

15. Jaubert-Miazza L, Green E, Lo FS, Bui K, Mills J, & Guido W. (2005). Structural and functional composition of the developing retinogeniculate pathway in the mouse. Visual Neuroscience, 22, 661–676.

16. Jeffery G, & Erskine L. (2005). Variations in the architecture and development of the vertebrate optic chiasm. Progress in Retinal and Eye Research, 24, 721–753.

17. Jeffery G, Levitt JB, & Cooper HM. (2008). Segregated hemispheric pathways through the optic chiasm distinguish primates from rodents. Neuroscience, 157, 637–643.

18. Kolb H, Linberg KA and Fisher SK 1992. Neurons of the human retina: Golgi study. J. Comp. Neural, 318, 147.

19. Ogden T. 1989a. The glin of retina, in 'Retina' (eds. SJ Ryan and T Ogden), CV Mosby, St. Louis, p. 53.

20. Ogden T. 1989b. Topography of the retina, in 'Retina' (eds. SJ Ryan and T Ogden), CV Mosby, St. Louis, p. 32.

21. Sigelman J. and Ozanics V. 1982. Retina in ocular anatomy, embryology and teratology (ed. F. Jakobiec), Harper and Row, Philadelphia, p. 441.

22. Tripathi RC and Tripathi BJ 1984. Anatomy of the human eye, orbit and adnexa. In 'The Eye', 3rd edition (Ed. H. Davson), Academic Press, London, pp. 40, 145.

23. Williams RW 1991. The human retina has a cone-rich rim. Vis. Neurosci, 6, 403.

24. Zinn KM and Benjamin-Henkind, J. 1982. Retinal pigment epithelium in 'Ocular Anatomy, Embryology and Teratology (ed. F. Jakobiec), Harper and Row, Philadelphia, p. 553.

PHYSIOLOGY OF RETINA

AK Khurana, Indu Khurana,
Aruj K Khurana, Bhawna Khurana

METABOLISM AND PHYSIOLOGICAL ACTIVITIES OF RETINA

RETINAL METABOLISM

The respiratory rate of the retina is twice that of the brain. Half of the respiratory rate is accounted for by the ellipsoid regions of the photoreceptors, which are rich in mitochondria. Unlike the brain, the retina does not require insulin for glucose to enter the cells. Müller's cells possess glucose-6-phosphatase activity, which enables them to release glucose from their stores into the neuroretina.

Nourishment and oxygen required by the retina are supplied to its tissues from the bloodstream. It is well known that the retina ceases to function a few minutes after its blood supply is stopped. This shows how essential are the vegetative processes taking place in the retinal cells if vision is to operate.

Glucose, lipids, amino acids and other provisions such as vitamins and minerals, are all needed by the retina. An adequate oxygen supply is essential. These items come from the capillaries in the choroid and via the central retinal artery and also, to a small extent, through the circle of Zinn and (probably in trifling amounts) from the vitreous. Carbonic acid and other catabolites return via such routes. Carbohydrates are essential for the production of energy and the retina is sensitive to any fall in concentration within its tissues. It can tolerate a fall in concentration as low as 30 mg/100 ml without any disturbance of activity, but if the concentration becomes any lower, vision suffers. Deprivation of glucose for 8 to 10 minutes results in irreversible cellular damage. Since carbohydrates and oxygen have a close relationship, a similar situation is very likely to occur with a shortage of oxygen.

Production of energy in the retina proceeds in the same way as in other tissues. The most important method of carbohydrate breakdown is via glycolysis (the Embeden-Meyerhof process) to pyruvate and lactate, after that, via the Krebs cycle, to carbonic acid and water. In

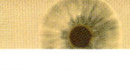

retina, glycolysis occurs even if there is a sufficient supply of oxygen, this is unlike other tissues where glycolysis occurs only if there is no oxygen present.

Glycogen is found stored in retina, essentially in the glial cells such as Müller's fibers. Such a store serves as a buffer against changes in the concentration of glucose in the tissues.

Lipids make up an insignificant source of energy for the retina. Some intermediate building blocks are needed in the process of anabolism. Amino acids are also essential for the cells. Above all, proteins are needed for enzymes and for anabolism and catabolism. In the elderly, retinal metabolic processes wane. In addition, external influences, such as ionizing radiation, may lower metabolism.

DISC MORPHOGENESIS

Disc morphogenesis has been studied mainly in rod-dominated retinas. This highly specialized process takes place in several stages:

Plate formation. Cytoplasm filled plates are formed by the accumulation of lipid and proteins within a budding of the outer segment membrane. Opsins are present in the membrane of these plates from the onset of disc morphogenesis.

Expansion. The plates expand to reach the width of the rod or cone outer segments. As each plate enlarges, a further plate develops proximally, so that a stack of expanding plates is formed.

Rim proteins are added at the cilium and loop outwards into the plasma membrane. The transmembrane proteins peripherin/rds and rom-I have been localized to the margins of photoreceptor discs. They have no enzymatic properties and are thought to act structural proteins.

Zipping up of upper and lower membranes is seen only in rods, and is followed by the internalization of the newly formed discs.

Maturation and stabilization of the discs-interactive homodimers between peripherin/rds molecules, and between rom-I molecules at the hairpin/disc lamellae junction are thought to stabilize this region of the disc. Linkage of rhodopsin molecules in adjacent lamellae also contributes to disc stability.

SHEDDING AND PHAGOCYTOSIS OF PHOTORECEPTOR OUTER SEGMENTS

Shedding describes the sloughing of the apical sections of photoreceptor outer segments. In rods, it is maximal 1 hour after light exposure, and in cones shedding is maximal 2–3 hours after the onset of darkness. Mammalian rod outer segment disc shedding follows a light entrained, free running circadian rhythm. The signal to shed is not disrupted by optic nerve transection, so it is thought to originate within the retina and not within the central nervous system. The exact nature of the signal has yet to be determined. It could be transmitted via a neural pathway or be a paracrine effect of a diffusible substance. The leukotrienes LTC4, and a GABA induced reduction in Melatonin production are thought to participate in these effector pathways. The retinal pigment epithelial cells have specific receptors for rod outer segments at their apices, and the oligosaccharides on the N-terminal at these sites. The retinal pigment epithelium is able to phagocytose many different materials at different rates, suggesting that there are several phagocytic mechanisms in these cells. The ingestion of rod outer segments is thought to involve secondary messengers (possibly cAMP). This is followed by digestion, which is aided by the numerous lysosomal acid hydrolases found in the retinal pigment epithelium.

PHYSIOLOGY OF VISION

Physiology of vision is a complex phenomenon which is still poorly understood. The main mechanisms concerned with vision are:

- *Initiation of visual sensation (Transduction)*
- *Processing and transmission of visual sensation, and*
- *Visual perceptions.*

INITIATION OF VISUAL SENSATIONS

The rods and cones serve as sensory nerve endings for visual sensations. Stimuli for visual

sensations may be divided, in a purely physical sense, into two types: inadequate and adequate.

Inadequate stimuli produce glowing sensations called *phosphenes.* Mechanical stimulation by pressure on the sclera is an example of inadequate stimulus which produces *pressure phosphene* (which appears as a patch with contrasting border). Other examples of inadequate stimuli are rapid eye movements in dark (producing *movement phosphene),* passage of weak electric current through retina (producing *electrical phosphene)* and passage of X-rays or other ionizing radiations through the retina (producing *radiation phosphenes).*

Adequate stimuli to vision are formed by visible portion of the electromagnetic radiation spectrum, i.e. 'the light'. It lies between ultraviolet and infrared portions from 400 nm at the violet end of the spectrum to 750 nm at the red end. The white light consists of seven colors denoted by 'VIBGYOR' (violet, indigo, blue, green, yellow, orange and red). *Light ray* is the term used to describe the radius of concentric waveforms. A group of parallel rays of light is called a *beam of light.*

Light falling upon the retina is absorbed by the *photosensitive pigments* present in the rods and cones, and initiates *photochemical changes* which are described in detail under the section *Photochemistry of vision.* The photochemical changes trigger a sequence of events (electrical changes) that initiate the visual sensations. The retinal receptors are not just transducers of light into chemical and electrical signals; they are active processors of information. Thus the electrical potential changes produced and actively processed in the retina are transmitted through the ganglion cells and along the fibers of the optic nerve and other parts of the visual pathway to the visual cortex. The details of processes concerned are described as processing and transmission of visual sensation and *Electrophysiology of the retina.*

PHOTOCHEMISTRY OF VISION

INTRODUCTION

As mentioned earlier, the light falling upon the retina is absorbed by the photosensitive pigments in the rods and cones and initiates photochemical changes which in turn initiate electrical changes and in this way the process of vision begins. To understand the process of photochemistry it is mandatory to know in detail about the photosensitive compounds, i.e. the rod I pigments and the cone pigments. Further, pivotal to all photoreactions in animal tissue, is the presence of fat soluble compound, vitamin A. Therefore, the subject of photochemistry will be discussed under following heads:

• *Vitamin A and visual pigments*
• *Visual pigments*
• *Light-induced changes.*

VITAMIN A AND VISUAL PIGMENTS

The vitamin A cycle from its dietary intake to its transport to the eye is depicted in Fig. 2.1 and described below:

Dietary sources of retinol

Dietary sources of retinol for humans include animal foods and plant foods. *Animal foods* contain vitamin A as such (i.e. retinol); some foods are much richer in retinol than others. The liver, which stores retinol, is the best source. Milk products are also very rich in retinol. *Plant foods* do not contain vitamin A as such but in the form of precursors the carotenoid pigments (carotenes). The carotenes cannot be used directly in the photochemical process but must be converted into vitamin A (retinol) by metabolic activity in the wall of the small intestine. Three types of carotenes—the alpha, beta and gamma—are present in plant food. The beta carotenes yield 2 molecules of vitamin A, while the alpha and gamma yield one molecule each (I).

Absorption and storage

In the intestine, the vitamin A is esterified and reaches the bloodstream through the intestinal lymphatics. Most of this retinol from the bloodstream is transported to the liver, where it is stored. In the liver, retinol becomes bound with the retinol-binding protein (RBP). It is quite stable in this combination.

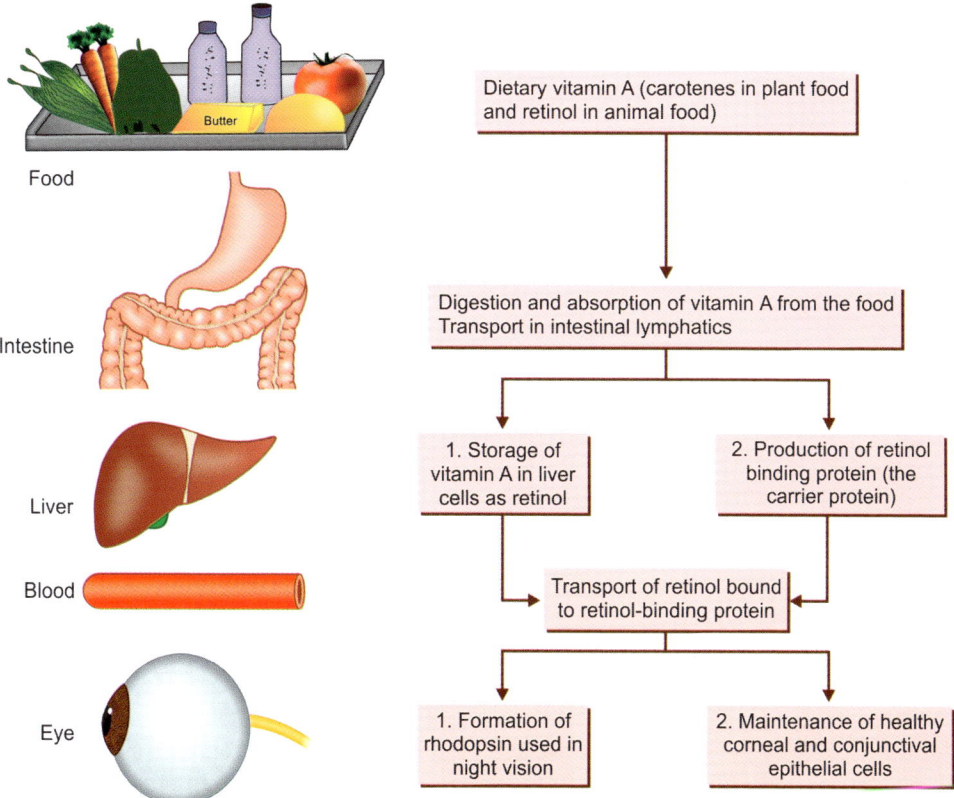

Food

Intestine

Liver

Blood

Eye

Dietary vitamin A (carotenes in plant food and retinol in animal food)

Digestion and absorption of vitamin A from the food Transport in intestinal lymphatics

1. Storage of vitamin A in liver cells as retinol

2. Production of retinol binding protein (the carrier protein)

Transport of retinol bound to retinol-binding protein

1. Formation of rhodopsin used in night vision

2. Maintenance of healthy corneal and conjunctival epithelial cells

Fig. 2.1 *Vitamin A cycle from its dietary intake to its transport to the eyes*

Transport from liver to the eye

The retinol-protein complex enters the circulation and reaches the target tissues where it is utilized. In the retina, it becomes attached to the specific receptors present on the basal surfaces of the retinal pigment epithelial (RPE) cells. Then, it is assumed that the RBP is left outside and the retinol is transported by a specific transport protein inside the RPE cells.

Utilization of vitamin A for
synthesis of rhodopsin (Fig. 2.2)

Inside the RPE cells, there occurs no change in the retinol (vitamin A). Thus the retinol passes through the RPE cells (unchanged) into the outer segments of the photoreceptor's. Inside the photoreceptor's outer segment, the retinol is oxidized to retinene by the enzyme retinene reductase. The retinene then combines immediately with the protein opsin to form the rhodopsin. The NAD oxidative system (present in the RPE) supports the reaction of rhodopsin formation by removing hydrogen. Therefore, for the formation of rhodopsin, it is essential that the RPE and photoreceptor outer segment must be closely opposed to each other. The freshly formed rhodopsin molecule is then incorporated into the newly forming double discs, which then assume their place in the innermost portion of outer segment of photoreceptors.

VISUAL PIGMENTS

Visual pigments are those substances which have the property of absorbing light (the visible portion of electromagnetic spectrum). When a substance absorbs all wavelengths of light equally, it appears gray or black. A green pigment absorbs light of all wavelengths except green and thus appear green. However, most of the pigments in the visual cells are not limited in their absorption to one small band of wavelengths but rather absorb, to a greater or

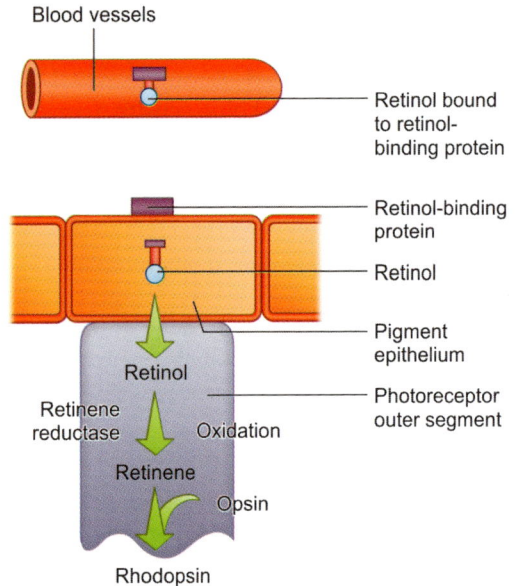

Fig. 2.2 *Utilization of vitamin A for synthesis of rhodopsin*

lesser extent, over a broad range of the spectrum. The peak of each pigment's absorption curve is called its *absorption maximum*.

The visual pigments in the eyes of humans and most other mammals are made up of a protein called *opsin* and retinene, the aldehyde of vitamin A. The term retinene is used to distinguish this compound from retinene *two* which is found in eyes of some animal species. Since the retinene are aldehydes, they are called *retinals.* The vitamin A as such is alcohol and thus called *retinol.*

Rhodopsin (visual purple)

Rhodopsin is the photosensitive visual pigment present in the discs of the rod outer segments. It consists of a protein opsin (called as scotopsin) and a carotenoid called retinal (the aldehyde of vitamin A). Rhodopsin is thus a membrane-bound glycolipid which is held in a rigid, highly organized arrangement, partially by the action of phospholipid present in the plasma membrane of the photoreceptor discs.

Human rhodopsin has a molecular weight of 40,000.[3] It is one of the many serpentine receptors coupled to G proteins (Fig. 2.3A and B). Rhodopsin protein is insoluble in water but can be taken into solution if detergent is added. The rhodopsin is essentially a solute in a two-

dimensional solution. It is sensitive to heat and chemical agents (ethanol, strong acids or alkalies) that denature the protein.

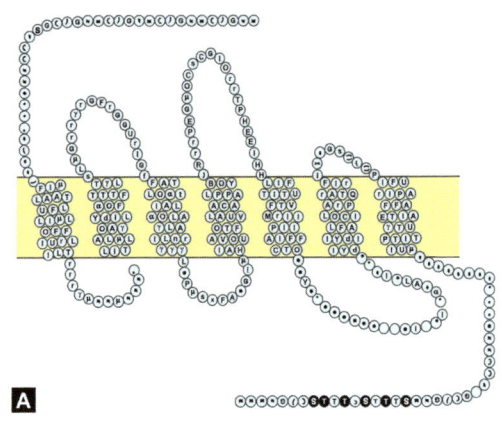

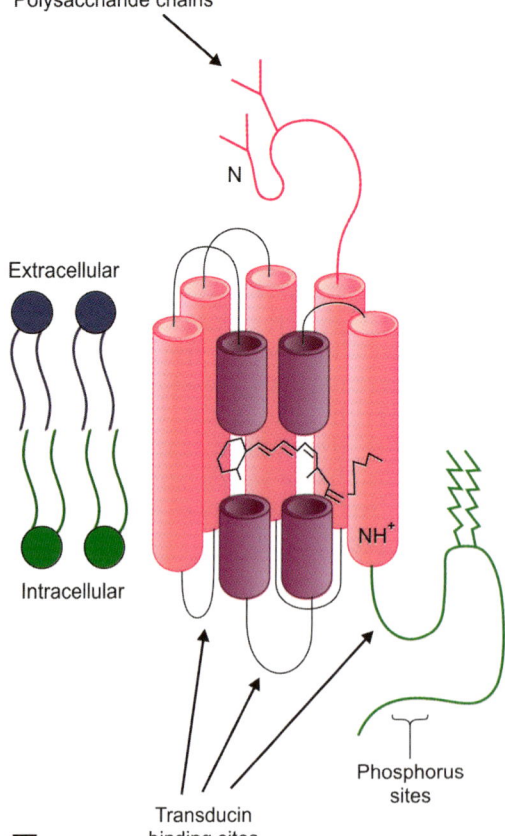

Fig. 2.3 *Schematic diagram of rhodopsin depicting:* **(A)** *Serpentine receptor coupled with G protein; and* **(B)** *Protein opsin crosses the disc membrane seven times*

The protein opsin of the human rhodopsin is a 348 amino acid protein that crosses the disc membrane seven times (Fig. 2.3). Two palmitate molecules are linked with cysteines via thioester linkages at the intracellular C-terminal. These fatty acids are anchored into the lipid bilayer forming a fourth intracellular loop. Oligosaccharide residues are located on the extracellular N-terminal; there is some evidence that these may help maintain the structural integrity of the disc. The amino acid sequences for all human cone opsins is almost identical, the difference in spectral absorbance being determined by a few different amino acids. The light absorbing form of vitamin A is retinal, which binds to opsin at a Schiff base linkage site to form rhodopsin.

The absorption spectrum of rhodopsin as shown in Fig. 2.4 depicts that its peak sensitivity to light lies within the narrow limits of 493–505 nm. It absorbs primarily yellow wavelength of light, transmitting violet and red to appear purple by transmitted light; it is, therefore, also called visual purple.

Cone pigments

The visual pigments present in the cones have not been so intensively studies as the rhodopsin. There are three kinds of cones in primates. Cone pigments are somewhat different from the rhodopsin, in that they respond to specific wavelengths of light, giving rise to color vision. These differences are present in the opsin portion of the molecule, whereas the chromophore 11-cis-retinal remains the same. The peak absorbance wavelength of the 'blue', 'green' and 'red' sensitive cones lie at about 435,

535 and 580 nm, respectively. The relative sizes of the populations of the three types of cones are not well established, through several lines of evidence indicate that blue-sensitive cones are the least prevalent. As yet the molecular details of the cone pigment protein remain obscure.

LIGHT-INDUCED CHANGES

As also mentioned earlier, the light falling upon the retina is absorbed by the photosensitive pigments in the rods and cones and initiates photochemical changes which in turn initiate electrical changes and in this way the process of vision sets in.

The photochemical changes occur in the outer segments of both the rods and the cones. These changes have been intensively studies in the rod's outer segments. However, similar reactions probably also apply to the cones. The photochemical reactions studied in the rod outer segments can be described under three headings:
- *Rhodopsin bleaching*
- *Rhodopsin regeneration*
- *Visual cycle.*

Rhodopsin bleaching

As discussed earlier, the rhodopsin consists of a protein called *opsin* and a carotenoid called retinene (vitamin A aldehyde or 11-cis-retinal). The light absorbed by the rhodopsin converts its *11-cis-retinal* into *all-trans-retinal*. These are isomers having same chemical composition but different shapes (Fig. 2.5). This light-induced isomerization of 11-cis-retinal into all-trans-retinal occurs through formation of many inter-

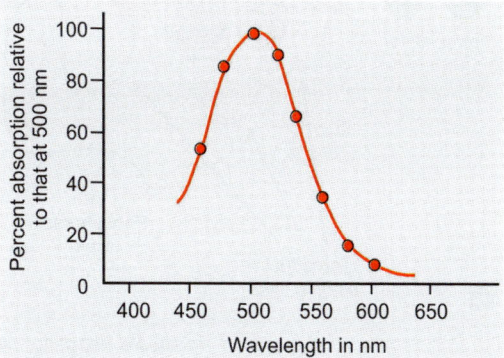

Fig. 2.4 *Absorption spectrum of rhodopsin cone pigments*

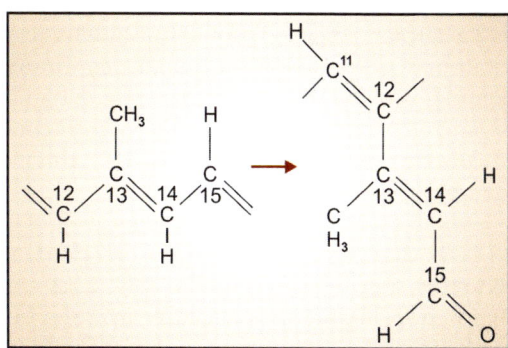

Fig. 2.5 *Isomerization of 11-cis retinal to all-trans-retinal*

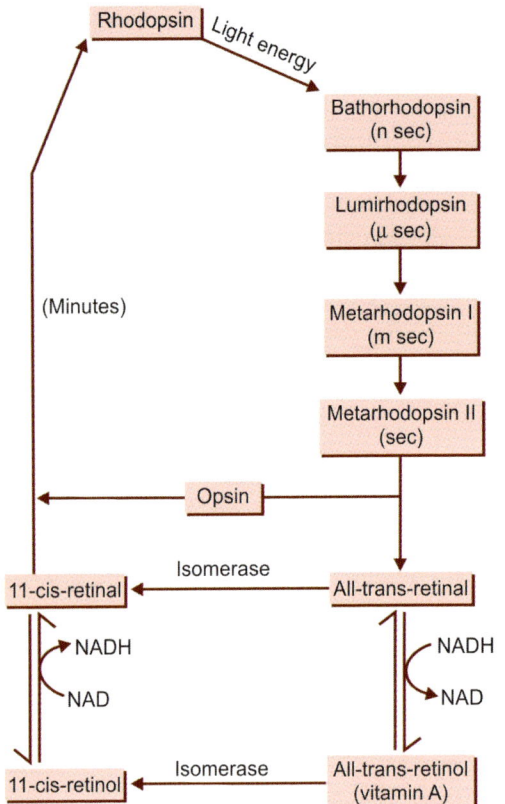

Fig. 2.6 *The scheme for the reactions set into motion by light falling on the rhodopsin*

mediates which exist for a transient period (Fig. 2.6). One of the intermediate compounds (*metarhodopsin II,* also called as activated rhodopsin) of the above isomerization chain reaction acts as an enzyme to activate many molecules of transducin. The transducin is a GTP/GDP exchange protein present in an inactive form bound to GDP in the membranes of discs and cell membrane of the rods. The activated transducin (bound to GTP) in turn activates many more molecules of phospho-diesterase (PDE) which catalyses conversion of cyclic guanosine monophosphate (cGMP) to GMP, leading to a reduction in concentration of cyclic GMP (cGMP) within the photoreceptor (Fig. 2.7). The reduction in cyclic GMP is responsible for producing the electrical response (receptor potential), which marks the beginning of the nerve impulse. Further details are described in the section on *electroneurophysiology of vision.*

The all-trans-retinal (produced from light-induced isomerization of 11-cis-retinal) can no longer remain in combination with the opsin and thus there occurs separation of opsin and all-trans-retinal. This process of separation is called *photodecomposition* and the rhodopsin is said to be bleached by the action of light.

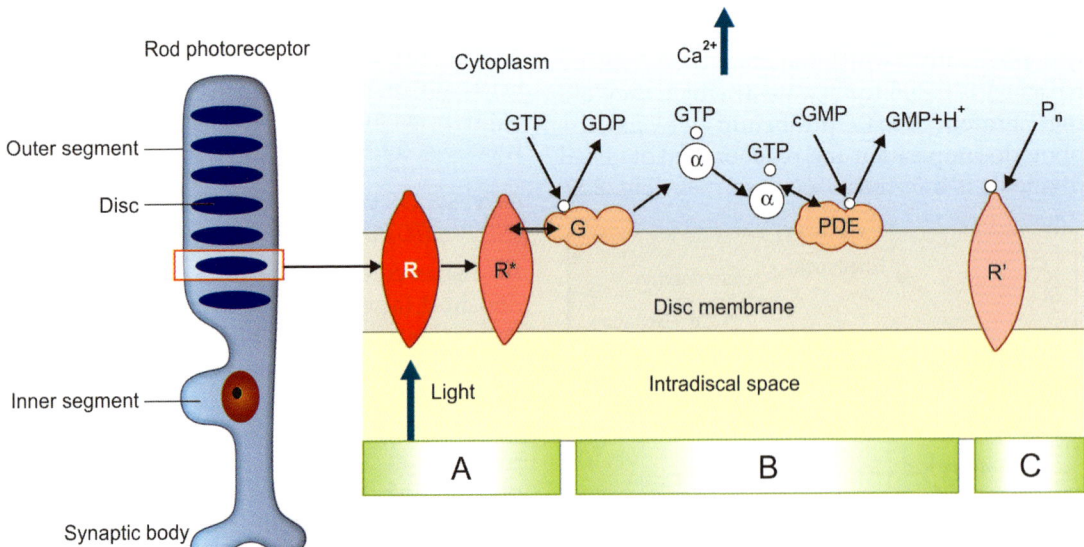

Fig. 2.7 *The scheme for reactions triggered by rhodopsin bleaching which affect cGMP:* **(A)** *Light-induced conversion of rhodopsin (R) into the active form (R*);* **(B)** *activation of G-protein (G), GTP/GDP exchange and activation of cGMP phosphodiestrase (PDE) protein; and* **(C)** *phosphorylation of photolysed rhodopsin (R')*

Rhodopsin regeneration

The all-trans-retinal separated from the opsin (as above), subsequently enters into the chromophore pool existing in the photoreceptor outer segment and the pigment epithelial cells (for this, close approximation of RPE and photoreceptor is must). The all-trans-retinal may be further reduced to retinol by alcohol dehydrogenase, then esterified to re-enter the systemic circulation.

The first stage in the reformation of rhodopsin, as shown in Fig. 2.8, is isomerization of all-trans-retinal back to 1-cis-retinal. The process is catalyzed by the enzyme *retinal isomerase*. Energy for the regeneration process is supplied by the overall metabolic pool of the photoreceptor outer segment. The 11-cis-retinal in the outer segments of photoreceptors reunites with the opsin to form rhodopsin. This whole process is called regeneration of the rhodopsin. Thus the bleaching of the retinal photopigments occurs under the influence of light, whereas the regeneration process is independent of light, proceeding equally well in light or darkness. The amount of rhodopsin in the rods, therefore, varies inversely with the incident light.

Visual cycle

In the retina of living animals, under constant light stimulation, a steady state must exist under which the rate at which the photochemicals are bleached is equal to the rate at which they are regenerated.[8] This equilibrium between the photodecomposition and regeneration of visual pigments is referred to as *visual cycle* (Fig. 2.8).

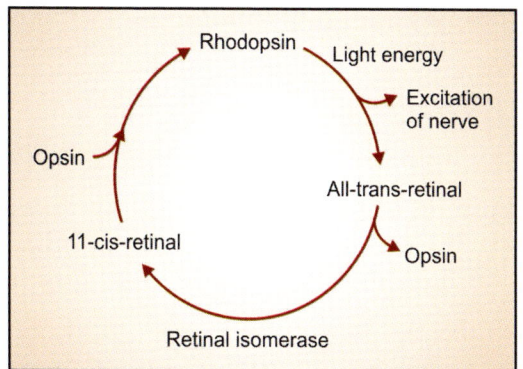

Fig. 2.8 *Visual cycle, showing rhodopsin bleaching and regeneration*

The bleaching regeneration equilibrium which is reached in either the rods or the cones during various conditions of incident light accounts for only a portion of the sensitivity change that is observed. The remaining portion of the adaptive mechanism occurs under the influence of neural elements within the retina and does not involve a photopigment mechanism. The exact level within the retina, at which this visual mechanism operates is unclear, although a gathering amount of evidence indicates that it is at the level of synapses of the photoreceptors with the dendrites of the bipolar cells and may involve activity of horizontal cells.

Photochemistry of photopic vision

Like rhodopsin, cone pigments also consist of the protein opsin (called photopsin) and the retinene (11-cis-retinal). Photopsin differs slightly from the scotopsin (rhodopsin). As mentioned earlier, there are three classes of cone pigments: red sensitive (erythrolabe), green sensitive (chlorolabe) and blue sensitive (cyanolabe), which have different absorption spectra.

It has been assumed that when light strikes the cones, the photochemical changes occur in the cone pigments which are very similar to those of rhodopsin. However, it has been noted that, nearly total rod bleaching occurs before significant bleaching can be observed in the cones. This differential bleaching quality sets aside the scotopic rod portion of the visual system from the photopic portion which functions during brightly lighted conditions.

GENESIS OF VISUAL IMPULSE IN THE PHOTORECEPTOR

As discussed earlier, the formation of metarhodopsin-II (also known as activated rhodopsin) triggers a cascade of biochemical reactions which results in reduction in the concentration of cyclic GMP in the photoreceptor; which in turn triggers the genesis of visual impulse by producing a generator potential in the photoreceptors. This process of translation of the information content of a light stimulus into electrical signals is known as transduction. The transduction process is highly quantum efficient, in that a single photon causes a response in the rod's membrane potential.

Normally, the inner segment of the photoreceptor continually pumps Na$^+$ from inside to outside, thereby creating a negative potential on the inside of entire cell. However, the Na$^+$ channels present in the cell membrane of the outer segment of photoreceptor are kept open by the cyclic GMP, in the dark. So, Na$^+$, from the extracellular fluid, flows inside the outer segment, i.e. in dark. As a result the cell membrane in the outer segment is hypopolarized with respect to the inner segment, i.e. the current flows from the inner to the outer segment (Fig. 2.9). Current also flows to the synaptic ending of the photoreceptor. This is called standing potential or dark current.

When light strikes the photoreceptor, the amount of cyclic GMP in the photoreceptor is reduced (as discussed in photochemistry of vision), so some of the Na$^+$ channels (which were kept open by cyclic GMP in dark) are closed, and the result is a hyperpolarizing receptor potential. Thus the photoreceptor potential is different from the receptor potentials in almost all other sensory receptors in that the excitation of photoreceptor causes increased negativity of the membrane potential (hyperpolarization), rather than decreased negativity (depolarization) which is characteristic of all other receptors. Normally, in dark the electronegativity inside the rod membrane is about 40 millivolts and after excitation it approaches about 70 to 80 millivolts. Further, the eye is unique in that the receptor potential of the photoreceptors is local graded potential, i .e. it does not propagate and does not follow the 'all or none law'.

The sequence of events in photoreceptors by which incident light leads to production of a nerve impulse (*phototransduction*) is summarized in Fig. 2.10.

Cone versus rod receptor potential

The cone receptor potential has a sharp onset and offset, whereas the rod receptor potential has a sharp onset and slow offset. The curve relating the amplitude of receptor potentials to stimulus intensity have similar shapes in rods and cones, but the rods are much more sensitive. Therefore, rod responses are proportionate to stimulus intensity at levels of illumination that

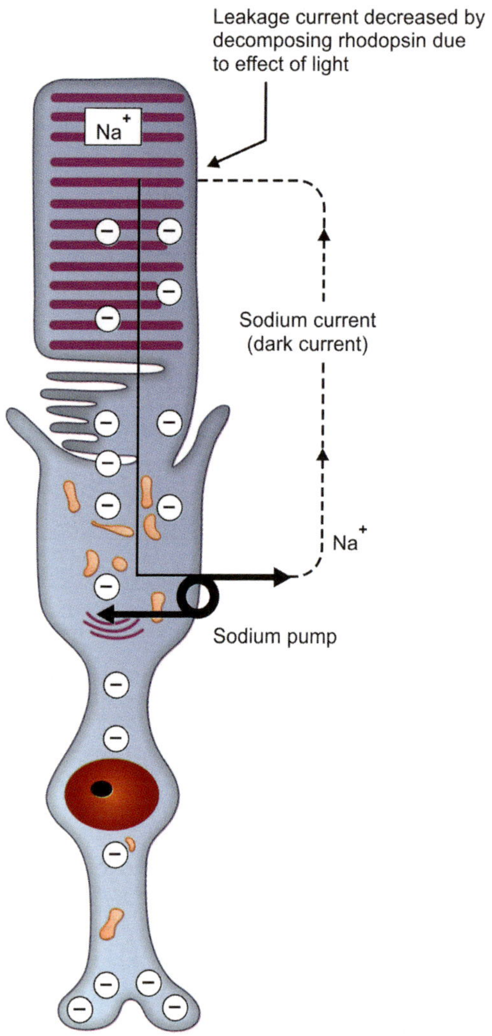

Fig. 2.9 *Basis of genesis of photoreceptor hyperpolarization*

are below the threshold for cones. On the other hand, cone responses are proportionate to stimulus intensity at high levels of illumination when the rod responses are maximal and cannot change. That is why cones generate good response to change in light intensity above background but do not represent absolute illumination well, whereas rods detect absolute illumination.

PROCESSING AND TRANSMISSION OF VISUAL IMPULSE IN THE RETINA

The *receptor potential* generated in the photoreceptors (as discussed above) is transmitted by

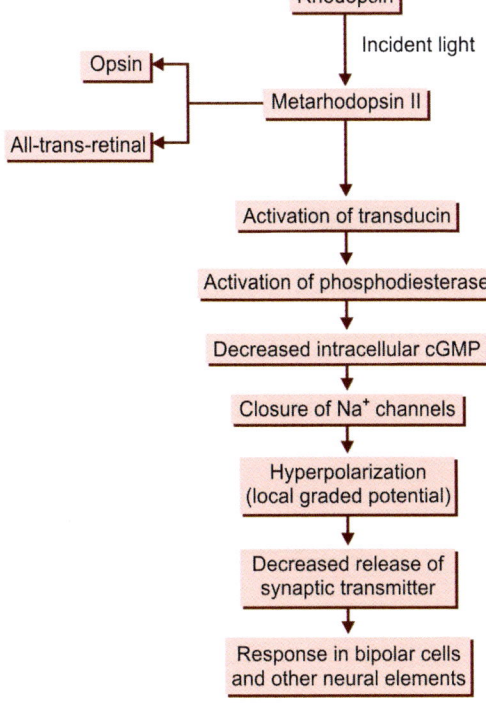

Fig. 2.10 *Sequence of events involved in phototransduction process in the photoreceptor*

electronic conduction (i.e. direct flow of electric current, not action potential) to the other cells of the retina viz. horizontal cells, bipolar cells, amacrine cells and ganglion cells. However, the ganglion cells transmit the visual signal by means of action potential.

NEUROTRANSMITTERS IN THE RETINA

Role of neurotransmitters employed for synaptic transmission in the retina still have not all been delineated clearly. However, a great variety of different synaptic transmitters are found in the retina. A few assumptions are as follows:

- *Glutamine*, an excitatory transmitter, is released by rods and cones at their synapses with bipolar and horizontal cells.
- *Amacrine cells* produce five different types of inhibitory transmitters. They include: gamma aminobutyric acid (GABA), glycine, dopamine, acetylcholine and indolamine.
- The transmitters of the bipolar cells and horizontal cells have still not been isolated.

- *Cholinesterase* has been found in the processes of Muller, horizontal, amacrine, and ganglion cells. In the human retina, only the true acetylcholinesterase has been found, suggesting that acetylcholine may be the dominant synaptic neurotransmitter in the human.
- *Carbonic anhydrase* has also been isolated from cones and RPE but not rods. Its exact role is also not clear.

PHYSIOLOGICAL ACTIVITIES IN THE RETINAL CELLS

The neurophysiological activities (concerned with the processing and transmission of visual signal) occurring in the different retinal cells can be summarized as below:

HORIZONTAL CELLS

Horizontal cells transmit signals horizontally in the outer plexiform layer from rods and cones to the bipolar cells. Their main function is *to enhance the visual contrast* by causing *lateral inhibitions*. This phenomenon of lateral inhibition has been observed by record of electrical activities occurring in the retina (Fig. 2.11), which shows that when a minute spot of light strikes the retina, the central most area is excited but the area around (called as surround) is inhibited. Thus, instead of the excitatory signal spreading widely in the retina because of the spreading dendritic and axonal trees in the plexiform layers, transmission through the horizontal cells puts a stop to this by providing lateral inhibition in the surrounding area. It has been found to be an essential mechanism which allows high visual accuracy in transmitting contrast borders in the visual image.

Thus, the principal purpose of the microcircuitry of the outer plexiform layer seems to be the processing of spatial information.

The concept of receptive field has been evolved to explain the processing of visual signal. In general sense, the receptive field is defined as the influence area of a sensory neuron. It is circular in configuration. It has been observed that receptive field of the horizontal cells is very large in contrast to the photoreceptor cell.

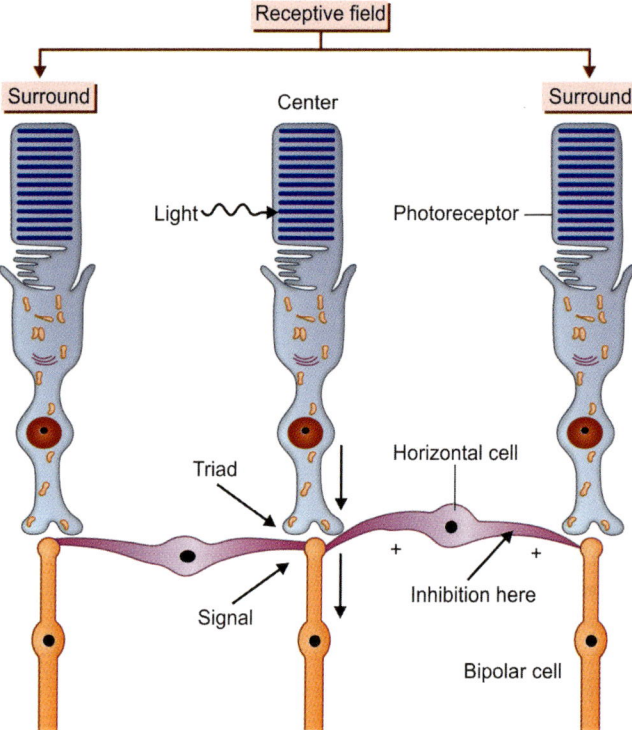

Fig. 2.11 *Phenomenon of lateral inhibition in the surround receptive plexiform layer. The central photoreceptor has been stimulated with light and the inner portion of the cell membrane has become more negative. The signal is transmitted upwards to the bipolar cell and also horizontally via the horizontal cells. This horizontal transmission results in inhibition of the photoreceptor-bipolar cell synapse of the neighbouring photoreceptor element. The stimulated bipolar cell may be hyperpolarized or depolarized*

BIPOLAR CELLS

The bipolar cells are neurons of the first order of visual pathway. Their dendrites are stimulated by the light-induced hyperpolarization of the photoreceptors.

The important points delineated regarding the physiological activities concerning the bipolar cells are as follows:

• Some bipolar cells *depolarize* while others *hyperpolarize* (Figs 2.11 and 2.12) when the photoreceptors are excited, i.e. the two different types of bipolar cells provide opposing excitatory and inhibitory signals in the visual pathway. Two possible hypotheses put forward to explain this differential response are as follows:

i. Perhaps the *depolarizing bipolar cells* respond to the excitatory neurotransmitter, glutamate and the hyperpolarizing bipolar cells do not.

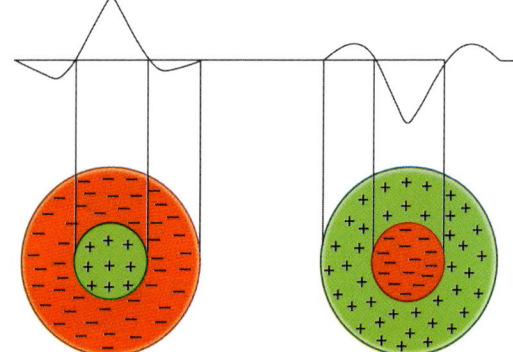

Fig. 2.12 *The centre-surround response to light in 'on' or centre depolarizing bipolar cell (left) and 'off' or centre-hyperpolarizing bipolar cell (right). Plus signs indicate regions giving a depolarizing response, minus signs, a hyperpolarizing one*

ii. Perhaps some bipolar cells receive direct excitation from the photoreceptors, whereas the others receive the signal indirectly

through the horizontal cells. Because horizontal cell is an inhibitory cell, this would reverse the polarity of the electrical response.

• *Receptive field* of the bipolar cell is also circular in configuration but has got a *centre-surround antagonism.* As shown in Fig. 2.12, in case of centre depolarizing cells (also called as 'on' cell) the light striking the center of receptive field activate and the light striking the 'surround' inhibits bipolar cell output. The reverse occurs in the center hyperpolarizing cell (also called as 'off cell'), i.e. the light striking the 'centre' is inhibitory and the light striking the 'surround' is excitatory to bipolar cell output. The size of the centre of the bipolar cell receptive field is determined by the reach of its dendrites and that of the much larger 'surround' is determined by the spread of interconnected horizontal cells.

• The importance of the above described reciprocal relationship between the depolarizing and hyperpolarizing bipolar cells is that it provides a second mechanism for lateral inhibition *(spatial information processing)* in addition to horizontal cell mechanism. Further, this reciprocal relationship allows half of the bipolar cells to transmit positive signals and the other half to transmit negative signals; both of these have a useful role in transmitting visual information to the brain.

AMACRINE CELLS

• Amacrine cells receive information at the synapse of the bipolar cell axon with ganglion cell dendrites (Fig. 2.13) and use this information for temporal processing at the other end of the bipolar cell (12–14). As shown in Fig. 2.13, at the synapse, the bipolar cells project onto both ganglion and amacrine cells. The amacrine cell then adjusts the bipolar cell in a *negative feedback arrangement* as to the subsequent response that will be projected onto the ganglion cell.

• Electrically, the amacrine cells produce *depolarizing potentials* and spikes that may act as generator potentials for the propagated spikes produced in the ganglion cells.

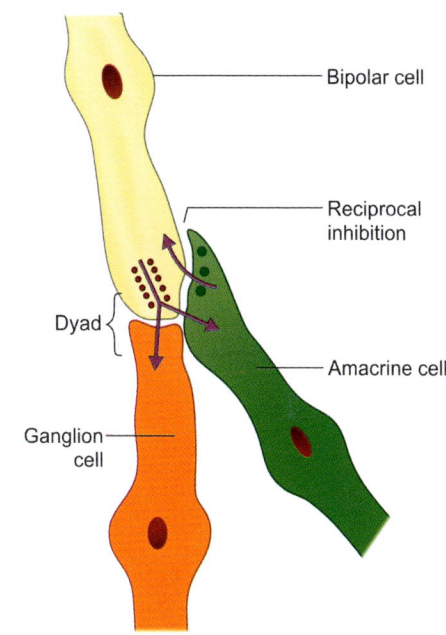

Fig. 2.13 *The bipolar-amacrine-ganglion cell interaction. For explanation see text*

• Various types of amacrine cells have been identified by morphological or histochemical means. Functions of some of the types of amacrine cells have been characterized as below:

– Some amacrine cells are part of the *direct pathway for rod vision,* i.e. the impulse travels from rod to bipolar cells to amacrine cell to ganglion cells.

– Some amacrine cells respond very strongly at the onset of a visual signal, but the response dies out rapidly.

– Other amacrine cells respond very strongly at the offset of the visual signal but again the response dies quickly.

– One type of amacrine cells respond both when a light is turned on or off signalling simply a change in illumination irrespective of direction.

– Another type of amacrine cells are direction sensitive and respond to movement of a spot across the retina in a specific direction. Thus the amacrine cells help in *temporal summation* and in the initial analysis of visual signals before they even leave the retina.

GANGLION CELLS

- The electrical response of bipolar cells (local graded potential) after modification by the amacrine cells is transmitted to the ganglion cells which in turn transmit their signals by means of action potential to the brain. Thus, the ganglion cell action potentials are similar to digital or frequency modulation (FM), while the slow graded potentials of the rest of retina are analogous to analog or amplitude modulation (AM) (Fig. 2.14).
- The ganglion cells which produce propagated spikes are of two types in terms of their centre response: "on-centre" cells that increase their discharge and "off-centre" cells that decrease their discharge upon illumination of the centre of their receptive fields.
- Three distinct groups of ganglion cells (W, X and Y) have been described depending upon the function they serve and are as follows:
  - W-ganglion cells are small (diameter >10 micrometre) and constitute about 40 per cent of all the ganglion cells. Their dendrites spread widely in the inner plexiform layer

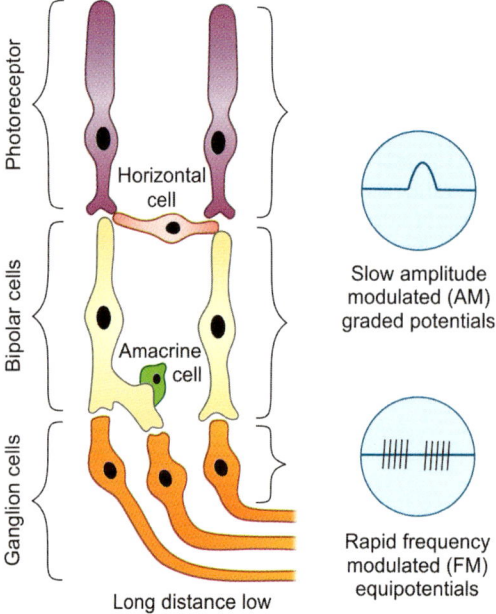

and thus they have broad fields in the retina. These cells receive most of their excitation from rods, transmitted by way of small bipolar cells and amacrine cells and are thus important for much of our rod vision under dark conditions. These cells are also especially sensitive for detecting directional movements anywhere in the field of vision.
  - X-ganglion cells: Most numerous (55 per cent of total cells), are of medium diameter (between 10 and 15 micrometre). They have very small fields, because their dendrites do not spread widely. Thus, their signals represent discrete retinal locations and so the visual image is mainly transmitted through these cells. Further, since every X-ganglion cell receives input from at least one cone cell, so probably they are responsible for the color vision as well.
  - Y-ganglion cells: These are the fewest (5 per cent of total) and largest (up to 35 micrometre in diameter) of all the ganglion cells. However, they have a very broad dendritic field and are thus able to pick up signals from a widespread retinal area. They respond to rapid changes in visual image, either rapid movement or rapid change in the light intensity.

    Cleland *et al* described X-cells as *sustained cells* and Y-cells as *transient cells*. The studies performed while recording from optic nerve fibers identify transient units as type I and sustained units as type II. The response of Y-cells (type I fibers) is phasic, with a transient excitation to a spot stimulus that decays quickly (Fig. 2.15). The X-cell (type II fibers) response has a tonic sustained component to a spot stimulus.

- *Ganglion cells* affect the relative sensitivity of different parts of the retina as follows:
  - The number of ganglion cells in the centre of fovea (about 35,000) is equal to the number of cones; this accounts for the high degree of visual acuity in the central retina in comparison with poorer acuity peripherally.
  - Peripheral retina has much greater sensitivity to weak light than the central retina. This results partly from the fact that rods are about 300 times more sensitive to light than are cones, but it is further magnified by the

Fig. 2.14 *The amplitude modulation (AM) and frequency modulation (FM), electrical responses from the retina. For explanation see text*

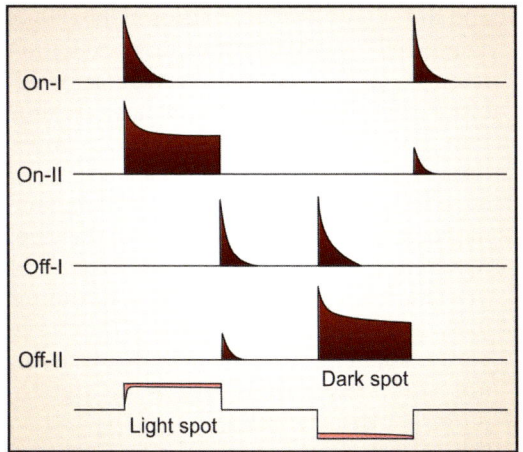

Fig. 2.15 *Diagrammatic illustration of four types of responses to light and dark spot stimuli in the cat optic nerve. From Satio et al.*

fact that as many as 200 rods converge on the same optic nerve fiber in the peripheral retina.

ELECTROPHYSIOLOGY OF RETINA

Applied aspect of electrophysiology of retina include:
- Electroretinogram (ERG)
- Electro-oculogram (EOG), and
- Visual evoked potential (VEP)

These have been described in detail in Chapter 8, Electrophysiological tests (page 129).

BIBLIOGRAPHY

1. Amer S. Akhtar M: The regeneration of rhodopsin from all trans retinal. Solubilization of an enzyme system involved in the completion of the visual cycle. Biochem J 128:987–989, 1973.

2. Arden GB: Receptor potentials. Br Med Bull 26: 125–129, 1970.

3. Blasie JK: The nef electric charge on photo-pigment molecules and frog retinal receptor disc membrane structure. Biophys J 12:205–213, 1972.

4. Bortqff A.: Localization of slow potential responses in the Necturus retina, Vision, Res. 4:627, 1964.

5. Daeman FJM, Rotmans JP, Bonting S: On the rhodopsin cycle, Exp Eye Res 18:97-103, 1974.

6. Daemen FJM: Vertebrate rod outer segment membranes. Biochem biophys Acta 300:255–288, 1973.

7. Fletcher RT, Chader GJ: Cyclic GMP: control of concentration by light in retinal photoreceptors. Biochem Biophys Res Commun 70:1297–1302, 1976.

8. Heller J, BokD: Retinol binding protein. Am J Ophthalmol 81:93–97, 1976.

9. Kaneko, A.: and Hashimoto, H.: Recording site of single cone response determined by an electrode marking technique, Vision Res. 7:847, 1967.

10. Koehn CJ: Relative biological activity of beta-carotene and vitamin A. Arch Biochem 17:337–344, 1948.

11. Nicol GD, and Miller WH: Cyclic GMP injected into retinal rod outer segments increases latency and amplitude of response to illumination, Proc. Natl. Acad. Sci. USA. 75:5217, 1978.

12. Poo MN, Cone RA: Lateral diffusion of rhodopsin in necturus rods. Exp Eye Res 17:503–510, 1973.

13. Wald G: The chemistry of rod vision. Science 113: 287–291, 1973.

14. Walloe L: Excitation of photoreceptors. Acta Ophthalmol 47:1163–1175, 1969.

15. Yoshikami S, Hagins WA: Control of the dark current in vertebrate rods and cones. In Langers H (ed): Biochemistry and Physiology of the Visual Pigments. Berlin, Springer-Verlag, 1970, pp 245–255.

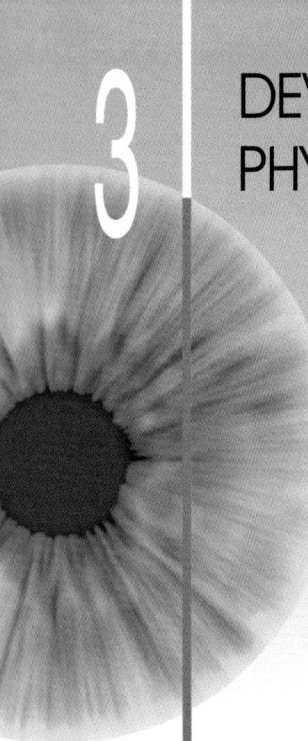

3

DEVELOPMENT, ANATOMY AND PHYSIOLOGY OF VITREOUS

**AK Khurana, Aruj K Khurana,
Indu Khurana, Bhawna Khurana**

DEVELOPMENT OF VITREOUS

Certain landmarks in the development of vitreous humour which need to be considered are:

FORMATION OF OPTIC VESICLE AND OPTIC STALK

The first evidence of primitive eye formation occurs during the third week of gestation. The region of neural plate (*see* Fig. 1.1A), which is destined to form the prosencephalon shows a linear thickened area on either side (*see* Fig. 1.1B), which soon becomes depressed to form the optic sulcus (*see* Fig. 1.1C).

Meanwhile the neural plate becomes converted into prosencephalic vesicle. As the optic sulcus deepens, the walls of the prosencephalon overlying the sulcus bulge out to form the *optic vesicle* (*see* Fig. 1.1D and E). The proximal part of the optic vesicle becomes constricted and elongated to form the *optic stalk* (*see* Fig. 1.1F to H).

FORMATION OF THE OPTIC CUP

During the fourth week of gestation (embryo 7.6–7.8 mm), while the lens vesicle is forming, simultaneously the optic vesicle is converted into a double-layered *optic cup*. It appears from Fig. 1.2 that this has happened because the developing lens has invaginated itself into the optic vesicle. However, this is not so. The conversion of the optic vesicle to the optic cup is due to differential growth of the walls of the vesicle. The margins of optic cup grow over the upper and lateral sides of the lens to enclose it. However, such a growth does not take place over the inferior part of the lens, and therefore, walls of the cup show deficiency in this part. This deficiency extends to some distance along the inferior surface of the optic stalk and is called the *choroidal* or *fetal fissure* (*see* Fig. 1.3). This embryonic ocular fissure closes by 6th week of gestation. When the lips of the fissure fail to fuse by 6th or 7th week, typical colobomas result. By the end of 7th week of gestation, most of the basic structures of the eye are present. Thereafter, ocular development is mainly a

process of differentiation and modification, of various parts of the globe.

ENTRAPMENT OF VASCULATURE

With the formation of optic cup, part of the inner vascular layer of mesenchyme is carried into the cup through the choroidal fissure. With the closure of this fissure, the portion of the mesenchyme which has made its way into the eye through the fissure is cut off from the surrounding mesenchyme and gives rise to hyaloid system of the vessels (Fig. 3.1).

DERIVATION OF VITREOUS

a. *Primary or primitive vitreous* is mesenchymal in origin and is a vascular structure having the hyaloid system of vessels. It is present in the first month of gestation (Fig. 3.1). Surface ectodermally derived elements that surround the lens during invagination are also thought to contribute to the primary vitreous. Thus the primary vitreous may be of mixed ectodermal and mesenchymal origin.

b. *Definitive or secondary or vitreous proper* is secreted by neuroectoderm of optic cup from 2nd month of gestation onwards. This is an avascular structure, basically an extracellular matrix, consisting mainly of a compact network of type II collagen fibrils and primitive hyalocytes. The precise origin of hyalocytes is presumed to be from the phagocytic monocytes of the primary vitreous. The content of hyaluronic acid is very low during the prenatal

period, but increases after birth. When this vitreous fills the cavity by 5th to 6th month of gestation, primitive vitreous is reduced to a small central space, *Cloquet's canal,* which courses between the optic nerve head and the posterior surface of the lens.

c. *Tertiary vitreous* is developed from neuro-ectoderm in the ciliary region during 4th month of gestation and is represented by the vitreous base and ciliary zonules.

ANATOMY OF VITREOUS

GENERAL FEATURES

- Vitreous humour is an inert, transparent, colorless, jelly-like, hydrophilic gel that serves the optical functions and also acts as important supporting structure for the eyeball.
- The vitreous cavity is bounded anteriorly by the lens and ciliary body and posteriorly by the retina.
- It weighs nearly 4 g and occupies a volume of almost 4 cc which is approximately two-thirds the volume of the entire globe.
- Vitreous is an extracellular material composed of approximately 99 per cent water.

STRUCTURE

The vitreous body is the largest and simplest connective tissue present as a single piece in the human body. However, for descriptive purposes, it may be divided into three parts—the hyaloid layer or membrane, the cortical vitreous and the medullary vitreous (Fig. 3.2).

1. *HYALOID LAYER OR MEMBRANE*

It is not a true membrane but the outermost surface layer or condensation of the vitreous body. It has a structure of connective tissue and shows striations due to its fibrils which run parallel with the surface.

A. ANTERIOR HYALOID MEMBRANE (ANTERIOR LIMITING MEMBRANE LAYER)

It covers the vitreous body anteriorly starting from a point approximately 1.5 mm from the ora serrata. The anterior hyaloid membrane, thus, lies in contact with the part of pars plana,

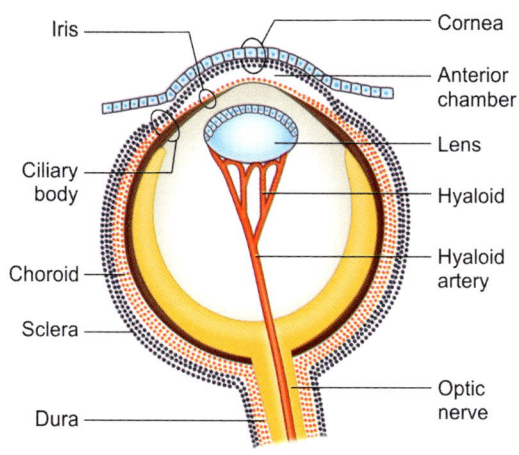

Iris — Cornea
— Anterior chamber
— Lens
Ciliary body — Hyaloid
— Hyaloid artery
Choroid —
Sclera —
— Optic nerve
Dura —

Fig. 3.1 *Derivation of various structures of the eyeball*

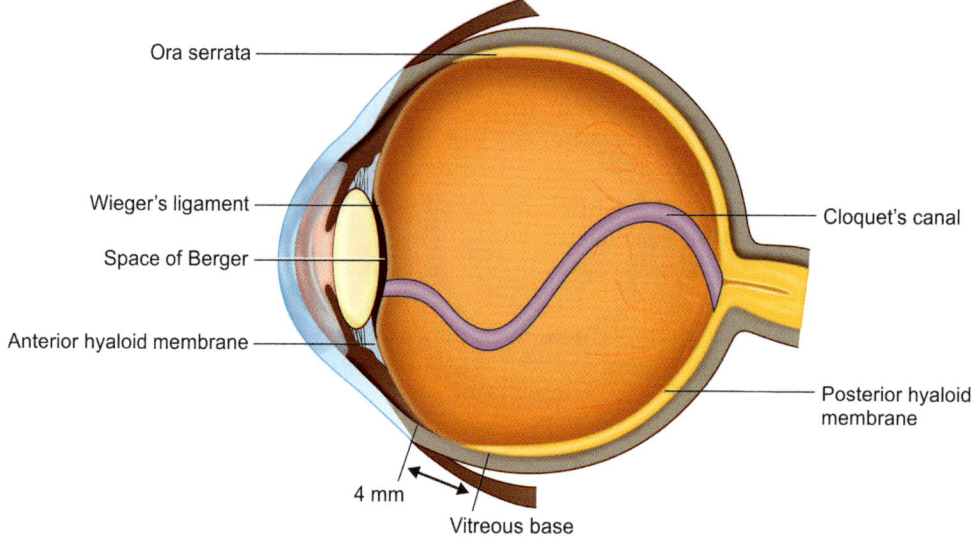

Fig. 3.2 *Gross anatomy of the vitreous*

ciliary processes, ciliary zonules and the posterior lens capsule. It is attached to the posterior lens capsule in the form of a ring about 9 mm in diameter. This attachment, which is especially firm in younger individuals, is known as the *hyaloideocapsular ligament of Wieger*. The central area within the 9 mm ring of attachment contains a potential space known an retrolental space or *Berger's space* or the patellar fossa. This space can be seen easily on slit lamp examination especially after the second decade of life. From the mid portion of Berger's space the anterior hyaloid membrane turns backward to form the anterior portion of the Cloquet's canal. Using specific staining techniques and a certain amount of traction, anterior hyaloid membrane has been shown to be connected with the other intraocular structures by following fine ligaments (Fig. 3.3):

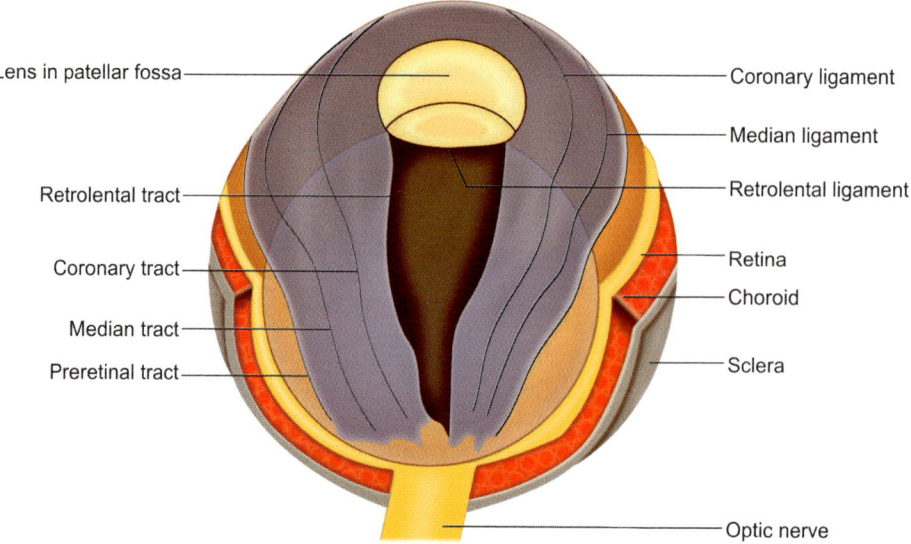

Fig. 3.3 *Vitreous tracts and ligaments in relation to anterior hyaloid membrane*

- *Hyalociliary zonules:* These fibers extend from the anterior hyaloid membrane to the valley between the ciliary processes.
- *Retrolental ligament* or the ligamentum hyaloideocapsulare attaches the anterior hyaloid membrane to the lens.
- *Coronary ligament:* Its fibers extend from the anterior hyaloid membrane to inner face of the posterior third of ciliary processes circumferentially.
- *Median ligament:* It also runs circumferentially from the anterior hyaloid membrane at the level of the mid-zone of pars plana.

B. POSTERIOR HYALOID MEMBRANE (POSTERIOR LIMITING MEMBRANE)

It extends back from the vitreous base up to the optic disc. It lies in contact with the internal limiting membrane of the retina, from which it is clinically distinguishable normally. Clinically, it becomes evident in the presence of preretinal (subhyaloid) hemorrhage and in posterior vitreous separation or detachment. The term *posterior hyaloid face* is usually applied for the detached posterior hyaloid membrane.

2. CORTICAL VITREOUS

Vitreous cortex refers to the entire peripheral zone, approximately 100 µ in width, of the main vitreous mass. It consists of a relatively more condensed fibrillar vitreous.

The vitreous gel consists of a delicate meshwork (reticular) of type II collagen fibrils interspersed with the sodium hyaluronate mucopolysaccharide molecules, which provide a considerable viscosity, elasticity and tensile strength to it.

Although the cortical vitreous represents only 2 per cent of the total vitreous volume, it is the metabolic center of the vitreous body, as it contains the *vitreous cells—the hyalocytes.* These cells are found in the entire cortical vitreous except in the retrolental part. The vitreous cells synthesize the hyaluronic acid and also act as phagocytes in special circumstances.

Microscopically, the hyalocytes are fusiform or stellate-shaped cells with prominent nuclei. Their cytoplasm contains PAS-positive granules, large amount of smooth surface endoplasmic reticulum, prominent Golgi apparatus, and lysosomal granules containing enzymes essential for phagocytic activity. In addition to the hyalocytes, about 10% of the total vitreous cells are fibrocytes and glial cells which are present in the vitreous cortex near the ciliary processes and optic disc.

3. MEDULLARY VITREOUS

The majority of the vitreous body is formed by the central medullary vitreous. Structurally, it is similar to the cortical vitreous except that it has a less fibrillar structure and is essentially cell-free, i.e. does not contain hyalocytes. Microscopically, the vitreous body is homogenous, but exhibits wavy lines as of watered silk in the slit lamp beam.

Running down the center of the vitreous body from the optic disc to the posterior pole of the lens is the *hyaloid canal (Cloquet's canal)* of doubtful existence in the adults. It represents the remnants of the primary vitreous. Down this canal runs the hyaloid artery of the foetus. Congenital remnants of the hyaloid arterial system may persist in different ways. A *Bergmeister's papilla* refers to the flake of glial tissue projecting from the optic disc. *Mittendorf dot* represents remnants of the anterior end of hyaloid artery, attached to the posterior lens capsule. It is essentially associated with a posterior polar cataract.

The Cloquet's canal is 1–2 mm in width and has a down turn in the central vitreous cavity. Its walls are formed by a vitreous condensation rather than a true membrane.

VITREOUS TRACTS AND TOPOGRAPHIC SUBDIVISION OF VITREOUS SPACE

VITREOUS TRACTS

Vitreous tracts are fine sheet-like condensations of vitreous tissue which radiate into the vitreous space from the ciliary body and anterior retina (Figs 3.3 and 3.4). These tracts give rise to the concentric 'onion-skin' arrangement of the adult vitreous. These tracts show a gentle curvature in younger eyes, which become more sinuous and extensive in adults. Vitreous tracts seen in the adult vitreous space are as follows:

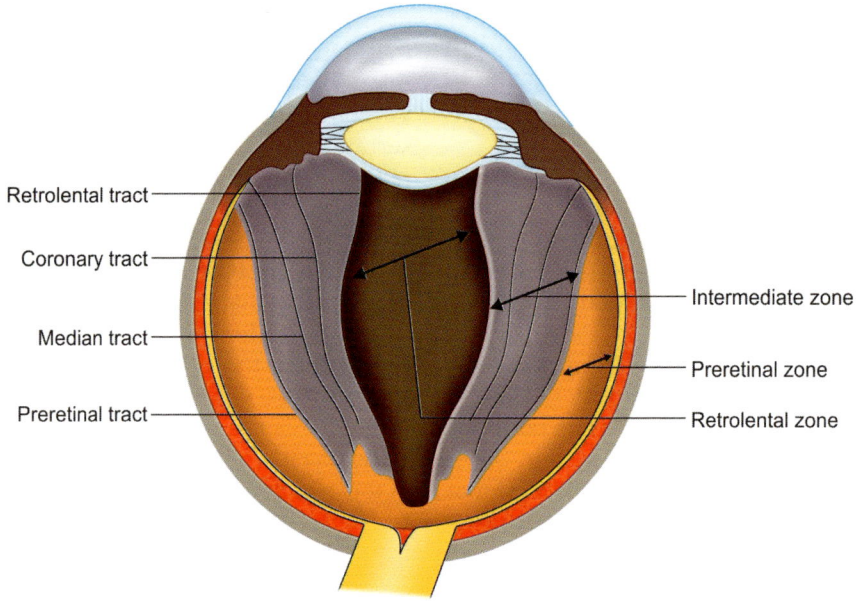

Fig. 3.4 *Vitreous tracts and zones of vitreous space*

1. *Retrolental tract (tractus retrolentalis).* It is the innermost vitreous tract which is attached anteriorly to the posterior lens capsule just near to hyaloideocapsular ligament at the boundary of patellar fossa. It runs backwards and terminates in front of the optic disc. It forms a reflecting membrane also called the membrana plicata of Vogt.

2. *Coronary tract (tractus coronaries).* It is attached anteriorly to the coronary ligament which is a circumferential band binding the inner face of the posterior third of ciliary processes to the anterior hyaloid membrane. It runs backwards in the central vitreous around the tractus retrolentis. It is not so distinct optically.

3. *Median tract (tractus medianus).* It is inserted anteriorly on the median ligament which is a circumferential band binding anterior hyaloid membrane to the mid zone of pars plana. It extends backwards as faint veil, around the tractus coronaries, into the central vitreous.

4. *Preretinal tract (tractus preretinalis).* It is outermost the vitreous tract which is attached anteriorly at the ora serrata circumferentially. It is a comparatively more reflecting mem brane extends backwards around the tractus medianus.

TOPOGRAPHIC SUBDIVISIONS OF VITREOUS SPACE

Vitreous space can be divided into three zones by the two optically distinct vitreous tracts—the tractus retrolentis and tractus preretinalis (Fig. 3.4). The three vitreous zones are as follows:

1. *Retrolental zone.* This zone of vitreous space is bounded anteriorly by the patellar fossa of the lens and circumferentially by the tractus retrolentis. The so called Cloquet's canal runs in the center of this zone of vitreous space.

2. *Intermediate zone.* It is bounded anteriorly by the epiciliary portion of the anterior hyaloid membrane and by the ciliary epithelium of the posterior pars plana. It is delineated from the retrolental zone by the tractus retrolentis and from the preretinal zone by the tractus preretinalis. The two optically indistinct and faint veil-like vitreous tracts—the coronary tract and the median tract—are present in this zone of the vitreous space.

3. *Preretinal zone:* This zone of the vitreous space is bounded on the outer side by the retina and on the inner side by the tractus preretinalis.

ATTACHMENTS OF THE VITREOUS

The vitreous is firmly attached to the surroun-ding structures around the ora serrata, the optic

disc, back of the lens (by margins of hyaloid capsular ligament of Wieger) and foveal region. The strongest attachment of the vitreous is to the pars plana and retina in the region of ora serrata and is called vitreous base.

1. Vitreous base

Vitreous base or origin of the vitreous refers to approximately 4 mm wide zone of the vitreous which is most firmly attached to the region of ora serrata, 1.5 to 2 mm area of the adjoining pars plana anteriorly and about 2 mm adjoining region of the peripheral retina posterior to the ora serrata temporally and about 3 mm posterior to the ora serrata nasally (Fig. 3.5A and B). In fact, the vitreous base is a three-dimensional zone and thus the functional base of the vitreous extends several millimetres into the vitreous body in this region. In some eyes, the vitreous base may have posterior extensions of firm attachment which may act as points of high vitreoretinal traction and may produce retinal tears.

In the regions of vitreous base, the collagen fibers from the cortical vitreous get inserted into the internal limiting membrane of the retina and pars plana part of ciliary body at right angles to their surface. It is this right angle attachment of the collagen fibers, which makes the vitreous base a three-dimensional zone, while in the posterior part the fibers, are nearly parallel to the internal limiting membrane of the retina. The microscopic details of the firm attachment of vitreous base are different anterior to the ora serrata when compared with the attachment posterior to the ora. Anteriorly, the attachment consists of complex interdigitations of vitreal collagen fibers with the reticular fibrillar material of the basement membrane of the non-pigmented ciliary epithelium. Some zonular fibers also blend into this junction. While posterior to the ora serrata the microscopic feature of the vitreous base firm attachment to the retina is characterized by a process called as *degenerative remodelling* of the retina, that is, in this region the internal limiting membrane of the retina shows focal ruptures through which the vitreous fibers are attached firmly with the plasma membrane of the retinal glial cells. Further, the presence of hemidesmosomes between the internal limiting membrane and Müller's cells located at vitreous base also contribute to the firm attachment.

The vitreous base attachments remain all through the life and are so strong that in traumatic detachment of the vitreous base, the vitreociliary or vitreoretinal junctions are not broken, rather the vitreous base is detached along with the underlying ciliary epithelium and retina.

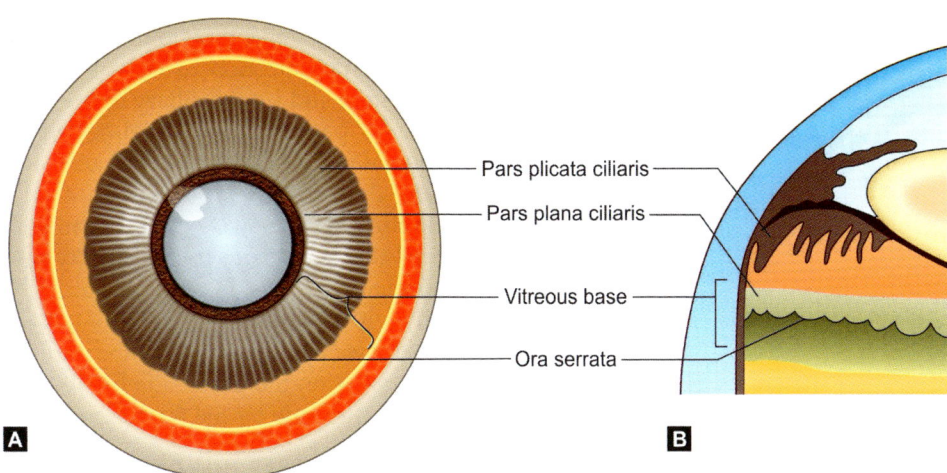

Pars plicata ciliaris

Pars plana ciliaris

Vitreous base

Ora serrata

A   **B**

Fig. 3.5 *Region of vitreous base: **(A)** As seen from inside the eyeball posteriorly; and **(B)** as seen in transverse section of the eyeball*

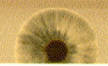

2. Hyaloideo-capsular ligament

The anterior vitreous surface (anterior hyaloid membrane) is attached to the posterior lens surface along a circular zone 1–2 mm wide and 8–9 mm in diameter just central to the insertion of the posterior zonular fibers. This attachment is called as hyaloideocapsular ligament of Wieger. The space between anterior hyaloid membrane and posterior capsule is called as Berger's space which is continuous with Cloquet canal a remanant of primary vitreous. Cloquet canal continues posteriorly in a serpentine fashion and open up into the space of Martegiani that is present over the optic nerve head.

3. Optic disc attachment

Posteriorly the vitreous is attached to optic nerve head. This attachment is invisible in young individuals. However, in older individuals beyoond 50 years as the process of degeneration of vitreous sets in and posterior hyaloid detaches itself from the optic nerve head, the ring of tissue is observed in the vitreous cavity which is termed as Weiss ring. It is a surest sign of posterior vitreous detachment (PVD).

4. Attachment to macular

The attachment of vitreous in the macular area occurs in an irregular, annular 3 to 4 mm diameter which is again invisible clinically. However, in the process of PVD a tenuous attachment of viterous may be seen at foveola by optical coherent tomography (OCT). Infact the advent of OCT has made it possible to monitor the process of PVD and ovserve the detachment of vitreous at the macula.

5. Paravascular attachments

The vitreous may have more than usual firm attachments to the retina along major vessels which is suspected mainly because of avulsions sometimes seen in retinal vessels in the process of PVD causing vitreous hemorrhage. Some authors have termed it as vitreo-retino-vascular bands.

BIOCHEMISTRY OF VITREOUS

BIOCHEMICAL COMPOSITION

The vitreous body is composed of three major structural components: water, collagen-like fibers, and hyaluronic acid a glycosaminoglycans (GAGs), and a few other minor components. *Water* forms 99% of the wet weight of the vitreous. The turnover of the vitreous water is very high, half of that present is replaced every 10–15 minutes. All the *solids* combined form the remaining 1% of the vitreous wet weight. The solids present in the vitreous can be discussed under two heads: macromolecular constituents and the low molecular weight constituents.

MACROMOLECULAR CONSTITUENTS

COLLAGEN

The insoluble proteins in the vitreous are present in the form of fine fibers which are most concentrated in the anterior portion of the vitreous body, particularly adjacent to the ciliary body, i.e. the vitreous base and in the cortical area adjacent to the retina but decrease toward the center and posterior portions of the eye. These fibrils are probably collagen in nature. Like the collagen, the vitreous insoluble proteins demonstrate typical X-ray diffraction pattern, is degraded by collagenase, has some typical amino acids characteristically of collagen, is soluble in boiling water and may be hydrolyzed to form a gel.

Type II collagen is the predominant (90%) collagen in the vitreous; the type II molecules are arranged in a staggered array with lysine-derived cross-links between molecules. Type IX collagen accounts for about 10% of vitreous collagen; cross-links also exist between type I and type II collagen. Type V and type XI collagens were thought to be separate collagen types but are now placed in the same family. Type VI/XI collagen is found in small amounts in the vitreous. Type IV collagen is a basement membrane collagen and is, therefore, not found in the vitreous. Immunohistochemical and ultrastructural studies of the posterior hyaloid membrane, from patients noted to have had a premortem posterior vitreous detachment

(PVD), have shown that this structure is a distinct membrane that stains for type IV and that the arrangement of collagen fibrils is markedly different from that of posterior vitreous cortex. These studies suggest that the posterior hyaloid membrane is wholly, or part of, the internal limiting membrane of the retina, and is not, as traditionally thought, condensed vitreous cortex. Stickler syndrome is a multi-system autosomal dominant disorder of type II collagen. Patients have characteristic vitreous abnormalities and have a high risk of developing giant retinal tears and retinal detachment.

HYALURONIC ACID

Hyaluronic acid, at the usual physiologic pH, occurs in the vitreous gel as a salt (sodium hyaluronate). It is a mucopolysaccharide (glycosaminoglycan or GAGs) macromolecule composed of equivalent amounts of two monosaccharides—the N-acetyl-glucosamine and glucuronic acid. Its molecular weight is between one to two million. The hyaluronic acid molecule presents as an unbranched linearly arranged polymer (linear hyaluronic chain of molecular length 2000–4000Å) which coils upon itself producing a large sponge-like spheroidal network interwined amongst the collagen fibers. The hyaluronic chains add the physical property of viscocity to the elasticity of collagen fibers. These hyaluronic chains interwined with the vitreous collagen fibers form a water binding meshwork which can bind water more than 50 times its weight. The great number of negative charges cause an electrostatic repulsion between the coils of the hyaluronic molecules and contributes to its ability to adsorb water.

The concentration of hyaluronic acid is highest in the posterior cortex, lesser in the central vitreous and lowest in the anterior periphery. The hyaluronic acid concentration increases from childhood (33 mg/ml) to adult levels (400 mg/ml) at the age of 13 years. The hyaluronic acid is produced by the hyalocytes which initiate its production through utilization of extracellular glucose. The continuation of the polymerization process may occur outside hyalocytes in the extracellular matrix of vitreous.

SOLUBLE PROTEINS

The soluble protein concentration of the vitreous is very low (about 10% of the serum concentration) and thus does not scatter light. This definitely indicates a barrier between the vitreous body and the vascular system. An interruption of this barrier as occurs during paracentesis or inflammation causes an inflow of serum proteins which may lead to vitreous turbidity, similar to the observation of aqueous flare in the anterior chamber during such events.

Soluble proteins in the vitreous are found in highest concentration in the epiretinal cortical layer and lowest in the vitreous base paralleling the hyaluronic acid distribution. Soluble protein of the vitreous mainly consist of *acid glycoprotein*. *Albumin* constitutes about one fourth of the total soluble proteins.

LOW MOLECULAR WEIGHT CONSTITUENTS

The vitreous levels of low molecular weight components are generally similar to the aqueous humour and plasma with some exceptions which can be explained on the basis of active transport in the aqueous humour (e.g. ascorbic acid) or metabolism (e.g. glucose).

SUGARS

The vitreous gel contains glucose, galactose, mannose, fructose, glucuronic acid and glucosamine. The latter two monosaccharides are predominantly conjugated into the hyaluronic acid molecule. Sugars diffuse into the vitreous primarily from the aqueous, or through the retinal and choroidal circulatory systems. The *glucose* content of the vitreous is approximately half of that present in aqueous humour or plasma because of its uptake and usage by the metabolically active retinal tissue. It is most likely also necessary for maintaining the metabolism of vitreous cells and lens.

ASCORBIC ACID

The concentration of ascorbic acid is higher in the vitreous than that of the plasma. It has been explained by the fact that the ascorbic acid, which is actively transported into the aqueous from the blood across the ciliary epithelium, freely diffuses into the vitreous. It has been

suggested that ascorbic acid forms a part of the oxidising systems that can depolymerize hyaluronic acid *in vitro*. This depolymerizing system may have a biologic role in vitreous hyaluronic acid turnover. It has been suggested that, if ascorbic acid is involved in breaking down of the hyaluronic acid molecules in pathophysiologic states, it may also be involved in condition necessary for creation of retinal detachment.

AMINO ACIDS

Twenty one, amino acids have been demonstrated in the vitreous humour of autopsied eyes. With the exception of glutamic acid and serine, levels of all the free amino acids were much lower than in the aqueous or plasma. This can be explained on the assumption that either the amino acids are uptaken and utilized by the retina and/or hyalocytes or they are actively transported from the vitreous into the retinal circulation.

ELECTROLYTE CONCENTRATION

Sodium concentration of sodium in the anterior vitreous is almost equal to that of plasma and aqueous humour indicating a passive diffusion. Penetration of Na^+ into the vitreous is slower than into the posterior chamber.

Potassium concentration of anterior vitreous and posterior chamber aqueous (9.5 mM/kg water) is higher than the plasma (5.6 mM/kg and the anterior aqueous (5 mM/kg water). This occurs because of an active transport of potassium across the ciliary body into the posterior chamber and also because of the active transport through the anterior capsule of the lens and passive diffusion (leak) through the posterior capsule of the lens into the vitreous. It has been observed that in the first 100 hours after death, the vitreous potassium level increases linearly and forms the basis of an accurate forensic test to determine time of death.

Calcium content of the vitreous humour is equal to that of aqueous humour and plasma.

Chloride concentration of the vitreous is higher than that of posterior chamber, anterior chamber and plasma. This is because the exchange of chloride seems to occur across both the retina and the posterior chamber.

Bicarbonate enters the eye through the ciliary body. It forms the buffer system of the eye. Its concentration is comparatively lower in the posterior vitreous.

Phosphate levels in the vitreous are lower than the aqueous humour indicating its utilization by the retina and the surrounding structures in formation of organic phosphates. These are involved in carbohydrate metabolism, maintenance of cell membrane integrity and continuation of activated Na^+-K^+ ATPase system for normal pumping activity.

Lactic acid is a by-product of metabolic activity. Its high levels in the posterior vitreous reflect retinal metabolism.

METABOLIC ACTIVITIES

Cortical vitreous, though represents only 2% of the total vitreous volume, is the metabolic center of the vitreous body. Hyalocytes present mainly in this part of vitreous are involved in the production of hyaluronic acid. It has been observed that when the hyaluronic acid is depolymerized by intravitreal injection of hyaluronidase in the rabbit, it is reformed within 6 weeks. The observation that the amount of labelled glucose incorporated into hyaluronic acid and its precursors is proportional to the number of hyalocytes present, confirm their metabolic activity.

PHYSIOLOGY OF VITREOUS

TRANSPORT PROCESSES

The active pump mechanisms located at the level of ciliary body, pigment epithelium and possible retinal vessels are concerned with active transport of materials across the vitreous. One such system is associated with removal of inorganic iodides and another with the outward transport of amino acids. A third such system has been shown to transport outward a great number of organic anions such as p-amino hippurate, probenecid, fluorescein and penicillin.

PHYSICOCHEMICAL PROPERTIES

WEIGHT AND VOLUME

Vitreous body weighs about 4 g and occupies a volume of almost 4 cc, which is approximately two-thirds the volume of the entire globe.

OPTICAL PROPERTIES

The fine random arrangement of vitreous fibers and high water content combine to maintain the gel in a high state of transparency. The presence of meager amount of soluble protein accounts for the absence of light scattering. The refractive index of the vitreous gel is about 1.33. It has been found to transmit almost 90% of light between 300 and 1400 nm with no transmission above or below these limits.

PLASTICITY

Plasticity of the vitreous body is provided by three-dimensional network of randomly oriented, road-like collagen fibers. The collagen fibers are electrostatically neutral because they are not cross-linked and thus allow the vitreous volume to expand, giving plasticity to the system.

VISCOELASTICITY

The property of viscoelasticity of the vitreous gel is provided by the network of hyaluronic acid molecular chains, entangled among the collagen fibers (Fig. 3.6). The sponge-like polymer coils of hyaluronic acid fold upon themselves. The numerous negatively charged groups in hyaluronic acid molecules precipitate extreme volume changes with change in physiochemical environment. Thus, the sponge-like coils of hyaluronic acid contribute viscoelasticity to the system.

GEL STABILITY

The combination of collagen fibers (supplying a basic structure) and the spongy hyaluronic

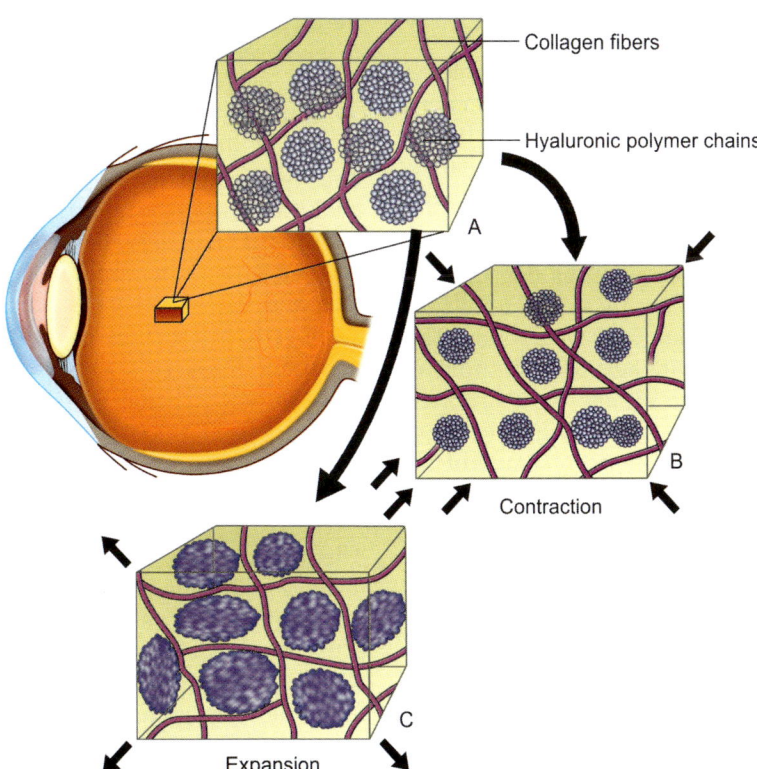

Fig. 3.6 *Dual network of hyaluronic acid molecular chains, entangled among the collagen fibers forming normal vitreous gel (**A**); contracted gel; (**B**) expanded gel (**C**)*

acid molecules (filling in the spaces between fibers) furnishes a *stable gel system* that can resist disorganizing forces such as centrifuga-tion or mechanical agitation. A collagen network alone collapses under such stress. The manner in which the collagen and hyaluronic acid interact to stabilize the system has been termed *frictional interaction*.

VITREOUS EXPANSION AND CONTRACTION

The property of *expansion and contraction* (volume changes) of the vitreous is a function of ionic charge of the vitreous structures as shown in Fig. 3.7A; the normal vitreous contains sodium ions, sodium chloride molecules and some positively changed protein molecules that neutralize the negatively charged hyaluronic acid. If the cationic molecules which neutralize the negatively charged hyaluronic acid molecules are removed by washing the gel with water or by neutralization, the residual nega-

tively charged hyaluronic acid molecules repulse each other with resultant *expansion of the vitreous gel* (Fig. 3.7B). On the contrary, if the sodium ions or sodium chloride molecules are replaced by positively charged protein molecules such as protamine sulfate or cationic dyes, the coils of hyaluronic acid cross-link and the gel system contracts (Fig. 3.7C).

Change in the vitreous volume has also been reported following transportive variation. Vitreous shrinkage correlates with rate of temperature rise, the duration of elevated temperature and the pH of vitreous. Heat from photocoagulation has been shown to experi-mentally cause vitreous shrinkage and contraction of posterior vitreous surface.

It has also been reported that the vitreous volume increases as the vitreous water content freezes. As thawing ensues, collagen fibers are disarranged and partial liquefaction occurs.

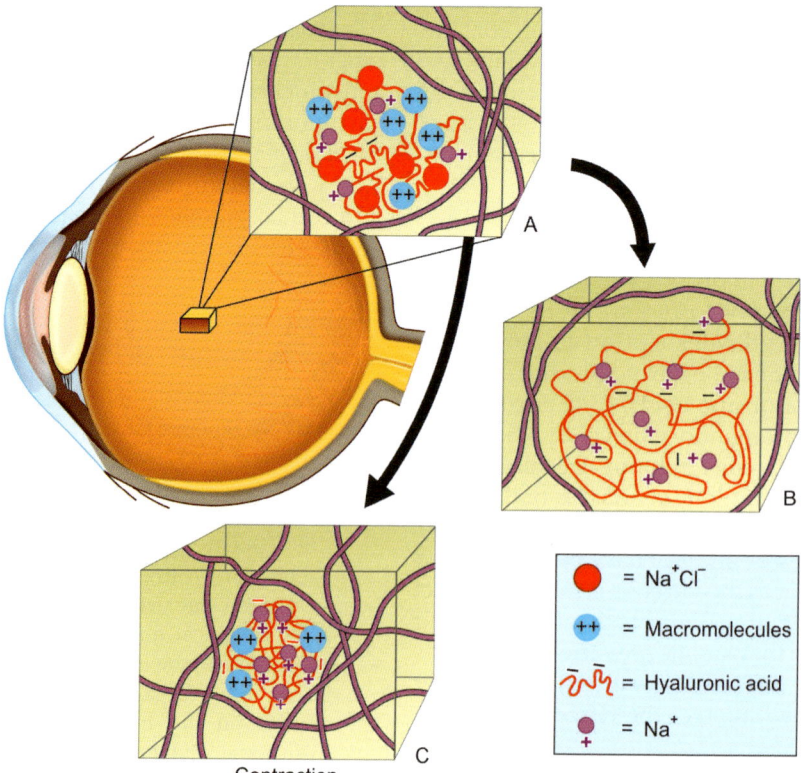

Contraction

Fig. 3.7 *Vitreous volume changes (a function of ionic charges of the vitreous): **(A)** Ionic charges of normal vitreous; **(B)** Ionic charges in vitreous expansion; and **(C)** Ionic charges in vitreous contraction*

EXCLUDED VOLUME CONCEPT OF THE VITREOUS

Excluded volume concept of the vitreous refers to the physical property of the collagen hyaluronic acid matrix of the cortical vitreous of effectively excluding most cells, proteins and often macromolecules by physically occupying the volume available. The low number of cells and the low concentration of soluble proteins contribute to a non-light scattering medium.

MOLECULAR SIEVE EFFECTS

Molecular sieve effect refers to the physiochemical property of the collagen hyaluronic acid matrix of the vitreous of selectively inhibiting the movement of water, large molecules and cells. The flow of water is retarded as much as 1000 times when it is forced to travel through a high concentration of hyaluronic acid. Movement of the positively charged solute molecules through the negatively charged hyaluronic acid matrix of cortical vitreous is markedly impeded. The dense, randomly oriented collagen network in the cortical vitreous may stop or trap the cells. Adjunctive to this vitreous effect is the basal lamina of the retinal-vitreous interface which retards passage of molecules larger than 150–200Å in diameter.

OSMOSIS

It has been shown by Duke Elder (1930) that the vitreous body will absorb water as a function of the water vapour pressure of its surroundings. This water absorption is partially a swelling phenomenon, related to the presence of GAG (hyaluronic acid), and partially an osmotic phenomenon caused by dissolved solids in the vitreous humour. Decrease in the vitreous following intravenous or oral administration of hyperosmotic agents such as mannitol, urea or glycerol have been explained by the fact that as the vitreous is in close contact with the internal vascular beds of the eye and any change in the osmotic pressure in the vessels will cause a transient osmotic flow of water (osmotic dehydration of the vitreous).

BLOOD-VITREOUS BARRIER

Blood vitreous or vitreoretinal barriers are the functional terms describing the inability of the vitreous constituents to equilibrate with blood and with surrounding fluids. Blood vitreous barrier consists of three components:

1. *Tight junctional complexes* at the level of retinal vascular endothelium, pigment epithelium of retina and non-pigmented epithelium of the ciliary body. It inhibits passage of high molecular weight constituents.

2. *Basal lamina of the vitreoretinal junction.* It physically blocks the passage of large molecules.

3. *Vitreous cortex.* The physiochemical characteristics of the vitreous hyaluronic acid network in the cortical vitreous effectively blocks or retards movement of cells, macromolecules and cations. Of the three components of the vitreoretinal barrier, the first (particularly the endothelial tight junctions) is of greatest importance. The vitreous-blood barrier restricts inflow of serum protein, reducing the Tyndall effect. When this barrier is broken down (as in trauma or inflammation) there occurs an inflow of proteins and consequently decrease in the vitreous transparency.

In addition to the vitreoretinal barrier, two other important factors also prevent the vitreous constituents to equilibrate with blood and the surrounding fluids. These are: (1) *Active transport pumping* mechanism located at the level of ciliary epithelium, retinal vascular endothelium and retinal pigment epithelium; and (2) small surface area to volume ratio of the vitreous.

BIBLIOGRAPHY

1. Balazs E. Molecular morphology of the vitreous body. In Smelser GK(ed): The Structure of the Eye. New York, Academic Press, 293, 1961.
2. Balazs EA, Sundblad L. Studies on the structure of the vitreous body. V. Soluble protein content, J Biol Chem 235:1973, 1960.
3. Balazs EA, Toth LZ, Eckl EA, Mitchell AP. Studies on the structure of the vitreous body. XII Cytological and histochemical studies on the cortical tissue layer. Exp Eye Res 3:57, 1964.
4. Balazs EA. Varga l, Gergely J. Comparative studies on the molecular characteristics of hyaluronic acid prepared from synovial fluid and some other tissues. Read before the Ninth International Congress on Rheumatic Diseases. Toronto. June 1957.

5. Balazs EA. Laurent UBG, DeRoche MH, Bunney DM. Studies on the structure of vitreous body. VIII. Comparative biochemistry Arch Biochem Biophys 81:464, 1959.

6. Balazs EA. Molecular morphology of the vitreous body. In Smelsen GK(ed): The Structure of the Eye. New York, Academic Press, 291, 1961.

7. Balazs EA. Physical chemistry of hyaluronic acid. Fed Proc 17:1086, 1958.

8. Balazs EA. Physiology of the vitreous body. In Schepens CL (ed): Importance of the Vitreous Body in Retina Surgery with Special Emphasis on Reoperations. St Louis, CVMosby, 29, 1960.

9. Balazs EA. Structure of the vitreous gel, XVII Concilium Ophthalmol (Acta) 2:1019, 1954.

10. Balazs EA. The molecular biology of the vitreous. In New and Controversial Aspects of Retinal Detachment. A McPherson. (ed.) New York. Harper & Row, 1968,

11. Becker B. Iodide transport by the rabbit eye. Am J Physiol 200:804, 1961.

12. Becker B. The transport of organic anions by the rabbit eye; 1. In vitro iodopvracet (Diodrast) accummulation by ciliary body-iris preparations Am J Ophthalmol 50:862, 1960.

13. Berman ER, Michaelson 1C. The chemical composition of the human vitreous body as related to age and myopia, Exp Eye Res 3:9, 1964.

14. Boettner A, Wolter JR. Transmission of the ocular media. Invest Ophthalmol 1:776, 1962.

15. Christiansen J, Kollarits CR, Fukui H, Fistiman M, Michels R, Mikumi I. Intraocular irrigating solution and lens clarity (In press).

16. Dayson H. Luck CD. A comparative study of the total carbon dioxide in the ocular fluids, cerebrospinal fluid and plasma of some mammalian species. J Pysiol (Long) 132:454, 1956.

17. Duke-Elder S, Gloster J. Physiology of the Eye. In Duke-Elder, S (ed): Systems of Ophthalmology, Vol IV, Physiology of the Eye and Vision. London, H Kimpton 222, 1968.

18. Duke-Elder S, Wybar KC. The vitreous body. In Duke-Elder S (ed): System of Ophthalmology, Vol II, The Anatomy of the Visual System. London, H Kimpton, 294, 1961.

19. Fessler JH, Fessler LI. Electron microscopic visualization of the polysaccharide hyaluronic acid. Proc Natl Acad Sci USA 56:141, 1966.

20. Fine BS, Yanoff M. Ocular Histology. New York, Harper and Row, 110, 1972.

21. Foos RY. Anatomic and pathologic aspects of the vitreous body. Trans Am Acad Ophthalmol Otolaryngol 77:171, 1973.

22. Foos RY. Vitreoretinal juncture: topographical variations. Invest Ophthalmol 11:801, 1972.

23. Gartner J. The fine structure of the vitreous base of the human eye and the pathogenesis of pars planitis. Am J Ophthalmol 71:1317, 1971.

24. Gloor BP. The vitreous. In Adler's Physiology of the Eye. Clinical Application, ed 6 RA Moses, ed. St Louis, CV Mosby Co. 1975.

25. Hogan MJ, Zimmerma LE. Ophthalmic Pathology. An Atlas and Textbook. Philadelphia, WB Saunders, 638, 1962.

26. Hogan MJ. The vitreous, its structure, and relation to the ciliary body and retina. Invest Ophthalmol 2:418, 1963.

27. Kinsey VE, Reddy DVN. An estimate of the ionic composition of the fluid secreted into the posterior chamber, inferred from a study of aqueous humor dynamics. Doc Ophthalmol 13:7, 1959.

28. Last RJ. The vitreous. In Wolf E(ed): Anatomy of the Eye and Orbit. Philadelphia, WB Saunders 174, 1968.

29. Lie JT. Changes of potassium concentration in the vitreous humour after death. Am J Med Sci 254:136;1967.

30. Morner CT. Untersuchung der protein-sub-stanzen in den lichtbrechenden medien des auges, III, Die Glasmembranen der lechtbreche-uden medien. Z. Physiol Chem 18:233, 1894

31. Nordmann, J. Biology due corps vitre: chimie, physique et physicochimie, physiologie, bacteriologie, immunologie, physiopathologie. In Brini A, et al. (ed): Biologie et Chirurgie du corps vitre, Paris, Masson and Cie., Editeurs 1968.

32. Osterlin SE, Balazs EA. Macromolecular composition and fine structure of the vitreous in the owl monkey. Exp Eye Res 7:534, 1968.

33. Osterlin SE, Jacobson B. The synthesis of hyaluronic acid in vitreous II. The presence of soluble transferase and nucleotide sugar in the acellular vitreous gel. Exp Eye Res 7:511, 1996.

34. Pirie A, Schmidt G, Waters JW. Ox vitreous humor. I. The residual protein. Br J Ophthalmol 32: 321, 1948.

35. Reddy DVN, Kinsev VF. Studies on the crystalline lens: IX. Quantitative analysis of free amino acids and related compounds Invest Ophthalmol 1:635, 1962.

36. Reddy DVN, Kinsey VE. Composition of the vitreous humor in relation to that of plasma and aqueous humors. Arch Ophthalmol 63:715, 1960.

37. Reddy DVN, Kinsey VF. Transport of alpha aminoisobutyric acid into ocular fluids and lens Invest Ophthalmol 1:44, 1962.

38. Reddy DVN, Rosenberg C, Kinsey VE. Steady state distribution of free amino acids in the aqueous humour, vitreous body and plasma of the rabbit. Exp Eye Res 1:175, 1961.

39. Reddy DVN, Rosenburg C, Kinsey VE. Steady state distribution of free amino acids in the aqueous humors, vitreous body and plasma of the rabbit. Exp Eye Res 1:175, 1969.

40. Straatsma BR, Alien RA. Retinal and vitreous abnormalities related to retinal detachment. Trans Pac Coast Otoophthalmol Soc 41:329, 1960.

41. Tolentino FI, Schepens CL, Freeman HM. Vitreo-retinal disorders. Philadelphia, WB Saunders, 1976.

42. Walker F, Patrick RS. Constituent monosaccharides and hexosamine concentration of normal human vitreous humor. Exp Eye Res 6:227, 1967.

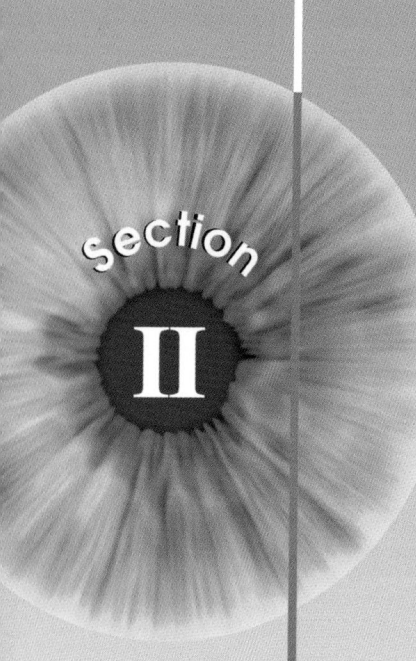

4 EXAMINATION OF POSTERIOR SEGMENT

AK Khurana, Subina Narang, Shaveta Bhayana
Aruj K Khurana, Bhawna Khurana

INTRODUCTION

Though the conventional direct and indirect ophthalmoscopies are still the most commonly used techniques, the ophthalmic imaging technology has undergone explosive growth in the past few years. Current techniques of posterior segment evaluation and imaging have contributed significantly to the understanding of pathophysiology and treatment of a variety of posterior segment disorders. Some of the common optical instruments and techniques for posterior segment evaluation include the following:
- Ophthalmoscopy
- Slit lamp biomicroscopic examination of the fundus
- Fundus camera
- Wide-field imaging system (retinal camera)
- Scanning laser ophthalmic techniques
  - Scanning laser ophthalmoscopy (SLO)
  - CSLO or scanning laser tomography (SLT)
  - Retinal thickness analyser
  - Scanning laser polarimetry (SLP) (retinal nerve fiber analyser)
- Optical coherence tomography
- OCT ophthalmoscopy

OPHTHALMOSCOPY

Ophthalmoscopy is a clinical examination of the interior of the eye by means of an ophthalmoscope. It is primarily done to assess the state of fundus and detect the opacities of ocular media. The ophthalmoscope was invented by Babbage

in 1848; however, its importance was not recognized, till it was reinvented by *von Helmholtz* in 1850. Ophthalmoscopic methods of examination in vogue are:

- Distant direct ophthalmoscopy
- Direct ophthalmoscopy
- Monocular indirect ophthalmoscopy
- Binocular indirect ophthalmoscopy.

DISTANT DIRECT OPHTHALMOSCOPY

It should be performed routinely before the direct ophthalmoscopy, as it gives a lot of useful information (vide infra). It can be performed with the help of a self-illuminated ophthalmoscope or a simple plain mirror with a hole in the center.

Procedure

The light is thrown into the patient's eye – with the patient sitting in a semidark room – from a distance of 20–25 cm, and the features of the red glow in the pupillary area are noted.

Applications of distant direct ophthalmoscopy

1. *To diagnose opacities in the refractive media*. Any opacity in the refractive media is seen as a black shadow in the red glow. The exact location of the opacity can be determined by observing the parallactic displacement. For this, the patient is asked to move the eye up and down while the examiner is observing the pupillary glow. The opacities in the pupillary plane remain stationary, those in front of the pupillary plane move in the direction of the movement of the eye and those behind it will move in opposite direction (Fig. 4.1).

2. *To differentiate between a mole and a hole of the iris*. A small hole and a mole on the iris appear as a black spot on oblique illumination. On distant direct ophthalmoscopy, the mole looks black (as earlier) but a red reflex is seen through the hole in the iris.

3. *To recognize detached retina or a tumour arising from the fundus*. A greyish reflex seen on distant direct ophthalmoscopy indicates either a detached retina or a tumour arising from the fundus.

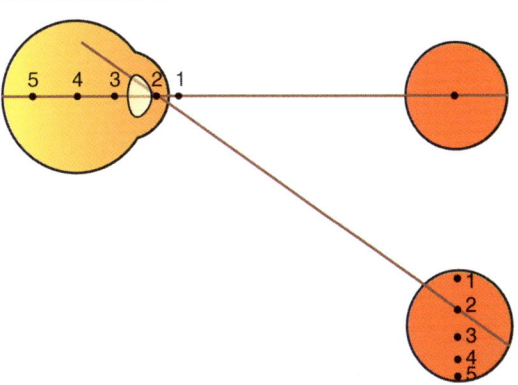

Fig. 4.1 *Parallactic displacement on distant direct ophthalmoscopy*

DIRECT OPHTHALMOSCOPY

It is the most commonly practised method for routine fundus examination.

OPTICS AND CHARACTERISTICS OF IMAGE

Optics

The modern direct ophthalmoscope (Fig. 4.2) works on the basic optical principle of glass plate ophthalmoscope introduced by *von Helmholtz*. Optics of direct ophthalmoscopy is depicted in Fig. 4.3.

A convergent beam of light is reflected into the patient's pupil (Fig. 4.3, dotted lines). The emergent rays from any point on the patient's fundus reach the observer's retina through the viewing hole in the ophthalmoscope (Fig. 4.3, continuous lines). The emergent rays from the patient's eye are parallel and brought to focus on the retina of the emmetropic observer when accommodation is relaxed.

- *In a hypermetropic patient*, the emergent ray from the illuminated area of retina will be divergent and thus can be brought to focus on the observer's retina, if the latter accommodates, or by the help of a convex lens (Fig. 4.4).
- *In a myopic patient*, the emergent rays will be convergent and thus can be brought to focus on the observer's retina by the help of a concave lens (Fig. 4.5).

Therefore, if the patient or/and the observer is/are ametropic, a correcting lens (equivalent to the sum of the patient's and observer's

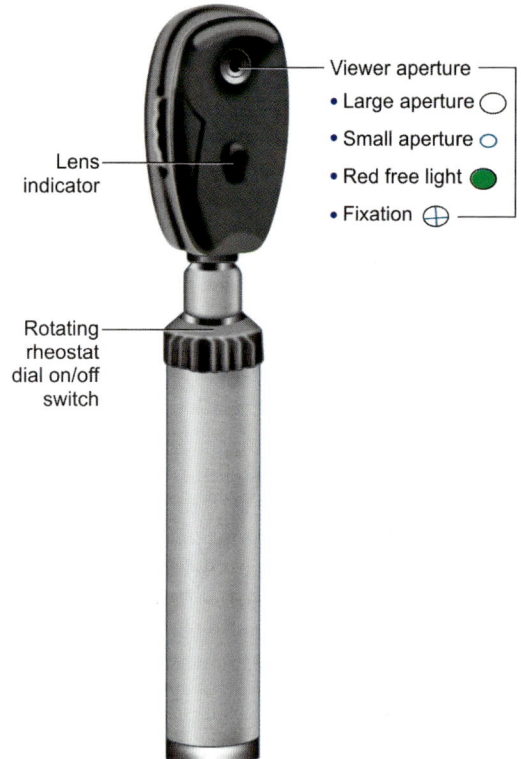

Lens indicator

Rotating rheostat dial on/off switch

Viewer aperture
- Large aperture
- Small aperture
- Red free light
- Fixation

Fig. 4.2 *Direct ophthalmoscope showing viewing aperture above illuminating aperture and lens indicators*

refractive error) must be interposed (from the system of plus and minus lenses, in-built in the modern ophthalmoscopes).

Characteristics of the image formed

In direct ophthalmoscopy, the image is erect, virtual and about 14–15 times magnified (Table 4.1) in emmetropes (more in myopes and less in hypermetropes).

Magnification of the direct ophthalmoscope for an emmetropic patient viewed by an emmetropic observer is 15x. If the patient and observer have refractive errors, then the axial length and refractive power of both eyes, plus the compensating lenses of the ophthalmoscope, all influence the resultant magnification. If the patient is myopic, then the eye has plus power and the ophthalmoscope requires a minus lens for viewing a clear images. The combination results in a **Galilean telescope**, which enlarges fundus detail. The opposite effect is seen in a hyperopic eye (reverse telescope).

If neither the patient nor the observer is emmetropic, then power of a single lens in the ophthalmoscope must be equal to the mathematical sum of the patient's and the observer's refractive errors. It is important to understand that when one or both of the participants have a large refractive error or a high degree of astigmatism, it is more advantageous to use the glasses to view the fundus.

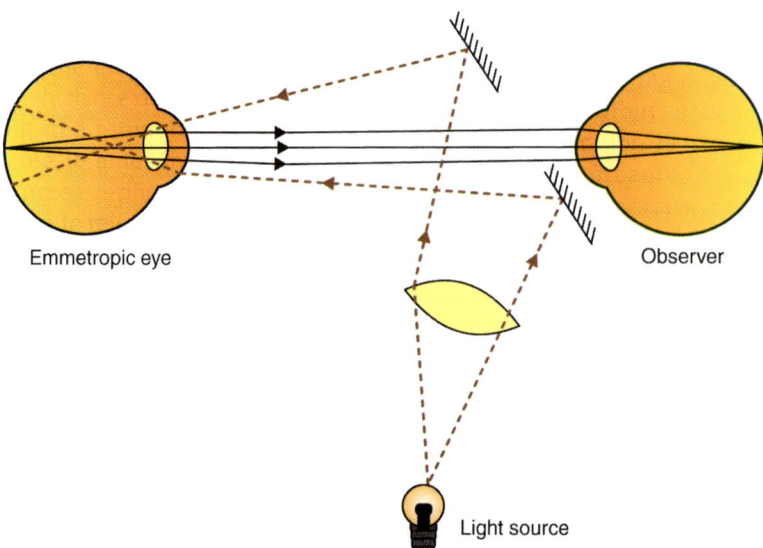

Emmetropic eye

Observer

Light source

Fig. 4.3 *Optics of direct ophthalmoscopy in an emmetropic patient*

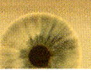

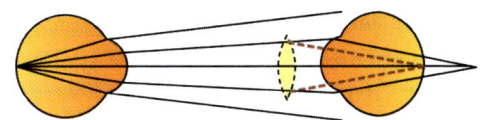

Fig. 4.4 *Optics of direct ophthalmoscopy in a hypermetropic patient*

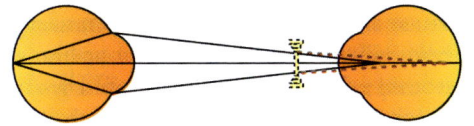

Fig. 4.5 *Optics of direct ophthalmoscopy in a myopic patient*

Field of view

The ophthalmoscopic field of vision (Table 4.1) is always smaller than the field of illumination in direct ophthalmoscopy. It is affected by the following factors:

- It is directly proportional to the size of the pupil of observed eye.
- It is directly proportional to the *axial length* of the observed eye.
- It is inversely proportional to the distance between the observed and the observer's eye.

focused by twirling the dial for the Reskoss disc, which has several plus- and minus-powered lasers. The optimal focusing lens on the Reskoss disc depends on the patient's refractive error, the examiner's refractive error (including unintended accommodation) and the examination distance (Table 4.2).

Once the retina is focused, the details should be examined systematically starting from disc, blood vessels, the four quadrants of the general background and the macula by utilizing the various illumination options and apertures provided in the direct ophthalmoscope (Table 4.3 and Fig. 4.6A).

Note. The problem is obtaining adequate illumination of the patient's fundus as the light source only illuminates that part of the fundus which is struck directly by light; the rest of the fundus remains dark. Therefore, the fundus can be adequately viewed only if the observed areas and the illuminated areas coincide. This can take place only if the light source and the observer's pupil are closely aligned optically (Fig. 4.6B). Most direct ophthalmoscopes (Fig. 4.2) have the illuminating beam situated below the viewing

Table 4.1. *Magnification, field of view and characteristics of the image formed with different techniques of fundus examination*

Technique	Magnification	Field of view	Characteristics of image	Principal use
Direct ophthalmoscopy	14X	5°	Erect, virtual	Routine view of disc and surrounding area
Indirect ophthalmoscopy				
• With 114 D	4X	40°	Inverted, reversed and real	Fundus lesion inspection
• With 120 D	3X	45°	Inverted, reversed and real	Routine examination
• With 130 D	2X	50°	Inverted, reversed and real	Routine examination
Biomicroscopic examination				
• With 178 D	10X	30°	Inverted, reversed and real	Posterior pole observation
• With 190 D	7.5X	40°	Inverted, reversed and real	Posterior pole observation
• With Hruby lens	12X	10°	Erect, virtual	Optic disc and vitreous observation
• With Goldmann fundus contact lens	10X	20°	Erect, virtual	Optic disc and macula inspection
Fundus camera	2.5X	30°	Erect, virtual Photodocumentation	

Table 4.2 *Direct ophthalmoscope's refractive power versus patient's spherical equivalent while focusing**

Direct ophthalmoscope's refractive power	Patient's refractive error
230 D	215 D
220 D	212 D
210 D	28 D
25 D	24 D
20	2Plano
15 D	16 D
110 D	115 D

*When the examiner's eye is emmetropic or corrected and the examination distance between the ophthalmoscope and cornea is 20 mm

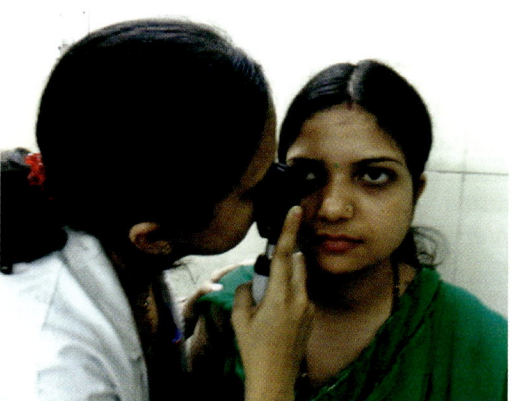

Fig. 4.6A *Technique of direct ophthalmoscopy*

Table 4.3 *Various apertures and illumination options with direct ophthalmoscope*

Aperture description	Use
Large spot	For viewing through a dilated pupil
Small spot	For viewing through a small pupil
Red-free fibre	Useful in detecting changes in the nerve fibre layer and identifying microaneurysms and other vascular anomalies
Slit	For evaluating contour of retinal lesions
Reticule or grid	For measuring vessel caliber or diameter of a small retinal lesion (marked in 0.2 mm increments)
Fixation target	For testing fixation pattern (central or eccentric)
Reskoss disc	Plus and minus lenses are for focusing the retina

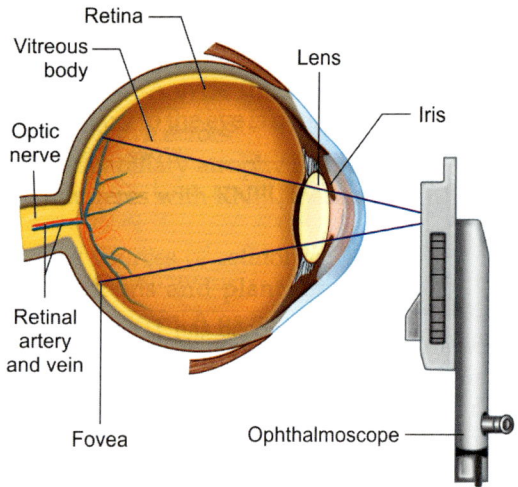

Fig. 4.6B *The light source and the observer's pupil are closely aligned optically and that part of the fundus which is properly illuminated can be adequately viewed*

aperture. Modern ophthalmoscopes have a condensing lens to intensify the light Beam and a diaphragm and projecting lens to limit the size of the light beam.

Problems faced during viewing

Unwanted reflections. To avoid both scattering and reflection of light rays into the viewing beam, both the illuminating and viewing beams must be maximally separated so that interference and hence reflections do not occur. Therefore, separation of the two beams must be maintained through the cornea and lens, yet overlap onto the retina. Thus, with a dilated pupil, reflex-free viewing is more easily obtained.

Peripheral viewing with a direct ophthalmoscope is limited because the pupil becomes too narrow for the viewing and illumination beams. The equatorial region is usually the limit in peripheral viewing with the direct ophthalmoscope. A technique to aid in peripheral viewing has to do with the change in the pupil configuration on extreme eyes gazes. When the patient looks to the right or left, the pupil is elongated vertically. In this situation the

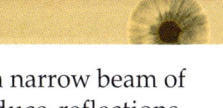

ophthalmoscope should be held vertically to facilitate the entrance of both beams into the eye. Likewise, a horizontal elongation of the pupil results during up or down gaze, and a horizontal orientation of the scope may be helpful.

Interpretation

Generally, an ophthalmoscopic examination of the fundus starts at the optic nerve head because localization of this structure provides immediate orientation. The image is virtual and upright. The optic disc should be examined for the cup-to-disc ratio, color, clarity of margins, spontaneous venous pulsations, and any abnormalities. The tissue around the disc is studied, with emphasis placed on the blood vessels, especially the superior and inferior temporal arcades. The vessels should be evaluated for their arteriovenous ratio, color, diameter, and course. The background retinal tissue is also examined. The macula is usually examined last because of the dazzling and discomfort that is experienced by the patient. The macula should be examined for the foveal reflex, color, pigmentation, and any abnormalities.

The size of any abnormal lesion is described in terms of disc areas and distance from disc or macula is described in terms of disc diameters. For depth of the lesion a 3-D difference in focal planes for focusing the lesion in an emmetropic eye converts into a linear depth equivalent of approximately 1 mm in a phakic eye and into approximately 2 mm in an aphakic eye. This is especially useful for documenting raised lesions, e.g. disc edema.

Accessory functions of direct ophthalmoscope

Accessory functions have been built into the ophthalmoscope to widen the diagnostic capabilities.

Slit diaphragm can produce a narrow slit beam, which can be used to detect elevation or depression of retinal lesions. Here, a distortion of the beam occurs when it travels across an elevation or depression. The beam bows toward the observer on an elevated area and away from the observer in a depressed area.

Pinhole diaphragm produces a narrow beam of light that can be used to reduce reflections, which is especially helpful when viewing through a small pupil. A small circle of light allows observation of fine retinal detail seen in the zone adjacent to the directly illuminated retina. This zone consists of areas of indirect illumination that enhance observation.

Fixation reticle can be used to discover eccentric fixation or eccentric viewing by the patient. This may be helpful in the evaluation of strabismic patients or for measuring the size of macular lesions.

Filters of different types can be very helpful while performing ophthalmoscopy. A cobalt blue filter can be used to enhance fluorescence angiography. A red free (green) filter to absorb red light; therefore, red objects appear very dark. This is helpful when studying blood vessels and hemorrhages. Defects in the nerve fiber layer and retinal edema are more easily seen with red-free light because of shorter wavelengths that are readily scattered by superficial retinal layers.

Cross polarizing filters reduce reflection because light reflected back from the cornea is depolarized and blocked by the viewing filter, but light reflected from the retina (except for the internal limiting membranes) is polarized and remains visible. The chief drawback of polarizing filters is the substantial reduction in illumination and hence less bright view of the fundus.

MONOCULAR INDIRECT OPHTHALMOSCOPY

Structural features

The monocular indirect ophthalmoscope consists of (Fig. 4.7):
- *Illumination rheostat* at its base,
- *Focusing lever* for image refinement,
- *Filter dial* with red-free and yellow filters,
- *Forehead rest* for steady proper observer head positioning, and
- *Iris diaphragm lever* to adjust the illumination beam diameter.

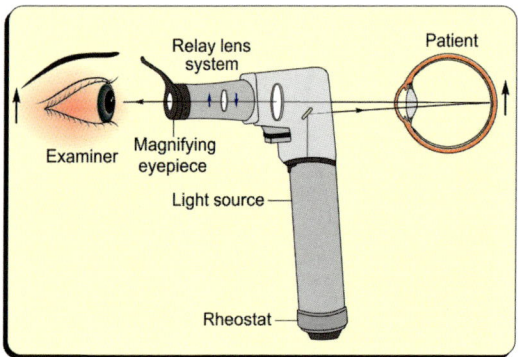

Fig. 4.7 *The optical principle of monocular indirect ophthalmoscopy, demonstrating the resultant erect magnified image*

Optics

An internal relay lens system re-inverts the initially inverted image to a real erect one, which is then magnified. This image is focusable using the focusing lever/eyepiece system (Fig. 4.7).

Indications and view of extent

Indications for use of monocular indirect ophthalmoscopy include:

- Need for an increased field of view
- Small pupils
- Uncooperative children
- Patient's intolerance of bright light of binocular indirect ophthalmoscope
- Basic fundus screening

Extent of view. Although vitreous base views are possible with monocular indirect ophthalmoscopy, its greatest effectiveness extends anteriorly to the peripheral equatorial region. The 40+ degree field of view of the monocular indirect ophthalmoscope is approximately the same as that of binocular indirect ophthalmoscope.

Advantages and disadvantages

Advantages of monocular indirect ophthalmoscopy include:

- Increased field of view similar to indirect ophthalmoscopy.
- Erect real imaging similar to direct ophthalmoscopy.

Disadvantages include:

- Lack of stereopsis
- Limited illumination
- Fixed magnification
- Fair to good resolution.

BINOCULAR INDIRECT OPHTHALMOSCOPY

Indirect ophthalmoscopy, introduced by Nagel in 1864, is now a very popular method for examination of the posterior segment. Indirect ophthalmoscopy was considered as an elementary part of examination by only the posterior segment or the retinal surgeons in yesteryears. It was the eagerness on the part of the examiner, who used only direct ophthalmoscopy, so as to come to a hasty diagnosis. He used to organize his thoughts on this cursory examination of the retina, and assumptions were made for the final diagnosis. However, in this modern era, indirect ophthalmoscopy is of great general use in ophthalmology and requires much effort and practice by the anterior as well as the posterior segment surgeons.

OPTICS OF INDIRECT OPHTHALMOSCOPY
Optical principle

The principle of indirect ophthalmoscopy is to make the eye highly myopic by placing a strong convex lens in front of patient's eye so that the emergent rays from an area of the fundus are brought to focus as a real inverted image between the lens and the observer's eye, which is then studied (Fig. 4.8A).

Optical system of binocular indirect ophthalmoscope

Optics of modern binocular indirect ophthalmoscopy is shown in Fig. 4.8B. Binocularity is achieved by reducing the observer's interpupillary distance from about 60 mm to approximately 15 mm by prisms/mirrors (Fig. 4.9). Even this artificial reduction of interpupillary distance requires larger patient's pupils for binocular viewing than those for the monocular viewing.

Field of illumination as shown in Fig. 4.10. The field of illumination is more in myopia and less in hypermetropia compared to emmetropia.

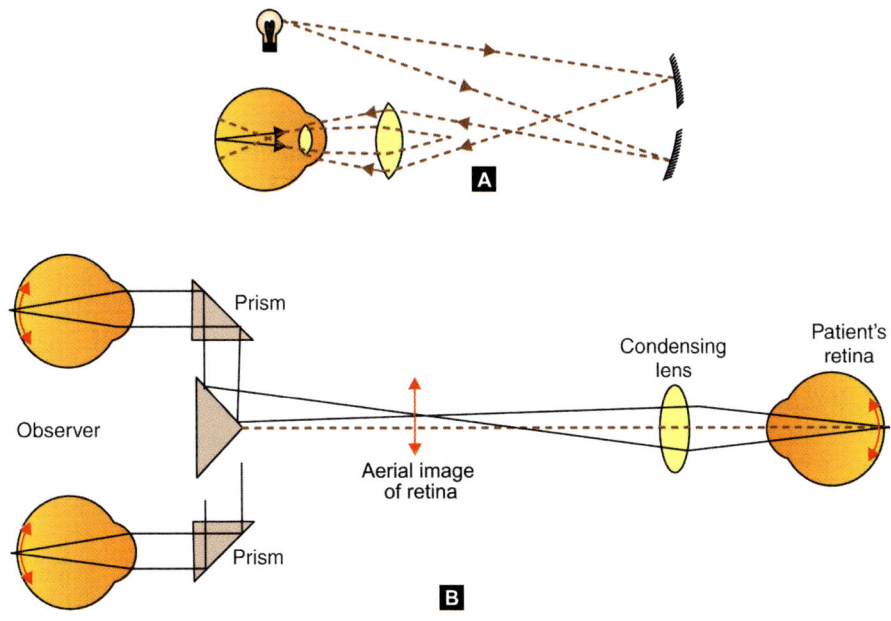

Fig. 4.8 *(A) Optics of indirect ophthalmoscopy; and (B) optical system of a modern binocular indirect ophthalmoscope*

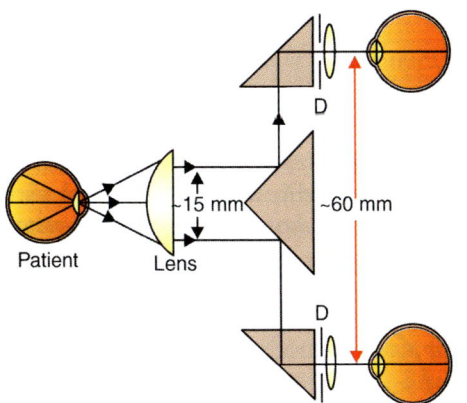

Fig. 4.9 *Stereopsis is produced by the binocular indirect ophthalmoscope. Note how the two prisms widen the incoming beams so that they are incident to the eyes of the observer*

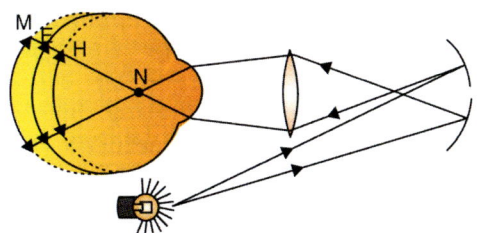

Fig. 4.10 *Field of illumination in various refractive errors*

Image formation

1. *Image formation in emmetropia.* The emergent rays from the illuminated area of retina are parallel in emmetropic patients and are, therefore, brought to focus by the condensing lens at its principal focus (Fig. 4.11). Thus an inverted image of the retina is formed in the air between the condensing lens and the observer.

2. *Image formation in hypermetropia.* The emergent rays from the illuminated area of retina are divergent in hypermetropic patients and thus appear to come from an imaginary enlarged upright image situated behind the eye (Fig. 4.12). The condensing lens, therefore, uses this as an object and forms an inverted image of it. Since the rays are divergent, the final image is situated in front of the principal focus.

3. *Image formation in the myopic eye.* The emergent rays from the illuminated area AB of retina in a myopic patient are convergent and, therefore, an inverted image A_1B_1 of it is formed in front of the eye. The condensing lens forms the final image A_2B_2 situated within its own focal length (Fig. 4.13).

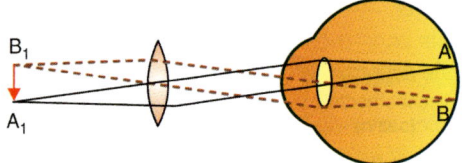

Fig. 4.11 *Image formation on indirect ophthalmoscopy in emmetropia*

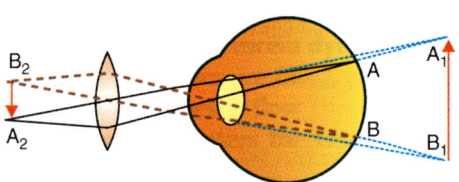

Fig. 4.12 *Image formation on indirect ophthalmoscopy in hypermetropia*

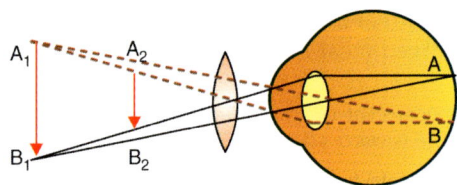

Fig. 4.13 *Image formation on indirect ophthalmoscopy in myopia*

Characteristics of the image

The image formed in indirect ophthalmoscopy is real, inverted and magnified. Magnification of image depends upon the dioptric power of the convex lens, position of the lens in relation to the eyeball and refractive state of the eyeball. About 53 magnification is obtained with a 113 D lens. With a stronger lens, image will be smaller but brighter and field of vision will be more. The important characteristics of the image formed by an indirect ophthalmoscope are as follows:

1. Relative position of images formed in emmetropic, myopic and hypermetropic eye. The relative positions of the images formed in emmetropic, myopic and hypermetropic eye, when the condensing lens used is situated at its own focal distance from cornea, are shown in Fig. 4.14.

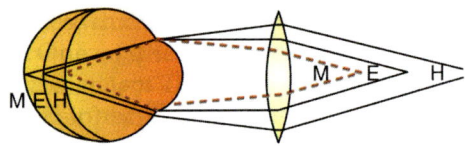

Fig. 4.14 *The relative positions of the images in indirect ophthalmoscopy in emmetropia (E), hypermetropia (H) and myopia (M)*

- *In emmetropia,* the emergent rays are parallel and thus focused at the principal focus of the lens, i.e. at E.
- *In hypermetropia,* the emergent rays are divergent and are, therefore, focused farther away from the principal focus, i.e. at H.
- *In myopia,* the emergent rays are convergent and are, therefore focused near to the lens than its principal focus, i.e. at M.

2. Size of the image vis-a-vis refractive condition of the eye.

i. *In an emmetropic eye,* the size of image always remains the same and is situated at its principal focus, because the rays emerging for such an eye are parallel (Figs 4.11 and 4.15).

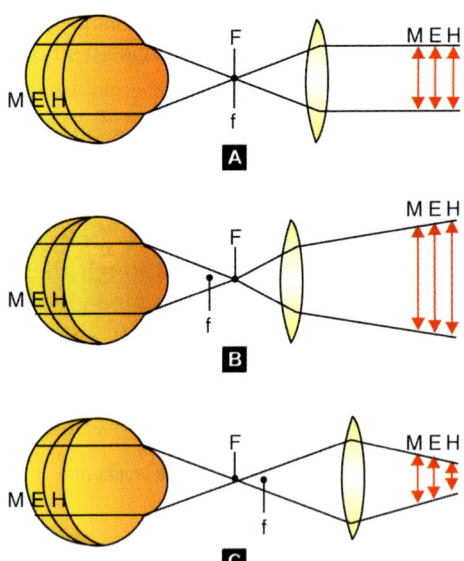

Fig. 4.15 *The size of the image in different refractive states (M): myopia; E: emmetropia; H: hypermetropia), when the condensing lens is held at such a distance that its principal focus (f): (A) Corresponds to the anterior focus of the eye (F); (B) is nearer than the anterior focus of the eye; and (C) is farther away from the anterior focus of the eye*

ii. In hypermetropia, the size of image will be:
- *Equal to an emmetropic eye,* if the condensing lens is held at such a distance that its principal focus (f) corresponds to the anterior focus of eye (Fig. 4.15A).
- *Larger than the emmetropic eye,* if the condensing lens is held at such a distance that its principal focus (f) is nearer than the anterior focus of the eye (F) (Fig. 4.15B).
- *Smaller than the emmetropic eye,* when the principal focus of the condensing lens (f) is farther away than the anterior focus of eye (Fig. 4.15C).

iii. In myopia, the size of image will be:
- *Equal to an emmetropic eye,* if the condensing lens is held at such a distance that its principal focus (f) corresponds to the anterior focus of eye (F) (Fig. 4.15A).
- *Smaller than the emmetropic eye,* if the condensing lens is held at such a distance that its principal focus (f) is nearer than the anterior focus of the eye (F) (Fig. 4.15B).
- *Larger than the emmetropic eye,* when the principal focus of the condensing lens (f) is farther away than the anterior focus of eye (Fig. 4.15C).

3. Image magnification in indirect ophthalmoscopy. Lateral (transverse, linear) magnification in an indirect ophthalmoscope is a function of the power of the condensing lens and power of the patient's eye. It may be expressed as power of the eye (60 D) to the power of the condensing lens. Therefore, a 20 D lens produces 33 lateral magnification and a 30 D lens produces 23 magnification (Table 4.1). Although the axial image remains constant in size for a given lens, if it is viewed from more than 25 cm (the reference point for the designation of magnification) the perceived magnification decreases proportionately to the viewing distance.

Field of illumination and observation

The field of observation is always larger than the field of illumination in indirect ophthalmoscopy. The size of the pupil does not affect the size of field of observation, provided it is larger than the image of the observer's pupil formed by the condensing lens in the observed pupil.

The field of observation is in fact a function of magnification and the condensing lens

diameter. An X-fold decrease in magnification equals an x^2 increase in the field of observation (Table 4.1).

Practice of indirect ophthalmoscopy

Prerequisites
- Indirect ophthalmoscope
- Dark room
- Convex lens 14 D/120 D/128 D/30 D (nowadays commonly employed lens is of 120 D)
- Pupils of the patient should be dilated.

Technique

The procedure is explained to the patient and is made to lie in the supine position, with one pillow on a bed or couch and instructed to keep both eyes open. The examiner throws the light into the patient's eye from an arm's distance (with the self-illuminated ophthalmoscope). In practice, binocular ophthalmoscope with head band or that mounted on the spectacle frame is employed most frequently (Fig. 4.16). Keeping the eyes on the reflex, the examiner then interposes the condensing lens (120 D, routinely) in the path of beam of light—close to the patient's eye and then slowly moves the lens away from the eye (towards himself or herself) until the image of the retina is clearly seen. The examiner moves around the head of the patient to examine different quadrants of the fundus. He or she has to stand opposite the clock hour

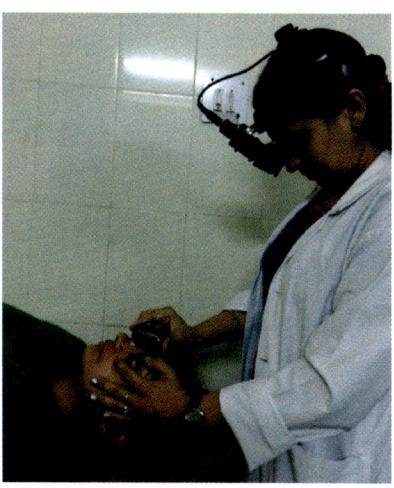

Fig. 4.16 *Technique of indirect ophthalmoscopy*

position to be examined; e.g. to examine inferior quadrant (around 6 o'clock meridian) the examiner stands towards patient's head (12 o'clock meridian) and so on. By asking the patient to look in extreme gaze, and using scleral indenter, the whole peripheral retina up to ora serrata can be examined.

Scleral indentation

This is done with the depressor placed on the patient's lids. This helps in making prominent the just or barely perceptible lesions. One can better appreciate the different tissue colors and densities.

- The examiner should move the scleral depressor in a direction opposite to that in which he or she wishes the depression to appear.
- The scleral depressor should be rolled gently and tangentially over the eye surface.
- The patients are most sensitive to scleral depression in superonasal quadrants.
- Sometimes a topical anaesthetic may be applied and scleral depressor is placed directly on the medial conjunctiva, causing little patient discomfort.
- The temporal part of the upper lid is sufficiently lax so that depressor can be placed inferiorly in the horizontal meridian.
- Sometimes when more posterior areas of fundus are to be examined, the examiner asks the patient to look slightly towards his or her position.

Small pupil ophthalmoscopy

In cases where the pupils do not dilate or if media opacities are enough so as to allow only few rays to enter the retina through a small clear media, small pupil ophthalmoscopy is required. Theoretically, it is possible to see the retina binocularly through 0.6 mm pupil with the 30 D lens. Indirect ophthalmoscopy can be performed through a small pupil without small pupil ophthalmoscope by using 30 D lens held as far as possible. When looking through a small pupil, it is convenient to visualize the retina, if light source is directed high in examiner's field of vision. Slight blurring can occur.

Fundus drawing

The image seen with the indirect ophthalmoscope is vertically inverted and laterally reversed; the top of the retinal chart is placed towards the foot end of the patient (i.e. upside down) (Fig. 4.17). This corresponds to the image of the fundus obtained by the examiner. The fundus drawing is made on a special Amsler's chart, which has 12 clock hours marked and has three concentric circles made on it. The innermost circle represents to the equator, the middle circle the ora serrata and the outermost circle the midpoint of pars plana.

Normal anatomical landmarks. For mapping of the finding, it is very useful to note the position of any lesion with respect to the *normal anatomical landmarks* on the retina (Fig. 4.18):

- *Vortex veins ampulla* are seen along the equator.
- *Long ciliary veins* may be seen at 3 o'clock and 9 o'clock positions.
- *Branching vessels* may also be used and marked to draw the pathology seen.

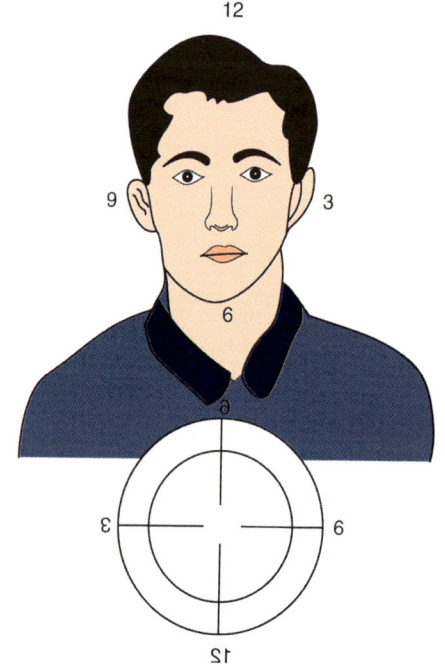

Fig. 4.17 *Position of the chart for drawing during indirect ophthalmoscopy*

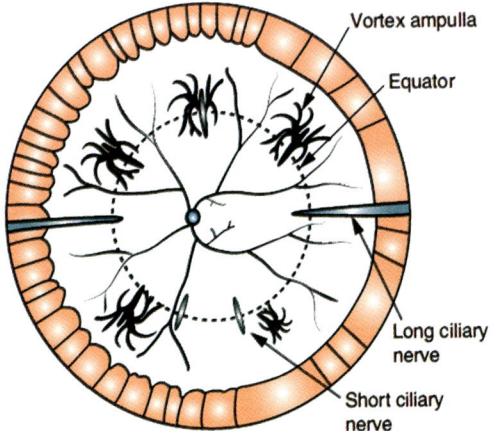

Fig. 4.18 *Normal anatomical landmarks which can be used as aids to draw the location of design seen on fundus examination*

Labels: Vortex ampulla, Equator, Long ciliary nerve, Short ciliary nerve

Symbols and color codes used to draw the fundus, as accepted internationally (Fig. 4.19), are as below:

- *Optic disc* is always shown with red margins.
- *Arteries* are drawn as red lines.
- *Veins* are drawn as blue lines.
- *Attached retina* is shown red.
- *Thin retina* is indicated by red hatching outlines in blue.
- *Detached retina* is drawn with blue color.
- *Retinal tears* are shown as red with blue outline. Flap of the retinal tear is also drawn blue.
- *Lattice degeneration* is shown as blue hatchings outlined in blue.
- *Retinal pigment* is shown as black.
- *Retinal exudates* are shown as yellow.

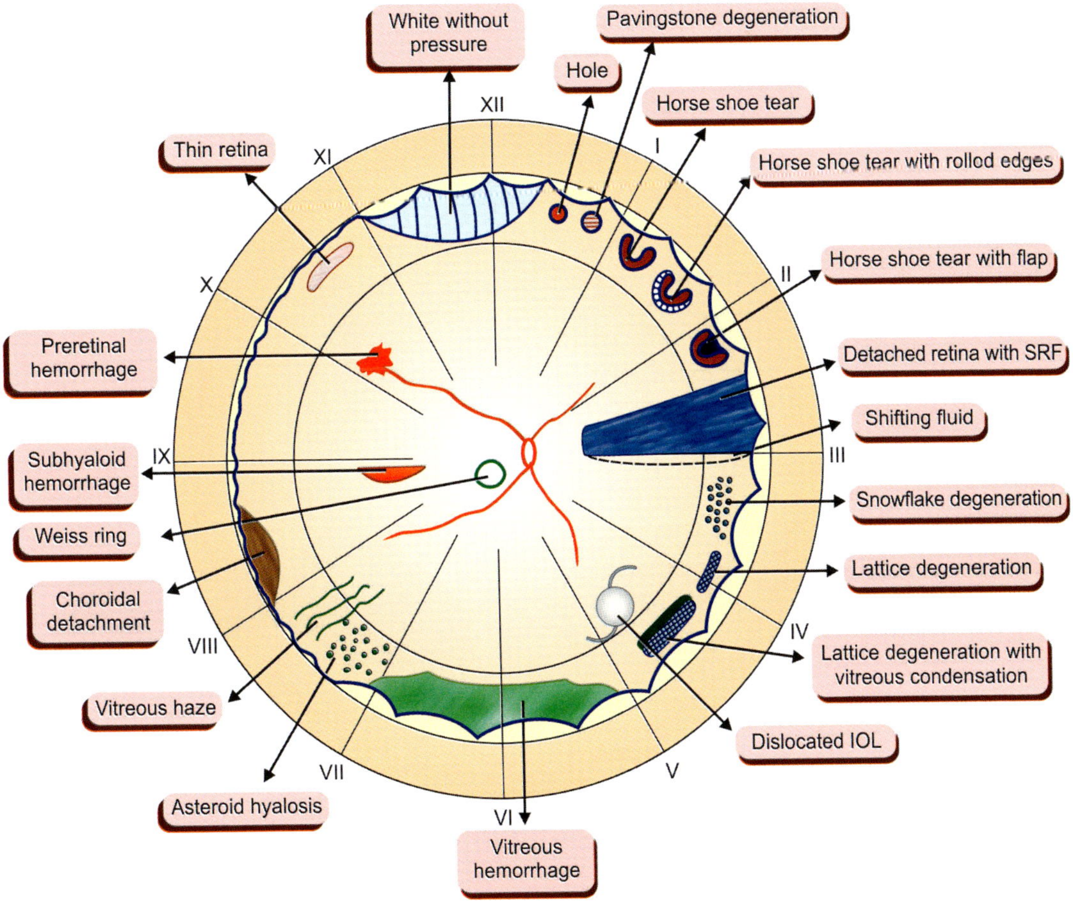

Labels (Fig. 4.19):
White without pressure — XII
Pavingstone degeneration
Hole
Horse shoe tear — I
Horse shoe tear with rolled edges
Thin retina — XI
Horse shoe tear with flap — II
Preretinal hemorrhage — X
Detached retina with SRF
Shifting fluid
Subhyaloid hemorrhage — IX
Snowflake degeneration — III
Weiss ring
Lattice degeneration
Choroidal detachment — VIII
Lattice degeneration with vitreous condensation — IV
Vitreous haze
Dislocated IOL
Asteroid hyalosis — VII
Vitreous hemorrhage — VI — V

Fig. 4.19 *A sample fundus diagram showing the universal color-coding system for a few common lesions and structures*

- *Choroidal lesions* are depicted brown.
- *Vitreous opacities* are depicted as green.

APPLICATIONS, DIFFICULTIES, ADVANTAGES AND DISADVANTAGES

Applications

It is essential for the assessment and management of retinal detachment and other peripheral retinal lesions.

Difficulties during viewing

Reflections and light scatter are problems ophthalmoscopy, and binocular viewing requires a larger pupil than monocular viewing to meet Gullstrand's original ophthalmoscope design. Moving the beams closer together will facilitate viewing through a **small pupil** but will increase reflections and reduce stereopsis. The advantage of the indirect ophthalmoscope is the ability to change the distance between the illuminating beam and viewing beams by tilting the mirror on the scope. During indirect ophthalmoscopy, the illumination is focused in the plane of the pupil to better satisfy Gullstrand's requirements, for this will be the smallest diameter of the beam. Because a +14 D condensing lens has a longer focal length, it is held a greater distance from the eye than a +30 D lens to place the smallest diameter of the beam in the pupil.

The indirect ophthalmoscopy lens design should be to decrease **peripheral aberrations** that increase with stronger and larger lens. To overcome this problem, most condensing lenses are made of an **aspheric** design. This results in a lens with two different curves, the steeper curve on the examiner side of the lens. The illumination beam produces reflections and scatter on the condensing lens surface that can be minimized by **antireflective coatings**. If the lens is held perpendicular to the line of viewing, it produces reflections on the front and rear surfaces in the center of the lens. These reflections can be directed out of the line of light by a **slight tilt of the lens**. Observation of the reflections can be helpful for determining the **proper orientation** of the condensing lens (i.e. the steeper curvature is on the examiner's side), when facing the proper direction, the two reflections will be approximately equal in size.

When opposite to this, one reflection will be significantly larger than the other. To help assist with proper orientation, modern condensing lenses have a silver or white ring painted on the edge of the lens holder's flange that faces the patient.

Excessive **lens tilt will induce astigmatic distortion** of the fundus image and should be avoided. However, this can be advantageous when viewing the peripheral fundus. By inducing astigmatism with the condensing lens at 90 degrees to the astigmatism produced during observation of the fundus periphery, it is possible to reduce peripheral optical distortions. The degree of induced astigmatism increases with greater lens tilt, and the observer can vary the tilt to obtain the clearest focus. Considerable practice is usually required before one becomes comfortable with the technique.

Peripheral viewing could be a problem. When viewing the periphery, the pupil becomes elliptical and much smaller in diameter along the short axis. This may make it impossible to direct both viewing beams and the illumination beam into the patient's pupil. This can be remedied by tilting the observer's head 45 degrees, which may allow the illumination beam and one viewing beam to enter the pupil. This will eliminate stereopsis, but will allow a more peripheral view of the fundus. Also, it is helpful to increase the viewing distance when examining through a small pupil by moving farther away from the condensing lens; the closer one is to the pupil, the less the chances of intercepting the angle of exiting rays.

Advantages of indirect ophthalmoscopy

1. Larger field of retina is visible. There is a 10-fold increase in the area of retina visible as compared to direct ophthalmoscopy.
2. Lesser distortion of the image of the retina.
3. Easier to examine, if the patient's eye movements are present and with high spherical or astigmatic refractive errors.
4. Easy visualization of the retina anterior to the equator, where most retinal holes and degenerations exist.
5. It gives a 3-D stereoscopic view of the retina with considerable depth of focus.

6. It is useful in hazy media because of its bright light and optical property.

Disadvantages of indirect ophthalmoscopy

1. Magnification in indirect ophthalmoscopy is 5 times, whereas in direct ophthalmoscopy it is 15 times.
2. Indirect ophthalmoscopy is impossible with very small pupils.
3. The patient is usually more uncomfortable with the intense light of indirect ophthalmoscope and with scleral indentation.
4. The procedure is more cumbersome, requires extensive practice both in technique and in interpretation of the images visualized.
5. Reflex sneezing can occur on exposure to bright light.

Effect of prolonged indirect ophthalmoscopy on patient's eye

Does prolonged indirect ophthalmoscope viewing affect eyes of patient? This is a commonly asked question by the patients before repeated examinations. Many technical advances in light sources have been made in modern ophthalmoscopes. These light sources can deliver high-intensity light to the subject's eye. A study by Robertson and Erickson of prolonged indirect ophthalmoscopy on human eyes failed to reveal any long-term retinal damage. However, there were some **short-term changes** consisting of irregular bending and twisting of photoreceptor outer segment and transient corneal edema. Attempts have been made to reduce the infrared radiation through the use of fiberoptics, dichroic mirrors, and tinted condensing lenses such as the Volk yellow-tinted lenses that absorb light in both blue and infrared wavelengths.

BIOMICROSCOPIC EXAMINATION OF FUNDUS

Biomicroscopic examination of the fundus can be performed after full mydriasis, using a slit-lamp and any one of the following lenses.

1. HRUBY LENS BIOMICROSCOPY

Hruby lens (Fig. 4.20A) is a planoconcave lens with dioptric power 58.6 D which neutralizes the optical power of the normal eye (160 D) and forms a virtual, erect image of the fundus (Fig. 4.20B). This lens provides a small field with low magnification and cannot visualize the fundus beyond equator.

2. CONTACT LENS BIOMICROSCOPY OF FUNDUS

Contact lens biomicroscopy combines stereopsis, high illumination and high magnification with the advantages of slit-beam. Following lenses are available for contact lens biomicroscopy of the fundus.

Modified Koeppe lens examination

Modified Koeppe lens, i.e. posterior fundus contact lens (Fig. 4.21A) can be used to examine the posterior segment. It provides a virtual and erect image (Fig. 4.21B).

Goldmann's three-mirror contact lens examination

Goldmann's three-mirror contact lens (Fig. 4.21C) consists of a central contact lens and three mirrors placed in the cone, each with different angles of inclination. With this, the central as well as peripheral parts of the fundus can be visualized. It also provides a virtual and erect image (Fig. 4.21B).

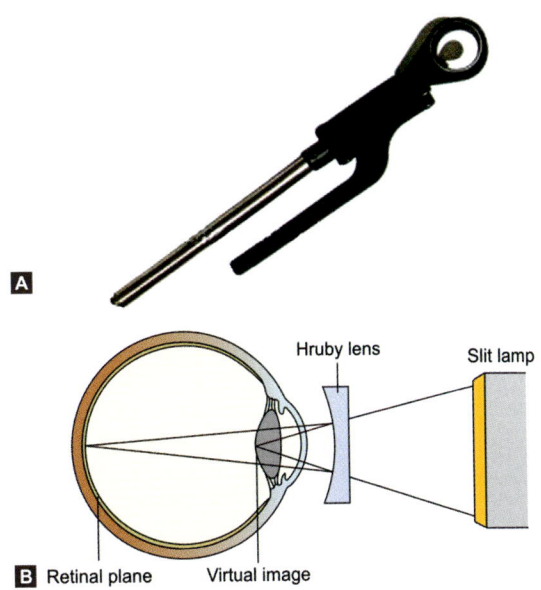

Fig. 4.20 *(A)* Hruby lens; and *(B)* optics of Hruby lens

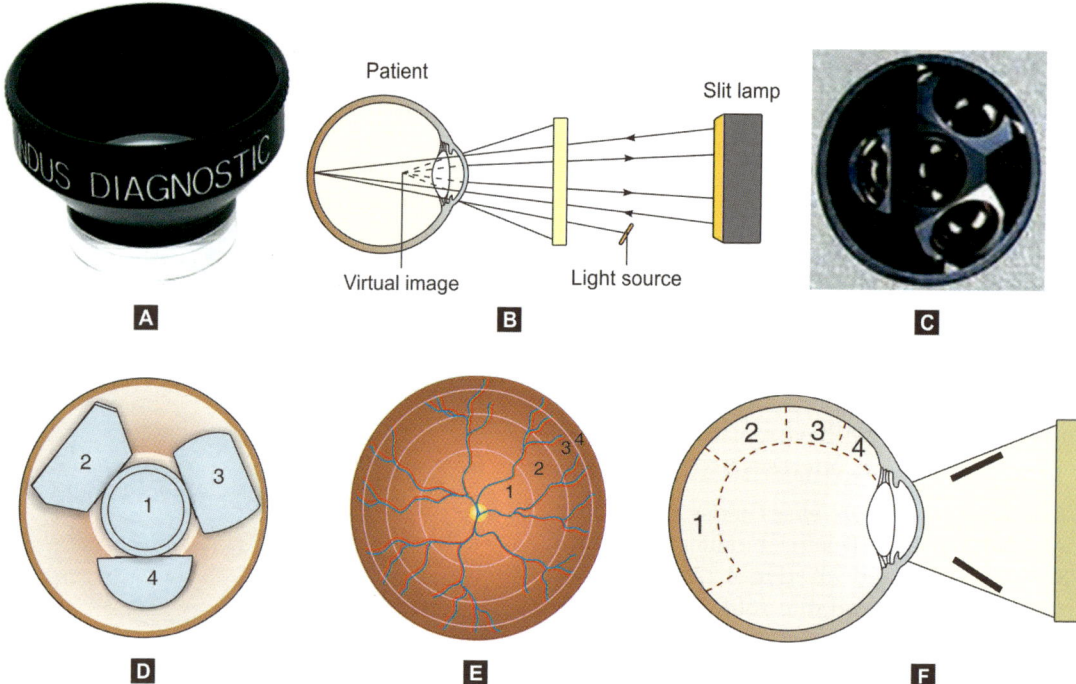

Fig. 4.21 *Contact lenses for biomicroscopy of fundus: (A) modified Koeppe lens; (B) optics of contact lens biomicroscopy; (C) Goldmann's three-mirror contact lens; (D) front view of the Goldmann's three-mirror lens with its four optical surfaces (1, for central posterior pole; 2, for equatorial area; 3, for anterior peripheral fundus; 4, for ora serrata and pars plana); (E) diagrammatic projection of viewing range for each component of Goldmann lens; and (F) panoramic diagram of specific viewing range for each lens component*

Technique

- Dilate the pupils as for indirect ophthalmoscopy.
- Instill topical anaesthetic drops.
- Insert coupling fluid into the cup of the contact lens, but do not overfill.
- Ask the patient to look up, insert the inferior rim of the lens into the lower fornix and press it quickly against the cornea.
- Always tilt the illumination column except when viewing the 12 o'clock position in the fundus (i.e. with the mirror at 6 o'clock).
- When viewing the different positions of the peripheral retina, rotate the axis of the beam so that it is always at right angles to the mirror.
- To visualize the entire fundus, rotate the lens for 3608 using the 59, 67 and 738 tilted mirrors to give views of the peripheral retina, the equatorial fundus and the area around the posterior pole, respectively (Fig. 4.21D to F).

- To obtain a more peripheral view of the retina, tilt the lens to the opposite side and ask the patient to move the eyes to the same side. For example, to obtain a more peripheral view of 12 o'clock position (with mirror at 6 o'clock), tilt the lens down and ask the patient to look up.
- Examine the vitreous cavity with the central lens, using a horizontal and a vertical slit-beam, and then examine the posterior pole.

Note. Since examination with contact lens biomicroscopy involves anaesthetizing the cornea and a direct touch, so it is neither liked much by the patients nor by the examiners. Therefore, presently, fundus contact lenses are primarily used for therapeutic purposes (retinal photocoagulation, etc.) and not for diagnostic purposes except for certain special circumstances. Nowadays examination with fundus non-contact lenses is being preferred for diagnostic purposes.

Wide-field (panfundoscopic) indirect contact

Wide-field (panfundoscopic) indirect contact lenses with a field of view up to 1308 are available for fundus examination and for performing laser photocoagulation. The image produced by such lens is inverted.

3. INDIRECT FUNDUS BIOMICROSCOPY

Indirect fundus biomicroscopy, also known as non-contact fundus biomicroscopy, has become quite popular in the last decade or so—to the extent that it has become an integral part of routine eye examination. As mentioned earlier, the non-contact lenses have replaced the contact lenses for diagnostic purposes.

Fundus non-contact lenses most commonly used for indirect slit lamp biomicroscopy are 78D (Fig. 4.22A) and 90D (Fig. 4.22B), but other lenses are also available (60D, 130D, etc.). Almost all condensing lenses used with slit-lamp are double-aspheric lenses, so it does not matter which side is held towards the patient.

Optics of indirect fundus biomicroscopy is exactly similar to that of indirect ophthalmoscopy (*see* page 58, Fig. 4.8A). Thus, a real, inverted image is formed between the condensing lens and objective lens of slit lamp.

Magnification provided by fundus non-contact lenses is calculated by dividing power of the eye by the power of lens. For example, 90D lens provides a magnification of 60/90 = 0.66, i.e. a minification of the image. However, the magnified image is seen because of the magnification provided by the slit lamp. Thus, 7.5X magnification seen with 90D lens (Table 4.1) is due to 10X of slit lamp.

Field of view. High-powered lens provides larger field of view but lesser magnification, e.g. the 190 D lens provides bigger field of view but gives lesser magnification than 178D lens (Table 4.1).

Technique of indirect fundus biomicroscopy is summarized below (Fig. 4.22C):
Tell patient about the procedure. Make patient comfortable on slit lamp. A quick look at anterior segment is a must before any fundus examination as it could give additional information many a times. Illumination system and microscope are preferably in click position or full alignment. Adjust slit lamp at magnification of 10X, low illumination and slit width of 2–3 mm. Give fixed target to the patient (e.g. examiner's ear for other eye). Focus slit lamp on cornea, introduce the lens into the beam

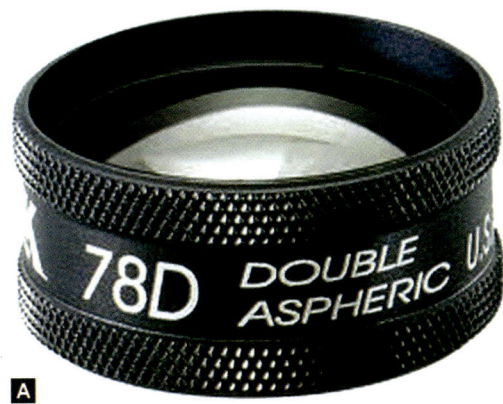

A

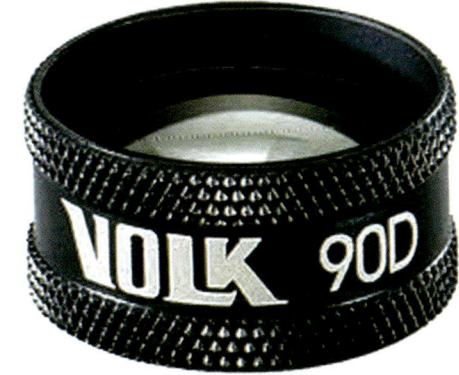

B

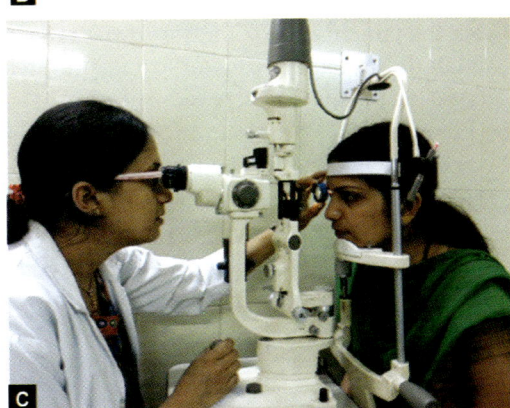

C

Fig. 4.22 *Indirect fundus biomicroscopy:* **(A)** *78D lens;* **(B)** *90D lens; and* **(C)** *technique of examination*

illuminating the patients eye by holding it in forefinger and thumb, using middle finger to widely open the upper lid of patient's eye or to stabilize the hand on the forehead band of the slit lamp. Now pull slit lamp backwards by approximately 2 inches. There is no correct direction for holding the lenses due to the aspheric nature of these lenses; either side can face the patient. Before seeing the retina vitreous must also be studied as important information can be got from it. Align the image in the center of the lens. As the image is inverted tell the patient to look in the direction opposite to the part of image what you want to view (Fig. 4.23).

Like slit lamp biomicroscopy we can examine a lesion by direct illumination on the lesion, indirect illumination adjacent to lesion and retroillumination from reflected light from within the lesion. The contours of chorioretinal lesions are more apparent with narrow beam projected onto the lesion's surface. The contour of the thin slit gives us clue to elevation or depression for subtle lesions in addition to stereopsis (Fig. 4.24).

Start the fundus examination from the peripheral fundus to ensure patient cooperation. Inferior most part of lens corresponds to anterior most part of superior fundus. Hold the lens with index finger and thumb while the middle or ring finger is used to retract the upper lid. The suggested protocol for sequence of examination (1 to 7) of fundus is shown in Fig. 4.25. For documentation the easy way is to reverse the file and draw as you see.

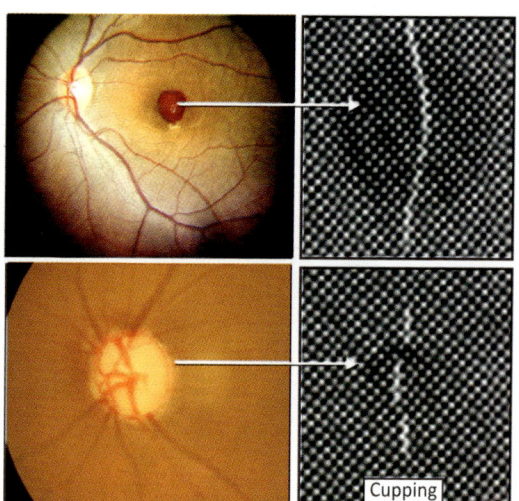

Fig. 4.24 *Kinking of narrow slit on retina helps to identify subtle contour changes in fundus*

To deal with reflection in line of sight we can tilt lens slightly, rotate lens around rotational axis, get illumination system slightly out of click position and further dilate the pupil (Fig. 4.26).

Certain tests like Watzke Allen sign are diagnostic for macular hole. We shine the slit of light on the hole and the patient sees kinking of slit or breaking of slit in center (Fig. 4.27).

The yellow tint lenses are also available and these filter the wave-lengths below 480 nm,

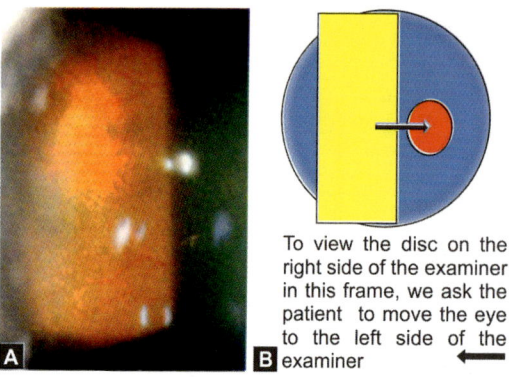

To view the disc on the right side of the examiner in this frame, we ask the patient to move the eye to the left side of the examiner

Fig. 4.23 *Align image in center of lens and to view that part of image which is not in field the patient is asked to move eye in opposite direction*

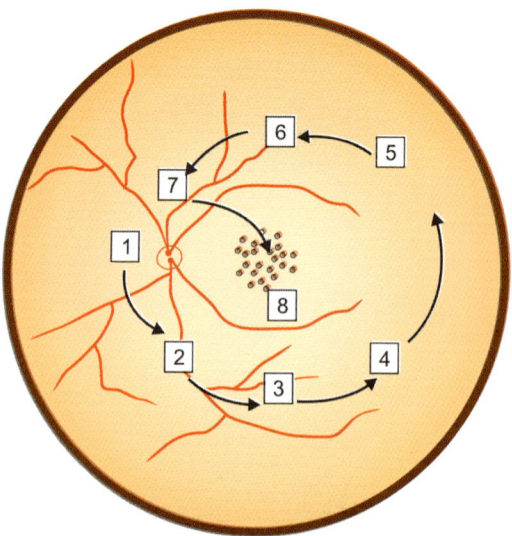

Fig. 4.25 *Suggested protocol for sequence of examination of fundus*

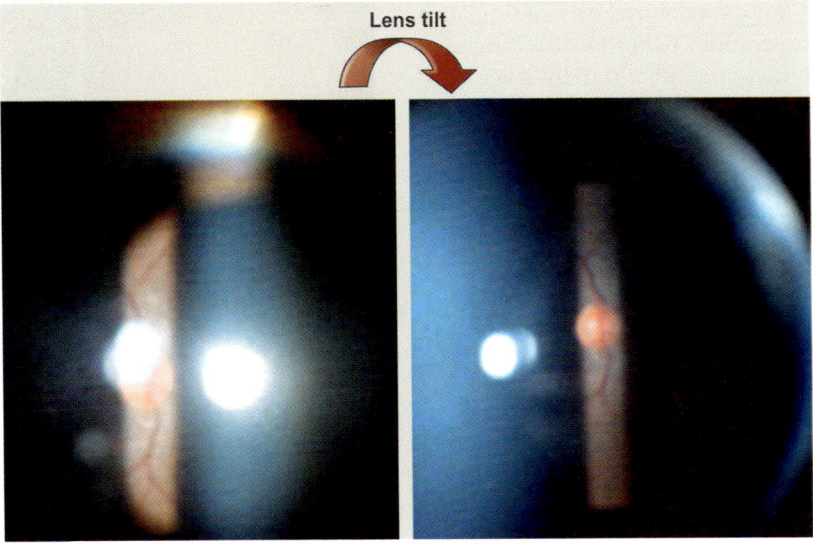

Fig. 4.26 *Demonstrating that mild lens tilt could take care of reflections causing problem in retinal examination*

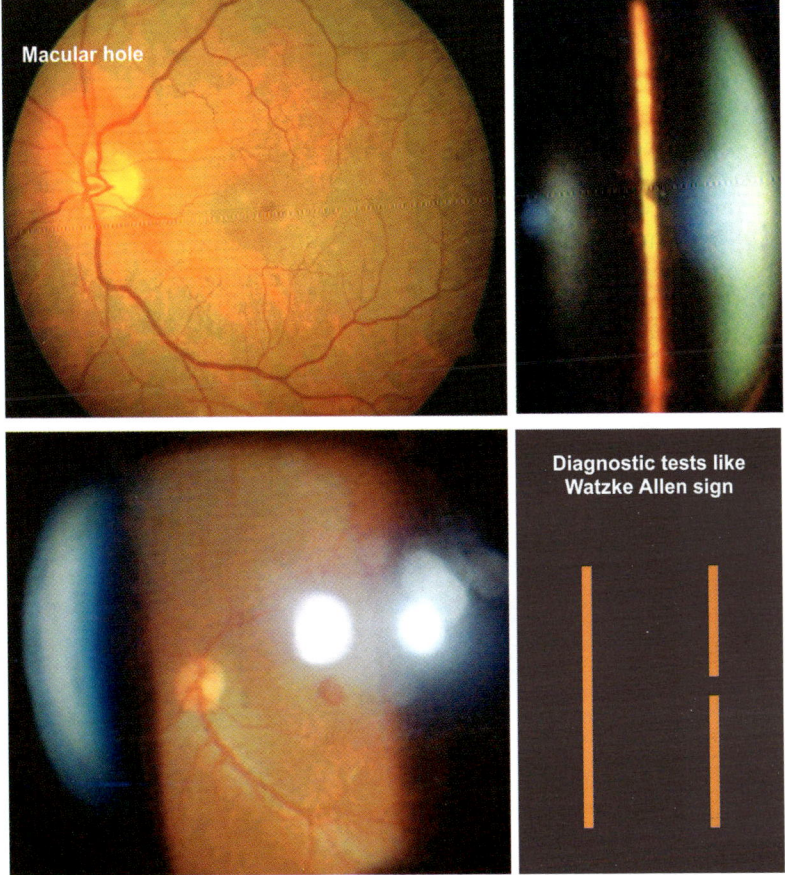

Fig. 4.27 *Watzke Allen sign in a case of macular hole could be diagnostic. The patient might identify a kink or break in continuity of the slit of light projected in the region of macular hole*

enhancing patient comfort and acceptance. The yellow tint may cause a slight color shift in the appearance of the retina which could cause misinterpretation of optic nerve pallor and makes detection of the macular edema more difficult.

Interpretation

Of major importance is the description of fundus lesions, which includes color, shape, size, elevation, and location. Size estimation of a lesion is usually accomplished by comparing it with a structure of known dimensions, such as the optic disc.

Most fundus lesions are described relative to disc diameters (DDs) in size (e.g. a choroid nevus is "2 DDs by 3 DDs"). This is often done by viewing the optic disc first and then quickly relocating the lesion and comparing the two. Since the horizontal diameter of a normal optic disc is 1.5 mm, it is possible to translate DDs into millimeters. For future comparison, the size of a lesion can also be compared with the reticle dimensions in direct ophthalmoscope projected on the fundus.

USES OF DIFFERENT FUNDUS EXAMINATION LENSES

Uses of different fundus examination lenses are summarised in Table 4.4.

FUNDUS CAMERA

OPTICAL PRINCIPLE

All fundus cameras are technically indirect ophthalmoscopes, and currently they are all based upon the principles of Gullstrand's ophthalmoscope. That is, the illumination and observation pathways pass through different portions of the patient's pupil to avoid reflections from the cornea and from the surfaces of the crystalline lens. Also, an inverted aerial image of the fundus is formed within the fundus camera, and this aerial image, in turn, is reimaged on to the film plane.

OPTICAL SYSTEM

The optical system of the fundus camera thus consists of two major components: the illumination system and the observation and photography system. Each of these components occupies its own independent pathway within the apparatus and shares with the other only one common point, the front or ophthalmoscopic lens (Fig. 4.28).

Illumination system

The fundus cameras employ two light sources: a low-intensity incandescent lamp for viewing the fundus and focusing the instrument and a high-powered electronic flashtube for taking the photograph. In the Zeiss fundus camera, these two light sources are optically combined

Table 4.4 *Uses of different fundus examination lenses*					
Lens	*To view and laser*	*Image*	*Relative mag*	*Spot mag*	*Field view*
Goldman	Macula equator periphery	Virtual errect	1.00	1.08	36°
Volk area centralis	Macula equator	Real inverted	1.13	0.95	82°
Mainster standard	Macula equator	Real inverted	1.03	1.05	90°
Mainster widefield	Equator periphery	Real inverted	0.73	1.47	125°
Volk quardr Aspheric	Equator periphery	Real inverted	0.56	1.82	130°
Volk superquad	Equator periphery	Real inverted	0.56	1.92	160°
Panfundoscope	Equator periphery	Real inverted	0.76	1.41	120°

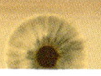

through the semireflecting surface (Fig. 4.28). In most of the other commercially available fundus cameras, the incandescent lamp and electronic flashtube are mounted on to a common base, and a transillumination method is used to combine the pathway of the two lights.

From this point onwards, the light from two light sources following a common pathway passes through a diaphragm, the adjustment of which controls the size of illuminated patch upon the patient's retina. This diaphragm is imaged at the surface of a holed mirror, which is itself imaged by the ophthalmoscopic lens in the plane of the patient's pupil. These two optical elements confine the illuminating beam to an annulus (a ring of light), the width of which is controlled by the diaphragm.

Observation and photographic system

The holed mirror, which is imaged by the ophthalmoscope lens in the plane of the patient's pupil, forms the entrance pupil of the viewing system. It confines the viewing beam to central region of the pupil. It also confines the illuminating beam to an annulus that surrounds the viewing beam. The illuminating and viewing paths are, therefore, separated in

the plane of the patient's pupil, thereby making the instrument reflex-free.

The ophthalmoscopic lens produces an image of the fundus between the holed mirror and the ophthalmoscopic lens. This image is viewed through the hole with a compound microscope. The objective of this microscope forms an image of the fundus, via a flip mirror, upon the ground glass screen that is placed at the focal point of the viewing eyepiece. When the photograph is taken, the flip mirror that diverts the image into the eyepiece for observation swings out of the optical pathway, thus permitting the image to be projected on to the film for photography (Fig 4.28).

The photographic component of the early instruments consisted of a small film carrier and a shutter mechanism. However, with the advent of fluorescein angiography, the simple film carrier has been replaced by a sophisticated, electronic motorized 35 mm camera system.

MODIFICATIONS IN FUNDUS CAMERA

1. *Fluorescein angiography system.* Fundus cameras have been modified for fluorescein angiography by addition of appropriate filters in the illumination and observation pathways

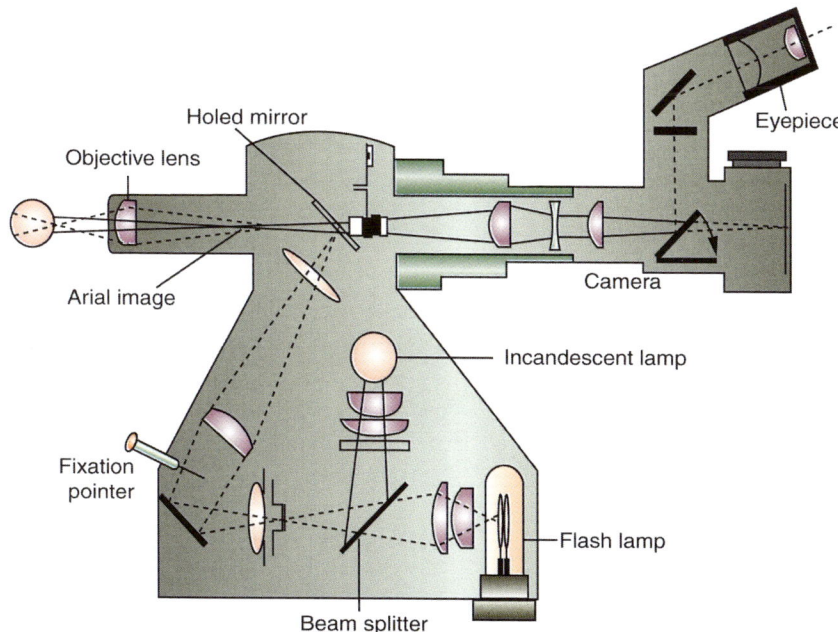

Fig. 4.28 *Schematic view of the Zeiss fundus camera to show outlines of the optical system*

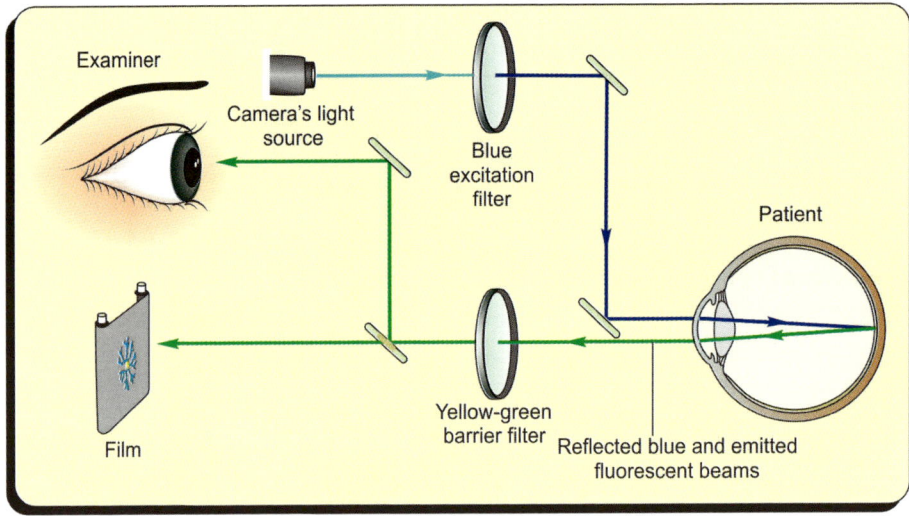

Fig. 4.29 *Blue excitation filter in the fundus camera produces blue light, which excites the unbound fluorescein molecules. The reflected blue light is absorbed by the yellow-green filter allowing only the fluorescing particles to be recorded on the film*

(Fig. 4.29). Special power supplies are necessary to allow multiple exposures per second.

2. *Digital fluorescein angiography system*. Recently, digital fluorescein angiography (DFA) is being used increasingly. The DFA system uses a CCD detector in the camera in place of a film. One of the commercially available digital fluorescein angiography system manufactured is shown in Fig. 4.30.

Advantages of DFA
• The images can be instantaneously viewed on a high-resolution monitor. This allows the

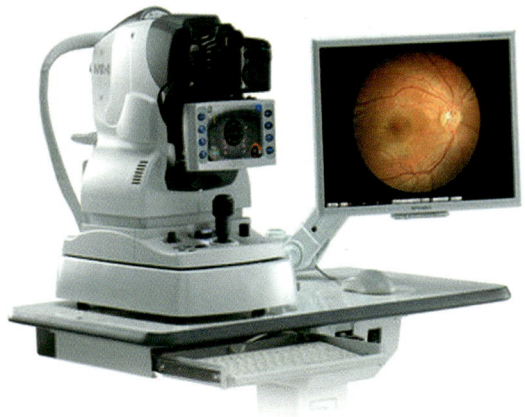

Fig. 4.30 *Digital fluorescein angiography system*

observer to manipulate the parameters (e.g. light intensity, centration of photography) while the study is in progress to obtain the optimum image.
• The images are recorded either on a computer hard drive or CD-ROM. The electronic recording allows immediate viewing of images and permits prompt management of the disease process.
• The angiograms can be electronically transmitted or printed form the digital data.

Disadvantage of DFA
The quality of the DFA is inferior to the film-based photographs; however, it is adequate for clinical purposes.

3. *Wide-field digital fundus fluorescein angiography* has also been introduced, specially for use in children.

4. *Non-mydriatic fundus cameras.* These use infrared light and semi-automatic or automatic focusing systems to allow fundus photography without dilating drops. The infrared light is invisible to the patient, and the pupil dilates physiologically. After alignment and focusing are completed, the white light flash is triggered, and the photograph is taken before the pupil has a chance to constrict.

5. *Wide-angle fundus cameras* up to 608 have appeared, having large diameter and aspheric objective lenses. Wide-angle photographs even up to 1488 are possible, but a contact type of objective lens and special illumination system are necessary for such photographs.

6. *Television ophthalmoscopy.* Several attempts at television ophthalmoscopy have been made, using fundus camera optics. In general, excessive illumination is required, and resolution is poor.

7. *Scanning laser ophthalmoscopy.* A promising new system is the SLO, where only a single spot of laser light is scanned over the fundus, with each point being recorded as it is illuminated. The primary advantage of this system is the extremely low level of total light required. (For details *see* page 74).

WIDE-FIELD RETINAL IMAGING SYSTEMS

Wide-field retinal imaging systems have been developed with the capability of capturing up to 2008 field of view with one picture as compared to only 30–608 field of view with current standard fundus photography system. The salient features of the following three commercially available wide-field retinal imaging systems are described here in brief:

- Retcam II and Retcam III
- Panoret 1000A
- Panoramic 200

RETCAM II AND III

Retcam II (Retinal camera II) is the advanced version of Retcam 120 (manufactured by Massie Research Lab., Dublin, CA).

Components of Retcam II. It is a mobile wide-field digital imaging system comprising following major components (Fig. 4.31):

- *Three-chip CCD medical grade digital video cameras* is the heart of Retcam II. It is light-weight (so easy to position) and is attached to the light source and image capture unit.

- *Hand-held image capture unit* is attached with the camera by a long cable for easy patient access.

- *High-index corneal contact lenses* form the essential part of the image-capturing unit. These lenses allow capturing of oblique rays emerging from the peripheral retina. The changeable lenses (nose pieces) available to be attached to the image-capturing unit of Retcam II are as follows (Fig. 4.32):

ROP (retinopathy of prematurity) lens, for premature infants which allows 1308 field of view.

Standard children lens, a 1208 field-of-view lens for pediatric to young adult patients.

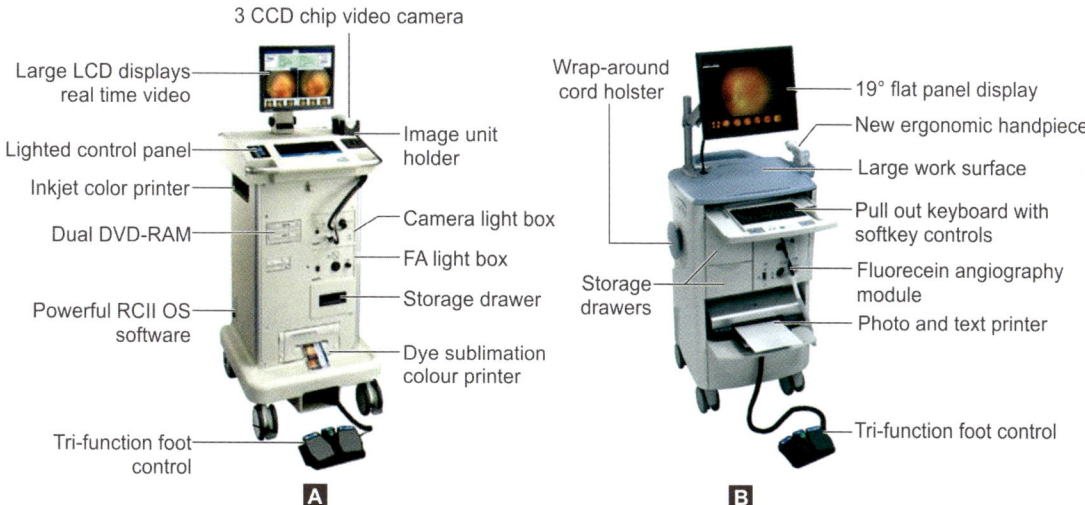

Fig. 4.31 *(A) Retcam II, the wide-field retinal imaging system and (B) Retcam III*

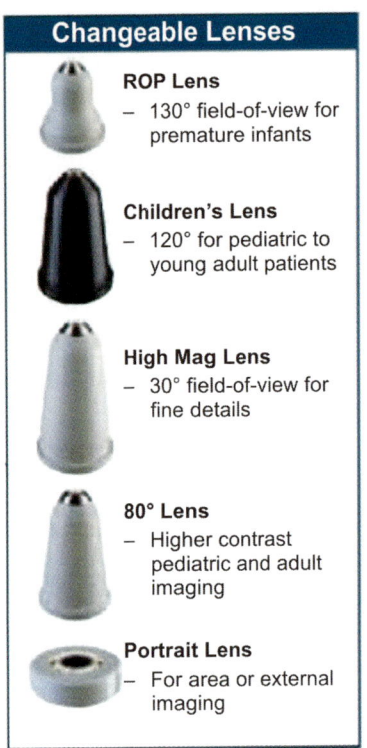

Changeable Lenses

ROP Lens
- 130° field-of-view for premature infants

Children's Lens
- 120° for pediatric to young adult patients

High Mag Lens
- 30° field-of-view for fine details

80° Lens
- Higher contrast pediatric and adult imaging

Portrait Lens
- For area or external imaging

Fig. 4.32 *Changeable high-index lens available for attaching with image-capturing unit of Retcam II*

High magnification lenses, a 308 field-of-view lens for fine details.

808 lens for higher contrast pediatric and adult imaging.

Portrait lens or external lens for area or external imaging.

- *Image processing unit, comprises* a Windows or T computer system which gets the information from the camera. This unit is equipped with a new multipurpose software.
- *Flat LCD color display* on 17 inch monitor allows the images to be viewed in real-time motion during acquisition.
- *Tri-function foot control* connected to the camera controls image focus, illumination and capture.

Special features of Retcam II

- *Cone-shaped lens* provided with it is very handy to hold while scanning the retina.
- *Wide, 130 and 120°, real-time image* of the fundus is particularly useful in diagnosis and

documentation of diseases such as retino-blastoma and ROP.

- *Images are stored in digital format*, thus are retrievable easily.
- *Camera has a large storage device* with good facility of transferring the images in other media like CD, USB and in other DVD device. The data can be shared with others for seeking an opinion.
- *Comprehensive database* keeps track of each imaging section for the patients, allowing for later or side by side review of the cases. This is particularly useful in assessing response to treatment as in chemoreduction for retino-blastoma and laser photocoagulation for ROP.
- *Fluorescein angiography can also be performed with it. It is* another major feature of this equipment. It is provided with a barrier filter, which helps to take the angiogram by still mode and continuous video for 20 seconds.
- In-built color printer allows the print images and the detailed case report of the patient.

Features of Retcam III

Additional features of Retcam III (Fig. 4.31B) are summarized below.

Procedure

It involves following steps:
- *Pupils* are dilated fully.
- *Anesthesia.* Neonates and infants can be easily examined under topical anesthesia achieved with proparacaine eyedrops. Older children may be given short-term sedation for the procedure.
- *Separation of lids* is done with the help of a pediatric lid speculum, after placing the patient in supine position.
- *Fixation of the head* is then achieved.
- *Coupling solution* like methylcellulose gel is applied to the cornea.
- *Image capture unit* with desired lens is then positioned with gentle contact to the anterior corneal surface. Illumination and focus are controlled by the operator with the foot switch. Often a quick scan of the entire retina can be performed in live video motion before acquisition of images. Once the desired field of view has been identified, the images can be captured with the foot switch control.

Limitations of retcam

- *Pupillary dilation* is extremely important for it, so not useful where pupillary dilation is a problem.
- *Other limitations* include need for camera lens–cornea contact, need for eyelid speculum and technical limitations of the camera.
- *Lack of stereopsis* and some loss of magnification of retinal field in exchange for a wide-angle field of view may also be seen as a limitation.
- *Cannot be used in adults* because with lens opacities that begin in adolescence and accumulate with age, the entering light is scattered more widely, causing decreased contrast sensitivity.

Advantages

- *Mobile, self-contained system* for use in nursery, ICU, operating rooms, etc.
- *Easy to use* – even technicians or nurses can operate.
- *Avoids stress and expertise* of indirect ophthalmoscopy and scleral indentation.
- *Interobserver variability* is eliminated.
- *Teaching tool for students*, and parents can be counselled.
- *Easy case management* with access to images, video clips, patient data, instant retrieval and side by side comparison.

Applications of wide-field imaging system

- *Pediatric retinal disorders* can be easily diagnosed, followed and objectively documented. Especially useful in ROP, retinoblastoma, shaken baby syndrome.
- *Pediatric anterior segment imaging*, gonio-imaging for glaucomatous damage, iris lesions.
- *Fluorescein angiography* can also be performed with advances in the technique.

PANORET 1000 AA
Principle

This wide-field imaging system employs the principles of trans-scleral illumination propagated by Pomerantzeff.

Advantages

Because a trans-scleral light source provides diffuse illumination, so this system:
- Can be used in the presence of media opacities
- Can be used in cases where pupillary dilation is a problem
- Can also be used in adults
- Both fluorescein angiography and indocyanine green angiography can also be performed.

Limitations

- Patients with heavily pigmented uvea are not well imaged.
- Since it is introduced recently, so there is limited clinical experience with its use.

PANORAMIC 200 NON-MYDRIATIC SLO
Principle

It is a non-contact non-mydriatic system based on the use of both a green (532 nm) and red (633 nm) laser to produce a digital image of 2000 by 2000 pixels. The resolution of image ranges from 20 to 40 m per pixel.

Applications

It is often used as a screening tool for diabetic retinopathy, age-related macular degeneration (ARMD) and glaucomatous disc changes.

Advantages

Field of view is 2008 in a single image.

Limitations

Being a table-mounted non-mobile unit, it cannot be used in small children and uncooperative patients.

LASER SCANNING IMAGING TECHNIQUES

- Scanning laser ophthalmoscopy
- Confocal scanning laser ophthalmoscopy
- Retinal thickness analyser
- Scanning laser polarimetry

SCANNING LASER OPHTHALMOSCOPY (SLO)

The scanning laser ophthalmoscopy was invented by Webb, Pomerantzeff and Hughes

in 1979. The word scanning here refers to the illumination system, which samples the retina point by point rather than capturing the image as a whole, as is done with a conventional fundus camera.

Principle

The SLO operates essentially as an inverted indirect ophthalmoscope. This means that a small illumination aperture is used to illuminate the eye while a large viewing aperture collects all the light emitted by the eye (Fig. 4.33). The small aperture creates a very narrow moving beam of light which can bypass most ocular media opacities (i.e. corneal scars, cataracts, vitreous hemorrhage) to reach the surface of the retina and record its surface detail. A live video image of the retina is displayed on a computer monitor and test results are digitally recorded (Fig. 4.34).

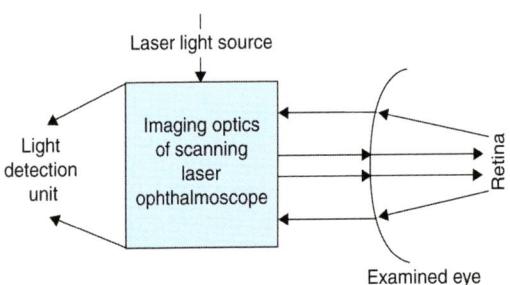

Fig. 4.33 *Optics of scanning laser ophthalmoscope as inverted indirect ophthalmoscope. Note that the light enters the eye through a small illumination aperture and the returned light is collected over a large viewing aperture*

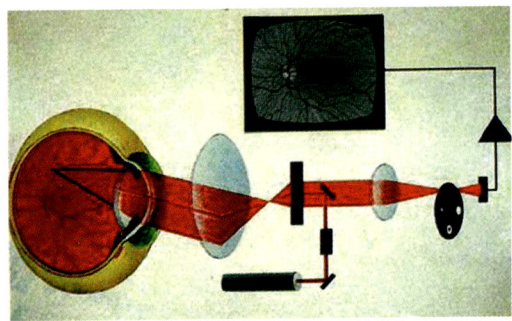

Fig. 4.34 *Optical path of recording of scanning laser ophthalmoscope (SLO)*

Applications of SLO

1. *Scanning laser acuity potential test.* The letter E corresponding to different levels of visual acuity (ranging from 20/1000 to 20/60) is projected directly on the patient's retina. The examiner can direct the test letters to foveal and/or extrafoveal location within the macula and determine a subject's potential visual acuity. This may be especially helpful in individuals who have lost central fixation but who may still possess significant eccentric vision. It is also useful in separating out the component of retinal function from anterior segment contributions to overall visual dysfunction when contemplating surgical interventions.

2. *Microperimetry/scotometry.* The SLO can visualize a particular area of the retina and test its sensitivity to visual stimuli, thereby generating a map of the seeing and non-seeing areas. If central vision is lost, the patient can potentially be trained to use an adjacent retinal site to substitute for central visual function.

3. *Hi-Speed FA/ICG.* Fluorescein and indocyanine green angiography (FA/ICG) performed using the SLO is recorded at 30 images per second, producing a real-time video sequence of the ocular blood flow. The standard fundus camera sequence is limited by flash recycling to one to two frames per second, and is unreliable in its ability to document details of choroidal filling which occurs over a 1–2-second span of time.

The higher speed of image acquisition more completely captures the chorioretinal filling sequence, and can be used to accurately identify the choroidal feeder vessels of neovascular membranes. Guided by high-speed FA/ICG results, laser treatment of sight-threatening diseases like exudative ARMD can be carried out with pinpoint accuracy.

SLO versus conventional fundus camera

1. SLO samples the retina point by point while the fundus camera captures the image as a whole.
2. In SLO, a single point on retina is illuminated for less than 1,000,000th of a second while the conventional fundus camera illuminates the eye for several milliseconds during flash capture.

3. The SLO captures a temporal image while conventional fundus camera captures a spatial image.
4. In SLO, light source is always laser, so it can achieve white light imaging comparable to conventional white light fundus photography.

Advantages of SLO over conventional fundus camera

- Low light level
- Highly light efficient
- Continuous imaging
- Large depth of field
- Instantaneous image availability for review
- The high capture speed allows dynamic image studies such as blood flow
- Allows excellent imaging even in the presence of media opacities

CONFOCAL SCANNING LASER OPHTHALMOSCOPY

The confocal scanning laser ophthalmoscopy, or CSLO, also known as scanning laser tomography, or SLT, was introduced by Webb and associates in 1987. The term *confocal* has been derived by combining the terms *conjugate* and *focal*, and it describes that the locations of the focal plane in the retina and the focal plane in the image sensor are located in conjugate positions. Confocality of the system is achieved by placing a pinhole in front of the detector, which is conjugate to the laser focus (Fig. 4.35). The size of the pinhole determines the degree of confocality, such that a small pinhole aperture will give a highly confocal image. Commercially available CSLOs include:

- HRT
- Top SS

HEIDELBERG RETINA TOMOGRAPHY

Heidelberg retina tomography (HRT), the most popular instrument, is available in two models– the HRT I (introduced in November 1991) and the HRT II C (introduced in April 1999). For both the models, the laser source is a *helium–neon diode laser* of wavelength 670 nm. The laser raster scans the x–y plane to obtain confocal optical sections of the retina. Once one plane has been scanned, the laser changes focus to scan a slightly deeper plane of the retina. This continues until a series of confocal optical sections through the depth of the fundus are obtained.

INSTRUMENT PROFILE

The instrument is small, light, portable and is table-mounted along with a notebook computer (Fig. 4.36). Press of signal button acquires optical

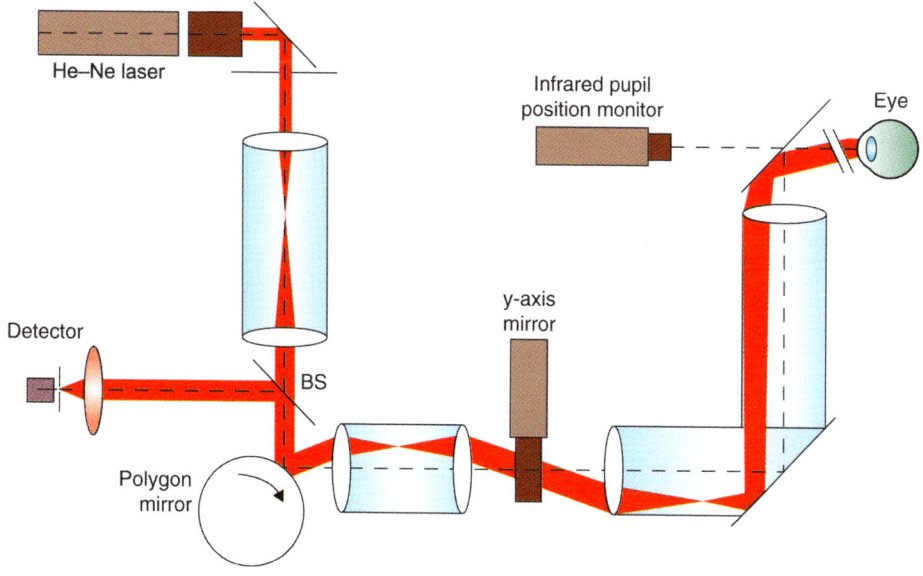

Fig. 4.35 *Optics of confocal scanning laser ophthalmoscope (CSLO)*

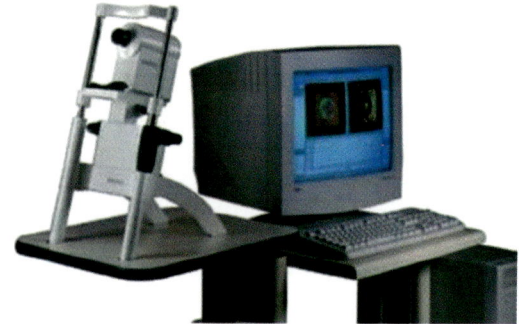

Fig. 4.36 *The Heidelberg retinal tomograph II*

section images within 32 milliseconds and with a repetition rate of 20 Hz two-dimensional. From the images obtained in this pre-scan of 4–6 mm depth, the software computes and automatically sets the correct location of the focal plane, the required scan depth for that eye and the proper sensitivity to obtain images with correct brightness. The Heidelberg retinal tomograph operation software automatically defines a reference plane for each individual eye. The reference plane is defined parallel to the peripapillary retinal surface and is located 50 m posteriorly to the retinal surface at the papillomacular bundle. The reason for this definition is that during development of glaucoma the nerve fibers at the papillomacular bundle remain intact longest and the nerve fiber layer thickness at that location is approximately 50 m. We can, therefore, assume to have a stable reference plane located just beneath the nerve fiber layer. All structures located below the reference plane are considered to be cup; all structures located above the reference plane and within the contour line are considered to be the rim.

ACQUISITION AND GENERATION OF TOPOGRAPHY IMAGE

HRT I

Image acquisition. The HRT I makes *32 scans through the retina resulting in a stack of optical sections* which represent both an area (x–y) and depth (z) image of the retinal structure under investigation (Figs 4.37 and 4.38A). The field of view can be set to three levels—108 × 108, 158 × 158 or 208 × 208. The depth to which the laser scans varies between 0.5 and 4.0 mm in 0.5 mm

steps. Thirty-two optical sections are generated at all of these depth levels, so the spacing between sections is closer at the lower depth levels and greater at the higher depth levels. The camera must be placed 15 mm from the examined eye, and the operator centers the optic disc on the monitor. The HRT I software has a quality control mechanism which informs the operator whether the image series is of good quality. Changes in focus and depth setting are advised until the series acquired is optimum. However, the operator has to examine the image series to establish whether there are any image-distorting eye movements. In such cases, the series have to be rejected. Generally, three optimum image series are obtained for each eye under examination (Fig. 4.38B). The topography images are then generated (Fig. 4.38C).

Generation of the topography image. Each confocal section of the 32-image series consists of 256 × 256 pixels. Each pixel location (x, y) has a varying brightness through the series. The distribution of reflected light intensity of each pixel through the 32 series is called the z-profile (Fig. 4.37). The z-profile is a symmetric distribution with a maximum at the location of the light-reflecting surface. By determining the position of the profile maximum, the height of each pixel can be determined (Fig. 4.38). The topography map is a color-coded representation of each pixel position within the 32 series. Each of the 32 confocal sections has been designated an arbitrary red value. Section 1 is dark red, section 32 is saturated white and the sections in between decrease in redness from 1 down to 32 in equal steps.

Alongside the topography image is a reflectivity image, which gives the most visual information about the optic disc under examination similar to a fundus photo (Fig. 4.37).

HRT II

Image acquisition. The HRT II differs quite considerably from the HRT I. There is one field of view (158), and each optical section has a resolution of 384 × 384 pixels. In contrast to the HRT I, which can be used for the acquisition of both optic nerve head (ONH) and macular images, the HRT II has been designed specifically for the grabbing of ONH images alone.

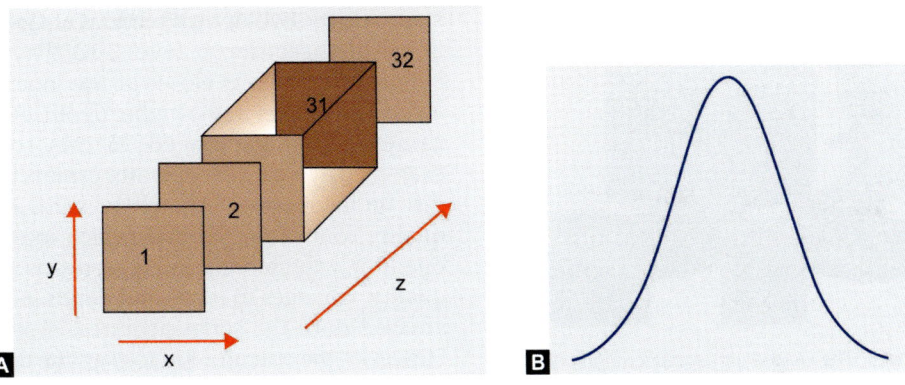

Fig. 4.37 *HRT I-image acquisition: (A) a stack of 32 image series; and (B) z-profile of pixel (x, y) in image series*

In image acquisition, the operator enters the patient's details and a rough setting of the examined eye's refraction. The patient is instructed to look at an internal fixation light, which results in an automatic centration of the ONH on the monitor. The acquisition button is activated, and the CSLO proceeds with image acquisition.

An automatic pre-scan with 4–6 mm depth is performed, and from the images obtained from this pre-scan, the software computes and automatically sets the correct location of the focal plane – the required scan depth for that eye and the sensitivity to obtain images with correct brightness. Following this, the system automatically acquires three image series with the predetermined acquisition parameters. The number of image planes acquired per series depends on the required scan depth – 16 images per millimetre scan depth are acquired. There is an automatic quality control during image acquisition, and so if one or more of the acquired image series cannot be used for any reason, additional images are acquired automatically until three good quality image series have been obtained. After image acquisition, the images are saved on the hard disc and the three topography images and the mean topography image are computed automatically.

This semi-automated image acquisition of the HRT II means that in busy practice situations, staff with minimal experience of using the instrument should be able to acquire images.

IMAGE ANALYSIS AND EXAMINATION OF RESULTS

I. SLT in glaucoma

The applications of SLT in glaucoma are:

1. Initial examination to discriminate between the normal eyes, glaucoma suspects and glaucomatous eyes

The printout of initial report has following details (Fig. 4.39).

Topography and reflectivity image. As described earlier (Fig. 4.37), the topography image is a color-coded map. The red areas are on the surface and the white areas are deeper in the scan (Fig. 4.39).

The reflectivity image approximates a mean brightness of all images. In the reflection image, the ONH is divided into six sectors. These sectors are compared to a normal database and then classified. Moorfield's regression analysis means that the rim (green and blue) and the disc area (green, blue and red) for each sector are compared to a normal database. Depending on the patient's age and overall disc size, the eye is then statistically classified as 'within normal limit', 'borderline' or 'outside normal limit'.

Horizontal/vertical height profile, i.e. height profile along the white horizontal and the white vertical line in the tomography image. The subjacent reference line (red) indicates the location of the reference plane (separation between cup and neuroretinal rim). The two black lines perpendicular to the height profile denote the

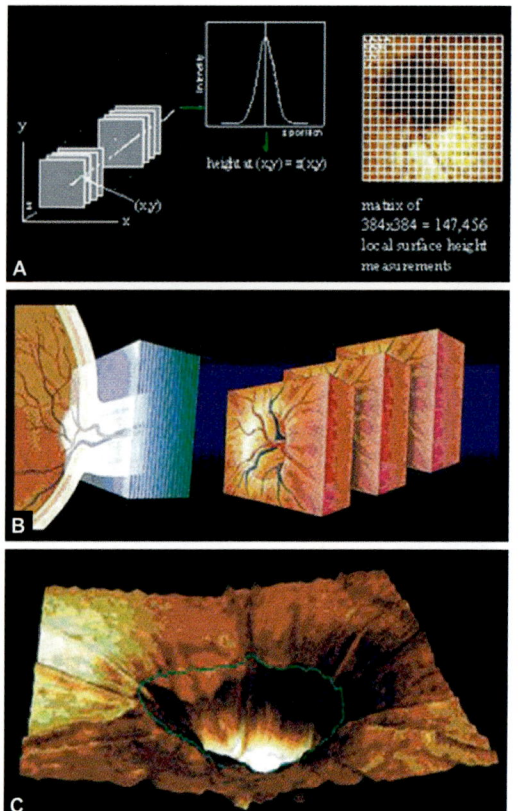

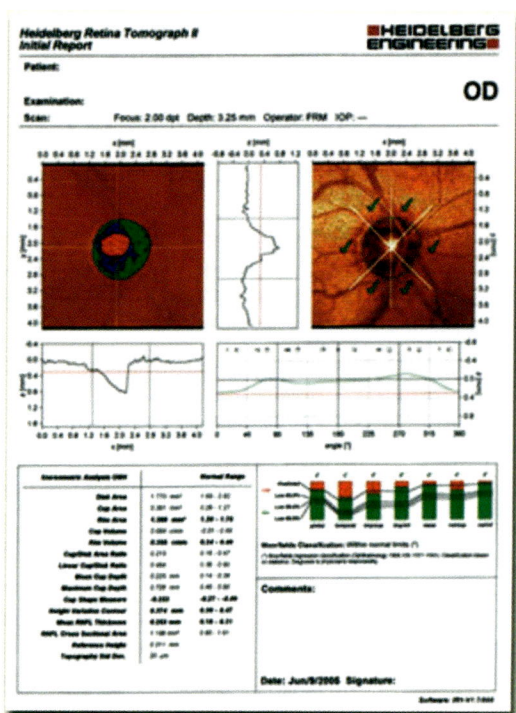

Fig. 4.39 *Initial examination report with the HRT II*

Fig. 4.38 *Principle of scanning laser tomography–concept of 3-D image composition based on 32 confocal sections: (A) A stack of 32 confocal sections (the software aligns the images but only compensates for small eye movements) the axial intensity distribution for each of the 256 × 256 pixels is plotted and the axial location of the maximum is coded into a 2-D image with 256 × 256 pixels; (B) Three separate image series acquired; and (C) 3-D image of optic nerve head*

borders of the disc as defined by the contour line.

Mean height contour graph. The height difference between the reference line (red) and the height profile corresponds to the retinal nerve fiber layer (RNFL) thickness along the contour line.

Stereometric analysis of ONH. For both instruments, an operator has to define the edge of the ONH, and this is done using the mouse. Once the ONH margin, i.e. contour line which matches the inner edge of scleral ring (Elschnig's ring) has been defined, area and volumetric information about the ONH are obtained.

The result of this analysis is a set of stereometric parameters. The most important parameters are disc area, cup and rim area, cup and rim volume, and mean and maximum cup depth, a measure for the 3-D shape of the cup and for the mean thickness of the RNFL along the contour line (Fig. 4.39). Most of the stereometric parameters provided by the Heidelberg retinal tomograph change significantly with progression of glaucoma; the standard errors of the means in the visual field groups are very small, and the means differ significantly between groups. The parameters are useful, therefore, to follow the progression of the disease. But the physiologic variability of the ONH configuration is high and so are the standard deviations of the parameter values. The distributions of the parameter values of the different groups overlap each other. Hence, it is difficult (except in advanced cases) to classify an individual eye as being normal or glaucomatous, based on individual stereometric parameters.

Disc analysis with HRT II – Moorfield's analysis feature. Once the contour line has been drawn, there is the option of using the Moorfield's regression feature. This compares the optic disc imaged to a normal database and predicts the normality of the disc.

Variability in acquisition can occur due to manual contour line drawing, inter- and intratest examinations. To overcome this, Moorfield's study revealed the advantage of examining the rim area in sectors. This graphic visualizes the result of the Moorfield's regression analysis. The whole column represents the total ONH area in this specific sector. It is divided into the percentage of rim area (green) and percentage of cup area (red). The age-dependent limits of the confidence intervals are as follows:

- If the percentage of the rim is larger than or equal to the 95% limit, the respective sector is classified as 'within normal limit'.
- If the percentage of the rim is between the 95 and the 99.9% limits, the respective sector is classified as 'borderline'.
- If the percentage of the rim is lower than the 99.9% limit, the respective sector is classified as 'outside normal limit'.

2. Follow-up examination to study the progression

Glaucoma is a progressive disease, and there is significant individual variability which makes labelling an eye glaucomatous after one single test hazardous. Therefore, proven progression of the disease becomes critical to the diagnosis and management. The baseline measurements are extremely important, since those parameters alone are taken for further retesting. Therefore, the image quality (as ascertained by standard deviation) should be good and it should be ensured that ONH is centerd, illumination is even, refractive error is incorporated and eye movements are minimal. It is claimed that disc changes are more frequent than field changes. Progression requires three consecutive readings (Baseline 1 three follow-up) to perform a topographic change analysis.

Topographic change analysis can be done by two methods:

i. *Change probability maps* (Fig. 4.40) are independent of the reference plane and the contour line

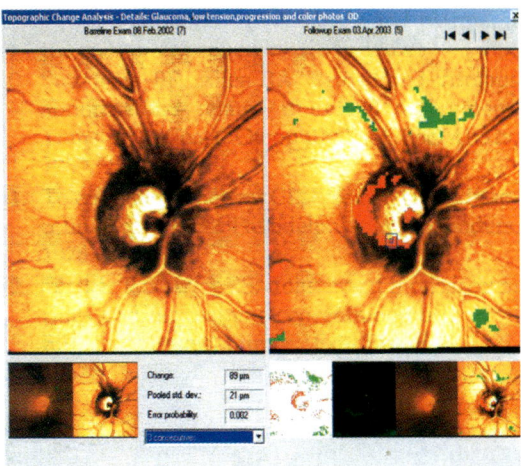

Fig. 4.40 *Change probability maps*

and are calculated automatically, comparing mean topography images.

- Red signifies 'significant' depression.
- Green signifies 'significant' elevation.
- The change is calculated by local change in surface height, measured in microns, at the location selected. A height change is considered significant:

If it is repeated in at least two (better is three) consecutive follow-up examinations.

If it is region of at least 20 connected superpixels.

ii. *Parametric change* is evaluated in the follow-up diagram that plots normalized stereometric values versus time. If average normalized parametric value decreases by more than 20.05 significant in two consecutive examinations, it is deemed 'suspected' and if it appears in three consecutive examinations, it is considered 'confirmed' progression (Fig. 4.41).

Frequency of examinations. Time determines the speed of progression, and repeated examinations cannot detect disease. High-risk cases on basis of race, age, family history and raised intraocular pressure should undergo a 6 monthly examination and other patients may be followed up annually. Examinations may be done more frequently for the first 18 months in patients showing signs of clinical progression so as to start detecting statistical 'change'.

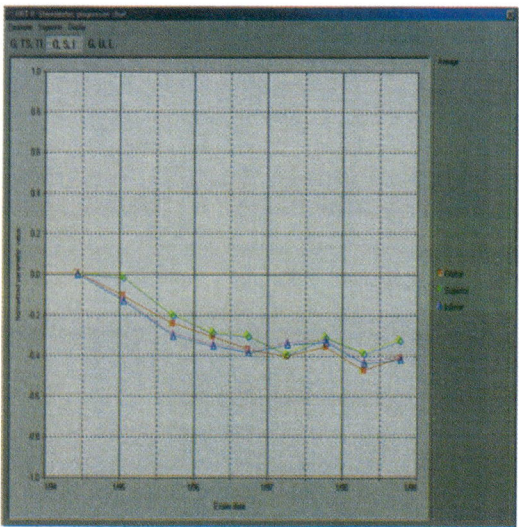

Fig. 4.41 *Parametric changes*

II. SLT in macular diseases

Researchers have developed a software algorithm that analyses the axial intensity distribution and computes a thickness-equivalent map of the retina. This is useful in macular pathologies such as macular edema or macular cysts. The researchers concluded that this analysis offers non-invasive, objective, topographic and reproducible index of macular retinal thickening. The scanning laser thicksness analyser using HRT II uses 147, 456 points while in OCT only 600–768 points are used.

RETINAL THICKNESS ANALYSER

Retinal thickness analyser (RTA) from Talia Technology (Fig. 4.42A) is an ophthalmic imaging device for the mapping and quantitative measurement of optimal thickness and disc topography (Fig. 4.42B). It uses a computerized laser slit lamp to measure retinal thickness at the central 208 of the macula, and overlaps a map of measurements on the patient's retinal image.

A vertical narrow green He–Ne (543.3 nm) laser slit-beam is projected at an angle on the retina while a CCD camera records the back-scattered light. Due to the oblique projection of the beam and the transparency of the retina, the backscattered light returns two peaks corresponding to the vitreoretinal and the chorio-

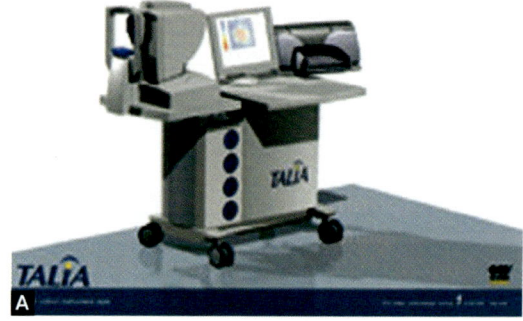

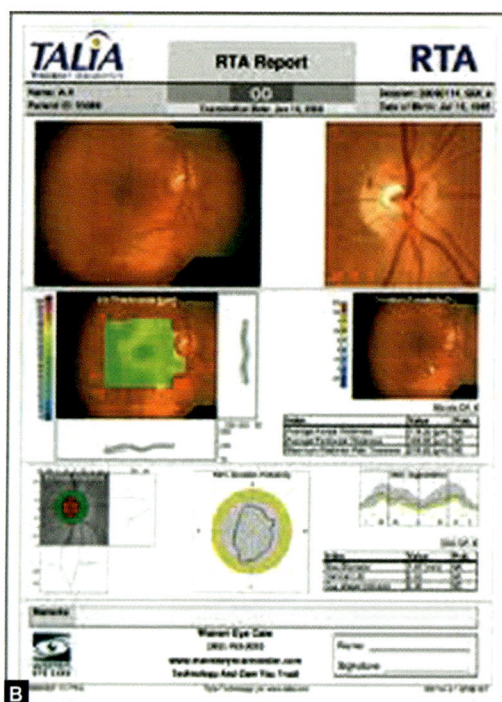

Fig. 4.42 *(A)* *Retinal thickness analyser (RTA); and* *(B)* *Talia, RTA report print out (Courtesy: Talia Technology)*

retinal interfaces. A 3 × 3 × 3 mm scan consisting of 16 optical cross-sections is acquired within 0.3 seconds. Five such scans are obtained at the macula, three scans at the disc and additional five scans cover the peripapillary area (Fig. 4.43).

Clinical applications

Retinal thickness analysis

As the CCD camera records the reflected image of the retinal cross-sections, a thickness algorithm identifies the location of the anterior and posterior retinal borders (Fig. 4.44).

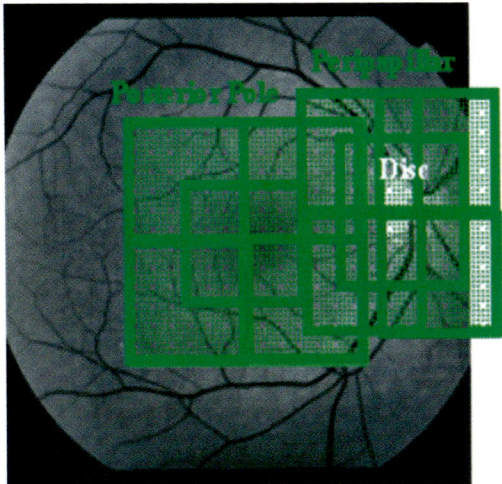

Fig. 4.43 *Thirteen RTA-scanned areas*

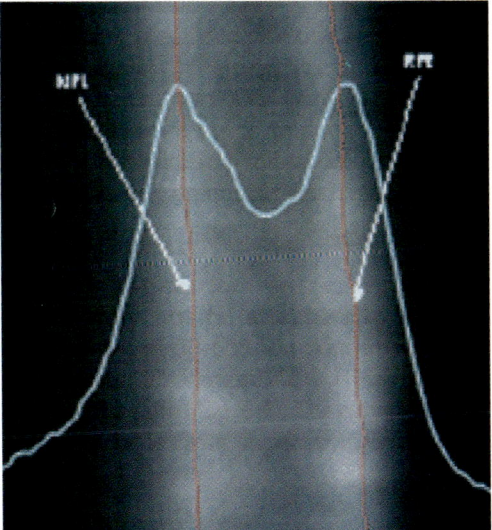

Fig. 4.44 *Light intensity profile as detected by the RTA's thickness algorithm*

The calculated distance between the two light peaks determines the retinal thickness at a given point. The algorithm measures 16 data points on each slit, 187.5 m apart, totalling 2560 thickness measurement points.

Indications of retinal thickness analysis include:
- Diabetic macular edema
- ARMD
- Cystoid macular edema
- Macular holes
- Epiretinal membrane, etc.

ONH topography analysis

The RTA acquires three scans over the disc covering a 3 3 3 mm area. Each of the 16 slit images represents the disc topography along a vertical line. Using edge detection analysis, the topography algorithm identifies the left border of the light, corresponding to the vitreoretinal surface, and calculates the disc topography (Fig. 4.45).

In order to obtain quantitative stereometric measurements, the operator is required to draw a contour line along the disc edge. The same contour line is used in follow-up visits to ensure accurate monitoring of subtle changes. The disc topography report displays a rim/cup area map (Fig. 4.46A) and a pseudo 3-D representation of the disc topography (Fig. 4.46B).

Thus the RTA may be used to assess the optic nerve in terms of the cup to disc (C:D) ratio as well as other ONH parameters. It is also able to monitor progression of nerve fiber layer thinning in glaucoma. Findings are presented in numerical values and may be shown in 2- or 3-D representation.

RTA: Clinical applicability in glaucoma. Early detection of glaucomatous damage is critical for successful treatment. Glaucoma is associated

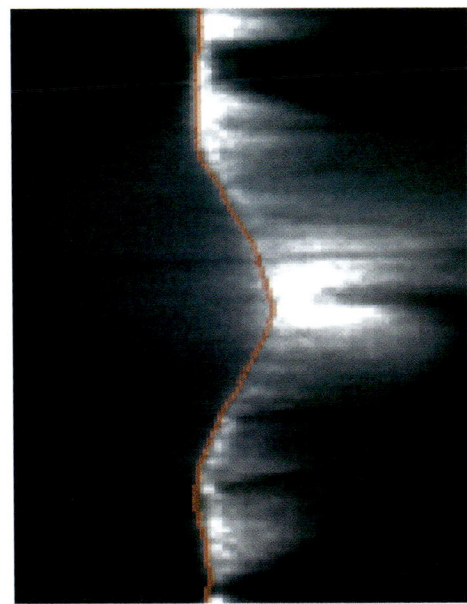

Fig. 4.45 *The vitreoretinal surface as detected by the RTA's topography algorithm*

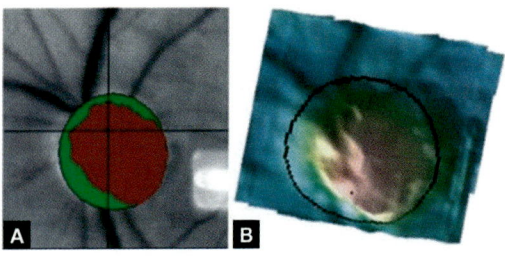

Fig. 4.46 *RTA – disc topography map:* **(A)** *Rim/cup area map and* **(B)** *pseudo 3-D representation*

with ganglion cell and nerve fiber layer loss. Today we know that up to 50% of the total number of ganglion cells are located in the macula. The loss of these two layers is directly reflected in retinal thickness.

None of the other automated imaging tools has emerged as a new gold standard for early glaucoma diagnosis and monitoring. The RTA, however, in addition to imaging the optic disc cupping, identifies and quantifies the anatomical damage in the macula and the peripapillary region even before the symptoms appear.

The RTA is the only tool that provides objective assessment of all three key components of glaucoma-associated changes in the fundus of the eye: macula, peripapillary region and disc area.

Anatomy imager 3-D rendering

Recently, the RTA has incorporated an anatomy imager into the device. The anatomy imager allows 3-D rendering of retinal thickness measurements over the fundus photo captured by the device. Alternatively, the programme allows easy importation of an external image (such as a fluorescein angiography study). The 3-D block may be rotated and cleaved as necessary to appreciate the relationship between abnormalities in retinal thickness and pathologies seen on fluorescein angiography.

SCANNING LASER POLARIMETRY (SLP)

SLP provides on objective quantitative assessment of the peripapillary RNFL, and thus is also called *RNFL analyser* GDx; the commercially available RNFL analyser has two models: the GDx FCC (old model) and GDx VCC (new model). RNFL analyser with variable corneal compensation (available as GDx VCC) is the most appropriate structural test for early detection of glaucomatous damage as it quantifies the morphology of RNFL.

PRINCIPLE AND OPTICS

The RNFL analyser works on the principle of SLP. The operating principle of SLP by which it determines the RNFL thickness is the measurement of the *retardation* of a polarized laser light passing through tissues possessing the physical property of *form birefringence* (explained below).

Form birefringence refers to splitting of a light wave by a polar material into two components. These components travel at different velocities, which creates a relative *phase shift*, also termed as retardation. The amount of phase shift or retardation is proportional to the thickness of polar tissue. The polar tissues are composed of parallel structures, each of which is of smaller diameter than the wavelength of the light used to image it. The RNFL behaves as a polar tissue because of the microtubules (with diameters smaller than the wavelength of light) present in the highly ordered parallel axon bundles. The greater the number of microtubules, the greater the retardation of the polarized laser light, indicating the presence of more tissue; thus giving an assessment of RNFL.

Optics. Figure 4.47 depicts the optics of SLP. The near-infrared laser light (780 nm) enters the eye at specific orientation. As the laser double passes the RNFL, it is split into two parallel rays by the birefringent microtubules (present in the

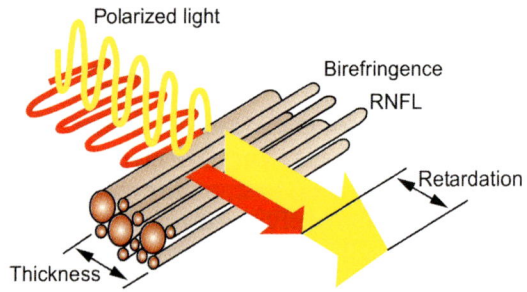

Fig. 4.47 *Optical principle of scanning laser polarimeter (SLP) (nerve fiber layer analyser)*

axons forming RNFL). The two rays travel at different speeds, and this difference (called retardation) is measured.

Total birefringence, anterior segment birefringence and RNFL birefringence

Total birefringence-associated retardation is the sum of anterior segment birefringence (from cornea and lens) and RNFL birefringence.

RNFL birefringence can be isolated from the total birefringence by compensating for the anterior segment birefringence.

Fixed versus variable corneal compensation

- *Fixed corneal compensation (FCC)* was employed in the earlier models of nerve fiber layer analysers (e.g. GDx FCC), ensuring that all individuals had a slow axis of corneal birefringence (corneal polarization axis) 158 nasally downward with a magnitude of 60 nm (corneal polarization magnitude). However, recently it has been shown that there exists a wide variation in the axis and magnitude of corneal polarization in healthy and glaucomatous eyes.
- *Variable corneal compensation (VCC)* is required to exactly measure the RNFL birefringence. The modified version of nerve fiber layer analyser (GDx VCC) measures and individually compensates for anterior segment birefringence for each eye and thus allows the exact measurement of RNFL birefringence.

GDX VCC NERVE FIBER LAYER ANALYSER

The new modified version of nerve fiber analyser, i.e. GDx VCC (Fig. 4.48) is an SLP, which basically consists of a confocal scanning laser ophthalmoscope with an integrated ellipsometer to measure retardation.

Procedure of measurement

The measurement is performed with an undilated pupil of at least 2 mm diameter. A 780 nm infrared laser is used to scan the parapapillary area to give the RNFL measurements. Time taken is about 0.7 seconds. Total chair time is less than 3 minutes for both eyes. First the eye is imaged without compensation. The uncompensated image presents total retardation

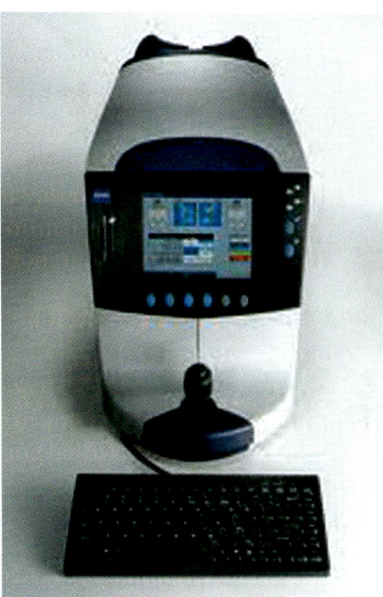

Fig. 4.48 *Commercially available nerve fiber layer analyser (GDx VCC) (Courtesy: Carl Zeiss Meditec AS)*

from the eye. The macular region of this image is then analysed to determine the axis and magnitude of the anterior segment birefringence. The macular region birefringence is uniform and symmetric due to radial distribution of Henle's fiber layer.

Interpretation of the GDx VCC printout

The measurements are compared with a *normative database* (from healthy volunteers of different races) to determine any significant deviations from normal limits which are flagged as abnormal with a p value. Most of the parameters on GDx VCC printout are calculated from the calculation circle. This is the area of 8 pixels between two concentric circles centerd around the optic disc. The GDx VCC printout is interpreted as below (Fig. 4.49):

1. *Color fundus image* is seen at the top of the printout. It is depicted as 208 3 208 image of the disc and parapapillary area (Fig. 4.49A). It is produced by more than 16,000 data points from the scanned area.

2. *Thickness (polarization) map* shows the RNFL thickness in a color-coded format in the 208 3 208 parapapillary area as below (Fig. 4.49B):

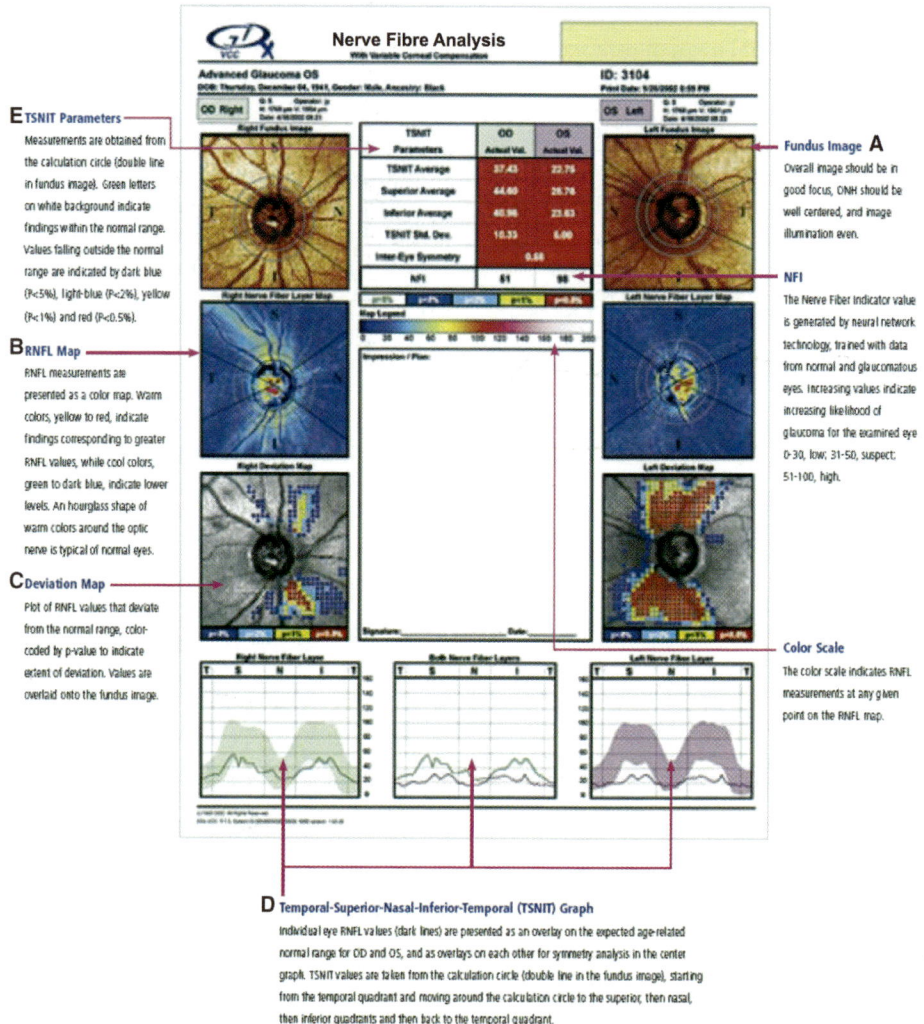

Fig. 4.49 *A representation printout of GDx VCC retinal nerve fiber layer analyser*

- *Thick RNFL areas* are indicated by bright colors: yellow, orange and red.
- *Thin RNFL areas* are indicated by dark color (dark blue, blue and green).
- *Typical normal pattern* is characterized by bright yellow and red colors (thicker areas) in the superior and inferior sectors and dark blue and green (i.e. thinner areas) in the nasal and temporal sectors.

Abnormal patterns of thickness map include:
- *Diffuse loss of RNFL* leads to its decreased thickness, seen as yellow instead of red.
- *Focal defects* are seen as concentrated dark areas.

- *Asymmetry* between superior and inferior quadrants of RNFL.
- *Asymmetry* between the RNFL of two eyes.
- *Increased thickness* of RNFL in nasal and temporal quadrants of RNFL (seen as red and yellow instead of blue).

3. **Deviation map.** It shows the location and magnitude of RNFL defects over the entire thickness map. It tells how the patient's RNFL thickness compares with values derived from the normative database in a 128 3 128 pixel (208 3 208) region centerd on the optic disc. Small color-coded squares indicate the amount of deviation from normal at each given location

and are presented over a black and white fundus image to provide a visual form of reference (Fig. 4.92C). Dark blue squares represent areas where the RNFL thickness is below the 5th percentile of the normative database; i.e. there is only 5% probability that the RNFL thickness in this area is within the normal range. Light blue squares represent deviation below the 2% level, yellow represents deviation below 1% and red represents deviation below 0.5%. Thus, a quick look at the deviation map gives an idea of the wedge defects of RNFL and the pattern of defects.

4. *The TSNIT graphs* (Fig. 4.49D). The TSNIT, i.e. 'temporal-superior, nasal-inferior-temporal' graph displays the range and the patient's values of RNFL thickness along the calculation ellipse in TSNIT order separately for right (OD) and left (OS) eyes.

- In a normal eye, the typical TSNIT graph shows a typical 'double-hump' pattern.
- A flat TSNIT graph indicates loss of RNFL.
- *TSNIT symmetry graph* is obtained by displaying the graphs of two eyes together. Normally, the curves from two eyes overlap. However, in glaucoma, one eye often has more advanced RNFL loss and, therefore, the two curves will have less overlap. A dip in the curve of one eye relative to another is indicative of RNFL loss.

TSNIT serial analysis graph and deviation from reference map for a given eye, for analysis of serial changes between visits can also be obtained from GDx VCC. This is very useful to demonstrate progression over a period of time.

5. *TSNIT parameters.* These are displayed in a table on the center of printout (Fig. 4.49E). The TSNIT parameters are summary measures based on RNFL thickness values within the calculation ellipse and include TSNIT average, superior average, inferior average, TSNIT standard deviation, intereye symmetry and the nerve fiber indicator (NFI).

- *TSNIT average* refers to average RNFL thickness around the entire calculation ellipse.
- *Superior average* is the average RNFL thickness in the superior 128 region of calculation ellipse.

- *Inferior average* is the average RNFL thickness in the inferior 1208 region of calculation ellipse.
- *TSNIT standard deviation* indicates the modulation (peak to trough difference) of the double-hump pattern. A normal eye has high and a glaucoma eye has low modulation in the double-hump pattern.
- *Intereye symmetry* measures the degree of symmetry between the right and left eyes. Normal eyes have good symmetry with values around 0.9.
- *NFI.* It is the most important parameter, since it is an indicator of the likelihood that an eye has glaucoma. NFI is generated from the patient's scanned data obtained from within and outside the calculation circle.

The output of NFI is a single value that ranges from 1 to 100 and indicates the overall integrity of the RNFL. The higher the NFI the more likely that the patient has glaucoma. The values of NFI are generally interpreted as:

- Normal: 1–30 (less likelihood of glaucoma)
- Glaucoma suspect: 30–50
- Abnormal: >50 (high likelihood of glaucoma)

Normal versus abnormal values of TSNIT parameters

Normal values of TSNIT parameters reported from Indian population are:

- TSNIT average: 54.8 6 4.1 (45.6 – 66.8) μ
- Superior average: 66.8 6 6.70 (55.1 – 85) μ
- Inferior average: 62.1 6 6.6 (38.9 – 74.3) μ
- NFI: 17.2 6 6.9 (4–35) μ

Abnormal values. Although there is no consensus on definition of abnormal scan, the following guidelines have been recommended for TSNIT average, superior average, inferior average, TSNIT standard deviation, intereye symmetry and NFI:

- Abnormal at p, <1% level
- Borderline at p, <5% level

Additional diagnostic parameters

Additional diagnostic parameters available in the machine for an extended analysis include the following:

- **Symmetry.** It is the ratio of the average of the 1500 thickest pixels each in the superior and

inferior quadrants. The values closer to 1 indicate more symmetry and thus more chances of normal scan.

- *Superior ratio.* It is the ratio of superior quadrant thickness (average of 1500 thickest pixels) and temporal quadrant thickness (average of 1500 median pixels).
- *Inferior ratio.* It is the ratio of inferior quadrant thickness (average of 1500 thickest pixels) and temporal quadrant thickness (average of 1500 median pixels).
- *Superior nasal.* It is the ratio of superior quadrant thickness (average of 1500 thickest pixels) and nasal quadrant thickness (average of 1500 median pixels).
- *Maximum modulation.* It is ratio of thickest quadrant versus thinnest quadrant. Normally the maximum modulation is more than 1, since superior and inferior quadrants are thicker than nasal and temporal quadrants. Value of 1 or less indicates RNFL loss.
- *Superior maximum.* It is the average of the 1500 thickest pixels in the superior quadrant.
- *Inferior maximum.* It is the average of the 1500 thickest pixels in the inferior quadrant.
- *Ellipse modulation.* It is the ratio of the thickest quadrant and the thinnest quadrant within the ellipse area.
- *Ellipse average.* It is the average thickness (in microns) of RNFL in the ellipse surrounding the ONH.

Advantages and limitations of GDx VCC

Advantages of GDx VCC
- Easy to operate
- Does not require pupillary dilation
- Good reproducibility
- Does not require a reference plane
- Can detect glaucoma on the first examination
- Early detection before standard visual field
- Comparison with age-matched normative database.

Limitations of GDx VCC
- Does not measure actual RNFL thickness (inferred value).
- Low sensitivity and specificity for detection of pre-perimetric glaucoma in clinical studies.
- Does not differentiate true biological change from variability.
- Limited use in moderate and advanced glaucoma.
- No database from Indian population.
- Affected by anterior and posterior segment lesions such as:
  - Ocular surface disorders
  - Macular pathology
  - Cataract and refractive surgery
  - Refractive errors
  - Peripapillary atrophy (scleral birefringence interferes with RNFL measurement)

BIBLIOGRAPHY

1. Matthew T. Witmer, MD, Szila´rd Kiss, MD. Wide-eld Imaging of the Retina. Surv Ophthalmol 2013;58;2:143–154.
2. Rosenthal ML, Fradin S: The technique of binocular indirect ophthalmoscopy. Highlights Ophthalmol 1966;9:179–257.
3. Rubin ML : Magnification; practical instruments: the indirect ophthalmoscope. In: Optics for clinicians. 2nd edn.
4. Saine P, Tyler M. Ophthalmic Photography. A Textbook of Retinal Photography. Angiography and Electronic Imaging. Boston, MA, Twin Chimney Publishing; 1997.

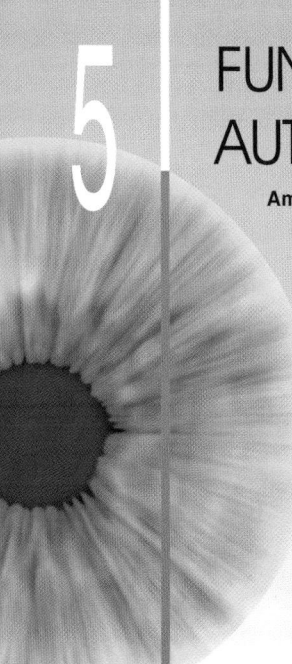

5 | FUNDUS ANGIOGRAPHY AND AUTOFLUORESCENCE

Amod Gupta, Subina Narang, Pradeep Venktesh, Mohit Dogra, Reema Bansal, MR Dogra

FUNDUS FLUORESCEIN ANGIOGRAPHY

BASIC PRINCIPLE, EQUIPMENT AND TECHNIQUE

Fundus fluorescein angiography (FFA) is the backbone of the retina services of any institute. It was first used in eye in 1961. A careful evaluation and interpretation of FFA are essential to diagnose, treat and follow up the disease. The most important is its role in guiding laser treatment of the retinal vascular and choroidal diseases.

BASIC PRINCIPLE

Sodium fluorescein is used for fluorescence. It absorbs light energy which is blue (465–490 nm) and fluoresces at green yellow (520–530 nm) (Fig. 5.1A). In addition to green yellow light reflected back by sodium fluorescein, there is blue light reflected back from structures that do not contain sodium fluorescein. This blue reflected light and green yellow light falls on the filter (barrier filter) which allows green yellow light to pass and keeps away blue reflected light. Failure of this filter leads to pseudofluorescence which may cause difficulty in interpretation and decreased resolution of FFA pictures (Fig. 5.1A).

EQUIPMENT

Both digital and film angiography can be used. Trends are shifting towards use of digital angiography in view of low incurring expenditure and immediate results. Camera with flash unit, timer and matched fluorescein filter form an important part of equipment (Fig. 5.1B). Timer is most important for arm to retina circulation time in diseases with decreased arterial perfusion. Fluorescein dye reaches the eye through systemic circulation after injecting in brachial vein. The exciter filter of the equipment transmits blue light from 465–490 nm which excites the sodium fluorescein dye and barrier filter transmits light from 525–530 nm which is reflected back by sodium fluorescein dye. The transmission of both filters should have

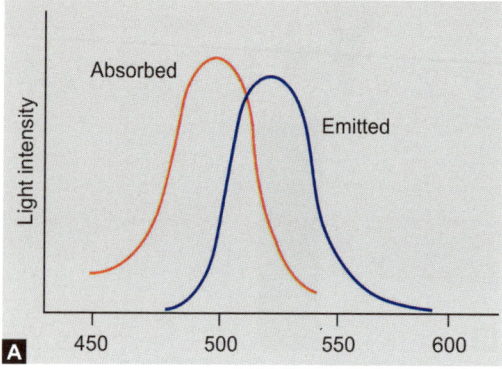

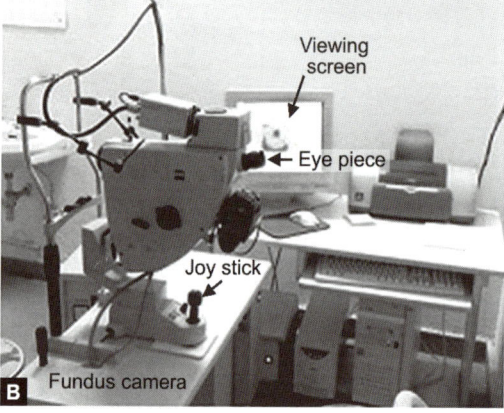

Fig. 5.1 (A) *Graph depicting fluorescein absorption and emission spectra; and* **(B)** *Fundus digital imaging system showing screen for simultaneous view of the acquired data and various parts*

minimum overlap. If there is overlap, pseudo-fluorescence will result. After the machine becomes old, the filters become thin, and transmission of more light is there leading to pseudofluorescence compromising the quality of FFA.

Sodium fluorescence is a low molecular weight dye (376.27 daltons) $C_{20}H_{12}O_5Na$ used for fundus fluorescein angiography. It diffuses through most of the body fluids and choriocapillaris. When injected, 80% of sodium fluorescein is protein bound and only 20% is available for flurescence. Inner and outer blood retinal barrier are impermeable to it in healthy state. It is eliminated through liver and kidney in less than 24 hours. Urine and skin may develop yellowish tinge.

PROCEDURE

Before proceeding with the test, photographer must settle the field that is to be centered, whether he wants 30° or 60°. Detailed macular evaluation is done by 30° FFA and wider pathologies need 60°. The camera must be adjusted for vertical adjustment and the eyepiece for accommodation keeping cross hair in sharp focus. The photographer ascertains pupillary diameter also by moving camera from side to side. This also helps him to ascertain focusing peculiarities of particular cornea and lens. By doing this he finds out the best position for a clear fundus photograph.

Before starting the procedure one must ensure availability of emergency tray including hydrocortisone vial, inj adrenaline 1:1000, inj phenargan, inj atropine, venous cannula, at least three 5 cc and 10 cc syringes with needles intravenous fluid bottles of normal saline as well as dextrose, Guide airways of pediatric and adult sizes, laryngoscope with both small and large blade, working battery cells, endotracheal tubes, oxygen cylinder with flow meter and transparent face mask (Fig. 5.2A to D). There should always be supply of light sources. Fluorescein dye used could be in 10 ml (5%), or 5 ml (10%) or 3 ml (25%) vials.

Informed consent has to be taken before the procedure and the procedure and adverse reactions must be told. Apart from discoloration of skin and urine, anaphylactic reaction and vasovagal shock are the other rare complications (Fig. 5.3D).

Position the patient with chin at chin rest and forehead touching the head bar. Inject dye slowly with syringe and 23 gauze scalp vein set and start timer. The most frequently accessed vein is antecubital vein and we expect to see the dye in the eye in 9 seconds after injection. The injection must be given in 4–6 seconds and too fast an injection may lead to nausea though it gives better picture.

Fluorescein injection has to be coordinated with fundus photograph. This must be injected after identification and control picture. The first frames should be area of interest which we call primary eye/macula. Initially, capture primary macula every 2 seconds after the dye is visible

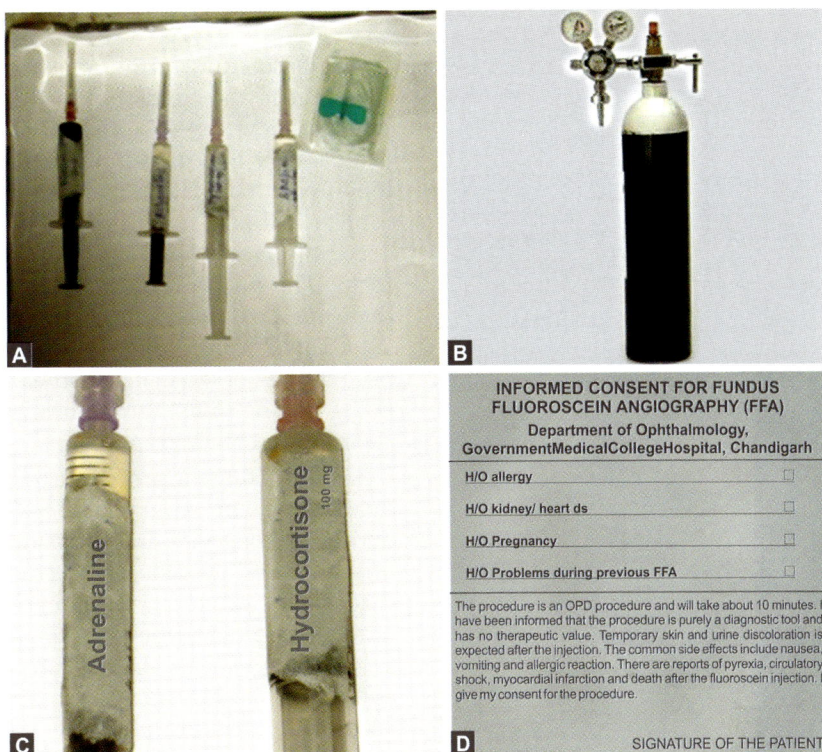

Fig. 5.2 *Emergency equipment tray including oxygen cylinder before start of FFA*

in choroidal circulation for 30 seconds. The secondary macula is clicked after primary macula followed by disc. The time interval between frames is increased. The periphery

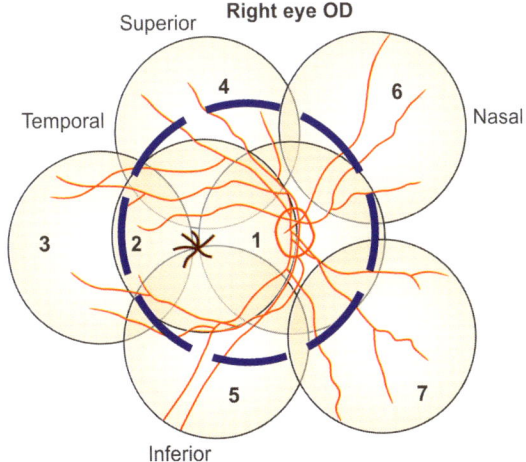

Fig. 5.3 *The 7 airlie house fundus fields to ensure proper clicking of all fields to include relevant data especially in diabetes mellitus*

should be recorded by tilting the camera. Pictures of other important areas can be taken as evident from clinical examination. We must cover all fields in both eyes in diabetic retinopathy according to airlie house classification as shown in Fig. 5.3. The eye is moved with the help of fixation light. FFA takes 4–10 minutes. Late pictures after 10 minutes are rarely required except CSCR, CME, etc. to note dye pooling.

CONTRAINDICATIONS

It should be avoided in first trimester of pregnancy. However, there are no contraindications in heart disease and cardiac pacemaker. Avoid FFA in cases with severe kidney disease as dye is excreted by the kidneys. Its better to avoid FFA in cases known to have allergy to dye. A sensitivity test is done to check allergy to dye before full dose of dye is injected in vein may be done in these patients. For patients having cardiac, respiratory disease, test can be done under anaesthetist doctor's supervision.

NORMAL AND ABNORMAL FUNDUS FLUORESCEIN ANGIOGRAM

NORMAL FUNDUS FLUORESCEIN ANGIOGRAM

In normal FFA, **choroidal flush** (Fig. 5.4A) appears first and arm to retina time for the dye is 10–12 seconds in normal adult . It could be faster in young and delayed in elderly. It is faint, patchy and irregularly scattered throughout posterior fundus. This also fills cilioretinal artery simultaneously, if present. Central retinal artery begins to fill with fluorescein dye 1–3 seconds later. After the arteries are filled, **early venous phase** is seen as lamellar flow phase (Fig. 5.4B) as fluorescein dye enters the veins along the walls. The flow of fluorescein is lamellar and it flows faster in the center of the vessel than on the sides (trilaminar flow). The dark central lamella is nonfluorescent blood that comes from periphery and which takes longer to fluorescene because of its more distant location. The laminae become thicker in next 5–10 seconds and finally merge to give complete fluorescence to the veins. **Arteriovenous phase** starts after this and fluorescene reaches peak in 20–25 seconds (Fig. 5.5A and B). The dye starts to empty from eye circulation after 30 seconds of dye injection. After this **recirculation phase** starts in which lower dye concentration continues to flow in eye circulation. The retinal circulation is completely free of dye in ten minutes. The dye might be retained in some eye tissues leading to pooling

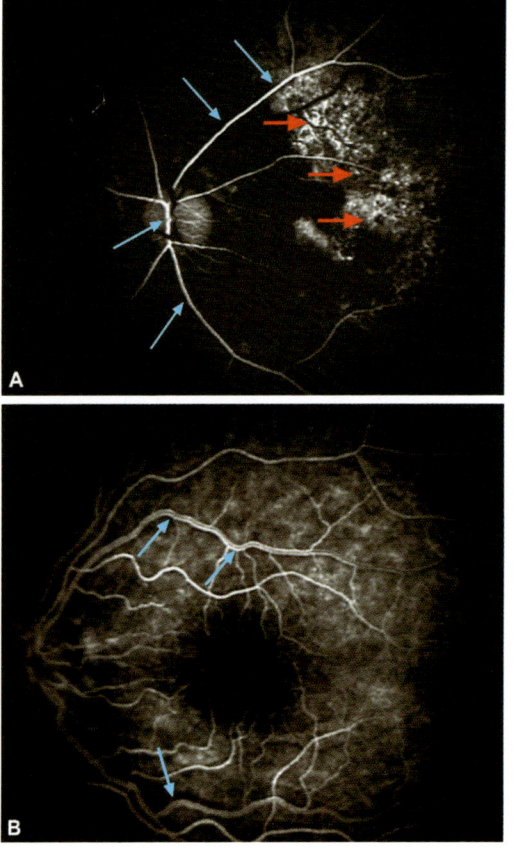

Fig. 5.4 *(A)* Choroidal flush appears as irregular patchy hyperfluorescence at posterior pole seen very early and increases over subsequent frames; and *(B)* early venous phase shows lamellar flow due to differential blood flow velocity in vessel and increase in choroidal hyperfluorescence

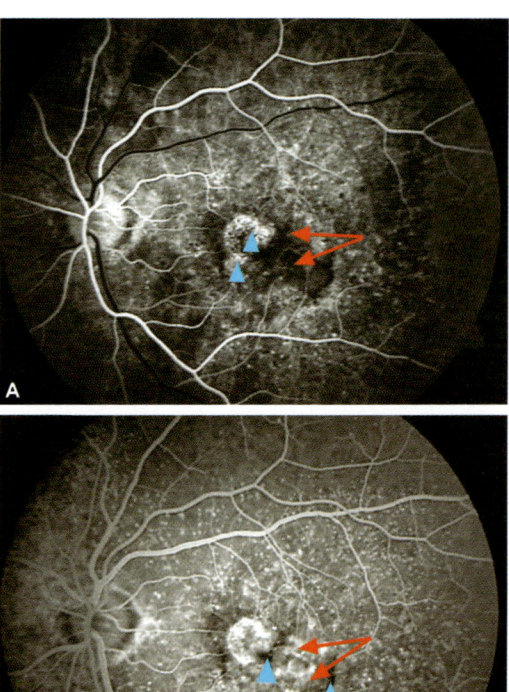

Fig. 5.5 *(A)* Early venous phase shows trilaminar flow and abnormal finding of hyperfluorescence (arrow heads) in foveal area with adjacent area of hypofluorescence (arrows); and *(B)* arteriovenous phase shows increase in fluorescence which peaks in 20–25 seconds (arrows). There is increase in hyperfluorescence in macular area along with block fluorescence (arrow heads) corresponding to CNVM with retinal hemorrhages

of dye (Fig. 5.6A and B) or staining like bruch's membrane, choroid, sclera, disc and adjacent visible sclera. We see a dark foveal avascular zone because of high columnar retinal pigment epithelial cells and more xanthophylls here than rest of fundus. There is also absence of vessels in center 400–500 microns. Anatomically we know that there are only 4 rows of retinal cells here (ILM, OPL, ONL, rods and cones). This helps us to understand stellate pattern of edema in macula and honey comb appearance +90 D slit lamp biomicroscopy.

Optic disc FFA needs to be understood clearly. It has a dual blood supply from the retinal vascular system and posterior ciliary vascular system. We see extensive vascular anastomotic channels between these two circulations in case of disease. There are many layers of nerve fibers and glial tissue. The lamina cribrosa portion of

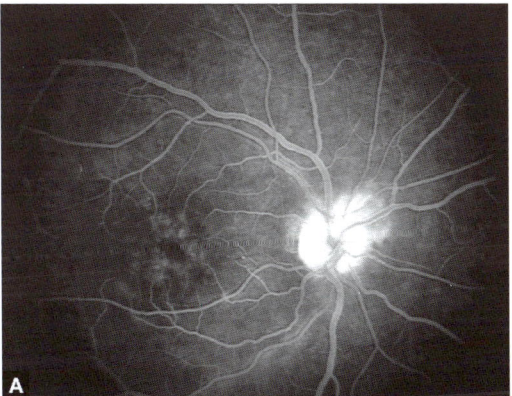

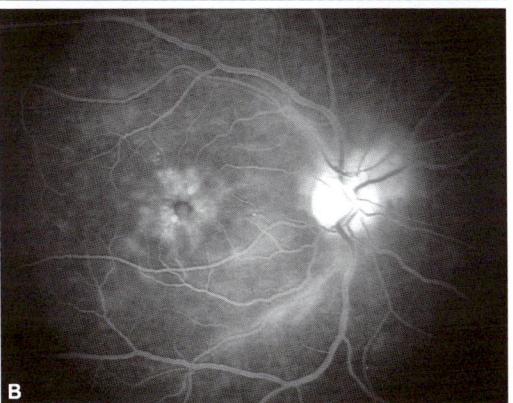

Fig. 5.6 (A) *Arteriovenous phase shows decrease in fluorescence and abnormal finding of macular hyperfluorescence; and* **(B)** *which increases in late phase suggestive of dye pooling in patelloid pattern in a case of cystoid macular edema*

nerve is supplied by short posterior ciliary arteries (SPCA) and prelaminar portion is supplied by centripetal braches from peripapillary choroid. There are small branches of retinal arterioles at peripapillary region. As most of the disc is supplied by ciliary system fluorescein dye at disc is seen much before retinal vessels fill up. Main venous drainage is into central retinal vein and peripapillary choroid.

ABNORMALITIES IN FUNDUS FLUORESCEIN ANGIOGRAM

These appear as hypo- and hyper-fluorescent areas which may be traced over subsequent angiogram frames to give proper diagnosis.

HYPERFLUORESCENCE

To interpret abnormal hyperfluorescence check the phase of angiogram in which it first appears and then look at it in subsequent phases. Hyperfluorescence could due to:

- Autofluorescence/pseudofluorescence, i.e. abnormal preinjection fluorescence
- Leakage of dye
- Transmission defect
- Staining

Abnormal preinjection fluorescence

- *Pseudofluorescence* will be visible at beginning of FFA in red free pictures or due to defect in filter matching which is unusual in modern machines and with frequent change in filters.
- *Autofluorescence* is seen in optic nerve head drusens and astrocytic hamartoma.

Leakage of dye

Hyperfluorescence which appears early in FFA and then increases in subsequent phases both in size and intensity due to leakage from abnormal vessels in retina or choroid as in CNVM.

Thus leakage is any hyperfluorescence that persists 15 minutes after injection after retinal or choroidal vessels are emptied of fluorescence (Figs 5.7 and 5.8). Leakage could be into vitreous as diffuse white haze in inflamed eye. It could also be in case of intraocular tumors or flat/raised neovascularisation.

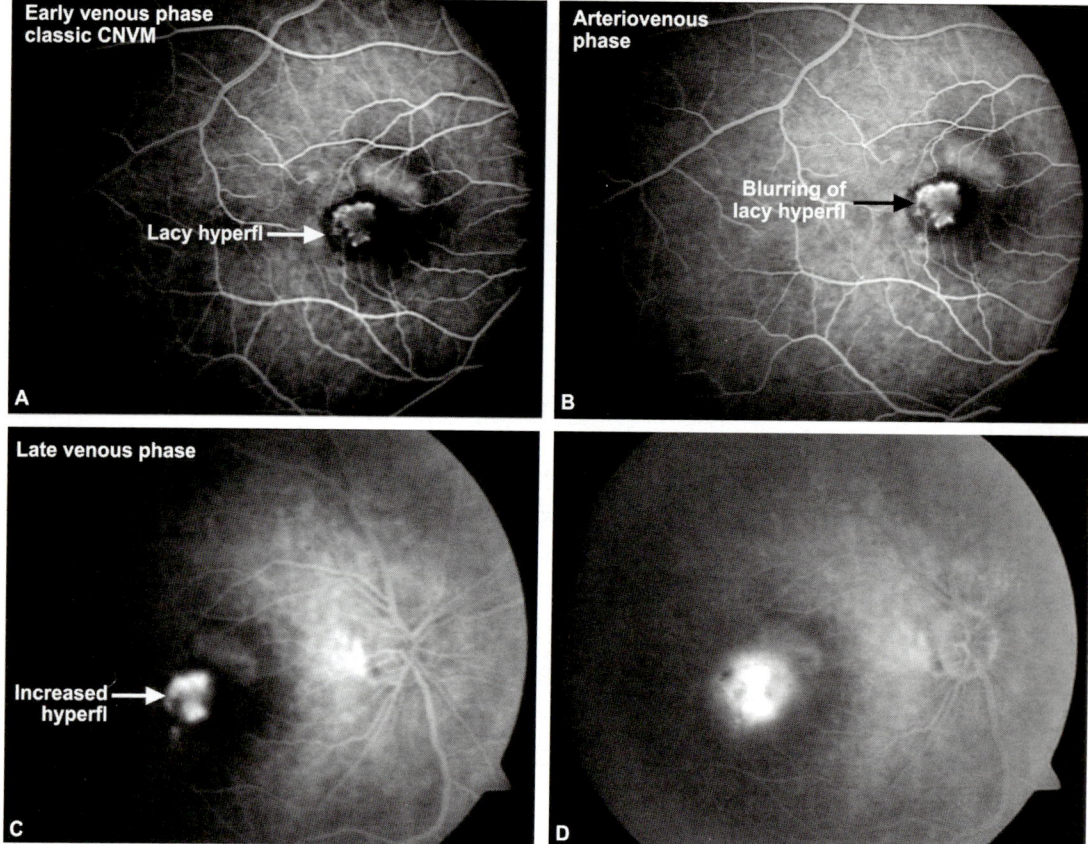

Fig. 5.7 *(A) Early venous phase showing juxtafoveal lacy heperfluorescence; (B) arteriovenous phase showing blurring of lacy hyperfluorescence; (C) late venous phase showing increase in hyperfluorescence; and (D) late phase of FFA showing increase in hyperfluorescence suggestive of classic CNVM*

Transmission hyperfluorescence (Fig. 5.9)

Hyperfluorescence which matches the background choroidal fluorescence, i.e first increases in AV phases and then decreases in recirculation phase, e.g. RPE atrophy in dry AMD.

Thus, transmission hyperfluorescence occur due to RPE atrophy leading to window defect which increases visibility of choroidal fluorescence. Normally pigment epithelium forms a barrier for choroidal fluorescence to be visible. Transmission hyperfluorescence starts in early frames along with choroidal flush and then increases as choroidal fluorescence increases in arteriovenous phase and decreases in late phases as choroidal flush decreases with washing away of dye. It neither increases in size nor changes in shape.

Staining

Some tissues take up the dye and this hyperfluorescence does not increase over time but persists in late phases which is called staining (Fig. 5.10). Hyperfluorescence which increases in subsequent phases in intensity but not size, e.g. staining of scar tissue.

Disc leakage should be differentiated from normal disc hyperfluorescence due to late staining of lamina cribrosa and leakage from peripapillary choroid.

Pooling of dye

Pooling of dye under sensory retina after breakdown the outer blood-retinal barrier. The pattern of hyperfluorescence in some diseases could be diagnostic like central serous chorioretinopathy(CSCR) (Fig. 5.11).

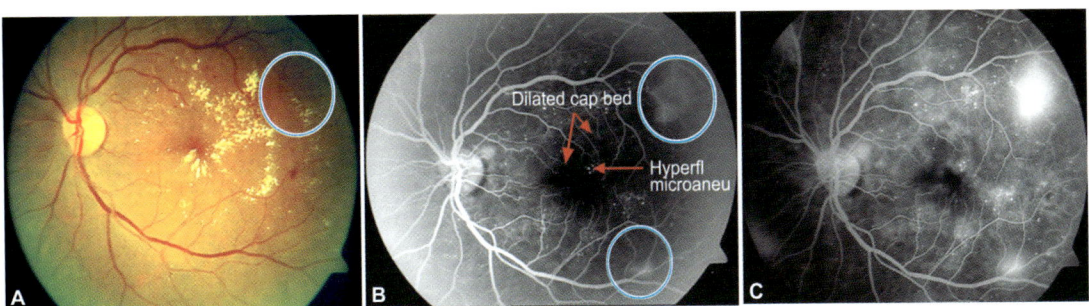

Fig. 5.8 (A) *Fundus picture showing clinically significant macular edema (CSME) encroaching the fovealcentre;* **(B)** *arteriovenous phase shows hyperfluorescent dots corresponding to microaneurysms and dilated capillary bed and also hyperfluorescence corresponding to neovessels. There is increase in hyperfluorescence in late phases and* **(C)** *the patient has proliferative diabetic retinopathy and CSME involving the foveal centre*

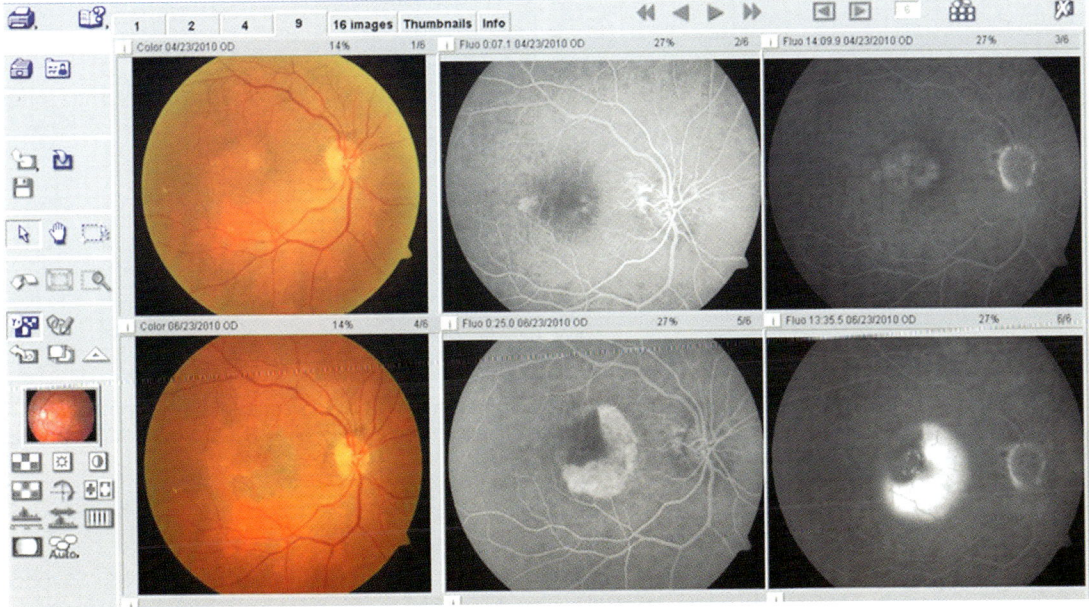

Fig. 5.9 *Case of occult CNVM: The top row showing patchy macular hyperfluorescence increasing in late phase. The bottom row is after injection bevacizumab leading to RPE rip. Hypofluorescence corresponds to RPE folded on itself. Hyperfluorescence is transmission defect due to absent RPE*

HYPOFLUORESCENCE

Hypoflurescence refer to decrease or absence of fluorescence during the course of FFA. Depending upon whether it is due to barrier effect or due to nonperfusion it can be classified as blocked fluorescence or vascular filling defect.

Blocked fluorescence

The transmission of fluorescence could be decreased in choroid or retina. In choroid it can be decreased by retinal hemorrhages and vitreous opacities. In retina the fluorescence can be decreased by preretinal bleed or vitreous hemorrhage (Fig. 5.12) or preretinal pigment clump. This can be differentiated from vascular filling defect by sequential study of FFA. There will be no change in fluorescence of an area with blocked fluorescence. The depth of lesion can be seen by vessels it blocks. If it is in nerve fiber layer it will block all vessels and if it is in inner nuclear layer, only retinal capillaries are

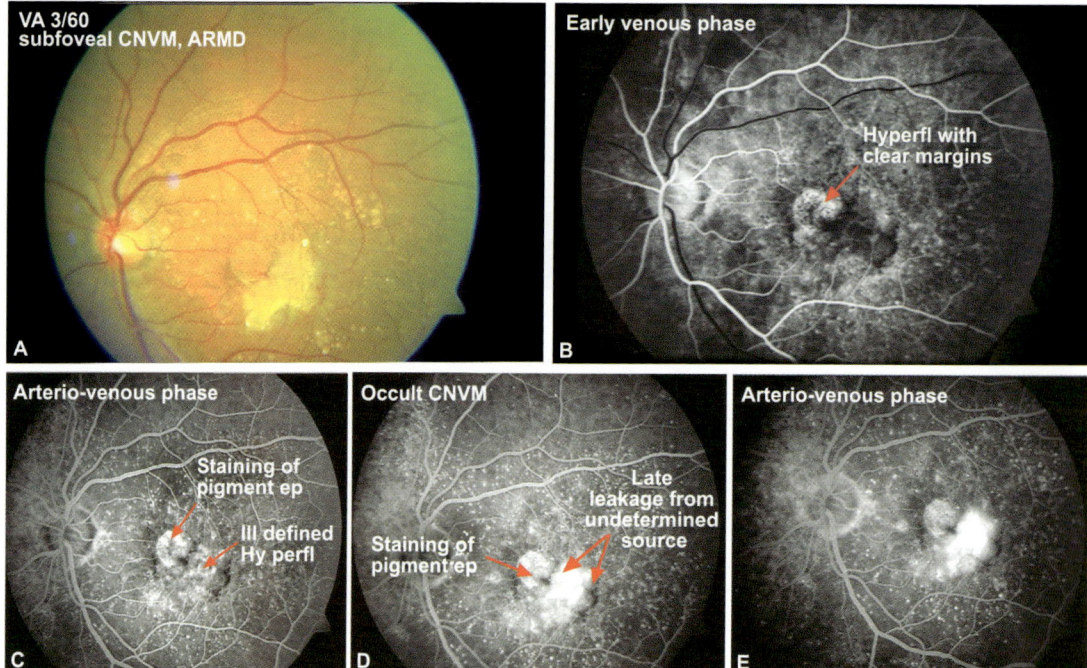

Fig. 5.10 *Scar of old CNVM with fresh recurrence at temporal edge seen as grayish membrane. Early hyperfluorescence with well defined borders which increases in intensity on late phases with adjacent late leakage from undetermined source (Figs A to E) suggestive of occult CNVM*

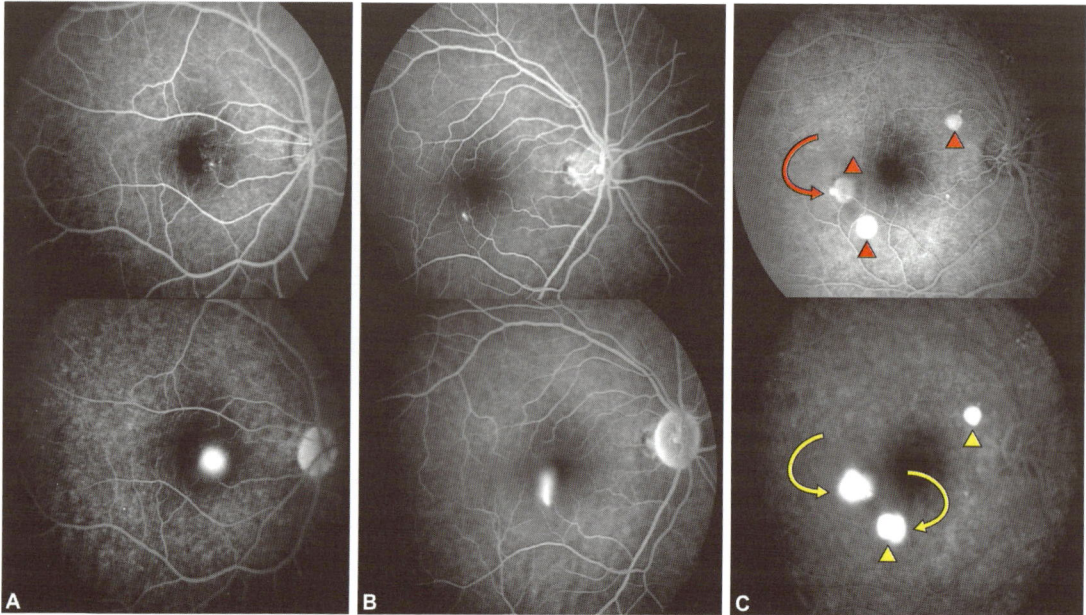

Fig. 5.11 *Top row shows early phase of FFA and bottom row shows corresponding late phases showing various patterns of leakage in CSCR: (A) expanding dot sign; (B) smoke stack sign; and (C) multiple leaks with fuzzy borders (curved arrow) and PED with well defined borders (arrow heads)*

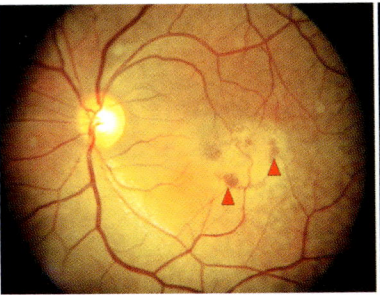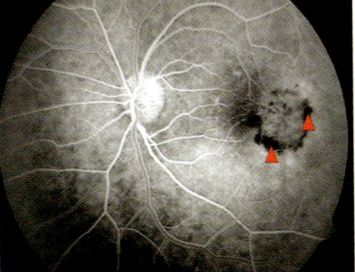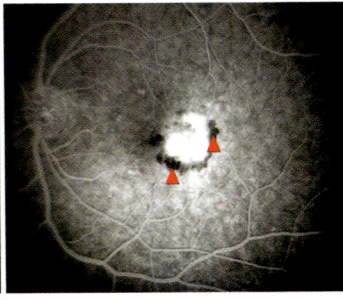

Fig. 5.12 *A case of CNVM showing increasing hyperfluorescence suggestive of active disease surrounded by hypofluorescent area persistent throughout the FFA sugestive of blocked fluorescence due to hemorrhage*

blocked. In blocked fluorescence, hypofluorescence persists in all phases of angiogram.

Nonperfusion or vascular filling defect

Hypofluorescence due to non perfusion, atrophy, absence of circulation or vascular insufficiency is present in early phases of angiogram but it may not persist after some time. If the vessel obstruction is complete or there is total tissue atrophy, it may persist through all phases of angiogram (Figs 5.13 and 5.14). In partial obstruction the filling is delayed or reduced compared to other areas with normal fluorescence. The level could be retinal or choroidal. Choroidal vascular filling defects are most difficult to pick. Early FFA frame should be seen. Normally in choroidal diseases due to nonperfusion, RPE is depigmented or atrophied and it becomes easier to discern choroidal filling defect. Normally RPE forms a barrier for choroidal fluorescence to be visible. Hypofluorescence in choroidal circulation appears in early phase and disappears in late phases due to pooling of dye from surrounding lobules 2–5 seconds later (Fig. 5.15). In some cases even large choroidal vessels are nonperfused and there is total choroidal hypofluorescence staining at edge later from surrounding choriocapillaris. The blocked fluorescent areas continues to be hypofluorescent throughout the angiogram (Fig. 5.16).

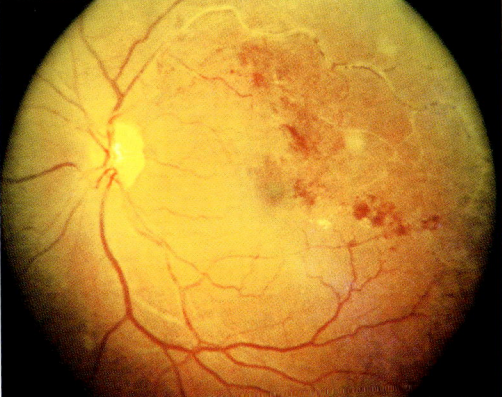

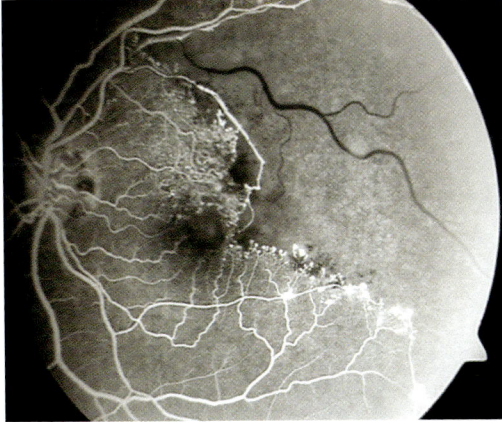

Fig. 5.13 *In a case of branch retinal vein occlusion, hypofluorescence in quadrant of retina corresponding to venous distribution of superotemporal BRV which appears in early frames persists throughout suggestive of both arterial and venous block*

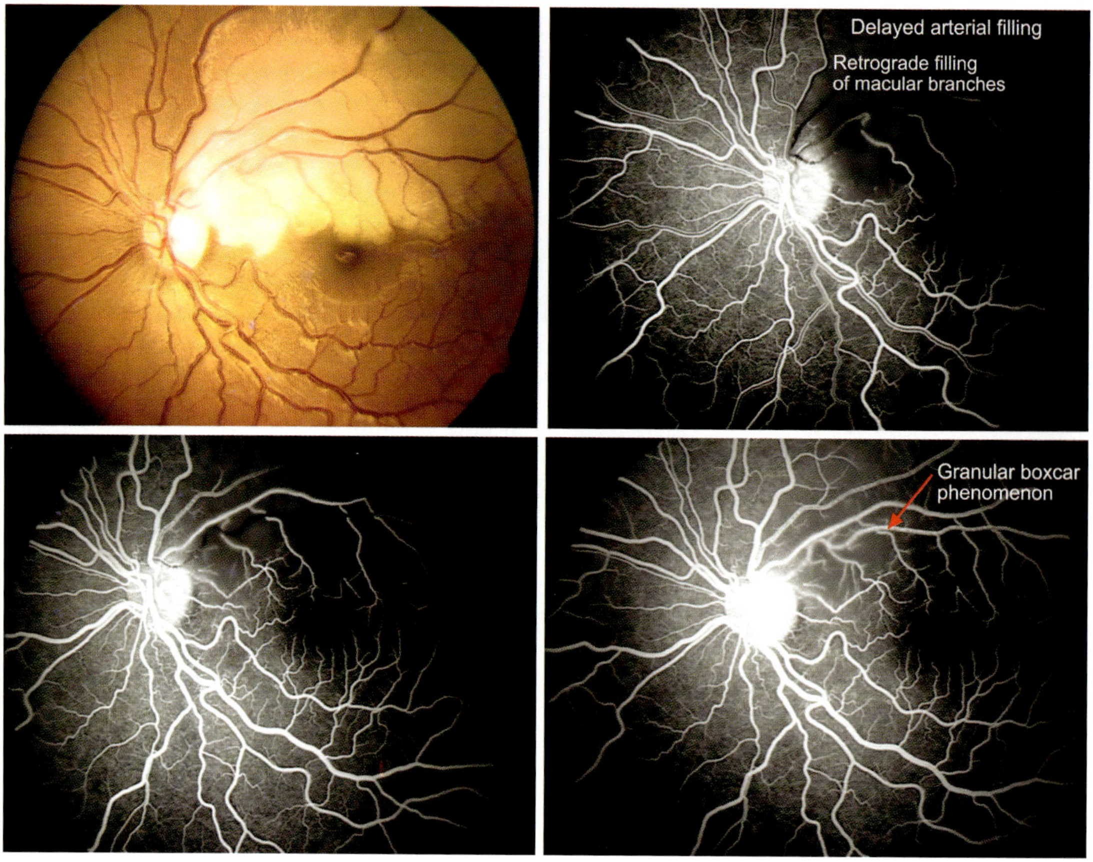

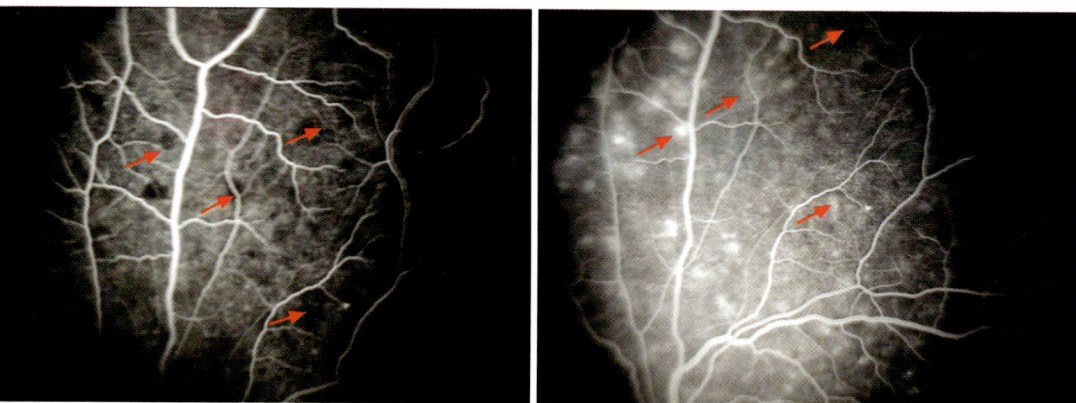

Delayed arterial filling

Retrograde filling
of macular branches

Granular boxcar
phenomenon

Fig. 5.14 *In a case of branch retinal artery occlusion there is delayed arterial filling and retrograde filling of macular branches. We can appreciate the granular boxcar phenomenon in late phases (arrow)*

Fig. 5.15 *A case of active multifocal choroiditis showing well defined hypofluorescence seen in early phases and pooling of dye from adjacent lobules in late phases leading to hyperfluorescence of the same area*

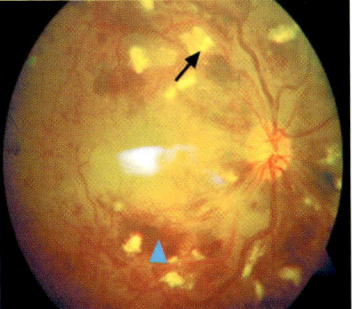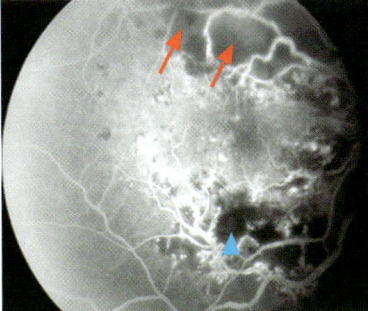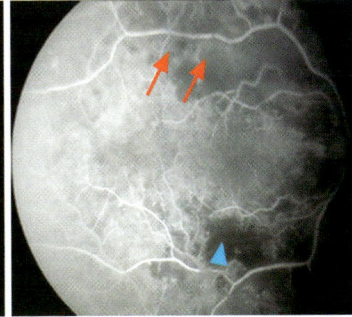

Fig. 5.16 *A case of severe non-proliferative diabetic retinopathy showing retinal hemorrhages leading to blocked fluorescence(arrowheads) and areas of capillary non-perfusion (arrows)*

COMPLICATIONS AND THEIR MANAGEMENT

Complications

In case of problem during FFA, it can be repeated at 30–60 minutes after first injection.

1. *Extravasation of fluorescein dye* can occur rarely. It is extremely painful and may lead to problem like superficial phlebitis, painful granuloma, toxic neuritis, sloughing of skin and necrosis. Local anesthetic and ice packs at the site of extravasation might help. If the whole dye extravasates choose another vein and reinject full dose and if the extravasation is at end then there is no need to reinject.

2. *Nausea* (5%)which occurs for 30–120 seconds and disappears slowly. Nausea usually occurs after initial pictures are already taken.

3. *Vomiting* is seen in 0.3–0.4% patients and usually 4 hours fasting is recommended before FFA to decrease nausea. In case of history of vomiting in a patient during previous FFA procedure, 25–50 mg of promethazine can be administered prior to procedure.

4. *Vasovagal attacks* can be there in anxious patients. A more severe form of vasovagal attack is syncopal attack (sweating, fainting, hypotension, bradycardia, decreased cardiovascular perfusion)

5. *Anaphylactic reaction* which is characterized by hypotension, tachycardia, bronchospasm, hives and itching) need to be differentiated from syncopal attack. The treatment for both vasovagal and anaphylactic shock lies in treating hypotension as a priority as prolonged hypotension will affect the perfusion of vital organs. It might be difficult to find intravenous access later thus maintain intravenous line till the end of the procedure.

6. *Allergic reaction* usually appears 2–15 minutes after injection of the dye in form of hives and itching. FFA sometimes gives rise to diffuse hypersensitivity reaction which occurs 48 hours later with diffuse rash and fever.

7. *Death and acute pulmonary edema after FFA* have also been reported.

Treatment of anaphylactic shock/ vasovgal reaction/allergic reaction

- Attach oxygen with face mask immediately.
- Start a normal saline infusion through the prior established intravenous access.
- If no IV access, then dilute the 1cc inj adrenaline to 10 cc so that the effective concentration is 1:10000. Ideally the injection should be ready before the start of procedure. Take one cc from this and inject subcutaneously or intravenous to the patient. It should bring the blood pressure (BP) to higher side in no time. Once the BP is achieved, have a iv access immediately, now start fluid through this.
- *Give inj hydrocortisone* 100 mg immediately
- Monitor blood pressure regularly at one minute interval

Treatment of vasovagal reaction

- *Supine position.* Make sure the patient is lying the supine position
- *Attach* oxygen with face mask immediately
- *Start a normal saline infusion* through the prior established intravenous access.
- *Monitor blood pressure* regularly at one minute interval

INDOCYANINE GREEN ANGIOGRAPHY (ICGA)

INTRODUCTION

Indocyanine green is a water-soluble tricarbocyanine dye, which was used to measure hepatic blood flow and cardiac output. Developed for use in photography during the Second World War, it got FDA approval in 1959 for human use. Its use in ophthalmology is mainly to image the posterior segment, especially the layers deeper to the retina. Due to its fluorescence spectrum in the infrared region, it is ideally suited to image the choroid.

PROPERTIES OF ICG MOLECULE

1. Molecular weight of 775 Daltons
2. Fluorescent molecule with peak absorption at 790–805 nm and peak emission at 830 nm
3. 98% protein bound (mainly to alpha-1 lipoprotein)-does not leak under normal conditions and stays in the intravascular compartment
4. Eliminated exclusively in bile by the liver
5. Half-life of 3–4 mins.
6. Has 5% sodium iodide to enhance solubility
7. Infrared spectrum of fluorescence enables it to image the choroid through blood, lipid and melanin.

PROCEDURE

Indocyanine green dye is injected in the antecubital vein and flushed. This is followed with a 5 ml bolus of saline. 25 mg of dye as lyophilized powder is available for dilution with 5 ml of aqueous solvent, giving a concentration of 5 mg/ml. Extravasation of dye does not lead to pain and burning.

Two types of imaging systems are used to do ICGA:

1. *Conventional high resolution digital imaging systems*
2. *Scanning laser ophthalmoscope (SLO) based systems* — Provide better quality images as compared to conventional imaging systems. Simultaneous FFA and ICGA are also possible. Same syringe can be used to inject both fluorescein and indocyanine green.

Colour, red free, green free and control photographs are taken before dye is injected. ICG is then injected and images are clicked after 8–10 seconds. As ICG fluoresces beyond the visible spectrum, images are difficult to focus. It is difficult to visualise vasculature and hence, visible pathology should be focused. Images are clicked every 8–10 seconds till blooming occurs. Blooming occurs when retinal and choroidal vessels have same concentration of dye and image quality deteriorates. Following this, images are taken at 3, 5, 7.10 and 25–30 mins.

ADVERSE EFFECTS

Adverse effects occur in only 0.15% patients and are both mild and transient. ICG has a better safety profile than fluorescein. Hot flushes, urticaria, hypotension, tachycardia, nausea and vomiting seldom occur. Death is reported to occur in 1 in 333333 patients.

PHASES OF ICGA

1. *Early phase*—Occurs at 2–3 mins and shows superimposed retinal and large choroidal vessels (Fig. 5.17).
2. *Intermediate phase*—Occurs at about 10 mins and shows maximal choroidal stromal fluorescence due to impregnation with indocyanine green dye (Fig. 5.18).
3. *Late phase*—Occurs at 28–30 mins and shows dark choroidal vessels against background stromal fluorescence (Fig. 5.19).

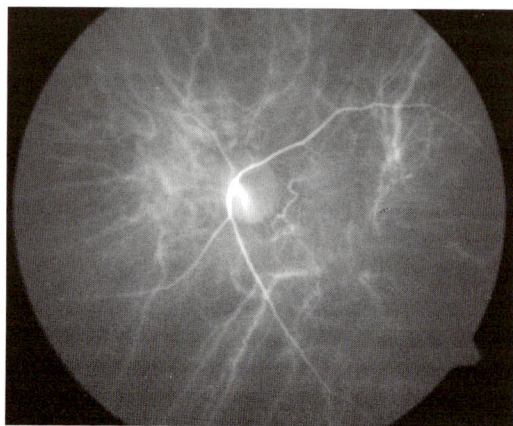

Fig. 5.17 *Early phase—Filling of both retinal and large choroidal vessels*

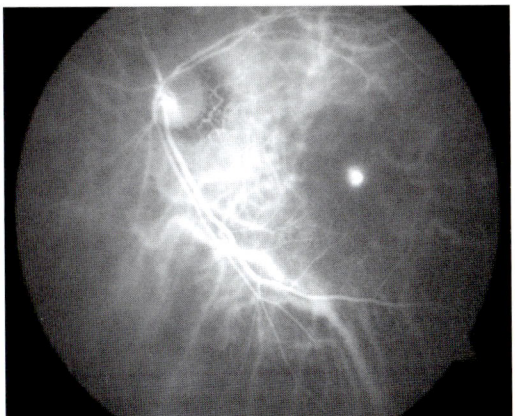

Fig. 5.18 *Intermediate phase—Choroidal vessels with stromal background fluorescence*

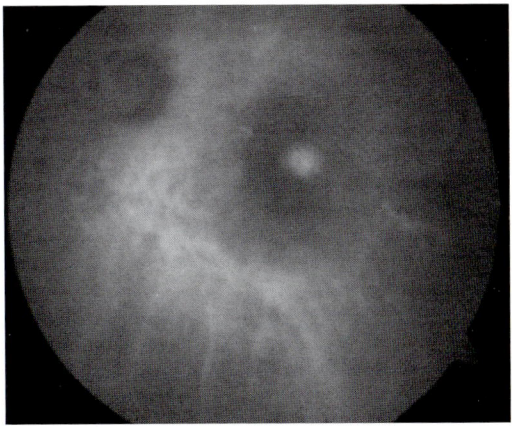

Fig. 5.19 *Late phase—Washout of dye from the circulation, showing dark optic disk and vessels on the background of stromal fluorescence*

INTERPRETATION OF ICGA

Interpretation of ICGA is more difficult as compared to FFA as both retinal and choroidal circulations are superimposed on each other. Transmission fluorescence is not applicable to ICGA, as retinal pigment epithelium does not act as a barrier to ICG imaging. Standard angiograms for ICGA do not exist. The resolution of ICGA is 11 microns. Two patterns of fluorescence are noted—hypofluorescence (Fig. 5.20) and hyperfluorescence (Fig. 5.21).

INDICATIONS

1. *Choroidal neovascular membrane (CNVM)* —
   Occult CNVM, pigment epithelial detachment

(PED), ICGA is used in suspected cases of occult CNVM. Subtle membranes, which are undetectable on FFA, can be easily picked up. Imaging of PEDs on FFA shows increasing fluorescence in late phases and hence obscures the detection of underlying pathology. ICGA is able to image the choroid below the PED and aids in arriving at a morphological diagnosis. Serous, fibrovascular or hemorrhagic PEDs can be equally well imaged using this modality. ICGA mediated photodynamic therapy (PDT) is used to reduce the need for recurrent injections of Anti-VEGFs in non-responsive patients (Fig. 5.22).

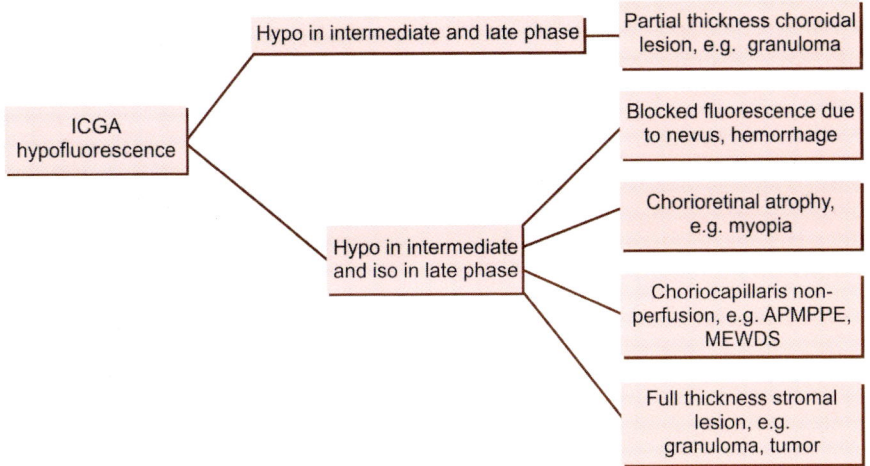

Fig. 5.20 *Causes of hypofluorescence of IGCA*

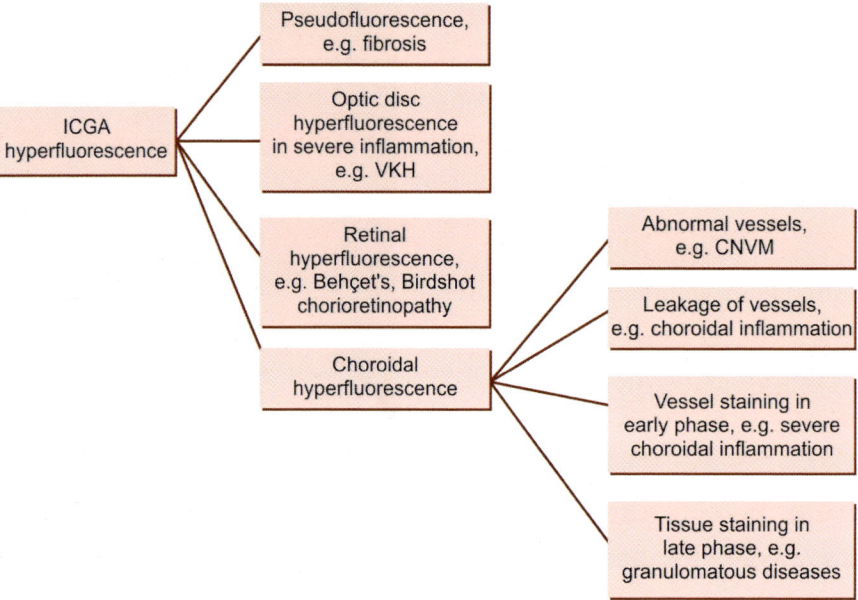

Fig. 5.21 *Causes of hyperfluorescence of IGCA*

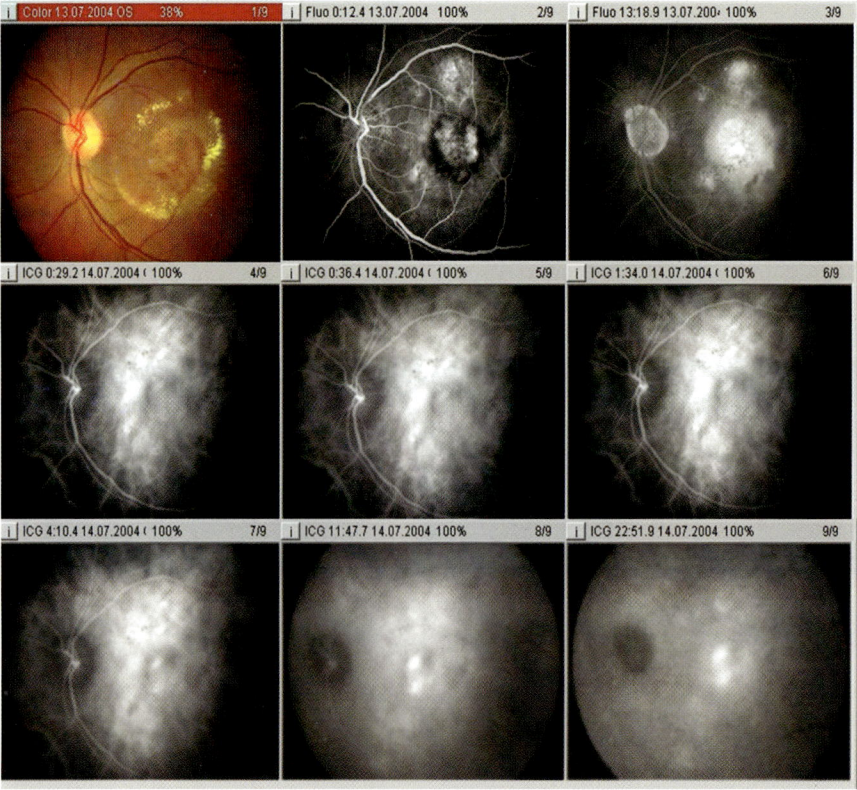

Fig. 5.22 *Top row shows a CNVM with lacy hyperfluorescence in early phase and late leakage on FFA. Middle and bottom row show ICGA images of hyperfluorescence from abnormal vessels which persists in the late phase*

2. *Retinal angiomatous proliferation (RAP)* — It is a relatively recently recognized entity and classified as type 3 CNVM. Retinal circulation is said to be the site of origin of blood vessels, instead of the choroidal circulation in types 1 and 2 CNVM. ICGA has helped stage this entity into 3 stages: stage 1–Intraretinal neovascularisation (IRN), stage 2– Subretinal neovascularisation (SRN) and stage 3– retinochoroidal anastomosis (RCA). Laser photocoagulation of retinal vessel is recommended for stages 1 and 2. ICGA mediated PDT and anti-VEGF agents are recommended for stage 3 RAP.

3. *Polypoidal choroidal vasculopathy (PCV)* — PCV is increasingly being considered as a type of CNVM. Up to 50% cases of CNVM are said to be due to PCV in Asian patients. Presentation is generally with subretinal hemorrhage or PED (hemorrhagic or fibrovascular). FFA is unable to pick up the lesion. ICGA outlines the areas of polyp like outgrowths of the choroidal vessels responsible for the symptoms. ICGA mediated PDT + anti-VEGF is recommended as the treatment of choice for this condition (Fig. 5.23).

4. *Central serous chorioretinopathy (CSC)* — It is generally a self-resolving disease, with spontaneous recovery in 60–70% cases. However, recurrent and non-resolving cases cause permanent vision loss and metamorphopsia. ICGA has a role in demarcating the points of choroidal hyperpermeability, which are more in number than points of leakage on FFA. These points of choroidal leakage, are subjected to low-fluence or half dose PDT and lead to decrease of leakage on ICGA. Hence, ICGA is used to demarcate areas for application of PDT and prognosticate patients of chronic CSC. Those patients showing clear areas of choroidal leakage respond better to therapy as compared to those showing diffuse choroidal leakage (Fig. 5.24).

5. *Choroidal tumours* — Longer wavelength of ICGA makes it ideally suited to image mass lesions of the choroid. Choroidal melanoma, choroidal metastais and choroidal hemangioma are common tumours. ICGA aids in diagnosis of all of the aforementioned. In cases

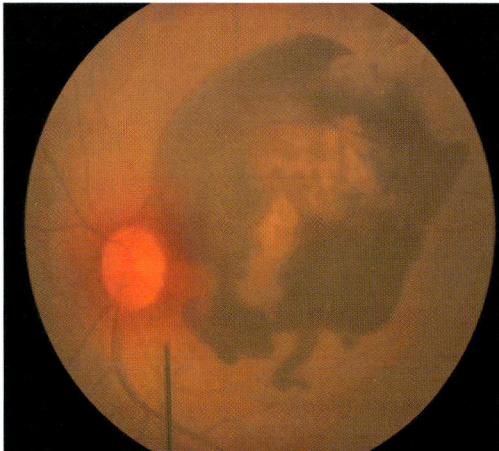

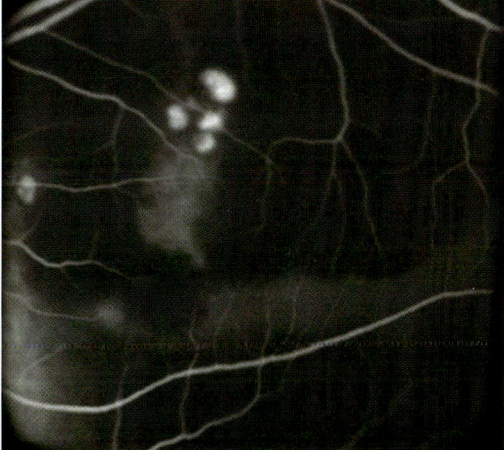

Fig. 5.23 *Fundus photo showing subretinal bleed in macular area with corresponding ICGA showing 4 grape like hyperfluorescent structures, suggestive of polypoidal choroidal vasculopathy*

of circumscribed choroidal hemangioma, ICGA shows early filling of the vessels in the tumour with late washout of dye surrounded by a hyperflourescent rim. ICGA mediated PDT has now become the treatment of choice for circumscribed hemangiomas, and leads to regression of the tumour and resolution of surrounding subretinal fluid.

6. *Choroidal inflammation*—Choriocapillaropathies , stromal choroiditis. Pattern of early and late phases of ICGA are the cornerstone for diagnosis of inflammations of the choroid. Inflammation of the choriocapillaris is characterized by hypofluorescence in the early phase, which persists in the late phase.

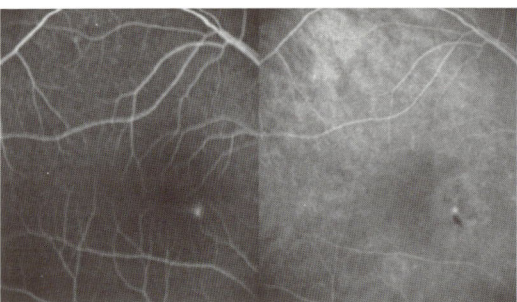

Fig. 5.24 *FFA, on the left, showing point of RPE leakage nasal to the optic disc. ICGA image, on the right, shows a greater area of hyperfluorescent choroid surrounding the point of retinal leakage. Widespread areas of choroidal hyperpermeability are characteristic of central serous chorioretinopathy*

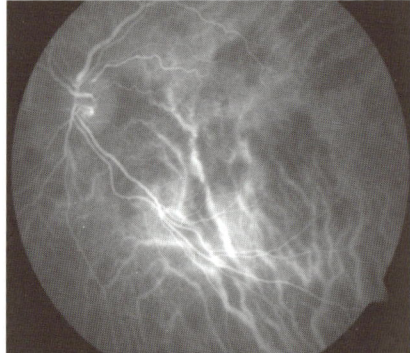

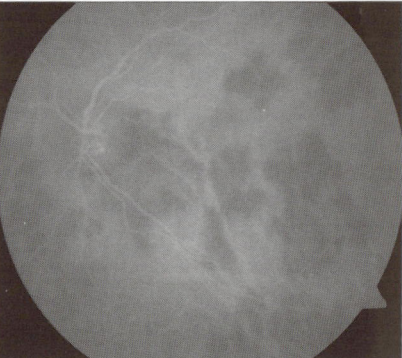

Fig. 5.26 *ICGA showing hypofluorescence in the intermediate and late phases, due to choriocapillaris non-perfusion*

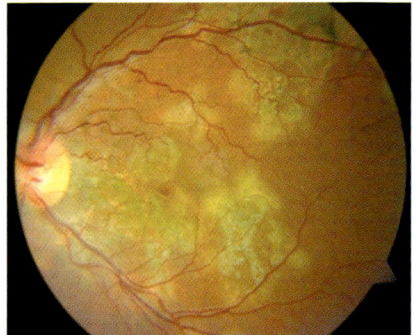

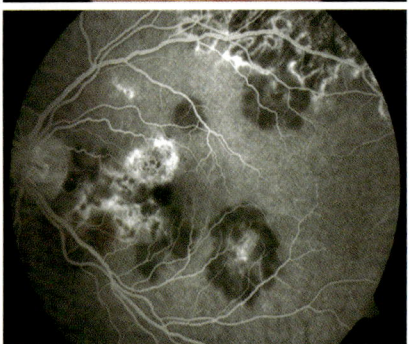

Fig. 5.25 *Fundus photo showing active and healed serpiginous choroiditis lesions with corresponding FFA showing hypo- and hyper lesions*

Choroidal stromal inflammations are characterized by leakage from choriocapillaris in the early phase, with hypofluorescence in the intermediate phase, which may (full thickness granulomas) or may not (partial thickness granulomas) persist in the late phase (Figs 5.25 and 5.26).

CONTRAINDICATIONS

1. Documented allergy to iodine
2. Liver disease
3. Pregnancy (Group C drug)
4. Previous allergy to ICG

FUNDUS AUTOFLUORESCENCE

INTRODUCTION

Fundus photography, fundus fluorescein angiography (FFA), indocyanine green angiography (ICG) and optical coherence tomography (OCT) have been conventionally used as end-points for diagnosing and monitoring retinal diseases in routine clinical practice for several years. Fundus autofluorescence (FAF) is a newer imaging modality for assessing retinal health by allowing metabolic mapping of the fluorophores present in the fundus. It is a non-invasive, and an in vivo imaging method that is now being increasingly used for diagnosing retinal diseases.

The dominant fluorophores are lipofuscin (LF) granules that accumulate in the postmitotic retinal pigment epithelium (RPE) cells as a by-product of the incomplete degradation of photoreceptor (PR) outer segments during a normal visual cycle. Lipofuscin consists of a mixture of pigments, including A2E, isomers of A2E and all-transretinal dimer. According to Eldred and Katz, the RPE LF contains at least 10 different fluorophores with discrete emission spectra in the green, golden yellow, yellow-green, and orangered emitting range. Lipofuscin accumulates naturally in the RPE cells and its pattern of distribution in the retina decides its normal FAF pattern. It is the stimulated emission of light chiefly from the LF in the RPE from which the autofluorescence images of the fundus arise. The metabolic activity within the RPE-PR complex can be indirectly judged by the LF content in the RPE. The RPE cells have no means to degrade or transport LF material and these granules are trapped in the cytoplasmic space. Minor fluorophores such as collagen and elastin in choroidal blood vessel walls may become visible in the absence or atrophy of RPE cells.

PRINCIPLE

The FAF signals are emitted across a broad-spectrum ranging from 500 to 800 nm. Ultraviolet light is routinely used to visualize LF with fluorescence microscopy ex vivo or in vitro. However, its transmission to the retina is limited in the living eye due to the absorption characteristics of the ocular media. The LF molecules exhibit a broad range of excitation (300–600 nm). Hence, visible light can be used to elicit its fluorescence in vivo. The emission spectrum is broad (480–800 nm) and maximal in the 600–640 nm region of the spectrum. The crystalline lens contributes to normal autofluorescence signal. Hence, modifications are made in the flashlight and detector to minimize the contribution of autofluorescence from the lens, and to allow absolute measurements of FAF. Excitation when using the fundus camera is usually done in the green spectrum (535 to 580 nm) and emission is recorded in the yellow-orange spectrum (615 to 715 nm) (Fig. 5.27A). With the confocal scanning laser ophthalmoscope (cSLO), excitation is usually induced in the blue range (488 nm), and an emission filter between 500 and 700 nm is used to detect emission of the FAF signal (Fig. 5.27B). Because of the difference in excitation and emission spectra, in addition to technical differences between the cSLO and the fundus camera, the types of detected FAF signal may vary between the systems, and it may be possible to visualize different fluorophores. In a normal subject, the fundus shows a diffuse normal FAF signal. Typically, marked hypo-autofluorescence of the optic nerve head (absence of autofluorescent material) and of retinal blood vessels (absorption phenomena by blood contents) are observed. Decreased autofluorescence is also seen in the foveal secondary to absorption from luteal (lutein and zeaxanthin) pigments. The parafoveal area shows mildly decreased intensity compared with the normal background signal at the outer macula (Fig. 5.27A and B).

CLINICAL APPLICATIONS

Abnormal accumulation of LF produces abnormally increased FAF (hyperauto-fluorescence). Accumulation of A2E is toxic and interferes with normal cell functioning. Diseases of the retinochoroid that cause an increased shedding of PR outer segments, disrupted RPE phagocytic function or an inability of the RPE to recycle metabolites produce hyper fluorescence due to LF accumulation as seen in age-related macular degeneration (ARMD) and inherited retinal

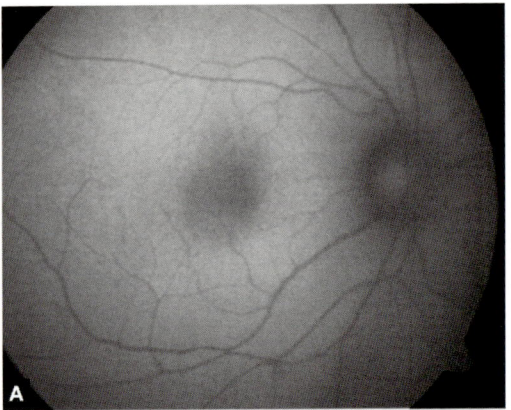

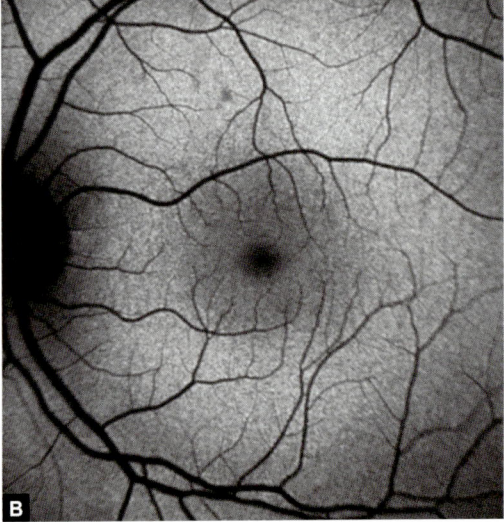

Fig. 5.27 *Fundus autofluorescence photograph of a normal right eye using fundus camera. (A) Where excitation is usually done in the green spectrum (535 to 580 nm) and emission is recorded in the yellow-orange spectrum (615 to 715 nm). Fundus photograph of a normal left eye using the confocal scanning laser ophthalmoscope; and (B) where excitation is usually induced in the blue range (488 nm), and an emission filter between 500 and 700 nm is used to detect emission of the fundus autofluorescence signal*

diseases. With the death of PR cells causing disruption of the visual cycle, there is atrophy of the RPE cells and a reduced metabolic turnover leading to decreased FAF (hypoautofluorescence). Deep hypoautofluorescence is observed over areas with advanced atrophic AMD, melanin pigment migration, or fibrotic scar tissue, suggesting RPE atrophy. This finding on FAF denotes extensive damage to the RPE, leading to compromised PR function.

1. Age-related macular degeneration (AMD)

Early AMD

A key role has been attributed to RPE in the disease process. Early manifestations include focal hypopigmentation and hyperpigmentation at the RPE level and drusen with extracellular material accumulating in the inner aspects of Bruch membrane. An international workshop on FAF phenotyping in early AMD reported an analysis of the variability of FAF findings in early AMD. Eight different FAF patterns were classified, including normal, minimal change, focal increased, patchy, linear, lacelike, reticular, and speckled patterns. A relatively poor correlation exists between visible alterations on fundus photographs and notable FAF changes. In early AMD, FAF findings may indicate more widespread abnormalities and diseased areas than clinically seen (Fig. 5.28A and B). The changes seen by FAF imaging may precede the occurrence of visible lesions as the disease progresses and may help to identify specific high-risk characteristics for disease progression as well as to design and monitor future interventional trials.

Geographic atrophy

It represents the atrophic late-stage manifestation of "dry" AMD. Due to loss of LF, outer retinal atrophy is characterized by severe hypoautofluorescence. Areas of increased intensity signals are observed in the junctional zone surrounding the atrophic patches by FAF imaging, which do not correlate well with funduscopically visible pigmentary changes (Fig. 5.29A and B). The identification of elevated levels of FAF intensities in the junctional zone of atrophy is of particular interest because these changes precede cell death and, therefore, absolute scotoma.

Pigment epithelial detachment (PED)

Most PEDs demonstrate a marked, evenly distributed hyper autofluorescence corresponding to the lesion surrounded by a well-defined, less autofluorescent halo delineating the entire border of the lesion. Some PEDs may also show an intermediate or decreased FAF signal over the lesion that may or may not correspond to areas of RPE atrophy or fibrovascular scaring.

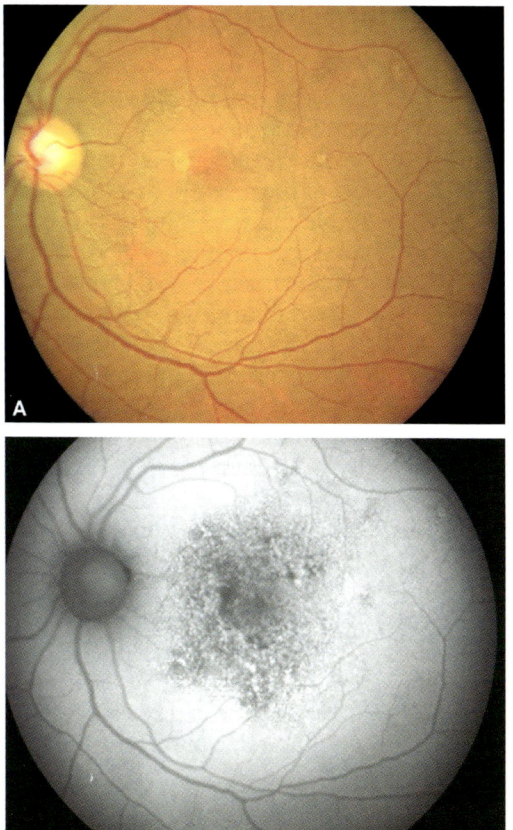

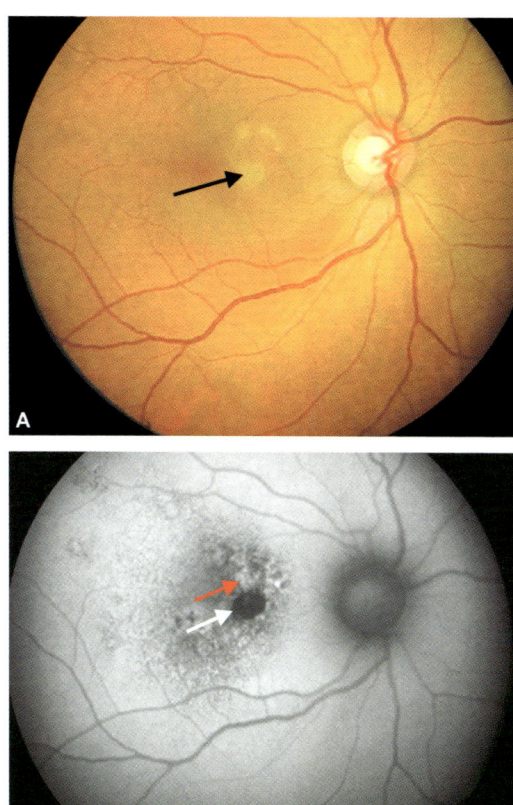

Fig. 5.28 *Fundus photograph.* **(A)** *Showing early age-related macular degeneration which are seen as more widespread abnormalities and diseased areas on fundus autofluorescence and* **(B)** *than clinically seen*

Fig. 5.29 **(A)** *Fundus photograph. Showing geographic atrophy. Fundus autofluorescence* **(B)** *showing severe hypoautofluorescence corresponding to outer retinal atrophy (white arrows). Areas of increased intensity signals (red arrow) are observed in the junctional zone surrounding the atrophic patches by FAF imaging, which do not correlate well with fundoscopically visible pigmentary changes*

Choroidal neovascular membrane (CNV)

Patches of "continuous" or "normal" autofluorescence corresponding to areas of hyperfluorescence on FFA are seen in early CNV secondary to AMD. This indicates that RPE viability is preserved at least initially in CNV development. By contrast, eyes with long-standing CNV typically have increasing hypoautofluorescence, suggesting PR loss, RPE atrophy, development of scar, and increased melanin deposition (Fig. 5.30A and B). Abnormal FAF signals typically extend beyond the edge of the angiographically defined lesion, indicating a more widespread involvement than seen in other imaging studies. Increased FAF signal around the edge of lesions may reflect the proliferation of RPE cells around the CNV.

2. Central serous chorioretinopathy (CSR)

It is characterized by idiopathic leaks at the level of the RPE leading to serous retinal detachment. The FAF findings correspond well with the disease stage and are in accord with RPE involvement. Patients with acute leaks show minimal abnormalities with a mild hyperautofluorescence of the serous detachment. Over time, irregular hyperautofluoresence increases in the area of detachment, corresponding to pinpoint subretinal precipitates seen clinically. Mixed pattern of autofluorescence appears in eyes with chronic disease with atrophic areas showing marked hypoauto-

fluorescence (Fig. 5.31A and B). Visualization of fluid tracks in the inferior retina ia a typical finding.

3. Macular hole

In early stages (1 and 2) of macular hole, mild to moderate hyperautofluorescence is noted centrally in the area of the hole. In stage 3 full thickness macular hole, a central hyperauto-fluorescence is noted. In stage 4 full thickness macular holes, an increased autofluorescence is noted corresponding to the hole with a surrounding ring of hypoautofluorescence corresponding to the cuff of subretinal fluid

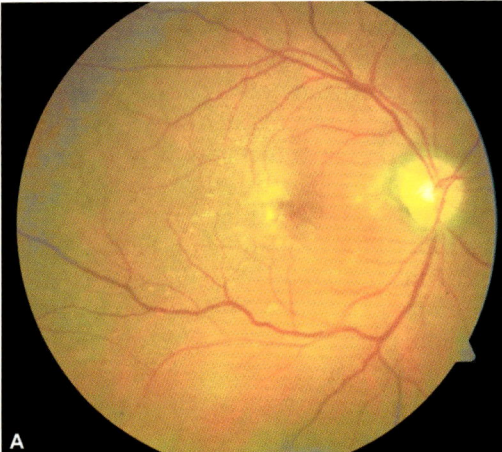

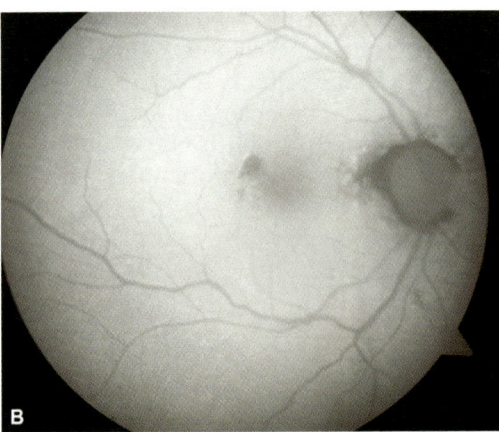

Fig. 5.30 *Fundus photograph. (A) Showing a long standing choroidal neovascular membrane which is seen as increased hypoautofluorescence on fundus autofluorescence imaging and (B) suggesting photoreceptor loss, retinal pigment epithelium atrophy, development of scar, and increased melanin deposition*

(Fig. 5.32A and B). This hyperautofluorescence of the macular hole is no longer visible following a successful surgery (Fig. 5.32C).

4. Retinal dystrophies

Localized abnormalities of FAF intensities are observed in many dystrophies. In patients with retinitis pigmentosa (RP) and cone dystrophies, parafoveal rings of hyperautofluorescence have been identified in absence of funduscopically visible correlates. As the disease progresses, these tend to shrink in RP or enlarge in cone dystrophies. These rings demarcate areas of preserved PR function. In patients with RP, these hyperautofluorescent rings correlate with results from visual function testing. Larger rings tend to correlate with a smaller peripheral visual field defect. In Stargardt disease, focal hyper-autofluorescent areas correspond to flecks seen on FP suggesting excessive localized LF accumulation. The FAF imaging also allows detection of the abnormal phenotype in some disorders when it is not otherwise clinically evident.

5. Chloroquine/Hydroxychloroquine toxicity

Early RPE alterations can be detected by FAF imaging or multifocal electroretinography when ophthalmoscopy and FFA are less sensitive. A pericentral ring of hyperautofluorescence is seen on FAF imaging in mild toxicity. As it advances, a pericentral mottled hypoauto-fluorescence is seen. In more advanced cases, a complete pericentral hypoautofluorescence develops (Fig. 5.33A to D).

7. Optic nerve head drusen

Optic nerve head drusens are sometimes not visible on clinical examination because they are subpapillary in nature. They get partially calcified from accumulation of axoplasmic derivatives of degenerating retinal nerve fiber and become increasingly visible with age. They must be differentiated from acquired disc edema, which warrants immediate neurological evaluation and treatment. These bodies are highly autofluorescent that can be detected on FAF imaging, besides B-scan ultrasonography (Fig. 5.34A to D).

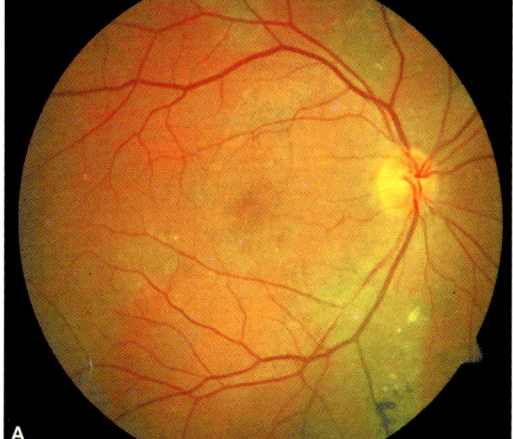

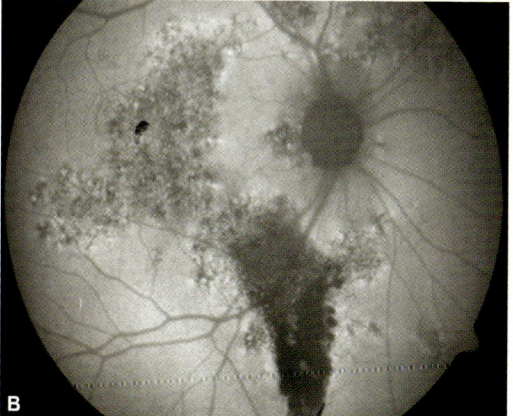

Fig. 5.31 *Fundus photograph. (A) Chronic central serous retinopathy and fundus autofluorescence and (B) mixed pattern of autofluorescence, with atrophic areas showing marked hypoautofluorescence*

8. Chorioretinal inflammatory disorders

In multifocal choroiditis, macular hyperautofluorescence is seen in areas of active chorio-

retinitis that completely disappears and becomes hypoautofluorescent with resolution of the disease activity after therapy. In APMPPE, placoid areas of hypoautofluorescent corresponding to areas of RPE scarring have been shown in the quiescent phase of the disease. Fundus AF changes have been described in other chorioretinal disorders, including acute syphilitic posterior placoid chorioretinitis which is a rare entity that may mimic APMPPE. Increased FAF corresponds to active geographic lesions at the posterior pole. In multifocal choroiditis and panuveitis (MCP), Haen and Spaide found that all chorioretinal scars visible by autofluorescence imaging were not visible by colour fundus photography. The FAF revealed that patients with MCP have much more widespread involvement of the RPE than would be suspected by any other means of imaging. During an exacerbation of disease activity in a previously quiescent eye with serpiginous choroiditis, a hyperauto-fluorescent signal on FAF imaging may highlight the active lesion which may be very subtle on FFA. We have described four stages of changing patterns of autofluorescence in tubercular serpiginouslike choroiditis as the lesions evolve from an acute stage to the stage of complete healing.

SUMMARY

FAF is a novel imaging modality that provides critical information in various retinal diseases. It is easy, simple, quick, efficient, and non-invasive, and is promising in improving the quality of care for patients with retinal disorders. It provides information over and

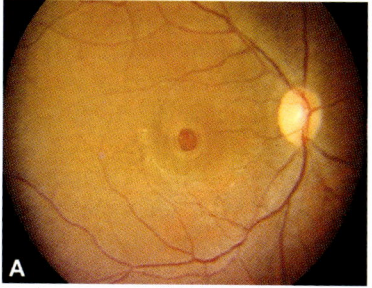
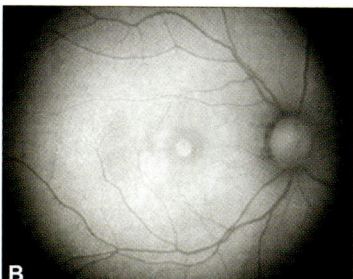
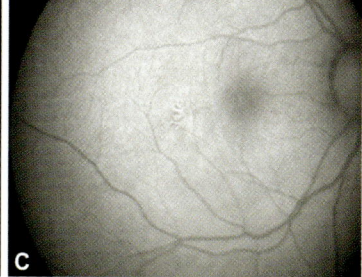

Fig. 5.32 *Stage-4 full thickness macular hole (A and B) showing an increased autofluorescence corresponding to the hole with a surrounding ring of hypoautofluorescence corresponding to the cuff of subretinal fluid; and this hyperautofluorescence of the macular hole is no longer visible following a successful surgery (C)*

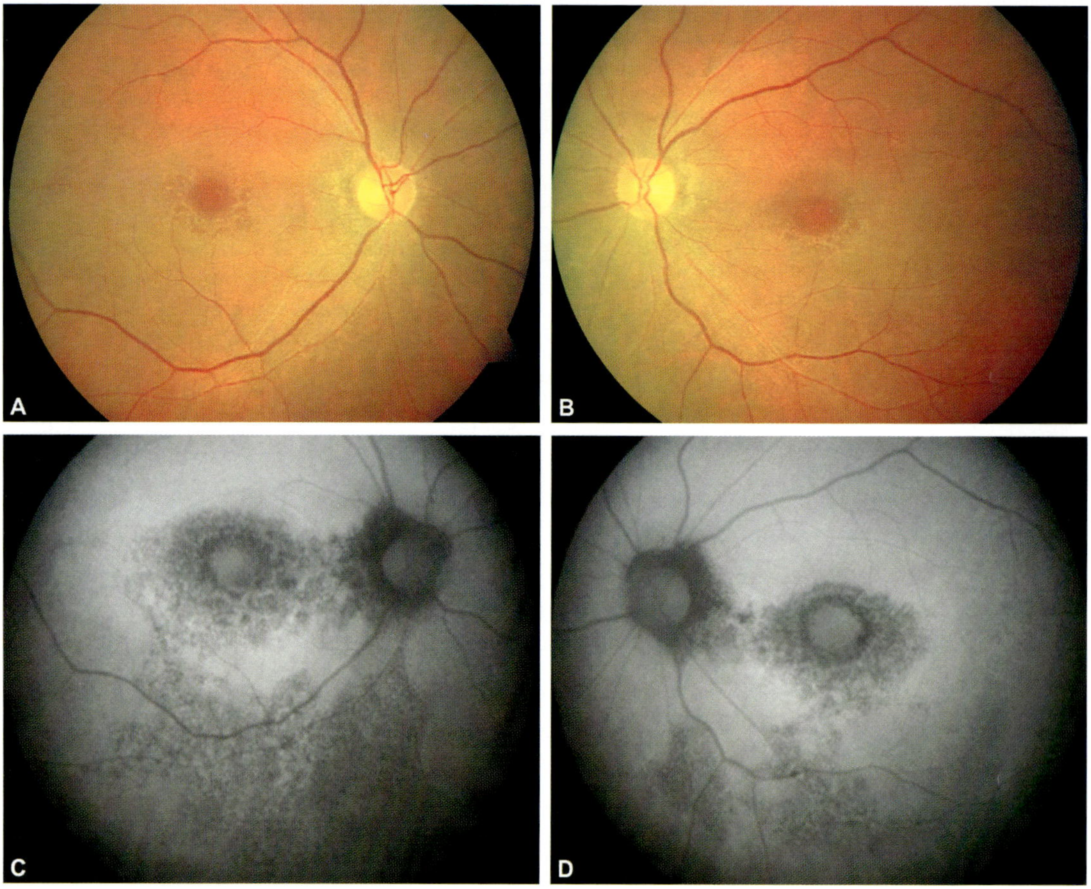

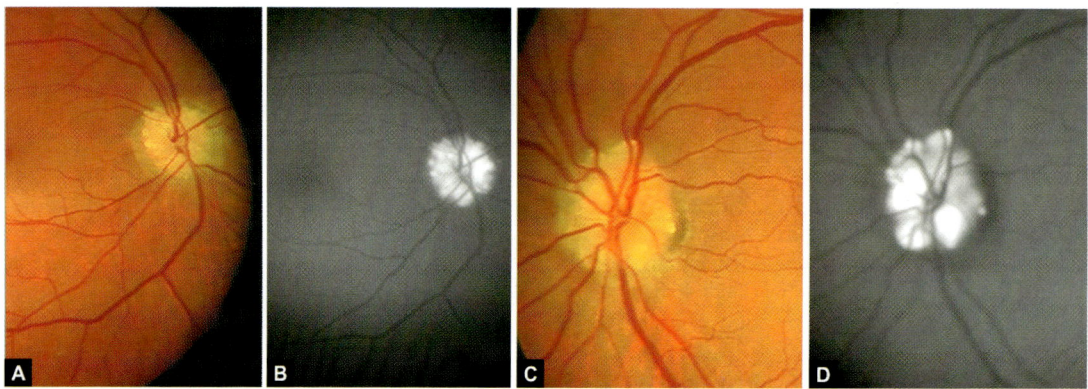

Fig. 5.33 *In advanced stages of chloroquine/hydroxychloroquine toxicity (A and B) and a complete pericentral hypoauto-fluorescence develops with surrounding mottled hypoautofluorescence (C and D)*

Fig. 5.34 *Optic nerve head drusens may not be clinically apparent (A and C), but can be easily detected on fundus autofluorescence imaging as highly autofluorescent lesions on the optic nerve head (B and D)*

beyond conventional imaging techniques, and is a reliable tool for disease monitoring.

BIBLIOGRAPHY

Fundus Angiography and Autofluorescence

1. Early Treatment Diabetic Retinopathy Study Research Group. Classification of Diabetic Retinopathy from Fluorescein Angiograms: ETDRS Report Number 11. Ophthalmology 1991:98(5):807–22
2. Kunimoto, Derek; KunalKanitkar, and Mary Makar (2004). The Wills eye manual: office and emergency room diagnosis and treatment of eye disease. (4th ed.). Philadelphia, PA: Lippincott Williams & Wilkins. p. 365
3. Schatz Howard. Fluorescein angiography: basic principles and interpretation. in Retina Volume 2 (Eds) Ryan SJ. St Louis C.V.Mosby Company 2006 p 3.

Indocyanine Green Angiography

1. Carl P Herbort. Fluorescein and Indocyanine Green Angiography in Uveitis. Middle East Afr J Ophthalmol 2009 Oct-Dec; 16(4):168–187.
2. Herbort CP, Guex-Crosier Y, LeHoang P. Schematic interpretation of indocyanine green angiography. Ophthalmology. 1994; 2:169–76
3. Lim JI, Flower RW. Indocyanine green angiography. Int Ophthalmol Clin. 1995; 35:59–7
4. Stanga Paulo E; Lim Jennifer I; Hamilton Peter. "Indocyanine green angiography in chorioretinal diseases: Indications and interpretation: An evidence-based update". Ophthalmology; (2003)110(1):15–21.

Fundus Autofluorescence

1. Bellmann C, Holz FG, Breitbart A, Völcker HE. Bilateral acute syphilitic posterior placoid chorioretinopathy-angiographic and autofluorescence characteristics. Ophthalmologe 1999; 96(8):522–8.
2. Bindewald A, Bird AC, Dandekar SS, et al. Classification of fundus autofluorescence patterns in early age-related macular disease. Invest Ophthalmol Vis Sci 2005; 46:3309–14.
3. Bird A. Age-related macular disease. Br J Ophthalmol 1996; 80:2–3.
4. Delori FC, Dorey CK, Staurenghi G, et al. In vivo fluorescence of the ocular fundus exhibits retinal pigment epithelium lipofuscin charac-

teristics. Invest Ophthalmol Vis Sci 1995; 36:718–29.
5. Delori FC. Spectrophotometer for non-invasive measurement of intrinsic fluorescence and reflectance of the ocularfundus. Appl Optics 1994; 33:7429–52.
6. Eandi CM, Ober M, Iranmanesh R, et al. Acute central serous chorioretinopathy and fundus autofluorescence. Retina 2005; 25:989–93.
7. Eldred GE, Katz ML. Fluorophores of the human retinal pigment epithelium: separation and spectral characterization. Exp Eye Res 1988; 47:71–86.
8. Feeney L. Lipofuscin and melanin of human retinal pigment epithelium. Invest Ophthalmol Vis Sci 1978; 17(7):583–600.
9. Fishkin NE, Sparrow JR, Allikmets R, Nakanishi K. Isolation and characterization of a retinal pigment epithelial cell fluorophore: an all-trans-retinal dimer conjugate. Proc Natl Acad Sci USA. 2005; 102:7091–96.
10. Framme C, Walter A, Gabler B, et al. Fundus autofluorescence in acute and chronic-recurrent central serous chorioretinopathy. Acta Ophthalmol Scand 2005; 83:161–7.
11. Gupta A, Bansal R, Gupta V, Sharma A. Fundus autofluorescence in serpiginouslike choroiditis. Retina 2012; 32:814–25.
12. Haen SP, Spaide RF. Fundus autofluorescence in multifocal choroiditis and panuveitis. Am J Ophthalmol 2008; 145:847–853.
13. Holz FG, Bellman C, Staudt S, et al. Fundus autofluorescence and development of geographic atrophy in age-related macular degeneration. Invest Ophthalmol Vis Sci 2001; 42:1051–56.
14. Kellner U, Renner AB, Tillack H. Fundus autofluorescence and mfERG for early detection of retinal alterations in patients using chloroquine/hydroxychloroquine. Invest Ophthalmol Vis Sci 2006; 47:3531–38.
15. Kurz-Levin MM, Landau K. A comparison of imaging techniques for diagnosing drusen of the optic nerve head. Arch Ophthalmol 1999; 117(8):1045–49.
16. McBain VA, Townend J, Lois N. Fundus autofluorescence in exudative age-related macular degeneration. Br J Ophthalmol 2007; 91:491–6.
17. Robson AG, Michaelides M, Saihan Z, et al. Functional characteristics of patients with retinal dystrophy that manifest abnormal parafoveal annuli of high density fundus autofluorescence; a review and update. Doc Ophthalmol 2008 Mar; 116(2):79–89.

18. Robson AG, Saihan Z, Jenkins SA, et al. Functional characterisation and serial imaging of abnormal fundus autofluorescence in patients with retinitis pigmentosa and normal visual acuity. Br J Ophthalmol 2006; 90:472–9.

19. Schmitz-Valckenberg S, Holz FG, Bird AC, Spaide RF. Fundus autofluorescence Imaging. Review and perspectives. Retina 2008; 28:385–409.

20. Spaide RF, Klancnik JM Jr. Fundus autofluorescence and central serous chorioretinopathy. Ophthalmology 2005; 112:825–33.

21. Sparrow JR, Boulton M. RPE lipofuscin and its role in retinal pathobiology. Exp Eye Res 2005; 80:595–606.

22. Vaclavik V, Vujosevic S, Dandekar SS, et al. Autofluorescence imaging in age-related macular degeneration complicated by choroidal neovascularization. A prospective study. Ophthalmology 2008; 115:342–6.

23. Von Rückmann A, Fitzke FW, Gregor ZJ. Fundus autofluorescence in patients with macular holes imaged with a laser scanning ophthalmoscope. Br J Ophthalmol 1998;82:346–51.

24. Weiter JJ, Delori FC, Wing GL, Fitch KA. Retinal pigment epithelial lipofuscin and melanin and choroidal melanin in human eyes. Invest Ophthalmol Vis Sci 1986; 27(2):145–52.

25. Wing GL, Blanchard GC, Weiter JJ. The topography and age relationship of lipofuscin concentration in the retinal pigment epithelium. Invest Ophthalmol Vis Sci 1978; 17(7):601–7.

26. Yeh S, Forooghian F, Wong WT, et al. Fundus auto fluorescence imaging of the White Dot syndromes. Arch Ophthalmol 2010; 128(1):46–56.

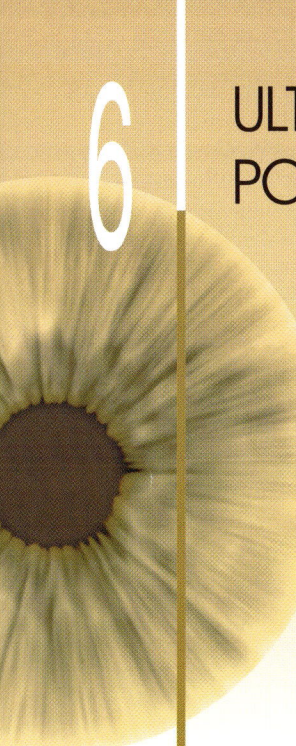

6

ULTRASONOGRAPHY OF THE POSTERIOR SEGMENT

Subina Narang, Mohit Dogra

PRINCIPLE AND TECHNIQUE

PRINCIPLE

Ultrasonography (USG) consists of high frequency sound waves with frequency greater than 20,000 Hertz (Hz) or 20 KHz. Sounds audible to healthy humans range from 20 to 20,000 Hz, thus ultrasound are beyond the audible range of humans.

It is based on the piezo-electric principle. This principle states that change in the polarity of electric current passing through a quartz crystal causes change in shape and size of the crystal, and vise versa. Thus, electric energy is transformed to sound energy.

These sound waves pass through the ocular structures and are reflected back to the probe from the various interfaces within the eye. These sound waves are converted by the transducer into electric signals and reconstructed into images using a computer software.

TECHNIQUE

To interpret the USG brief understanding of the modes and the scans of USG is required.

Modes of USG

A-Scan (amplitude scan)

It is of two types—biometric A-scan and standard diagnostic A-scan.

The standard diagnostic A-scan uses a probe with 8 MHz frequency and is designed to display a echo intensity of 100% for retina when the sound waves are perpendicular to it. Choroid and sclera also produce 100% echo intensity. All other intraocular structures have less than 100% echo intensity.

B-Scan (brightness scan)

It is a 2-dimensional display which uses the horizontal and vertical axis. A 10 to 20 MHz probe may be used and the echo intensity of the structure is determined by the brightness of the dots on the screen.

Most conventional ultrasound machines have a combination of B-scan and standard diagnostic

A-scan. The vector of the B-scan corresponds with the central transducer of the probe and the echo intensity of various points on the vector can be seen in the corresponding A-scan.

Convention

The pointer of the probe marks the point which will appear superior on the screen. The probe by convention is never kept temporal or inferior.

Types of scans

1. *Axial.* Probe faces perpendicular to the cornea and bisects the optic nerve. If the tip of the probe is superior, it is the vertical axial scan and if it faces nasally, then it is the horizontal axial scan (Fig. 6.1A).
2. *Horizontal.* The probe produces a lateral cross-section of the eye as it is moved from the center of the cornea to the equator. It is used as a screening scan to pick up foreign bodies (Fig. 6.1B).
3. *Longitudinal.* The probe is placed at the limbus along different clock hours and the opposite clock hour of the retina is seen. The anterior retina is seen superiorly and the optic nerve is seen inferiorly in every scan. It is used to precisely localize the foreign body (Fig. 6.1C).

INTERPRETATION OF SCANS

The monitor of the machine displays the following parameters which need to be understood for scan interpretation

PARAMETERS FOR SCANS

Gain. Amplification of intensity of echoes displayed. Increased gain causes increased penetration and low resolution

Time gain compensation (TGC). There is loss of sound waves as they pass through media. Increased TGC is used to image posterior structures to compensate for the lost signal

Sector angle. This angle of moving transducer determines the area of eye imaged—40 mm, 60 mm

Display. B-scan displayed by grey scale spread over range selected

Probe position. Indicated by position of the marker.

Eye. Whether right or left eye is examined is shown as OD or OS.

SPECTRUM OF USG IN POSTERIOR SEGMENT PATHOLOGY

Vitreous hemorrhage

Multiple point like echoes in the posterior vitreous cavity on B-scan and of low to moderate amplitude echogenicity on A-scan suggestive of retrohyaloid bleed (Fig. 6.2). In long-standing vitreous hemorrhage, the point like echoes get settled inferiorly and the vitreous cavity is clear. It gives information about posterior vitreous detachment (PVD).

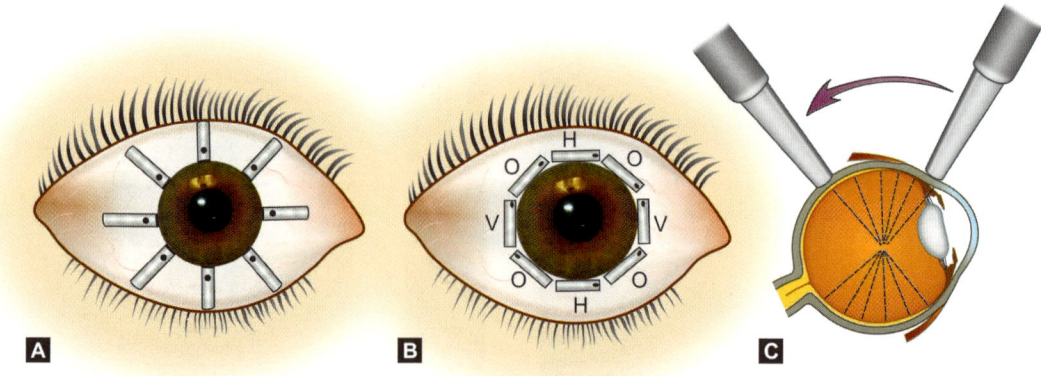

Fig. 6.1 *(A) Longitudinal B-scan approaches showing various probe marker orientation, which is always oriented towards centre of cornea; (B) transverse B-scan approaches showing horizontal probe positions (H),oblique probe position (O) vertical probe positions (V); and (C) technique of screening from limbus towards fornix to evaluate the topography of lesion*

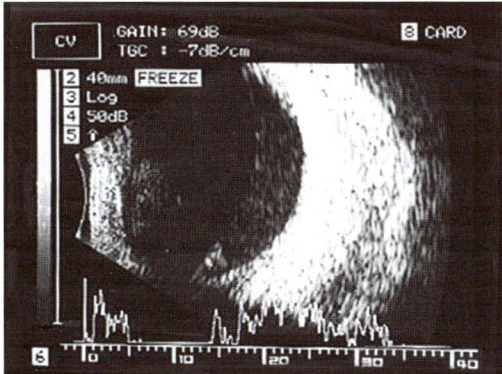

Fig. 6.2 *Moderate echogenicity point like echoes in posterior vitreous bound by thin membrane anteriorly (PVD), consistent with diagnosis of retrohyaloid bleed*

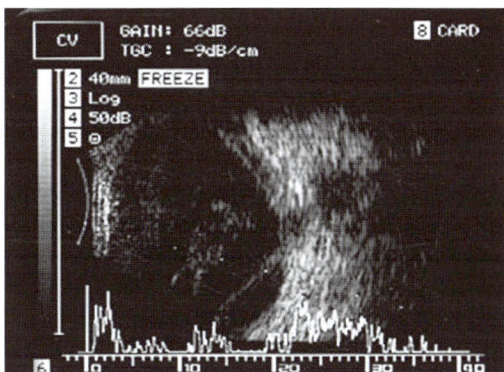

Fig. 6.4 *Membrane like structure attached to disc with low to moderate echogenicity, suggestive of incomplete PVD with vitreous haemorrhage*

Endophthalmitis

Multiple point like echoes of low to moderate echogenicity, similar to vitreous hemorrhage in vitreous cavity. Clinical scenario helps to differentiate the two. Membrane like structure picked on B-scan helps to prognosticate the patient. It also picks up retinal detachment (RD) and PVD, as in vitreous hemorrhage (Fig. 6.3).

Posterior vitreous detachment (PVD)

Membrane like structure seen on B-scan which may or may not be attached to the disc. Echogenicity of 50–60% on A-scan with after movements. The membrane disappears on reducing the gain (Fig. 6.4). The echogenicity of PVD is variable from superior to inferior part of globe.

Intraocular foreign body (IOFB)

Metallic foreign bodies appear as hyperechoic dots with a back shadowing on B-scan and have 100% echo intensity on A-scan. Longitudinal scans, at various clock hours are used to localize IOFBs (Fig. 6.5). The shape and size of IOFB will appear to vary in different scans, however, round air bubble will be 100% echoic but same size and shape in all scans and will assume the highest position.

Dislocated crystalline lens

Posterior dislocation of the crystalline lens in the vitreous is seen as a cyst like structure on B-scan with the anterior and posterior surfaces having high echogenicity on A-scan and the interior having moderate echogenicity.

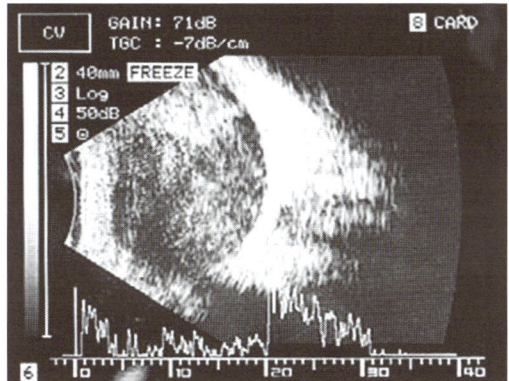

Fig. 6.3 *Multiple moderate to high echogenicity point like echoes in vitreous cavity suggestive of vitreous exudates in endophthalmitis*

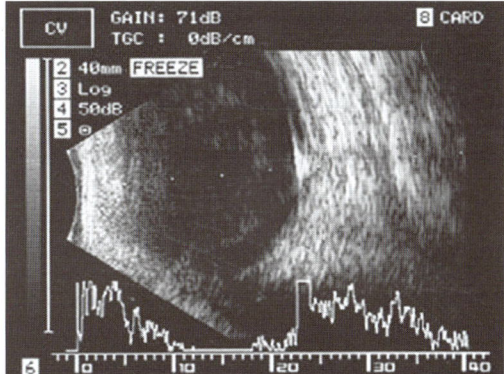

Fig. 6.5 *Hyperechoic structure with after shadow seen on the retina suggestive of metallic intraocular foreign body*

Associated PVD may be noted in some cases (Fig. 6.6).

Retinal detachment (RD)

Retinal detachments appear as membrane like structures attached to the optic disc (Fig. 6.7). The echo intensity is 100% on A-scan and it does not fade away on decreasing the gain. Old RDs loose mobility and appear to have no after movements. They may be associated with retinal cysts.

Associated giant retinal tears and retinal dialysis can be made out as defects in the membrane and on following the vector, the A-scan has low echo intensity in the area of the break.

Choroidal detachment

Choroidal detachment appear as dome shaped elevated membranes not reaching the disc. They may be touching each other, when they are called kissing choroidals (Fig. 6.8). Hemorrhagic choroidals have bright dots on B-scan and steeply rising double peaked echoes on A-scan in their interior, whereas serous choroidals have echo free interiors on B-scan. Serial ultrasounds are done in cases of hemorrhagic choroidals to look for clot liquefaction and appropriate time for surgery.

Post surgical changes

Scleral buckles are seen as indentations at the equator and cause elongation of the eyeball.

Silicon oil filled eyes appear longer as the ultrasound waves take longer to travel in silicon oil. The vector speed needs to be reduced to 980 m/s in order to accurately measure axial lengths.

Air or gas filled eyes impede the ultrasound waves from passing through them. The patient must be made to sit so that gas rises up and then the inferior part of the retina can be visualized with the probe kept superiorly.

Posterior scleritis

The classic T-sign clinches the diagnosis. It signifies fluid in the tenon's space and is seen as a hypoechoic band seen all around the outer wall of the globe (Fig. 6.9).

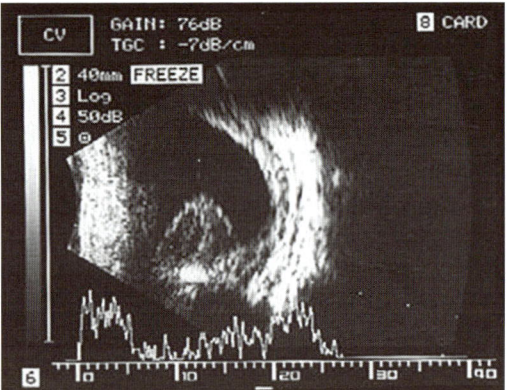

Fig. 6.6 *Cyst like structure with moderate to high echo-genicity suggestive of crystalline lens in the vitreous*

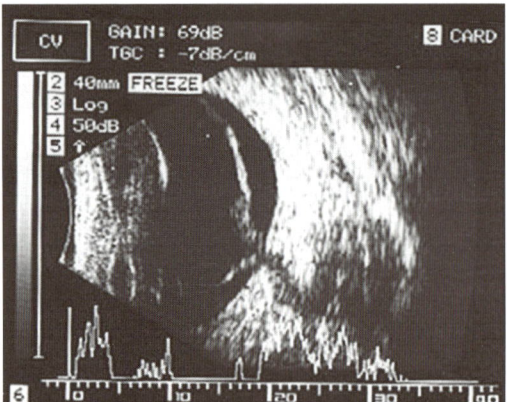

Fig. 6.7 *Membrane like structure with high echogenicity attached to the disc, suggestive of retinal detachment*

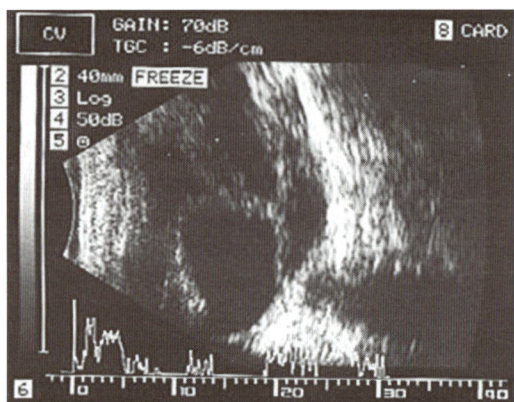

Fig. 6.8 *Two dome shaped cyst like structures with moderate echogenicity walls not reaching disc, suggestive of choroidal detachment, giving appearance of kissing choroidals*

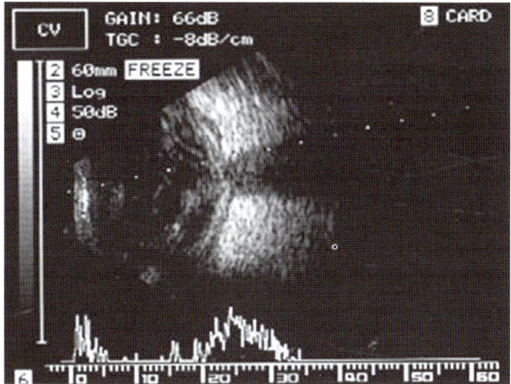

Fig. 6.9 *Echolucent area around globe and optic nerve, suggestive of fluid in the subtenon's space seen in posterior scleritis, giving it T-sign appearance*

Retinoblastoma

Ultrasound is used to look for intratumoral calcification in order to clinch the diagnosis in cases of retinoblastoma. High reflectivity with back shadowing is highly suggestive of calcification (Fig. 6.10).

Ultrasound is also used to measure the dimensions of the tumor and monitor response to chemotherapy or radiotherapy.

Increased axial length and calcification help to differentiate this entity from other causes of leucocoria like PHPV, Coat's disease and Stage 5 ROP.

Choroidal melanoma

Collar stud appearance is classic for choroidal melanoma and signifies rupture of Bruch's membrane. However, small melanomas may not be seen as classic mushroom shaped (Fig. 6.11) and appear as dome shaped elevations.

There is low to medium internal echogenicity with sound attenuation on A-scan. B-scan shows internal vascularity and acoustic hollowing.

Surrounding serous RD and choroidal excavation may or may not be seen.

Choroidal hemangioma

Dome shaped on B-scan and shows high internal echogenicity on A-scan.

Lack of internal vascularity and no acoustic hollowing help to differentiate from melanoma.

Uveitis

Ultrasound is used to look for vitreous hemorrhage, tractional RDs, exudates, serous RD and choroidal thickening.

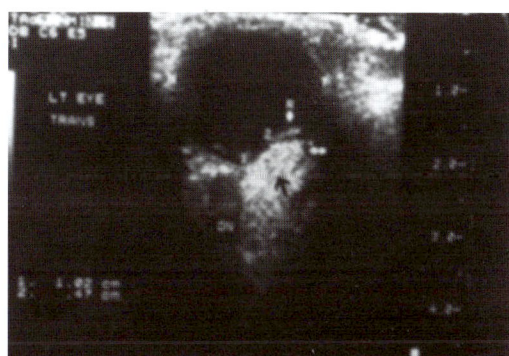

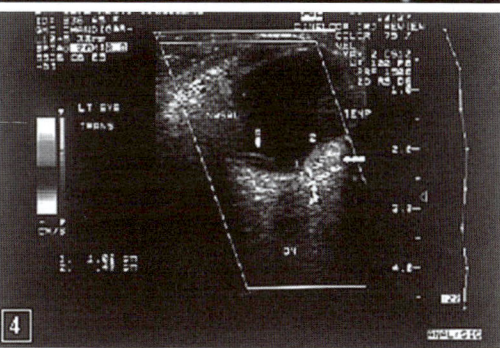

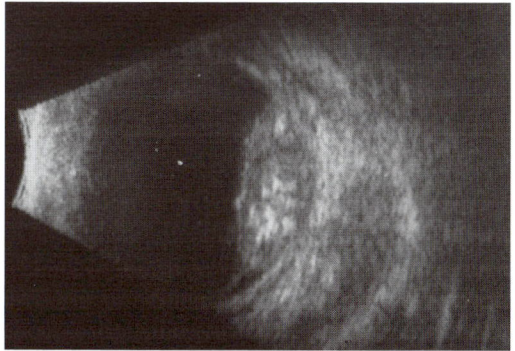

Fig. 6.10 *A 2-year-old baby with leucocoria showing mass lesion in the posterior pole with areas of high echogenicity corresponding to calcification suggestive of retinoblastoma*

Fig. 6.11 *A well circumscribed dome shaped subretinal mass of moderate echogenicity temporal to the optic disc with acoustically quiet areas along with retinal detachment suggestive of choroidal melanoma. Colour Doppler imaging shows increased vascularity of the lesion with a double circulation pattern due to visibility of both choroidal and retinal vessels*

Sympathetic ophthalmia and VKH disease are diagnosed when retinochoroid is thickened. Ultrasound can also be used to monitor response to therapy by showing decrease in retinochoroid thickness (Fig. 6.12).

Parasitic cysts

Cyst like structure with high echo intensity scolex in the center. There may be surrounding low to moderate point like echoes, suggestive of inflammatory reaction (Fig. 6.13).

COMMON PATTERNS OF POSTERIOR SEGMENT ULTRASONOGRAPHY AND THEIR DIFFERENTIAL DIAGNOSIS

Common USG patterns

Common patterns seen on posterior segment ultrasonography are:

• Point like echoes,
• Membrane like structure, and
• Cyst like structure

Table 6.1 depicts the causes of common USG patterns.

Differential diagnosis

Differential diagnosis of membrane like structures seen on posterior segment USG is depicted in Table 6.2.

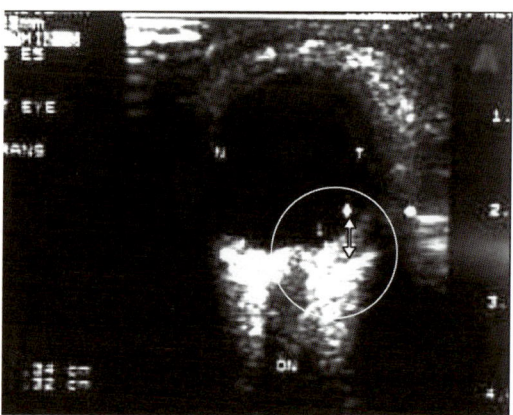

Fig. 6.12 *Thickened retinochoroid suggestive of VKH disease*

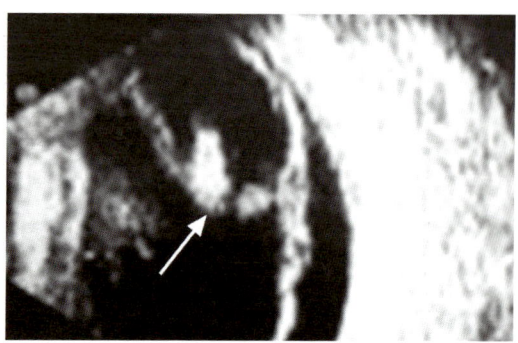

Fig. 6.13 *Cyst with hyperechoic focus at one end, suggestive of scolex in parasitic cyst with retinal detachment*

Table 6.1 *Common B-scan patterns*

Point like echoes	Membrane like structure	Cyst like structure
Vitreous hemorrhage	PVD	Crystalline lens
Vitreous exudates	Retinal detachment	Parasitic cysts
Vitreous degeneration	Choroidal detachment	Tumours

Table 6.2 *Differentiating diagnosis of membrane like structures*

Posterior vitreous detachment	Retinal detachment	Choroidal detachment
Smooth membrane with or without disc attachment with open funnel configuration	Open or closed funnel membrane with attachment at disc	Smooth dome shaped or flat membrane without disc attachment
Marked after movements	Moderate after movements in fresh RD and none in old RD	Minimal after movements
Echo intensity <100% which disappears on low gain	Echo intensity of 100% which persists on reducing gain	Thick, double peaked 100% echo intensity

Table 6.3 *Differential diagnosis of choroidal lesions*

Melanoma	Dome shaped or collar button shaped arising from choroid	Low to medium echo intensity, acoustic hollowing and choroidal excavation
Metastasis	Diffuse or irregular mass arising from choroid	Medium to high intensity echo intensity with irregular structure
Choroidal hemangioma	Dome shaped arising from choroid	High echo intensity with regular internal structure
Choroidal nevus	Dome shaped arising from choroid	High echo intensity without acoustic hollowing or excavation
Choroidal haemorrhage	Dome shaped arising from the choroid	Moderate to high echo intensity which decreases over 7–10d

Differential diagnosis of cyst like structures seen on posterior segment ultrasonography in given in Table 6.3.

BIBLIOGRAPHY

1. Examination techniques of globe. In Byrne SF, Green RL.(eds). Standardized echography of the eye and orbit. St. Louis, Mosby –Year Book, Inc. 1992, p-19

2. Green RL, Byrne SF. Diagnostic Ophthalmic ultrasound. in Ryan SJ(ed)Retina. Basic Science, Inherited retinal disease, and tumors. Volume 1. Philadelphia. Elsevier Inc. 2006, p-65.

3. Yannuzzi LA, Ober MD, Slakter JS, Spaide RF, Fisher YL, Flower RW, Rosen R. Ophthalmic fundus imaging: today and beyond. Am J Ophthalmol. 2004;137:511–24.

7 MACULAR OPTICAL COHERENCE TOMOGRAPHY

Subina Narang, Mohit Dogra

INTRODUCTION AND PRINCIPLE OF OCT

INTRODUCTION

There are changing trends in imaging of retina. Earlier fluorescein angiography was regarded as gold standard and then the trends shifted to doing optical coherence tomography (OCT) in conjunction. As the understanding of OCT increased trends shifted to preference of OCT due to non-invasive nature of procedure. But the recent trends are for multi-modality imaging (OCT, FFA, ICG, autofluorescence) to achieve a comprehensive description of retinal morphology and function. Diverse retinal images acquired by different modalities at the same time and different time instants must be mutually registered. Retinal autofluorescence provides information about retinal pigment epithelium. Indocyanine green angiography tells about choroidal vasculature and OCT provides overview of neurosensory retina, Retinal pigment epithelium (RPE) and chorio-capillaris. OCT has become the most important adjunct tool for diagnosis, assessment and management of macular diseases. Leakage is quantified and this is important for monitoring disease progression and seeing response to treatment. Increased resolution of OCT with newer machines gives us insight into well-being of photoreceptors and functional outcome also.

PRINCIPLE OF OCT

The basic principle of OCT is low coherence interferometry (Fig. 7.1).

Time domain (TD) OCT

In time domain OCT the light beam is split into reference beam and measurement beam and both travel different path but with same length before these are picked up by a detector to produce interference signal. In the reference beam a single echo is generated after reflection from the mirror and in the measurement beam various micro structures reflect these at variable intervals giving rise to multiple echoes. The intensity of echoes and time interval between

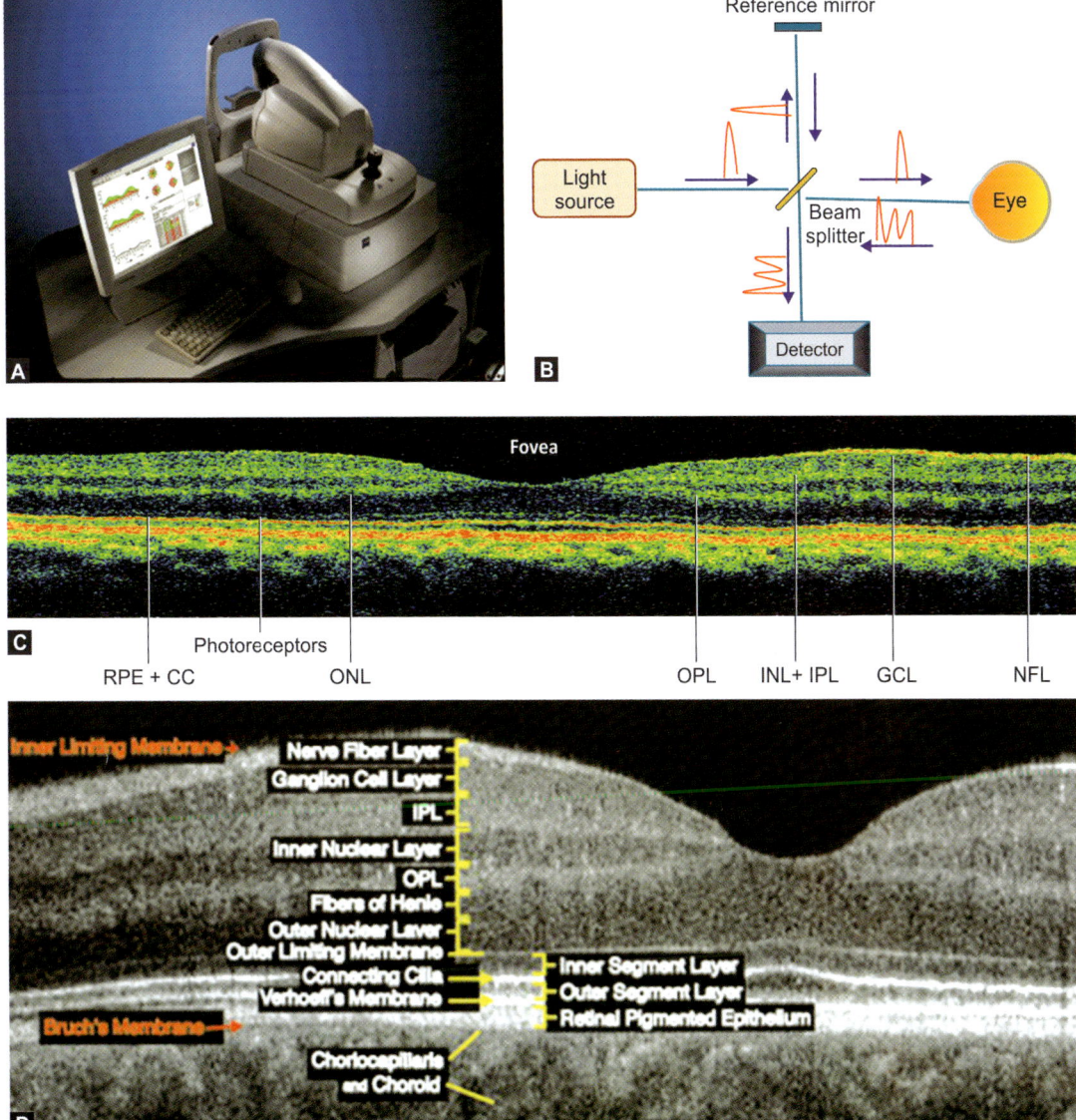

Fig. 7.1 **(A)** Photograph of stratus OCT machine (Carl Zeiss meditech) showing simultaneous viewing screen; **(B)** Line diagram showing principle of the OCT machine; **(C)** OCT scan of normal macula on stratus OCT showing correlation with various histological layers; and **(D)** OCT scan on spectral domain OCT showing correlation with different layers on histological examination

these generate 2-D anteroposterior view of different layers of retina which is compararable to in vivo histology of retina. This was first demonstrated by Huang in 1991. With the advent of new machines the resolution has improved and the time required has also decreased. In time domain OCT (TD OCT-stratus by Zeiss) the mirror of reference beam moves back and forth so the image acquisition time is more. Various retinal layers appear as hypo- and hyper- reflective layers on OCT as shown in Fig. 7.1C.

Images are now obtained by newer machines in 2–3 dimensions.

Spectral domain OCT

Spectral domain OCT (SD OCT) is based on the principle of Fourier transform mathematical equation (1807), where movement of mirror in the path of reference beam is not required and interference signal is a function of wavelength and all echoes of light from various tissue interfaces are analysed simultaneously. SD OCT is 50 times faster than TD OCT. SD OCT gives us best visualisation of various layers of retina.

- Examination can be simultaneously performed in different planes and 3D reconstruction and more precise quantitative measurement is possible.
- SD OCT gives clearer visualization and differentiation of each layer as compared to TD OCT.
- **Nerve fiber layer** is inner most layer and borders are sharper than on TD OCT.
- **Ganglion cell layer** can identify single hyperfluorescent spots as corresponding cells.
- **Nuclear layers** are hyporeflective. Intraretinal vessels are hyperreflective with posterior shadowing in TD OCT but vessel wall and lumen clarity is seen on SD OCT.
- **Outer layers of retina** can be analysed more clearly on SD OCT due to high speed and volume and appear as three bands. This helps in functional information on these tissues especially photoreceptors.
  - **External limiting membrane** is a moderately reflective membrane under ONL. It is almost always seen with SD OCT while it is seen with difficulty on TD OCT.
  - The first hyperreflective band under ONL is inner segment/outer segment junction (IS/ OS junction) of photoreceptors.
  - **The outer layer is RPE,** composed of two distinct hyperreflective bands separated by thin hyporeflective strip. The outer band is composed of RPE but the inner band origin is unclear, which sometimes is thought to be Verhoef's membrane (constituted by tight junctions of RPE cells) (Fig. 7.1C and D).
- Due to longer wavelength with spectral domain OCT even choroid can be visualized. In SD OCT the moderately hyperreflective outermost structure corresponds to sclera.
- **Newer OCT machines acquire retinal cube sections** (512 vertical, 528 horrizontal in cirrus

OCT in approximately 11 seconds) which can simultaneously show tomography in 3 sections. The acquisition time with newer software is so short that even motion artifact can also be removed. RPE and ILM can further be isolated from other retinal layers. Retinal thickness can further be evaluated in 3 D maps. White and red are the colors for thicker area and green and blue represent thinner areas.

COMPARISON OF CURRENTLY AVAILABLE OCT MACHINES

Currently available OCT machines include:
- Stratus OCT
- Cirrus OCT
- Spectralis OCT.

Comparison of some commercially available OCT machines is summarized in Table 7.1.

Different scan protocols with stratus OCT

1. *Line.* This protocol allows one to take a scan through a specified area of retina. The angle and length of the line can be altered. The longer the length of the lesser is the resolution.
2. *Radial lines.* This protocol contains 6 to 24 line scans which pass through a common axis. It is useful to measure the retinal thickness in a given area.
3. *Raster lines.* Multiple parallel line scans are taken to cover a larger rectangular area. The default setting is 6 lines with 3 mm rectangle.
4. *Macular thickness and fast macular thickness.* They are the same as radial line scans, but the aiming circle has a fixed diameter of 6 mm. The fast macular scan reduces the time taken to acquire scans.

Different scans protocols with cirrus and spectralis OCT

1. *Raster lines.* Similar to the protocol in time domain OCT.
2. *Raster lines HD.* Higher density images are acquired for better tissue detail.
3. *Macular cube (512×256).* Multiple scans are taken in a rectangle of set dimensions and retinal thickness can be calculated at any point within the rectangle. 3-dimensional reconstruction can

Table 7.1 *Comparison of different OCT machines available*

	Stratus (time domain)	Cirrus (spectral domain)	Spectralis (spectral domain)
Axial resolution	10 μ	5 μ	3.9 μ axial resolution 14 μ transverse resolution
Scan velocity	400 axial scan/sec	27,000 axial scan/sec	40,000 axial scan/sec
Enhanced depth imaging	Not possible	Not possible	Possible
Scanning time	Slower scanning time	0.017–0.25 sec	0.005–0.01 sec
Tracking eye movement	Absent	Absent	Present
Simultaneous ICG, FFA, red free picture and auto-flouresence	Not possible	Not possible	Possible
Central macular thickness measurement	Measures between RNFL and inner boundary of RPE	Measures between RNFL and outer boundary of RPE	Measures between RNFL and outer boundary of RPE
Central macular thickness	230 ± 33.2 microns	270 ± 43.7 microns	

also be done to look for anteroposterior traction in addition to transverse changes.

4. *Macular cube HD.* Similar to the macular cube protocol, but high density images are taken to improve tissue detail.

INTERPRETATION OF OCT IMAGING

LAYER WISE INTERPRETATION OF OCT

We must look at OCT layer wise, in addition to determining the central macular thickness, maximum retinal thickness and looking at the foveal contour, as below.

1. Retinal pigment epithelium (RPE)

For proper OCT interpretation we must try to trace RPE and its separation from Bruch's membrane. Normally these two are in close association with each other and RPE has very high reflectivity. In diseased state we can see RPE as separate from Bruch's membrane. In serous pigment epithelial detachment (PED) we can see RPE lifted up and Bruch's membrane appears as moderately reflective band under RPE (Fig. 7.2A and B). If posterior reflectivity is blocked then it is hemorrhagic PED (Fig. 7.3). It is also blocked in deposits of Best's disease. Drusens appear as PED filled with moderately reflective homogenous material. There is no serous detachment or cystic spaces associated with it (Fig. 7.4A and B).

Follow RPE band and look for any irregularity, thickening in contour, or fragmentation all of which are suggestive of occult CNVM (Fig. 7.5A to C). Associated neurosensory detachment/sensory macular detachment (SMD) and cystic spaces can be seen (Fig. 7.6A and B). Hyperreflective dots represent inflammatory reaction and are present in active CNVM

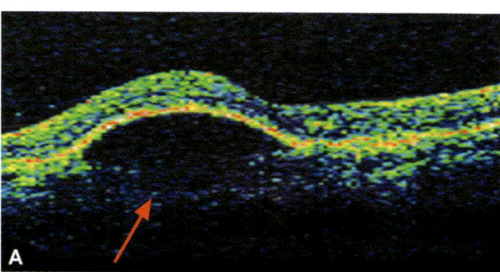

Serous PED

Fig. 7.2 *(A)* Retinal pigment epithelial detachment showing optically clear center and Bruch's membrane (arrow) is visible suggestive of serous pigment epithelial detachment (PED) and *(B)* serous PED with nerosensory detachment in a case of CSCR, subretinal space shows moderate reflectivity suggestive of fibrin (arrow)

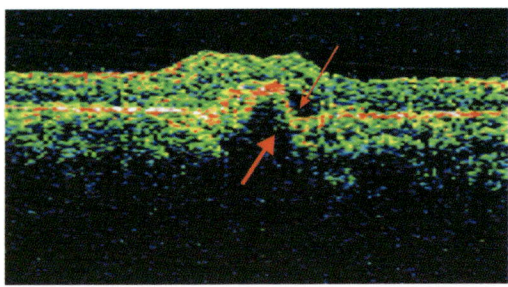

Fig. 7.3 *Retinal pigment epithelial detachment with fibrovascular proliferation in the PED (thick arrow) and block reflectivity posteriorly (thin arrow) and the Bruch's membrane is not seen*

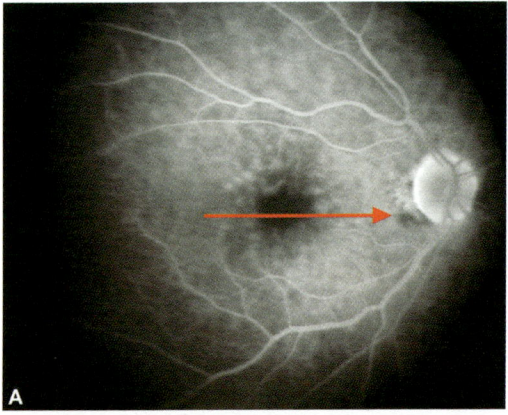

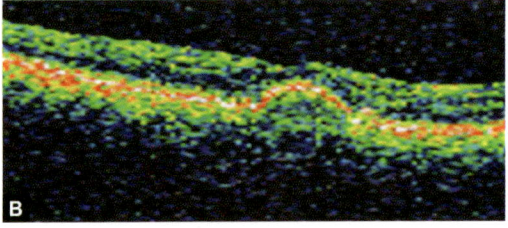

Fig. 7.4 (A) *FFA arteriovenous phase shows point like hyperfluorescence not increasing in late phases consistent with drusens and* **(B)** *OCT horizontal scan shows RPE detachment with moderately reflective homogenous material in the PED, suggestive of drusen*

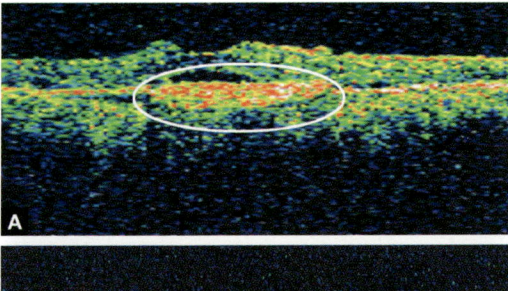

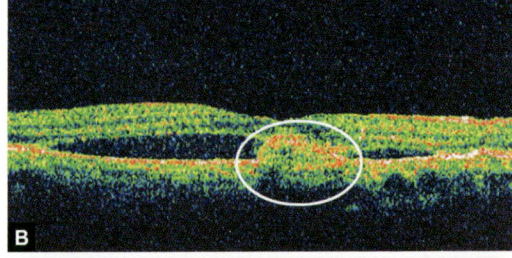

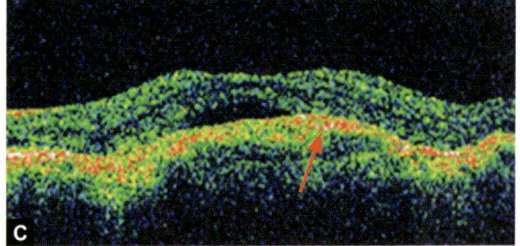

Fig. 7.5 (A) *RPE is irregular and thickened with overlying serous detachment suggestive of CNVM;* **(B)** *type 1 (classic) CNVM, hyperreflective membrane anterior to RPE with serous detachment; and* **(C)** *fibrovascular PED with serous detachment anterior to it suggestive of Type 2 (occult) CNVM*

Three main landmarks for outer retinal layers (outer nuclear layers ONL external limiting membrane ELM, inner segment outer segment junction IS/OS junctions) help us to prognosticate the patient. The integrity of photoreceptors is important for good functional outcome. Ischemic damage may lead to disruption of these layers. Branch retinal vein occlusion is a good example of disruption of these layers in the region of ischemia (Figs 7.9 to 7.11).

2. Evaluate structures anterior to RPE

The neuro-sensory retina anterior to RPE is evaluated for vitreous and vitreo-retinal adhesions, foveal depression/contour, various retinal layers, presence of cavities and deposits, serous macular detachment (SMD) (Figs 7.12 to 15). Any hyporeflective structures or hyper-reflective structures are looked for. Hyper-

(Fig. 7.7). Sometimes effraction of RPE is seen and retinochoroid anastomosis is seen clearly suggestive of retinal angiomatosis proliferans (Fig. 7.8). Numerous PEDs are seen in idiopathic polypoidal choroidovasculopathy (IPCV) and some choroidal polyps are seen reaching till inner retinal layers also. PEDs in IPCV are more steep and abrupt.

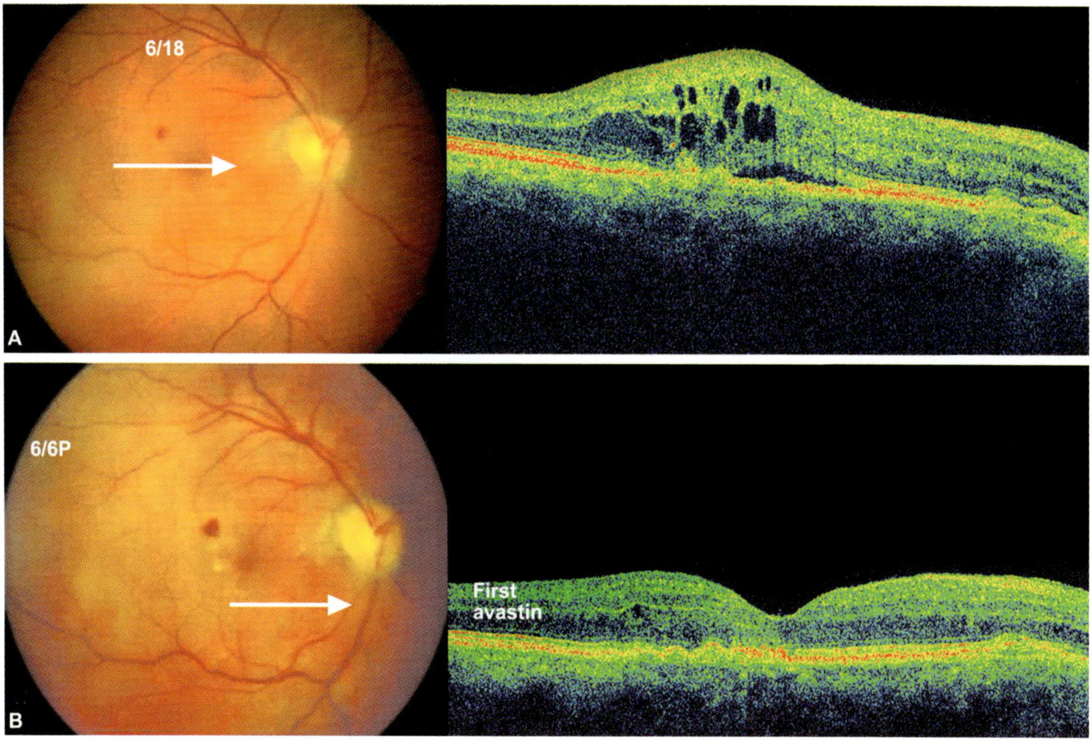

Fig. 7.6 **(A)** *Horizontal OCT scan shows fragmented and disrupted RPE without any thickening with overlying cysts in occult CNVM;* and **(B)** *Horizontal OCT scan after intravitreal bevacizumab showing resolution of serous detachment and cysts. (Courtesy: Professor MR Dogra)*

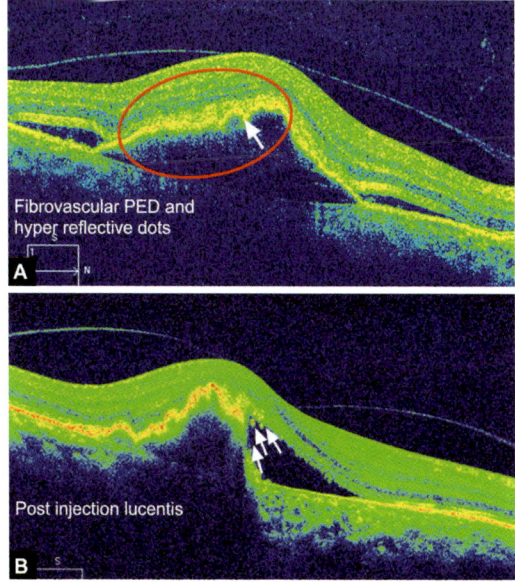

Fig. 7.7 **(A)** *RPE detachment with fibrovascular proliferation with hyperreflective dots suggestive of inflammation seen in active membrane and* **(B)** *same pattern RPE rip after injection lucentes. (Courtesy: Professor MR Dogra)*

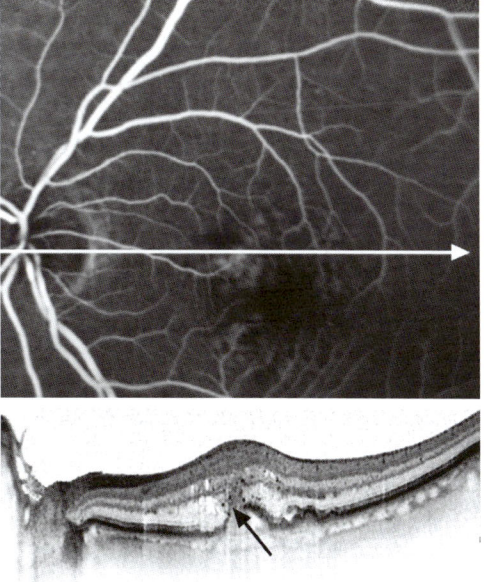

Fig. 7.8 *Effraction of RPE and retinochoroid anastomosis seen in retinal angiomatosis proliferans (Courtesy: Dr. Ethan Priel)*

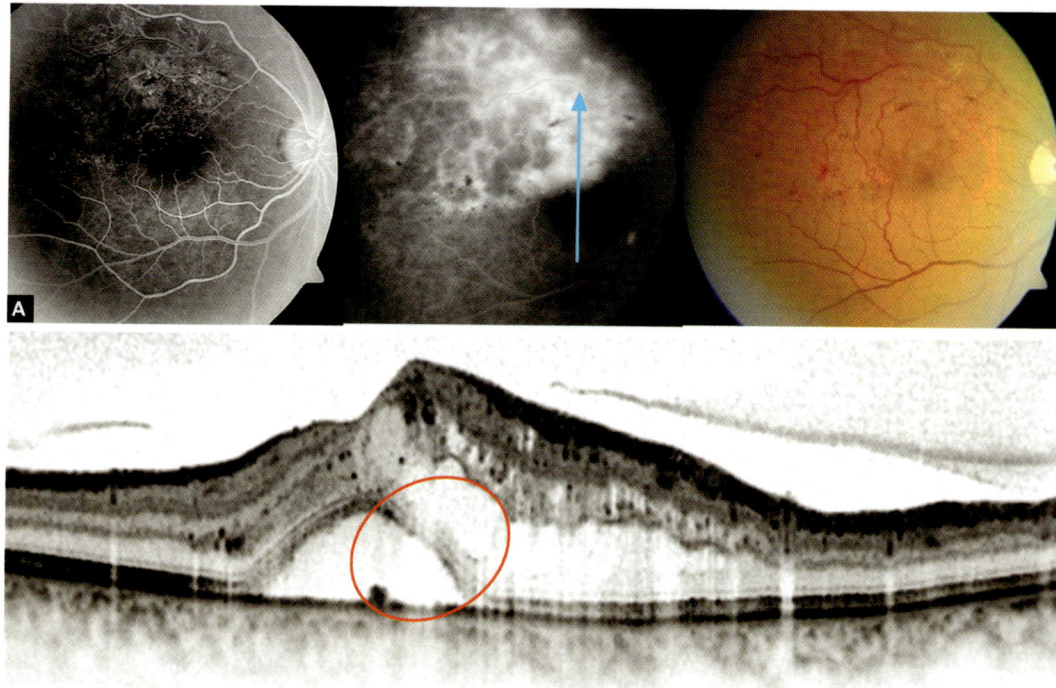

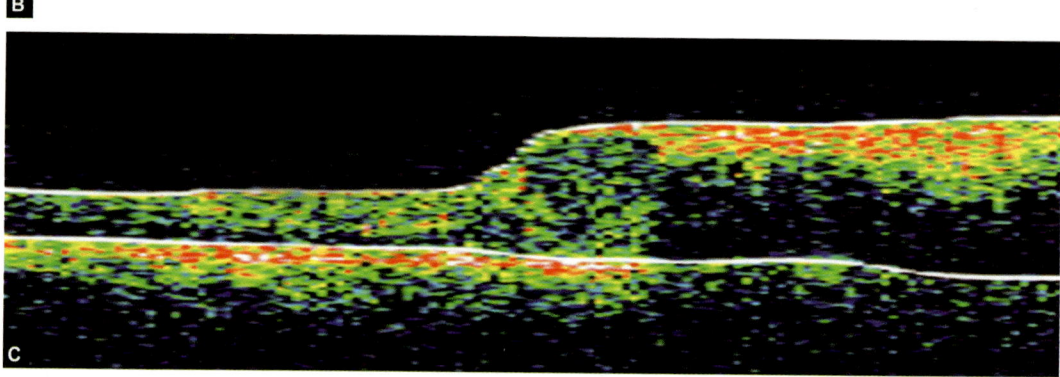

Fig. 7.9 *Case of BRVO. (A) Showing leakage on FFA; (B) Spectralist OCT scan showing increase in thickness with disruption of ELM, IS/OS junction; and (C) Stratus OCT scan of the same patient showing differential increase in thickness and loss of foveal dip*

reflective lesions could be linear beneath neurosensory retina or within retinal layers (pigment, hemorrhage, fibrous scar) or dots hyperreflective dots (HRD) suggestive of active inflammation especially in active CNVM.

3. Evaluate structures posterior to RPE band

Hyperreflectivity is suggestive of atrophy and hyporeflective is shadowing due to structures in anterior layers (Figs 7.16 and 7.17).

4. Thickness measurement

It is done by an inbuilt software. For reliable thickness measurement, we must evaluate the scan quality and center the measurement at the fovea (Fig. 7.18). Automated segmentation in high resolution OCTs gives more accurate retinal thickness measurements.

SD OCT measures thickness by incorporating RPE. The posterior line selected is line representing bruch's membrane. The Cirrus

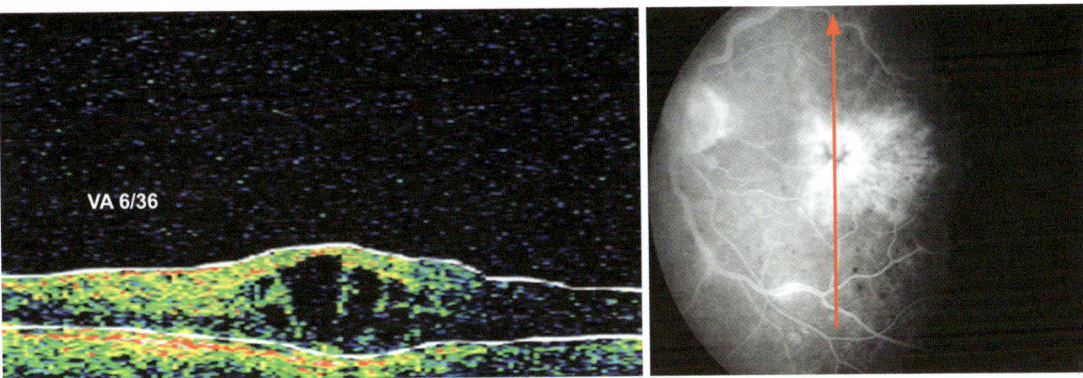

Fig. 7.10 *Vertical OCT scan in a case of CRVO showing cystoid macular edema separated by hyperreflective septa*

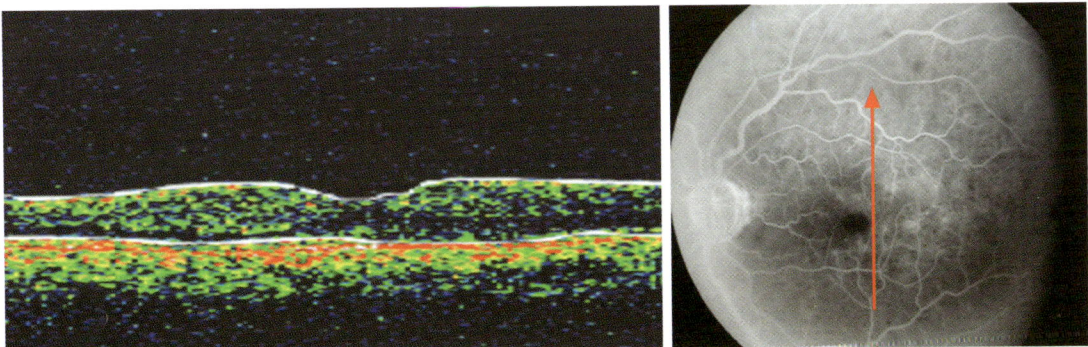

Fig. 7.11 *Resolution of macular edema and restoration of foveal contour after injection bevacizumab in the same patient as seen in Fig. 7.12*

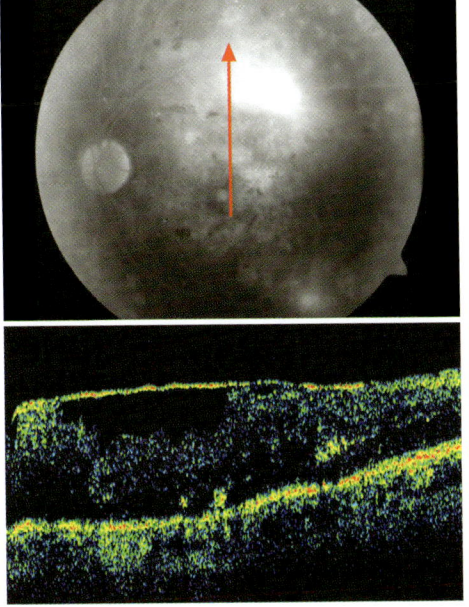

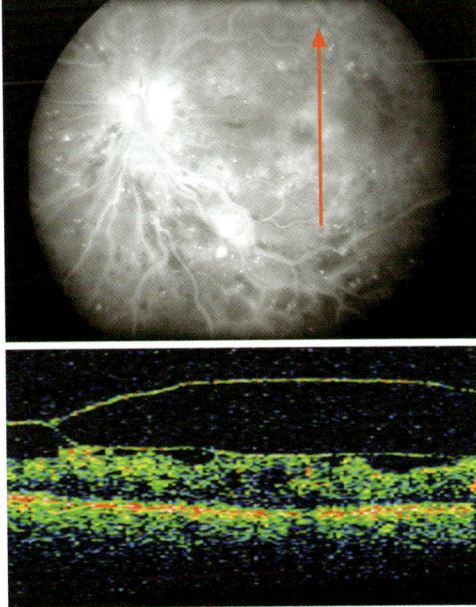

Fig. 7.12 *Vertical macular scan showing vitreomacular adhesions in a case of refractory CSME*

Fig. 7.13 *Vertical scan showing taut posterior hyaloid and vitreoschisis in a case of refractory CSME*

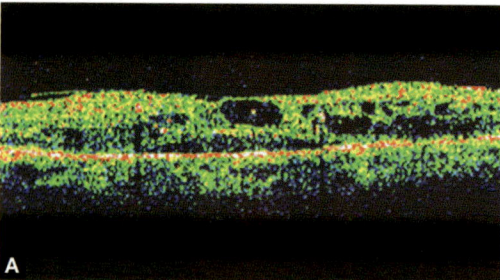

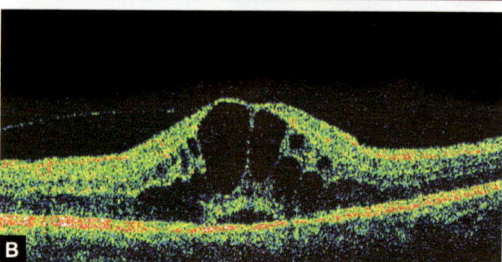

Fig. 7.14 (A) Horizontal OCT scan of CSME patient showing increased foveal thickness, loss of foveal contour, spongiform pattern of retinal thickening with submacular detachment; and **(B)** Horizontal OCT scan of CSME patient showing increased foveal thickness, loss of foveal contour, cystoids pattern of macular edema with hyperreflective septa separating cysts

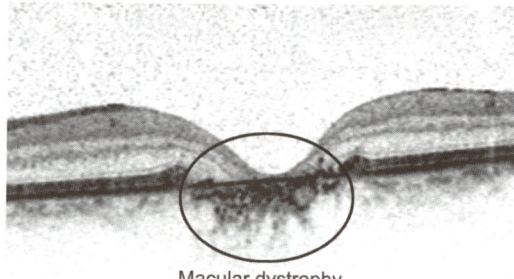

Macular dystrophy

Fig. 7.16 OCT scan showing marked decrease in foveal thickness and hyperreflectivity under fovea suggestive of foveal atrophy

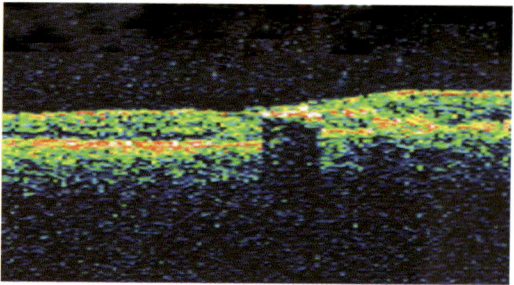

Fig. 7.17 OCT scan showing hyperreflectivity from pigmented scar and blocked reflectivity posterior to it

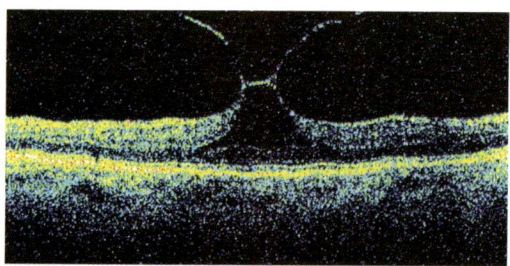

Fig. 7.15 OCT scan showing clinically significant macular edema with vitreo-macular traction

OCT FINDINGS IN COMMON MACULAR LESIONS

- Central serous retinopathy (*see* page 383)
- Cystoid macular edema (*see* page 399)
- Age related macular degeneration (*see* page 366)
- Macular hole (*see* page 353)

CONCLUSION

OCT is easy to perform and can give a lot of information besides the retinal thickness if read carefully layer wise. With OCT the disease is diagnosed and activity assessed by numerous direct and indirect signs. OCT cannot actually demonstrate vascular component, neovascular network or analyse whether it is an active CNVM or prefibrotic CNVM. Interpretation of OCT should be after correlation with other imaging modalities.

HD-OCT segmentation algorithm identifies the thickness of the retina from the retinal pigment epithelium (RPE) to the internal limiting membrane (ILM). Stratus OCT segmentation algorithm identifies the thickness of the retina based on the distance between the ILM and junction of the outer segments (OS) and inner segments (IS) of the photoreceptors. SD OCT thickness measurement are 40–80 µ higher than TD OCT.

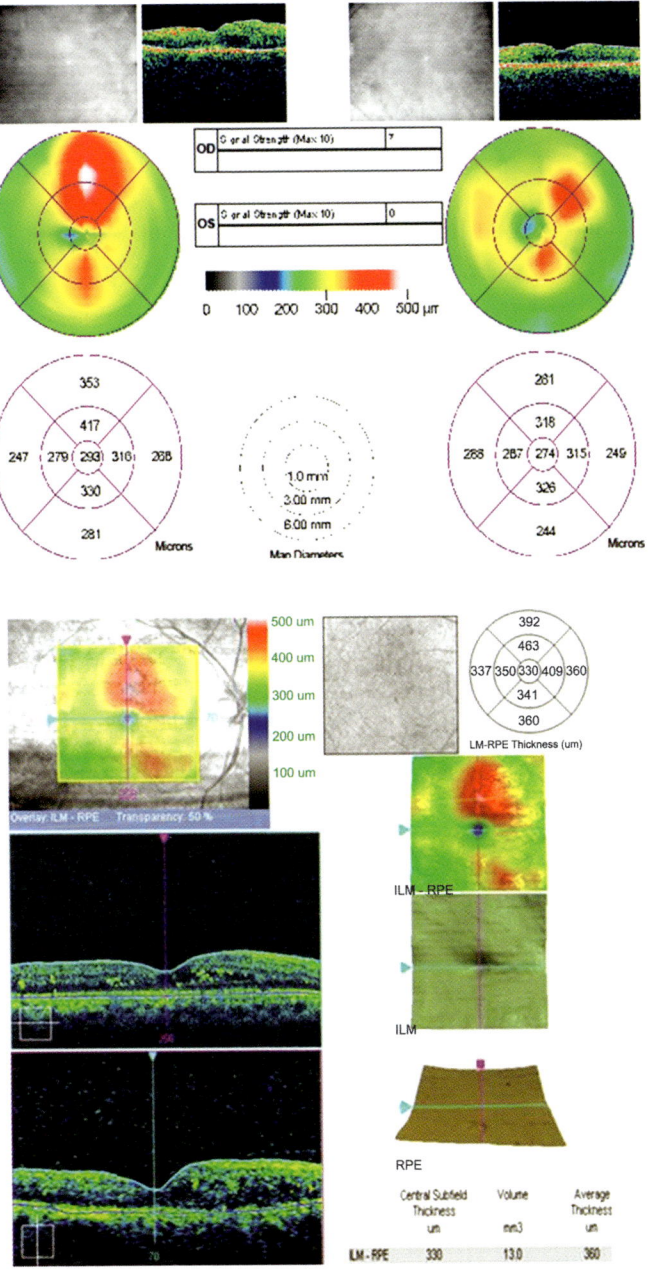

Fig. 7.18 *OCT scans showing retinal thickness measurement by stratus and cirrus OCT (Courtesy: Prof. MR Dogra)*

BIBLIOGRAPHY

1. AF Fercher, CK Hitzenberger, W Drexler, G Kamp, H Sattmann. In Vivo Optical Coherence Tomography. Am J Ophthalmol 1993:116:113–14.
2. Interpretation of OCT scans. In: Gupta V, Gupta A, Dogra MR. (Eds) Atlas Optical Coherence tomography of macular diseases and Glaucoma. Jaypee Brothers Medical Publishers(P) Ltd. 2006,17.
3. Keane PA, Patel PJ, Liakopoulos S, Heussen FM, Sadda SR, Tufail A. Evaluation of age-related macular degeneration with optical coherence tomography. Survey of Ophthalmology 2012; 57(5):389–414.

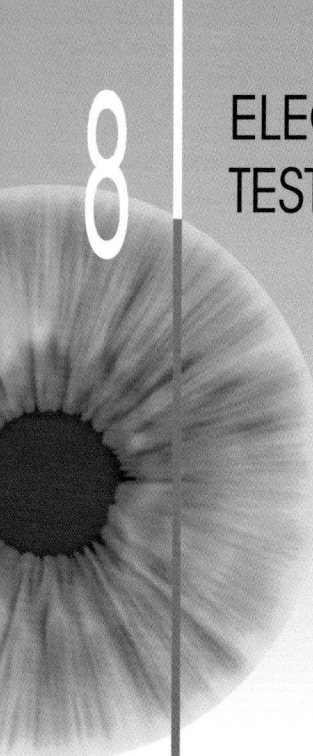

8 | ELECTROPHYSIOLOGICAL TESTS

Parul Ichhpujani, Shibal Bhartiya

GENERAL CONSIDERATIONS

Visual electrophysiology is an indispensable diagnostic support service to clinical ophthalmology as it helps to ascertain the functional integrity.

We have come a long way since 1849 when DuBois-Reymond first time described how to measure the electrical activity in the visual system. He discovered that excised fish eyes had a potential difference of about 6 mV between the cornea and posterior scleral surface. Einthoven and Jolly, and later, Granit, described the electroretinogram (ERG) in considerable detail in animal eyes using galvanometers (Einthoven, 1908; Granit, 1947) in the early years of the twentieth century. With the advancement in technology for recording, in early 1940s the human ERG was carried out in the clinical setting.

Marked improvements in equipment for generating and recording electrophysiological responses such as solid-state electronics, microprocessors and light emitting diodes

(LEDs) have led to a greatly increased understanding of the workings of the visual system in health and disease.

Which Electrophysiological Test Tells What?

The visual electrophysiology tests follow a hierarchal pathway along the various cell layers of the visual system.

Full field Electroretinogram (ERG). It measures the mass response generated from the cells of entire retina.

Flash Electroretinogram (fERG). Electrical responses from retinal photoreceptors and the inner retinal cells are ascertained by the a- and b-wave components of the flash ERG.

Pattern Electroretinogram (pERG). Pattern ERG tells about the macular photoreceptor function and the ganglion cells function is revealed and separated by the technique of recording.

Electro-oculogram (EOG). Examines the function of the retinal pigment epithelium (RPE).

Visual Evoked Potential (VEP). Tells the integrity of the visual pathway from optic nerve via optic chiasma to the occipital cortex.

A clear understanding of the nature of each of these tests is essential to derive a valid interpretation. This chapter gives an overview of various tests available and some idea of basic interpretation.

When do we order electrophysiological tests?

In some cases, even the detailed clinical examination of the eye cannot explain the exact cause of vision loss. These tests help to provide a piece of *"diagnostic jigsaw"* to detect and categorize the site of lesion in the visual pathway.

Common uses of visual electrophysiology in the clinical setting include the following:
- To provide evidence to confirm or exclude a specific diagnosis
- To indicate the level in the visual system at which a problem lies
- To monitor the progress of a known condition
- To provide an approximate objective measurement of visual acuity
- To provide an indication of the maturity of the visual system in infants
- To detect early disease or carrier status in relatives of an affected individual
- To provide an indication of visual potential in an injured or diseased eye.
- To detect a drug or metal toxicity.
- To assess the extent of ischemia of the inner retinal layers in a vascular pathology.

Standards for electrophysiological tests

For each of these recordings in the clinic, certain minimum standards have been laid down by the International Society for Clinical Electrophysiology of Vision (ISCEV). In 1989, they published the first internationally agreed standard for ERG. Standards for other electrophysiological tests and for calibration of recording equipment have been published more recently. These are available on the website www.iscev.org.

The adage *"Man before the machine"* holds very true for visual electrophysiology as the visual electrophysiologist is the key component of the system. The process of recording electrophysio-

logical responses requires special training and meticulous attention to detail. Factors which can influence responses include:
- Placement of recording electrodes
- Ambient lighting levels
- Pupil size
- Extraneous electrical interference
- Calibration errors of the recording equipment

Each laboratory should maintain their own database of normal values for each test, which must be updated if the equipment is changed or testing protocols revised.

ELECTRORETINOGRAM

Electroretinogram (ERG) is a measurement of retinal electrical response to a light stimulus. It measures the generalized loss of rods or cones or both.

PRINCIPLE

Due to selective transport of ions, the inside of the photoreceptor cells is more negative than the outside resulting in a standing membrane potential in the dark. Once light falls on the retina, it induces a change in the transmembrane movement of especially sodium and potassium ions, making the cells hyperpolarized, that is, they become more negative to the extracellular space than in the dark. These voltage changes are reflected in various ERG components.

TYPES OF ERG

The electrical response of retinal cells to light can be ascertained by the following forms of ERG:
- Full-field flash ERG
- Pattern ERG (pERG)
- Macular or Focal ERG
- Multifocal ERG (mfERG)
- Direct-current ERG
- Long-duration flash ERG (on-off responses)
- Bright-flash ERG
- Double-flash ERG

Flash ERG generates data appropriate for whole-eye disorders. The basic mfERG result is based on the calculated mathematical average of an approximation of the positive deflection component of traditional ERG response, the

b-wave. Multifocal ERG programs measure electrical activity from more than a hundred retinal areas per eye, in a few minutes. The enhanced spatial resolution enables scotomas and retinal dysfunction to be mapped and quantified.

TECHNIQUE OF ERG

- Recordings can be made from both eyes simultaneously and a common earth electrode is usually placed in the middle of the forehead. The corneal electrode may consist of a conducting foil or fiber placed at the lid margin in contact with the cornea or may be mounted in a special contact lens.
- The pupils are dilated and the subject's head is positioned within a bowl with a white, reflective inner surface and a radius that allows the whole retina to be evenly illuminated by light reflected from the surface. This is known as a Ganzfeld stimulus. The light source for the ISCEV standard ERG is a xenon discharge tube, but arrays of bright LEDs may also be used.
- The subject is dark-adapted for 20 min.
- *Scotopic threshold response (STR).* Initially recordings are made of the response to very dim flashes of white light. STR is a negative deflection of a few microvolts in amplitude. The response from many flashes must be averaged in order to detect the response above background noise.
- *Scotopic b-wave.* Flashes of progressively higher intensity are shown. As the flash intensity increases in intensity the implicit time decreases.
- *Scotopic a-wave.* At higher intensities, the a-wave appears and also increases in amplitude with increasing flash intensity. The earliest part of the a-wave originates from the photoreceptors, but the later part reflects the activity of Müller cells.
- *Oscillatory potential.* Next, a bright white flash (the 'standard flash') is used, which produces a mixed rod and cone response with a large a-wave and b-wave, and wavelets or oscillatory potentials superimposed on the ascending limb of the b-wave. The oscillatory potentials can be recorded separately by repeating the recording with a filter to remove the lower-frequency components of the response.

- *Single flash cone response; Cone a-wave and b-waves.* The subject is now light-adapted for 20 minutes to suppress rod activity, and a response is recorded to a bright light flickering at 30 Hz. This is a pure cone response. A recording is made of responses to single flash of bright light. The cone a-wave and b-wave so generated are of smaller amplitude and are faster than their rod counterparts. There is often a distinct peak (I-wave) on the descending limb of the cone b-wave.
- *30 Hz Flicker Cone Response.* Under the photopic condition repetitive standard flashes are presented at a frequency of 30 stimuli per second.

NEWER NOMENCLATURE FOR BASIC ERG RESPONSES

As per the revisions made in 2008 an ISCEV Standard ERG includes the following responses, named according to conditions of adaptation and the stimulus (flash luminosity) (Fig. 8.1):
- Scotopic 0.01 ERG (formerly "rod response") (Fig. 8.1A)
- Scotopic 3.0 ERG (formerly "maximal or standard combined rod-cone response") (Fig. 8.1B)
- Scotopic 3.0 oscillatory potentials (Fig. 8.1C)
- Photopic 3.0 ERG (formerly "cone response") (Fig. 8.1D)
- Photopic 3.0 flicker (Fig. 8.1E)

INDICATIONS

Inherited retinal degenerations in which the ERG can be useful include:
- Retinitis pigmentosa and related hereditary degenerations
- Retinitis punctata albescens
- Leber's congenital amaurosis
- Choroideremia
- Goldman-Favre syndrome
- Gyrate atrophy of the retina and choroid
- Congenital stationary night blindness
- X-linked juvenile retinoschisis
- Achromatopsia
- Cone dystrophy
- Disorders mimicking retinitis pigmentosa
- Usher syndrome

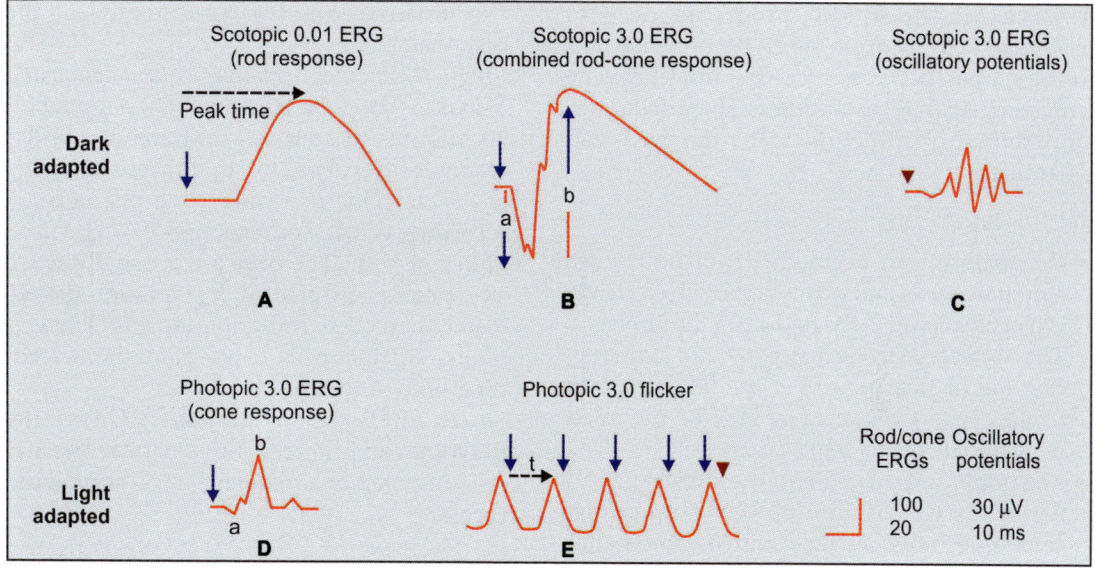

Fig. 8.1 *Exemplary waveforms of the six basic ERG responses*

Other ocular disorders in which the standard ERG provides useful information include:
- Diabetic retinopathy
- Other ischemic retinopathies including central retinal vein occlusion (CRVO), branch vein occlusion (BVO), and sickle cell retinopathy
- Toxic retinopathies, including those caused by plaquenil and vigabatrin.
- To monitor retinal toxicity in many drug trials.
- Autoimmune retinopathies such as Cancer Associated Retinopathy (CAR), Melanoma Associated Retinopathy (MAR), and Acute Zonal Occult Outer Retinopathy (AZOOR)

Note. Other ERG tests, such as the Photopic Negative Response (PhNR) and pattern ERG (PERG) may be useful in assessing retinal ganglion cell function in diseases like glaucoma.

INTERPRETATION OF ERG

Principal measures of the ERG waveform

Two measures are taken:
1) The amplitude (a) from the baseline to the negative trough of the a-wave, and the amplitude of the b-wave measured from the trough of the a-wave to the following peak of the b-wave; and 2) the time (t) from flash onset to the trough of the a-wave and the time (t) from flash onset to the peak of the b-wave.

Waveforms

- *a-wave*, sometimes called the "late receptor potential," reflects the general physiological health of the photoreceptors in the outer retina.
- *b-wave* reflects the health of the inner layers of the retina, including the outer nuclear bipolar cells and the Müller cells.
- ERG of a normal full-term infant looks similar to a mature ERG.
- ERG attains peak amplitude in adolescence and slowly declines in amplitude throughout life.

Abnormal ERG waveforms

- *Abnormal scotopic ERG*, the scotopic ERG is severely abnormal or unrecordable from an early stage and the photopic ERG is usually better preserved, but deteriorates as the disease progresses.
- *Negative ERG.* Preserved a wave, but reduced b-wave. This is found in conditions such as central retinal artery occlusion and congenital stationary night blindness.
- *No ERG response* is seen in Batten's disease, Leber's congenital amaurosis
- *Increased a wave* is seen in albinism

Note. If the full field ERG is normal and the patient has an unexplained visual loss then a focal or multifocal ERG should be done.

LIMITATIONS OF ERG

A limitation of traditional full-field ERG for the diagnosis of retinopathy is its lack of sensitivity. ERG results are normal unless more than approximately 20% of the retina is affected. So, a patient might be legally blind as a result of macular degeneration and still appear normal.

ELECTRO-OCULOGRAM

The Electro-oculogram (EOG), assesses the function of the outer retina; retinal pigment epithelium (RPE) and the interaction between the RPE and the rod photoreceptors. Since the test is carried under photopic-conditions, it cannot distinguish between photoreceptor and RPE dysfunction.

PRINCIPLE OF EOG

- The eye behaves like a dipole, and the cornea is positive in charge with respect to the back of the eye, and has a standing or resting potential of about 6 millivolts.
- Exposure of the retina to a steady light results an increase in this resting potential.
- EOG measures changes in the standing potential to light and dark conditions.

TECHNIQUE OF EOG

- The pupil is dilated after an informed consent.
- Skin electrodes are placed near the medial and lateral canthi. A ground electrode is placed at the forehead. Saccadic eye movements result in flow of current around orbit proportional to the magnitude of standing potential of each eye.
- A Ganzfield is used to illuminate the retina uniformly. The test recordings are initiated after allowing the patient about six minutes for light adaptation.
- The patient is then asked to move his eye first in one direction, and then the other for a fixed 30 degrees, using diode fixation lights (green fixation light in the center and red on the sides).

- The voltage changes so generated are recorded by the skin electrodes during 20 minutes of dark adaptation, and then during a 12–15 minute period of light adaptation.
- The voltage changes are amplified and displayed by the acquisition system of the machine.
- The interpretation of these voltage changes includes the calculation of the amplitude of the light peak in relation to the dark trough as a percentage, the Arden index (Fig. 8.2).

  An Arden index > 185% or an Arden quotient of >2, is considered as normal. An Arden quotient of <1.65 is significantly abnormal.

INDICATIONS OF EOG

Light response is affected in diffuse disorders of RPE and the photoreceptor layer of retina including some characterized by rod dysfunction, chorio-retinal atrophy and by inflammation. In most of these disorders, there is correlation between effects on the EOG and on the ERG, with exception of disorders of bestrophin gene, including Best vitelliform maculopathy, autosomal recessive bestrophinopathy and autosomal dominant vitreoretinochoroidopathy (AD-VIRC) in which the clinical EOG can be highly abnormal even with normal ERG.

CLINICAL INTERPRETATION OF EOG

- *Arden index* (light peak/dark trough × 100) of greater than 185 is considered as normal.
- *A normal ERG and abnormal EOG* are classically seen in patients, as well as asymptomatic carriers of Best's vitelliform macular dystrophy.
- *EOG abnormality is seen in RPE and rod-photoreceptor disorders* including retinitis pigmentosa, choroideremia and age-related macular degeneration.
- *EOG can be used to distinguish* between choroidal melanomas and nevi, since it is abnormal in the former.
- EOG abnormalities are also detected in drug and heavy metal toxicities.
- Oscillatory potentials are decreased when retinal ischemia is present.

LIMITATIONS OF EOG

- The test cannot be performed in patients with poor fixation, children, infants and unco-operative adults.

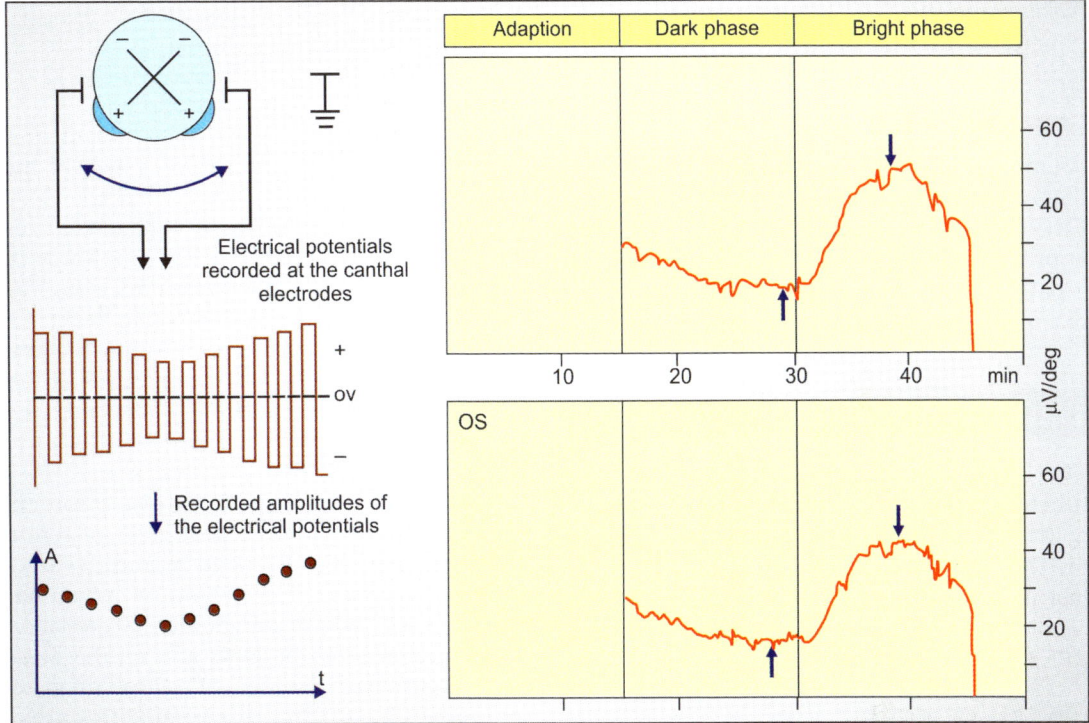

Fig. 8.2 *Light peak and dark troughs recorded during EOG*

• Media opacities and illumination levels can influence the voltage amplitude and therefore, EOG abnormalities must be interpreted with caution.

VISUAL EVOKED POTENTIAL

Visual evoked potential (VEP) is an evoked electrophysiological signal that can be extracted, using signal averaging, from the electro-encephalographic activity recorded at the scalp. It is a sensitive indicator of visual function, with the typical response measuring only 5–10 microvolts in amplitude, which are masked by the electroencephalographic (EEG) noise of 50 microvolts or greater.

TYPES OF VEP

VEP is classified into the following subtypes, depending on the visual stimuli used to elicit the response:
1. *Flash VEP.* Where standard ERG flash is used.
2. *Pattern VEP*

• *Pattern reversal.* Where the pattern of an isoluminant checkerboard or grating of various spatial frequencies is reversed to elicit the VEP. This is the preferred technique for most clinical purposes as the results of pattern reversal stimuli are less variable in waveform and timing than the results elicited by other stimuli.
• *Pattern onset/offset.* Where the VEP is recorded as the patterned stimulus of the pattern reversal is presented.
3. *Special VEPs.* Steady state VEP, sweep VEP, motion VEP, chromatic VEP, binocular VEP, multichannel VEP, LED google VEP, are other forms of VEP.

TECHNIQUE OF VEP

• Each eye is tested separately after an informed consent.
• Silver-silver chloride or gold disk electrode are placed using conducting paste on the scalp relative to bony landmarks in relation to the head size as per the international 10/20 system.

- The active electrode is placed on the midline over the visual occipital cortex (OZ), reference electrode is placed at the frontal pole (FZ) while the ground electrode is at the forehead or earlobe.
- Recordings are done with refractive correction without mydriasis using monocular stimulation.

  Extreme pupil sizes and any anisocoria should be noted.
- For pattern stimulation, the visual acuity of the patient should be recorded and the patient should be optimally refracted for the viewing distance of the screen.

INDICATIONS OF VEP

Flash VEP

- In difficult and uncooperative patients
- In patients with dense media opacities and very poor vision.

Pattern VEP

- Pattern-reversal for pre-chiasmal lesions and for patients with nystagmus
- Pattern-onset/offset VEP for malingerers

  VEP is a useful tool along with ERG and other clinical assessments to differentiate various conditions such as cortical visual impairment, delayed visual maturation and amblyopia.

INTERPRETATION

The VEP traces (two reproducible records of each) can be presented as positive upwards or negative upwards. The polarity convention and stimulus parameters used should be indicated in the report besides the amplitude and latency. Latency is measured from the stimulus onset to peak of the component measured. It must be remembered that interocular difference in the pattern-reversal VEP indicates dysfunction of the entire pre-chiasmal pathway and includes ocular, retinal and optic nerve causes (Fig. 8.3).

Normal waveforms

1. *Flash VEP.* It consists of a series of positive and negative peaks that are designated in numerical sequence. Commonest components recorded are N2 and P2 at 90 and 120 msec, respectively.

2. *Pattern-reversal VEP.* The peaks are named as negative or positive followed by the latency. Commonest wave used for clinical cases is the P100 component (positive peak at 100 msec) since it is a very robust measure with minimal interocular and inter-subject measurement variation.

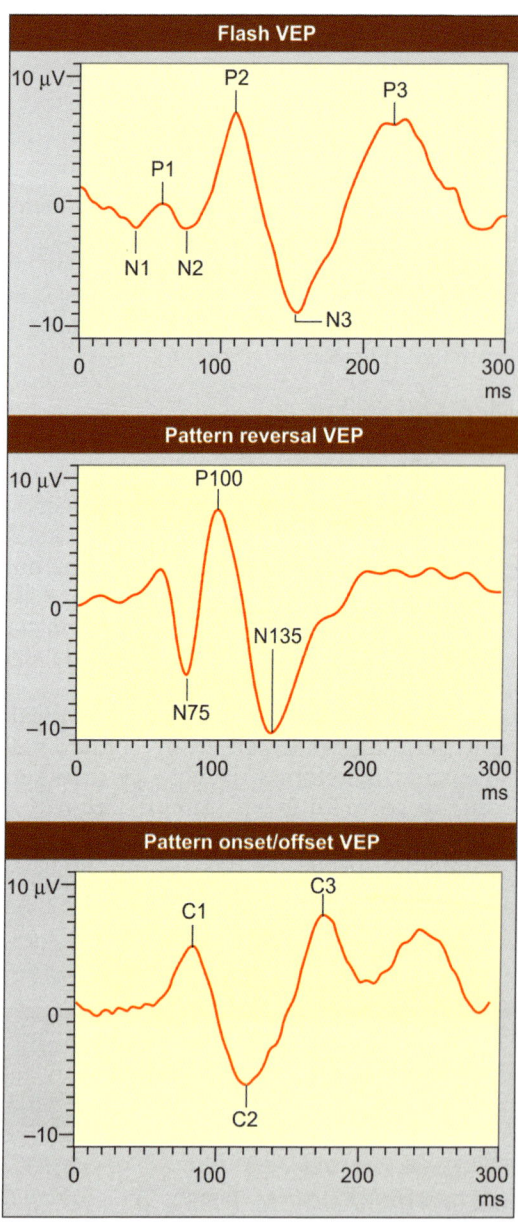

Fig. 8.3 *Normal waveforms for flash VEP, pattern VEP and pattern onset/offset VEP*

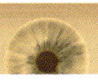

Table 8.1 *Outline of potential indications for specific electrophysiological tests*

Provisional diagnosis	EOG	ERG	Bright flash ERG	Pattern ERG	Flash VEP	Pattern VEP	Special VEP
Inherited retinal dystrophies	+	+					
Vascular diseases including diabetes		+		+		+	
Opaque media or trauma		+	+		+		
Retrobulbar neuritis				+		+	
Unexplained visual loss		+		+		+	
Infant with questionable vision		+			+		+
Albinism		+					+
Toxic and nutritional eye disease	+	+		+	+		
Glaucoma				+			
Suspected intracranial lesion				+		+	+

3. *Pattern-onset/offset VEP.* Three components described are C1 (positive at 75 msec), C2 (negative at 125 msec) and C3 (positive at 150 msec). With a stimulated hemifield, the response will appear contralateral to the hemifield stimulated (Fig. 8.3).

LIMITATIONS OF VEP

VEP has following limitations:
- Age, refractive error, inattention and conscious defocusing of the pattern affect the VEP latency.
- Stimulus parameters such as contrast, luminance, check size and field size are important determinants of the waveform and it is essential for each laboratory to establish their own normal controls.
- Since the amplitudes of VEP are very small, surrounding noise can easily contaminate them and, therefore, strict vigil has to be kept on the recording equipment, recording technique and the stimulus parameters used.
- Numerous specialized types of VEP are being assessed and these are still used as investigational tools. Knowledge in these areas is still evolving.

ELECTROPHYSIOLOGICAL TESTS: TIME TAKEN, POTENTIAL INDICATIONS AND PRACTICAL STATUS

TIME TAKEN FOR VARIOUS ELECTROPHYSIOLOGICAL TESTS

Time taken for various electrophysiological tests is as follows.

- ERG: 60 minutes (40 min DA + drops)
- EOG: 45 minutes
- Pattern ERG: 30 minutes
- Flash or pattern VEP: 30–45 minutes
- Special VEPs: 30–60 minutes

In case of pediatric assessment (under 7 years), multiply time by 1.5.

POTENTIAL INDICATIONS OF VARIOUS ELECTROPHYSIOLOGICAL TESTS

Outline of potential indications of specific electrophysiological tests as summarized in Table 8.1.

PRACTICAL STATUS OF ELECTROPHYSIOLOGY

- *ERG* is an extremely helpful tool in detecting or confirming retinitis pigmentosa, even in the absence of typical bony corpuscles.
- *EOG* is useful in differential diagnosis of abnormalities of the retinal pigment epithelium such as Best's disease.
- *VEP* is a useful tool along with ERG and other clinical assessments to differentiate various conditions such as cortical visual impairment and delayed visual maturation.

BIBLIOGRAPHY

1. Brigell M, Bach M, Barber C, Moskowitz A, Robson J. Guidelines for calibration of stimulus and recording parameters used in clinical electrophysiology of vision. Doc Ophthalmol 2003;107:185–93.
2. Holder GE, Brigell MG, Hawlina M, Meigen T, Vaegan, Bach M. ISCEV standard for clinical

pattern electroretinography-2007 update. Doc Ophthalmol 2007,114:111–6.

3. Hood DC, Bach M, Brigell M, Keating D, Kondo M, Lyons JS, Marmor MF, McCulloch DL and Palmowski-Wolfe AM. ISCEV Standard for clinical multifocal electroretinography (2011 ed).

4. Jasper, HH. Report of Committee on Methods of Clinical Examination in Electroencephalo-graphy. Electroenceph. Clin. Neurophysiol., 1958;10:370-375.

5. Marmor MF, Brigell MG, Westall CA, Bach M. ISCEV Standard for Clinical Electro-oculo-graphy (2010 Update), Doc Ophthalmol 2011; 122:1–7.

6. Marmor MF, Fulton AB, Holder GE, Miyake Y, Brigell M, Bach M. Standard for clinical electro-retinography (2008 update). Doc Ophthalmol 2009;118:69–77.

7. Odom JV, Bach M, Brigell M, Holder GE, McCulloch DL, Tormene AP, Vaegan. ISCEV

standard for clinical visual evoked potentials (2009 update). Doc Ophthalmol 2010;120:111–9.

8. Perlman I. Relationship between the amplitudes of the b wave and the a wave as a useful index for evaluating the electroretinogram. Br J Ophthalmol.1983;67:443–448.

9. Regan D. Human brain electrophysiology. New York: Elsevier, 1989.

10. Sutter E E Noninvasive Testing Methods: Multifocal Electrophysiology. In: Darlene A. Dartt, editor. Encyclopedia of the Eye, Vol 3. Oxford: Academic Press; 2010. pp. 142-160.

11. Towle VL, Cakmur R, Cao, Y Brigell M Parmeggiani L. Locating vep equivalent dipoles in magnetic resonance images. 1995;80:105-116.

12. Wachtmeister L, Dowling JE. The oscillatory potentials of the mudpuppy retina. Invest Ophthalmol Vis Sci. 1978;17:1176–1188.

13. Weleber RG. The effect of age on human cone and rod ganzfeld electroretinograms. Invest Ophthalmol Vis Sci. 1981;20:392–399.

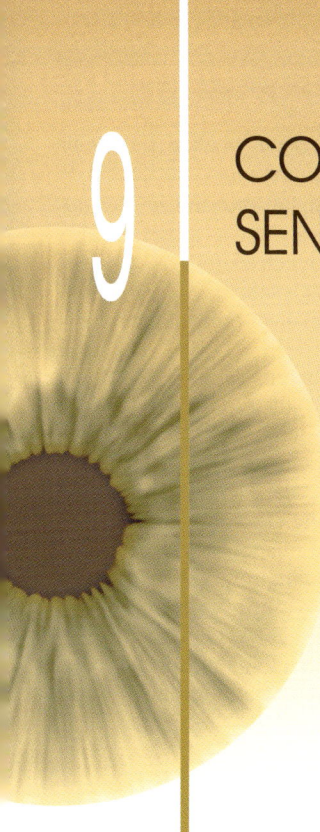

9

CONTRAST SENSITIVITY

AK Khurana, RK Bansal,
Aruj K Khurana, Bhawna Khurana

GENERAL CONSIDERATIONS

INTRODUCTION

Contrast sensitivity is the ability to perceive slight changes in luminance between regions which are not separated by definite borders and is just as important as the ability to perceive sharp outlines of relatively small objects. It is only the latter ability which is tested by means of the Snellen's test types. In many diseases, loss of contrast sensitivity is more important and disturbing to the patient than the loss of visual acuity. Further, contrast sensitivity may be impaired even in the presence of normal visual acuity.

The first measurement of contrast sensitivity function of the human visual system was reported by Schade, in forms of modulation transfer function (MTF). Campbell and Green in 1968 first measured contrast sensitivity using sinusoidal gratings and concluded that measurement of contrast sensitivity gives a more complete description of the function of retina.

TYPES OF CONTRAST SENSITIVITY

1. Spatial contrast sensitivity

Spatial contrast sensitivity refers to detection of striped pattern at various levels of contrast and spatial frequencies. In its measurement, patient is presented with sine wave grating of parallel light and dark bands (Arden gratings) and is asked to tell the minimum contrast at which the bars can be seen at each frequency. The width of the bars is defined as spatial frequency, which expresses the number of pairs of dark and light bars subtending an angle of 1 degree at the eye. A high spatial frequency implies narrow bars, whereas a low spatial frequency indicates wide bars.

2. Temporal contrast sensitivity

Here the contrast sensitivity function is generated for time-related (temporal) processing in the visual system by presenting a uniform target field modulated sinusoidal in time rather than as a function of spatial position.

Both temporal and spatial contrast sensitivity testing yield significantly more complete and

systematic data on the status of visual performance than the conventional tests.

MEASUREMENT OF CONTRAST SENSITIVITY

When a subject is presented with the grating frequencies and contrast below which resolution is impossible indicates the threshold level; and the reciprocal of this contrast threshold gives the contrast sensitivity.

Contrast sensitivity is measured as (L_{max} – L_{min}/ L_{max} + L_{min}); where L is the luminance recorded by photocells scanning across the gratings.

There are three variables in the measurement of contrast sensitivity:

1. Average amount of light reflected depends on illumination of paper and darkness of ink.
2. Degree of blackness in relation to the white background, i.e. contrast.
3. The distance between the grating periods or cycles per degree of visual angle.

Various methods have been developed to measure contrast sensitivity. Bodis Wollner introducing contrast sensitivity measurement in clinical practice, suggested the name *'visuogram'* analogue to an 'audiogram' to describe a patient's 'contrast sensitivity curve'. The deficits were expressed in terms of decibels; and three types of deficits were described:

1. *High frequency type* characterized by increasing loss at high frequency.
2. *A level loss type* characterized by a similar loss for all spatial frequencies.
3. *A selective loss type* characterized by deficits in a narrow band of spatial frequencies.

SINE WAVE VERSUS SQUARE WAVE GRATING

• *Sine wave patterns.* Visual scientist will describe contrast in terms of alternating bars of light and dark in terms of spatial frequency, the units are described as cycles per degree (cpd). One cycle consists of a black bar and white space next to it (Fig. 9.1).

• *Square wave or foucalt gratings* are also used to describe contrast sensitivity. However, in optics very few images can be described as

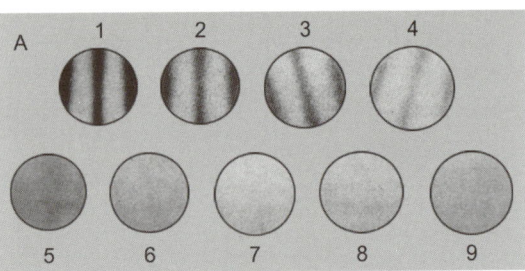

Fig. 9.1 *Sine wave patterns of different contrast used for testing contrast sensitivity*

perfect square wave gratings with perfect sharp edges. Sine wave patterns are considered essential element from which any pattern can be constructed. Combination of different sine waves can add up to produce a square pattern (Fig. 9.2). This trick of breakdown of any alternating pattern in to unique sum of sine waves is known as Fourier transformation (Fig. 9.3).

Visual system operates by breaking down observed patterns and scenes into sine waves of different frequencies. The brain then adds them up again to produce mental impression of a complete picture. Fourier transformations are the ways that the visual system encodes and records retinal images.

RECORDING OF CONTRAST SENSITIVITY

Recording of contrast sensitivity for a person is called as contrast sensitivity testing function (CSTF). A good optical system has high contrast sensitivity for low frequencies. It gradually decreases for the higher spatial frequencies as diffraction and other aberrasions make detection of finer details more difficult. Retina-brain tend to enhance the contrast of spatial frequencies of 2–6 cpd. CS also decreases with increasing age because of more diffraction by lens and decreased ability of retina-brain processing to enhance the contrast with increasing age. CS also decreases with decrease in retinal luminance.

As mentioned above, CS was first used by neurologist Dr. Ivan Bodis-Wollner 40 years back in patients of occipital lesions, who had disturbing visual symptoms but retained good visual acuity. In 1977 a British ophthalmologist Dr GB Arden introduced first commercially

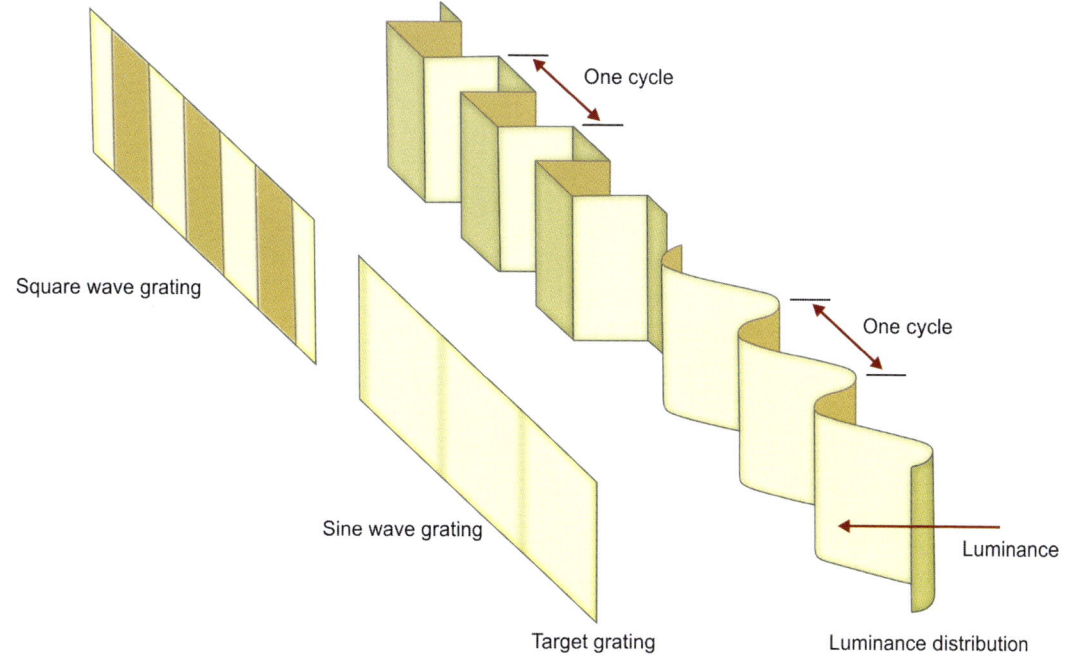

Fig. 9.2 *Square wave and sine wave grating pattern measured as cycles per degree*

available contrast sensitivity product. Later he and his colleagues published a number of papers in patients of glaucoma, cataract, optic neuritis, amblyopia, etc. FDA developed interest in CS in late 1980 and early 1990 when multifocals lenses became available and laser vision correction was introduced. Now testing of CS has been incorporated in routine clinical practice and FDA has approved its use in clinical trials. Now the standard of FDA trials is testing of four different frequencies under two different levels of lighting conditions; photopic and mesopic (85 cd/m² and 3 cd/m²).

CS testing has also been found to be useful in patients who retain good Snellen acuity but suffer from disturbing visual symptoms. Snellen acuity is also insensitive tool in patients who are developing cataract and have normal Snellen acuity. Its usefulness has been found in many other ocular diseases like; refractive surgery, multifocal intraocular lens implants, glaucoma, diabetic retinopathy, amblyopia, optic neuritis and age-related macular degeneration.

In general, the methods recommended to measure contrast sensitivity include: simple plates, cathode ray tube display on a screen letter acuity charts, laser interferometer which produces grating on the retina, visual field testing using low contrast rings on stimuli, pattern discrimination test, prototype for forced choice printed test, visually evoked cortical potentials to checker board pattern reversal dependent contrast threshold measurement, two alternative forced choice test, and many more.

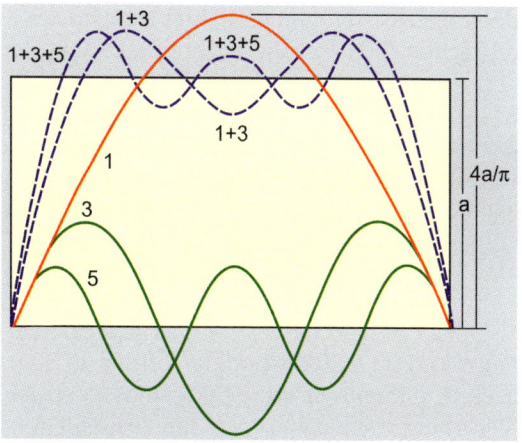

Fig. 9.3 *Fourier transformation; summation of sine waves gives square wave pattern*

Some of the simple, inexpensive but reliable methods of measuring contrast sensitivity are described in brief.

1. Arden gratings

Arden in 1978, introduced a booklet containing seven plates—one *screening plate* (No. 1) and six *diagnostic plates* (No. 2–7). The contrast changes from top to bottom and covers a range of approximately 1.76 log units. The plates are studied at 57 cm, with spatial frequency increasing from 0.2 cycles/degree to 6.4 cycles/degree, each being double the frequency of the previous one. A score of 1–20 is assigned to each plate, depending upon the amount of plate uncovered. Sum of six plates with an upper limit of 82 was established for normal subjects together with an interocular difference of less than 12.

2. Cambridge low contrast gratings

Cambridge low contrast gratings consist of a *'set of ten plates'* containing gratings in a spiral bound booklet. To perform the test, the booklet is hung on a wall at a distance of 6 metres. The pages are presented in pairs one above the other. One page in each pair contains gratings and the other is blank (Fig. 9.4), but have the same mean reflectance. The subject is simply required to choose which page, top or bottom, contains the gratings. The pages are shown in order of descending contrast and told to stop when the first error is made. Four descending series are shown separately to each eye. When no error is made at plate 10, then a score of 11 is given. Depending upon the total score of the patient from four series, the contrast sensitivity is noted from the conversion table (Fig. 9.5).

3. Pelli-Robson contrast sensitivity chart

This chart consists of letters which subtend an angle of 3 degrees at a distance of 1 meter. The chart is printed on both the sides. The two sides have different letter sequence but are otherwise identical. The letters on chart are organized as triplets, there being two triplets in each line (Fig. 9.6A and B). The contrast decreases from one triplet to the next. The log contrast sensitivity varies from 0.00 to 2.25.

To perform the test, the chart is hung on the wall, so that its center is approximately at the level of subject's eye. The chart is illuminated as uniformly as possible so that the luminance of the white areas is between the acceptable range of 60 to 120 cd/m, which corresponds to a photographic exposure between 1/15 and 1/30 second at f/5.6 with an ASA of 100. The luminance is determined with the help of a light meter. While recording, the subject sits directly in front of the chart at a distance of one metre (with the best distance correction) (Fig. 9.7). The subject is made to name or outline each letter on the chart, starting from the upper left corner

Fig. 9.4 *Cambridge low contrast gratings. From Wilkins et al*

CAMBRIDGE LOW CONTRAST GRATINGS
SCORE SHEET

Total score	Contrast sensitivity
4	10
5	13
6	16
7	20
8	24
9	28
10	33
11	37
12	43
13	49
14	55
15	62
16	70
17	78
18	88
19	99
20	110
21	120
22	130
23	140
24	150
25	170
26	180
27	190
28	210
29	230
30	250
31	270
32	290
33	310
34	340
35	370
36	400
37	440
38	480
39	520
40	560

Patient's Name .... Date of Birth ....

Record Number .... Date of Testing ....

Examined by ....

Summary of procedure

1. Test each eye separately.
2. Show Demonstration pages and instruct patient to choose which page ("top" or "bottom") contains the stripes.
3. Show subsequent pairs of pages in numberical order.
4. Encourage patient to respond, guessing if necessary.
5. Stop when the first error occurs (or at No. 10).
6. Note number on which error occurred in the table below; enter 11 if no errors.
7. Go back four plates from where you stopped (or to Demonstration).
8. Repeat steps 3–7 until four series have been completed.
9. Add the four scores together and enter total in table below.
10. Convert total score to contrast sensitivity using table overleaf.
11. Repeat steps 3–10 for the otehr eye, beginning the first series with stimulus No. 1.

Left eye	Right eye
Error on :	Error on :
Series 1	Series 1 ....
Series 2	Series 2 ....
Series 3	Series 3 ....
Series 4	Series 4 ....
Total	Total ....
Contrast Sensitivity	....

Percentile limits of normal performance on the published version of the Cambridge Low Contrast Gratings

Age range	90th percentile	95th percentile	97.5th percentile
10–19	24	22	20
20–29	29	27	28
30–39	29	28	27
40–49	28	25	24
50–59	21	18	18
60–80	24	23	22

Total scores lower than those tabulated may be considered abnormal, i.e. poorer than those expected form 90,95 and 97.5% of the normal population.

Fig. 9.5 *Cambridge low contrast gratings score sheet and conversion table*

and reading horizontally across the line. Subject is made to guess, even when concluded, when the subject guesses two of the three letters of the triplet incorrectly. The subject's sensitivity is indicated by finest triplet from which two of the three letters are named correctly.

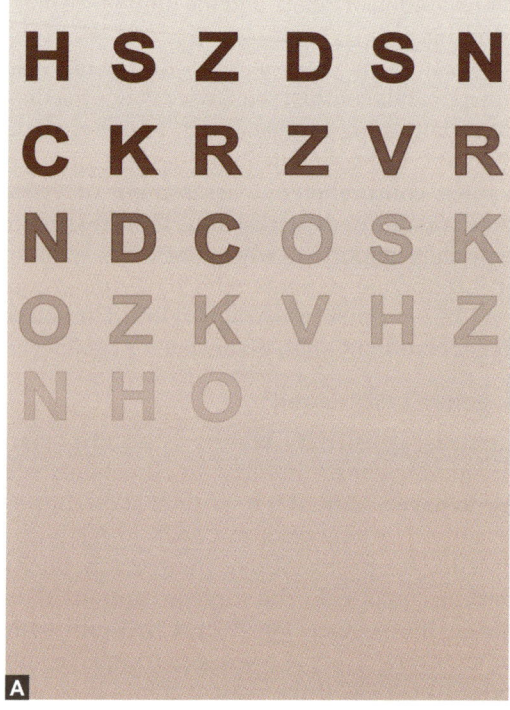

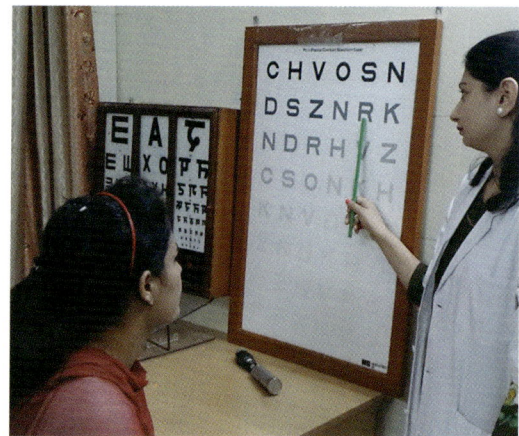

Fig. 9.7 *Measurement of contrast sensitivity with Pelli-Robson chart*

0.00	**H S Z**	**D S N**	0.15
0.30	**C K R**	**Z V R**	0.45
0.60	**N D C**	**O S K**	0.75
0.90	**O Z K**	**V H Z**	0.05
1.20	**N H O**	**N R D**	1.35
1.50	**V R C**	**O V H**	1.65
1.80	**C D S**	**N D C**	1.95
2.10	**K V Z**	**O H R**	2.25

Fig. 9.6 *Pelli-Robson contrast sensitivity chart: (A) Photograph; and (B) Log contrast sensitivity score of each triplet*

4. The visitech chart

This chart consists of sine wave gratings and is used at a distance of 3 m from the subject. In this test, contrast is assessed at several spatial frequencies (distance of separation of the grating bars) and the subject has to identify the orientation of the gratings, i.e. whether vertical or 15 degrees clockwise, or anticlockwise.

5. Vector vision charts

Vector vision CSV 1000 (USA) charts test frequency of 3, 6, 12 and 18 cpd.

6. Fact CS charts

The fact CS chart test for 1.5, 3, 6, 12 and 18 cpd.

NEURAL MECHANISMS AND FACTORS AFFECTING CONTRAST SENSITIVITY

NEURAL MECHANISMS OF CONTRAST SENSITIVITY

Campbell and Green gave the concepts *of different visual channels* for handling information about different bands of spatial frequencies. This concept indicates that retina is non-uniform. Fovea is specialized for high acuity and is responsible for high spatial frequencies. In the retinal periphery, only low frequency channels are represented. For coarse grating, central and peripheral retina have equal contrast sensitivity per unit area of retina, but larger the retinal area stimulated greater is the sensitivity. Thus, contrast sensitivity will be reduced in peripheral retinal diseases, and the use of low frequency grating would provide rapid check of peripheral retinal function.

Further, Campbell and Robson proposed the existence within nervous system of linearly operating independent mechanisms selectively sensitive to limited range of spatial frequencies.

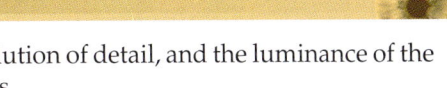

The orientation to limited range of spatial frequencies, the orientation selectivity and the interocular transfer of the adaptation effect implicated the visual cortex as the site of these neurons. They attempted to explain the preliminary and essential role of such interactions in the recognition of complex images and generalization for magnification.

FACTORS AFFECTING CONTRAST SENSITIVITY

1. *Refractive errors.* Visibility of low spatial frequencies is not limited by the refractive property of the eye; the refractive errors affect only the higher frequencies.

2. *Age.* There occurs a definite decrease in contrast sensitivity with increasing age. It has been reported that from twenties onwards, contrast sensitivity scores for normal population decline with age by about 10% each decade of life. The average decline over the lifespan is similar to the range of sensitivity within the normal population at any given age.

3. *Lenticular changes.* Early lens changes can reduce contrast sensitivity essentially for low spatial frequencies. This decrease in contrast sensitivity is not related to the visual acuity.

4. *Ocular and systemic diseases.* Contrast sensitivity is also found to be affected by various ophthalmic as well as systemic diseases. It is decreased in cases with retinal, optic nerve and visual pathway diseases, glaucoma, ocular hypertension, retrobulbar neuritis, multiple sclerosis, amblyopia, diabetes mellitus, and pituitary adenoma, etc.

DIAGNOSTIC APPLICATIONS

The contrast sensitivity function in recent years has become of interest as a possible diagnostic indicator of visual function. Deviations from normal standards have been reported in a number of conditions; some of which are listed above. It has been reported that contrast sensitivity (modulation transfer functions) may provide a fairly complete statement of the relations among spatial frequency or the fineness of visual details, the contrast required

for resolution of detail, and the luminance of the stimulus.

Visual acuity is the least indicative of visual function. It is contrast sensitivity that is the most important thing to measure in terms of visual function. Contrast sensitivity testing provides a more comprehensive assessment of vision than visual acuity testing. This testing is especially important when assessing, treating, and following patients who have undergone LASIK or those with age-related macular degeneration (AMD), glaucoma, or cataracts.

1. Before LASIK surgery

Contrast sensitivity testing is an important preoperative measurement for all patients who are to have LASIK. It is important to do contrast sensitivity testing prior to LASIK to establish a baseline for postoperative comparison. Such a finding could make the surgeon cautious about doing the surgical procedure without some other testing to explain reduced contrast results prior to LASIK. If the patient comes back after LASIK with reduced contrast, there would be no explanation as to why this would happen after LASIK. One should know this beforehand in any patient. After LASIK, contrast sensitivity is usually reduced for 2 to 3 months. Although immediate contrast sensitivity testing can be done, it is best to wait a few months, with a follow-up contrast sensitivity test completed 3 months after LASIK as it returns to normal after 3 months of LASIK surgery.

2. Age-related macular degeneration

Patients with treatable macular disease should have contrast sensitivity testing as part of the preoperative evaluation to assess the effectiveness of treatment. CS testing can indicate how far AMD has progressed in terms of how much the contrast has been damaged by this macular process. Hence CS testing is imperative as a guideline and as a follow-up test in these patients. This is particularly true in patients who are to undergo photodynamic therapy or intraocular steroid treatment. The Snellen visual acuity measurement does not provide the whole story. It is recommended that CS testing is done immediately after treatment

and again at 6 weeks and 3 months in patients with AMD. If these patients have fairly good contrast, they will do better with low vision aids also.

3. Glaucoma

Standard visual field testing does not reveal early progression of glaucoma. Patients with glaucoma have a specific response to contrast sensitivity testing. Everything else can seem to be normal in these patients. The acuity is stable, pressures are normal, the fields seem to be stable, however the contrast can gradually decrease. Contrast tests that provide mid-frequency information are the most useful in glaucoma management because they test the frequency most at risk from cell damage. Patients with glaucoma who are at risk should be tested for contrast sensitivity every 6 months.

4. Cataract

Typical high-contrast visual acuity testing is not accurate in patients with cataracts. A patient can have a cataract and yet see dark letters on the Snellen chart, which gives a false impression. Different types of cataract may respond differently to contrast sensitivity testing. Depending upon the type of cataract, one will want to do a contrast test as part of the initial examination as it gives an edge on when to order surgery. A reduced contrast sensitivity test usually indicates the need for surgery before a visual acuity test will.

5. Diabetic retinopathy

Visual acuity testing does not provide sufficient information towards retinal function in patients of diabetic eye disease. CS has been widely studied in patients of diabetic eye disease.

Patients of diabetes show lowering of CS before they actually develop diabetic retinopathy and have normal visual acuity. Dissociation in visual acuity and CS occurs early in the diabetic eye disease. Disturbance in foveal avascular zone has been found to be associated with lowering of CS for 6 and 12 cpd. Panretinal photo-coagulation in proliferative diabetic retinopathy and macular treatment in macular edema can reduce the CS, hence it is important that patients undergo CS testing before photocoagulation.

BIBLIOGRAPHY

1. Arden G, Jacobsen J. A simple grating test for contrst sensitivity-glaucoma screeing. Inv Ophthal Vis Sci 1978;17:23–32.

2. Bodis-Wollner I. Visual acuity and contrast sensitivity in patients with cerebral lesions. Sci 1972;178:769–71.

3. David Miller, Optics and Refraction.Ed. Podos M, Yanoff M. Gower Medical Publishing. New York 1991. 7.14–7.24.

4. Karz G, Levkovitch-Verbin H, Treiter G, Belkin M, et al. Mesopic foveal contrast sensitivity is impaired in diabetic patients without retino-pathy. Graefes Arch Clin Exp Ophthalmol 2010;248:1699–703.

5. Lorente-Velázquez A, Nieto-Bona A, Collar CV, Mesa AG. Straylight and contrast sensitivity after corneal refractive therapy. Optom Vis Sci. 2011;88:1245–51.

6. Sukha AY, Rubin A. High, medium, and low contrast visual acuities in diabetic retinal disease. Optom Vis sci 2009;86:1086–95.

7. Tran TH, Despretz P, Boucart M. Scene perception in age-related macular degeneration: the effect of contrast. Optom Vis Sci. 2012;89: 419–25.

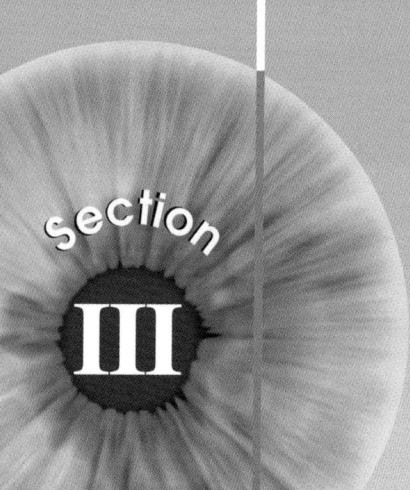

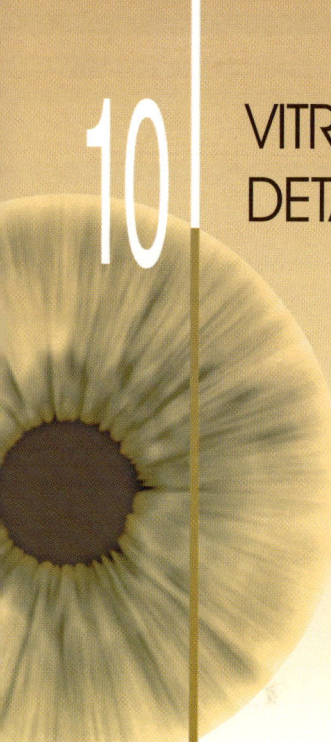

VITREOUS LIQUEFACTION, DETACHMENT AND OPACITIES

Sunandan Sood

APPLIED ANATOMY
Gross Anatomy
Histology
Attachments
- Vitreous base
- Hyalaideo-capsular ligament
- Optic disc attachment
- Attachment to macula
- Paravascular attachment

AGE-RELATED VITREOUS CHANGES
- Age-related liquefaction
- Posterior migration of vitreous base

DISORDERS OF VITREOUS
- Posterior vitreous detachment
- Asteroid hyalosis
- Vitreous amyloidosis
- Cholesterolosis bulbi
- Intraocular lymphomas
- Familial vitreoretinal disorders
  - Stickler syndrome
  - Wagner syndrome
  - Jansen syndrome

APPLIED ANATOMY

GROSS ANATOMY

Vitreous is the largest organ of the eye that occupies the four fifth of its volume. It is gel like structure which is mostly acellular having a volume of about 4.0 ml and weighing about 4 gm. Embryologically it is the secondary vitreous which becomes the definitive vitreous of infants and adults, primary vitreous contributing the hyaloid system whereas the tertiary vitreous develops into zonnules and suspensory ligaments in an adult. Vitreous body is somewhat spherical posteriorly and has a cup-shaped depression anteriorly known as patellar fossa. Thus it conforms to the contours of retina behind and lens infront. Grossly the peripheral vitreous is known as cortex and central vitreous is termed as medulla.

HISTOLOGY

Histologically as well as histochemically three components of the vitreous body can be discerned. The fibrillar framework providing structure to the vitreous is composed of type II collagen which is concentrated in the cortical areas. The second component is hyaluronan which intertwines with the collagen fibrillar framework of vitreous and is responsible to keep it in gel form. The molecules of third component is the hyalocytes which are very few in number and are loacated in the cortical layers only. The vitreous does not have any true membrane, however, peripherally the condensed cortical vitreous behaves like a membrane which is known as anterior hyaloid membrane/face anteriorly and posterior hyalloid face/membrane posteriorly.

ATTACHMENTS

The vitreous body is attached to all contiguous structures, however the firmness of its attachment varies. It has the following attachments in the decreasing order of its firmness: Vitreous base, lens, optic disc, macula and paravascular (Fig. 10.1).

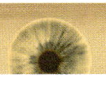

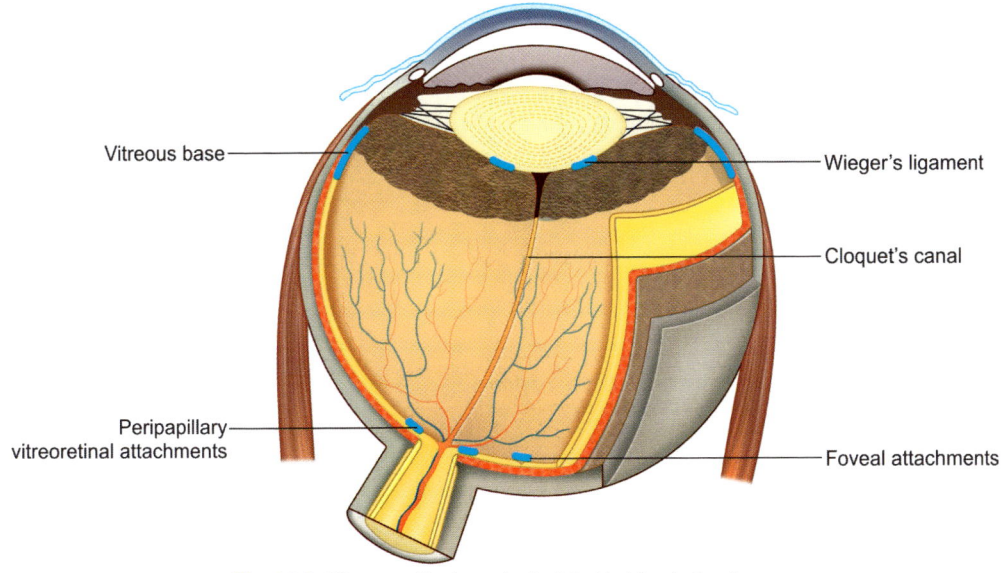

Fig. 10.1 *Vitreous attachments depicted in blue in the figure*

Vitreous base

Vitreous is most firmly attached to the vitreous base, a circumferential zone where the vitreous is attached to the epithelium of pars plana and to the peripheral retina. It is 2–6 mm wide and it straddles oraserrata, 2–3 mm infront and 2–3 mm behind the ora serrata. Here the density of collagen is the greatest and the fibers are oriented at right angle to the retinal plane, whereas elsewhere the orientation is tangential to this plane. The posterior border of the vitreous base is located more posteriorly in older individuals as compared to young since it is said to extend posteriorly with age, however, it is more anterior nasally than temporally. Thus following PVD this posterior location of posterior border of the vitreous base temporally may be responsible for increased frequency of retinal breaks temporally as compared to other locations in the peripheral retina.

Hyaloideo-capsular ligament

The anterior vitreous surface (anterior hyaloid membrane) is attached to the posterior lens surface along circular zone 1–2 mm wide and 8–9 mm in diameter just central to the insertion of the posterior zonular fibers. This attachment is known as hyaloideo-capsular ligament of Wieger. The space between anterior hyaloid membrane and posterior capsule is known as Berger's space which is continuous with cloquet canal a remanant of primary vitreous. Cloquet canal continues posteriorly in a serpentine fashion and open up into the space of martegiani that is present over the optic nerve head.

Optic disc attachment

Posteriorly the vitreous is attached to optic nerve head, this attachment is invisible in young individuals. However, in older individuals beyond 50 years the process of degeneration of vitreous sets in and posterior hyaloid detaches itself from optic nerve head, the ring of tissue is observed in the vitreous cavity which is termed as Weiss ring (Fig. 10.2). It is a surest sign of posterior vitreous detachment (PVD).

Attachment to macula

The attachment of vitreous in the macular area occurs in an irregular, annular 3 to 4 mm diameter which is again invisible clinically. However, in the process of PVD a tenuous attachment of vitreous may be seen at foveola by optical coherent tomography (OCT). In fact the advent of OCT has made it possible to monitor the process of PVD and observe the detachment of vitreous at the macula (Fig. 10.3).

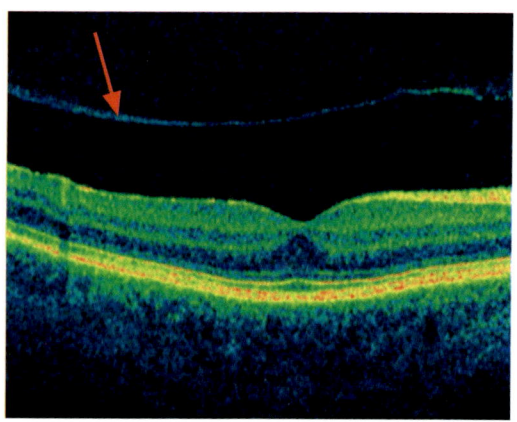

Fig. 10.2 *Fundus photograph showing PVD with Weiss' ring*

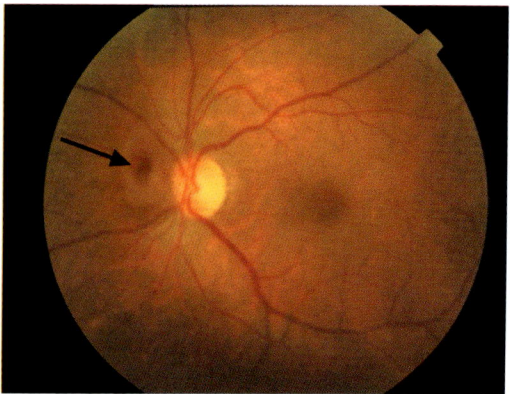

Fig. 10.3 *OCT picture showing PVD*

Paravascular attachment

The vitreous may have more than usual firm attachments to the retina along the major vessels which is suspected mainly because of avulsion, sometimes seen of retinal vessels in the process of PVD causing vitreous hemorrhage. Some authors have termed this attachment as vitreo-retino-vascular bands.

AGE-RELATED VITREOUS CHANGES

AGE-RELATED LIQUEFACTION

In the adulthood the vitreous is in gel form. However, with the increasing age mostly by 45 to 50 years the liquefaction of the gel sets in, which is basically because of breakdown of normal hyaluronic acid and collagen association. The process of liquefaction has been termed as synchisis. Initially small synchitic cavities develop in the center of the vitreous body which coalesce to form bigger cavity. Simultaneously this leads to the collapse of collagen fibrillar network of vitreous body, the process known as syneresis. In due course of time through a defect in the posterior hyaloid surface the synchitic fluid escapes behind this surface thus separating the posterior hyaloid surface from internal limiting membrane of retina which is termed as posterior vitreous detachment (Fig. 10.4A and B). Synchisis and

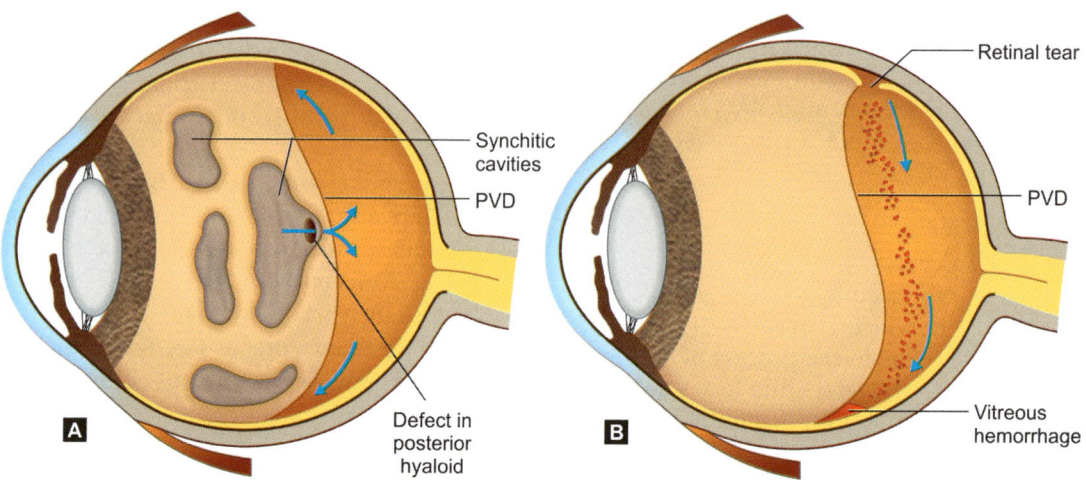

Fig. 10.4 **(A)** *Showing PVD and* **(B)** *PVD with vitreous hemorrhage*

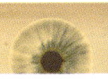

syneresis of vitreous body although is a age-related process but it occurs earlier and is more extensive in myopic eyes as compared to hyperopic and emetropic eyes. It is accelerated with intraocular inflammation, surgical aphakia, trauma and in Wagner's and Stickler's hereditary syndromes.

POSTERIOR MIGRATION OF VITREOUS BASE

It has been observed that the width of the vitreous base posterior to ora serrata increases with age from about 2 to 3 mm in the radial dimension particularly in temporal periphery. It is reported that the posterior migration of vitreous base and collagen fibril aggregation within the vitreous base may play an important role in the pathogenesis of peripheral retinal breaks and RD due to increased traction on peripheral retina following PVD.

DISORDERS OF VITREOUS

POSTERIOR VITREOUS DETACHMENT (PVD)

The pathogenesis of PVD has been discussed above which is largely an age-related change in the vitreous. It was first recognized by Goldmann in 1954 and the relationship between synchisis, syneresis of vitreous and PVD was established by Foos and Wheelor in 1982.

PVD is more common in females than in comparably age matched males. It is present in less than 10% of patients under the age of 50 years, in about 27% of patients aged 60–69 and in about 63% of patients above age 70.

It is also more common in aphakic eyes and in modern day surgery after YAG capsulotomy, and these eyes have an increased risk of developing RD.

Clinical features

It usually occurs as an acute event. Patient suddenly starts complaining of flashes in subdued light which is because of mechanical irritation of retina in the process of separation and complain of floaters due to the casting of shadows of the collapsed collagen fibrillar network of vitreous on the retina (entoptic phenomenon). In majority about 90% the vitreoretinal attachment is weak at this age and the

process of separation of posterior hyaloid surface from internal limiting membrane (ILM) of retina is completed with in few days to few weeks time. The detached vitreous retracts forward and sits quietly behind the lens when the symptoms of flashes and floaters disappear.

However, in 10% patients the process of separation is not uneventful. Instead there may be formation of retinal breaks with or without vitreous hemorrhage occurring when the detached vitreous reaches a point of firmer vitreoretinal adhesion. The traction at such points induce retinal tears and avulsion of vessels leading to vitreous hemorrhage (Fig. 10.4). The abnormal firmer attachments of vitreous with retina are usually seen at Lattice degeneration, enclosed oral bays, retinal tufts and at posteriorly advancing vitreous base.

Diagnosis

The diagnosis can be made with either on 90D biomicroscopy or on 20D indirect ophthalmoscopy. The ring of attachment of posterior vitreous to the optic nerve head can be seen on these examinations known as Weiss ring (Figs 10.2 and 10.3), when present is a surest sign of PVD. Shallow PVDs may be difficult to demonstrate on biomicroscopy, however, the posterior vitreous face may be seen a few millimetetres infront of retinal surface or else one should look for collapsed vitreous gel anteriorly behind the lens and an empty fluid space behind the gel especially in the superior quadrants in order to diagnose PVD. In the absence of above signs if one can demonstate condensation of collapsed collagen fibrillar network of vitreous body, that is also an evidence of PVD.

These days one can diagnose PVD on OCT as well which starts as posterior perifoveal vitreous detachment spreading radially to involve larger areas (Fig. 10.4A and B).

On contact B-scan ultrasonography the detached posterior vitreous face is seen as thin white line bounding the vitreous gel (p-114).

Management

In 90% of patient the patients are asymptomatic. Symptomatic PVD is a most important clinical

condition because of an increased risk of retinal detachment. Hence each symptomatic patient warrants exhaustive and painstaking indentation indirect ophthalmoscopy to rule out retinal breaks, and if any are found, need immediate prophylactic laser/cryotherapy in order to prevent RD.

Complications

In addition to vitreous hemorrhage and retinal break, PVD may cause tractional distortion and elevation of macula called as vitreomacular traction syndrome. It may also progress to foveal cavitation and macular hole formation.

Adherent plaques of vitreous on the macula may cause epiretinal membrane formation.

Vitreous traction also plays a role in the pathogenesis of some instances of CME and macular cyst formation.

ASTEROID HYALOSIS

- It used to be called as asteroid hyalitis, now it is amply clear that, it is not an inflammatory condition, hence asteroid hyalosis is a preferred term. It is benign condition characterized by small yellow-white spherical opacities throughout the vitreous cavity (Fig. 10.5).
- The prevalence of asteroid hyalosis is 0.8–2% in adult population of more than 50 years and it increases with age. It is unilateral in >75% without any gender predominance, no racial predisposition and generally not heritable. Clinical studies have reported a relationship with diabetes and hypertension.

- On 90D biomicroscopy examination the asteroid bodies appear small round to oval opacities suspended in the vitreous. These bodies move as vitreous moves and tend to settle back to their original position. Gravity does not affect their location. The size of granules varies from 3–100 μm.
- The presence of asteroid in the vitreous hardly affect patient's vision since the small proportion of light rays are scattered by the asteroid bodies that is in contrast to the effect of irregular or diffuse vitreous opacities, such as vitreous inflammation or hemorrhage which significantly degrade retinal image. However, rarely when it is very dense it may affect vision.
- The asteroid bodies have been shown to be composed of calcium containing phospholipids.
- So far the etiopathogenesis of asteroid hyalosis is unclear. Unilaterality in vast majority rule out systemic factors and it appears that some unknown local factors come into play in this condition.
- The condition do not require any treatment, however, in some situations, extremely dense asteroid may hinder the view of retina particularly in the assessment of diabetic retinopathy. Surprisingly in this eventuality FFA provides an excellent view of the fundus and of retinal vasculature when USG and OCT provide a very limited view.
- The patient may be subject to PPV in the following circumstances only:
  – Poor visualization of the fundus.
  – Inability to localize retinal breaks in rhegmatogenous RD.
  – Rarely if there are visual symptoms.

PVD rate in eyes with asteroid hyalosis is low compared to age matched persons from the population. It is difficult to induce PVD in asteroid hyalosis implying thereby stronger vitreoretinal attachments. Several authors reported retinal tears while removing vitreous in eyes with asteroid hyalosis. Thus one should be careful and avoid itrogenic breaks during PPV in patients of asteroid hyalosis.

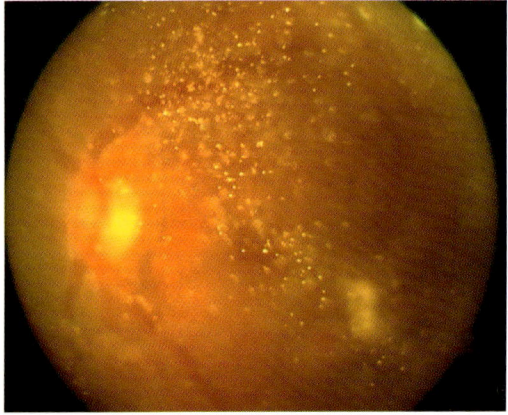

Fig. 10.5 *Fundus photograph showing asteroid hyalosis*

VITREOUS AMYLOIDOSIS

The term implies as if there is deposition of amyloid material only in vitreous. The deposition involves all the ocular as well as orbital tissues. Since the amyloid deposits can be clearly discerned in the vitreous body and once the clinical diagnosis is established by vitreous biopsy, it is said to be pathognomic of familial amyloidotic polyneuropathy (FAP). Thus vitreous amyloidosis is part of FAP.

FAP is rare subtype of amyloidosis caused by mutations in transthyretin gene (TTR), which leads to aggregation of beta pleated sheet of proteins in various tissues. FAP is characterized by:

- Vitreous opacities
- Cardiomyopathy
- Neuropathies-peripheral, autonomic, central

The systematic disease is of interest to the vitreoretinal specialist since it is the only amyloidosis with vitreal involvement. It is typically transmitted in an autosomal dominant fashion. FAP has four types, all share peripheral neuropathy as a clinical feature but vitreal involvement is seen in types I and II only.

Ophthalmic features

Symptoms. The onset of symptoms usually begins after the third decade characterized by dysfunction of three major organ systems, either in isolation or in combination, however, the involvement of the vitreous is often a presenting feature. Patient experiences progressive deterioration of vision usually of both eyes, one eye may be more involved than the other but rarely it is unilateral (Fig. 10.6).

Signs. Ophthalmic findings are varied as amyloid is deposited in various ocular and orbital tissues:

- *Dry eyes* because of amyloid deposit in lacrimal glands.
- *Perilimbal microaneurysm* in the conjunctiva.
- *Reduction of coreal sensitivity.*
- *Pupillary change.* The pupillary margin have a scalooped configuration. The pupil may be unequal in size and in some cases nonreactive to light and near reflex.
- *Fleck deposits* on the anterior surface of lens and pupillary margin like pseudoexfoliation.

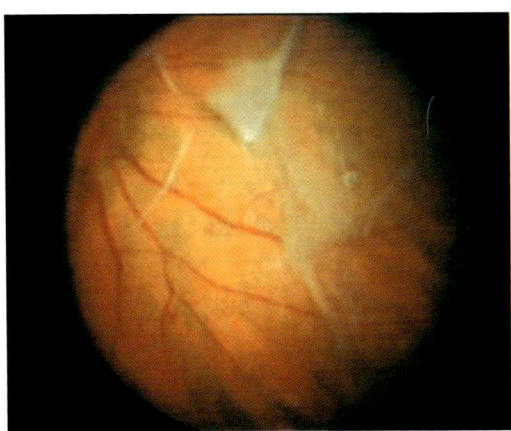

Fig. 10.6 *Fundus photograph showing amyloid deposits in vitreous cavity*

Multiple small dots or footplates are formed on the posterior lens surface known as pseudopodiolentis which is hallmark of vitreous amyloidosis.

- *Raised IOP* and glaucomatous optic nerve damage.
- *Diffuse deposits of fibrillar opacities throughout the vitreous.* These whitish or grey opacities have 'cobweb', 'glasswool' or 'cotton wool' appearance.
- Retina show *perivascular infiltrates and sheathing,* perifoveal intraretinal amyloid deposit forming a grey ring. Multiple superficial grayish retinal lesion resembling cotton wool spots are indivative of intraretinal amyloid infiltration. Dot and blot hemorrhages are occasionally seen in the equatorial region.
- *On FFA* arteriolar filling defects are seen, macula edema, multiple microaneurysmal abnormalities and staining of cotton wool like infiltrates are seen.
- *EOG* may display reduced dark or light troughs. ERG may depict reduced scotopic response or may be normal. VEP may demonstrate prolongation of the P 100 latency in some of the cases.

Prognosis, diagnosis, differential diagnosis and treatment

Prognosis of FAP is poor, the course of the disease is relentlessly progressive and leads to death within 5–15 years of the onset of symptoms:

Diagnosis. Classical clinical picture as above. Vitreous biopsy is confirmatory

Differential diagnosis is depicted in Table 10.1

Treatment. Pars plana vitrectomy helps in visual rehabilitation, however, there is higher recurrence rate of amyloid deposits in 20–25% cases. The vitrectomy should be as complete as possible in order to avoid recurrence. The visual acuity may improve to 6/12 in 50% of cases after 3 years of follow up.

CHOLESTEROLOSIS BULBI (SYNCHYSIS SCINTILLANS)

Benson in 1984 was the first to distinguish between asteroid hyalosis and synchisis scintillans. In this condition vitreous is laden with numerous, yellowish white, gold or multicolored, glistening, angular and crystalline bodies formed of cholesterol. These float freely in the usually liquid vitreous and tend to settle inferiorly. These are stirred up with the movement of the eye to settle down again with every pause. This phenomenon appears as a beautiful shower of golden rain on ophthalmoscopic examination, hence the name synchisis scintillans (Fig. 10.7).

The condition occurs almost exclusively in eyes that have undergone repeated or severe accidental or surgical trauma with large intraocular hemorrhages. The origin of these cholesterol crystals is not known but probably come from leaking retinal vessels. The vision is usually spared but there is hardly any treatment of the condition.

Difference between synchisis scintillans and asteroid hyalosis are depicted in Table 10.2.

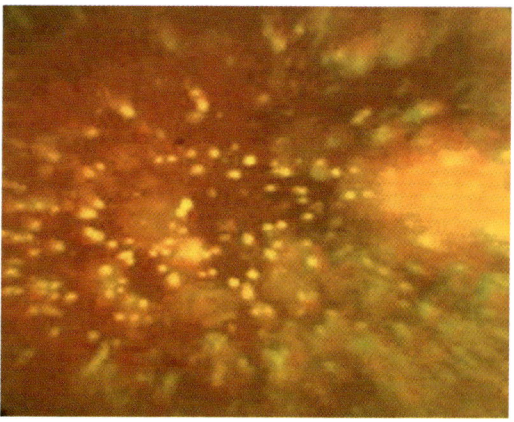
Fig. 10.7 *Fundus photograph showing synchisis scintillans*

INTRAOCULAR LYMPHOMAS

Several types of lymphoma can involve the eye and mimic uveitis and thus rightly termed as masquerade syndrome:
- Non-Hodgkin's lymphoma of CNS
- Systemic non-Hodgkin's lymphomas metastatic to eye.
- Hodgkin's lymphoma.

Characteristic features

- The involvement of eye is relatively rare in Hodgkin's lymphoma and occurs late in the course of disease. The involvement of eye is more frequent in the other two distinct forms of non-Hodgkin's lymphoma. Patients with systemic non-Hodgkin's lymphoma metastatic to the eye are usually quite sick with fever, lymphadenopathy and weight loss. The diagnosis of ocular lymphoma in this type is usually not difficult. However, non-Hodgkin's lymphoma of CNS may present first with ocular findings often posing a diagnostic dilemma.

Table 10.1 *Difference between asteroid hyalosis and vitreous amyloidosis*		
Features	*Asteroid hyalosis*	*Vitreous amyloidosis*
Laterality	Unilateral	Bilateral
Effect on vision	None	Decreased vision
Progression	Slow	Rapid
Appearance of deposits	Small yellow white spherical opacities	Cobweb, glass wool
Systemic association	None	Neuropathy Cardiomyopathy

Table 10.2 *Differences between asteroid hyalosis and synchisis scintillans*

Asteroid hyalosis	Synchisis scintillans
1. Vitreous is formed	1. Vitreous is liquefied and PVD is present.
2. The opacities are greyish white in color, small round or oval in shape and are suspended in the vitreous.	2. The bodies are golden yellow, angular, crystalline and glistening in color. These move like a shower of golden rain.
3. Most of the patients are diabetic	3. Occur in severely traumatized eyes with intraocular hemorrhages.
4. These are calcium-containing phospholipids.	4. Cholesterol crystals.

- The median age of presentation is between 50 and 60 years. Mostly the disease starts in one eye and the other eye is involved in due course of time.
- The patient has typical signs and symptoms of panuveitis. Vitreous cells, occurring in sheets are typical of the disease.
- Panuveitis along with history of seizures, headaches, focal weakness, sensory deficits, confusion, difficulty in gait are all strong indications of CNS involvement.
- MRI and lumbar puncture should be ordered to clinch the diagnosis of NHL-CNS.
- Vitreous biopsy may be sent for cytological analysis.
- Treatment of the condition is the treatment of NHL-CNS which is beyond the preview of this book.

Thus a strong suspicion of neoplastic condition such as large cell lymphoma should be considered in the differential of a case of panuveitis with collection of vitreous cells occurring in sheets. If there are associated CNS symptoms it may be NHL-CNS or if the patient is quite sick with lymphadenopathy and weight loss, it may be systemic non-Hodgkin's lymphoma metastatic to eye. Nevertheless when in doubt vitreous biopsy can clinch the diagnosis.

FAMILIAL VITREORETINAL DISORDERS

There are certain inherited conditions which have almost similar if not identical ocular features, however, the relative frequency of retinal detachment varied among pedigrees. The hall mark of these group of conditions is:
- An optically empty vitreous cavity with sparse intravitreal membranes and strands.
- Degenerative pigment epithelial alterations.
- Lattice like changes in the retina.
- The elctroretinogram may be subnormal.

These are classified into two groups. One group is having ocular features exclusively, e.g. Wagner syndrome and Jansen syndrome. The 2nd group in addition to ocular features also have associated systemic features like Stickler syndrome. In general ophthalmic practice one may come across these, thus the salient features of the following syndromes with optically empty vitreous cavity will be discussed:
- Stickler syndrome
- Wagner syndrome
- Jansen syndome

Stickler syndrome

It was first reported by Gunner B Stickler in 1965. It has an incidence of 1 in 10000 population and both sexes are equally affected. Stickler termed it as hereditary progressive arthro-ophthalmo-pathy and is variably severe connective tissue disorder. It is characterised by distinctive facial abnormalities, ocular features, hearing loss and bone and joint involvement. COLZA1 is the gene responsible in majority (75%) of patients of Stickler disease. Gene COL 11A1 is responsible for Type II and gene COL 11A2 cause Stickler like syndrome. It is transmitted by autosomal dominant inheritance meaning thereby that if there is one affected parent then the chances of passing on the syndrome to the offspring is 50%.

Clinical features

- Ocular features include optically empty vitreous cavity with sparse intravitreal membranes and strands. Additional features are high myopia, developmental cataract, open angle glaucoma and characteristically patient is highly prone to retinal detachment (Fig. 10.8).
- Oro-facial abnormalities included flattening of middle third of the face inclusive of nasal

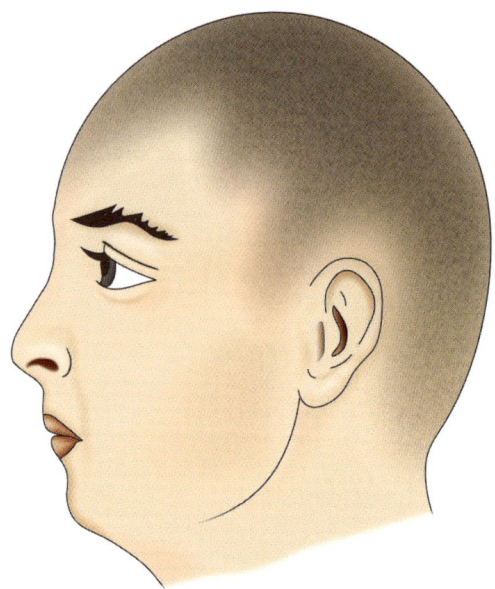

Fig. 10.8 *Face of the patient of Stickler syndrome having relative mandibular hypoplasia*

bridge and maxilla. The patients have Pierre Robin malformation complex of micrognathia, cleft palate and glassoptosis.
- Some degree of sensorineural deafness is seen in 40% patients.
- The skeletal abnormalities may not be that obvious but one must keep a high index of suspicion in order to diagnose these. These include joint hyperextensibility, precocious arthritis and mild spondyloepiphyseal dysplasia.
- It is important to recognize this condition because of high incidence of RD. The RD once occurs, is difficult to repair due to multiple posterior and large breaks and propensity to have PVR. Patient with a Stickler syndrome is a candidate for prophylaxis before he develops RD which is difficult to treat. It is common cause of giant retinal tear (GRT) in a young child.
- Perivascular pigmentation, a variety of lattice may be seen. It may extend posteriorly in a radial fashion.
- ERG is normal initially but may be reduced with the progress of the disease. Visual fields are normal initially but may get constricted later in the course of disease.

Mangement
- Periodic fundus examination of all family members in order to localize breaks if there are any and to subject these to prophylactic laser retinopexy.
- Cataract extraction is required relatively early in life.
- RD if any is treated by bucking or by vitreo-retinal surgical technique, however, the prognosis is poor.
- The other systemic features are treated by specialists of that discipline.

Genetic counselling and examination of family members at high risk are mandatory in this disease. If one of the parents is affected there is 50% chance of passing on the disease to the offspring. Each sib of an affected individual has 25% chance of being affected, 50% chance of being asymptomatic carrier and 25% chance of being unaffected.

Wagner syndrome

It is a rare hereditary vitreoretinal disease described by Hans Wagner in 1938. It is a connective tissue disorder affecting the collagen. It is autosomal dominant in inheritance with 100% penetrance and without any sex predilection. The main feature is optically empty vitreous lacking normal structure. The gene responsible for it has recently been found. It is the vesicant gene (CSPG2) on the long arm(q) of the 5th chromosome (5q 13–14).

Clinical features
- Ocular findings are similar but not identical to Stickler. The two conditions are now considered distinct entities both genetically and phenotypically.
- The characteristic feature is optically empty vitreous with some strands and veils of vitreous which is best examined by indirect ophthalmoscopy or Goldmann three mirror contact lens.
- Anterior or posterior cortical cataracts are common mostly in the third decade of life and it progress with age. Mild to moderate myopia is present.
- Contrary to earlier reports, on recent analysis of original predigree it has been observed that

Features	Wagner/Jansen syndrome	Stickler syndrome
1. Inheritance	Autosomal dominant.	Autosomal dominant
2. Visual acuity	Deteriorates slowly after 20 years due to posterior chorioretinal atrophy	Usually good unless affected by RD or foveal atrophy
3. Prevalence	1 : 1000000	1 : 10000
4. Retinal detachment	Common in Jansen rare in Wagner	50% have RD
5. Other features	Anterior chamber dysgenesis Cataract Optically empty vitreous Optic nerve dysmorphism Chorioretinal atrophy Glaucoma Nyctalopia	Cataract Glaucoma Optically empty vitreous Radial perivascular retinal Degeneration Radial and circumferential/ Lattice
6. Systemic features	None	Cleft palate, flat mid face Hearing loss Epiphyseal dysplasia Osteoarthritis
7. ERG	ROD response affected first, reduced in older partients	Normal
8. Gene	CSPG2	COL2A1
9. Genetic Loci	5q 13–14	COL11A1 12q14, 1P21

Table 10.3 *Wagner/Jansen syndrome versus Stickler syndrome*

patients of Wagner disease are also predisposed to RD but the risk is relatively less than that of Stickler. The RDs are simpler and managed by buckling successfully.

- Bone spicule perivascular pigmentation along both artery and veins can occur and optic atrophy may be present.
- Contrary to Stickler the Wagner disease do not have any systemic features of bones, joints, face and ears.
- ERG is normal initially but it is reduced and correspond with the chorioretinal findings.

Management

- Cataract correction may be required early in life.
- Prophylactic treatment of retinal breaks should be performed.
- All the family members be examined and genetic counselling is imperative.

Jansen syndrome

This syndrome has exactly the same ocular features as the Wagner syndrome even the responsible gene has also been detected to be same (vesican gene). The difference is that Wagner studied the condition in Swiss family whereas Jansen studied in the dutch family. The

other difference is that RD is always associated in the pedigree of Jansen disease and the RD has poor prognosis while the incidence of RD is very low in Wagner and RD is simple and can be treated successfully by buckling procedure only.

Wagner/Jansen syndrome versus stickler syndrome

Table 10.3 depicts the cardinal features.

BIBLIOGRAPHY

1. Cuilla TA, Tolentino F, Morrow JF, et al. Vitreous amyloidosis in familial amyloidotic poly-neuropathy. Report of a case with the Val 30 met tranthyretin mutation. Surv Ophthalmol 1995; 40:197–206.
2. Fawzi AA, VoB, Kriwanek R, et al. Asteroid hyalosis in an autopsy population: The UCLA experience. Arch. Ophthalmol 2005; 123: 486–90.
3. Monteiro JG, Martins AFF, Figuera A, et al. Ocular changes in FAP with dense vitreous deposits. Eye 1991; 5: 99–105.
4. Tina RMHR, Donald JD, Robert BB. Diseases of vitreous. In: Albert DM, Miller JW, Azar DT, Blodi BA, (eds). Alber and Jakobiec's Principles and Practice of Ophthalmology. Philadelphia: Saunders; 2008: chap 188; p. 2387.

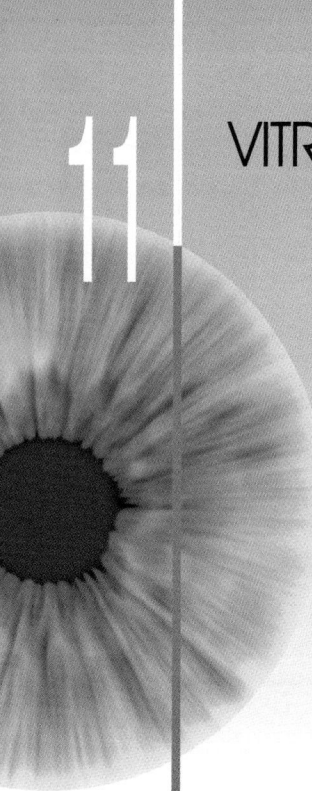

VITREOUS HEMORRHAGE

Sunandan Sood, Panchmi Gupta

GENERAL CONSIDERATIONS AND ETIOPATHOGENESIS

Introduction
- Blood-vitreous barrier
- Etiopathogenesis vitreous hemorrhage

CLINICAL PROFILE AND MANAGMENT
- Clinical features
- Fate of vitreous hemorrhage

- Diagnosis
- Treatment

COMPLICATIONS AND VITREOUS HEMORRHAGE IN VITRECTOMIZED EYES
- Complications
- Vitreous hemorrhage in vitrectomized eyes

GENERAL CONSIDERATIONS AND ETIOPATHOGENESIS

INTRODUCTION

Vitreous is transparent and one of the most delicate connective tissue of the body. It forms almost 80% volume of the eyeball. A healthy vitreous is in gel form and is devoid of blood vessels. However, blood may extravasate into it either from retinal or uveal source. Mostly hemorrhage into the vitreous leads to sudden painless diminutions of vision. Total or near total vitreous hemorrhage leads to a condition where neither patient sees anything nor doctor can see the fundus detail.

BLOOD-VITREOUS BARRIER

Normally the vitreous constituents do not equilibrate with the surrounding retina. The mechanisms which maintain this barrier are as under:
- *The tight junctions of retinal vascular endo-thelium,* pigmented and nonpigmented

epithelium of ciliary body, these form blood-vitreous barrier. These tight junctions inhibit the passage of high molecular weight blood constituents into vitreous.
- *An active transport pump mechanism* located at the above mentioned sites.
- *At the vitreoretinal interface there is presence of basal lamina* which causes physiological blockage of transport of large molecular weight molecules.
- *The vitreous hyaluronic acid network* has physiochemical properties which retard or actually block the movement of cations, cells and macromolecules.

By virtue of these barriers vitreous remains transparent and free of blood and its consti-tuents. However, this barrier can be broken by many pathological conditions mentioned below causing vitreous hemorrhage.

ETIOPATHOGENESIS OF VITREOUS HEMORRHAGE

- *In blunt trauma* the retina may be torn and the blood vessels bridging the tear may bleed into the vitreous. In addition there may be avulsion

159

of superficial retinal vessels and rupture of ciliary body causing vitreous hemorrhage.

- *In proliferative retinopathies* like PDR and following CRVO, BRVO and vasculitis, new vessels grow on the surface of retina (NVE) and on to the posterior hyaloid and surface. PVD induced by loss of ionic equilibrium exerts traction at these fragile and delicate new vessels, which bleed and cause vitreous hemorrhage. Even the movement of eyeball cause movement of vitreous body causing traction on these, new vessels which rupture and bleed (Fig. 11.1).
- *PVD* occurring as a result of aging process in the vitreous or due to trauma may tear the adherent retina and adjoining blood vessels causing vitreous hemorrhage (Terson's syndrome) (*see* Fig. 10.4).
- *Rise of subarachnoid pressure* as in sub-arachnoid hemorrhage may cause subhyaloid hemorrhage (Terson's syndrome) (Fig. 11.2).
- Chronic uveoretinal inflammation may cause neovascularisation resulting in vitreous hemorrhage.
- Intraocular tumors may invade the retinal vessels and cause vitreous hemorrhage.
- Blood dyscrasias can also result into vitreous hemorrhage as anywhere else in the body.
- *Retinal neovascularisation* due to any other cause.
- *Parsplanitis.*

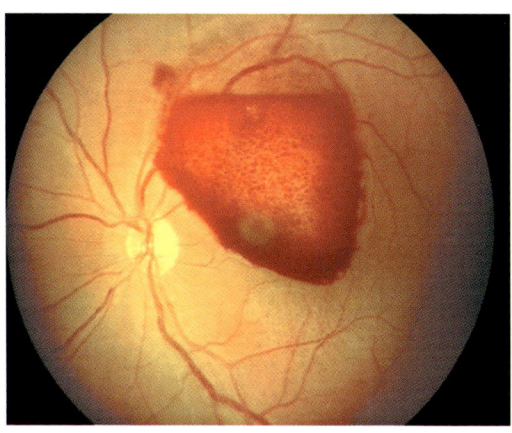

Fig 11.2 *Fundus photograph showing a boat shaped subhyaloid hemorrhage*

CLINICAL PROFILE AND MANAGEMENT

CLINICAL FEATURES

- *Sudden painless loss of vision* the severity of which depends on the size and location of the vitreous hemorrhage. If the hemorrhage is small and trickles inferiority then the loss of vision might be of few lines and the patient may complain of only foggy vision. However, large hemorrhage involving the whole of vitreous leads to drastic loss of vision which may be finger counting close to face. Thus a proper record of the vision should be made.

- *Direct pupillary reaction* may vary from almost normal to sluggish, ill sustained reaction. In a dense vitreous hemorrhage relative afferent pupillary conduction defect (RAPD) may be present.

- *Iris should be examined* for rubeosis iridis.

- *Fundus detail after dilating pupil* should be carried out either by 90 D slit lamp or by 20D indirect ophthalmoscopy with brightest light. It is common experience that in spite of dense vitreous hemorrhage the peripheral retina may be visible by indirect ophthalmoscopy with sclera indentation and the cause of vitreous hemorrhage may become obvious.

- If no view is possible then the diagnosis is made by *B-scan ultrasonography.*

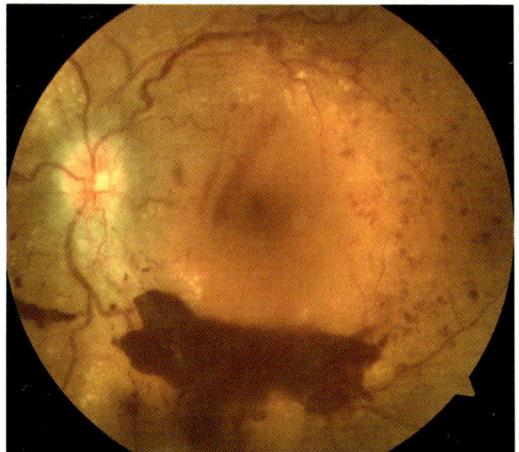

Fig 11.1 *Fundus photograph showing PDR with vitreous hemorrhage*

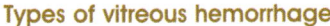

Types of vitreous hemorrhage

Intravitreal hemorrhage. If the hemorrhage occurs with in the vitreous body it is called as intravitreal hemorrhage. It can be complete or incomplete. In later type it can be anterior, central or posterior vitreous hemorrhage.

Subvitreal hemorrhage. If the hemorrhage is present with in the posterior hyaloid face and internal limiting membrane of retina it is called as subvitreal hemorrhage. Clinically it is also called as subhyaloid or preretinal hemorrhage.

Appearance of vitreous hemorrhage

It depends upon the following:
- Whether vitreous is gel/liquid.
- The amount of bleeding.
- Changes that occur in vitreous due to the presence of blood in it.

1. *If the bleeding is small and occurs in a formed vitreous,* the blood readily clots along the vitreous fibers, looks red and forms finger like intravitreal projections. In the gel vitreous the blood remains stationary and hardly moves with the movement of the eye. With time the hemolysis of erythrocytes occur, blood in vitreous also promotes liquefaction and cavity formation. With the synchisis of vitreous the blood tends to accumulate in the dependent part of the globe due to gravity. The red colored opacities may transform to yellowish fluffy vitreous opacities and membranes. It takes few months to years for the hemorrhage to clear. The posterior hemorrhage in the vicinity of retina clears earlier than the central and anteriror vitreous hemorrhage.
2. *If the bleeding occurs in a synchitic vitreous (fluid),* the blood remains unclotted because the clotting factors are diluted by the fluid vitreous. It accumulate in the dependent part of the globe. It disperse with the movement of globe leading to fluctuating vision, i.e. patient may tell that vision is better in the morning than other part of the day.
3. *If the bleeding is massive hardly* any glow is appreciated. In this eventuality one has to wait for few weeks to ascertain the appearance of hemorrhage and to evaluate the retina by 20 D indentation indirect ophthalmoscopy.

4. *The diagnosis of subvitreal or subhyaloid hemorrhage* is very easy. It is typically described as boat shaped hemorrhage with a straight superior horizontal configuration and semicircular inferior border. Sometimes layering of blood is seen which consists of a thin yellow top layer of plasma components and thick red cell layer at the bottom. It may trickle inferiorly in the eventuality of posterior vitreous detachment. It is commonly seen in Terson's syndrome and in diabetes (Fig. 11.2).

FATE OF VITREOUS HEMORRHAGE

Resolution of vitreous hemorrhage occurs. The rate of resolution depends upon the following factors:
- *Amount of blood.* Small vitreous hemorrhage resolve earlier.
- *State of vitreous.* The hemorrhage in formed vitreous takes longer to absorb than in the fluid vitreous.
- *Proximity to retina.* Posterior hemorrhages close to the retinal circulation resolve earlier than anterior and central vitreous hemorrhage.

The blood in the vitreous undergoes fibrinolysis, RBC hemolysis and absorption of breakdown products of blood by macrophage assisted phagocytosis. The small vitreous hemorrhage may resolve completely whereas in large vitreous hemorrhage the vitreous may lose its transparency and become opaque because of organisation of vitreous hemorrhage.

DIAGNOSIS

- In most instances if not immediately but with the passage of time complete fundus examination by scleral depression indirect ophthalmoscopy can help in the establishment of cause of vitreous hemorrhage.
- The history of diabetes, hypertension and clues from the examination of the fellow eye may also help in the diagnosis.
- The history of trauma is important and fundus may depict choroidial ruptures and other evidence of trauma.
- In case of NVE/NVD, rule out causes of proliferative retinopathies like, vasculitis BRVO, CRVO and diabetes.

- In dense vitreous hemorrhage **B-scan ultrasonography** may help. It can also help in ruling out RD and intraocular tumor. In these cases bilateral patch and sleeping with head end raised for about 7–10 days may help in clearing the hemorrhage and fundus visualization. In case cause is not detected, repeated indirect ophthalmoscopy and ultrasonography may help in arriving at the diagnosis in due course of time.
- Utrasonography is useful adjunct to the clinical examination. This technique may not pick up fresh unclotted blood, but as the cellular accumulation occurs, reflectivity increases proportionately.
- In mild hemorrhage a chain of low amplitude spikes is seen on A-scan and dots and short lines are displayed on B-scan. In more dense hemorrhage higher reflectivity on A-scan and greater the number of opacities on B-scan are seen. The gray scale display is better perceived at 80–90 dB and when the sensitivity is reduced from 80–70 dB the majority of echoes disappear (Fig. 11.3).
- If the blood gets organised, larger interfaces are formed resulting in higher reflectivity on A-scan and membranous surface on B-scan.
- PVD is common with vitreous hemorrhage. In B-scan the PVD is usually smooth with or without any attachment to the optic nerve. It may become thick particularly inferiorly and posteriorly due to aggregation of cells on its surface. Accordingly reflectivity may vary

from extremely low to extremely high spikes, thus difficult to differentiate from RD. It is the kinetic echography on B-scan which clinches the diagnosis. In PVD B-scan shows typically a very fluid after movements where as in RD these after movements are slow and less mobile (p. 114 and 115).

TREATMENT

- Small vitreous hemorrhage resolves spontaneously within few week to few months.
- It is imperative to wait for at least two months for the hemorrhage to resolve. However, if it does not resolve, it is labelled as nonclearing vitreous hemorrhage and the treatment is vitrectomy and treatment of underlying pathology.
- *Early parsplana vitrectomy* is considered if there is associated rehagmatogenous or tractional RD. Diabetic retinopathy vitrectomy study (DRVS) also recommended early vitrectomy in diabetic vitreous hemorrhage with TRD. In indicated cases endophotocoagulation is also carried out in order to prevent recurrence.
- *In traumic vitreous hemorrhage vitrectomy is recommended within 14 days* of injury. The goals of the vitrectomy are to clear the media, to remove the vitreous scaffold from the scleral laceration site, to remove the posterior hyaloid, to identify and treat retinal breaks and RD.
- *Retinal laser photocoagulation* following vitrectomy act as prophylaxis against recurrent vitreous hemorrhage in patients of diabetes, CRVO , BRVO and vasculitis.
- *Laser hyaloidotomy.* In patients of subhyaloid hemorrhage which cause substantial visual loss when present in the macular area can be drained with YAG laser (Laser hyaloidotomy). The blood trickles down to the dependent part of the vitreous cavity with immediate visual improvement.
- *Enzymatic vitreolysis.* Enzyme hyaluronidase in its pure form is being tried in patients of vitreous hemorrhage. It has the capacity to liquefy vitreous thereby settling the blood inferiorly. Resultant clear media allows the examination of the fundus which helps in arriving at the diagnosis and subsequent treatment, eventually the hemorrhage undergo natural absorption.

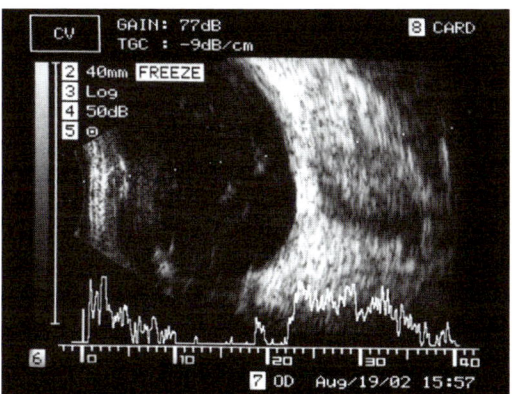

Fig 11.3 *Ultrasound B-scan showing mild to moderate intensity echoes in mid-vitreous cavity suggestive of vitreous hemorrhage*

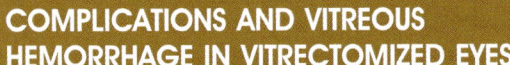

COMPLICATIONS AND VITREOUS HEMORRHAGE IN VITRECTOMIZED EYES

COMPLICATIONS

- *Vitreous syneresis.* Blood affects the collagen fibrillar framework of vitreous and promotes vitreous syneresis.
- *Bands and membranes.* The blood may organise to form bands and membranes, the later may cover the inner surface of neurosensory retina, particularly macula causing cellophane retinopathy. The bands may cause tractional retinal detachment.
- *Secondary glaucoma.* Long-standing vitreous hemorrhage may produce glaucoma by any of the following mechanisms:
  - The RBC lose their elasticity and become khaki colored and rigid known as ghost cells. These cells block the trabecular meshwork (TBM) and cause ghost cell glaucoma particularly when anterior hyaloid face is broken.
  - The RBC debris, haemoglobin aggregate and macrophages may obstruct TBM causing glaucoma known as erythroclastic glaucoma.
  - The hemosiderin released from RBCs sticks to collagen frame work of TBM leding to its inflammation thus embarrassing aqueous outflow and causing glaucoma.
- *Complicated cataract.* The long-standing vitreous hemorrhage can cause complicated cataract.
- *Siderotic change.* The long-standing vitreous hemorrhage can cause siderotic changes in the cornea and retina.
- *Optic atrophy.* Subsequently it may cause necrosis of ganglion cell layer of retina and optic atrophy.

VITREOUS HEMORRHAGE IN VITRECTOMIZED EYES

- With the introduction of AntiVEGF drugs it is a matter of routine to inject AntiVEGF drug intravitrealy before posting the patient for PPV. This drug has made the life of vitreo-retina surgeon easy by remarkably lowering down the incidence of intraoperative bleeding thus the surgeons these days rarely ever comes across an instance of abandoning the surgery because of intractable intraoperative bleeding.

In addition the improvised vitreoretinal surgical techniques, expertise and state of the art equipments further help in achieving adequate intraoperative hemostasis. Still there is small group of patients who can have hemorrhage after parsplana vitrectomy. It can occur in immediate postoperative period or within few months time.

- The one occurring within a week of surgery is mostly due to inadequate intraoperative haemostasis or due to release of RBCs entrapped in the still uncut vitreous base. The hemorrhage in the vitrectomized eyes clears spontaneously and the absorption of blood in aphakic or pseudophakic eyes is thought to be faster than the phakic eyes, as the lens in later acts as a barrier against the anterior migration of RBCs and blood by-products.
- The delayed type hemorrhage occurs either from the rapidly growing neovascular tissue or from fibrovascular ingrowth at the internal aspect of sclerotomy sites or from iris neovascularisation. This type of hemorrhage can be prevented by endolaser or immediate postoperative PRP. Fibrovascular growth is dealt with laser indirect ophthalmoscope. One may observe for few weeks or can either attempt vitreous lavage or sequential fluid gas exchange. If the observation period of about two months does not help then repeat vitrectomy and intraoperative identification and treatment of bleeding sites is recommended. It is preferred that fluid air exchange should be followed by air silicone oil exchange since silicone oil has hydrophobic property and can prevent recurrent post-operative hemorrhage.

BIBLIOGRAPHY

1. Butner RW, McPherson AR. Spontaenous vitreous hemorrhage Ann Ophthalmol 1982; 14: 268–70.
2. DiBernardo C, Blodi B, Byrne SF. Echographic evaluation of retinal tears in patients with spontaneous vitreous hemorrhage. Arch Ophthalmol 1992;110:511–4.
3. Ogawa T Kitaoka T, Dakey, et al. Terson's Syndrome: a case report suggesting the mechanism of vitreous hemorrhage. Ophthalmology 2002;108:1654.
4. Winslow RL, Taylor BC. Spontaneous vitreous hemorrhage: etiology and management South Med J 1980;73:1450–2.

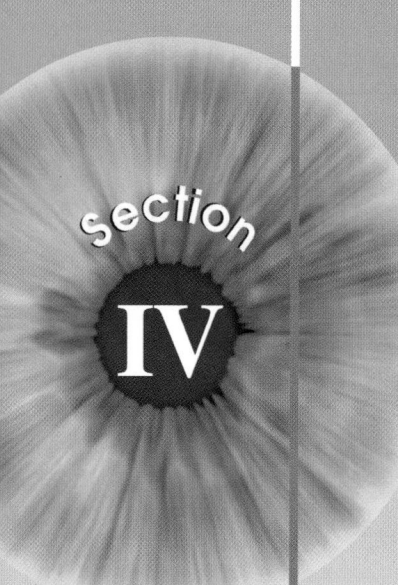

Disorders of Retina

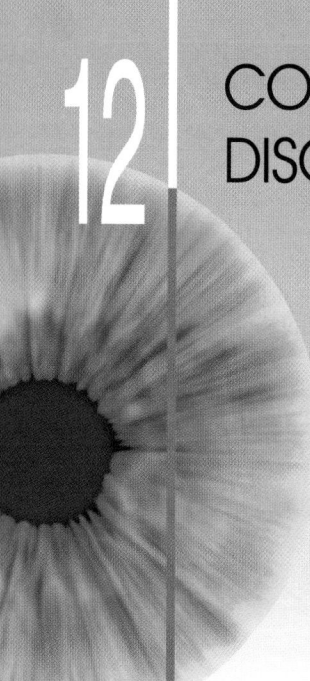

CONGENITAL AND DEVELOPMENTAL DISORDERS OF THE RETINA

Michael T. Trese, Amir H Kashani

INTRODUCTION

There are many named developmental and congenital disorders of the retina. There are also eyes that present with definite vitreoretinal abnormalities that may not fall into a named category of disease, but still behave in a similar fashion of aberrant-formed vitreoretinal adhesion or vitreoretinal juncture and retinal dysplasia of varying degrees. This chapter cannot be encyclopedic, but will focus on familial exudative vitreoretinopathy (FEVR), persistent fetal vasculature syndrome (PFVS), Coats' disease, Norrie's disease, and congenital retinoschisis (CRS). The examination of children is common to all of these diseases and requires close attention to visual behavior since conventional visual acuity measurements may not be possible or reflective of visual potential. It also requires frequent use of examination under anesthesia in this population of children which often cannot be contained and examined in the office.

Although prevalence is an important feature in congenital and developmental disorders of the retina, particularly relative to the merit of screening newborns, it is very difficult to get a prevalence that is reliable in diseases that are considered rare.

COMMON CONGENITAL DISORDERS OF RETINA

FAMILIAL EXUDATIVE VITREORETINOPATHY

Familial exudative vitreoretinopathy (FEVR), originally described by Schepens and Cheswick in the 1969 is a disease that has often been thought of as looking like retinopathy of prematurity, but occurring in full-term infants and without a history of oxygen supplementation. That is a reasonable way to start thinking about familial exudative vitreoretinopathy, but many other features factor into its appearance and behavior that help to make the diagnosis. Eighty-five percent of the time FEVR involves both eyes, although it certainly can be

asymmetric. Mostly it occurs in early age but the disease can reactivate throughout patient's lifetime.

Etiopathogenesis

For many years, it has been known that the initial events of familial exudative vitreo-retinopathy, which involve a malformation of the normal retinal vasculature, leave a variable area of avascular peripheral retina. This avascular peripheral retina has been thought to drive VEGF expression, much like ROP, leading to neovascularization, leakage, exudation, and sometimes combined exudative and tractional retinal detachments. This disease can often lead to blindness or severe visual impairment.

Genetics

Familial exudative vitreoretinopathy is associated with genetic mutations involving frizzled-4 mutations, LRP-5 and 6, Norrie's disease gene, and in T-span-12. Each mutation has been associated with phenotypically recognizable FEVR. These mutations affect WNT signaling and WNT signaling certainly is involved in vascular and neural tissue development. It may be that therapeutic approaches to FEVR may be developed along the lines of WNT signaling control.

Clinical features and staging

In 1998 Pendergast reported a staging of FEVR ranging from stage 1 to stage 5 (Table 12.1 and Fig. 12.1A to E)

Table 12.1 *Clinical classification of familial exudative vitreoretinopathy*

Stage	Clinical feature
1	Avascular retinal periphery without extraretinal vascularization
2	Avascular retinal periphery with extraretinal vascularization—Without exudate—With exudate
3	Retinal detachment-subtotal, not involving fovea—Primarily exudative—Primarily tractional
4	Retinal detachment-subtotal, involving fovea—Primarily exudative—Primarily tractional
5	Retinal detachment-total—Open funnel-Closed funnel

The staging also breaks down the disease into eyes that have little or no exudate and eyes that have larger amounts of leakage or exudate.

Diagnosis

In the past, FEVR has been diagnosed through clinical examination alone looking for features such as a dragged disc, exudative retinal detachment, tractional retinal detachment, radial folds, and folds that contact and adhere to the posterior lens. Today, however, it is impossible to diagnose or manage FEVR, particularly in its more early stages, using wide-field angiography. In a younger individual, this may require an exam under anesthesia and contact wide-field angiography. In older patients, non-contact based wide-field angiography is available in at least a few commercial designs.

Reactivation

One of the most disturbing features of FEVR, which is a lifelong potentially active vitreo-retinal disease, is that it can reactivate throughout a patient's lifetime. We now know that posterior capillary dropout can be an early warning sign of FEVR activation. Posterior capillary dropout precedes exudation and at this time can be treated with appropriate photo-coagulation therapy, much as is done in diabetes and vein occlusions.

Treatment

The current treatment for familial exudative vitreoretinopathy involves peripheral laser ablation of avascular periphery, as well as in some circumstances intravitreal anti-VEGF therapy. The latter course must be approached with caution given the fact that this disease may be diagnosed in developing young children. The other therapeutic possibility is that vitrectomy with the use of ocriplasmin enzyme to cleave the vitreoretinal juncture and silicone oil may be an effective way to manage long term suppression of familial exudative vitreoretinopathy activity.

Future management of this disease may very likely include pharmacotherapy to manipulate blood vessel loss. In summary, the understanding of familial exudative vitreoretinopathy has expanded greatly over the last several years and

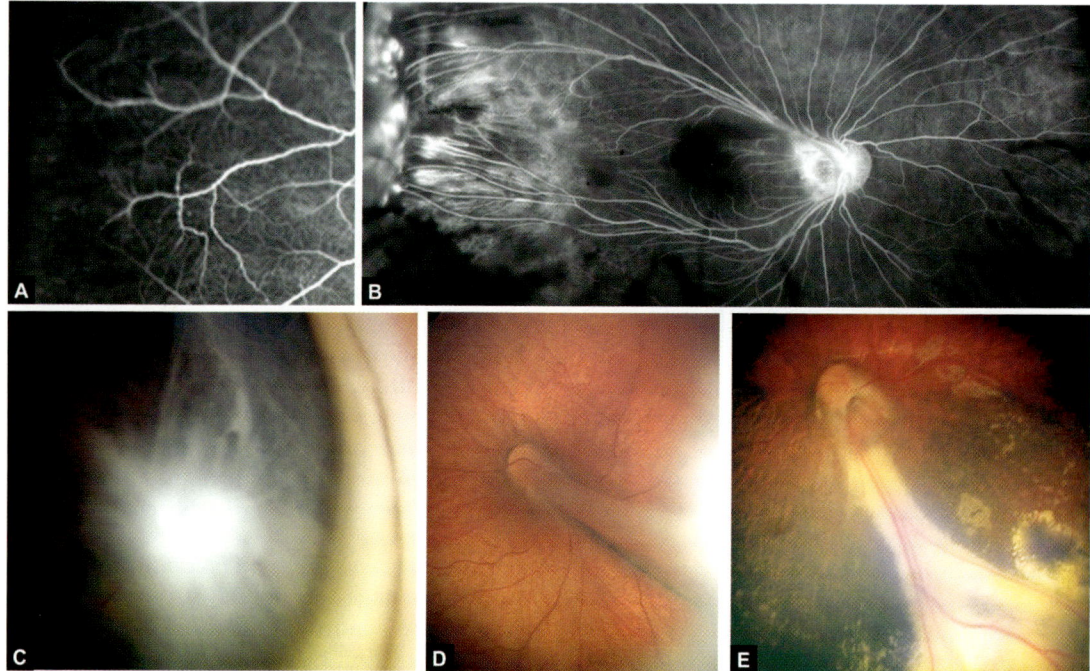

Fig. 12.1 *Image of Familial Exudative Vitreoretinopathy (FEVR).* **(A)** *peripheral avascular areas of Stage 1 FEVR. No leakage is noted in late phase of fluorescein angiography;* **(B)** *wide Field Angiography in Stage 2 FEVR with peripheral laser treatment. Peripheral avascular areas with central vascular and macular dragging. Note the peripheral avascular areas and leakage in late phase angiography indicative of Stage 2 disease;* **(C)** *anterior hyaloidal opacification commonly seen in Stages 3–5 FEVR. Unlike persistent fetal vasculature, this opacification usually does not involve the capsule or lens substance;* **(D)** *classical dry fold of Stage 4 FEVR and* **(E)** *Stage 4 FEVR with prominent exudation suggestion of concurrent active disease or recent disease activity*

hopefully management for the future will be much better for children and families affected by this disease.

PERSISTENT FETAL VASCULATURE SYNDROME

Persistent fetal vasculature syndrome (PFVS) previously referred to as persistent hyperplastic primary vitreous (PHPV) was nicely described by Dr. Goldberg in a Jackson lecture several years ago. In his Jackson lecture, Dr. Goldberg pointed out that the vasculature that persisted in children with this disease was not solely that of the hyaloid system, but also the tunica vasculosa lentis.

Clinical profile

Clinical features

PFVS is unilateral in 90% of cases and children often present with an anterior form, a posterior form or some combination of both (Fig. 12.2A).

- *In cases with anterior involvement the involved eye is commonly smaller eye.* The involved eye often has elongated ciliary processes and a plaque with vessels that can extend to the ciliary processes. These vessels generally tie into the hyaloid vessel and stalk tissue, which customarily extends from the posterior aspect of the opaque material in the area of the lens to the optic nerve (Fig. 12.2B). It is important to note that this opaque material replaces the lens capsule and therefore cannot be peeled from the lens surface.
- *The posterior form* can have a clear posterior lens capsule and have vessels remaining in the posterior pole, most often located at the optic nerve. These vessels can be either very small in the diameter or can be rather stout with a diameter of 1–1.5 millimeters.
- *The combined form* of PFVS has a plaque anteriorly as well as stalk tissue that extends

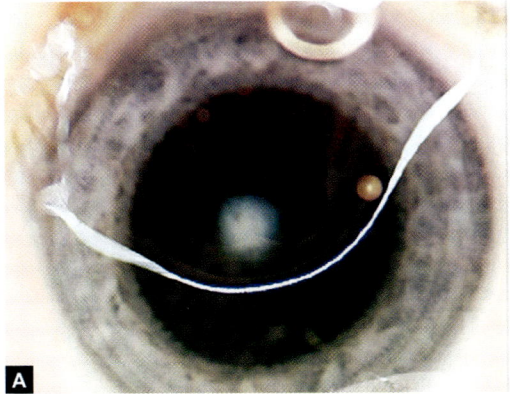

A

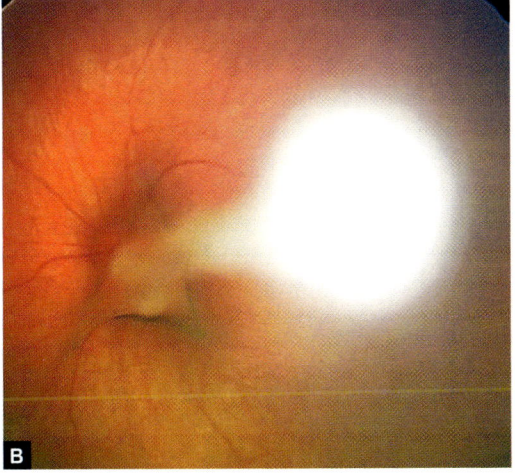

B

Fig. 12.2 *Photographs of persistent fetal vasculature (PFV). (A) external color picture of posterior capsular opacification in PFV. This opacification is intrinsic to the capsular material; and (B) color fundus photograph of remnant stalk tissue extending from the disc to the posterior aspect of the lens. This was a unilateral finding in this child as is common in PFV*

out other life threatening diseases such as retinoblastoma (which uncommonly occurs in smaller eyes) before proceeding with therapy for potential amblyopia and other morphologic features of persistent fetal vasculature syndrome.

The second presentation is in children that have much less of a retrolenticular plaque and have an eccentric insertion in the lens away from the visual axis. This allows them to function visually for several years before presenting in the 6 to 10 year age range with strabismus. These children often have dragging and tractional retinal detachment in the posterior pole making their surgical correction much different than the first mentioned presentation. This will be discussed somewhat later in this chapter.

Unilateral versus bilateral presentation A very large percentage of children with persistent fetal vasculature syndrome have been unilateral in presentation, but there is a small percentage of children who do present with bilateral persistent fetal vasculature syndrome. The bilateral presentation is often misdiagnosed since ophthalmologists are mostly attuned to a unilateral presentation. In addition, the bilateral presentation is often accompanied by a larger amount of retinal dysplasia than the unilateral cases. However, unilateral persistent fetal vasculature syndrome can have very severe gross retinal dysplasia as well. Whenever, the diagnosis of bilateral persistent fetal vasculature syndrome is entertained, Norrie's disease, which will be discussed later in this chapter, must be ruled out. Genetic testing for Norrie's disease is available in a number of centers. As we will see later in this chapter, Norrie's disease has more systemic issues than persistent fetal vasculature syndrome even in its bilateral form as it is currently understood.

posteriorly and often involves a tractional retinal detachment in the area of the optic nerve.

Presentations

Patients can be divided into two categories that present in different ways.

The first presentation is customarily observed around birth and usually involves leukocoria in one eye that is also usually smaller than the other. This leukocoria often brings the child to the attention of the pediatrician performing a red reflex test prior to discharge from the hospital. The investigation then needs to rule

Treatment

Management of persistent fetal vasculature syndrome for the more common presentation at birth is lensectomy, division of stalk tissue, and sometimes diathermy to the stalk vessel if necessary. There are several reasons to divide the stalk cautiously. The most important reason is that retinal tissue can be adherent along the

side of the stalk contributing to the formation of tractional retinal detachment.

The child that presents with an eccentric stalk can be managed with lens-sparing vitrectomy, but the order of division of the stalk appears to be important to avoid damage to the posterior lens capsule and subsequent flocculent cataract formation. In those eyes it is better to divide the stalk with sharp dissection before vitrectomy while being very careful to avoid retinal folds along the side. This can often lead to dramatic retraction of the stalk, which usually is under a large amount of strain. The anterior stalk remaining behind the lens can regress in its entirety leaving a clear lens capsule. The child who presents with the condition of eccentric stalk often presents with strabismus. Many of the children following retinal surgery will have resolution of their strabismus as their tractional retinal detachment resolves.

There are two more severe variations of persistent fetal vasculature syndrome. Persistent fetal vasculature syndrome can be associated with posterior coloboma and this association needs to be ruled out relative to foveal involvement and potential visual acuity results. A second syndrome, microcornea, posterior lenticonus, persistent fetal vasculature and coloboma (or MPPC) has been recently described. This posterior lenticonus can be enormous with the lens itself filling 50 per cent of the vitreous cavity. The surgical results can be rewarding with some of these children achieving very good vision depending on the retinal dysplasia and coloboma in the posterior pole.

A genetic cause of persistent fetal vasculature syndrome has not been identified at this time. However, many of the features of persistent fetal vasculature syndrome seem to be common to other genetically driven diseases such as Norrie's disease. However, at this point Norrie's disease mutations have not been seen in bilateral persistent fetal vasculature syndrome.

Future management of persistent fetal vasculature syndrome in large part involves detection. As screening of newborns is improved, perhaps with photographic screening detection, an earlier intervention will most likely be possible.

Summary

Successful surgical intervention of PFVS involves either clearing the media and/or resolve any tractional retinal detachment. The rate-limiting step in visual prognosis following surgery for PFVS is the amount of retinal dysplasia. We divide retinal dysplasia into two categories:

Gross category, meaning that it is easily visible when the retina can be observed; or

Microscopic category, meaning that there are changes in the retina that are not easily seen with ophthalmoscopy. The prognosis is relatively better in the latter.

COATS' DISEASE

Clinical profile

Coats' disease described by George Coats involves what has been called telangiectatic vessels generally in the periphery. These telangiectatic vessels leak exudative material and can contribute to an exudative deposit in the foveal macular area, which can be devastating to vision. Coats' disease has a very large spectrum from small one-half to one clock hour involvement in the periphery to all 12 clock hours being involved and total exudative retinal detachment (Fig. 12.3A). The peripheral retina beyond the area of the telangiectatic vessels is often avascular and may contribute to the drive from VEGF for this exudative process (Fig. 12.3B). The classic presentation of Coats' disease is unilateral involvement in males but bilateral cases can occur mostly in the first decade of life. It is important to consider retinoblastoma in the differential diagnosis of cases that have a very large exudative retinal detachment. Retinoblastoma must be distinguished from Coats' disease as the management is both different and can be devastating to the child's well-being.

Treatment

Coats' disease has been managed with destructive therapy to the peripheral retina using either cryo or laser therapy to the telangiectatic vessels. These vessels often require repeated treatment and it is important to make this point with the family when the child is initially seen

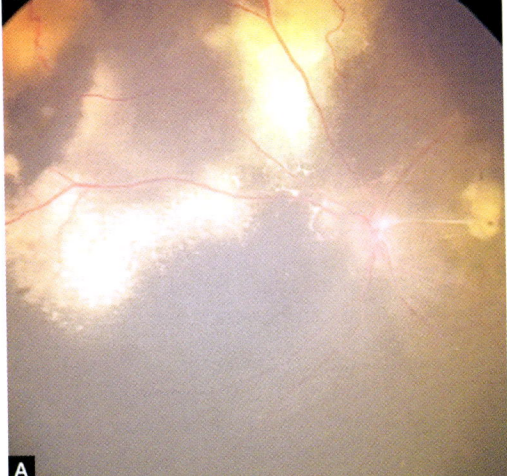

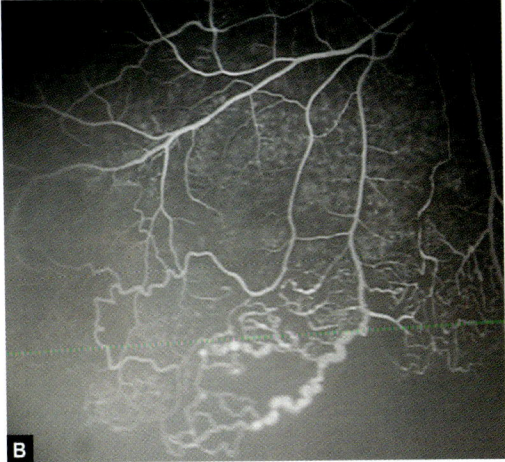

Fig. 12.3 *Representative photographs of a patient with advanced Coats' disease. **(A)** Note the prominent lipid exudation in the periphery as well as the macula in this case. The lack of RPE granularity suggests a very large exudative retinal detachment involving nearly the whole retina and **(B)** fluorescein angiography reveals large avascular areas in the periphery with characteristic telangiectasias*

so the family does not leave with the impression that one treatment will leave the child completely treated. It is important to follow these children regularly in clinic throughout their lives.

In the era of anti-VEGF therapy, the role of anti-VEGF injections has been explored by Jumper who feels that the central macular lesion may be able to be suppressed by the use of repeated anti-VEGF therapy. This needs to be confirmed by other investigators.

The management of Coats' disease can include destruction by cryotherapy, laser, photodynamic therapy, and can involve direct vascular destruction with diathermy during vitrectomy in very refractory cases.

The visual acuity in Coats' disease is entirely dependent upon avoiding the characteristic central lipid deposit. This lipid deposit appears to occur without contiguous lipid deposition from the periphery, much like a macular star.

The exact pathophysiology of this is not well understood, but this process may be avoided by vigilant destruction of the telangiectatic vessels, which can reopen following treatment.

Glaucoma can result with Coats' disease and management of intraocular pressure is often an issue in Coats' patients. Control of the retinal telangiectatic vessels and avascular retina by destructive retinopexy may help with the management of glaucoma.

The bilateral features of Coats' disease are indeed uncommon as is presentation of what is called "Coats' reaction" in a female. These are managed in the same fashion as described above.

NORRIE'S DISEASE

Clinical profile

Norrie's disease is a complex ocular and systemic disease. Norrie's disease has malformation of vasculature and neural tissue. In its most complicated form Norrie's disease also involves ocular structures, the ear, and central nervous system. Norrie's disease has been reported in multiple children in single families and is the result of mutations in the Norrie's disease gene. The mutations in the Norrie's disease gene can present with a familial exudative vitreoretinopathy phenotype as mentioned above as well as the Norrie's disease phenotype. Approximately 30 percent of children with Norrie's disease have the full-blown disease involving the central nervous system, hearing, and ocular structure malformations. The visual acuity results in Norrie's disease are greatly dependent on the level of retinal dysplasia. Previously it had been felt that no therapy was helpful for Norrie's disease; however, recently Walsh has reported that surgical intervention in Norrie's disease can lead to both preservation of the eye, as well as visual acuity, with the best reported

acuity of 20/200, which is truly remarkable vision in what can be a very devastating retinal disease.

Presentations

Norrie's disease has a variety of ocular presentations. **One presentation** is with a very thin avascular peripheral retina and an oval appearing structure of retina in the vitreous cavity with a stalk extending from the center of this oval retinal structure to the posterior aspect of the lens (Fig. 12.4). Interestingly, this avascular peripheral retina in Norrie's disease does not seem to drive the same type of VEGF response that several other pediatric retinal diseases with avascular peripheral retina do, possibly because the retina is so thin that it can receive oxygenation and nutrients from the choroidal circulation. Therefore, in Norrie's disease peripheral laser ablation is not generally suggested. In fact with peripheral laser ablation a multitude of peripheral retinal holes can be generated. Although it is not known for sure, it is possible that the child may achieve at least some light perception with this avascular peripheral retina.

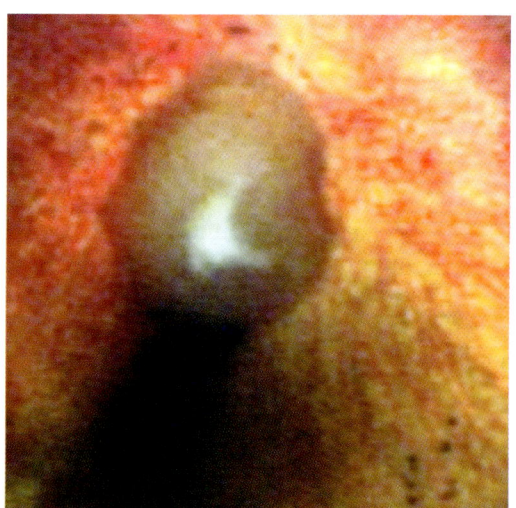

Fig. 12.4 *Representative photograph of patient with Norrie's disease. Note the typical large dysplastic appearing tissue in the posterior pole that is assumed to be retina. Note the dense appearing white stalk tissue that is emanating from the globular, dysplastic retinal mass towards the viewer. The atrophic peripheral retina is characterized by black areas representing pigmentary changes*

End-stage Norrie's disease may mimic severely dysplastic persistent fetal vasculature syndrome, and perhaps even very severe familial exudative vitreoretinopathy. Differentiation may be very difficult as all the three diseases can be bilateral and all three can involve subretinal hemorrhage and exudate. As one possible clue to differentiating them, the retinal dysplasia and vascular changes of Norrie's disease and persistent fetal vasculature syndrome seem to be worse than those of familial exudative vitreoretinopathy. So the FEVR total retinal detachment may have relatively normal appearing retinal tissue, whereas Norrie's disease and persistent fetal vasculature syndrome, tend to have retinal tissue that appears greatly disorganized.

Treatment

Norrie's disease is a classic example of a defect in WNT signaling (gene controlling signaling pathways that affect the way the cells and tissue develop) and involves very severe tissue changes of both neural and vascular tissue in the central nervous system, auditory, and the ocular structures. This type of disease can be prevented in animal models by driving WNT signaling using the protein Norrin as has been shown by a number of authors.

Future improvements in the diagnosis and management of Norrie's disease would seem to be based on prenatal detection, which is uncommonly performed at this time. The management of Norrie's disease currently consists of childhood screening and possible surgical therapy for gross changes in ocular structures based on the work of Walsh et al.

CONGENITAL RETINOSCHISIS

Clinical profile

Congenital retinoschisis (CRS) has been described for many years and involves a six exon gene in which well over a hundred mutations have been described. The classic teaching originally based on Congenital X-linked retinoschisis was that 100 percent of eyes had foveal schisis and 50 percent had peripheral retinoschisis. In these cases schisis was thought to involve the nerve fiber layer splitting from the

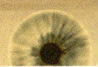

neurosensory retina. CRS tends to be a bilateral disease that primarily affects males while females are usually silent carriers.

The electrophysiology of this disease has been consistent and well-known to affect the b-wave. Interestingly, the b-wave is primarily a reflection of mid-retinal structure, which we know is perhaps the common area of retinal destruction based on more recent optical coherence tomography (OCT) studies.

Classification system

Classification system of congenital retinoschisis has been developed that focuses on three features. (Table 12.2 and Fig. 12.5).

Previous to OCT testing, it had been felt that the retina had been split primarily in the nerve fiber layer. Now with OCT testing, we know that much of the retinal splitting occurs in the mid-retina, which is supportive of the b-wave electrophysiologic changes mentioned above. The classification system includes foveal schisis, lamellar schisis (which is difficult to see clinically), and peripheral retinoschisis presenting as a large splitting of the retina in the periphery with either an intact inner wall or an inner wall with very large retinal breaks. The classification systems refers to Type 1 as foveal schisis alone, Type 2 as foveal and lamellar schisis, Type 3 as foveal, lamellar, and peripheral schisis, and Type 4 as foveal and peripheral schisis. We know that Type 1 and Type 4 are very rare and that 92 percent of patients have lamellar schisis. The very large majority of patients with known retinoschisis mutations have foveal schisis as well, although recently Luo reported a patient with many years of observation and positive genetic testing for

retinoschisis without foveal schisis, but with large areas of peripheral retinoschisis. This child also had electrophysiologic changes consistent with the b-wave reduction. Also in the area of exceptions to the rule, female patients have been described with findings of retinoschisis. It is important in taking the family history of patients with retinoschisis to make sure to ask about amblyopia and strabismus as retinoschisis is often under-diagnosed.

Clinical presentation

There are basically two types of populations of children with congenital retinoschisis

• *First presentation* is in population of children who generally present in the late first decade of life or in the teens with a reduction in visual acuity sometimes mistaken as amblyopia or even strabismus. This child generally has visual acuities that may be as bad as 20/200 but proceed to stay generally at that level. These children may retain a visual acuity even in the 20/50 to 20/60 range throughout later life and as they age and develop an atrophic macular lesion, which is sometimes misdiagnosed as macular degeneration.

• *A second presentation* is of more severe type. This population of children present with large schisis cavities that impede vision with full-thickness retinal detachment and recurrent vitreous hemorrhage.

Treatment

The management of congenital retinoschisis has changed recently. In the past congenital retino-schisis had been recognized as a problem which generally reduced the vision to 20/200, but may not have reduced the vision beyond that.

Table 12.2 *Classification system for congenital X-linked retinoschisis*			
CXLRS type	*Foveal cystic schisis (clinical examination)*	*Lamellar macular schisis (OCT testing)*	*Peripheral schisis*
Type 1 foveal	+	−	−
Type 2 foveolamellar	+	+	−
Type 3 complex	+	+	+
Type 4 foveoperipheral	+	−	+

CXLRS: congenital X-linked retinoschisis; OCT: optical coherence tomography

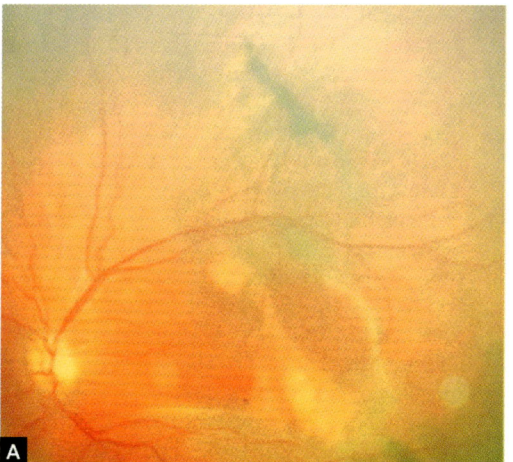

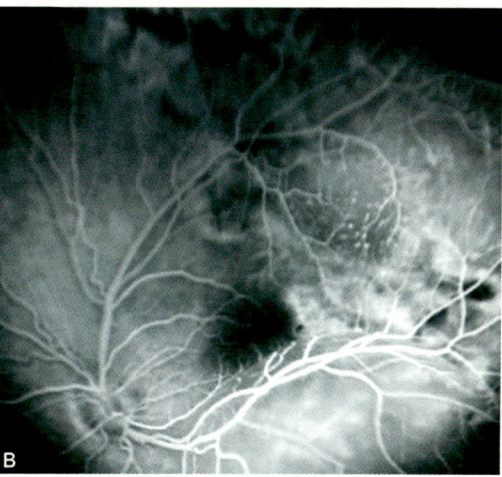

Fig. 12.5 *Photographs of congenital X-linked retinoschisis (CXLRS). **(A)** Color fundus photograph of CXLRS with macular schisis, lamellar schisis and peripheral schisis. Note the pigmentary changes indicative of the chronic nature of the disease and **(B)** late phase fluorescein angiogram with prominent dye pooling in the inferior schisis cavity as well as the pooling in the areas of macular and lamellar schisis more centrally*

Surgical management of retinoschisis is limited to two circumstances – the combined schisis full-thickness retinal detachment as well as the schisis cavity that over hangs the macula and does not allow light to easily get to the macular area. In both of these cases, an ocriplasmin-assisted vitrectomy in eyes with intact inner walls, drainage of schisis cavity fluid through a small retinotomy in the inner wall and a small 39 gauge cannula to drain what is very thin intraschisis fluid can be performed. Notably this intraschisis fluid has been found to be deficient

in retinoschisis, which is consistent with the primary disease process. The intraschisis fluid does have Tenascin-C, which degrades extra-cellular matrix and may contribute to the continued progression of schisis cavities.

In current surgical techniques for treatment of congenital retinoschisis, we leave a silicone oil bubble to help prevent reformation of schisis cavities and blockage of light to the macula. We try to leave approximately a 70–80 percent silicone oil bubble such that face-down positioning allows bathing the posterior lens surface in fluid and maintains lens clarity. We have seen lenses that have remained clear now for greater than a decade. The second mechanism of management of full-thickness retinal detachment can involve both scleral buckling and vitrectomy techniques. The management of inner and outer wall retinal breaks has been well-described in other places, and fundamentally involves closure of the retinal break common to the principles of any rhegmatogenous retinal detachment repair. Localizing the outer wall breaks can be quite challenging since they often occur at the posterior junction of the schisis cavity and can be very small in nature. It is possible to treat these breaks alone and leave the inner schisis layer untreated. Also it is possible to do an inner wall retinectomy, especially in eyes in which there are large inner wall breaks. We prefer trying to preserve the inner wall since we hope in the future that something like retinoschisin may be available to revitalize these two leaflets.

Certainly when leaflets are approximated, gene therapy may be a very reasonable approach in this disease. Currently, the exact cycle of retinoschisin reduction and degradation is not well described, but we hope that in the future a combination of surgical therapy, synthetic retinoschisin, and gene therapy may lead to therapeutic intervention that would be available to both prenatal as well as postnatal children.

Future treatments for retinoschisis hopefully may include gene therapy. Gene therapy is unlikely to effectively treat large areas of peripheral schisis cavities, particularly in the periphery. It is possible that the outer and inner leaflets of retinoschisis cavities may be viable and

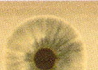

therefore, they may be reconnected using a synthetic retinoschisin that appears to be the glue and perhaps neurotransmitter that is missing in these children's eyes.

CONCLUSION

Congenital and developmental disorders of the retina continue to remain a challenge to the vitreoretinal surgeon. The importance of early screening and detection cannot be over emphasized. Currently, management often involves end stage disease because children tend to ignore ocular problems until a second eye is involved. The types of screening mechanisms which have become popular for retinopathy of prematurity may at some point be extended to include all newborns in which case discovery early of congenital retinal diseases, retinoblastoma, and other vision threatening issues may be easily discovered and managed in a fashion that salvages much more in the way of vision for these children.

BIBLIOGRAPHY

1. Alexandrakis G, Scott IU, Flynn HW Jr, et al, Visual acuity comes with and without surgery in patients with persistent fetal vasculature. Ophthalmology 2000;107:1068–72.
2. Azzolini C, Pierro L, Codenotti M, et al. OCT images and surgery of juvenile macular retinoschisis. Eur J Ophthalmol 1997;7:196–200.
3. C and Tenascin-C in schisis cavities of patients with congenital X-linked retinoschis. Retina 2007 Oct;27(8):1086–9.
4. Criswick VG, Schepens CL. Familial exudative vitreoretinopathy. Am J Ophthalmol 1969;68: 578–94.
5. Dass AB, Trese MT. Surgical results of persistent hyperplastic primary vitreous. Ophthalmology 1999;106:280–4.
6. Drenser KA, Trese MT, Capone A Jr, Hartzer M, Dailey W. Elevated levels of Cystatin
7. Eadie JA, Luo CK, Trese MT. Novel clinical manifestation of congenital X-linked retinoschisis. Arch Ophthalmol 2012 Feb: 130(2):255–7.
8. Goldberg MF. Persistent fetal vasculature (PFV): an integrated interpretation of signs and symptoms associated with persistent hyperplastic primary vitreous (PHPV). LIV Edward Jackson Memorial Lecture. Am J Ophthalmol 1997;124:587–626.
9. Jumper JM, Pomerleau D, McDonald HR, Johnson RN, FuAD, Cunningham ET Jr. Macular fibrosis in Coats' disease. Retina 2010 April;30 (4 Suppl):S9-14.
10. Pendergast SD, Trese MT. Familial exudative vitreoretinopathy. Results of surgical management. Ophthalmology 1998;105:1015–23.
11. Prenner JL, Capone A Jr, Ciaccia S, Takada Y, Sieving PA, Trese MT. Congenital X-linked retinoschisis classification system. Retina 2006 Sep; 26(7 suppl):S61-4.
12. Ranchod TM, Quiram PA, Hathaway N, Ho LY, Glasgow BJ, Trese MT. Microcornea, posterior megalolenticonus, persistent fetal vasculature, and coloboma. A new syndrome. Ophthalmology 2010 Sep;117:1843–47. Epub 2010 Apr 24
13. Recchia FM, Capone, Jr., A, Trese MT. Coats' Disease. In: Hartnett ME, Trese MT, Capone A, et al, (Eds). Pediatric Retinal Diseases: Medical and Surgical Approaches. Philadelphia: Lippincott Williams & Wilkins; 2005 Chp. 29, pp 429–36.
14. Sieving PA, MacDonald IM, Trese MT. Congenital X-Linked Retinoschisis. In: Hartnett ME, Trese MT, Capone A, et al. Eds. Pediatric Retinal Diseases: Medical and Surgical Approaches. Philadelphia: Lippincott Williams & Wilkins 2005; Chp. 25, pp 377–85.
15. Trese MT, Capone A Jr, Persistent fetal vasculature syndrome (persistent hyperplastic primary vitreous). In: Hartnett ME, Trese MT, Capone A, et al. Eds. Pediatric Retinal Diseases: Medical and Surgical Approaches. Philadelphia: Lippincott Williams & Wilkins; Chp 30, p 440, 2005.
16. Trese MT, Capone, Jr., A. Familial Exudative Vitreoretinopathy. In: Hartnett ME, Trese MT, Capone A, et al. Eds. Pediatric Retinal Diseases: Medical and Surgical Approaches. Philadelphia: Lippincott Williams & Wilkins; Chp. 28, pp 425–28, 2005.
17. Trese MT, Capone, Jr., A. Persistent Fetal Vasculature Syndrome (Persistent Hyperplastic Primary Vitreous). In: Hartnett ME, Trese MT, Capone A, et al. Eds. Pediatric Retinal Diseases: Medical and Surgical Approaches. Philadelphia: Lippincott Williams & Wilkins 2005 Chp. 30, pp 437–2.
18. Walsh MK, Drenser KA, Capone A Jr., Trese MT. Early vitrectomy effective for Norrie disease. Arch Ophthalmol 2010; 128(4):456–60.
19. Walsh MK, Drenser KA, Capone A, Trese MT. Early vitrectomy effective for bilateral combined anterior and posterior persistent fetal vasculature syndrome. Retina 2010 Apr;30:S2–S8.

TRAUMATIC LESIONS OF POSTERIOR SEGMENT

Subina Narang, Ritu Gera

RETINAL LESIONS DUE TO DIRECT TRAUMATIC IMPACT
- Commotio retinae/Berlin's edema
- Choroidal rupture
- Retinal tears
- Retinal and vitreous haemorrhage
- Retinal detachment
- Scleral rupture and optic nerve injury
- Retinitis sclopeteria

RETINAL LESIONS SECONDARY TO TRAUMA ELSEWHERE
- Purtscher retinopathy
- Valsalvas retinopathy
- Terson's syndrome
- Fat embolism syndrome
- Shaken baby syndrome

RETINAL LESIONS DUE TO DIRECT TRAUMATIC IMPACT

Blunt trauma of eye leads to certain lesions in retina due to direct impact, or indirect impact, or secondary to trauma to other parts of body. Retinal lesions due to direct impact are as below.

COMMOTIO RETINAE/BERLIN'S EDEMA

Commotio retinae is a countrecoup contusive injury to the retina after blunt trauma to anterior segment of eye. It may or may not be accompanied by choroidal rupture. It was first described by Berlin in 1873. It can occur centrally or peripherally, and when it involves the macula, it is called Berlin's edema.

The retina appears normal on examination although the patient may complain of decreased vision. The affected area becomes white and opaque usually hours after the trauma. "Berlin's edema" is not a true edema. Swelling and disorganization of the outer retinal layers cause the opaqueness. There are various contradictory studies for intracellular and extracellular edema. The studies have shown disruption of photoreceptor outer segment and retinal pigment epithelium (RPE) which is outer blood-retinal barrier.

The visual acuity in commotio retinae varies from 20/20 to 20/400 and does not always correlate with the degree of retinal opacification. The prognosis is usually excellent except in the cases with associated subfoveolar choroidal rupture and/or subfoveolar hemorrhage. Poor outcome is seen in severe retinal pigment epithelial damage involving hyperplasia or migration of RPE and serous retinal detachment. Late manifestations of blunt injury to the RPE vary from minor atrophic changes to massive hyperplasia and migration resulting in bone corpuscular and granular pigmentation that resembles retinitis pigmentosa. In rare cases cystoid macular edema is seen which can progress to a macular hole. Berlin's edema is usually self-limited and resolves without sequelae, and there is no known intervention that alters its course and prognosis (Fig. 13.1).

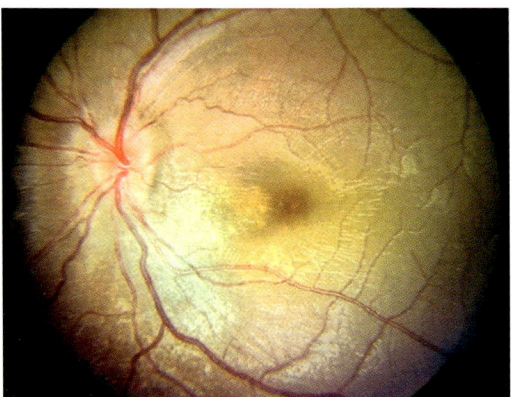

Fig. 13.1 *Fundus picture showing Berlin's edema characterised by white opacification at level of deep sensory retina, mild disc edema and internal limiting membrane folds*

CHOROIDAL RUPTURE

Approximately 5–10% of patients with blunt trauma develop a choroidal rupture. Choroidal rupture can be secondary to indirect or direct trauma. Cases secondary to direct trauma tend to be located more anteriorly and at the site of impact and parallel to the ora, whereas those secondary to indirect trauma occur posteriorly. Most eyes have a single rupture, but up to 25% of eyes have multiple ruptures. These ruptures have a crescent shape and are concentric to the optic disc (Fig. 13.2). Indirect choroidal ruptures are almost 4 times more common than direct ruptures. Mostly ruptures occur temporal to the disc, and 66% involve the macula.

After blunt trauma, the ocular globe undergoes mechanical compression and then sudden hyperextension. the sclera has tensile strength to resist this insult; the retina is also protected because of its elasticity. The bruch membrane neither has elasticity nor tensile strength; therefore, it breaks.

During the acute phases the small capillaries in the choriocapillaris are damaged, leading to subretinal or sub-RPE hemorrhage, which in conjunction with retinal edema may obscure the choroidal rupture. The deep choroidal vessels are usually spared. As the blood clears, a white, curvilinear, crescent-shaped streak concentric to the optic nerve is seen. Fibroblast activity is seen by 4–14 days. During the healing phase, choroidal neovascularization (CNV) is a universal phenomenon (Fig. 13.3). In most cases, it involutes spontaneously but in 15–30% of

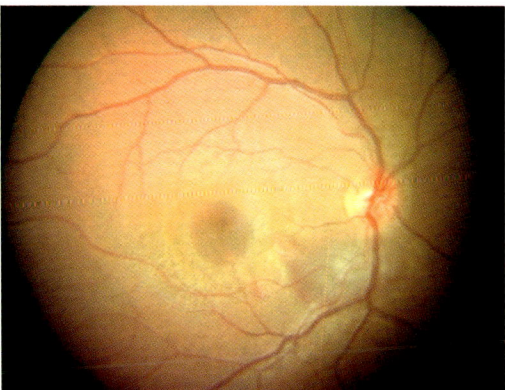

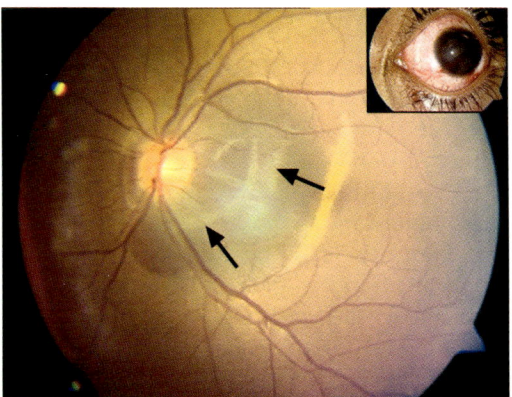

Fig. 13.2 *Fundus photograph of two crescent shaped choroidal ruptures concentric to disc and subretinal bleed (arrows). Inset shows anterior segment picture of the same patient showing iridodialysis*

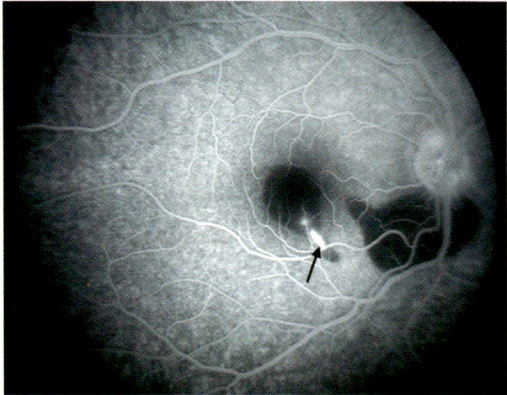

Fig. 13.3 *Colored picture and FFA showing choroidal rupture, resolving subretinal bleed and FFA showing hyperfluorescence due to choroidal neovascular membrane (black arrow)*

patients, CNV may arise again and lead to a hemorrhagic or serous macular detachment with concomitant visual loss.

Older age and macular rupture, the length of the rupture, and the distance of the rupture to the center of the fovea may be risk factors for CNV. If fovea is not involved prognosis is good.

The ocular examination must be thorough to rule out orbital fractures or globe ruptures. Consider CT scan and MRI of the eye and orbit under appropriate circumstances. Fluorescein angiography and Indocyanine green ICG may be a useful adjunct to detect CNV. If CNV is extrafoveal, it may be treated successfully with laser photocoagulation and anti-VEGF therapy for subfoveal CNVM.

RETINAL TEARS

Acute posterior vitreous detachment (PVD) and retinal tears immediately after a blow to the head have been seen in patients who were predisposed to retinal tears because of high myopia, lattice degeneration, or other abnormalities.

Various types of tears

1. Necrotic tears

When a blunt object strikes the eye posterior to the ora serrata, the direct coup effect on the retina may cause full-thickness retinal necrosis with subsequent retinal detachment. The underlying RPE is usually damaged as well.

2. Vitreous traction tears

Giant retinal tear (GRT) is defined as peripheral break extending through 90 or more of the retinal circumference in which the vitreous gel is attached essentially to the anterior flap thereby allowing independent mobility of the posterior edge of tear. GRT are idiopathic in 70%, traumatic in 20% and in 10% occur at the posterior edge of chorioretinal degeneration. GRT needs to be differentiated from dialysis. Dialyses is disinsertion of retina from ora serrata which could be of variable extent. Vitreous is attached to the posterior margin of the dialysis and posterior vitreous detachment is absent thus preventing it from inversion whereas in giant tear vitreous remains strongly attached to the anterior margin of the tear and the posterior

flap, without any vitreous adhesion is free to move and inverts towards disc due to gravity.

3. Avulsion of the vitreous base

This is pathognomonic of blunt trauma The avulsed vitreous base looks like a ribbon floating in the vitreous cavity. Unfortunately, the vitreous base does not separate cleanly from the retina and pars plana epithelium The retina can be torn along the posterior margin of the vitreous base, or the nonpigmented pars plana epithelium can be torn along the anterior margin of the vitreous base, or both can be torn simultaneously. Similarly, if the vitreous is strongly adherent to either lattice degeneration or a vitreoretinal scar posterior to the vitreous base, a posterior flap tear may occur. These tears can cause a retinal detachment (Fig. 13.4A and B).

4. Tears along the anterior and posterior margins of the vitreous base

Tears along the anterior and posterior margins of the vitreous base are most common inferotemporally followed by superonasally, the former is by direct injury and the later is because of countercoup injury. When located superonasally, they are nearly always caused by trauma. All dialysis, even inferotemporal ones, are traumatic. However, many are familial, bilateral, or found in patients with no historical or histopathologic evidence of injury. In these cases, there is probably a developmental abnormality of the inferotemporal peripheral retina and vitreous base.

5. Stretch tears

Occasionally, rapid horizontal expansion of the eye can produce a stretch tear of the retina. These curvilinear breaks are usually concentric to the optic nerve. They can cause retinal detachment, but they are self-sealing.

6. Traumatic macular holes

Usually occur following blunt ocular trauma, also reported with, accidental laser injuries, lightening and electrical shock. The pathogenesis is not well established, possibly the acute compression-decompression force exerted on the globe cause local posterior vitreous detachment, leading to dehiscence in the fovea or to avulsion of a small operculum.

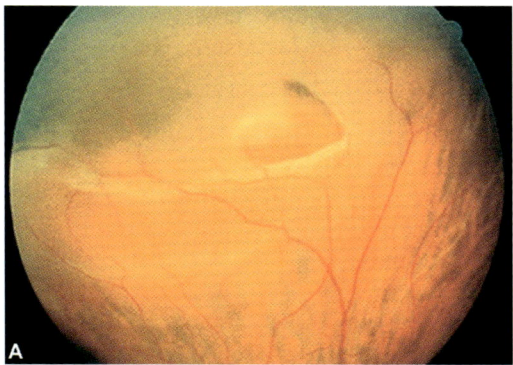

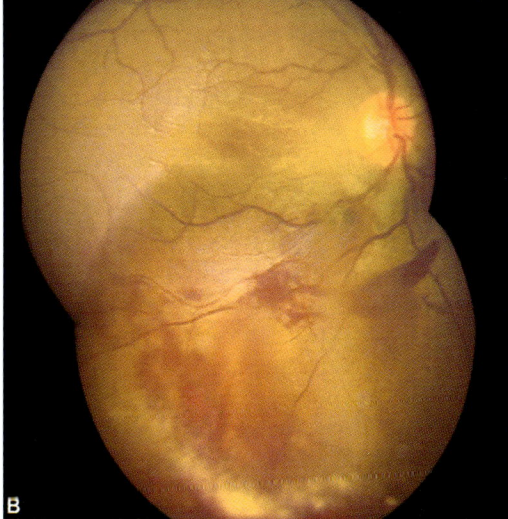

Fig. 13.4 (A) *Fundus photograph showing retinal tear with retinal detachment,* **(B)** *another case of resolving vitreous hemorrhage who on follow up showed inferior retinal detachment after trauma*

In laser the macular hole caused by coagulation necrosis following the intense laser burn, and the hole can develop in the days or weeks following the injury.

The surgical management of traumatic macular holes is similar to that of idiopathic macular holes, and includes—vitrectomy, ILM peeling, and fluid-gas exchange (Fig. 13.5). Selection of cases and timing of surgery are important, and outcomes often depend on associated trauma-related ocular pathologies. Spontaneous closure of the hole can occur but is not common, and surgery should not be deferred for too long, as long-standing holes are associated with poor prognosis.

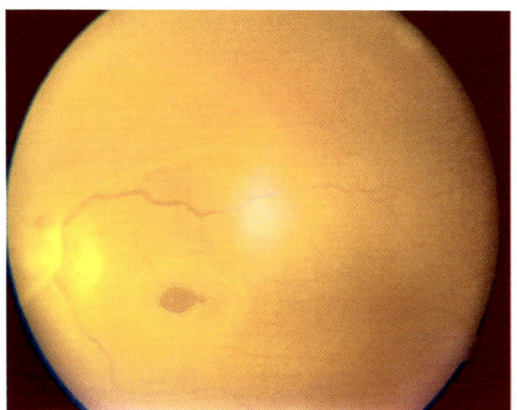

Fig. 13.5 *Fundus photograph showing full thickness traumatic macular hole*

RETINAL AND VITREOUS HEMORRHAGE

When the retina is torn, blood vessels that bridge tears may bleed into the vitreous. Vitreous hemorrhage can also result from acute PVD, avulsion of superficial retinal vessels and possible mechanism is rupture of the ciliary body. Ultrasound examination is indicated if the posterior segment is obscured by hemorrhage to rule out retinal tear or detachment, choroidal detachment, posterior vitreous detachment, or occult ruptured globe. Bed rest with head end elevation is recommended, as it encourages the blood to settle and improves the view to the fundus. Early intervention by pars plana vitrectomy is desired in case of associated retinal detachment.

RETINAL DETACHMENT

Blunt trauma is the leading cause of retinal detachment in children and adolescents. Men and boys are most likely to be engaged in fighting or contact sports, and they form at least three-fourths of the patients with traumatic retinal detachment. The affected patients have a formed vitreous, traumatic retinal detachments typically progress slowly unless a giant tear is present. Sometimes, the trauma occurs months before the detachment is diagnosed which is because of the time taken in the liquefaction of vitreous after blunt trauma in young patients. On examination demarcation lines, atrophy of the underlying pigment epithelium, subretinal precipitates, retinal

macrocysts, and extensive vitreous "tobacco dust" are all commonly seen. Proliferative vitreoretinopathy is uncommon, so the prognosis for reattachment is excellent, provided, of course, there is no missed break. In 87% of traumatic retinal detachments, the causative tear is found at the vitreous base. Superonasal breaks at the anterior vitreous base are commonly overlooked. Because many traumatic retinal breaks cause subsequent retinal detachment, they should all be treated with laser or cryotherapy.

SCLERAL RUPTURE

The two most common locations for scleral rupture are at the limbus (under intact conjunctiva) and parallel to the muscle insertions between the insertion and the equator in the eyes that have not undergone prior surgery. Radial and posterior ruptures are relatively uncommon.

The hallmarks of scleral rupture are severe reduction in visual acuity, an afferent pupillary defect, hypotony (although a normal intraocular pressure does not rule out a small rupture), an abnormally deep anterior chamber, decreased ocular ductions, severe subconjunctival edema, hyphema, and vitreous hemorrhage.

The diagnosis can rarely be confirmed by ophthalmoscopy because severe vitreous hemorrhage, hyphema, or both nearly always accompany scleral rupture. Ultrasonography and computed tomography (CT) scanning may be helpful. Both show a shrunken globe. In addition, the CT scan shows subconjunctival edema and also useful in identifying any intraocular foreign bodies. In cases where subconjuctival hemorrhage is dense surgical exploration can be done

The prognosis for recovery of useful vision in a ruptured globe is very poor, as choroid and retina are also torn leading to fibrovascular tissue proliferation into the eye and severe massive periretinal proliferation.

OPTIC NERVE INJURIES

The optic nerve can be severely damaged by blunt trauma. The common injuries are optic nerve sheath hemorrhage, fracture optic canal, bony chip impinging on optic nerve and optic

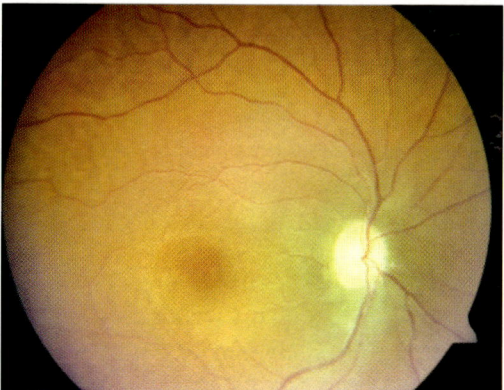

Fig. 13.6 *Fundus picture showing disc pallor after indirect optic nerve injury*

nerve avulsion. There is generation of direct shock-waves due to trauma The intrasheath hemorrhage and edema cause indirect compression of optic nerve. The management of traumatic optic neuropathy is controversial. Recommendations are high-dose intravenous steroids in indirect injury, especially if they can be started within 8 hours. In case of direct injury, based on CT findings surgical decompression of optic nerve sheath hematoma and neurosurgical decompression of the optic canal is done (Fig. 13.6).

Minor direct trauma or even a blow to the occiput can cause severe complication of avulsion of the optic nerve which usually is accompanied by severe damage to other ocular tissues as well.

RETINITIS SCLOPETERIA

Retinitis sclopeteria is due to shock waves generated by passage of a high-velocity missile through the orbit without directly striking the eye. This causes rupture of the choroid or retina and leads to irregular ragged holes. The holes are result of mechanical disruption and fragmentation of retina. Initially a subretinal or vitreous hemorrhage may be seen. Profoundly decreased vision is seen in optic nerve damage. In severe cases, massive amounts of fibrous tissue proliferate into the eye. A claw-like break is often seen in Bruch's membrane and in the choriocapillaris. It is tempting to intervene due to frightening size and posterior location of the breaks but retinal detachment rarely occurs due to inflammation at the edges of necrotic retina

which causes firm chorioretinal adhesions, but late detachment from a break at a distal site can occur.

RETINAL LESIONS SECONDARY TO TRAUMA ELSEWHERE

PURTSCHER RETINOPATHY

Purtscher retinopathy has been associated with traumatic injury, primarily blunt thoracic trauma and head trauma, and numerous non-traumatic diseases. Purtscher retinopathy is hemorrhagic and vaso-occlusive vasculopathy syndrome of severe vision loss with multiple patches of superficial retinal whitening and retinal hemorrhages.

Pathogenesis

The most accepted mechanism is leuko-embolization that causes arteriolar occlusion and infarction of the microvascular bed. Leukocyte aggregation, which is induced by complement 5a, is believed to be the most likely mechanism of embolization. Traumatic chest compression and increased intracranial tension after blunt head trauma are common causes. Besides trauma it is also seen in cases of acute pancreatitis, long bone fractures, postpartum period, pre-eclampsia shock, disseminated intravascular coagulopathy, fat embolization and vasculitic diseases. The degree is not necessarily indicative of the risk of developing retinopathy.

Clinical features

The patients may present with unilateral or bilateral vision loss (possibly severe) generally within 2 days. Decreased vision occurs in the affected eyes, generally in the range of 20/200 to counting fingers. Vision often improves over several months to a range of 20/30 to 20/200, depending on the severity of the retinal damage. The retinal findings in Purtscher retinopathy are cotton-wool spots, areas of retinal whitening around the optic nerve, and intraretinal hemorrhages. Less common reported findings include serous detachment of the macula, preretinal hemorrhages, dilated vessels, and

optic disc edema. Confluence of cotton-wool spots in the central macula may simulate the cherry-red spot that is seen in central retinal artery occlusion. Macular cotton-wool spots and intraretinal hemorrhages in patients with this history of trauma are diagnostic of the condition. Typically, there is sparing of the retinal whitening immediately adjacent to the larger retinal vessels (Fig. 13.7A and B).

Differential diagnosis

Differential diagnoses of Purtscher retinopathy includes central retinal artery occlusion, giant cell arteritis, hypertension, ocular manifestations of HIV, syphilis, Sjögren syndrome and Terson syndrome. If the patient has a history of head trauma or thoracic trauma, obtain appro-

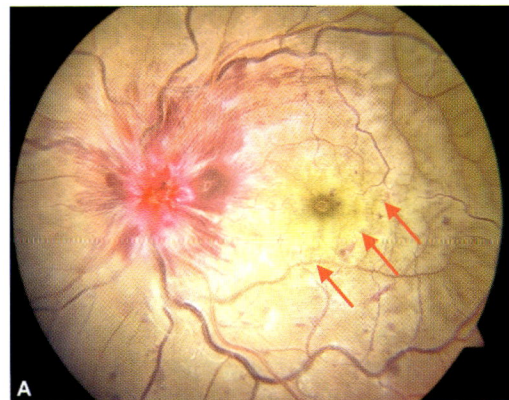

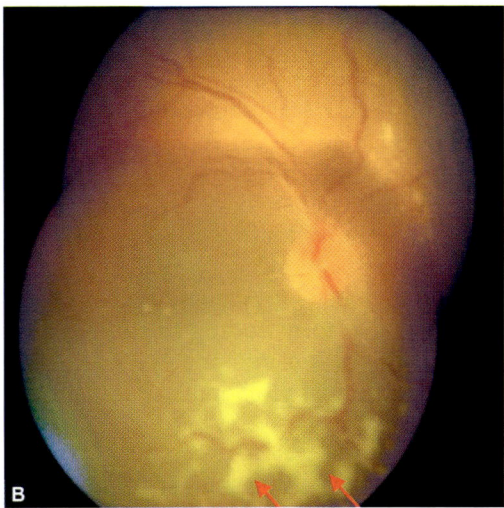

Fig. 13.7 *(A)* Fundus picture showing superficial retinal hemorrhages and *(B)* retinal whitening surrounding optic disc suggestive of Purtscher's retinopathy

priate X-ray films or imaging studies-skull or rib fractures may be present. These injuries may require more extensive investigations. Fundus fluorescein angiography studies (early in the disease) demonstrate capillary leakage and staining of the retinal arterioles, venules and capillaries. In severe disease nonperfusion of the small arterioles that surround the central macula, perivenous staining, venous dilation are often noted.

Treatment

- *No proven treatment* exists for Purtscher retinopathy that occurs after traumatic injury.
- *Control of the underlying disease* with other medications may be indicated and provide surgical care as required for trauma (Fig. 13.7).

VALSALVA'S RETINOPATHY

The retinopathy is caused by increased intrathoracic pressure at Valsalva's manoeuvre which is forceful exhalation against closed glottis, like during straining at stools, coughing, heavy weight lifting.

This is characterised by well circumscribed red blood under internal limiting membrane, which is usually boat shaped, in or near macular region. The color of blood may alter with time. The individuals with tortuosity of 2nd or 3rd order arterioles are predispodsed to it which is inherited as autosomal dominant trait (Fig. 13.8A and B). It clears on its own and only reassurance is required. It is initially red but eventually loss of hemoglobin it may appear yellow. If it does not clear parsplana vitrectomy may be planned. Laser hyaloidotomy is not recommended as it invariably leads to epiretinal membrane formation.

TERSON'S SYNDROME

The syndrome of vitreous hemorrhage with subarachnoid bleed is called Terson's syndrome. 3–8% patients of subarachanoid bleed have vitreous hemorrhage. This usually is associated with numerous intraretinal and subretinal bleeds. The posterior hyaloid is partially detached and gives scaffold for raised epiretinal membrane over macular area.

The explanation for this is that acute rise in intracranial pressure is transmitted via

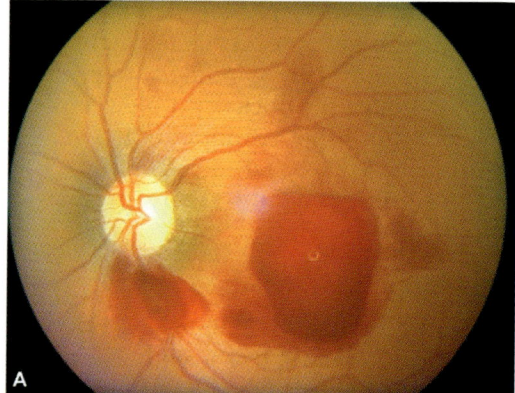
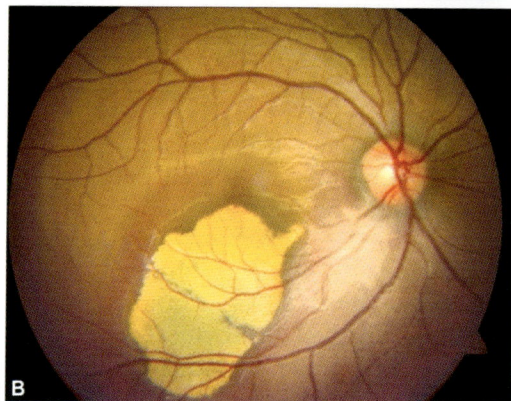

Fig. 13.8 *(A) Fundus picture showing preretinal bleeding— a case of Valsalva's retinopathy and (B) fundus picture of another case of Valsalva's retinopathy showing altered color of blood after 3 months*

intravaginal space to optic disc and causes venous stasis via compression of orbital veins. The spontaneous resolution may take an year. To prevent amblyopia, early vitrectomy is recommended in children. The incidence of epiretinal membrane is same in eyes undergoing vitrectomy or not. In adults the treatment could be guided by laterality, density of vitreous hemorrhage and epiretinal membrane, occupational needs of the patient. Observation of 3 months could be done to evaluate the clearing of vitreous hemorrhage. The patients should be subjected to ultrasonography to observe for retinal detachment during the period of observation.

FAT EMBOLISM SYNDROME

This was described in 1861 as spectrum of clinical findings in patient suffering fractures of

medullated bones especially fracture femur bone. It effects multiple organs and may be fatal in 20% cases. Systemic findings are petechial rash, respiratory insufficiency, CNS symptoms and Purtscher's like retinopathy in eye. The cause is believed to be fat embolism. The visual prognosis is good and rarely permanent scotomas may develop.

SHAKEN BABY SYNDROME

Shaken baby syndrome (SBS) is a severe form of child abuse caused by violently shaking an infant or child. Child abuse could be diagnosed by ophthalmologist primarily in 6% of the cases before other features are seen. There may be no associated soft tissue injury or fracture. The shaken baby syndrome is seen in children less than 3 years of age. It is typically caused by angular declaration associated with forceful striking of head against hard surface but if the surface is soft the visible signs of trauma could be missing. The CNS signs of trauma could be nystagmus, 3rd nerve palsy, cortical blindness. The signs could be lid ecchymosis, edema and fractures. There could be anterior segment hyphema, angle recession or cataract. Posterior segment signs could be vitreous hemorrhage, optic atrophy, intraretinal hemorrhages and peripheral avascular retina. Traumatic retinoschisis is a particularly diagnostic lesion caused by traction applied to the retina by the vitreous jelly as the child is submitted to repetitive acceleration-deceleration forces. The retina splits, creating a blood filled cystic cavity, not reported in otherwise healthy children except SBS victims. Peripheral retinal nonperfusion is also observed in SBS victims. Preretinal and/or vitreous hemorrhage may be associated with the development of retinal nonperfusion. The role of prophylactic laser treatment is unclear, and close observation for the development of neovascularization is warranted.

BIBLIOGRAPHY

1. Gross JG, King LP, de Juan E Jr, Powers T. Subfoveal neovascular membrane removal in patients with traumatic choroidal rupture. Ophthalmology 1996;103:579–85.
2. Han DP, Mieler WF, Schwartz DM, Abrams GW. Management of traumatic hemorrhagic retinal detachment with pars plana vitrectomy. Arch Ophthalmol 1990;108:1281–6.
3. Marr W, Marr E. Some observations on Purtscher's disease: Traumatic retinal angiopathy. Am J Ophthalmol 1962;54:693–705.
4. Ross W. Traumatic retinal dialyses. Arch Ophthalmol 1981;99:1371–74.
5. Schultz PN, Sobol WM, Weingeist TA. Long-term visual outcome in Terson syndrome. Ophthalmology 1991;98:1814–19.
6. Shapiro I, Jacob HS. Leukoembolization in ocular vascular occlusion. Ann Ophthalmol 1982,14: 60–262.
7. Sipperley JO, Quigley HA, Gass JDM. Traumatic retinopathy in primates: The explanation of commotio retinae. Arch Ophthalmol 1978;96: 2267–73.
8. Wood CM, Richardson J. Indirect choroidal ruptures: Aetiological factors, patterns of ocular damage, and finalvisual outcome. Br J Ophthalmol 1990;74:208–11.
9. Yanagiya N, Akiba J, Takahashi M, et al. Clinical characteristics of traumatic macular holes. Jpn J Ophthalmol 1996;40:544–47.

14 | RETINAL VASCULITIS

Sunandan Sood, Anjani Khanna

DEFINITION, ETIOLOGY AND TERMINOLOGY
- Definition
- Etiology
- Terminology

GENERAL CLINICAL FEATURES
Symptom profile
Staging of vasculitis
- Stage of active retinal vasculitis
- Stage of occlusions
- Stage of neovascularization
- Advanced stage of disease

SPECIFIC CLINICAL ENTITIES
Disorders associated with predominantly periphlebitis
- Tuberculosis
- Sarcoidosis
- Behçet's disease
- Multiple sclerosis

- HIV
- Eales' disease

Disorders associated with periarteritis predominantly
- Syphilis
- Acute retinal necrosis
- Systemic lupus erythematosus
- Polyarteritis nodosa

Disorders associated with both periarteritis and periphlebitis
- Toxoplasmosis
- Wegner's granulomatosis
- Frosted branch angitis
- Crohn's disease

MANAGEMENT
- Investigations
- Complications
- Treatment
- Prognosis

DEFINITION, ETIOLOGY AND TERMINOLOGY

DEFINITION

Inflammation of retinal vessel wall resulting in evident clinical manifestations such as vascular sheathing, leakage and occlusion is termed as retinal vasculitis.

ETIOLOGY

Retinal vasculitis can be either primary ocular disorder without any systemic disease or it can be a manifestation of a systemic disorder. It can be thus complication of infective, neurological or neoplastic disorder or in association with systemic inflammatory disease or else it can be idiopathic.

Retinal vasculitis without systemic disease (Idiopathic)

Eale's disease, frosted branch angiitis, pars planitis, birdshot retinochoroidopathy, idiopathic retinal vasculitis aneurysms and neuroretinitis (IRVAN).

Retinal vasculitis with systemic disease

Infectious disorders include:
- *Bacterial.* Tuberculosis, syphilis, brucellosis, Lyme disease, cat-scratch disease.
- *Viral disease.* Herper simplex, herpes zoster, cytomegalovirus, hepatitis -B, C; HIV.
- *Parasitic disease.* Toxoplasmosis, toxocariasis.

Neurological disorder. Multiple sclerosis.

Neoplastic disorders. Acute leukemia, ocular lymphoma.

Systemic inflammatory disorders. Behcet's disease, sarcoidosis, systemic lupus erythematosis, Wegner's granulomatosis, polyarteritis nodosa, rhemuatoid arthritis, relapsing polychondritis, HLA-27 associated uveitis, Crohn's disease, dermatomyositis, polymyositis, Takayasu's disease, Buerger's disease.

TERMINOLOGY

Although the term retinal vasculitis is popular world wide on the basis of available meager pathological data, it is more of retinal perivasculitis which can involve either veins predominantly or the arteries or the both. Accordingly on the basis of clinical examinations, veins (periphlebitis) are predominantly involved in tuberculosis, sarcoidosis, Behcet's disease, multiple sclerosis, Eales' disease and HIV. Predominantly retinal arteritis occur in association with SLE, PAN, syphilis, HSV (acute retinal necrosis) VZV (progressive outer retinal necrosis), IRVAN (idiopathic retinal vasculitis, aneurysm and neuroretinitis). Both retinal arteries and veins are involved in toxoplasmosis, frosted branch angiitis, relapsing polychondritis, Wegner's granulomatosis and Crohn's disease.

GENERAL CLINICAL FEATURES

SYMPTOM PROFILE

Retinal vasculitis can be asymptomatic, minimally symptomatic or sight threatening. This is the one condition where timely diagnosis and proper treatment can prevent sight threatening complications and provide gratifying results. Patient is asymptomatic initially if the peripheral vessel is involved without vitreous involvement. Mostly patient present with painless rapid decrease in vision which may be at times preceded with floaters. Patient may have large area of scotoma relating to the area of ischemia.

STAGING OF VASCULITIS

The retinal vasculitis mainly passes through four stages such as stage of active vasculitis, stage of occlusion, stage of neovascularization and advanced stage of the disease.

1. Stage of active retinal vasculitis

Active vascular disease is characterized by sheathing or cuffing of blood vessels and vitreous cells. The veins are dilated, tortuous with perivascular exudates along with superficial flame shaped and in more severe cases sheets of hemorrhages. Sheathing could

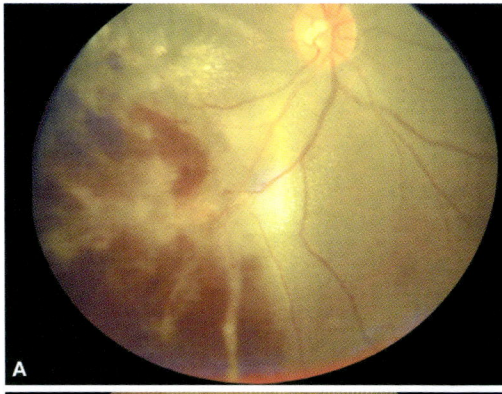

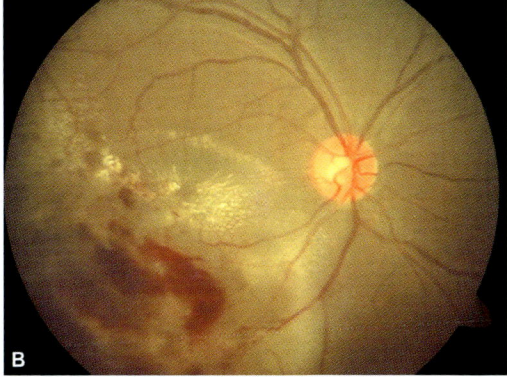

Fig. 14.1 **(A)** *Right fundus photographs showing sheathing of blood vessels, veins are dilated with perivascular exudates alongwith superficial hemorrhages suggestive of active periphlebitis and **(B)** Macular edema, however, the follow up picture shows some resolution*

vary from thin white lines to segmental heavy exudative sheathing. This could be associated with early signs of occlusion such as cotton wool spots, retinal edema and intraretinal hemorrhages (Fig. 14.1).

2. Stage of occlusion

The lesion of active vasculitis may progress further and get occluded and may develop variable degree of capillary nonperfusion (CNP). Junction between perfused and nonperfused retina may show telengiectatic vessels, microaneurysms, veno-venous shunts, hard exudates and cotton wool spots. Obliterated vessels may be seen as white lines.

3. Stage of neovascularization

CNP areas release VEGF (vascular endothelial growth factors) because of hypoxia leading to

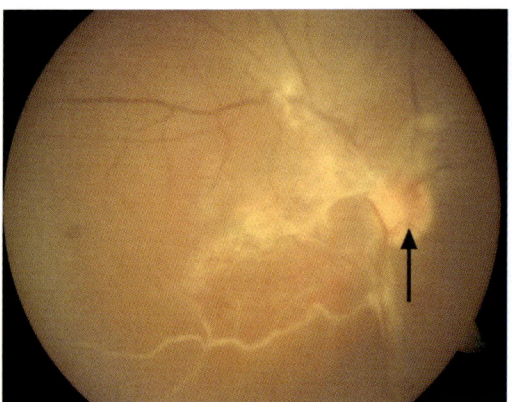

Fig. 14.2 *Right fundus photograph showing stage of neovascularization disc (NVD) in a case of vasculitis*

neovascularization. If less than 90° retina is hypoxic then NVE (neovascularization elsewhere) and if more than 90° retina is hypoxic then NVD(neovascularization disc) is likely to occur which is the nature's way of healing by reperfusing the hypoxic area. NVE occurs at the junction of perfused and nonperfused areas (Fig. 14.2). However, new vessels are fragile and likely to break with trivial trauma like the movement of eye causing vitreous hemorrhage and rapid painless dimunition of vision. In due course of time the hemorrhage may settle down with propped up posture and process of resolution starts. This may lead to improvement in vision to be followed by another recurrent bleed (Fig. 14.3). Eventually the fibrovascular gliosis may follow causing tractional retinal detachment (TRD).

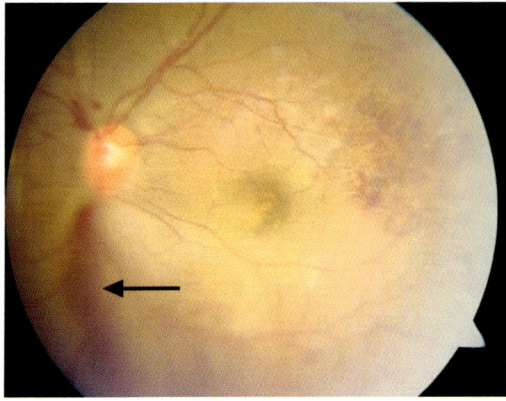

Fig. 14.3 *Left fundus photograph showing vitreous hemorrhage from NVD in a case of vasculitis*

4. Advanced stage of disease

Because of increasing hypoxia, the VEGF may permeate anteriorly causing rubeosis iridis leading to neovascular glaucoma (NVG). Further traction may cause break in the retina causing combined retinal detachment. Vision is mainly affected by CME, vitreous hemorrhage and TRD.

SPECIFIC CLINICAL ENTITIES

DISORDERS ASSOCIATED WITH PERIPHLEBITIS PREDOMINANTLY

1. Tuberculosis

Ocular tuberculosis may be due to organismal invasion or due to hypersensitivity to myco-bacterial antigens mostly in the absence of active systemic disease. Although the most common ocular manifestation of tuberculosis is choroiditis, but retinal periphlebilitis may be presenting sign of ocular tuberculosis. It manifest as an obliterative periphlebitis with thick perivenous sheathing affecting the retina in multiple quadrants starting at or anterior to equator and progressing posteriorly. The inflammation induced occlusion can lead to hypoxia and release of VEGF and consequent proliterative vascular retinopathy (Fig. 14.4).

The patient usually present with recurrent vitreal bleeding and in the advanced disease may develop TRD. It may be associated with focal choroiditis seen typically under the retinal vessel. Active periphlebitis may be associated with vitritis and mild to moderate AC reaction. The disease is mostly bilateral affecting healthy young adults in the 3rd and 4th decade of life involving men more often than women.

It is very uncommon to have associated active tubercular lesions but highly positive Mantoux test, positive PCR and quantiferon Tb gold test and characteristic vasculitis lesions with heavy exudation and patch of choroiditis usually clinch the diagnosis. The condition is treated with oral steroids and with appropriate anti-tubercular therapy. The proliferative stage of neovascularization is treated by laser photo-coagulation. Patients with nonresolving vitreous hemorrhage and with TRD are treated with

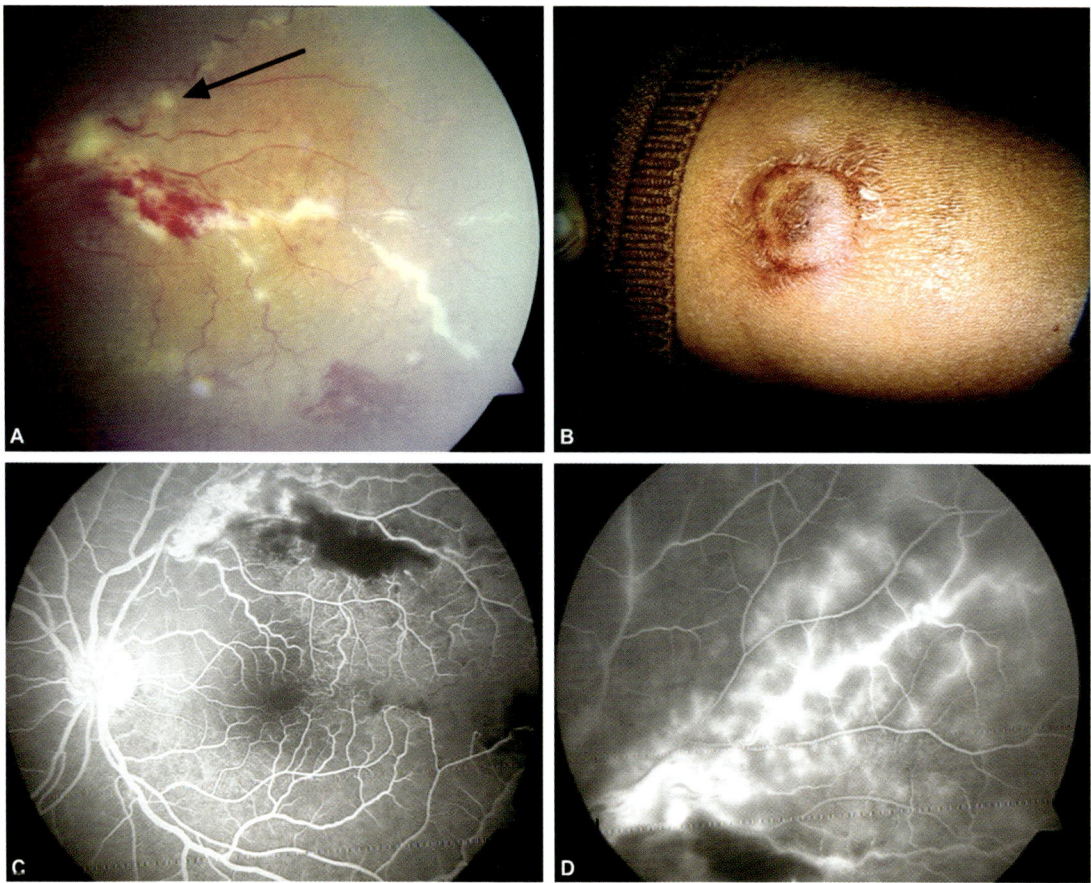

Fig. 14.4 *(A) Left fundus photograph showing active tubercular periphlebitis with choroiditis (black arrow) with superficial hemorrhages; (B) Mantoux test highly positive >15 mm; (C) FFA shows hypofluorescence because of hemorrhage, hyperfluorescence suggestive of active periphlebitis and (D) FFA showing areas of capillary nonperfusion (CNP) in the periphery*

early parsplana vitrectomy and adequate endo laser photocoagulation. The prognosis of vision is usually good unlike PDR vitrectomy.

2. Sarcoidosis

In addition to anterior granulomatous uveitis and conjunctival nodule, the characteristic posterior segment findings include, intermediate uveitis with vitritis and peripheral phlebitis. Retinal periphlebitis is of non-occlusive type with typical segmental cuffing. Sometimes there may be extensive sheathing and perivenous exudates which are termed as "Candle wax drippings". Multiple small round chorioretinal lesions are frequently seen in the peripheral fundus. The diagnosis is usually established

with X-ray chest, negative Mantoux test, raised serum Ca and ACE levels. The treatment is oral steroids in the active stage, lasers in proliferative stage and PPV in patients of non-clearing VH and TRD (Fig. 14.5).

3. Behçet's disease

It is a multisystem inflammatory disorder involving oral and genital ulcerations and inflammation of eye and skin. HLA-B51 is strongly associated with the susceptibility of the disease. Ocular involvement typically includes non-granulomatous panuveitis with or without hypopyon and retinal vasculitis. Veins are predominantly involved in the form of leaky periphlebitis and recurrent vaso-occlusive

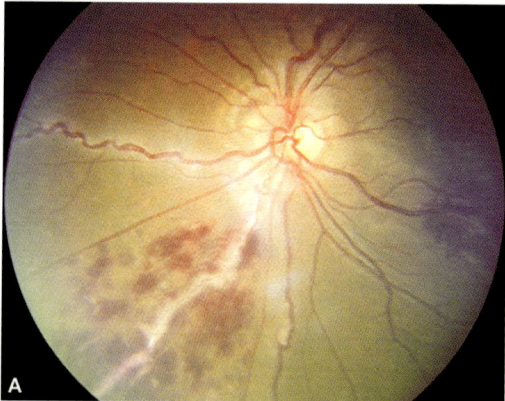

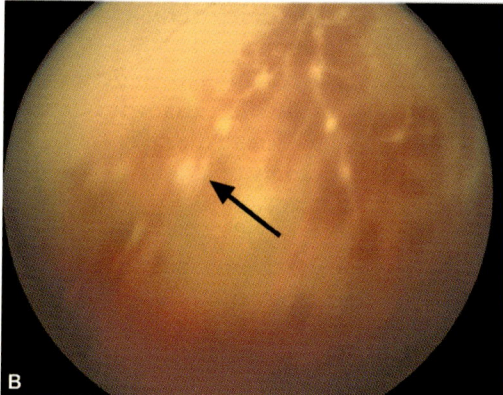

Fig. 14.5 (A) *Left fundus photograph showing active periphlebitis in patient of sarcoidosis and **(B)** perivenous exudates which are termed as candle wax drippings (black arrow)*

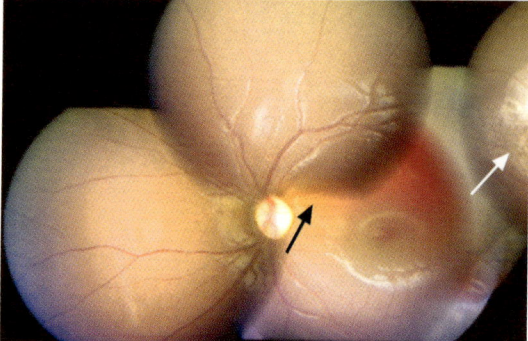

Fig. 14.6 *Left fundus photograph showing active periphlebitis (black arrow) and active parsplanitis (white arrow) in a case of multiple sclerosis*

described in multiple sclerosis inclusive of iridocyclitis, pars planitis, retinitis, periphlebitis and optic neuritis and some times these may be presenting sign of the disease. The disease is bilateral in 95%. Retinal periphlebitis may occur in 5–10% of cases of multiple sclerosis. In an active lesion perivenular infiltrates are present which can progress to occlusive peripheral vasculitis leading to neovascularization, vitreous hemorrhage and tractional retinal detachment (Fig. 14.6).

5. Human immunodeficiency virus (HIV)

Mostly perivasulitis in HIV patients is associated with cytomegalovirus (CMV) retinitis which is the most common opurtunistic infection in these patients. The classical CMV retinitis is associated with scattered yellow-white areas of necrotizing retinitis with hemorrhage described as "Pizza pie retinopathy". It is often associated with retinal phlebitis presenting as perivenous sheathing. However, in some cases of AIDS, perivasculitis of the peripheral vessels involving veins more often than arteries has been observed even without CMV retinitis (Fig. 14.7).

6. Eales' disease

Henry Eale in 1880 described five young men with recurring vitreal and retinal hemorrhages associated with constipation and epistaxis. The description has varied over the years, however, it is defined as an idiopathic inflammatory venous occlusive disease of young adult males, involving retina in multiple quadrants of both

episodes which are the major cause of visual morbidity. Course of disease is characterized with recurrent explosive attacks and spontaneous remissions. The diagnosis is established by following the criteria proposed by the international study group for Behçet's disease in 1990. The criteria require recurrent aphthous ulcers of oral mucosa as an essential symptom plus two or more symptoms of genital ulceration, eye lesions, skin lesion and positive pathergy test.

4. Multiple sclerosis

It is a chronic disease of unknown etiology characterized by demyelination and sclerosis in the central nervous system. The age of onset is typically between 20 and 40 years and females are more commonly affected than males. Various ocular inflammatory lesions have been

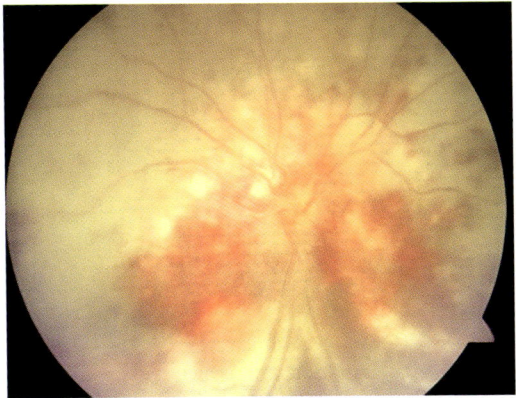

Fig. 14.7 *Right fundus photograph showing classical CMV retinitis in a HIV patient. It is associated with scattered yellow white areas of necrotizing retinitis with hemorrhage termed as "Pizza pie retinopathy". Patches of periphlebitis are also seen*

eyes commencing anterior to equator and progressing posteriorly. Non-perfusion leads to neovascularization causing recurrent vitreous hemorrhage and tractional retinal detachment. The disease is mostly without vitritis, uveitis and obvious systemic disease. The condition is in essence diagnosis of exclusion. Thus three hallmark of the disease are retinal phlebitis, capillary non-perfusion and neovascularization.

The disease is not common in American and European continent, however 1% of adult in India has been estimated to be suffering from this disease. There are reports from Indian subcontinent blaming hypersensitivity to tuberculo-proteins as the most probable

causative factor in the etiopathogenesis of the condition. The condition is treated in active stage by steroid, in stage of neovascularization by photocoagulation and non-clearing vitreous hemorrhage and TRD by PPV (Fig. 14.8A and B). In well equipped vitreoretinal centers the prognosis of vision is fairly good.

DISORDERS ASSOCIATED WITH PERIARTERITIS PREDOMINANTLY

1. Syphilis

It is sexually transmitted disease (STD) caused by spirochete *Treponema pallidum*. Although leutic vasculitis is predominantly arterial but it needs to be excluded in any patient with retinal vasculitis as it is a great imitator and can mimic wide variety of ocular disorders. Since treponema can thrive in all the layers of the eye thus it can cause variety of lesions such as focal or multifocal chorioretinitis, vitritis, retinal vasculitis, neuroretinitis, optic neuritis, intermediate and panuveitis and pseudoretinitis pigmentosa (Fig. 14.9A and B).

2. Acute retinal necrosis (ARN)

It is mainly caused by viruses such as varicella zoster, herpes simplex types 1 and 2. The Clinical features included peripheral necrotizing retinitis, retinal arteritis with severe vitritis and anterior chamber reaction. The necrosed retina appears greyish-white in color. The vision loss usually occur due to rhegmatogenous retinal detachment, macular involvement or optic neuropathy. Vasculitis is predominantly peri-

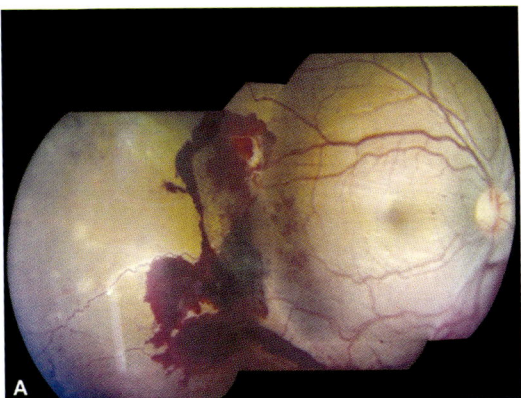

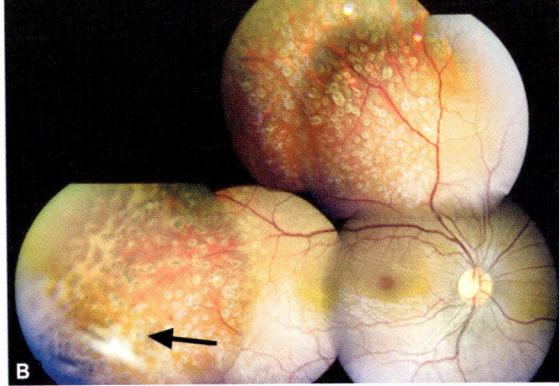

Fig. 14.8 *Right fundus photograph showing healed periphlebitis in a patient of Eales' disease. (A) Stage of neovascularization with preretinal bleeds and (B) regression (black arrow) after panretinal photocoagulation*

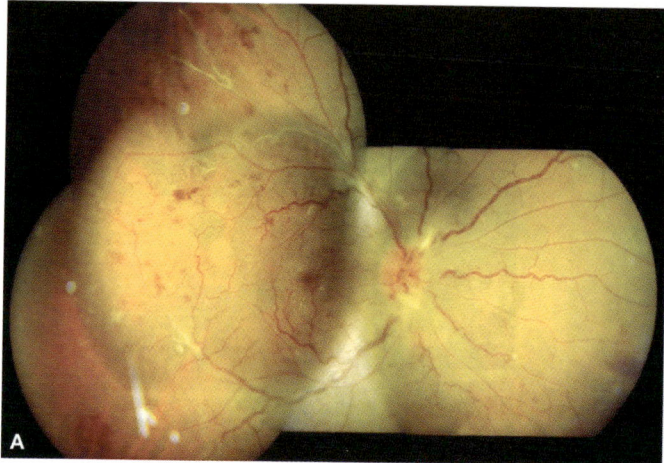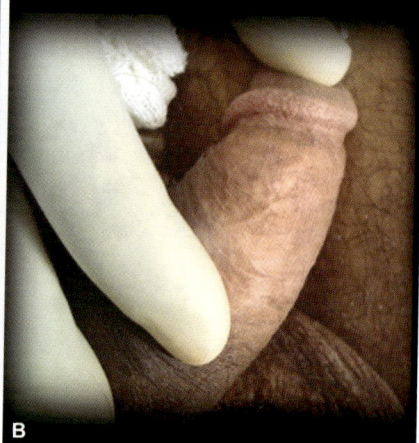

Fig. 14.9 *(A)* Right fundus photograph showing active vasculitis in a patient of syphilis and *(B)* chancre on the genitalia

pheral arteritis with closure probably at the beginning of the peripheral necrosis.

3. Systemic lupus erythematosus (SLE)

It is an autoimmune disease characterised by multisystem involvement causing small vessel occlusion in different organs. The prevalence ranges from 3 to 29% and retinal vascular lesions are the most common ocular manifestation of SLE. It is due to periarteritis leading to arteriolar occlusion. The retinopathy consists of cotton wool spots with or without retinal hemorrhages not associated with hypertension. It can be focal or diffuse vascular disease. The former is more common where retinal artery or vein occlusion may occur. The later is less common but more severe characterized by diffuse arteriolar occlusion with extensive capillary nonperfusion.

The patients with SLE and with raised anti-phaspholipid antibodies (APLA) have a higher risk of retinal vascular occlusive disease. Exacerbations of disease activity might manifest in retina as a retinal vascular occlusion. The clinical manifestations and higher titres of anti-double stranded DNA antibody, raised anti nuclear antibody, positive lupus erythematosus cell phenomenon, hypergammaglobulinemia, raised circulating immune complexes and reduced serum complement help in the diagnosis of SLE.

4. Polyarteritis nodosa (PAN)

It is a necrotizing vasculitis of small and medium sized arteries in various organs involving heart, kidney, liver, GIT and CNS. Ophthalmic involvement is observed in 10–20% of patients of PAN. Retinopathy which is primarily peri-arteritis consist of cotton wool spots, hemorr-hages, edema and central retinal artery occlusion. Other ocular manifestations include peripheral ulcerative keratitis, necrotizing scleritis, nongranulomatous iritis, vitritis, papilitis and ischemic optic neuropathy.

DISORDERS ASSOCIATED WITH BOTH PERIARTERITIS AND PERIPHLEBITIS

1. Toxoplasmosis

It is caused by the obligate intracellular parasite *Toxoplasma gondii*. Infection may occur by either congenital or acquired route primarily affecting the retina. The characteristic retinal lesion is focal necrotizing retinitis frequently involving the macula resulting into atrophic scar with pigmented borders. Reactivation is commonly seen adjacent to an old atrophic scar. There may be an associated vasculitis near to or distant to the active retino-choroiditis. Recently frosted branch angiitis and occlusive vasculitis secondary to toxoplasma has also been reported. In addition granulomatous anterior uveitis may be associated. Immunocompro-mised patients manifest more severe form of the disease (Fig. 14.10).

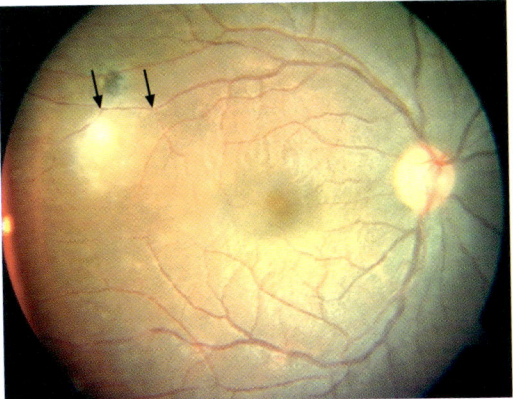

Fig. 14.10 *Right fundus photograph showing active lesion of retino-choroiditis adjacent to healed lesion of toxoplasmosis with adjoining perivasculitis*

2. Wegner's granulomatosis

It is a necrotizing granulomatous vasculitis classically involving the kidneys and upper and lower respiratory tract. Ocular involvement occurs in 28–58% patients which include retinal artery occlusion, choroidal arterial occlusion, retinal vein occlusion and optic nerve vasculitis. Other involvements are episcleritis, scleritis, corneal ulceration and paranasal granulomata. The diagnosis is established by antineutrophil cytoplasmic antibodies (ANCAs) and typical histopathological feature of inflammation of small vessels, necrosis and granuloma formation.

3. Frosted branch angiitis

It is an extreme form of diffuse perivasculitis involving both arteries and veins, however predominantly veins, mostly bilateral, without any sex preference and occurs in young healthy individuals who typically have acute bilateral visual loss associated with anterior and posterior segment inflammation. Fundus appearance include retinal edema, severe sheathing of retinal vessels resembling the appearance of frosted tree branches. In addition patient has retinal hemorrhages, hard exudates and serious retinal detachments of macula and periphery (Fig. 14.11A and B). Fundus fluorescein angiography demonstrates leakage of dye but no evidence of decreased blood flow or occlusion. Initially the condition was considered to be idiopathic and patients respond to systemic corticosteroids with rapid resolution.

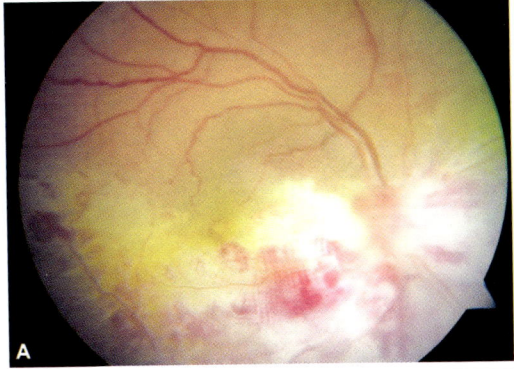

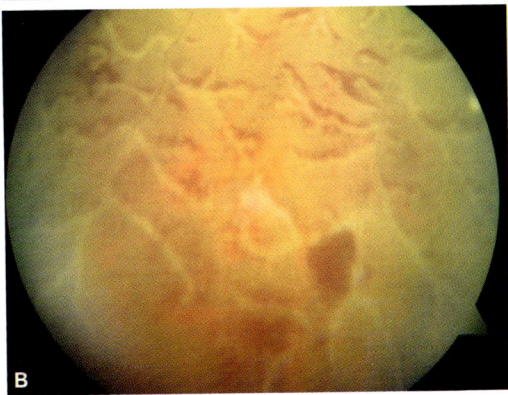

Fig. 14.11 *(A) Retinal edema, dilated tortuous vessels with severe sheathing and superficial hemorrhages in case of frosted branch angiitis; and (B) the sheathing of retinal vessels resemble the appearance of frosted tree branches, hence the name frosted branch angiitis*

However, sufficient evidence exist that it can be associated with wide variety of conditions like lymphoma and leukemia, viral infections and autoimmune diseases. It has also been reported to be associated with SLE, Crohn's disease, AIDS, HIV without CMV retinitis, HSV infection and with toxoplasma.

4. Crohn's disease

It is a chronic inflammatory bowel disease of unknown origin. The eye is involved in 4–10% of patients presenting with occlusive retinal arteritis and phlebitis.

MANAGEMENT

INVESTIGATIONS

The diagnosis of retinal vasculitis involves a multidisciplinary approach supported by

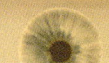

laboratory investigations, detailed history, review of systems and physical examination which may help us to rule out infectious etiology. Once the infectious etiology is believed to be unlikely then any associated systemic disease is considered and the diagnostic workout is tailored according to that disease. If, however, the patient has no signs and symptoms suggestive of systemic disease then the diagnosis of idiopathic retinal vasculitis is most likely. In this situation the basic work up of the patient include FFA, total and differential leucocytic count, ESR, VDRL, FTA-ABS, Mantoux test, HIV serology and X-ray chest.

Fundus fluorescein angiography

Fundus fluorescein angiography (FFA) demonstrates leakage of dye and staining of vessel wall during the active stage of the disease. Sometimes clinically normal looking vessels may show apparent disease on FFA. In addition CME, NVE, NVD, vascular occlusion and capillary nonperfusion (CNP) area, can be confirmed by using angiography.

Test for tuberculosis

Positive mantoux test, findings on X-ray chest, raised ESR point towards tuberculosis. In suspected ocular TB cases PCR from aqueous and quantiferon TB gold test from blood may clinch the diagnosis.

Test for sarcoidosis

Negative Mantoux test, raised serum calcium and serum ACE levels, CECT chest and transbronchial lung biopsy may help in obtaining the diagnosis of sarcoidosis.

Test for other infectious diseases

Serology for toxoplasmosis, PCR from aqueous tap for VZV, HSV 1 and 2 and CMV retinitis in case of vasculitis associated with acute retinal necrosis and progressive outer retinal necrosis may be ordered.

Test for systemic diseases

Patients with suspected systemic vasculitis can be diagnosed by ordering rheumatoid factor, antinuclear antibodies, antineutrophil cytoplasmic antibody, antidouble stranded DNA antibodies C-reactive proteins, LE cell phenomenon test.

Other tests

HLA-B51 point towards Behçet's disease and *HLA-DRS* towards SLE. *Vitreous biopsy* may help in suspected ocular lymphoma. *MRI and full neurological evaluation* may establish multiple sclerosis.

Finally young adults with no known cause of vasculitis (Eales' disease) are labelled as idiopathic and managed as per the stage of presentation.

COMPLICATIONS

These are cystoid macular edema (CME), vitreous hemorrhage, tractional retinal detachment (TRD), rubeosis iridis and neovascular glaucoma (NVG).

TREATMENT
Treatment of retinal vasculitis

In cases of active infective vasculitis oral steroids are started in the dose of 1 mg/kg/b.w and are gradually tapered over 3 months period under the cover of specific antibacterial, antiviral or anti-parasitic drugs.

Patients with tuberculosis or presumed ocular tuberculosis usually require ATT for 9 months with oral steroid. Similarly in cases of syphilis, appropriate antibiotics are instituted alongwith oral steroids.

In cases of active non-infective vasculitis such as sarcoidosis, Behçet's disease and systemic arteritis, oral steroids are given and these entities may require immunosupressives for the control of disease.

Treatment of complications of retinal vasculitis

- *CME* may be managed by using posterior subtenon kenacort.
- *Stage of neovascularization* may require sector laser in cases of NVE and scatter laser (PRP) in cases of NVD.
- *Advanced changes such as recurrent vitreous hemorrhage and tractional retinal detachment* can be managed by pars plana vitrectomy (PPV). AntiVEGF drugs may have role prior to PPV in order to reduce the chances of

intraoperative bleeding and for better visual prognosis after PPV.

- ***Rubeosis iridis and neovascular glaucoma*** is managed by PRP and glaucoma filteration surgery.

PROGNOSIS

Prognosis of vision is relatively better than diabetic retinopathy since the patients are younger in age group and the macula remains healthy. However, macular edema and macular ischemia are significant causes for poor visual prognosis. In addition inflammatory vascular occlusions are other factors detrimental to good visual prognosis. Recently it has been reported that adequate treatment of obliterative retinal vasculitis with systemic steroids and specific anti-infective therapy, laser application as and when required and early PPV when necessary, may result in improving the anatomic and visual outcome.

BIBLIOGRAPHY

1. Abu EI-Asrar AM, AL Kharashi SA. Full PRP and early vitrectomy improves prognosis of retinal vasculitis associated with tuberculo-protein hypersensitivity (Eales' disease). Br. J. Ophthalmol 2002: 86: 1248–51.
2. Biswas J, Mukesh BN, Narain S, Roy S, Madhavan HN. Profiling of HLA in Eales' disease. Int. Ophthalmol 1998;21:277–81.
3. Biswas J, Therese L, Madhavan HN. Use of PCR in detection of *Mycobacterium tuberculosis* complex DNA from vitreous samples of Eales' disease. Br. J. Ophthalmol 1999;83:994.
4. Biswas J. Eales disease—an update. Survey ophthalmol 2002:47:197.
5. Chang TS, Aylward W, Davis JL, et al. Idiopathic retinal vasculitis, aneurysms and neuro-retinitis. Ophthalmology 1995;102: 1089–97.
6. Curi ALL, Freeman G, Pavesio C, Aggressive retinal vasculitis in PAN. Eye 2001;15: 229–31.
7. Eales H. Primary retinal hemorrhages in young-men. Ophthalmol Rev 1882;1:41.
8. Elliot AJ. Thirty year observation of patients with Eales' disease Am J Ophthalmol 1975;80: 404.
9. Geier SA, Nase mann J, Klauss V, Kronawitter U, Goebel FD. Frosted branch angitis in a patient with AIDS. Am J Ophthalmol 1992;113:203–5.
10. Graham EM, Stanford MR, Sander MD, Kasp E, Dumonde DC. A point prevalence sudy of 150 patients with idiopathic retinal vasculitis: I. Diagnostic value of ophthalmological features Br J Ophthalmol 1989;73:714–21.
11. Gupta A, Gupta V, Arora S, Dogra MR, Bambery R. PCR-positive tubercular retinal vasculitis. Clinical characteristics and management. Retina 2001;21:435–44.
12. Herbort CP, Limino L, Abu El-asrar AM. Ocular vasculitis: a multidisciplinary approach. Curr Opin Rheumatol 2005;17:25–33.
13. Kumar A, Tiwari HK, Singh RP, et al. Comparative evalution of early vs deferred vitrectomy in Eales' disease. Acta Ophthalmol Scand 2000; 78:77.
14. Nakao K, Ohba N, Human T-cell lymphotropic virus type 1-associated retinal vasculitis in children. Retina 2003;23:197–201.
15. Perez VL, Chavala SH, Ahmed M, et al. Ocular manifestations and concepts of systemic vasculitides. Surv Ophthalmol 2004; 49:399–418.
16. Quillen DA, Stathopoulos NA, Blankenship GW, Ferriss JA. Lupus associated frosted branch periphlebitis and exudative maculopathy. Retina 1997;17:449–51.
17. Rothova A. Ocular involvement in sarcoidosis. Br J Ophthalmol 2000;84:10–6.
18. Samuel MA, Equi RA, Chang TS, et al. Idiopathic retinitis, vasculitis aneurysms and neuroretinitis (IRVAN): new obervations and a proposed staging system. Ophthalmology 2007;114:1526–9.
19. Spaide RF, Vitale AT, Toth IR, Oliver JM. Frosted branch angiitis associated with CMV retinitis. Am J Ophthalmol 1992;113:522–8.
20. Vine AK. Severe periphlebitis, peripheral retinal ischaemic, preretinal neovascularization in patients with MS. Am J Ophthalmol 1992;113: 28–32.
21. Ysasaga JE, Davis J. Frosted branch angitis with ocular toxoplasmosis. Arch Ophthalmol 1999; 117:1260–1.

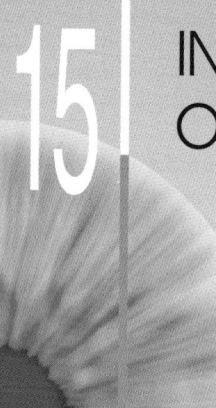

INFLAMMATORY DISEASES OF THE RETINA AND CHOROID

Subina Narang, Mohit Dogra, Anjani Khanna, Pratik Topiwala

RETINO-CHOROIDAL INFLAMMATORY DISEASES AS A PART OF SYSTEMIC DISEASES
- Tuberculosis
- Sarcoidosis
- Spirochaetal (Syphilis)
- Toxoplasmosis
- Ocular toxocariasis
- DUSN
- Ocular cysticercosis
- AIDs
- HIV
- ARN

- PORN
- CMV

CHOROIDAL INFLAMMATIONS
Primary Inflammatory Choriocapillaropathies
- Serpiginous choroiditis
- Acute posterior multifocal placoid pigment epitheliopathy

Primary stromal choroiditis
- VKH
- Sympathetic ophthalmitis

WHITE DOT SYNDROMES

RETINO-CHOROIDAL INFLAMMATORY DISEASES AS PART OF SYSTEMIC DISEASES

TUBERCULOSIS

INTRODUCTION

Tuberculosis is a clinical disease caused by infection with *Mycobacterium tuberculosis* and is characterized pathologically by the formation of granulomas. TB predominantly involves lung. It can also involve other body organs like gastrointestinal tract, genitourinary tract, cardiovascular system, skin, central nervous system and eyes. It may or may not be associated with pulmonary involvement. The disease is of prime importance in countries like India.

EPIDEMIOLOGY

Approximately one-third of the world's population (2 billion) are infected with *M. tuberculosis* and 10% of infected population may develop disease during lifetime. Ocular involvement was reported to occur in 1.4% cases of tuberculosis in 1967 while it was reported to occur in 18% cases of TB in 1997. The epidemic of human immunodeficiency virus (HIV) infection has had a significant impact on the global epidemiology of tuberculosis. Transmission of infection occurs predominantly due to aerosolized droplets. Most patients develop an asymptomatic infection that usually heals with granuloma formation. Sensitization is manifested by a positive skin test to an extract of the tuberculous bacillus (purified protein derivative, PPD). It occurs between period of 2 and 10 weeks. Disease usually is in quiescent stage but onset of symptoms can occur after a derangement of immune system due to age, disease, or the use of immunosuppressive therapy for other conditions.

OCULAR LESIONS

CLINICAL PROFILE

Ocular disease is mainly hypersensitivity reaction to sequestered tubercular antigen. TB

can involve both the anterior and posterior segments of the eye as well as the ocular adnexa and orbit. The most common clinical presentation appears to be posterior uveitis (46%), followed by anterior uveitis, panuveitis, and intermediate uveitis (11%). Clinical presentation of tubercular uveoretinal inflammation are summarized in Table 15.1.

ANTERIOR SEGMENT INVOLVEMENT

Anterior segment involvement is seen as granulomatous uveitis with large sized keratic precipitates, broad based synechiae and iris granulomas (Fig. 15.1A to D).

Rarely granulomas can be seen in angle or hypopyon may be seen. Tubercles may also rarely occur in the anterior chamber, lids conjunctiva, cornea, and sclera. Corneal involvement can present as interstitial keratitis

and phylectenular keratoconjunctivitis due to an immunologic response to the mycobacteria.

INTERMEDIATE UVEITIS

Intermediate uveitis may present as parsplanitis, snowballs, peripheral venular sheathing and cystoid macular edema (CME).

POSTERIOR SEGMENT INVOLVEMENT

Posterior segment involvement may be present as:
- *Tubercular uveitis and/or choroidal tubercles* (Fig. 15.2). In 28% of patients with miliary TB tubercles can be seen in the choroid, giving the impression of a unifocal or multifocal choroiditis. Choroidal tubercles are yellow discrete with indistinct borders with or without serous detachment. Histopathologically they are tubercular granulomas with

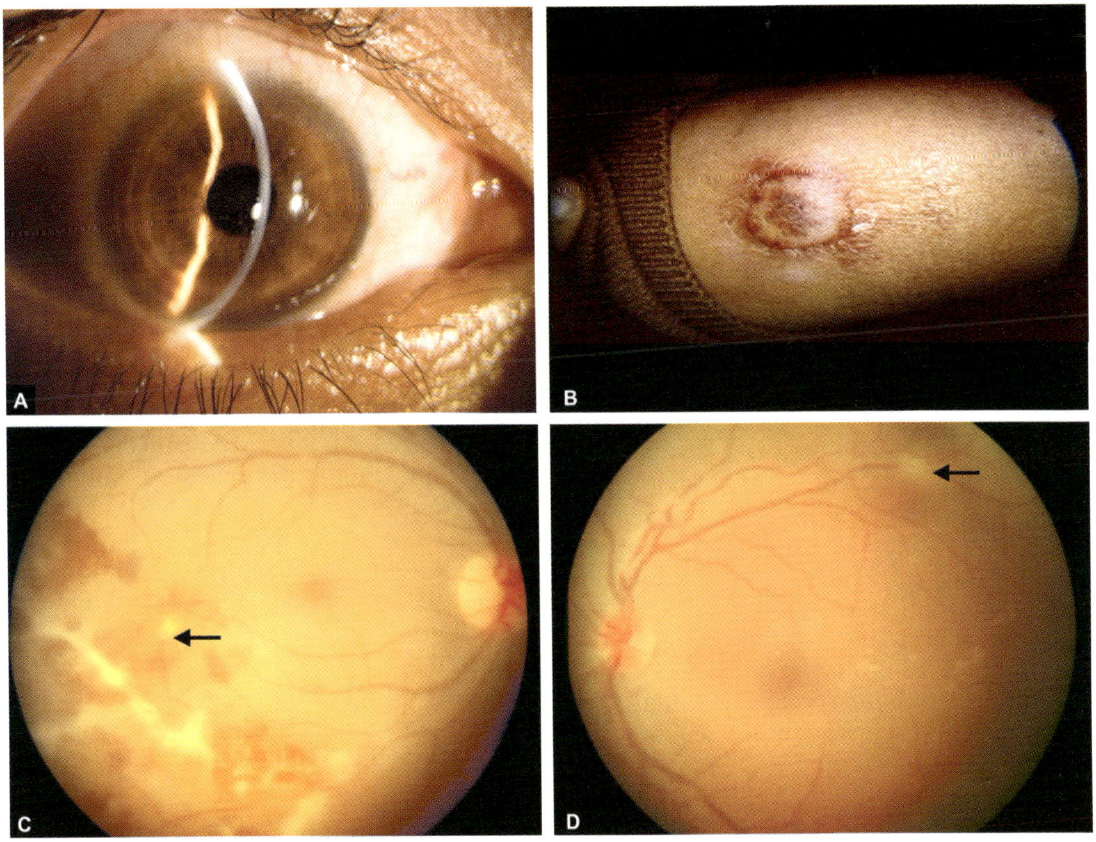

Fig. 15.1 *(A) Slit lamp picture of anterior segment showing large keratic precipitates; **(B)** Clinical photograph of left arm of the same patient showing necrotic Mantoux test; **(C)** Fundus picture of right eye of the same patient showing active vasculitis and choroiditis (arrow); and **(D)** Fundus picture of left eye showing patchy vasculitis (arrow)*

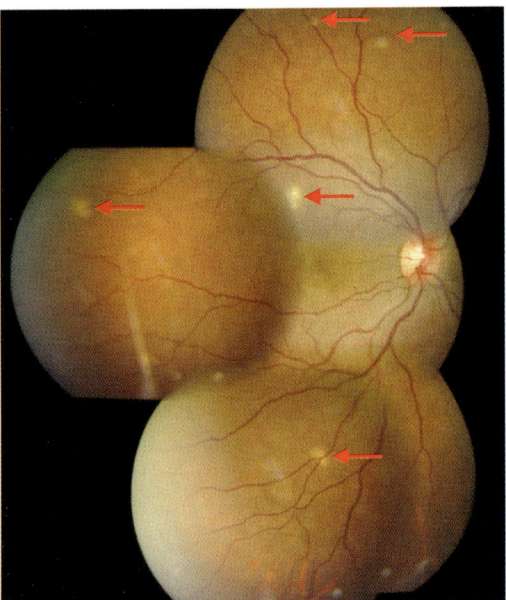

Fig. 15.2 *Fundus montage of a patient with miliary tuberculosis showing tubercles (arrow)*

caseous necrosis in the center with or without Acid Fast Bacilli. They have also been associated with the development of subretinal neovascularization.

- *The periphlebitis* is along with choroidits.
- Multifocal choroiditis could be active lesions yellowish lesions with fizzy margins and overlying retinal edema (Fig. 15.3) and inactive healed flat scars may also be seen.
- There are capillary non perfusion areas along with neovascularisation (Fig. 15.4).
- *Vitreous hemorrhage* may also be present.
- *Serpiginous like choroiditis* (Fig. 15.5A to D) could be seen with initial focal lesion and later confluent worm like progression. Diffuse large plaque with subretinal granulomas may also be seen (Fig. 15.6A to C). The age group is younger and mild vitritis is seen.
- *Neuroretinitis* may also be seen with macular star. Subretinal abscesses are also seen in tuberculosis.
- *Optic disc granuloma* can also be seen in tuberculosis. It usually is present with periphlebitis (Fig. 15.7).

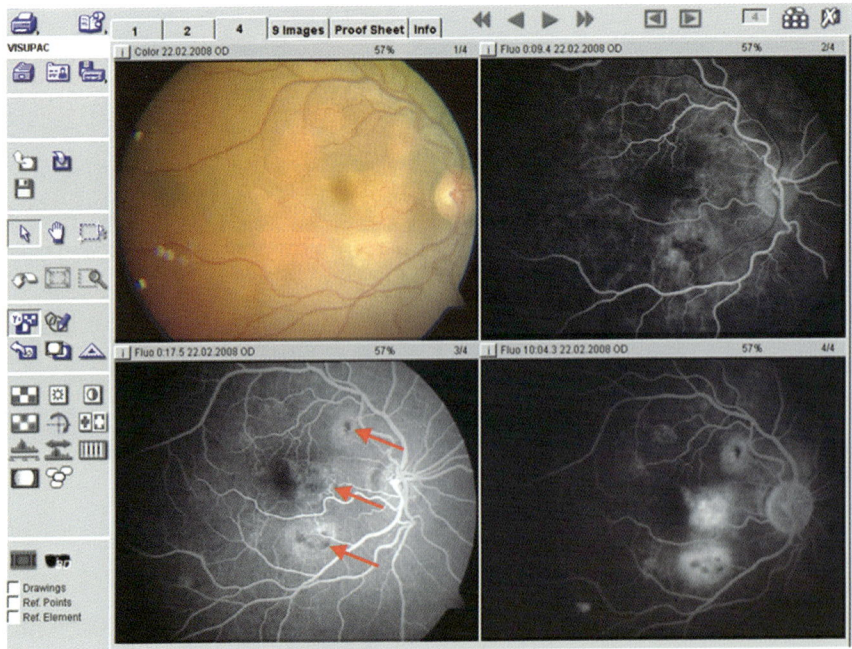

Fig. 15.3 *Fundus photograph showing multifocal active choroiditis in a case with positive Mantoux; fundus fluorescein angiography (FFA) confirms the activity by leakage in late frames of FFA*

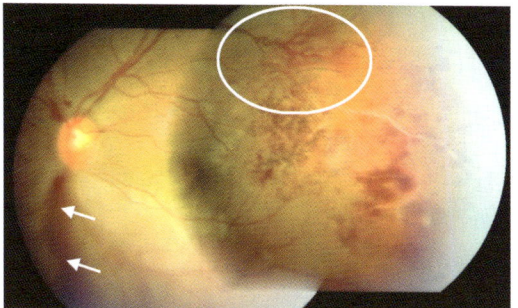

Fig. 15.4 *Fundus photograph showing inactive sheathing and neovascularisation (white circle) and vitreous hemorrhage (yellow arrows)*

DIAGNOSIS

Mantoux test. The diagnostic tool for ocular TB remains Mantoux test read after 48–72 hrs of injection of 5 tuberculin units. The reading of >10 mm is regarded as positive test in high risk cases like those in endemic areas and health care workers who are exposed to TB. In subjects with BCG vaccination strongly positive Mantoux test is regarded as positive.

An intermediate-strength tuberculin skin test should be used for most patients. The PPD test is not 100% sensitive or specific for the disease especially in countries where BCG vaccination is given in universal immunization programme. A positive PPD test result in a patient with uveitis does not necessarily imply TB, without other signs of TB.

Interferon-γ-release assays are new alternatives to the tuberculin skin test. QuantiFERON-TB Gold has excellent specificity and is unaffected by BCG vaccination. ESATb and CFPIU which are absent in all strains of BCG. It measures IFN-γ response of T cells to *Mycobacterium tuberculosis* antigen. It is highly specific but it is positive in only 30% of cases. This test used two proteins.

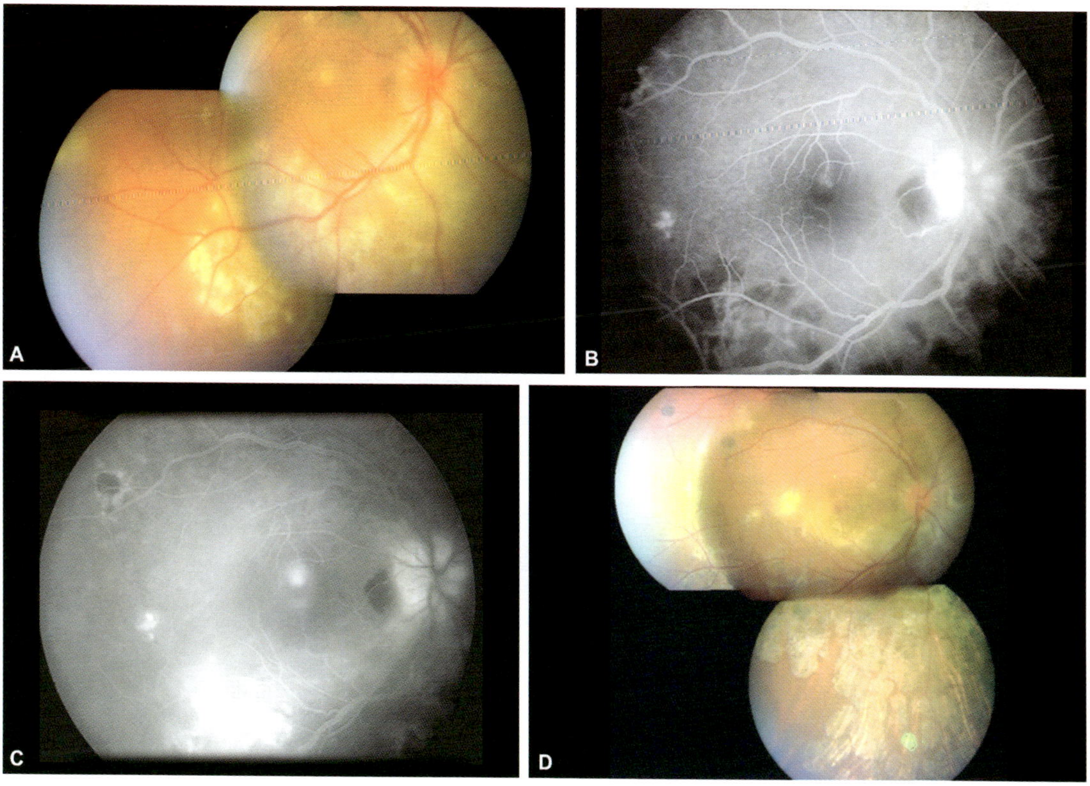

Fig. 15.5 *Biopsy proven case of abdominal tuberculosis, (A) Fundus picture showing serpiginous like choroiditis; (B and C) FFA showed classical hypofluorescence in early and hyperfluorescence in late phase; and (D) Fundus picture shows partial resolution after 3 weeks treatment of ATT and steroids*

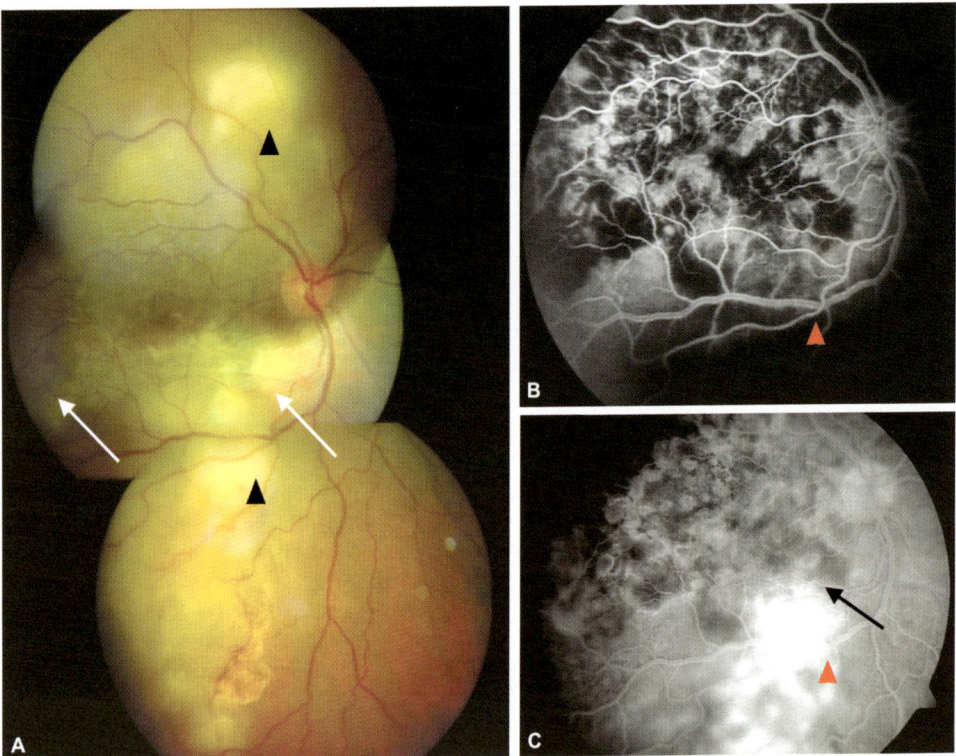

Fig. 15.6 *(A) Fundus picture of a case with necrotic Mantoux test showing serpiginous like choroiditis with granulomas (arrow head; (B and C) FFA shows early hypofluorescence and late hyperfluorescence*

Identification of Mycobacterium tuberculosis organisms in ocular tissues or fluids is the necessary requisite for diagnosis.

Systemic evaluation for evidence of the disease should be done.

Chest X-ray should be obtained and high resolution CT (HRCT) chest can pick up lung parenchymal involvement if chest X-ray is normal. Contrast enhanced CT (CECT) can detect mediastinal lymphadenopathy.

Polymerase chain reaction (PCR) of aqueous or vitreous aspirate has also been used to diagnose TB infection. It amplifies discrete DNA fragments in intraocular fluids.

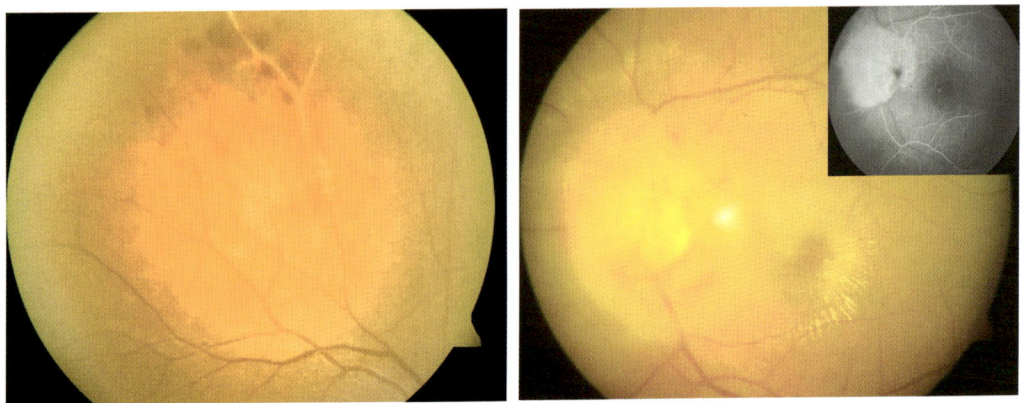

Fig. 15.7 *Fundus picture of a patient with Mantoux of 22X22mm shows periphlebitis in periphery and optic disc granuloma*

Histopathological examination has demonstrated AFB in RPE cells. It is difficult to get adequate samples but the definite proof is presence of AFB in ocular samples.

Table 15.2 summarizes the investigation required for a suspected case of ocular tuberculosis.

DIAGNOSTIC CRITERIA FOR INTRAOCULAR TUBERCULOSIS

Definitive intraocular tuberculosis. Any one or more signs listed in Table 15.1 with any ocular investigations (Table 15.2).

Presumed intraocular tuberculosis. Any one or more signs listed in Table 15.1 with any systemic investigations or positive response to 4 drug

Table 15.1 *Clinical presentation of TB*	
Anterior uveitis	Granulomatous
	Non-granulomatous
	Iris nodules/ciliary body trabeculoma
Intermediate uveitis	Granulomatous
	Non-granulomatous with organising exudates in pars plana/peripheral uvea
Posterior/panuveitis	Choroidal tubercle/tuberculoma
	Subretinal abscess
	Serpiginous like choroiditis
Retinitis and retinal vasculitis	
Neuroretinitis and optic neuropathy	
Endophthalmitis and panophthalmitis	

Table 15.2 *Investigations for ocular TB*	
Ocular investigations	Demonstration of AFB from ocular fluids (microscope/culture)
	Positive polymerase chain reaction (PCR) from ocular fluids
Systemic investigations	Mantoux test
	Radiography of chest: Healed or active TB
	Confirmed active extrapulmonary tuberculosis (microscopic exam/culture)
	Diagnostic criteria for intraocular tuberculosis

therapeutic trial test (isoniazid, rifampicin, ethambutol, pyrizinamide) over 4–6 wks.

TREATMENT

If the clinical findings support a diagnosis of TB, a complete course of antituberculosis therapy should be considered.

Most regimens contain isoniazid and rifampicin for 12–18 months. A third drug usually pyrazinamide added for the first 3 months to prevent resistance. Most regimens now include at least a 2 month course of four drugs, including isoniazid, rifampicin, pyrazinamide, and ethambutol, followed by an additional 12–18 months of isoniazid and rifampicin. Latent TB should also be treated by isoniazid and rifampicin.

The addition of antitubercular therapy to corticosteroids in uveitis patients with underlying latent or manifest TB appears to reduce the recurrences of uveitis. Corticosteroids are usually required for 6–12 weeks to control acute reaction. A history of exposure to TB, a history of inadequately treated TB, a positive PPD test result (induration >15 mm) or positive culture results all greatly increase the likelihood of disease.

Multidrug resistant (MDR) TB is the major issue nowadays and fatality rate with this is 20–80%. About 20% of isolates are MDR and 2% are extremely drug resistant. For these newer drugs like rifabutin, fluoroquinolones, linazolids and interferon gama are used.

Monitoring for complication and side effects

During the treatment period, the patients should be monitored for the side effects of ATT and steroids. Optic neuritis, peripheral neuropathy and hepatotoxicity may be seen.

There could sometimes be paradoxical worsening of ocular lesions after starting ATT (Fig. 15.8) due to enhanced delayed hypersensitivity of the host and the suppressor mechanisms are decreased in addition to increased exposure to mycobacterial antigens.

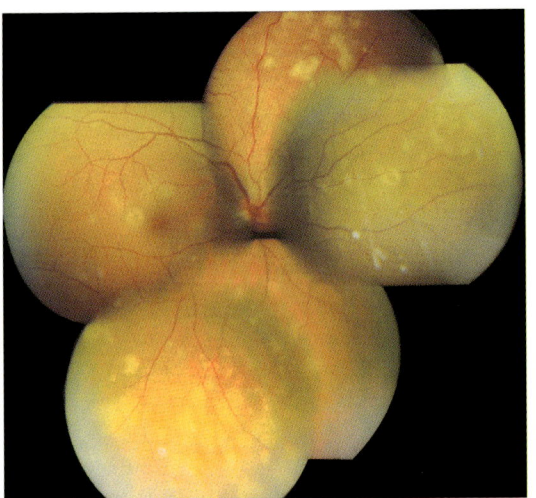

Fig. 15.8 *After ATT for chest TB patient showing paradoxical reaction as multifocal tuberculosis due to enhanced delayed hypersensitivity*

SARCOIDOSIS

Sarcoidosis is a chronic granulomatous disorder of an unknown etiology involving multiple systems. The eye involvement is seen in 25–50% of sarcoidosis patients.

EPIDEMIOLOGICAL FEATURES

It has worldwide distribution with greater prevalence in Northern European countries. Prevalence is high in 20–40 yrs of age in both sexes, females are commonly affected in 45–65 yrs of age. The disease appears in an acute and a chronic form. In elderly people, the chronic form is more common, whereas in young acute form is common. Acute panuveitis occurs in the acute, aggressive form of sarcoidosis, usually in association with Heerfordt syndrome, with uveoparotid fever. Bilateral disease is found in up to 50–70% patients. Sibling of affected patients have 5 times chance of developing disease.

Histopathological features include non-caseating granuloma which can appear in any organ of body. Granuloma is composed of epithelioid cells, Langhans' type multinucleate giant cells and lymphocytes. Giant cells may show inclusion bodies like Schaumann and asteroid bodies.

CLINICAL FEATURES

Sarcoidosis can involve any ocular tissue but uveitis is the most common ocular manifestation (85% of total ocular sarcoidosis).

ACUTE SARCOIDOSIS

Acute form presents suddenly and the presentations include:

1. *Lofgren syndrome* includes iridocyclitis, erythema nodosum, febrile arthropathy, bilateral hilar adenopathy.
2. *Heerfordt's syndrome* (uveoparotid fever) includes uveitis, parotitis, fever and facial nerve palsy.

CHRONIC SARCOIDOSIS

Chronic sarcoidosis has insidious onset with: *Chronic uveitis* with progressive pulmonary fibrosis and airway obstruction.

- It causes *granulomas of orbit and eyelid.*
- *Palpebral and bulbar conjunctival nodules* are known to occur.
- Lacrimal gland infiltration may lead to keratoconjunctivitis sicca.

ANTERIOR SEGMENT LESIONS

Anterior chronic granulomatous iridocyclitis is the most common ocular lesion.

Characteristic features include broad based synechiae, mutton-fat KPs (Figs 15.9 and 15.10), iris nodules (Koeppe' and Busacca's) occur in 12–15% of cases. Whitish oval aggregation of cells are seen as snowballs especially in inferior periphery (Fig. 15.10).

Acute anterior uveitis. 15% of cases may present as acute anterior uveitis or small KPs.

Corneal involvement occurs as limbal/corneal nodules, interstitial keratitis, nummular corneal infiltrates and corneal endothelial opacity. Band shaped keratopathy is the long-term complication or may be due to associated hypercalcemia.

Secondary glaucoma can occur due to extensive posterior synechia formation and resultant iris bombe. Angle might show granulomatous lesion of sarcoidosis.

POSTERIOR SEGMENT LESIONS

Posterior segment involvement is seen in 3% of cases. Posterior segment features include:

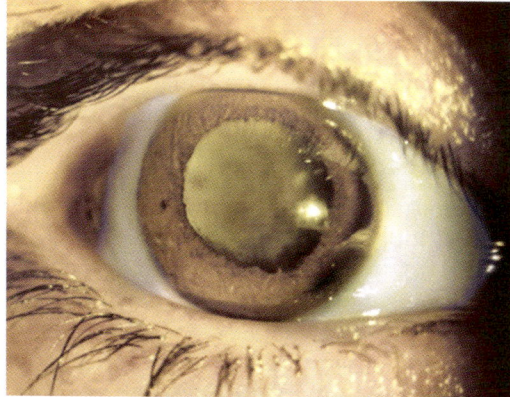

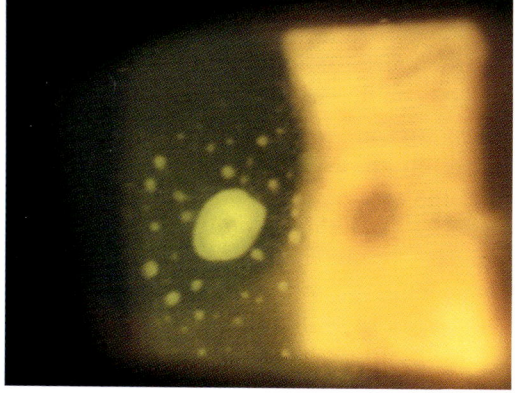

Fig. 15.9 *Case of granulomatous uveitis with negative Mantoux and hilar lymphadenopathy suggestive of sarcoidosis*

- *Classical white oval aggregates* (snowballs) (Fig. 15.10), when linearly arranged also called as 'string of pearls".
- *Perivascular sheathing* in the form of segmental phlebitis (Fig. 15.11).
- *Focal chorioretinitis* which later on heal with pigmentation is the predominant posterior segment manifestation.
  The irregular spherical conglomerates of epitheloid cells along vessels impart typical candle-wax dripping appearance.
- *Macular edema*, with presence of granuloma on and within substance of optic nerve. Occlusive involvement of veins may lead to vascular occlusion leading to subsequent capillary nonperfusion which eventually leads to neovascularisation and vitreous hemorrhage.
- *Granulomas of optic nerve* or elsewhere may also be seen in isolation (Fig. 15.12).
- *Optic neuritis* is seen as papillitis or retrobulbar neuropathy.

Note. Posterior segment involvement may be accompanied by CNS involvement in 25–30% of cases. There could be meningeal involvement, hydrocephalus and papilledema. A multiple arterial ectasias and macroaneurysms are characteristic of sarcoidosis. These could be seen at site of lesion.

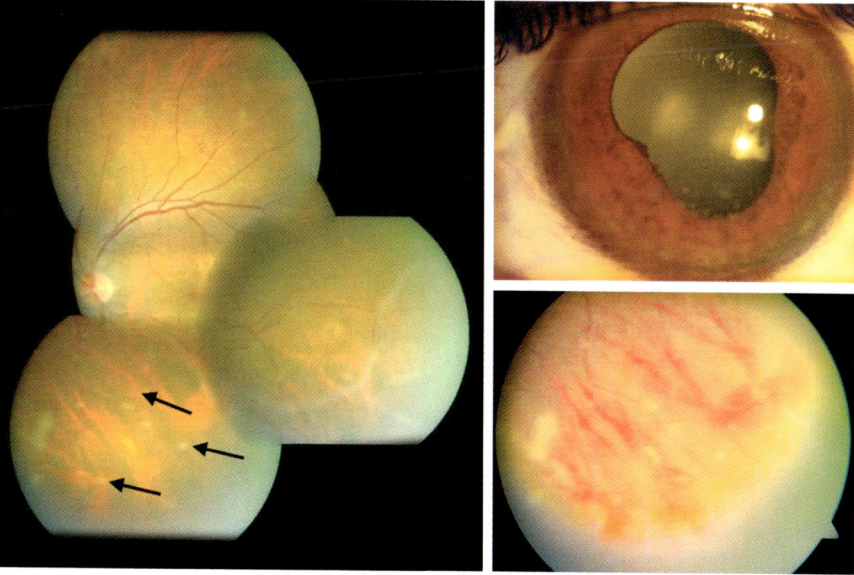

Fig. 15.10 *Case of granulomatous panuveitis with negative Mantoux, bronchoalveolar lavage (BAL) proven sarcoidosis, showing snowball opacities (arrows)*

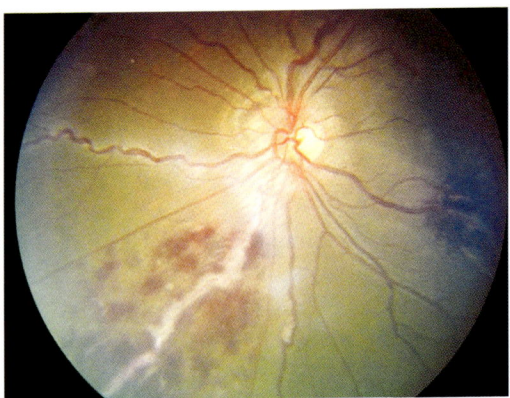

Fig. 15.11 *Fundus picture of a Mantoux negative patient showing segmental periphlebitis with candle-wax dripping suggestive of sarcoidosis*

DIAGNOSIS

Fundus fluorescein angiogrpahy (FFA) demon-strates leakage from clinical/subclinical periphlebitis. Disc leakage may be seen frequently. CNP is seen with adjoining areas of neovascularisation which show leakage. Choroidal vessel involvement could be seen on ICG.

Mantoux test: A negative Mantoux test in a previously BCG vaccinated patient depicts energy and likely diagnosis of sarcoidosis. Conversion of past positive reaction into negative reaction is highly significant.

Serum calcium levels are frequently raised. Hypercalcemia is seen in 10–15% of patients

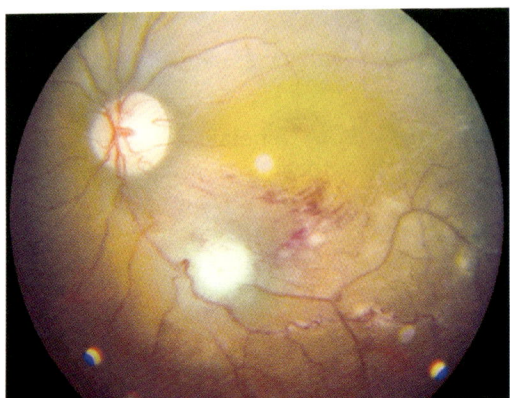

Fig. 15.12 *Fundus picture of a Mantoux negative male showing granuloma along inferior arcade*

with sarcoid. Levels suggestive are about 3 times elevated than normal.

Histopathological examination of involved tissue may show characteristic granuloma which is a confirmatory test of sarcoidosis. Transbronchial lung biopsy is positive in 60% of patients with normal chest X-ray.

Chest roentgenogram is highly sensitive screening tool positive in 50–89% of patients. CT scan of thorax can be ordered when there is high index of suspicion.

ACE levels and lysozyme levels can be used to support diagnosis both of them may give erroneous results. Serum ACE levels are increased in 60–80% of sarcoid patients and are suggestive of body marker of active granuloma. These test may be present in numerous other systemic conditions and is not useful in patients on ACE inhibitors.

Serum lysozyme test is recommended in patients on ACE inhibitors.

Gallium scan shows increase in uptake of Gallium at involved sites. It is highly sensitive test. Bronchoalveolar lavage (BAL) is sensitive test for sarcoidosis. The earliest finding is mononuclear alveolitis with elevated CD4/CD8 ratio.

DIAGNOSTIC CRITERIA FOR SARCOIDOSIS AS PER INTERNATIONAL WORKSHOP ON SARCOIDOSIS 2006, TOKYO, JAPAN

Four levels of certainty for the diagnosis of ocular sarcoidosis (diagnostic criteria)

Patients in whom other possible causes of uveitis have been excluded (Tables 15.3 and 15.4):

1. *Definite ocular sarcoidosis:* Biopsy-supported diagnosis with a compatible uveitis.
2. *Presumed ocular sarcoidosis:* If biopsy was not done but chest X-ray was positive showing BHL associated with a compatible uveitis.
3. *Probable ocular sarcoidosis:* If biopsy was not done and the chest X-ray did not show BHL but there were 3 of the above intraocular signs and 2 positive laboratory tests.
4. *Possible ocular sarcoidosis:* If lung biopsy was done and the result was negative but at least 4 of the above signs and 2 positive laboratory investigations were present.

Table 15.3 *Seven signs of ocular sarcoidosis*

1. Mutton-fat keratic precipitates (KPs)/small granulomatous KPs and/or iris nodules (Koeppe/Busacca)
2. Trabecular meshwork (TM) nodules and/or tent-shaped peripheral anterior synechiae (PAS)
3. Vitreous opacities displaying snowballs/strings of pearls
4. Multiple chorioretinal peripheral lesions (active and/or atrophic)
5. Nodular and/or segmental periphlebitis (+/– candle wax drippings) and/or retinal macroaneurysm in an inflamed eye
6. Optic disc nodule(s)/granuloma(s) and/or solitary choroidal nodule
7. Bilaterality.

Table 15.4 *Laboratory investigations or investigational procedures*

For diagnosis of ocular sarcoidosis in patients having the above intraocular signs included:

1. Negative tuberculin skin test in a BCG-vaccinated patient or in a patient having had a positive tuberculin skin test previously
2. Elevated serum angiotensin converting enzyme (ACE) levels and/or elevated serum lysozyme.
3. Chest X-ray revealing bilateral hilar lympha-denopathy (BHL)
4. Abnormal liver enzyme tests
5. Chest CT scan in patients with a negative chest X-ray result

TREATMENT

Steroid in various forms are the mainstay of therapy:

- *Oral prednisolone* at 1 mg/kg can be given.
- In intolerant patients *periocular depot steroids*, intravitreal implant fluocinolone acetonide or dexamethasone implant can be used.
- *Steroid sparing agents* like methotrexate, azathioprine, mycophenolate mofetil, or cyclosporin can be tried.
- *Topical cycloplegics* are used to prevent ciliary body spasm, photophobia and synechia.

Treatment of associated complications like:

- Cataract can be treated surgically after disease remains silent for more than 3 months.
- Glaucoma should be treated by medical or surgical therapy.

SPIROCHAETAL (SYPHILIS)

Treponema pallidum is a spirochete and is a great mimicker which can have variable ocular manifestations.

AETIOPATHOGENESIS

Syphilis is transmitted sexual contact and trans-placental (mother to fetus). Patients in stage of primary syphilis or secondary syphilis with skin lesions is infective. Latent syphilis and tertiary syphilis are not infectious.

   T. pallidum can penetrate intact mucous membranes or abraded skin. The **incubation period** ranges from 10–90 days. The lymphatics of the primary affected area carry organism to the bloodstream which leads to its dissemina-tion.

CLINICAL MANIFESTATIONS

Primary syphilis presents with painless ulcerated genital lesion called chancre, along with inguinal lymphadenopathy.

Secondary syphilis presents with fever, sore throat, diffuse macular rash and generalised lymphadenopathy generally after one to two months.

Tertiary syphilis. Disease then enters in quiescent stage. Patient may manifest *tertiary syphilis* after many years with aortitis, meningeal involvement and involvement of nervous system manifesting in several ways such as tabes dorsalis and generalised paralysis of insane.

OPHTHALMIC LESIONS

Primary syphilis chancres of lid and conjunctiva are found.

Secondary syphilis. Generalised maculopapular or pustular exanthematous involvement of lid with loss of brow and eyelashes. Conjunctivitis with papillofollicular reaction. Scleritis and episcleritis can occur. Interstitial keratitis with iridocyclitis and papules or nodules on iris. Granulomatous or non-granulomatous anterior uveitis. Posterior segment findings are chorio-retinitis with predominant involvement of peripapillary area and vitritis. The retinal necrosis here is indistinct unlike ARN. Resolution of

inflammatory reaction may lead to appearance simulating retinitis pigmentosa. Involvement of vessels, retinal detachment (exudative) and disc edema are rarer findings.

Tertiary syphilis. Gummas are characteristic lesions of tertiary syphilis. Gummatous involvement of lids can lead to severe blepharitis. Bilateral inflammatory involvement of periosteum of orbit can occur. Interstitial keratitis usually unilaterally is the most common corneal finding in tertiary syphilis. In addition to CNVM and diffuse fibrosis finding similar to secondary syphilis are seen.

Congenital syphilis leads to bilateral interstitial keratitis. Other features are pigmentary retinitis and glaucoma.

The Argyll Robertson pupil and disc edema are seen in cases of meningeal involvement oculomotor abnormalities. Optic atrophy is seen in long-standing cases.

DIAGNOSIS

VDRL test primarily a screening test has high false negative rate. It can also be used to monitor the activity of disease. It is also useful in evaluating patient's response to treatment.

Fluorescent treponemal antibody absorption, or FTA-ABS is most sensitive and specific in all stages of syphilis.

TPHA (*Treponema pallidum* hemagglutinin test) rated equal to FTA-ABS.

Concomitant screening for HIV should also be done.
Detection of IgM bodies in congenital syphilis has high diagnostic specificity (as these antibodies do not cross placenta).

TREATMENT

Ocular syphilis is treated like neurosyphilis.

PRIMARY AND SECONDARY SYPHILIS

- *Procaine penicillin,* 2.4 million units IM daily and probenecid, 500 mg PO qd × 14 days or aqueous crystalline penicillin G 3–4 million units IV every 4 hours for 10 to 14 days
- *Benzathine penicillin* G, 2.4 million units IM in a single dose (although treatment failures have been reported)

- Alternatives include:
  Doxycycline, 100 mg PO bid × 15 days or *tetracycline* 500 mg PO qid for 15 days. *Azithromycin* can also be used or ceftriaxone 2 g IV or IM for 10 to 14 days.

TERTIARY SYPHILIS

CDC recommends crystalline penicillin G IV infusion of penicillin G, 18 to 24 million units per day for 10 to 14 days in ocular syphilis or IM benzathine penicillin G, 2.4 million units given weekly for 3 weeks.

CONGENITAL SYPHILIS IN THE INFANT

- Procaine penicillin, 50 000 units/kg/day IM × 10 days
- Crystalline penicillin G, 50 000 units/kg/day IV in two divided doses × 10 days.

OCULAR TOXOPLASMOSIS

Ocular toxoplasmosis is an important cause of retinitis which is potentially blinding with multiple recurrences.

ETIOPATHOGENESIS

Life cycle of toxoplasm

Toxoplasma gondii is an obligate intracellular parasite found in a widespread distribution in both animals and humans.

It is a zoonosis with **cats being the definitive hosts**.

Strains. Toxoplasma gondii has three strains and there can be recombinants too.
- *Type 1* is highly virulent in mice. It can cause ocular toxoplasmosis in immunocompetent hosts.
- *Type 2 and Type 3* are relatively avirulent, and involve more common by the immunocompromised and congenital toxoplasmosis.

Forms. There are three forms of the parasite.
- *Tachyzoites* (trophozoites) which are invasive forms and can invade all mammalian cells except non-nucleated erythrocytes. The tachyzoites penetrate the cells, reside within the vacuoles and divide by endodyogeny forming **bradyzoites**
- *Bradyzoites* which elaborate a membrane and form tissue cysts of 10–200 microns size with

50–3000 bradyzoites in each cyst. These can develop in any organ and are responsible for latent infection. Rupture of these cysts can lead to reactivation of infection and in immuno-compromised patients can lead to dissemination of organisms.

- *Sporozoites (oocysts)* are produced in the epithelial cells of cat intestine who get infected after ingestion of raw meat, wild birds and mice. The organisms undergo schizogony (asexual division) followed by sexual cycle producing millions of oocysts which are released 3–21 days after ingestion. Oocysts remain viable in moist soil up to 2 years and are susceptible to dry heat and temperature >66°C.

Modes of transmission

- Ingestion of undercooked infected meat containing oocysts or tissue cysts.
- Ingestion of oocysts by contaminated hands or food.
- Transplacental transmission.
- Inoculation of tachyzoites through breaks in the skin.
- Blood transfusion or organ transplantation.
- Ingestion of raw milk.
- Contaminated water.

Pathogenesis

Most of the cases of ocular toxoplasmosis are acquired as is clear from Brazilian and American study.

- Acquired infection in immunocompetent hosts is mostly subclinical and asymptomatic limited by host's immune response.
- If the organism reaches the eye tachyzoites are released and cause retinitis and involve the choroid secondarily. Inflammatory response consists of lymphocytes, macrophages, epitheloid cells, plasma cells at the edge of the lesion.
- Encystment and conversion of tachyzoites to bradyzoites by host's immune response-persistence of latent infection in the cyst in the scar or adjacent to it for years.
- Reactivation of infection during immuno-suppression with rupture of cyst and release of organisms and direct injury to retinal tissue by Toxoplasma.

CLINICAL FEATURES

Acquired systemic toxoplasmosis

It is the most common form found in immuno-competent hosts. Mostly asymptomatic with 10–20% patients exhibiting a self-limited mild flu-like illness with fever, malaise, myalgia, maculopapular rash sparing palms and soles, lymphadenopathy, hepatosplenomegaly and atypical leucocytosis in peripheral blood.

In ocular toxoplasmosis, anterior segment shows a nonspecific granulomatous or non-granulomatous reaction. The characteristic lesion is a patch of retinitis adjacent to an inactive retinochoroidal scar (Fig. 15.14). There is retinal and choroidal necrosis with a sharp demarcation between affected and unaffected retina.

Congenital systemic toxoplasmosis

Transplacental transmission occurs if the mother acquires infection just before or during gestation and not in chronic infection. The earlier in the gestational period the mother gets infection, lesser the chances of transmission but graver the consequences. That is risk of transmission in first trimester is 15–20% and can cause abortion, stillbirth. In third trimester risk of transmission is 40% but most are asymptomatic.

The newborn can have three characteristic features:

1. Convulsions
2. Cerebral calcification
3. Retinochoroiditis is the most common manifestation of congenital toxoplasmosis present in 75–80% patients, bilateral in 85% and involves the posterior pole due to end artery anatomy of fetal macular circulation. In children with mild infection the disease might be detected on routine examination or evaluation of squint. Other features are hydrocephalus, microcephaly, psychomotor retardation, organomegaly, jaundice, rash, fever. This syndrome needs to be differentiated with congenital rubella, herpes simplex, syphilis and CMV.

Clinical features of ocular toxoplasmosis

It typically presents between 10 and 35 years of age. The patient presents with floaters due to vitritis or diminution of vision due to cataract,

CME, media opacities due to vitritis. The disease presents as granulomatous anterior uveitis, vitritis and focal necrotizing retinitis with secondary choroiditis and rarely scleritis (Fig. 15.13).

The characteristic lesion is an area of retinitis adjacent to an inactive healed lesion (Fig. 15.14). There is a focus of retinitis involving the inner layers of retina and presenting as whitish fluffy lesion with surrounding retinal edema and overlying intense vitritis. This is known as "Headlight in fog" appearance.

The retinal lesions can be large destructive lesions (>1DD in size, intense vitritis, always require treatment) inner punctuate retinitis (occur in periphery as punctuate lesions and overlying mild vitritis, do not require treatment, but will require treatment if involve macula) outer punctate retinitis (involve deeper layers of retina, RPE, do not cause vitritis, resolve and recur).

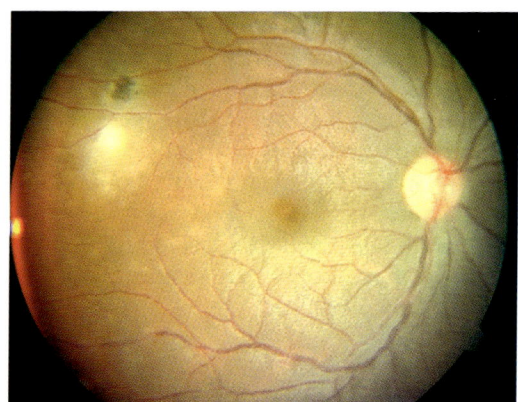

Fig. 15.14 *Fundus photograph showing active toxoplasma lesion adjacent to old toxo scar*

Secondary complications like cataract, glaucoma, band keratopathy, posterior synechaie formation, cystoids macular edema, retinal perivasculitis, chorioretinal vascular anastomosis, retinal detachment, branch artery obstruction and optic atrophy can occur.

Toxoplasma papillitis

It occurs in a few patients with infection in or near the optic nerve head with papillitis, adjacent retinal edema with healed toxoplasma scars in some patients and visual field defects in sectorial involvement. Resolution results in sectorial optic disc pallor and persistence of the associated visual field defect.

Toxoplasma in immunocompromised hosts

Toxoplasmosis is a common cause of morbidity and mortality in immunocompromised people with AIDS, organ transplant patients, patients on chemotherapy, etc. It can lead to pneumonitis, encephalitis and cardiac failure with patients with AIDS having cerebral toxoplasmosis more commonly. Ocular manifestations of the disease is due to direct damage to retinal tissue by invading organisms and consists of atypical and severe retinochoroiditis.

DIAGNOSIS

The diagnosis is clinical and based on characteristic lesion of active retinitis adjacent to an area of chorioretinal scar. To confirm the above various serologic tests done are indirect fluorescent antibody test and ELISA. Due to

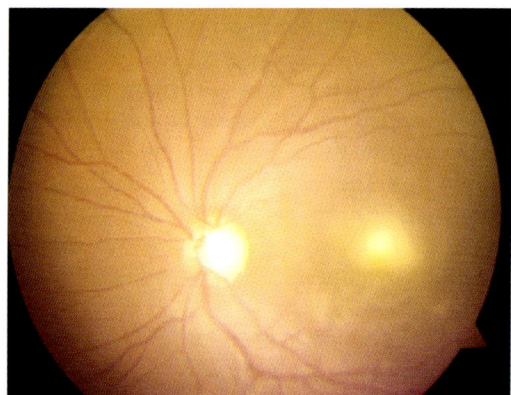

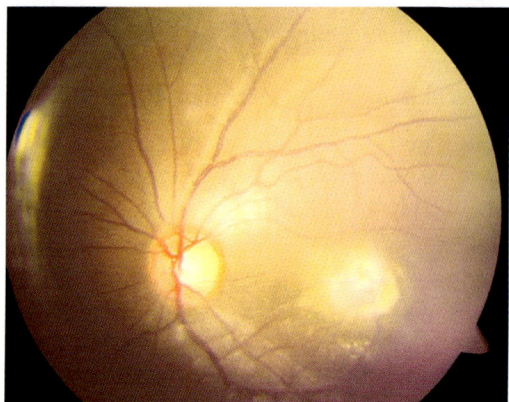

Fig. 15.13 *Fundus picture showing patch of macular retinochoroiditis with positive toxo titres. The patient responded to oral clindamycin and coticosteroids*

high prevalence of Toxoplasma antibodies in the general population if there is a characteristic lesion and positive titres, the diagnosis is taken to be toxoplasmosis but if there is an atypical lesion and positive titres it can only be presumed to be toxoplasmosis. Aqueous humor antibody and polymerase chain reaction is helpful in cases in which the disease is suspected but histology and serology yield negative results.

TREATMENT

Indications for treatment are:

Immunocompromised hosts, congenital toxoplasmosis, posterior pole lesions, vitreous reaction 3+, 4+, large >1DD lesions, persistence of disease >1 month, decrease in vision.

Various drugs used are:
- *Pyrimethamine* two 50 mg loading doses 12 hour apart, then 25 mg orally bd along with *Sulfadiazine* 2 g loading dose, then 1 g orally qid.
- *Oral corticosteroids* minimize the damage to ocular structures due to inflammatory response but are to be used only under the cover of antibiotics.
- *Folinic acid* is also given 3 to 5 mg orally twice weekly. Increased fluid intake is recommended to minimize sulfadiazine renal crystallization.
- *Other drugs* that can be used are Clindamycin as 300 mg qid, Azithromycin in combination with Pyrimethamine, Minocycline, Trimethoprim-Sulfamethoxazole, Atovaquone.

Topical corticosteroids and cycloplegics are used to treat anterior uveitis.

Photocoagulation can be considered for choroidal neovascularisation.

Duration of treatment is generally 4–6 weeks.

Recurrences are common and the risk is increased with cataract surgery.

Prophylaxis with double strength trimethoprim-sulfamethoxazole can be considered.

OCULAR TOXOCARIASIS

Ocular toxocariasis is an important cause of reduced visual acuity in young patients. It is more common in children than adults and is mostly asymptomatic.

ETIOPATHOGENESIS

Life cycle of toxocara

It is a common roundworm of dogs and the most common cause of ocular toxocariasis and visceral larve migrans. It does not complete its life cycle in humans.

Soil contaminated with faeces containing fertilised ova with infectious larvae

↓

Ingested by humans and dogs

↓

From intestinal epithelial cells, larvae enter lymphatics, systemic and portal circulation

↓

Ocular toxocariasis → heart, lungs, liver, brain, kidney and muscles

The life cycle is complete at this stage in humans and dogs wherein the organism is enclosed in an inflammatory granulomatous and eosinophilic response.

When the bitch becomes pregnant there is an alteration in immune response and the larvae start to migrate through the placental circulation to the fetus. They enter the lungs and pharynx of the newborn puppy and mature into adult worms in the intestine of the puppy and infectious ova are released in the faeces.

Routes of infection in puppies

1. *Prenatal infection* is the primary route of transmission
2. *Postnatal-faeces* and milk of infected nursing mother
3. Faecal matter of other canines, mice.

Note. The larvae do not mature in humans so there is no use testing the faeces for ova in human infections.

Toxocara canis is responsible for:
- Visceral larva migrans
- Ocular toxocariasis in humans.

VISCERAL LARVA MIGRANS

It affects young children ranging from 6 months to 4 years of age with average age 2 years. It can be a symptomatic with mild to moderate

eosinophilia, or a self-limiting illness with fever, irritability, pallor, anorexia, malaise, transient infiltrates in lungs, hepatomegaly being the most common sign. It can also have a fulminant and fatal course with pneumonia, seizures and congestive cardiac failure. Systemic disease is rarely associated with ocular disease.

CLINICAL PRESENTATIONS

It can present with any one of the following:

Chronic endophthalmitis

This form occurs in young children with no history of preceding trauma, intraocular surgery or any other cause of bacterial or fungal endophthalmitis. The anterior segment may have no signs of inflammation or can occasionally have a granulomatous anterior uveitis with hypopyon. The media clarity is poor due to intense vitritis and there can be fluffy yellowish exudates and underlying retinal detachment.

The vitreous reaction may dramatically resolve leaving a white mass representing primary focus of infection or site of the parasite or can evolve into cicatricial stage with developing fibrocellular membranes.

Posterior pole granuloma

In acute stage these present as vitritis and ill-defined hazy masses around vitreous inflammation. In late stages when the inflammation has subsided, the child may present with strabismus, clear media and well defined small (0.75–6 mm) subretinal or intraretinal inflammatory masses. These are white or gray in color with traction bands running from the mass to surrounding retina if inflammation has extended into the vitreous cavity. The prognosis for this condition is good, the central vision is compromised at the time of detection. Late complication can be choroidal neo-vascularisation.

Peripheral inflammatory mass

These may present in acute stages with inflammatory reaction or late stages with no inflammation and peripheral whitish masses with fibrocellular bands running from the mass to posterior retina and optic nerve. The bands can cause retinal folds or rhegmatogenous and tractional retinal detachment. These can also present as more diffuse snow banks and pars planitis. The prognosis is relatively good.

Atypical presentations

Inflammation and swelling of the optic nerve head, motile subretinal nematode, diffuse chorioretinitis. Anterior segment involvement can result in conjunctivitis, keratitis, iris nodules and lens changes.

DIFFERENTIAL DIAGNOSIS

A high index of suspicion is required to diagnose toxocariasis. It needs to be differentiated from retinoblastoma, retinopathy of prematurity, familial exudative vitreo-retinopathy, Coats disease, persistent fetal vasculature syndrome.

LABORATORY DIAGNOSIS

Enzyme-linked immunosorbent assay—If the patient has signs and symptoms of toxocariasis a serum titre of 1:8 is sufficient to support the diagnosis. ELISA titres are higher in aqueous and vitreous aspirates than in serum.

Cytology of aqueous aspirates or vitrectomy specimens can show eosinophils or occasionally remnants of toxocara organisms.

Biopsy of granuloma is diagnostic.

TREATMENT

- *Posterior pole or peripheral lesion* without inflammation may not be treated. In case of severe inflammation oral steroids have been found useful in active disease.
- *Topical steroids and cycloplegics* are used in anterior segment inflammation. Use of antihelmentic drugs like mebendazole is controversial.
- *Periocular injections* of steroids are used in severe inflammation of vitreous and retina.
- *Vitrectomy* is performed in vision threatening serve inflammatory disease. Scleral buckling or closed vitrectomy is done for retinal detachment with good anatomical outcomes.

Prevention can be done if all puppies are treated with antihelminthic drugs before they are 4 weeks old, frequent hand washing and general hygiene can be the strategies to prevent toxocariasis.

DIFFUSE UNILATERAL SUBACUTE NEURORETINITIS (DUSN)

Diffuse unilateral subacute neuroretinitis (DUSN) is a rare infectious disease due to worm infestation of subretinal space.

EPIDEMIOLOGY

Most commonly affects healthy young adults. Disease is prevalent in USA, Caribbean area and Latin America. Different nematodes like *A. caninum*, *Toxocara canis*, *Ancylostoma caninum* and *Baylisascaris procyonis* have been put forth as etiologic agent. It has been noted that *A. caninum*, a hookworm found in dogs causes cutaneous larva migrans which may precede DUSN in some patients.

PATHOGENESIS

Histopathological examination of eye reveals non-granulomatous vitritis, retinitis, retinal and optic nerve perivasculitis with extensive degeneration of the peripheral retina. Later progressive optic atrophy, narrowing of retinal arteries and degenerative changes in retina as well as pigment epithelium. It is assumed that pathogenesis involves mechanical disruption and inflammation of the outer retina.

CLINICAL FEATURES

- *Symptoms and signs during early stages include:* Decrease in visual acuity, ocular discomfort, conjunctival injection, nongranulomatous iridocyclitis, retinal perivenous exudation, sheathing, subretinal hemorrhage, serous exudation.
- *Disease is caused by two nematodes* which when examined ophthalmoscopically appear to have different sizes smaller one between 400 and 1000 micron and larger one measuring 1500–2000 microns.
- *Examination fundus* reveals cluster of multifocal, evanescent gray-white lesions at outer retinal level, usually with nematode in vicinity. Lesions appear in crops in one segment of retina. Lesions disappear only to reappear in another area associated with movement of nematode.
- *Fluorescein angiography* during early stages shows hypofluorescent spots and late frames show staining, along with perivascular leakage of dye. Leakage of dye from optic nerve head. FFA does not help in localisation of worm.

TREATMENT

- *Thermal laser application* on worm is the treatment of choice.
- *Antihelminthic agents* like ivermectin, albendazole and thiabendazole can be tried.

OCULAR CYSTICERCOSIS

Human infection in cysticercosis is caused by *Cysticercus cellulosae*, the larval stage of *Taenia solium* (pork tapeworm) and saginate. Eye is the most commonly affected organ though it can affect any organ. Neurocysticercosis is associated with significant morbidity and mortality.

LIFE CYCLE OF CYSTICERCUS CELLULOSAE

Humans are the only definitive hosts for *T. saginata* and *T. solium*. Eggs or gravid proglottids are passed with feces. The eggs can survive for days to months in the environment.

↓

Cattle (*T. saginata*) and pigs (*T. solium*) become infected by ingesting vegetation contaminated with eggs or gravid proglottids.

↓

In the animal's intestine, the oncospheres hatch, invade the intestinal wall, and migrate to the striated muscles, where they develop into cysticerci. A Cysticercus can survive for several years in the animal.

↓

Humans become infected by ingesting raw or undercooked infected meat. In the human intestine, the cysticercus develops over 2 months into an adult tapeworm, which can survive for years. The adult tapeworms attach to the small intestine by their scolex and reside in the small intestine The adults produce proglottids which mature, become gravid, detach from the tapeworm, and migrate to the anus or are passed in the stool (approximately 6 per day).

↓

Eggs produce larvae in the intestine which penetrate the intestinal wall and reach the eye via posterior ciliary arteries.

↓

Larvae can reside in the subretinal space causing exudative retinal detachment or can perforate and cuase retinal break and enter the vitreous cavity.

EPIDEMIOLOGY

It is mostly found in age groups 10–30 years with no sex predilection. *Taenia solium* is endemic to Southeast Asia, India, Mexico, Africa, Eastern Europe, Central and South America. It is associated with poor hygiene.

CLINICAL FEATURES

Cysticercosis can involve any ocular structure-eyelids, orbit, subconjunctiva, anterior chamber or posterior segment. Subretinal involvement is more common than vitreous involvement.

The patients may be asymptomatic with good vision or present with pain, redness, photophobia, moving sensations and diminution of vision. Neurocysticercosis presenting with seizures can have concomitant ocular involvement.

On ocular examination the characteristic appearance of a motile cysticercus in anterior chamber, vitreous or subretinal space is pathognomonic. There can be variable inflammatory reaction in the anterior or posterior segment.

45–50% patients have larvae in the vitreous or subretinal space. The classical appearance is of a globular or spherical translucent white cyst (1.5 to 6 disc diameters in size) with a scolex, that undulates in response to examining light. RPE atrophy can be seen around the area of entry of cysticercus in the subretinal space. There can be associated retinal detachment. B scan ultrasonography will reveal a sonolucent zone with well defined margins and a central highly reflective scolex.

INVESTIGATIONS

- *ELISA* for anticysticercus antibodies—positive in 60–70% patients with ocular or neural cysticercosis.
- *Eosinophilia* is seen in blood and aqueous. Stool examination may reveal eggs of *T. solium* in definitive hosts.
- *CT scan* may show intracerebral calcification, hydrocephalus.

TREATMENT

- *Surgery* is the treatment of choice for intraocular cysticercus.
- *Antihelminthic agents* like Albendazole are not given for intra-ocular cysticercosis. These can be given for orbital or optic nerve lesions under the cover of systemic corticosteroids to prevent worsening of disease by inflammation caused by larval death. The steroids should be started before Albendazole
- *Laser photocoagulation* may be done for small subretinal cysticerci.
- Removal of larvae from vitreous or subretinal space can be done by vitreoretinal surgery (Fig. 15.15).

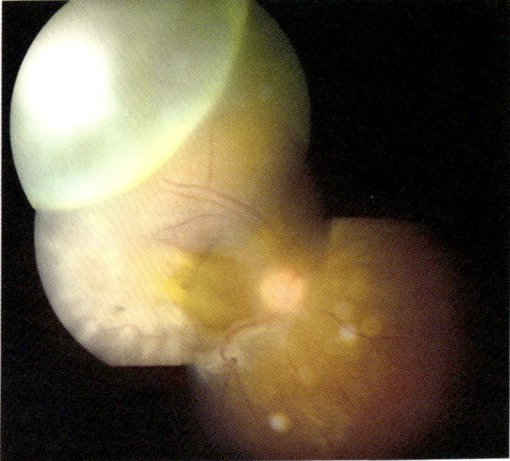

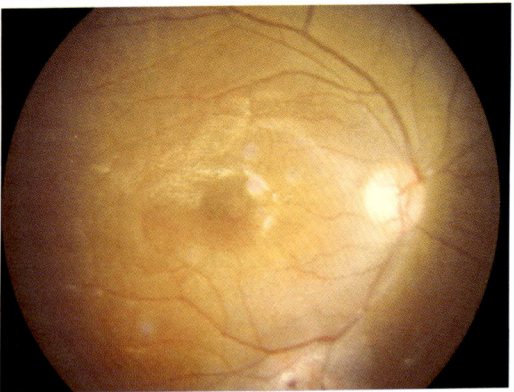

Fig. 15.15 *Fundus picture shows intraocular cysticercus in a 26-year-old male showing intravitreal cysticercus and retinal detachment. Postoperative picture after PPV with silicone oil temponade shows attached retina*

Note. If left untreated ocular cysticercosis can cause blindness, atophy and phthisis in 3–5 years.

ACQUIRED IMMUNODEFICIENCY SYNDROME

Two types of human immunodeficiency virus have been identified HIV1 and HIV2 both cause the same effects, HIV2 being found predominantly in Western Africa.

HIV is a retrovirus having a single stranded RNA as its genome and affects predominantly CD4+ helper T cells which are crucial for cell mediated immunity. Hence the infection leads to CD4+ cell death and severe immunosuppression.

PATHOGENESIS

HIV virion binds to the CD4+ cell and is internalized

↓

In the cell viral reverse transcriptase converts viral RNA to DNA

↓

Viral DNA is incorporated into host DNA with the help of viral integrase

↓

Viral DNA directs synthesis of new viral proteins using the infected cell's apparatus

↓

Proteases process proteins into new viral particles which are shed from the cell. Infected cell eventually dies.

EPIDEMIOLOGY

- *Sexual transmission* both homosexual and heterosexual routes account for transmission. It is more common in commercial sex workers, men who have sex with men.
- *Intravenous drug abuse* transmission is through shared needles.
- *Needle stick injury* accidental needle stick injuries in health care providers also accounts for transmission. Seroconversion to HIV after a needle stick injury is about 0.3%, 10–100 fold less than with hepatitis B or C.
- *Blood, blood product transfusion.*
- *Perinatal transmission* from infected mother to child—it can occur *in utero*, during delivery or by breastfeeding.

Note. HIV worldwide has caused approximately 20 million deaths and about 30 million people are infected.

DIAGNOSIS

The diagnosis of HIV is usually made by enzyme-linked immunosorbent assay (ELISA) and confirmed by Western blot when bands from Gag, Pol and Env proteins are detected on Western blot. The antibodies to viral antigens can be detected 2–8 weeks after infection. ELISA test is 100% sensitive but not 100% specific so false positives can result. The virus can also be cultured from blood, semen, saliva, tears and solid tissues. In the eye it is found in cornea, vitreous and retina.

HIV DISEASE

Acute retroviral syndrome

It occurs 1–6 weeks after HIV infection and consists of fever, rash, myalgia, headache or gastrointestinal symptoms. The patients have elevated liver enzymes and CD4+ count is reduced. The count decreases by 75 cells/microlitre/year.

ACQUIRED IMMUNODEFICIENCY SYNDROME

The time from initial infection to development of AIDS is about 10 years lesions in AIDS include:
- *Opportunistic infections* due to damage to immune system opportunistic infections like *Pneumocystis carinii, Cryptococcus neoformans,* cytomegalovirus, oral candidiasis.
- *Malignancy* like Kaposi's sarcoma can emerge.
- *Direct infection of brain by HIV* causes encephalopathy.

Note. Progression of the disease is accelerated by reducing CD+ count and increasing viral load. *Pneumocyctis carinii* infection occurs when CD4+ <200 cells/microlitre and CMV retinitis occurs when it is <50 cells/microlitre.

Ocular manifestations of HIV infection

Eyelids. Molluscum contagiosum, Kaposi's sarcoma.

Conjunctiva. Dry eye, Kaposi's sarcoma, microsporidial conjunctivitis, herpes virus conjunctivitis.

Cornea and lens. Ulcerative keratitis, dry eye, herpes simplex keratitis, herpes zoster ophthalmicus, microsporidiosis, cataract.

Optic nerve. Optic neuropathy.

Retina and choroid. Microvasculopathy, CMV retinitis, acute retinal necrosis, progressive outer retinal necrosis, syphilis, toxoplasmosis, pneumocystis choroidopathy, cryptococcosis, mycobacterial infection, intraocular lymphoma, candidiasis, histoplasmosis. All these have been dealt with in their respective chapters. Retinal manifestations would be elaborated further.

The most common findings are dry eye, a retinal microvasculopathy and CMV retinitis.

Retinal microvasculopathy

It occurs in 25–92% of patients and includes small dot retinal hemorrhages and cotton wool spots which are retinal nerve fiber layer infarcts. This is probably caused by antigen-antibody immune complexes which circulate in the body and deposit in the microvasculature of the eye. Superficial and deep retinal hemorrhages, retinal perivasculitis and vascular occlusions occur. The cotton wool spots can be distinguished from an area of infectious retinitis in that the cotton wool spots do not enlarge with time, they disappear over a period of time and new lesions appear.

Diminished lactoferrin and lysozyme lead to decreased tear production and **dry eyes** which can be treated with artificial tears.

HIV therapy. Highly active antiretroviral therapy (HAART), or "triple therapy", or AIDS cocktail" refers to a regimen with one protease inhibitor with two nucleoside reverse transcriptase inhibitors used in treatment of patients with CD4+ <350 cells/microlitre. Protease inhibitors are indinavir, nelfinavir, ritonavir, saquinavir, efavirenz the nucleoside reverse transcriptase inhibitors are zidovudine, stavudine, zalcitabine, didanosine, lamivudine. Lack of adherence to the drug regimen can lead to resistance or failure of therapy.

Opportunistic infections

The major ocular associations of HIV are as follows.

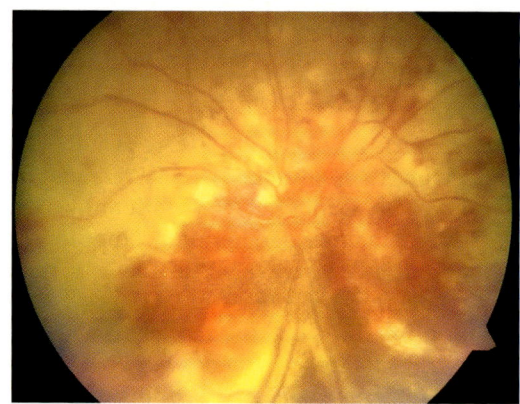

Fig. 15.16 *Fundus picture of a case of congenital HIV showing scattered hemorrhages and retinitis consistent with CMV retinitis*

Cytomegalovirus retinitis

CMV infection is an opportunistic infection in immune suppressed persons or in infants with congenital CMV infection. It is a herpes class virus with double stranded DNA and occurs when the CD4+ cell count is <50 cells/micro litre occurring in 15–20% of these patients during the course of disease.

CMV reaches the eye via hematogenous spread and begins as small white retinal infiltrates. It can appear as a perivascular fluffy white lesion with many scattered hemorrhages (Fig. 15.16) or as a more granular appearing lesion representing new foci of viral activity and a central area of clearing with atrophic retina and stippled retinal pigment epithelium. The disease grows at approximately 250 microns/week. There is low grade vitritis and there may be anterior chamber keratic precipitates. Vision is mostly normal as the lesions start in the periphery. Visual loss can develop as a absolute scotoma due to retinal necrosis and central visual loss with macular involvement. The disease progresses as the old lesion spreads at its borders to involve the uninfected retina, the center of the old lesion being replaced with glial tissue. Retinal detachment can develop in approximately 20% of patients with retinitis, 50% of whom develop detachment in the second eye if it has retinitis. The detachment is due to vitreous traction on the thin atrophic retina. Scleral buckling is done for retinal breaks near the vitreous base. For more posterior and multiple

breaks vitrectomy, endolaser surgery and application of long acting retinal tamponade is done.

CMV retinitis and HAART. Before HAART the median time to progression of CMV retinitis was approximately 2 months even with anti- CMV therapy and in untreated immunocompromised patients, it is 2–3 weeks. With the advent of HAART there is a decrease in HIV replication, elevation in CD4+ counts, reduced mortality, decrease in incidence and altered course and clinical appearance of CMV retinitis. However reactivation of CMV can occur if CD4+ counts fall below 50/microlitre. The treatment is 4 drugs regimen for ocular CMV are Ganciclovir, Foscarnet, Cidofovir, Fomivirsen.

- *Ganciclovir:* It is a virostatic agent which is triphosphorylated in the cell and inhibits viral DNA polymerase. It helps in halting the progression and development of a less active lesion in more than 90% of the patients. Recurrences are common unless underlying immunosuppression is altered by HAART. Induction is done with 5 mg/kg IV twice daily for 14–21 days followed by maintenance of 5 mg/kg once a day. A major side effect is neutropenia for which granulocyte colony stimulating factor can be given.
- Foscarnet inhibits DNA polymerase by a different mechanism from ganciclovir and also reverse transcriptase and replication of HIV. It is given intravenously with a 2–3 week induction dose of either 60 mg/kg three times a day or 90 mg/kg twice daily followed by maintenance dose of 90 mg/kg or 120 mg/kg daily. Foscarnet causes less bone marrow suppression than ganciclovir but is more nephrotoxic and also causes nausea, GIT disturbances and fatigue.
- Cidofovir is a cytosine derived nucleotide analogue given as 5 mg/kg intravenously once a week for two weeks as induction and 3–5 mg/kg once every other week as mainten- ance. Nephrotoxicity is a major adverse event and probenecid and adequate hydration is given with the therapy and it is never combined with foscarnet.
- Fomivirsen is an antisense oligonucleotide complementary to mRNA in CMV and inhibits

its replication. It is given intra-venously in a 330 µgm dose.

Presently in patients receiving HAART anti- CMV maintenance therapy is stopped if the patients have stable CMV retinitis and CD4+ are stable or increasing and have been >100 cells/ microlitre for >3 months. These patients are µl closely for reactivation or development of extraocular disease and if the CD4+ count falls <50 cells/µl restarting anti CMV therapy should be considered. Combined therapy with ganciclovir and foscarnet is being tried and intravitreal injections of ganciclovir, foscarnet and cidofovir have also been used. A ganciclovir intravitreal implant which releases 1 µg per hour for 8 months has been shown to increase the mean time to progression to 226 days but does not treat systemic infections.

Herpes zoster

Herpes zoster ophthalmicus occurs more frequently in HIV positive patients and may be the presenting sign of the disease. Cutaneous zoster occurring in AIDS patients is more likely to disseminate and is difficult to treat with acyclovir. Varicella zoster retinitis can present as acute retinal necrosis on next page and progressive outer retinal necrosis (described on next page) and the response to acyclovir is inconsistent. It is important to differentiate between CMV and VZV retinitis on the basis of clinical criteria, rate of progression and multifocality as CMV does not respond to acyclovir which is a treatment for VZV retinitis.

Pneumocystis carinii choroiditis

It is a form of extrapulmonary disease which used to be prevalent with the use of aerosolised pentamidine and has decreased with the disconti- nuation of its use. It manifests as multifocal white plaques in the choroid with minimal vitreous inflammation and rarely cause visual loss.

Mycobacterium avium—Intracellulare choroiditis

This disease gives an evidence of disseminated systemic infection and manifests as infiltrates of 50–100 µm size scattered throughout the fundus and causes no visual symptoms.

Other diseases

Other diseases like toxoplasmosis, B cell lymphoma and syphilis can also occur. Drug related inflammation with rifabutin (occurring as bilateral severe uveitis and responsive to steroids and reduction of rifabutin dose) can occur. Other drugs like didanosine and fomivirsen can also cause inflammation and RPE changes.

ACUTE RETINAL NECROSIS

Initially described in 1971 as Kirisawa's uveitis, acute retinal necrosis is now reported throughout the world. Typically thought to affect young adults it has been described in children and elderly too. It can be found in both the sexes with slight male preponderance. It affects both immunocompetent and immuno-suppressed patients.

ETIOLOGY

In 1986 Culbertson and colleagues demons-trated herpes zoster in two eyes with ARN by histochemical staining. Varicella zoster has been seen to account for most of the cases of ARN, herpes simplex 1, 2 and CMV account for the rest. PCR studies have demonstrated that varicella zoster and herpes simplex type 1 cause disease in patients older than 25 years while herpes simplex 2 affects patients younger than 25 years. A genetic predisposition has been demonstrated to mount an immune response against the virus in patients with HLA-DQw7 and phenotype Bw62.

CLINICAL FEATURES

Most cases begin as unilateral disease, in one-third of cases the second eye becomes involved within 1–6 weeks. There is acute onset of anterior uveitis with pain, redness, floaters, blurred vision, anterior chamber inflammation with or without keratic precipitates. There may or may not be a herpes infection at another site or history of the same.

Vitritis is caused by lymphocytes and plasma cells. The retinal lesions start as small, patchy, white yellow areas that tend to enlarge circum-ferentially (Fig. 15.17), increase in number and coalesce. The lesions start in the periphery, rarely in the posterior pole but do not follow the vessel architecture. The lesions begin to resolve after weeks leaving behind clear areas called the Swiss cheese pattern with perturbation of RPE.

Retinal vasculitis with severe retinal arteritis, capillary non-perfusion and retinal hemorr-hages is common (Fig. 15.15). Venous occlusions and neovascularisation is uncommon. The patients can also have optic neuropathy with afferent papillary defect and severe loss of vision with visual field defects and impaired color vision. Disc edema is common and optic nerve involvement can be due to vascular occlusive disease, viral infiltra-tion of nerve or optic nerve distension.

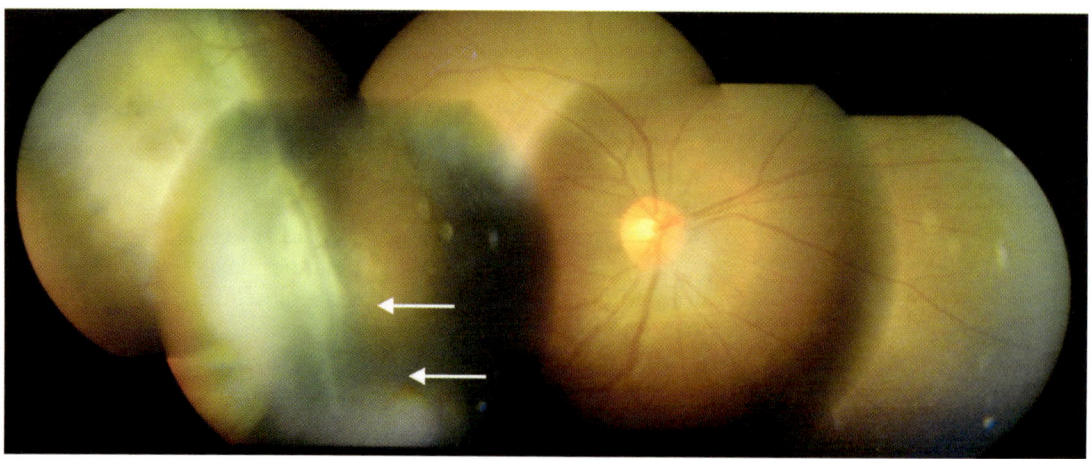

Fig. 15.17 *Fundus photograph showing circumferential retinitis of ARN (arrows)*

The diagnostic criteria for ARN syndrome given by American Uveitis Society are:

- One or more foci of retinal necrosis with discrete borders in the peripheral retina.
- Rapid progression of the disease if antiviral has not been given.
- Circumferential spread of disease.
- Evidence of occlusive vasculopathy with arteriolar involvement.
- A prominent inflammatory reaction in the vitreous and anterior chamber.

The acute inflammatory disease resolves with or without therapy in several months. The acute phase resolves in 2–3 months and tractional and rhegmatogenous retinal detachments can develop in around 86% of patients.

DIFFERENTIAL DIAGNOSIS

This includes all causes of intense vitritis like exogenous bacterial endophthalmitis, fungal endophthalmitis, Behçet's disease, Pars planitis, toxoplasmosis, syphilis, CMV retinitis, sarcoidosis, intraocular lymphoma, progressive outer retinal necrosis.

TREATMENT

Acyclovir 500 mg/m² IV 8 hrly for 10–14 days is the best initial therapy. Oral acyclovir 800 mg five times a day is continued for additional 6 weeks. The goal of therapy is to hasten the resolution and prevent involvement of contralateral eye. The side effects are nausea, vomiting, headache and a reversible increase in serum creatinine and liver enzymes which occur in less than 3% of patients. Valaciclovir 1 g tds orally and Famciclovir 500 mg tds orally have similar efficacy to acyclovir. Patients with severe progressive disease despite treatment can be given ganciclovir or foscarnet. Systemic corticosteroids can be added to treat severe disease after 24–48 hours of intravenous acyclovir.

The role of prophylactic laser at junction of diseased and healthy retina is questionable. Retinal detachment and optic neuropathy are causes of severe visual loss in patients with ARN. Vitrectomy with fluid gas exchange and endolaser have been done but the results are confounded by proliferative vitreoretinopathy.

Optic nerve fenestration and corticosteroids have been tried for optic neuropathy.

PROGRESSIVE OUTER RETINAL NECROSIS

Progressive outer retinal necrosis (PORN) is a variant of necrotizing herpetic retinopathy in immunocompromised patients. It presents as a rapidly progressive necrotizing retinitis with early patchy choroidal and deep retinal lesions which progress relentlessly involving the whole retina. There can be a history of cutaneous herpes zoster prior to the ocular disease and also optic nerve involvement with afferent pupillary defect can be present. There can also be a substantial destruction of inner retina later in the disease.

Etiology

Varicella zoster virus and herpes simplex virus have been implicated in the cause of PORN. Most of the patients are immunocompromised.

Clinical features

Table 15.5 shows PORN versus ARN.

Therapy

Intravenous ganciclovir and foscarnet with intravitreal foscarnet have been tried along with high dose intravenous acyclovir with inconsistent results. 70% of eyes have been reported to develop retinal detachment despite prophylactic retinopexy.

PORN should be differentiated from ARN.

CHOROIDAL INFLAMMATIONS

PRIMARY INFLAMMATORY CHORIOCAPILLAROPATHIES

SERPIGINOUS CHOROIDITIS

Serpiginous choroiditis is characterized by destruction of the inner layers of choroid and the retinal pigment epithelium (RPE) along with involvement of the retina.

Other names suggested for the disorder are geographic choroiditis, geographic choroidopathy, geographic helicoid peripapillary choroidopathy and macular geographic helicoid choroidopathy.

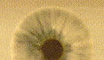
Table 15.5 Differentiating features of PORN and ARN

Progressive outer retinal necrosis (PORN)	Acute retinal necrosis (ARN)
Multifocal lesions with deep retinal opacification without granular borders and there may be areas of confluent opacification	One or more foci of full thickness retinal necrosis with discrete borders
Lesions are located in peripheral retina with or without macular involvement	Lesions located in peripheral retina
Extremely rapid progression of lesions	Rapid progression which can be halted with intravenous acyclovir therapy
No consistent direction of disease spread	Circumferential spread of disease around peripheral retina
Absence of vascular inflammation	Occlusive vasculopathy with arteriolar involvement
Minimal or absent intraocular inflammation	Prominent anterior and posterior chamber inflammation
Perivenular clearing of retinal opacification	Optic neuropathy/atrophy, scleritis, pain

Etiopathogenesis

Etiopathogenesis of this disorder is largely unknown. It is a morphological diagnosis and— various agents implicated in causation are herpes simplex virus (HSV), Epstein-Barr virus (EBV), cytomegalovirus (CMV), human herpes virus (HHV)-8, and varicella-zoster virus (VZV), tuberculosis syphilis sarcoidosis. It is also considered by some authors to be part of the white-dot syndromes.

It is relatively rare entity consisting of about 5% of total uveitis patients. Histologic examination shows an extensive loss of the RPE and destruction of the overlying retina. Choriocapillaris show lymphocytic infiltrate, suggesting that the disease has an inflammatory etiology.

Clinical features

Common age group 30–60 years. More common in whites. No sexual predilection is found. The patient presents with blurred vision, a central or pericentral scotoma in one eye. Disease progresses in a serpentine fashion, usually starting at the optic disc and winding through the posterior pole, hence the name. Acute lesions are gray-white, bit elevated and involve the choriocapillaris and RPE (Fig. 15.5). Progression may lead to involvement of the underlying large choroidal vessels. Thinning of the neurosensory retina and scarring with hyperplasia of RPE are common sequelae. Active lesions may occur adjacent to an area of choroidal and RPE atrophy. Hence, simultaneous presence of active and inactive lesions can be found. Neovascular

membrane formation can occur, if it involves macula visual disturbance can occur. Retinal vasculitis and branch vein occlusion have also been reported in these patients.

Fundus fluorescein angiography

Active lesion will show early blockage with late hyperfluorescent borders that spread toward the center of the lesion. The early hypofluorescence of active lesions may be due to blockage of the underlying choroidal fluorescence by swollen RPE cells or choroidal vasculature blockade. In inflammatory vascular involvement staining of vessels is found. ICG can demonstrate the area of involvement earlier than FFA and is more sensitive.

Treatment

Steroids form the mainstay of treatment during active stage. Immunosuppresive agents are less efficacious.

ACUTE POSTERIOR MULTIFOCAL PLACOID PIGMENT EPITHELIOPATHY (APMPPE)

It is an idiopathic disorder found in young adults with mean age of onset of 27 years. The pathogenesis of APMPPE is unknown. Occasionally, a viral prodrome occurs, and adenovirus 5 has been isolated in one patient with a concurrent viral infection. It is also associated with HLA-DR2 and HLA-B7. It presents with bilateral painless decrease in vision. Vitreous cells and multiple flat yellow-white placoid lesions in the posterior pole,

ranging in size from 0.5 to several disc diameters which become less opaque within 2–3 weeks and develop pigment changes at the level of the RPE. Additional findings may include optic disc edema and episcleritis. Rarely erythema nodosum has been described, which consists of painful subcutaneous nodules in the axilla and lower extremities and cerebral vasculitis also has been described.

Fluorescein angiography displays early hypofluorescence and late hyperfluorescence of the active lesions (Fig. 15.18). Inactive lesions may show window defects as a result of depigmentation of retinal pigment epithelium. ICG angiography displays decreased visibility of the larger choroidal vessels in the early phase.

In some patients atrophy and scarring of the retinal pigment epithelium develop with resultant poor visual acuity. The lesions usually resolve spontaneously in two weeks without significant choroidal atrophy hence has better visual prognosis. No treatment is required. 90% achieve a visual acuity of more than 20/25. In rare cases, recurrences may occur within 6 months of the initial episode. In cases of foveal involvement, corticosteroids may be considered, although their efficacy has not been proven in a controlled study. Corticosteroids may be beneficial in cases of associated cerebral vasculitis. Choroidal neovascularization is a rare complication of APMPPE.

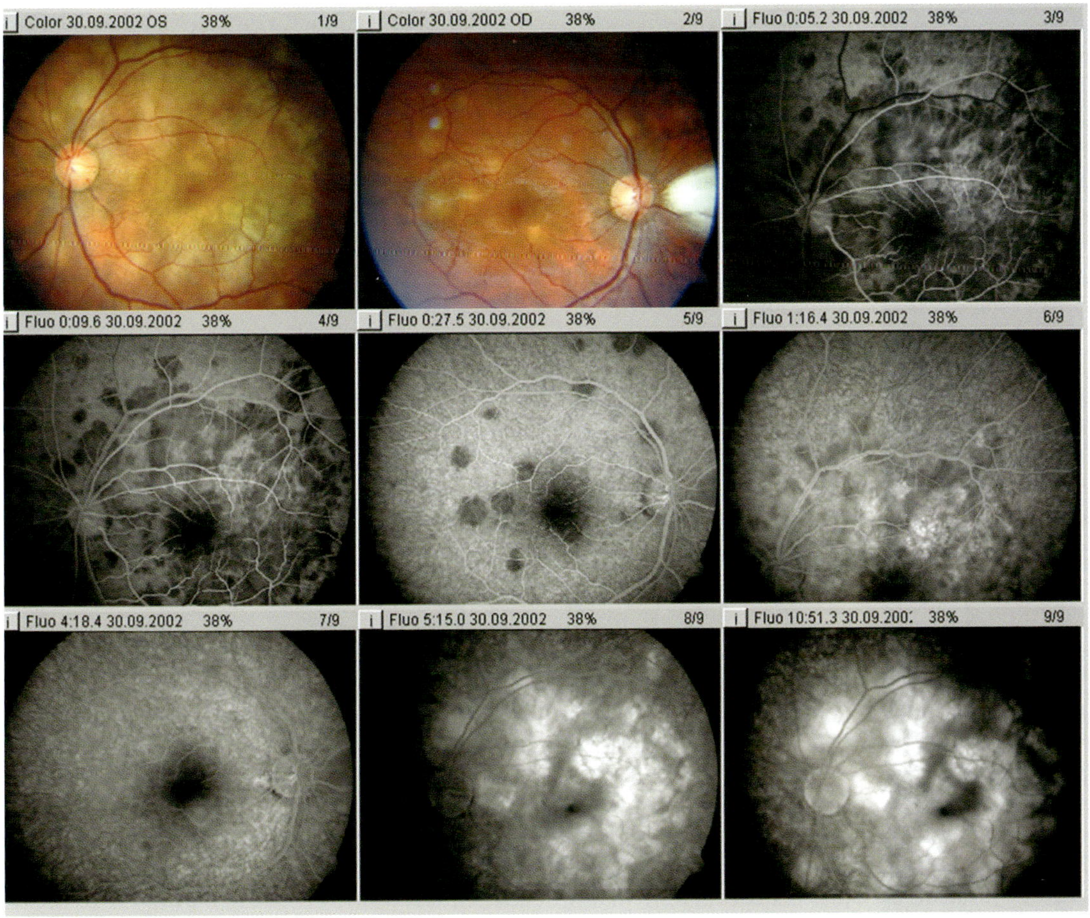

Fig. 15.18 *Young adult presenting with bilateral blurred vision showing bilateral multifocal yellowish lesions which showed early hypofluorescence and late hyperfluorescence on FFA consistent with APMPPE. The lesions healed without any pigmentation after a short course of steroids*

PRIMARY STROMAL CHOROIDITIS

VOGT-KOYANAGI-HARADA SYNDROME

It is an uncommon multisystem disease of autoimmune etiology characterized by chronic bilateral diffuse granulomatous panuveitis with accompanying integumentary, neurologic and auditory involvement.

Etiology and pathogenesis

The precise etiology and pathogenesis of this disease are presently unknown but clinical and experimental evidence suggests it to be autoimmune etiology in which T helper 1 cells are directed against self-antigens associated with melanocytes of all organ systems in genetically susceptible individuals. There is upregulation of interleukin 6, 8 and interferon gamma. The antigens implicated are tyrosinase or tyrosinase related proteins, an unidentified 75 kDa protein and S-100 which are targeted against on melanocytes.

It is common in Asians, Asian Indians, Hispanic, Native Americans and Middle Easterners and uncommon amongst whites and sub-Saharan Africans. The incidence is 8% in Japan and women are more commonly affected than men in the Japanese population. There has been a strong association with HLA-DR4 in Japanese population, the strongest risk is observed with HLADRB1*0405 and HLA-DRB1*0410 haplotypes.

There are four stages of VKH—prodromal, acute uveitic, convalescent and chronic recurrent. In acute uveitic stage there is diffuse, non-necrotizing, granulomatous inflammation consisting of lymphocytes, macrophages, epitheloid and multinucleate giant cells without involvement of choriocapillaris. There can be involvement of iris and ciliary body and there are focal aggregates of epitheloid histiocytes admixed with RPE, Dalen Fuch's nodules between Bruch's membrane and RPE. There can be proteinaceous fluid exudates beneath the neurosensory detachment. In convalescent stage the inflammatory reaction lacks epitheloid cells and loss of melanocytes causing "sunset glow fundus"(Fig. 15.20) . The chronic recurrent stage is characterized by granulomatous choroiditis with damage to choriocapillaris.

Clinical features

Prodromal stage

The patients present with headache, nausea, meningismus, fever, tinnitus, orbital pain, photophobia and hypersensitivity of skin and hair to touch several days before ocular disease. There can also be focal neurologic signs and cerebrospinal pleocytosis with normal glucose levels is seen in 80% of the patients and this may persist for 8 weeks. Auditory problems frequently coincide with ocular disease and are found in 75% of patients. Central dysacusia-involving higher frequencies or tinnitus occurs in about 30% of patients and improves within 2–3 months though there may be persistent deficits.

Acute uveitic stage

Bilateral granulomatous uveitis causing blurring of vision starts 2–3 days after the onset of CNS signs. There is anterior uveitis with mutton-fat KPs and iris nodules, vitritis, thickening of posterior choroid, hyperaemia and edema of optic nerve and multiple serous detachments which may coalesce to form large bullous exudative detachments (Fig. 15.19). IOP may be elevated with shallow anterior chamber due to ciliary body edema or hypotony due to ciliary body shutdown.

Convalescent stage

There is resolution of exudatuve retinal detachment and gradual depigmentation of choroid resulting in classic orange red discoloration or sunset glow fundus. Small round depigmented lesions develop in the inferior peripheral fundus.

Perilimbal vitiligo (Sigiura sign) is found more commonly in Japanese patients. Vitiligo, alopecia and poliosis develop along with development of fundus depigmentation giving it classic 'sunset glow' (Fig. 15.20).

Chronic recurrent stage

There are repeated bouts of granulomatous anterior uveitis with development of KPs, posterior synechiae, iris nodules, iris depigmentation and stromal atrophy. Posterior segment recurrences are uncommon but there may be subclinical choroidal inflammation. There can be

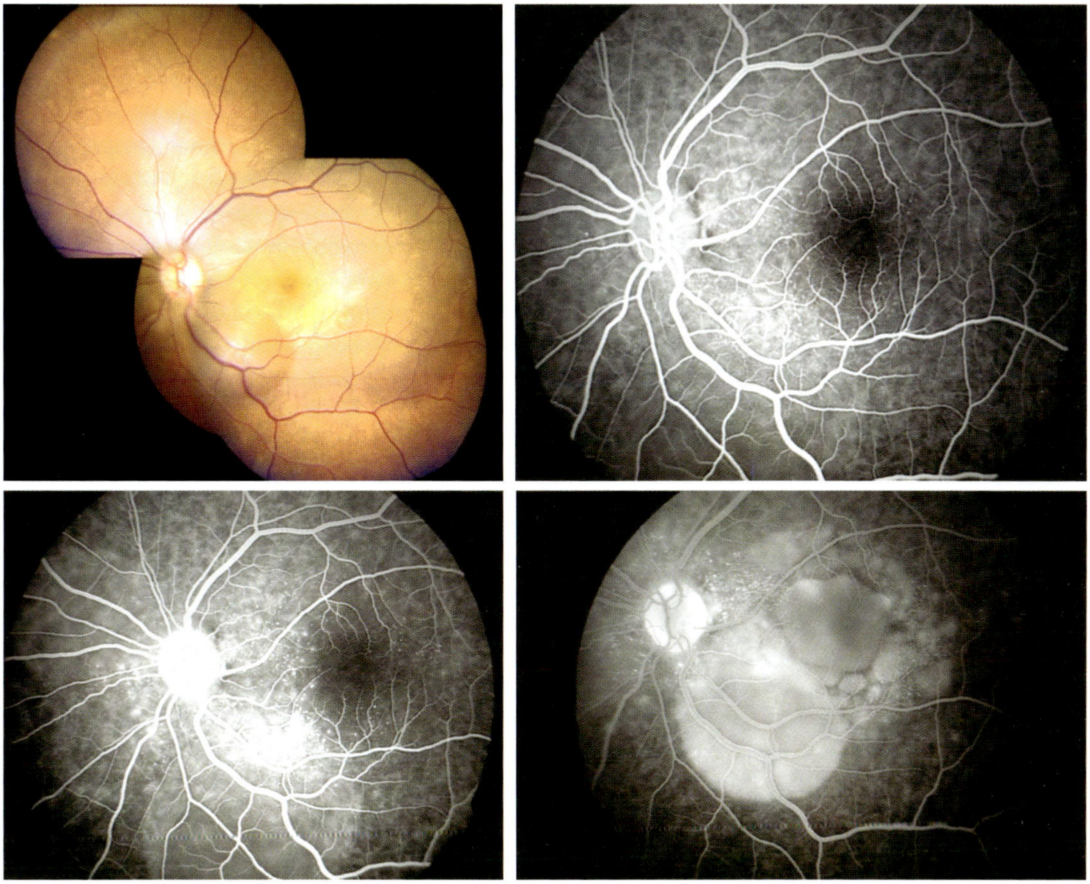

Fig. 15.19 *Case of limited haradas showing serous detachments in posterior pole and disc edema. Ultrasonography showed increased retinochoroid thickness and FFA showed multiple point like hyperfluorescent leaks at RPE level in arteriovenous phase and pooling of dye at late stages*

development of posterior subcapsular cataract, glaucoma, CNV and subretinal fibrosis.

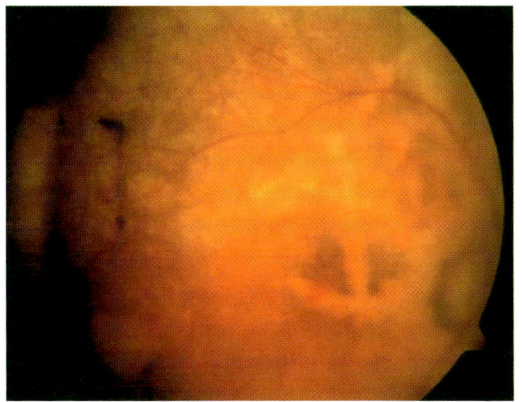

Fig. 15.20 *Sunset glow fundus in chronic phase of VKH*

Diagnosis

The diagnosis of VKH is essentially clinical. On FA there are numerous punctuate hyperfluorescent foci at the level of RPE in the early phases followed by pooling of dye in areas of neurosensory detachment in late phases. There may be disc leakage but CME and retinal vascular leakage is rare. ICG helps in detection and follow-up of subclinical choroidal inflammation. On ultrasonography there is thickening of posterior choroid most prominent in peripapillary area, exudative retinal detachment, vitreous opacification and posterior thickening of the sclera. OCT is used for monitoring serous macular detachment, CME and CNV (Table 15.6).

Table 15.6 *Diagnostic criteria for VKH syndrome*

Complete VKH syndrome
  I. No history of penetrating ocular trauma or surgery
  II. No clinical or laboratory evidence of other ocular or systemic disease
  III. Bilateral ocular disease (either A or B below must be met)

A. *Early manifestations*
1. Diffuse choroiditis as manifested by either focal areas of subretinal fluid or bullous serous subretinal detachments
2. With equivocal fundus findings then both FA showing focal delayed choroidal perfusion, pinpoint leakage, large placoidal areas of hyperfluorescence, pooling of dye within subretinal fluid and optic nerve staining; ultrasonography showing diffuse choroidal thickening without evidence of posterior scleritis

B. *Late manifestations*
1. History suggestive of findings from 3A, and either both 2 and 3 below or multiple signs from 3 below
2. Ocular depigmentation—sunset glow fundus or Sigiura sign
3. Other ocular signs—nummular chorioretinal depigmentation scarsor RPE clumping and/or migration or recurrent or chronic anterior uveitis
4. Neurologic/auditory findings (meningismus, tinnitus, CSF pleocytosis)
5. Integumentary findings (not preceding central nervous system or ocular disease)—alopecia, poliosis, vitiligo

Incomplete VKH syndorme. Criteria I to III and either 4 or 5 from late manifestal

Probable VKH syndrome. Criteria I to III must be present, isolated ocular disease

Treatment

In acute stage oral steroids 1–1.5 mg/kg prednisolone of 200 mg of intravenous methylprednisolone 3 doses are given followed by high dose oral corticosteroids which are slowly tapered over 6 months to 1 year according to response. Intravitreal steroid injections or flucinolone acetonide implant can also be used. In recurrent disease immunosuppressive drugs like cyclosporin, azathioprine, mycophenolate mofetil) can be used to achieve prompt inflammatory control and tapering of steroids.

Oral corticosteroids reduce the risk of CNV and subretinal fibrosis by 82% and risk of visual acuity decline to 20/200 in better seeing eye by 67%.

SYMPATHETIC OPHTHALMITIS

Sympathetic ophthalmitis also known as sympathetic uveitis is a rare bilateral diffuse granulomatous uveitis which occurs a few days to decades after a penetrating accidental or surgical trauma to the eye. The injured eye, the "exciting eye" and the other eye "sympathizing eye" both are affected and injury or incarceration of uveal tissue is common to all the cases.

Sympathetic ophthalmitis can occur 5 days to as long as 66 years after trauma or surgery but is rare before 2 weeks of trauma, 80% cases occurring within 3 months, 90% within 1st year with peak incidence about 4–8 weeks after trauma. The incidence is 0.19% following penetrating trauma, 0.007% after surgery and 0.01% after vitrectomy.

It can occur after keratectomy, iridectomy, cyclodialysis, releasing of iris adhesions, paracentesis, cataract extraction, retinal surgery, vitrectomy, laser cyclophotocoagulation, cyclocryotherapy, evisceration. The incidence has decreased due to aggressive surgical management of severly traumatized eyes.

In trauma cases there is a male preponderance while in cases following surgeries females are equally affected as males. There are two peaks in age groups with children and young adults and those in 6–7th decade of life being affected.

Aetiopathogenesis

It is hypothesized that sympathetic ophthalmia occurs from altered T cell response to one of the soluble proteins associated with the retinal photoreceptor membranes called the S antigen

or to othe retinal or choroidal melanocyte antigens. HLA associations are seen with HLA-A11, HLA-B40, HLA-DR4/DRw53, HLA-DR4/DQw3, HLA-DRB1*04, -DQB1*04, the last two also seen to be associated with VKH syndrome.

Pathologic alterations in both exciting and sympathizing eye are characterized by diffuse granulomatous inflammation and lymphocytic infiltration of uveal tract with nests of epitheloid and giant cells. The choroid is thickened with infiltration of lymphocytes, plasma cells, eosinophils and granulomatous non-necrotizing inflammation and epitheloid cells. The infiltrating lymphocytes are of CD4+ helper and CD8+ cytotoxic type. Dalen Fuchs nodules are present in 1/3rd patients and are made up of a mixture of Ia+, OKM1+ cells (histiocytes) and depigmented RPE cells which are Ia−, OKM1−. There is sparing of choriocapillaris and retinal inflammatory infiltrates, retinal perivasculitis and retinal detachment can be present. Scleral involvement can be around emissary veins, optic nerve and surrounding meningeal sheaths. There can be phacoanaphylaxis with zonal granulomatous inflammation around lens material.

Clinical features

There is further decrease in vision and photophobia in the exciting eye and the patient presents with pain, photophobia, increased lacrimation, blurring of vision, visual fatigue, paresis of accommodation in the sympathizing eye. Both the eyes show ciliary injection, partially dilated poorly responsive pupil, thickened iris, clouding of vitreous. Development of KPs is the most ominous sign in exciting eye (Fig. 15.21).

There is insidious or rapid onset of mild anterior or posterior uveitis in the sympathizing eye with tenderness of globe, mild ciliary flush, cells and flare and KPs and mild to moderate vitritis. There can be papillitis, generalized retinal edema (Fig. 15.22), small yellow-white deposits beneath the RPE which histopathologically correspond to Dalen Fuchs nodules. There can be choroiditis multiple choroidal granulomas, exudative retinal detachment.

Diagnosis

The diagnosis is clinical and no serologic/immunologic tests are available for the disease.

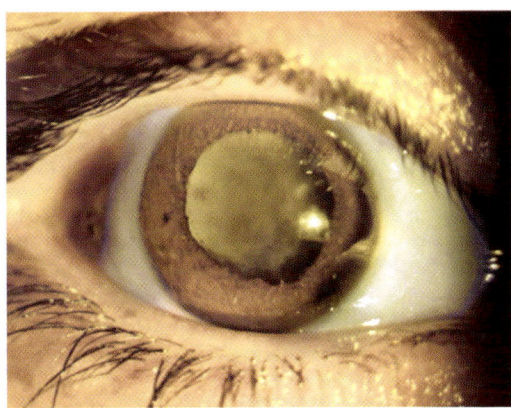

Fig. 15.21 *Young boy with sympathetic ophthalmia after surgery showing granulomatous reaction and exudative retinal detachment*

FFA shows multiple subretinal enlarging hyperfluorescent spots with pooling of dye and late staining of retinal vessels. Dalen Fuchs spots block fluorescence in early phases and are hyperfluorescent in late phases. In cicatricial stage these become atrophic and appear as window defects.

On ICG the active lesions show hypofluorescence in intermediate phase followed by fading and atrophic scars are hyperfluorescent throughout.

A few patients can have atypical cells in CSF, high frequency deafness, hair and skin changes similar to VKH syndrome.

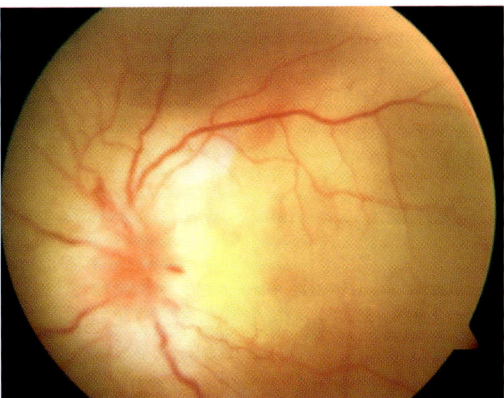

Fig. 15.22 *Another case of sympathetic ophthalmia after open globe injury presenting with disc edema and anterior uveitis*

Complications

Complications like cataract, secondary glaucoma, exudative retinal detachment, chorio-retinal scarring, choroidal neovascularisation, subretinal fibrosis, optic atrophy can develop.

Treatment

The most important strategy is to prevent the occurrence of sympathetic ophthalmitis by careful microsurgical wound toilet and prompt closure of all penetrating injuries and in eyes with no visual function and disorganisation of ocular contents enucleation within two weeks after injury should be done.

There has been seen no benefit to sympa-thizing eye from enucleation of exciting eye whether done briefly before, along with or subsequent to the development of sympathetic ophthalmitis at various elapsed intervals following injury. And the exciting eye may eventually provide better visual acuity so its enucleation then is not indicated.

Steroids form the mainstay of therapy, 100–200 mg prednisolone is given for the first week and gradually tapered and continued up to 6 months after resolution of inflammation. Subtenon injections of steroids, mydriatics and cycloplegics are used concurrently. Supplemental treatment with immunosuppressive agents like azathioprine (2–2.5 mg/kg/day), chlorambucil (6–8 mg orally once a day) or ciclosporin (5 mg/kg) can be used and they allow reduction in steroid therapy. Studies have reported visual acuity of 20/60 or better in 60–64% patients with prompt steroid treatment. Hence, with prompt treatment with steroids and immuno-suppressives many eyes can retain useful vision.

WHITE DOT SYNDROMES

DEFINITION AND CLASSIFICATION

White dot syndromes was the name given to group of idiopathic immunological disorders characterized by visual disturbances with multiple whitish sub-retinal lesions in the fundus. The lesions are located at level of outer retina, RPE and choroid. The etiology of these syndromes was unknown. This pot pourri of disorders has subsequently been replaced by the term choroidal inflammatory disorders. The advent of ICG angiography greatly assisted in localizing the site of primary involvement in these disorders as the choroid. Classification of choroidal inflammatory disorders into inflammatory choriocapillaropathies and stromal choroiditis is now widely recognized.

A. Inflammatory choriocapillaropathies

These are characterised by inflammation of the choriocapillaris and non-perfusion seen in early and late phases of ICGA. These can be primary seconds.

1. Primary inflammatory choriocapillaropathies

The primary site of inflammation is the choriocapillaris. These include:

- Multiple evanescent white dot syndromes (MEWDS)
- Acute idiopathic blind spot enlargement (AIBSE) (Fig. 15.23)
- Acute posterior multifocal placoid pigment epitheliopathy (APMPPE) (discussed earlier)
- Multifocal choroiditis (MFC) and pigmented inner choroidopathy (PIC) (Fig. 15.24)
- Serpiginous choroiditis (discussed earlier) (Fig. 15.25)
- Presumed tubercular serpiginous like choroiditis (discussed earlier)
- Rare and unclassified forms
- Acute zonal occult outer retinopathy (AZOOR).

2. Secondary inflammatory choriocapillaropathies

Involvement of the choriocapillaris is secondary to inflammation of the RPE or the choroidal-stroma. These includes:

- Toxoplasma retinochoroiditis (discussed earlier)
- Birdshot chorioretinopathy, etc.

B. Stromal choroiditis

These are characterised by inflammation of the stroma, which leads to leakage from the overlying choriocapillaris in the early phase and hypofluorescence in the intermediate and late phases, on ICGA. These can be primary or secondary.

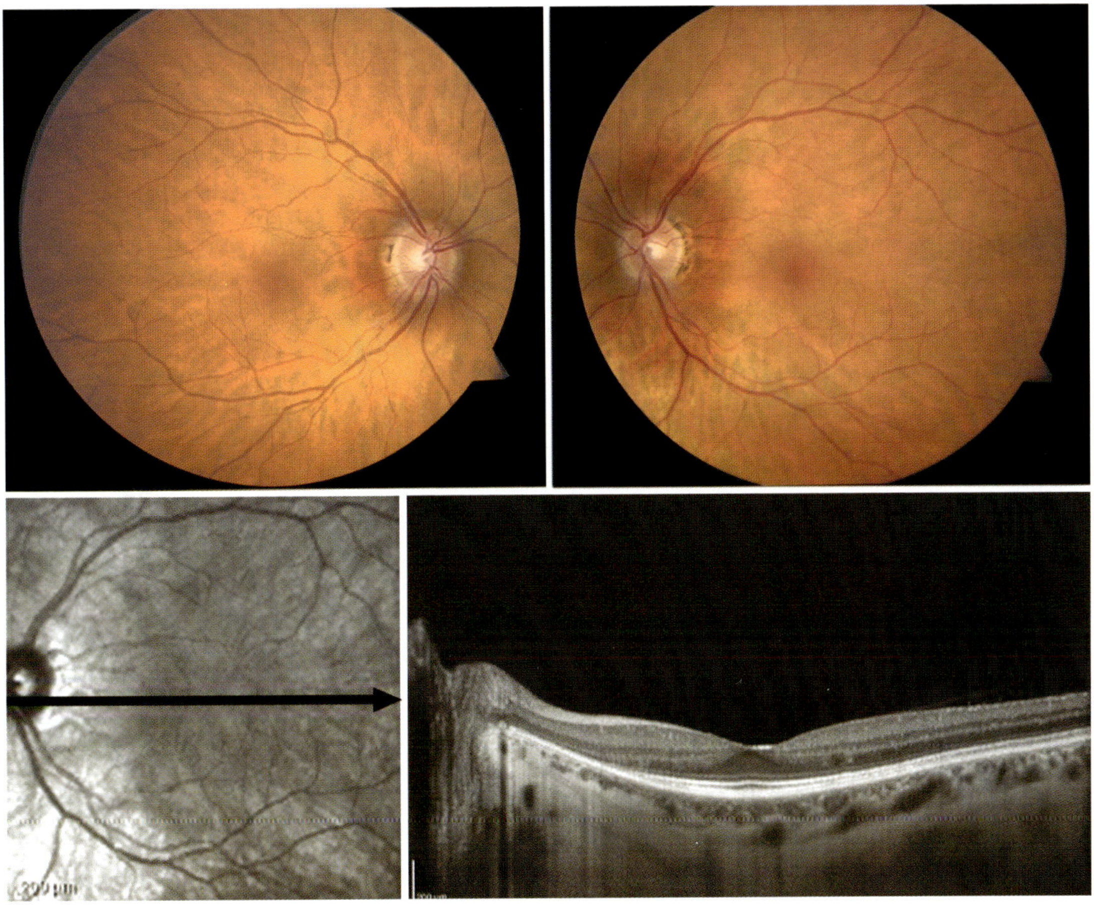

Fig. 15.23 *AIBSE: 36-year-old woman with temporal field defect and photopsias. VA 20/20 OU, normal fundus exam. Enlarged blind spot on left side with loss of peripapillary photoreceptors. (Courtesy: Dr Anita Aggarwal)*

1. Primary stromal choroiditis (discussed earlier)

Primary site of involvement is the choroidal stroma. These include:

- Vogt-Koyanagi-Harada (VKH) disease
- Sympathetic ophthalmia (SO)
- Birdshot chorioretinopathy (BC)

2. Secondary stromal choroiditis (discussed earlier)

Inflammation of the choroidal stroma is secondary to systemic diseases such as:

- Tuberculosis
- Sarcoidosis
- Syphilis

A. INFLAMMATORY CHORIOCAPILLAROPATHIES

Introduction

Characterised by inflammation of the choriocapillaris, leading to delayed perfusion or non-perfusion of the choriocapillaris and the outer retina. Symptoms of visual blurring, field loss and photopsiae hence result. Ocular signs can vary from no clinically detectable lesions (in MEWDS), multiple yellowish retinal lesions (APMPPE and MFC) to extensive chorioretinal scarring (serpiginous choroiditis).

Investigations

Visual field testing and ERG confirm the patchy nature of the disease and also elucidate outer retinal dysfunction.

ICG angiography is the gold standard for diagnosis, follow-up and characterization of these disorders. In the acute stage, patchy hypofluorescence is seen all over the fundus, due to choriocapillaris non-perfusion. This is seen in both the intermediate and late phases.

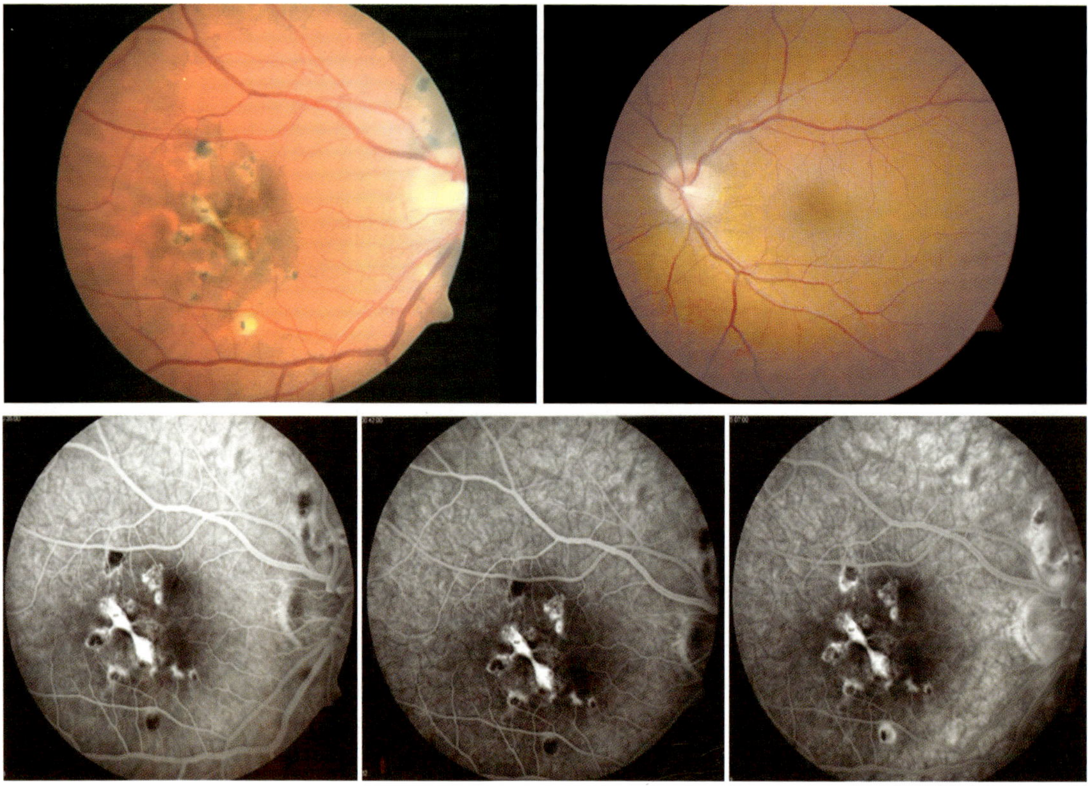

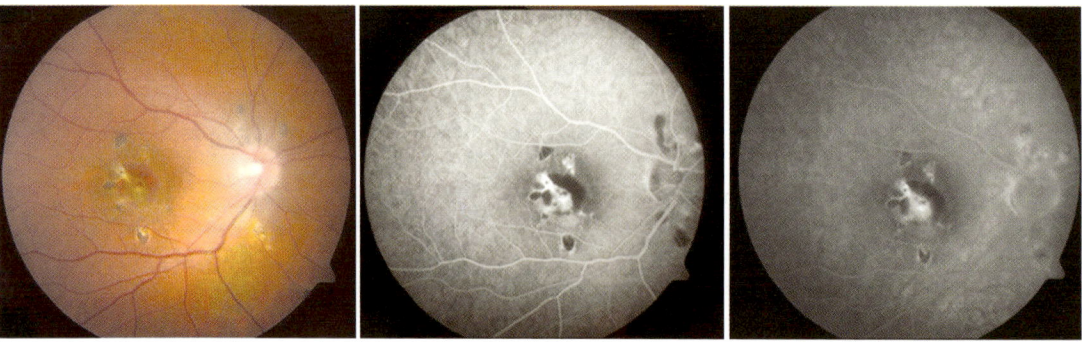

Fig. 15.24A *This patient is a 26-year-old woman with moderate myopia with PIC lesions in the right eye in 2003 (Courtesy: Dr Anita Aggarwal)*

Fig. 15.24B *She returned with central distortion , due to a type 2 CNVM with subretinal blood (Courtesy: Dr Anita Aggarwal)*

In the convalescent stage, the areas of hypo-fluorescence disappear (MEWDS) or persist (APMPPE, MFC), due to chorioretinal scarring.

FFA is not pathognomonic for these disorders as it images the retinal circulation, which is secondarily affected. However, delayed choroidal filling in the early phase is universally seen. Late phases may show no change (MEWDS), hyperfluorescence (APMPPE) or mixed hypo and hyperflourescence (MFC and serpiginous choroiditis). Late phase hyperfluo-rescence correspond to the level of choriocapillaris ischemia and hence inner retinal exudation. Cases of mixed fluorescence in the late phase

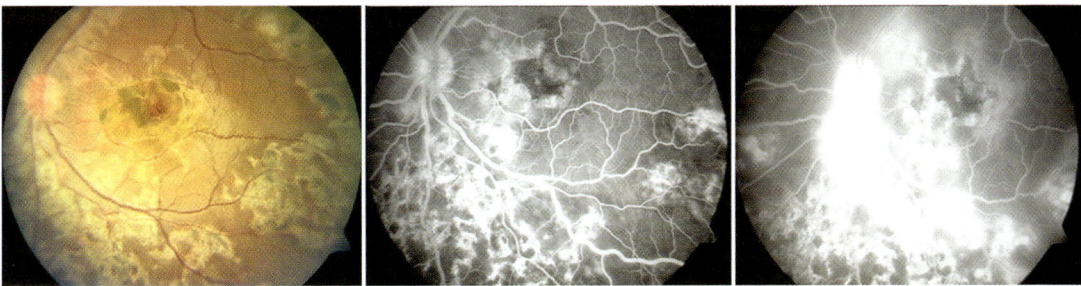

Fig. 15.25A *32-year-old male presented with decreased vision and peripherally helicoid confluent old and fresh choroiditis lesions consistent with serpiginous choroiditis*

are due to chorioretinal scarring and RPE pigmentation.

Characteristic features

Characteristic features of common inflammatory choriocapillaropathies are summarized in Table 15.7.

B. STROMAL CHOROIDITIS

Introduction

Characterised by inflammation of the choroidal-stroma, most commonly by granulomatous diseases. This leads to leakage of the normally non-fenestrated larger choroidal vessels. Choriocapillaris, RPE and outer retina are subsequently involved, leading to visual loss. Ocular signs may include disc edema, exudative retinal detachments, yellowish white subretinal lesions and hypopigmented scars.

Investigations

ICGA is the cornerstone for diagnosis, classification and follow-up. Early phases show leakage from choroidal vessels. Intermediate phases show hypofluorescent dark dots (HDD), due to the presence of granulomas, which prevent the leakage of ICG from the vessels in that area. These HDD may stay hypofluorescent in the late phase in case of full thickness granulomas or may become isofluorescent in the late phase in case of partial thickness granulomas. The surrounding choroidal vessels loose their distinct outline and have fuzzy borders, which lead to late diffuse hyperfluorescence. Disc hyperfluorescence may be seen in severe inflammation.

FFA is helpful to look at RPE and retinal changes. It shows pin point hyperfluorescent spots in the early phase (VKH, SO), pooling of dye in the late phase (VKH, SO), window defects (VKH, SO, BC) and pseudo delay of arterio-venous dye transit time (BC).

Characteristic features

Some characteristic feature of primary stromal are summarized below.

VKH disease (Figs 15.19 and 15.20)
- Bilateral granulomatous panuveitis.
- Prodrome of tinnitus, headache, meningismus, hearing loss and fever followed by acute uveitic stage of keratic precipitates, vitritis, disc edema, multiple exudative RDs. Convalescent stage has poliosis, vitiligo, sunset glow fundus and nummular hypo pigmented lesions.
- FFA shows pinpoint hyperfluorescence in early and pooling of dye in late phases and window defects in convalescent stage
- ICGA shows early choroidal vessel leakage, hypofluorescent dark dots, fuzzy choroidal vessels and disc hyperfluorescence
- Treatment is with long-term cortico-steroids and immunosuppressive agents

Sympathetic ophthalmia (Fig. 15.21)
- Bilateral granulomatous panuveitis associated with trauma or surgery.
- Similar to VKH disease in all other aspects. Trauma is the most important cause in developing countries, while post PPV is the most important cause in developed countries.

Table 15.7 *Inflammatory choriocapillaropathies*

MEWDS and AIBSE (Fig. 15.23)	APMPPE (Fig. 15.18)	MFC and PIC (Fig. 15.24A and B)
Young to middle aged females, unilateral	Young adults, bilateral 20–50 yrs, unilateral or bilateral	Recurrent disease, bilateral (MFC) or unilateral (PIC)
Symptoms include visual loss, photopsiae and field loss. Signs include normal fundus or discrete discoloration of midperipheral fundus	Symptoms include visual loss, field loss and photopsiae. Signs include yellowish white lesions in the posterior pole and mild to moderate AC and vitreous inflammation in the acute stage and chorioretinal atrophic scars in the convalescent stage	Symptoms include moderate to advanced vision loss, photopsiae and visual field loss. Signs include AC and vitreous inflammation and yellowish white retinal lesions of posterior pole and midperiphery. In convalescent stage chorioretinal scars
Preceded by viral flu-like illness in 50% cases	May be precede by a flu-like illness.	Secondary CNVM in 30–40%
ICGA shows patchy and peripapillary hypofluorescence which persists in the late phase	ICGA shows geographic hypofluorescence which persists in late phase	ICGA shows early hypofluorescence persisting in late phase, which is more than in MEWDS or APMPPE
FFA shows early hypofluorescence and late hyperfluorescence or absence of findings. AIBSE are said to be subclinical or resolved counterparts of MEWDS	FFA shows early hypofluorescence and late hyperfluorescence	FA shows early hypo and late hyperfluorescence in acute stage. Convalescent stage shows mixed hypo and hyper pattern
No treatment is needed as spontaneous recovery occurs in 6–10 weeks	Generally no treatment is needed, but some cases may result in scarring of the posterior pole and permanent visual loss in which case steroids may be considered	Systemic steroids for bilateral and sub-tenon steroids for unilateral disease along with immunosupression. CNVM requires Anti VEGFs and/or PDT
Serpiginous choroiditis	*Serpiginous like choroiditis Fig. 15.5*	*AZOOR*
Recurrent, progressive bilateral autoimmune disease	Recurrent, progressive, may be unilateral or bilateral, secondary to tubercular hypersensitivity	Rare, middle aged females.
Vision loss, visual field loss and photopsiae may occur	Vision loss and field loss	Sudden onset field loss with prominent photopsiae, which are worse in bright light and show movement
Peripapillary type is most common and begins as yellowish white lesions around the disc which spread in a amoeboid pattern. Macular type is rare but causes more severe visual loss. Ampiginous type starts a multifocal AMPPE like lesions but gradually coalesce to classic serpiginous lesions	Multifocal type is most common and begins as discrete yellowish white subretinal lesions in the posterior pole and periphery which later coalesce to form SC like lesions. Diffuse type is similar to SC right from the start. Mixed type has both types in two eyes	Fundus shows no abnormality in acute stage. In late stages, sectoral retinitis pigmentosa type picture may be seen
Lesions heal with extensive RPE pigmentation and cause diffuse chorioretinal atrophy and CNVM formation	Lesions heal with less RPE pigmentation and AC and vitreous inflammation is more marked	ICGA and FFA are normal if the fundus is normal. In late stages, FFA may show window defect in areas of RPE loss
ICGA shows early hypofluorescence persisting in the late phase	ICGA shows early hypofluorescence persisting in the late phase	Stabilization and partial recovery is seen at 4–6 months
FFA shows early hypo and late hyperfluorescence in acute stage and window defect in chronic stage	FFA shows early hypo and late hyperfluorescence in acute stage and window defect in chronic stage	
Pulse steroids in the acute stage along with immunosupression are strongly recommended to prevent severe vision loss. Anti-VEGFs and PDT are needed for CNVMs	Oral steroids are needed to control the inflammation and anti-tubercular drugs (ATT) are needed to prevent recurrences. 4 drug ATT is started and isoniazid and rifampicin are continued for 9–12 months. Pyrazinamide and ethambutol are stopped after 2–3 months.	No treatment is found to be particularly effective, however anecdotal reports of improvement with steroids are there

Birdshot chorioretinopathy

- Bilateral granulomatous posterior uveitis, with primary involvement of both choroidal stroma and retina in individuals with HLA A29.
- Retinal findings include vasculitis of small and large vessels, CME and disc edema. Choroidal involvement leads to granulomas in the stroma in the periphery of the fundus. In the healed stage, yellowish white depigmented lesions in the periphery and a pseudoretinitis pigmentosa like picture may be seen.
- FFA shows pseudo delay of arteriovenous transit, due to massive dye leakage, CME and disc hyperfluorescence.
- ICGA shows numerous HDDs which become isofluorescent in the late phase and fuzzy choroidal vessels. Convalescent stage shows disappearance of HDDs and hypo-fluorescent areas (chorioretinal atrophy)
- Treatment is with long-term steroids and immunosuppressive agents

BIBLIOGRAPHY

1. Gass JD, Agarwal A, Scott Iu. Acute zonal occult outer retinopathy: a long-term follow-up study. Am J ophthalmol 2002;134:329–39.
2. Gupta V, Aggarwal A, Gupta A, Bambery P, Narang S. Clinical characteristics of serpinginous choroidopathy in North India. Am J Ophthalmol 2002;134:47–55.
3. Gupta V, Gupta A, Arora S, Bambery P, Dogra MR, Agarwal A. Presumed tubercular serpiginous like choroiditis: Clinical presentation and management. Ophthalmology 2003;110:1744–49.
4. Gupta V, Gupta A, R Narsing. Intraocular tuberculosis-an update. Surv Ophthalmol 2007;52: 561–87.
5. Gupta V, Agarwal A, Gupta A, Bambery P, Narang S. Clinical characteristics of serpiginous choroidopathy in North India. Am J Ophthalmol 2002;134:47–56.
6. GuptaV, Gupta A, Arora S, Bambery P, Dogra MR. Agarwal A. Presumed tubercular serpiginous like choroidopathy. Clinical presentation and management. Ophthalmology 2003;110: 1744–9.
7. Herbert CP, Guex- Crosier Y, LeHoang P. Schematic interprewtation of indocyanine green angiography. Ophthalmology 1994;2:169–176.
8. Herbort CP, Rao NA, Michizuki M. International criteria for diagnosis of ocular sarcoidosis: results of first international wporkshop on ocular sarcoidosis IWOS. 2009;17:160–9.
9. Howa Kimyam A, Cunningham ET (Jr). Ocular Toxoplasmosis. Ophthalmol Clin North Am 2002;15:327–2.
10. Jampol LM, Becker KG. White dot syndromes of retina: a hypothesis based on common genetic hypothesis of autoimmune/inflammatory disease. Am J Ophthalmol 2003;135:376–9.
11. Jampol LM, Sieving PA, Pugh D, Fisherman GA, Gilbert H. Multiple evanescent white dot syndrome. 1. Clinical findings. Arch Ophthalmol 1984:671–4.
12. Muthiah MN, Michaelides M, Child CS, Mitchell SM. Acute retinal necrosis: a national population-based study to assess the incidence, methods of diagnosis, treatment strategies and outcomes in the UK. Br J Ophthalmol 2007;91:1452–5.
13. Narang S, Handa U, Kochhar S, Kumar S, Sood S. Submacular hydatid cyst: a case report. Retina cases and brief reports Oct. 2009.
14. Narang S, Handa U, Nanda A, Bansal R, Nahar R, Sood S. Primary Intravitreal hydatid cyst: diagnosis on cytological examination. Ann Trop Med Parasitol 2006 Jun;100(4):371–4.
15. Narang S, Sood S. Probable Vogt-Koyanagi-Harada's syndrome associated with tonic pupils. Nep J Oph 2010;2(2):154–6.
16. Rao NA, Sukavatcharin S, Tsai JH. Vogt-Koyanagi-Harada disease diagnostic criteria. Int Ophthalmol 2007;27:195–9.
17. Tabbara KF. Tuberculosis. Curr Opin Ophthalmol 2000;11:493–501.

16 RETINAL VEIN OCCLUSIONS

Sunandan Sood, Mohit Dogra, Soniya Bhalla

CENTRAL RETINAL VEIN OCCLUSION

INTRODUCTION

Retinal vein occlusion is the second most common retinal vascular disease following diabetic retinopathy. It can be classified anatomically as central retinal vein occlusion (CRVO) and Hemi central retinal vein occlusion (HCRVO). Venous occlusion occurs behind lamina cribrosa in CRVO. Vision loss varies from minimal to complete blindness. Causes for vision loss are macular edema, epiretinal membrane, dense intraretinal hemorrhages, macular ischemia, vitreous hemorrhage, tractional retinal detachment or neovascular glaucoma. Hayreh reported that after RVO in one eye incidence of developing a second vein occlusion in the next 4 years was 2.5% in the same eye and 11.9% in the fellow eye.

INCIDENCE AND DEMOGRAPHICS

Most patients with CRVO are male and older than 65 years. Most cases are unilateral, and approximately 6–14% of cases are found to be bilateral. Branch retinal vein occlusion is 3 times more common than central retinal vein occlusion. Contrary to CRVO, men and women are affected equally in BRVO with the bulk of presentations between age 60 and 70 years. Little documentation exists regarding race and RVOs; however, they are thought to be rare in the Asian and West Indian populations.

PATHOGENESIS

The central retinal artery and vein share a common adventitial sheath as they exit the optic nerve head and pass through a narrow opening in the lamina cribrosa. Due to this narrow entry in the lamina cribrosa, the vessels are in a tight compartment with limited space for displacement. This anatomical position predisposes to thrombus formation in the central retinal vein by various factors, including slowing of the bloodstream, changes in the vessel wall, and changes in the blood (Virchow's Triad). Occlusion of the central retinal vein leads to building up of back pressure in the retinal venous

system and increased resistance to venous blood flow which cause stagnation of the blood and ischemic damage to the retina. Ischemic damage to the retina stimulates increased production of vascular endothelial growth factor (VEGF) in the vitreous cavity. Increased levels of VEGF stimulate neovas-cularization of the posterior and anterior segment (responsible for secondary complications due to CRVO). Also, it has been shown that VEGF causes capillary leakage leading to macular edema.

Site of occlusion in the CRVO in nonischemic type is neither in the lamina cribrosa nor in the adjacent retrolaminar region but further back. The severity of retinopathy would depend on the site of occlusion-the farther back the occlusion, the milder the retinopathy, because of the availability of more and more collateral channels. However, in ischemic type of CRVO the thrombus is adjacent to lamina and it is more complete (Fig. 16.1A and B).

Number of **risk factors** for CRVO have been identified and out of these the advancing age is the most important risk factor. Common systemic diseases associated with CRVO are hypertension, diabetes, heart disease and atherosclerosis. **Hypertension** is present up to 64% of patients over the age of 50 years and in

25% of younger patients with retinal vein occlusion. **Hyperlipidemia** is present in about 35% of patients of vascular occlusion. **Diabetes mellitus** is present in 10% of patients over the age of 50 years but is uncommon in younger patients. In general further work up is not indicated in patients older than 50 years with known systemic vascular risk factors for CRVO. However, other diseases should be considered in patients younger than 50 years and in patients with bilateral CRVO. Amongst the haemato-logical abnormalities hyperhomosysteinemia is the most common and significant thrombophilic risk factor for the development of CRVO. The other less important factors are, factor V Leidan mutation, protein C and S deficiency, abnormal fibrinogen level, antiphospholipid antibodies and lipin anticoagulant factor. Hyperviscosity states like polycythemia, leukemia, sickle cell disease, multiple myeloma, Waldenström macroglobulinemia, dehydration and elevated hematocrit have been found to be associated with CRVO.

Ocular condition like OAG has an increased risk of developing CRVO. Similarly, conditions like ischemic optic neuropathy, tilted disc, optic nerve head drusen, thyroid related ophthal-mopathy, etc. are predisposed to have CRVO.

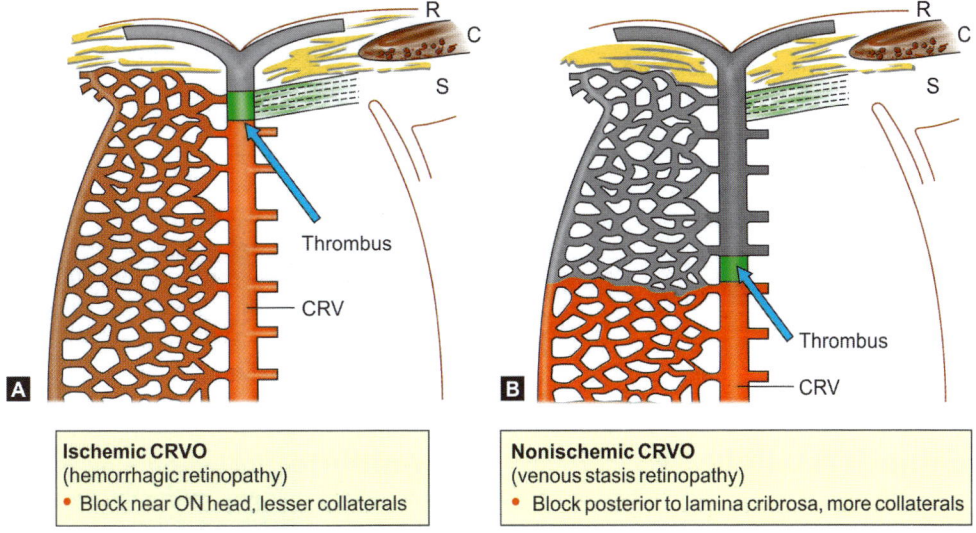

Ischemic CRVO
(hemorrhagic retinopathy)
• Block near ON head, lesser collaterals

Nonischemic CRVO
(venous stasis retinopathy)
• Block posterior to lamina cribrosa, more collaterals

Fig. 16.1 (A) *Site of thrombus (arrows) which is just behind the lamina cribrosa in ischemic CRVO; and **(B)** Further back in non-ischemic CRVO which allows the availability of collaterals in the latter condition*

Oral contraceptives, diuretics and rarely hepatitis B vaccine have been blamed in the causation of CRVO.

CLASSIFICATION, CLINICAL FEATURES, COURSE AND COMPLICATIONS

1. Nonischemic CRVO (venous stasis retino-pathy) 80%
2. Ischemic CRVO (haemorrhagic retinopathy) 20%

Multiple of terms have been used in an attempt to classify two ends of the spectrum of the disease. The term non-ischemic is coined when the thrombosis of central retinal vein is incomplete and retina is still partially perfused and the disease is mild, hence labeled as venous stasis retinopathy. Conversely when the thrombosis is complete, retina is non-perfused, the condition is severe and the term used is ischaemic CRVO. An intermediate or indeterminate form may also exist but 80% of those eyes eventually progress to the severe ischemic type.

NONISCHAEMIC CRVO

- 80% of the CRVOs are non-ischemic type.
- Non-ischemic CRVOs characterized by rapid unilateral painless diminution of vision which is usually better than 6/60 without any RAPD.
- *Fundus examination* shows mild dilatation of veins with few dot as well as flame shaped hemorrhages in all the quadrants of retina. Macular edema lowering visual acuity and mild disc edema may or may not be present. If disc edema is prominent in younger patients, a combined inflammatory and occlusive mechanism may be present that has been termed as papillophlebitis (Fig. 16.2).
- *FFA* usually demonstrates prolongation of the retinal circulation time with breakdown of capillary permeability, but minimal area of non-perfusion (Fig. 16.3B). In patients of nonischaemic CRVO having cilioretinal artery (cilioretinal artery is normally present in 20% eyes only) there occurs functional blockade of cilioretinal artery blood flow because of raised retinal venous pressure which do not allow the choroidal arterial circulation to pump blood in cilioretinal artery (p 252) (Fig. 16.3 A to F).

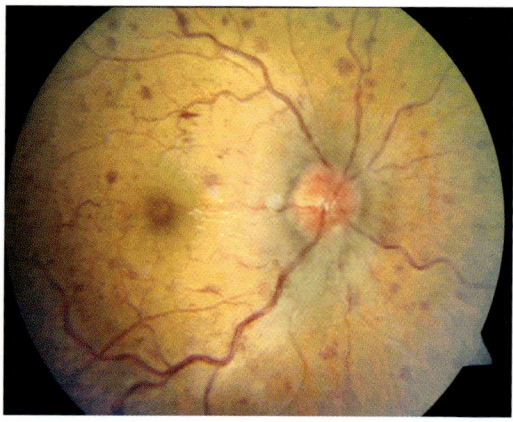

Fig. 16.2 *Right fundus photograph of nonischaemic CRVO showing mild disc edema, dilated veins and multiple scattered superficial hemorrhages*

- *Perimetry* do not show any field defect.
- *ERG* is also nearly normal.

ISCHAEMIC CRVO

- 20% of CRVO are of ischemic type.
- Ischaemic CRVO is usually associated with sudden painless profound loss of vision which is mostly unilateral. The vision is usually worse than 6/60.
- *Relative afferent pupillary conducion defect (RAPD)* and one or the other field defect mostly dense central scotoma is present.
- *Fundus on examination* shows marked venous dilatation and tortuosity. Widespread superficial, flame shaped and sheets of hemorrhages in all four quadrants and the appearance has been rightly termed as tomato ketch up retinopathy. Multiple cotton wool spots are seen because of non perfusion. Macula is markedly edematous, disc edema is usually present to a varying degree and breakthrough vitreous hemorrhage may also be observed (Fig. 16.4A).

In due course of time the hemorrhages may decrease or resolve completely with resultant RPE alterations. However, macular edema often persists despite resolution of the retinal hemorrhages.

- *FFA* at this stage is likely to be of value in assessing the state of perfusion of retina. If CNP areas are more than 10 disc area (DA) on the posterior pole it points towards ischemic CRVO (Fig. 16.4B).

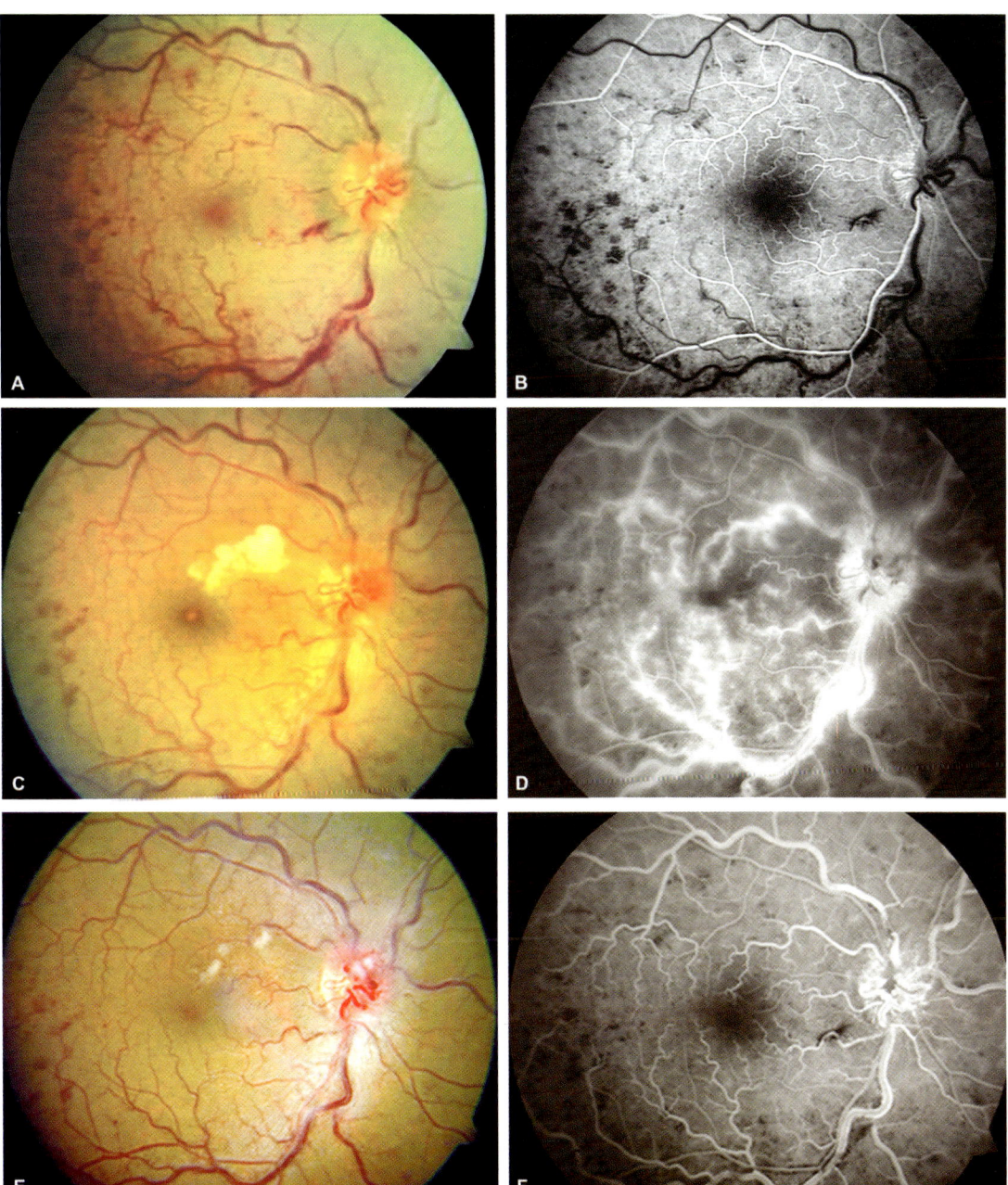

Fig. 16.3 *(A) Fundus photo of right nonischaemic CRVO; (B) Shows delayed arm to retina time; (C) Shows cilioretinal artery occlusion in the same case occurring in due course of time; (D) Shows blocked fluorescence in the area of blood supply of cilioretinal artery (papillomacular bundle); (E) Resolution of cilioretinal artery occlusion; and (F) Shows FFA picture showing nearly normal perfusion of centrocaecal area as seen on further follow-up*

- *ERG* may be helpful in distinguishing between ischemic and nonischemic CRVO since b/a wave amplitude ratios, photopic and scotopic b-wave amplitudes and flicker amplitude are significantly smaller in eyes with significant capillary non-perfusion.

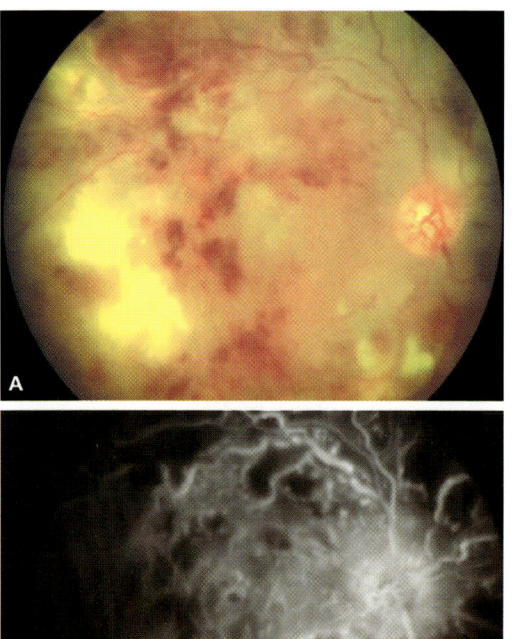

Fig. 16.4 **(A)** *Fundus photograph of right ischaemic CRVO, showing disc edema markedly dilated veins, multiple superficial and sheets of hemorrhages (tomato ketch up retinopathy) and soft exudates; and* **(B)** *Shows areas of capillary nonperfusion (CNP) on FFA done 6 weeks later*

COURSE OF CRVO

It has been reported that about one-third of non-ischemic CRVOs convert to ischemic by 3 years of follow-up, which is basically because of progression of thrombus from proximal to distal part of retrolamina and due to incomplete thrombosis becoming more complete. Neovascularization of iris (NVI) develops in 45–80% of cases of ischemic CRVO while it is less than 5% in non-ischemic, however, out of 45–80% only one-third cases of NVI develop neovascular glaucoma. The future risk of development of CRVO is 2.5% in the same eye and 11% in the fellow eye.

COMPLICATIONS

These are more frequently seen after ischemic CRVO.

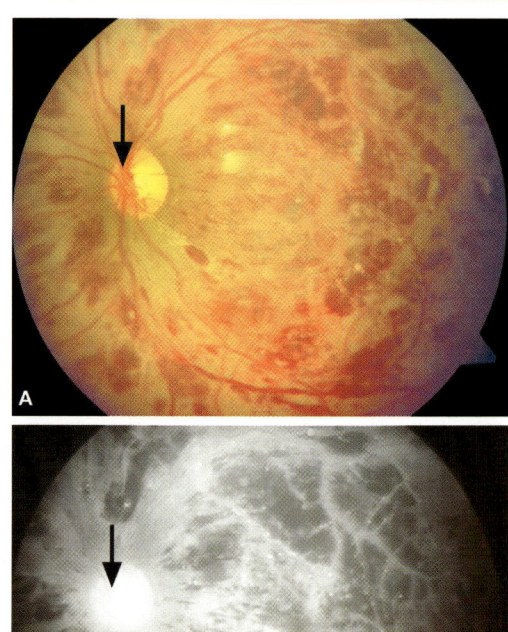

Fig. 16.5 **(A)** *Fundus phtograph of right ischaemic CRVO showing NVD; and* **(B)** *NVD seen on FFA with CNP areas*

- *Iris and angle neovascularization* (NVI + NVA) which typically occur in CRVO are the dreaded complications because of the risk of development of neovascular glaucoma (NVG).
- *Neovascularization of the disc (NVD) and retina (NVE)* may also develop. Neovascularization mostly occurs within 7 months of development of CRVO (Fig. 16.5A and B).
- *Cystoid macular edema* (CME) is common following CRVO which is said to be intractable in ischemic CRVO. However, with the introduction of intravitreal anti-VEGF drugs the response has been observed to be encouraging in the recent reports (Fig. 16.6A to E).
- *Vitreous hemorrhage* and *epiretinal membranes* may also develop.
- *Optociliary shunt vessels* may develop on the optic nerve head, a sign of newly formed

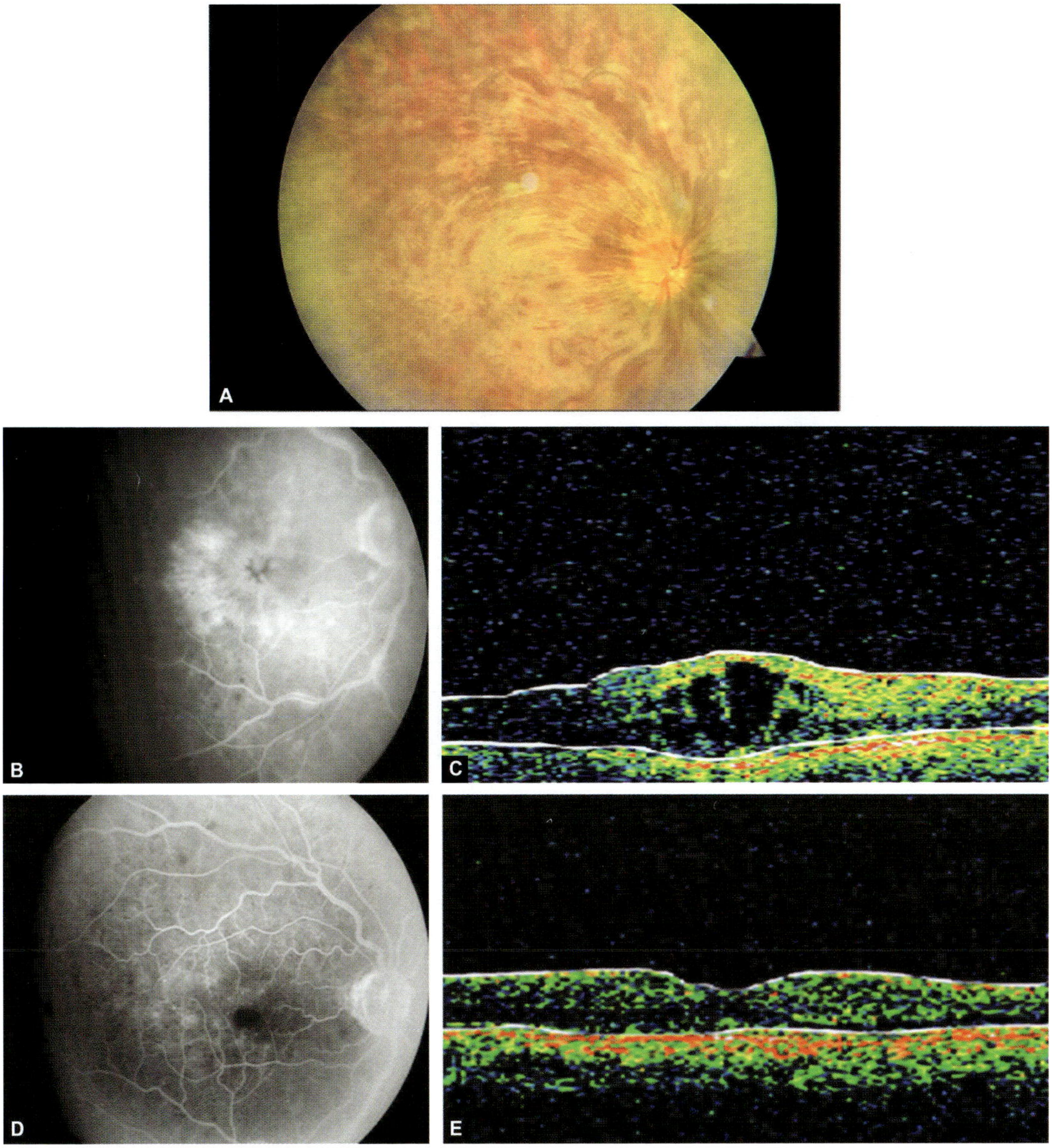

Fig. 16.6 *(A) Shows classic features of right ischaemic CRVO; (B) Petaloid hyperfluorescence in the macula on FFA suggestive of CME; (C) OCT of macula shows, loss of foveal contour, increase in central foveal thickness with hyperreflective septa and hyporeflective spaces suggestive of CME; (D) Injected anti-VEGF intravitreally, show resolution of CME on FFA; and (E) resolution of CME on OCT with improved VA*

collaterals with the choroidal circulation. These disc collaterals are larger in caliber than NVD and do not leak on FFA and may protect the eye from anterior segment neovascularization (Fig. 16.7).

MANAGEMENT AND PROGNOSIS

CLINICAL EVALUATION

- *Ocular history* will determine the onset and duration of the occlusion.
- *History of systemic diseases,* such as hypertension, diabetes, heart disease and personal

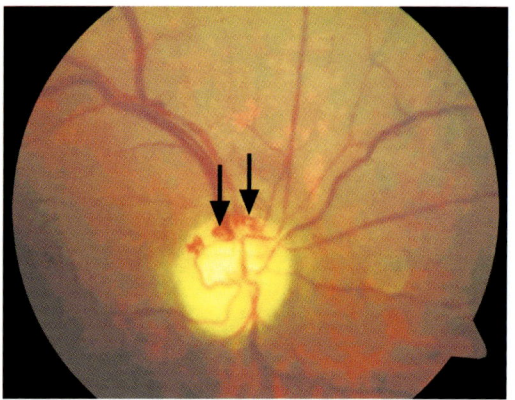

Fig. 16.7 *Right fundus phtograph of old CRVO showing disc collaterals (black arrows) and pale disc*

and family history of thrombosis or hypercoagulable state should be determined.
- *Ocular examination* should include visual acuity, pupillary reaction and record of IOP. Undilated slit lamp examination to detect NVI and undilated gonioscopy to rule out NVA. The fundus examination should be carried out with 90D slit lamp examination in case the media is clear and with 20D indirect ophthalmoscopy if media is relatively hazy.
- *Goldmann perimetery and ERG* evaluation is very important in order to decide whether CRVO is nonischaemic or ischemic since this will determine treatment option and the follow-up schedule. It can be done in early stage of presentation of the patient even in the presence of retinal hemorrhages.
- *FFA* in early stages of CRVO can only confirm the diagnosis of occlusion in doubtful cases by finding out a significatnt delay in arteriovenous transit time, however, it cannot assess the status of perfusion when the retina is splattered with retinal hemorrhages. One has to wait for about 4 weeks for the hemorrhages to resolve, so that capillary nonperfusion (CNP) areas can be assessed. Hence ERG and perimetry are better tools than FFA in determining the type of CRVO in acute stage.
- *Optical coherent tomography (OCT):* It is helpful in evaluating and monitoring macular edema and subretinal fluid accumulation following CRVO. It can also aid in the diagnosis of epiretinal membrane (ERM).
- *Systemic workup* is usually not indicated in persons older than 50 years. with known systemic risk factors for CRVO. Younger patients are more likely to have predisposing conditions resulting in CRVO. Thus in such cases initial laboratory investigation may include ESR, ANA, APLA and fasting plasma homocysteine levels. Individual with B/L simultaneous CRVO should have detailed evaluation for hypercoagulable conditions. Differentiation of non-ischaemic CRVO from ischaemic CRVO is shown in Table 16.1.

DIFFERENTIAL DIAGNOSIS

- *Diabetic retinopathy* which is generally bilateral while CRVO is unilateral.
- *Ocular ischaemic syndrome (OIS)* due to carotid occlusive disease has only dilated veins and these are not as tortuous as seen in CRVO. The retinal hemorrhages are seen typically in OIS in the midperiphery and these patients may have a history of amaurosis fugax, TIA or orbital pains.

TREATMENT

It can be discussed in the following heads:
- Medical therapy
- Laser therapy

S no.	Test	Non-ischaemic CRVO	Ischaemic CRVO
	Table 16.1 *Differentiation of non-ischaemic CRVO from ischaemic CRVO*		
1.	Visual acuity	>6/60	<6/60
2.	RAPD	Absent/minimal	Present
3.	ERG	Normal	Delayed
4.	Goldmann perimetry	Normal	Central scotoma/one or other field defect
5.	Risk of NV	Low risk	High risk

- Intravitreal anti-VEGF drugs
- Intravitreal steroids
- Surgical therapy
- Intravitreal TPA

A. Medical therapy

- *Treatment of associated medical* conditions such as hypertension, diabetes mellitus, dyslipidaemia and hyperhomocysteinemia should be carried out. *Smoking* should be avoided.
- OAG, if detected, should be treated.
- *Role of systemic anticoagulation* is unclear as there is no evidence that agents such as aspirin, heparin or warfarin prevent or alter the natural course of CRVO.
- *Role of hemodilution* and/or pentoxifylline (lowering blood viscosity) in improving visual acuity and macular edema and in reducing the risk of progression to ischemic CRVO is yet not fully established.

B. Laser therapy

CRVO study is the largest multicentric trial carried out to answer questions like role of grid pattern laser photocoagulation in perfused macular edema and role of early or delayed PRP in prevention of NVI and NVA causing neovascular glaucoma (NVG) which is one of the most feared complication of CRVO.

- The CRVO study did not recommend the grid laser photocoagulation for CRVO associated macular edema. However, in the younger patients there was trend towards improved visual acuity in the treatment group. A dense central scotoma is common in ischaemic CRVO and laser PRP may add peripheral scotoma possibly leaving less useful retina and visual field. Therefore CRVO study recommended PRP in patients of ischaemic CRVO after waiting for the development of NVI for at least two clock hours on undilated gonioscopy (Fig. 16.8). However, PRP should not be delivered prophylactically. Prophylactic placement of PRP may be considered in Indian scenario where CRVO is ischemic and compliance and follow-up of the patient is doubtful.
- *Chorioretinal venous anastomosis* has been tried by delivering laser energy (argon or Nd-YAG systems) at a branch retinal vein to rupture the posterior vein wall and Bruch's

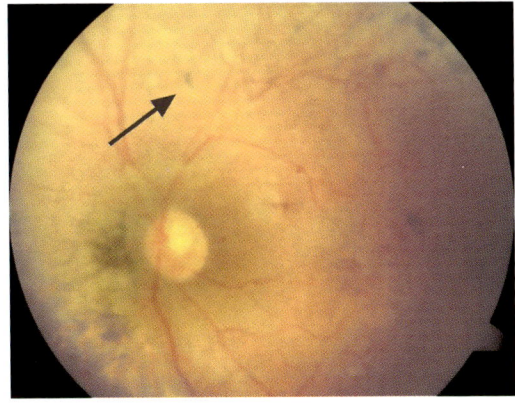

Fig. 16.8 *Left fundus photograph of old CRVO with NVI of more than two clock hours showing marks of panretinal photocoagulation (PRP)*

membrane. Success rate has been reported to be 10–54%. Complications of this technique include immediate intraretinal, subretinal or vitreous haemorrahage and late fibrovascular proliferation and CNVM. Visual recovery has been found to be limited inspite of successful anastomosis. Because of increased risk of complication (67%) and poor visual recovery, it is not a recommended treatment option.

C. Intravitreal anti-VEGF drugs

Injection of Bevacizumab (0.05 ml/1.25 mg) into vitreous cavity through pars plana in patients with macular edema has been shown to be effective not only in resolving the edema but also in corresponding improvement in vision. Although the exact mechanism of action of intravitreal injection of bevacizumab is not known, bevacizumab probably reduces VEGF concerntrations in the vitreous cavity. This leads to a reduction in capillary permeability and thereby macular edema. But action is again short lasting like triamcinolone. Repeated injections are required. Complications are similar to Triamcinolone injection. However, glaucoma and cataract do not occur.

In a study of 29 consecutive eyes with macular edema secondary to BRVO (21 eyes) and CRVO (8 eyes) 1.25 mg bevacizumab was injected intravitreally over a period of 12 months and an average of 8 injections were administered. The decrease in central retinal thickness and gain in vision of 16 letters at 12 months was statistically

significant and the injections were safe and effective. However, the main limitation was short-term effectiveness and high recurrence rate requiring repeat injections (Fig. 16.6 D and E).

Intraocular injection of 0.3 mg or 0.5 mg ranibizumab (Leucentis) FDA approved drug provides rapid improvement in 6 months visual acuity and macular edema following CRVO, with low rates of ocular and nonocular side effects (Cruise study-2010). Long-term follow-up of these patients is needed to know the persistence of these gains for more than 6 months. These drugs are presently under investigation and may prove to be valuable adjunct in the pharmacotherapy of CRVO.

Also in patients with neovascular glaucoma, a similar dose has shown to significantly decrease angle neovascularization and improved intra-ocular pressure control, both medically and surgically.

D. Intravitreal steroids

In patients with macular edema injection of triamcinolone acetonide (1 mg/0.1 ml) into the vitreous cavity (IVTA) through pars plana has been shown to be effective not only in resolving the edema but also in corresponding improve-ment in vision. The improvement in vision is observed more in non-ischemic than in ischaemic CRVO. Triamcinolone reduces VEGF concentra-tions in the vitreous cavity which leads to a reduction in capillary permeability and macular edema. This treatment modality has not yet been evaluated in a prospective randomized controlled clinical trial (Score study-2009). The main drawback of an injection of triamcinolone is transient effect leading to recurrences of macular edema, requiring repeat triamcinolone injections, typically every 3–6 months. In addition, other significant complications due to the injection of triamcinolone include cataract, glaucoma, retinal detachment, vitreous hemorrhage and endophthalmitis.

Sustained Release Dexamethasone Intravitreal Implant

OZURDEX implant is composed of a biodegra-dable copolymer of lactic acid and glycolic acid containing 700 µg of micronized dexamethasone. The drug-copolymer complex gradually releases the total dose of dexamethasone over 4–6 months after insertion into the eye through a small pars plana puncture using a customized applicator system. The peak effect occurs in 60 days. The advantage is repeated injections are avoided. The disadvantage is raised IOP and cataract formation and the high cost. However, it is a good choice in aphakic, pseudophakic and steroid non-responders (Geneva study-2011).

E. Surgical therapy

Pars plana vitrectomy (PPV) has been often employed to address the complications of CRVO like nonclearing vitreous hemorrhage. PPV can be combined with the removal of ERM if any and placement of laser if indicated. PPV with posterior hyaloid removal might also improve the persistent macular edema. In eyes with NVG, PPV may be combined with endolaser (PRP) and pars plana placement of a seton glaucoma drainage device.

Recently, Opermach proposed combining PPV with transvitreal incision of the nasal scleral ring to release pressure and thus to surgically decompress CRV at the level of scleral outlet. The procedure has been termed as **Radial optic neurotomy**. The procedure addresses the "compartment syndrome" that may exist in these eyes where CRV, CRA and optic nerve traverses through a 1.5 mm diameter area just like carpal tunnel syndrome at the wrist. The results reported by the authors are variable some showing visual improvement with resolution of hemorrhages and macular edema while others did not observe any improvement. However, to date the procedure is not accepted as a treatment option since the efficacy is unproven and safety profile is also questionable.

F. Intravitreal tissue plasminogen activator (thrombolytic agent)

Tissue plasminogen activator (TPA) has been tried intravitreally without beneficial effect. However, in some reports improvement in visual acuity has been observed with retinal vein cannulation and infusion of tissue plasminogen activator. Since the efficacy and the safety profile of the drug is still unproven, therefore, this treatment option is not a acceptable modality of treatment.

FOLLOW-UP

The follow-up of the patient is guided by the visual acuity (VA) at the initial presentation. If the initial VA is 6/12 or better the patient should be followed up 1–2 months for 6 months. In case the VA is worse than 6/60, these eyes should be examined monthly for 6 months and than bimonthly for another six months since these eyes are at a higher risk of developing NVI and NVA. Eyes with VA between 6/18 and 6/60 should also be examined monthly for 6 months since these eyes are at intermediate risk of developing NVI and NVA.

During the examination, VA, RAPD, undilated slit lamp examination, ERG, Goldmann perimetry and IOP should be recorded. If at any time during follow-up VA drops below 6/60, assessment of perfusion status by FFA and follow-up for an additional 6 months is recommended.

PROGNOSIS

The visual acuity at the time of presentation is an important prognostic indicator of final visual outcome. The patients with VA 6/12 or better, majority maintain this vision. The patients with poor VA at the onset (worse than 6/60) the prognosis is poor since there is only 20% chance of improvement. Those with intermediate VA (6/18 to 6/60) the outcome is variable; 20% may improve to 6/12, 40% stay in intermediate group and 40% may worsen to <6/60. In other words nonischaemic has much better prognosis than ischaemic CRVO. Eventual improvement depends on the availability and development of collaterals.

CONCLUSION

CRVO is a sight threatening condition with significant ocular morbidity during the natural course of the disease owing to the development of macular edema and neovascularization. Early diagnosis, prompt identification of complications and their management may help in limiting the visual loss. Ongoing research and application of newer modalities of the therapy may throw more light in the proper management of the condition.

TRIALS IN CENTRAL VEIN OCCLUSIONS

Important trials conducted in central retinal vein occlusions are depicted in Table 16.2.

HEMICENTRAL RETINAL VEIN OCCLUSION (HCRVO)

In approximately 20% of the humans two independent trunks of central retinal vein enter and traverse the optic nerve before joining to form single central retinal vein. The upper trunk drains the upper half of retina and lower trunk drains the lower half. When thrombosis occur in one of the trunk it is labeled as hemi-central retinal vein collusion. It is the least common type of venous occlusive disease (Fig. 16.9A).

Pathogenesis of HCRVO is similar to that of CRVO and accordingly is of ischemic and non-ischemic type and former is seen in about 20% and latter in 80% cases.

CLINICAL FEATURES

It is characterized by superior or inferior field defect as well as central visual loss from macular involvement. The involved half of the retina will have similar features as in CRVO except that corresponding part of the disc will show disc edema. In differentiation from ischemic to non-ischemic HCRVO the various test discussed above in CRVO do not help except that the visual fields with a Goldmann perimeter show in addition to central scotoma, a dense segmental defect with larger isopter and FFA shows CNP areas in involved retina (Fig. 16.9B).

DIFFERENTIAL DIAGNOSIS

It is also imperative to differentiate HCRVO from major BRVO. The latter is always ischaemic type while former can be ischaemic (20%) and non-ischemic type (80%). The site of occlusion in BRVO is at A/V crossing where as in HCRVO it is with in the optic nerve. Disc is normal in BRVO where as in HCRVO the corresponding part of the disc is edematous. The location of collaterals in BRVO are located on the retina away from disc where as in HCRVO are located on the optic disc or with in optic nerve.

Neovascularization seen in ischemic HCRVO is different from the one seen in ischemic CRVO. NVE and NVD is commonest in ischemic HCRVO where as NVI and NVA is commonest in ischemic CRVO. Hence the NVG is rare in HCRVO. Lastly in HCRVO collaterals may form

Table 16.2 *Trials in central retinal vein occlusions*

CRVO trials	No. of patient	Year	Interventions	Outcome	Clinical implication	Follow-up
Copernicus	189	2012	VEGF-trap eye 2 mg intravitreal every month vs sham injection	Effect on VA, CMT and progression to neovascularization	VEGF trap eye reduces CMT and improves VA	Ongoing
Geneva study	1256	2011	Sustained release dexamethasone intravitreal implant (Ozurdex) 0.7 mg vs sham injection	0.7 mg implant increase VA in 30–32% patients, 12.4–15.6% rise in IOP	0.7 mg ozurdex is an effective modality to reduce CMT and improve VA for up to 5 to 6 months	1 year
CRVO Bypass study	113 (Non-ischemic CRVO)	2010	Laser induced chorioretinal anastomosis (L-CRA) in patients of non-ischemic CRVO	Progression to ischemic CRVO occurred in 9.8% eyes vs 20.8% (sham group)	L-CRA is a helpful measure in patients of non-ischemic CRVO to improve VA and retard progression	18 months
Cruise study	392	2010	0.3 mg ranibizumab vs 0.5 mg ranibizumab vs sham	44% in 0.3 mg and 46–47% in 0.5 mg group. Patients gained > 15 letters of VA by intravitreal ranibizumab	0.3 and 0.5 mg ranibizumab improves VA and CMT	6 months
Score study	241	2009	1 mg triamcinolone vs 4 mg triamcinolone vs observation for macular edema secondary to CRVO	26–27% patients gained >15 letters in both triamcinolone groups. Rates of increased IOP lower in 1 mg grouped as compared to 4 mg group	1 mg intravitreal steroid should be initiated to reduce CMT and improve VA in patients with CRVO and macular edema	12 months
CRVO study	711	1995	1. Effect of laser photocoagulation on macular edema 2. Effect of PRP to retard NVA/NVI or conversion to NVG	1. No difference in VA between laser and observation groups 2. Extensive PRP done at the time of appearance of NVA or >2 clock hours of NVI led to resolution in 80–90%	1. Observation alone is needed for CRVO in macular edema 2. PRP to be instituted as soon as NVI/NVA are detected, not before	Concluded

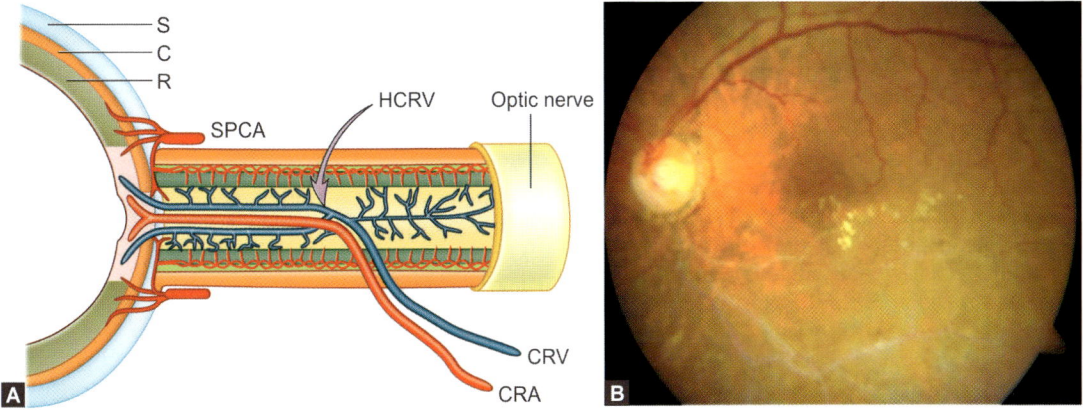

Fig. 16.9 *(A)* Dual trunk of CRV is seen in the substance of optic nerve in about 20% of cases normally; and *(B)* Left fundus photograph of old inferior HCRVO with CME

at the disc. Differential diagnosis is usually from major BRVO as discussed above.

MANAGEMENT

The clinical evaluation and investigations are the same as has been suggested in CRVO. As regards to treatment, the risk factors should be looked after as defined in CRVO. The treatment of macular edema and NV is on the same lines as that of CRVO.

PROGNOSIS

Visual prognosis appears to be better in HCRVO than in CRVO. Prognosis appears to correlate with the extent of retinal perfusion.

BRANCH RETINAL VEIN OCCLUSION

The exact incidence of branch retinal vein occlusion (BRVO) in Indian population is not known however, in Blue Mountains Eye study in Australia, of all the RVOs, 70% were BRVO, 25% CRVO and 5% were HCRVO. Usually it is U/L but may be bilateral in 5% cases. It is reported that after any RVO in one eye, the incidence of developing a second vein occlusion in the next 4 years was 2.5% in the same eye and 12% in the fellow eye. The overall incidence of BRVO was 1.1% seen most commonly in seventh decade with no gender predilection. It is also well known that BRVO is seen more frequently in the temporal than nasal part of the retina, and

of the temporal retina more commonly in the superior than inferior quadrant.

The risk factors for BRVO are the same as that for CRVO, i.e. hypertension, diabetes, dyslipidemia, age related atherosclerosis and open angle glaucoma.

BRVO has been classified into major BRVO and macular BRVO.

PATHOGENESIS

BRVO is always of ischaemic type. The precise mechanism causing the venous occlusion is poorly understood, multiple theories often contradictory exist. Most acceptable theory is that at AV crossings the artery and vein share a common adventitial sheath. Histopathological studies have shown that BRVO at AV crossings has been associated with arteriosclerotic changes in the overlying retinal arterioles. The resultant thickening of the artery could cause compression of adjacent vein, resulting in turbulence of blood flow, endothelial cell damage and thrombotic occlusion of the vein leading to elevation of venous pressure. This in turn lead to macular edema and ischemia of involved quadrant. Unrelieved pressure can also result in rupture of vein wall causing intraretinal hemorrhage and breakthrough vitreous hemorrhage.

CLINICAL FEATURES

Patient usually present with sudden painless loss of vision depending upon the extent of

macular involvement or else patient may present with blind spot in his field of vision. In addition to macular edema the other causes of loss of vision in BRVO are macular non-perfusion, dense intraretinal hemorrhage, vitreous hemorrhage, neovascular glaucoma, epiretinal membrane and traction retinal detachment. VA in BRVO is comparatively less affected than CRVO. 50–60% of untreated patient will have a final visual acuity of 6/12 or better. However, 20–25% patients have 6/60 or worse. Final VA of <6/60 is uncommon. VA may remain unaffected if branch involved is nasal.

Complete ocular examination should be performed including evaluation for iris and angle neovascularization (NVI and NVA) and a dilated fundus examination with 90D slit lamp. Fundus findings include dilatation and tortuosity of obstructed vein, superficial hemorrhages, retinal edema and cotton wool spots (NFL infarcts) in the sector of retina drained by the affected vein. The site of occlusion is mostly at AV crossing. In case of superior or inferior temporal vein involvement, the macula show edema. However, if BRVO is nasal, peripheral and small, it may produce findings which are subtle and difficult to detect on examination (Fig. 16.10).

The intraretinal hemorrhages resolve months after the occurrence of BRVO. In chronic phase after the resolution of hemorrhages, the ophthalmoscopic diagnosis may be difficult. The diagnosis at this stage can be aided by FFA on noting a segmental distribution of retinal vascular abnormalities like capillary nonper-

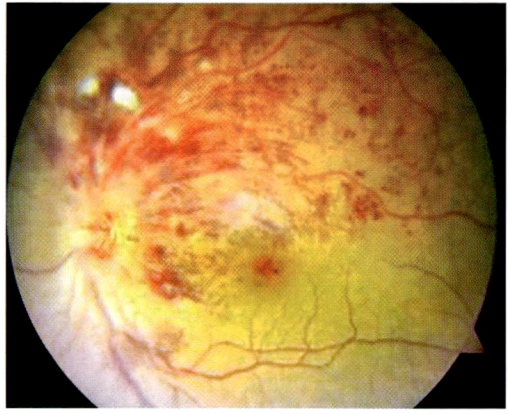

Fig. 16.10 *Left fundus photograph of BRVO showing dilated superotemporal vein with multiple hemorrhages and soft exudates along the superotemporal arcade and CME*

fusion, dilatation of adjacent capillaries, microaneurysms and collateral vessels formation (Fig. 16.11A to C).

COMPLICATIONS

- *Macular edema* is the most common complication and is leading cause of vision loss associated with BRVO. The visual recovery is more likely to occur in perfused macula as compared to nonperfused as seen on FFA (Fig. 16.12 A to C).

- *Neovascularization* occurs most commonly in the retina (NVE). NVD is much less common and NVI is rare in BRVO. It occurs in response to the release of VEGF from hypoxic retina 6–12 months following BRVO. Numerous study has reported the incidence of NVE from 20–30% (Fig. 16.13).

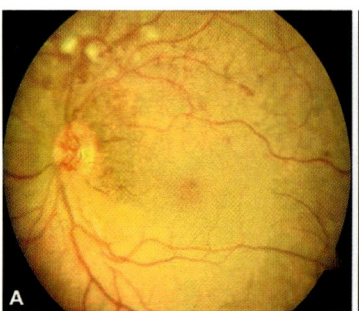
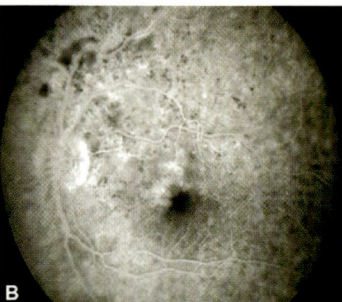
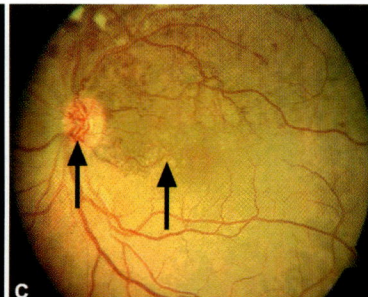

Fig. 16.11 *(A) Left fundus phtograph of the same patient as Fig. 16.10 after 3 months showing resolving retinal hemorrhages and cotton wool spots; (B) Late phase FFA shows CME (petaloid hyperfluorescence) with well perfused macula; and (C) Grid laser was done for CME (arrow). Disc show collaterals (arrow)*

- *Vitreous hemorrhage* typically occurs later in the course of the disease following the rupture of friable and thin neovascular vessels.
- *Tractional retinal detachment* (TRD) can occur following BRVO if fibrovascular proliferation develops.
- *Collateral vessels* may develop at the junction of nonperfused and perfused retina. Collateral vessels are distinct from neovascular vessels in that collaterals are flat while neovascular vessels are elevated, the former do not leak on FFA while the latter leak (Fig. 16.11C).
- *Other visually significant complications of BRVO* include ERM, RPE irregularity and subretinal fibrosis.

DIFFERENTIAL DIAGNOSIS

It is important to differentiate between HCRVO and BRVO since HCRVO is of ischaemic and non-ischemic type while BRVO is always ischemic type. The site of occlusion in BRVO is at the AV crossings while in HCRVO it is with in the optic nerve.

In HCRVO the corresponding part of the disc is edematous while disc is normal in BRVO unless AV crossing is situated on the disc. The location of collateral in major BRVO is on the retina away from the disc while in HCRVO these are on the disc or within the optic nerve.

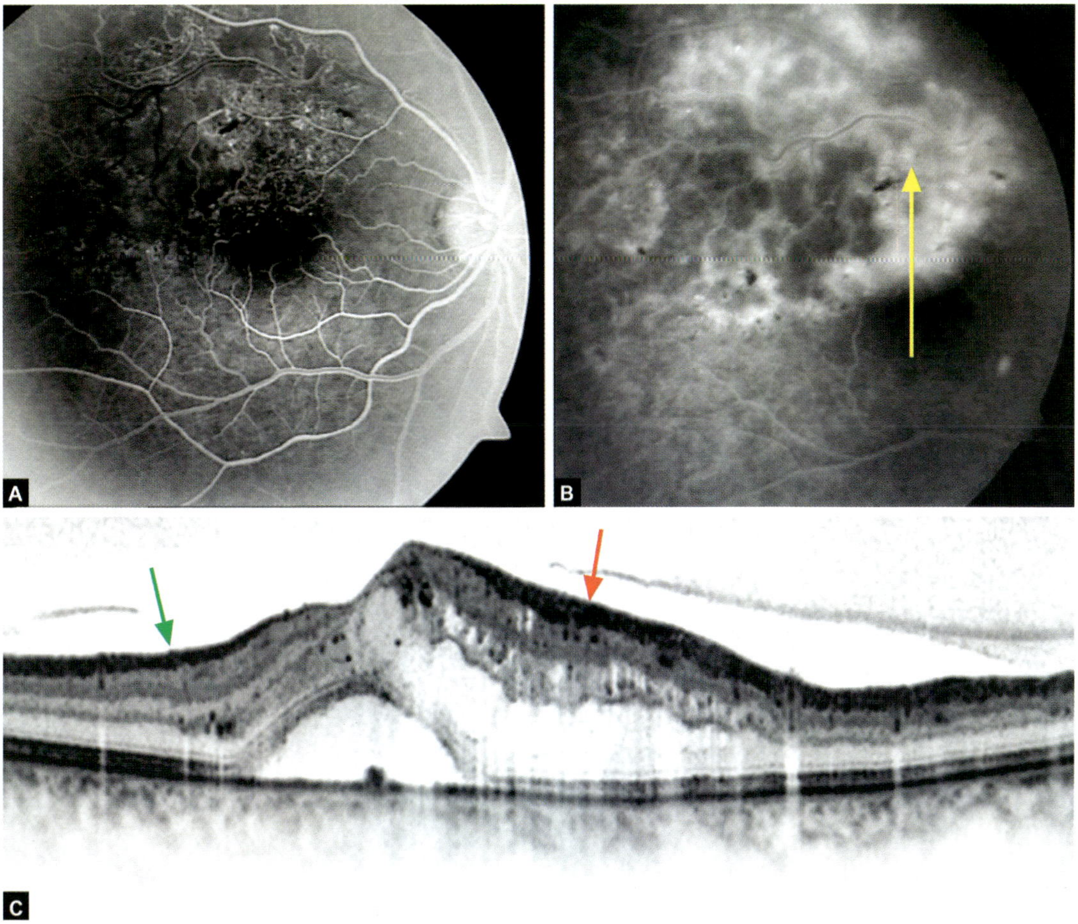

![Fundus fluorescein angiography and OCT images labeled A, B, and C]

Fig. 16.12 *(A) FFA of old case of right BRVO showing well perfused macula; (B) with CME; and (C) vertical high resolution OCT scan shows presence of differential retinal edema, more in the superior area (red arrow) however normal retinal thickness in the inferior area (green arrow). (Photographs Courtesy: Dr. Ethan Priel)*

MANAGEMENT

FFA has hardly any role in the acute stages because of masking by the presence of retinal hemorrhages. However, in doubtful cases it can help in the diagnosis of BRVO since the affected vein fills very slowly. In the late stages after the resorption of hemorrhages, one can see areas of capillary non-perfusion, numerous dilated collateral vessels at the junction of perfused and non-perfused retina and well perfused fovea may show flower petal hyperfluorescence (petaloid) due to CME (Fig. 16.11B). In addition, leakage of dye in the late frames may suggest NVE. However, enlarged and irregular FAZ may suggest ischemia. OCT may be performed in order to diagnose CME and to monitor the progress and resolution of CME (Fig. 16.14).

Treatment modalities include:
• Medical treatment
• Laser therapy
• Anti-VEGF therapy
• Intraocular corticosteroid
• Surgical treatment.

Medical treatment

Systemic evaluation of commonly associated risk factors like hypertension, diabetes, dyslipidemia, age related atherosclerosis, glaucoma

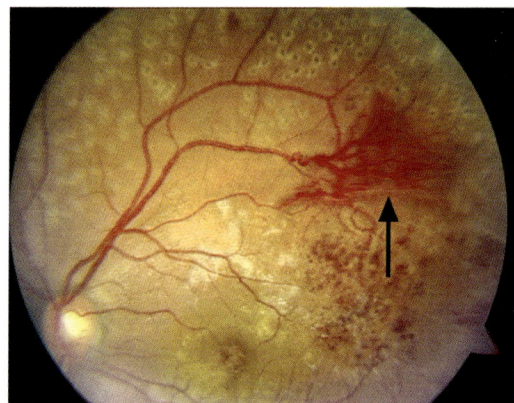

Fig. 16.13 *Left eye fundus photograph of old case of superotemporal BRVO showing NVE (black arrow) with scatter laser spots in superotemporal quadrant*

and smoking are an integral part of history taking and examination. It is essential to identify and treat these risk factors in consultation with internist in order to treat and to prevent the risk of future RVO in older, individuals. However, in patients under 50 years of age extensive workup following BRVO is often necessary inclusive of investigations for hypercoagulable and hyperviscosity states and to treat these in case detected. Systemic anticoagulation has been found to be of no benefit in the therapy of BRVO.

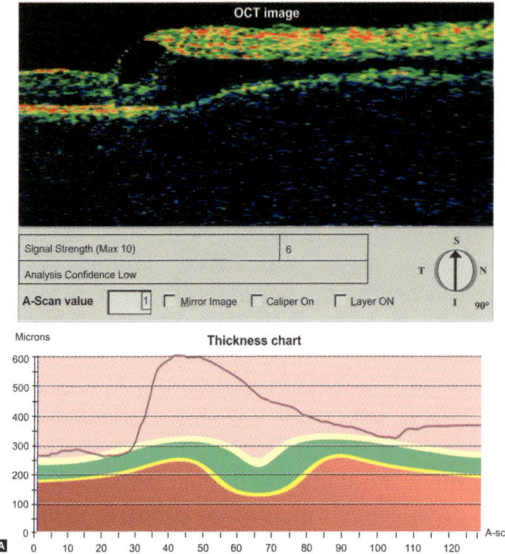

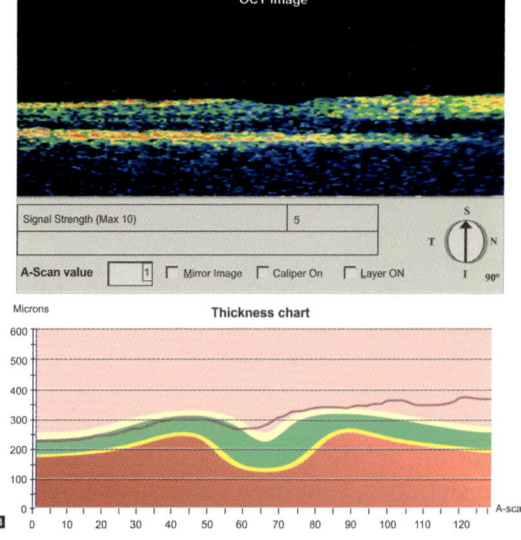

Fig. 16.14 *(A) OCT scan of a patient of BRVO showing differential macular edema (412 μ); (B) resolved to 290 μ after intravitreal anti-VEGF injection*

Laser therapy

It is required for treating the BRVO associated complication of cystoid macular edema (CME) and neovascularization (NV) leading to vitreous hemorrhage. The collaborative branch vein occlusion study, a multicentric, randomized clinical trial recommended grid pattern laser photocoagulation for the treatment of CME persisting even three months after BRVO provided the fovea is perfused as seen on FFA and vision is less than 6/12. Foveal avascular zone (FAZ) should be avoided in laser therapy and all the intraretinal hemorrhages should have resolved before laser treatment. Recommended laser parameters included a duration of 0.1 second, 100 µ diameter spot size and power setting sufficient to produce a medium white burn (Fig. 16.15). After 3 years of follow-up 63% of treated eyes gained two or more lines of vision compared to 35% of untreated group. Retreatment of residual CME is advised after waiting at least for a period of 3 months that too after performing FFA. Most probably grid pattern laser photocoagulation act by producing a thinning of the retina so that choroidal vasculature supplies some of the inner retinal needs, producing a consequent autoregulatory constriction of the retinal vasculature in the leaking area and thereby decreasing the edema. Laser treatment is not recommended since it does not improve vision if macular non-perfusion accounts for visual loss.

NVE and NVD following BRVO leads to vitreous hemorrhage. The BRVO study recommended scatter laser photocoagulation only after the development of NVE which reduces the risk of vitreous hemorrhage from 60 to 30%. If the patient present with vitreous hemorrhage, staged sessions of scatter laser photocoagulation may be necessary depending upon the clearing of vitreous hemorrhage. The scatter laser photocoagulation is applied with green laser (double frequency Nd:YAG Laser) to achieve 'medium' white burns 200–500 micron in diameter, spaced one burn width apart covering the entire area of capillary non- perfusion (CNP), as identified by FFA in the concerned quadrant (Fig. 16.13).

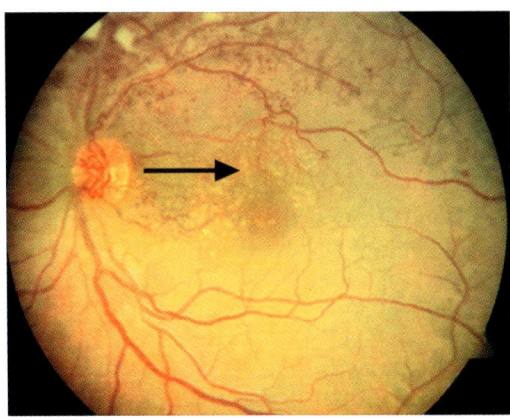

Fig. 16.15 *Left fundus photograph of BRVO, the patient underwent grid laser superiorly for CME*

Anti-VEGF therapy

There are sufficient reports in the available literature recommending the role of intravitreal Ranibizumab (Leucentis) and Bevacizumab (Avastin) in the acute stage of BRVO. It is said that anti-VEGF agents mop off the VEGF released owing to the hypoxia caused by BRVO. The VEGF release lead to increased capillary permeability, thereby causing macular edema. Anti VEGF drugs help in relieving the macular edema in acute stage and in late stage resolves neovascularization (NV). However, the effect is short-term, therefore, repeated injections are required after about 4 weeks. Nevertheless anti-VEGF drugs are adjunct to the therapy of BRVO (Fig. 16.14).

Intraocular corticosteroids

Before the advent of anti-VEGF therapy Intravitreal Triamcinolone Acetonide (IVTA) 2–4 mg used to be given for controlling macular edema associated with BRVO. Triamcinolone has been shown experimentally to reduce the break down of blood retinal barrier by inhibiting factors such as prostaglandins, interleukins, VEGF and protein kinase C. IVTA may give favourable response in reducing macular edema as reported by small case studies. Also this treatment modality has not yet been evaluated in a prospective randomized controlled clinical trial. However, visual acuity (VA) improvement is more likely to occur in perfused rather than nonperfused macular edema. Again the effect

is transient lasting for approximately 3 months. There are reported side effects of IVTA, e.g. accelerated cataract formation, raised IOP, endophthalmitis, vitreous hemorrhage, lens injury and retinal detachment. Since, glaucoma and cataract do not occur with anti-VEGF drugs and these drugs are more specific, therefore, intravitreal anti-VEGF drugs are preferred over IVTA in the treatment of macular edema associated with BRVO. However, laser photo-coagulation remain the standard of care in CME of BRVO, whereas these drugs are adjunct to laser therapy so far.

Surgical treatment

- *Pars plana vitrectomy (PPV)* is performed for treating the complications of BRVO. Surgical indications include nonclearing vitreous hemorrhage, TRD involving macula, epiretinal membrane and complication of ghost cell glaucoma.
- *Pars plana vitrectomy with creation of posterior vitreous detachment (PVD)* has been reported to be effective in reducing CME and improving VA in patients of BRVO. Possible explanation for the clinical improvement include removal of vitreous traction and increased oxygenation of macula. Another theory postulates that PPV may facilitate diffusion of harmful cytokines such as VEGF away from the retina.
- *Arteriovenous adventitial sheathotomy* is an attempt to decompress the involved venule by separating the overlying retinal artery from the underlying vein at AV crossing by sectioning the shared adventitial sheath during PPV. This may be performed in patients having recalcitrant CME even after grid laser photo-coagulation. Although the result reported are favourable but the procedure is not fraught from complications and it has not been investigated in prospective, randomized controlled large scale trials. Hence, as of now it is not recommended as one of the treatment option for BRVO.

FOLLOW-UP AND PROGNOSIS
Follow-up

BRVO patients should be followed every month. On every follow-up visit VA and IOP should be recorded. Dilated fundus examination should be carried out to look for resolution of retinal hemorrhages and macular edema. The later can be quantified and monitored by OCT. Base line FFA may be done after about 4 weeks once hemorrhages resolve. On 2nd and 3rd follow-up visit FFA may also help in discerning CNP (capillary nonperfusion) areas and NVE if any. Once laser therapy is indicated the monthly follow-up is carried out for a minimum of 6 months. Associated systemic conditions if any are controlled under the supervision of internist.

Prognosis

The prognosis of BRVO is usually good. 50% of eyes develop efficient collaterals within 6 months and visual acuity returns to at least 6/12. Eventual recovery depends upon the amount of venous drainage hampered by the occlusion. Cystoid macular edema is the main cause of persistent low vision after BRVO. The prognosis of vision is guarded if the macula is not perfused and FAZ is enlarged. NVD develops in about 10% and NVE in about 25% of the eyes and it usually appears within 6–12 months but may develop anytime within first 3 years. However, timely placement of scatter laser photocoagulation can prevent the complication of vitreous hemorrhage.

MACULAR BRVO

When one of the tributary vein draining the macula is blocked it is called Macular BRVO. Invariably it is thrombosis of one of the branches of either superior or inferior temporal vein draining the macular area. Similar tributary vein blockage elsewhere in the periphery may remain undetected, however, in macula it is important since it causes sudden diminution of central vision. It has the same pathogenesis as of major BRVO.

Clinical Features

Patient usually presents with sudden painless loss of central vision. Anterior segment inclusive of pupillary reaction is normal. However, on 90D dilated slit lamp examination a patch of variable size in the macular area is observed with few superficial hemorrhages and one or two cotton wool spots along with retinal edema involving

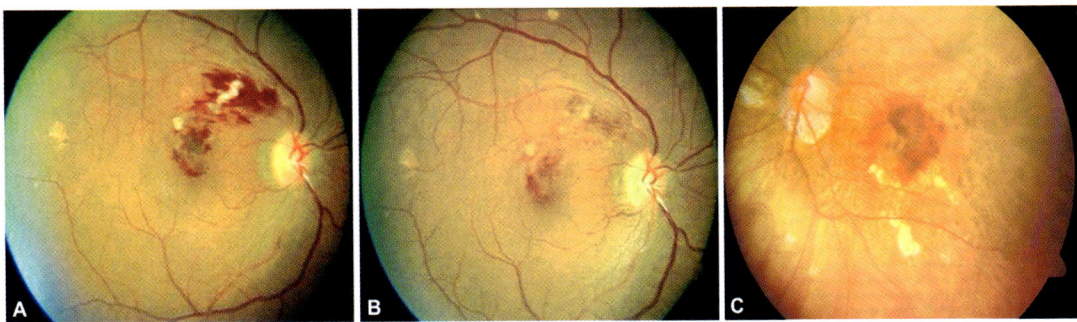

Fig. 16.16 *(A) Right fundus photograph of case of macular BRVO showing superficial hemorrhages and cotton wool spots on the macula in the area of drainage of occluded macular vein; (B) Resolution of hemorrhages in the same patient after 3 months; and (C) Left fundus photograph of a patient of wet ARMD showing subretinal hemorrhage and exudates*

the fovea centralis (Fig. 16.16A and B). In due course of time the hemorrhages absorb, cotton wool spots resolve, but macular edema may persist. FFA at this stage may depict area of capillary non-perfusion along with incomplete circle of petalloid hyperfluorescence in the area of macular edema. Since area involved is small and hypoxia caused is so little that neovascularization does not occur.

Differential Diagnosis

Since macular BRVO occurs in older age group therefore it needs to be differentiated from exudative ARMD (Table 16.3 and Fig. 16.16A to C).

Treatment

- *Common systemic associations* as in major BRVO need to be identified and treated under the care of internist.
- *Anti-VEGF drugs* like Leucentis or Avastin when given intravitreally help as adjunct in the faster resolution of associated macular edema.
- *Grid pattern laser photocoagulation* is avoided in the era of anti-VEGF drugs.

TRIALS IN BRVO

Important trials conducted in BRVO are depicted in Table 16.4.

S.no.		Macular BRVO	Exudative ARMD
		Table 16.3 *Macular BRVO versus exudative ARMD*	
1.	Laterally	Usually unilateral	Usually bilateral
2.	Associated systemic disease	Usually there	May not be there
3.	Clinical picture	A patch of superficial hemorrhages, cotton wool spots with macular edema	A subfoveal/juxtafoveal patch of subretinal haemorrhage, exudates, neurosensory and RPE detachment along with soft drusen
4.	FFA	Show CNP area, microaneurysms and dilated capillary at the junction of perfused and non-perfused retina along with incomplete pettaloid hyper-fluorescence	Lacy pattern of hyperfluorescence in early frames which increase in size and intensity in late frames. May be late hyperfluorescence from undeter-minate source along with RPE detach-ment
5.	OCT	Increased thickness at the site of lesion and cystoid spaces	Suggestive of classic or occult CNVM

Table 16.4 *Clinical trials in BRVO*

BRVO trials	No of patient	Year	Interventions	Outcome	Clinical implication	Follow-up
Geneva study	1256	2011	0.35 mg dexamethasone implant vs 0.7 mg dexamethasone implant vs sham	0.7 mg implant improved VA in 30–32% patients	0.7 mg ozurdex should be used in patients with CRVO and macular edema	1 year
BRVO study	387	2010	0.3 mg vs 0.5 mg ranibizumab vs sham injection	61% patients gained >15 letters VA in 0.5 mg ranibizumab group, compared to 29% in sham group	0.5 mg ranibizumab injection reduce CMT and improve VA in patients with macular edema and BRVO	6 months
AV sheathotomy vs IVTA for macular edema in BRVO	40	2008	AV sheathotomy vs IVTA for BRVO macular edema		Due to equal efficacy of both IVTA is preferred as it is cost effective	6 months
BRVO study		1984	1. Macular laser photocoagulation for macular edema 2. Scatter laser for NVD/NVE	1. 65 % patients with grid laser improved >15 letters of vision compared to 37% of sham 2. Scatter laser reduced the chances of vitreous hemorrhage when the patient had NVD/NVE from 60 to 30%	1. Macular grid laser to be done for perfused macula in BRVO with VA <6/12 after 3 months 2. Scatter laser to be started when NVD/NVE develop to reduce chances of vitreous hemorrhage	
BRVO score study	411	2009	1 mg triamcinolone vs 4 mg triamcinolone vs laser photocoagulation for BRVO macular edema	26–27% patients gained >15 letters in all groups but cataract and raised IOP were more in both triamcinolone groups	Laser photocoagulation remains the standard of care for BRVO macular edema	1 year

BIBLIOGRAPHY

Central Retinal Vein Occlusion

1. A randomized clinical trial of early PRP for ischaemic CRVO. The central vein occlusion study group N report. Ophthalmology 1995; 102:1434–44.

2. Brown DM, Campochiaro PA, Singh RP, Li Z, Gray S, Saroj N, Rundle AC, Rubio RG, Murahashi WY. CRUISE Investigators. Ranibizumab for CME following CRVO: six month primary end point results of a phase III study. Ophthalmology 2010 Jun; 117(6):1124–33. el. Epub 2010 Apr 9.

3. Campochiaro PA, Heier IS, Feiner L, Gray S, Saroj N, Rundle AC Murahashi WY, Rubio RJ. Ranibizumab for CME following BRVO: six month primary end point results of a phase III study. BRAVO investigators.

4. Evaluation of grid pattern photocoagulation for macular edema in CRVO. The central vein occlusion study group M report Ophthalmology 1995; 102:1425–33.
5. Gottlieb JL, Blice JB, Mestichelli B, et al. Activated protein C resistance factor V laiden and CRVO in young adults. Arch Ophthalmol 1998;116: 557–79.
6. Hayreh SS, Klugman MR, Beri M, et al. Differentiation of ischaemic from non ischaemic CRVO during the early acute phase. Graefes Arch Clin Exp Ophthalmol 1990;228:201–17.
7. Hayreh SS, Zimmerman MB, McCarthy MJ, et al. Systemic diseases associated with various types of retinal vein occlusion. Am J Ophthalmol 2001:131:61–7.
8. Hayreh SS, Zimmerman MB, Padhajsky P. Incidence of various types of retinal vein occlusion and their recurrence and demographic charac- teristics. Am J Ophthalmol 1994; 117:429–41.
9. Hayreh SS. Central vein Occlusion. Ophthalmol Clin North Am 1998;11:559–90.
10. Heyreh SS, Zimmerman MB, Podhajsky P. Hematological abnormalities associated with various types of retinal vein occlusions. Graefes Arch Clin Exp Ophthalmol 2002;240:180–96.
11. Lahey JM, Tunc M, Kearney J, et al. Laboratory evaluation of hypercoagulable states in patients with CRVO who are less than 56 yeas of age. Ophthalmology 2002;109:126–31.
12. McAllister IL, Douglas JP, Constable JJ, et al. Laser induced chorioretinal venous anastomosis for non-ischaemic CRVO: evaluation of the complications and their risk factors. Am J. Ophthalmol 1998;126:219–29.
13. Park CH, Jaeff GJ, Fekrat S. IVTA in eyes with CME associated with CRVO. Am J Ophthalmol 2003;136:419–25.
14. Risk factors for CRVO. The eye disease case- control study group. Arch. Ophthalmol 1996; 114:545–54.
15. Weinberg DV, Wahle AE, Ip MS, Scott IU, Vanveldhuisen PC, Blodi BA; for the SCORE Investigator group. Score study report 12: Development of venous collaterals in Score study. Retina. 2012 Sept 11 (Epub ahead of print).

Branch Retinal Vein Occlusion

1. Argon laser photocoagulation for prevention of neovascularization and vitreous hemorrhage in branch vein occlusion: a randomized clinical trial. Branch vein occlusion study group. Arch Ophthalmol. 1986;104:34–41.
2. Branch vein occlusion study group. Argon laser photocoagulation for macular edema in branch vein occlusion. Am J Ophthalmol 1984; 98:271–82.
3. Cahill MT, Stinnett SS, Fekrat S. Meta-analysis of plasma homocysteine, serum folate, serum vitamin B_{12}, and thermolabile MTHFR genotype as risk factors for retinal vascular occlusive disease. Am J Ophthalmol 2003; 136:1136–50.
4. Campochiaro PA, Heier IS, Feiner L, Gray S, Saroj N, Rundle AC. Murahashi WY, Rubio RJ. Ranibizumab for CME following BRVO: six month primary end point results of a phase III study. BRAVO investigators.
5. Cohill MT, Kaiser PK, Sears JE, et al. The effect of ateriovenous sheathotomy on CME secondary to BRVO. Br. J Ophthalmol 2003; 87:1329–32.
6. Hauer JA, Bandello F, Belfort R (Jr), Blumenkranz MS, Gillies M, Heier J, et al. Dexamethasone intravitreal implants in patients with macular edema related to branch or central retinal vein occlusion twelve-month study results Geneva Trial Ophthalmology 2011;118:2453–60.
7. Lahey JM, Kearney JJ, Tunc M. Hypercoagulable states and central vein occlusion. Curr Opin Pulm Med 2003;9:385–92.
8. Martidis A, Duker JS, Greenberg P, et al. Intra- vitreal triamcinolone for refractory diabetic macular edema. Ophthalmology 2002;109: 920–7.
9. Risk factors for branch retinal vein occlusion. The eye disease case-control study group. Am J Ophthalmol 1993;116:286–96.
10. Scott IU, Ip MS, Vanveldhuisen PC, Oden NL, Blodi BA, Fisher M. et al. The Standard Care vs Corticosteroid for Retinal Vein Occulsion (SCORE) study report 6. Arch Ophthalmol 2009; 127:1115–28.

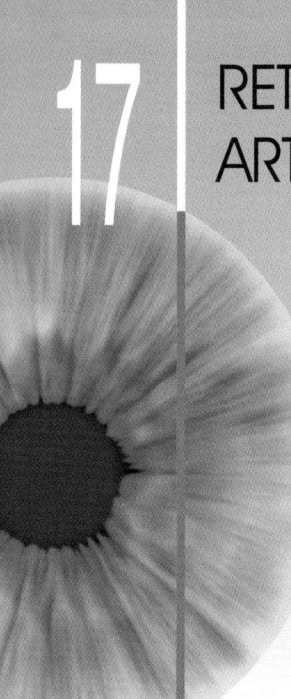

17 RETINAL ARTERY AND OPHTHALMIC ARTERY OCCLUSIONS

Sunandan Sood

RETINAL ARTERY OCCLUSIONS

INTRODUCTION

The retinal artery occlusive disease can be classified as central retinal artery, branch retinal artery and cilioretinal artery occlusion leading to acute loss of vision in the distribution of the affected retina. Central retinal artery occlusion (CRAO) constitutes 57%, branch retinal artery occlusion (BRAO) 38% and cilioretinal artery in 5% of all the cases of retinal artery occlusive disease. In 1859, von Graefe was the first to describe CRAO secondary to emboli related to bacterial endocarditis. Since, then the understanding of the retinal artery occlusion has vastly increased. The CRAO has the worst visual prognosis, whereas branch and cilioretinal artery occlusions have better visual prognosis.

INCIDENCE AND DEMOGRAPHY

Data concerning the incidence of CRAO in Indian population are not available but as per the information gathered from the western literature it has been estimated to occur with a frequency of about one per 10000 out patients visits. It may occur at any age but has been seen most frequently in 7th decade of life. There does not appear to be racial predilection although there is male predominance. The right and left eyes appear to be involved equally. In approximately 1–2% of patients there is bilateral involvement. Systemic risk factors include hypertension, diabetes, lipid disorders, cardiac valvular disease, giant cell arteritis and other vascular inflammatory diseases.

ETIOPATHOGENESIS

Mechanisms of occlusions are embolic, thrombotic, vasculitic and vasospastic; more than one mechanism may be operative at the same time in a patient. In general, age is an important factor in determining the mechanism of occlusion. Patients aged 50 and above usually have occlusion associated with embolic disease whereas younger patients have occlusion secondary to thrombosis.

1. Embolism

Since, CRAO disease is primarily a disease of elderly, embolic occlusion is the most common mechanism. Atherosclerosis of the great vessels of the neck is responsible for the source of emboli in 80% of cases of retinal arterial disease which can be evaluated by color doppler imaging (CDI). The heart and major vessels are another important source of emboli in condition like valvular abnormalities, atrial fibrillation and atrial myoma which can be evaluated by echocardiography. These emboli which can be cholesterol, calcific or platelet fibrin emboli are sometimes clinically visible in 20 to 40% of cases on 90D slit lamp examination. These block the central retinal artery at the level of lamina since it has the narrowest lumen there or at the bifurcation of the artery where it cause branch retinal artery occlusion (BRAO).

2. Thrombosis

Virchow's triad regarding the pathogenesis of thombus consisting of vessel wall abnormalities, stasis of blood flow and changes in blood components holds true in arterial occlusive disease of retina as well, although it is of more relevance in venous thrombosis. Structural abonormality in a vessel wall like prepapillary arterial loop can contribute to retinal arterial occlusion by thrombosis. Abnormalities of blood components which can be hereditary or acquired typically lead to venous thrombosis but in the presence of other local or systemic hyper-coagulable factors like pregnancy, oral contraceptives, trauma and malignancy, cigarette smoking may lead to arterial thrombosis. These should be considered in patients with a positive family history of thrombotic events occurring at a younger age. The conditions that are genetically determined and increase the likelihood of vascular thrombosis like anti-thrombin deficiency, protein C and S deficiency, hyper-homocystinemia, antiphospholipid syndrome and activated protein C resistance and factor V Leiden may be associated with retinal artery occlusive disease.

3. Vasculitic

Classically it occurs in giant cell arteritis where combined mechanism of vascultis and throm-bosis play a role in retinal artery occlusive disease. Elevated ESR, C reactive protein and confirmation by temporal artery biopsy clinches the diagnosis. In addition other systemic vasculitis associated with rheumatoid, SLE and Behçet's disease may lead to CRAO/BRAO.

CLINICAL FEATURES

Central retinal artery occlusion (CRAO)

Patient mostly present with the history of sudden painless profound loss of vision in one eye. Visual acuity of less than 3/60 occurs in more than 90% of eyes at the time of presentation. In some cases there is preceding history of transient monocular loss of vision (amaurosis fugax) which is suggestive of an embolic cause of occlusion.

Anterior segment examination, relative afferent pupillary defect (RAPD) is positive.

Fundus examination show yellowish white appearance of the posterior pole owing to the ischaemic edema of the retina except at foveola where a cherry red spot is seen because of intact choroidal circulation (Fig. 17.1A). Arteries are markedly attenuated with segmentation or box carring of the blood column seen both in arteries and veins. Absence of light perception is rarely encountered and if it is there then one should suspect the presence of concomitant choroidal circulatory compromise due to ophthalmic artery blockage or optic nerve damage.

Approximately 25% of acute CRAO have a patent cilioretinal artery that supplies part or all of the papillomacular bundle (Fig. 17.1B). Depending upon the involvement of the papillo-macular bundle the vision may vary from 6/36 to 6/12 however, only a small island of central vision may remain in these cases.

In about 20–40% of eyes with CRAO, emboli are visible with in retinal artery system mostly at bifurcation (Fig. 17.2). The presence of embolus is associated with poorer vision. These can be cholesterol, or calcific emboli, the former being more common and smaller than the later. The cholesterol embolus is smaller, yellowish and glistening (Hollenhorst plaque) in appearance and arise from atherosclerotic carotid arteries, aortic arch and ophthalmic artery. The calcific emboli originate from cardiac valves.

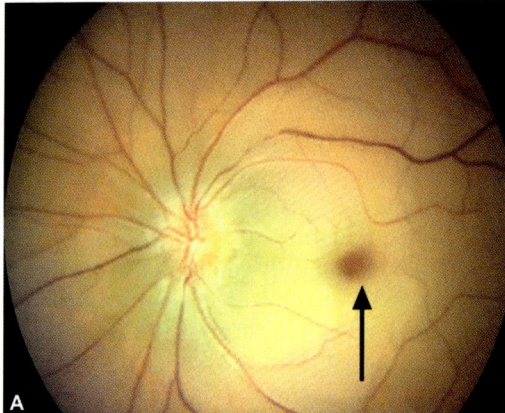

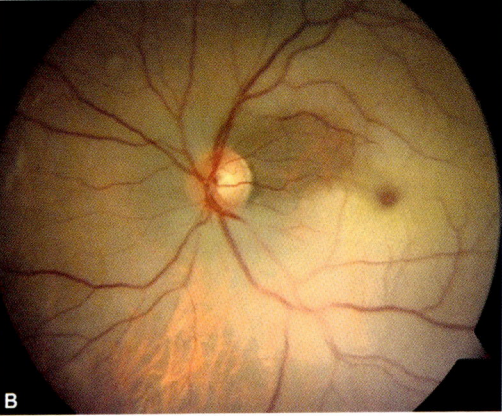

Fig. 17.1 *(A) Left fundus photo of a case of CRAO showing generalized whitening of retina, attenuated arterioles with presence of chery red spot (black arrow) in the centre of macula; and (B) Showing a patch of normally perfused retina in the area of blood supply of cilioretinal artery (papulo macular bundle) surrounded by generalized whitening of retina suggestive of sparing of cilioretinal artery in a case of CRAO*

In most cases the retinal opacification resolves over a period of 4–6 weeks, usually leaving a pale disc, narrowed retinal vessels and atrophic appearing retina. The pigmentary changes are usually absent unless there is involvement of choroidal circulation. The most devastating complication of retinal occlusive disease is neovascular glaucoma. It develops at a mean of 8–9 weeks after the event unlike eyes with CRVO in which rubeosis iridis develop at a mean of 5 months after the obstruction. It has been reported to occur in 2–16% of these eyes.

The diagnosis of CRAO is clinched by funduscopic findings and in doubtful cases by FFA which show an intact choroidal flush with absent, incomplete or delayed filling of the dye in the retinal circulation. A marked prolongation of choroidal filling along with delayed filling of retinal circulation should arouse suspicion of ophthalmic artery obstruction.

Branch retinal artery occlusion (BRAO)

It presents as an acute painless loss of visual field in the distribution of occluded artery. Visual acuity may range from 6/6 to 3/60 depending upon the nasal or temporal branch and on the degree of foveal involvement. RAPD may be present depending upon the extent of retinal involvement. Funduscopically, branch retinal artery occlusion appear as a localized region of superficial retinal whitening which is most prominent in the posterior pole along the distribution of occluded vessel (Fig. 17.3).

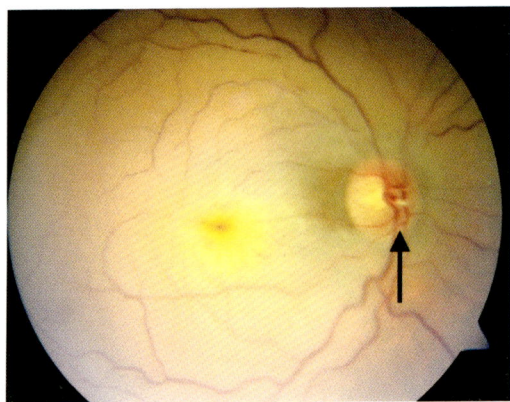

Fig. 17.2 *Right fundus photo showing small, yellowish, glistening cholesterol embolus (Hollenhorst plaque) at the disc (black arrow)*

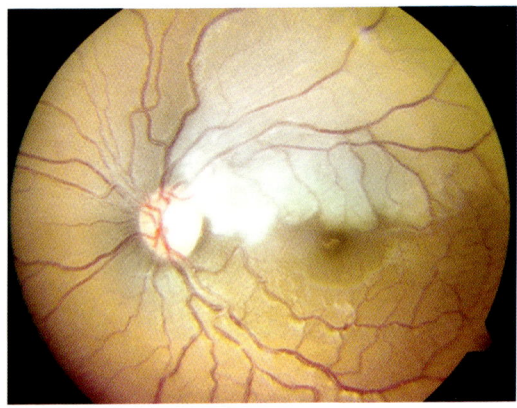

Fig. 17.3 *Left fundus photo showing whitening of supero-temporal quadrant of left eye of a case of superotemporal BRAO*

Emboli may be seen in 30% of cases when the obstruction is observed at bifurcation. It is indeed not clear whether temporal arteries are more commonly affected, or whether nasal BRAO is common. The nasal BRAO is often asymptomatic, and thus, may not be detected. FFA show delayed transit of the dye through the affected vessel and often retrograde filling of the vessel can be observed in the late frames of the angiograms (Fig. 17.4A and B).

Visual prognosis in eyes with BRAO is usually good provided the foveal vasculature maintains normal perfusion. About 80% of eyes eventually improve to 6/12 or better, however, visual field defect persists. The fundus appearance may return to near normal weeks to months following the acute episode.

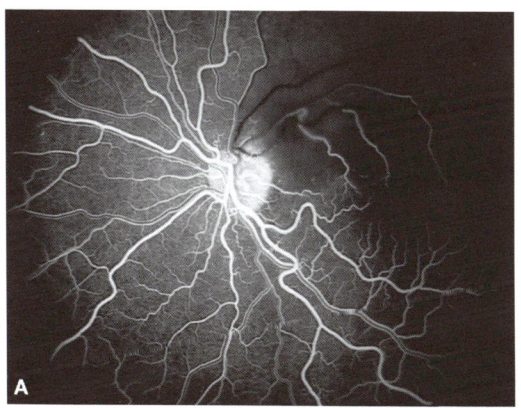

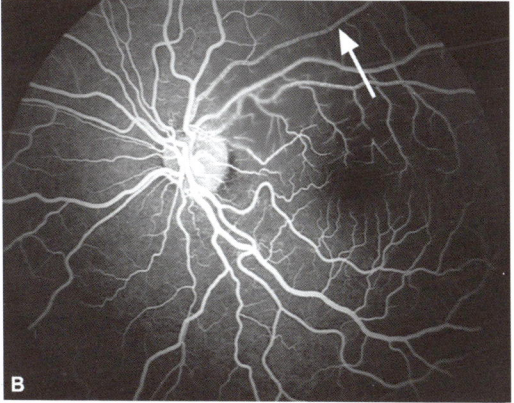

Fig. 17.4 *(A) FFA of the same case as in Fig. 17.3 show blocked retinal fluorescence in early frame and retrograde filling of the area in late frame in figure; and (B) Supero-temporal artery show segmentation of blood column (arrow) termed as box carring or cattle truck appearance*

Cilioretinal artery occlusion

Cilioretinal artery arises from short posterior ciliary arteries and is present in 30% of eyes entering the retina from temporal aspect of the disc. In normal course of FFA cilioretinal artery fills simultaneously with choroidal circulation, about 1 or 2 seconds earlier than the filling of the retinal circulation.

Ophthalmoscopically cilioretinal artery occlusion can occur as an isolated entity (>40%), in conjunction with non-ischemic Central Retinal Vein Occlusion (CRVO) 40% and in association with Anterior Ischemic Optic Neuropathy (AION) 15%.

Typically the patient with cilioretinal artery occlusion present with subtle pericentral scotoma. RAPD is usually not present since the area involved is very small. The fundus show superficial retinal whitening over the distribution of cilioretinal artery (Fig. 17.5). Isolated cilioretinal artery occlusion usually has good visual prognosis. 90% of affected eyes improve to 6/12 or better vision. The visual prognosis in patients of cilioretinal artery occlusion in conjunction with non-ischemic CRVO is also good since 70% of eyes achieve 6/12 or better vision. However, the visual prognosis is quite poor in the group of eyes with cilioretinal artery obstruction in association with AION.

MANAGEMENT

Management needs to be discussed under following heads:

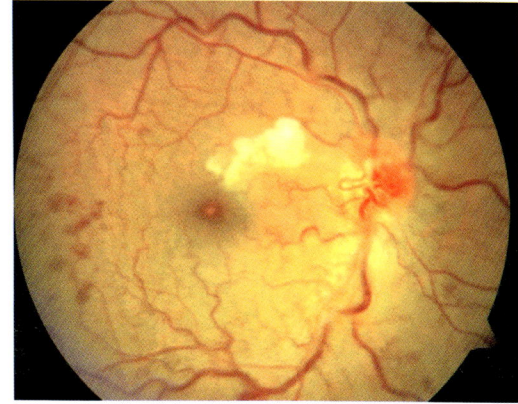

Fig. 17.5 *Right fundus photo showing cilioretinal artery occlusion in a case of nonischaemic CRVO*

1. Work up for associated Systemic Condition to Establish Etiology

As regards to work up for associated systemic condition, hypertension, diabetes needs to be ruled out but this should not delay treatment of RAO. We must start treatment immediately and systemic work up can follow. Color Doppler imaging can be done to assess carotid artery circulation and atherosclerosis. transthoracic/transoesophageal echocardiography should be ordered to assess cardiac status. ESR and C reactive protein levels for giant cell arteritis. Complete blood count, platelet count to rule out various vasculitic and thrombosis type syndromes. In addition, protein C, protein S, activated protein C, factor V Leiden, fasting plasma homocysteine and antiphospholipid levels may be done to complete the total work out. Despite the above investigations in about 20–30% patients no systemic association is documented.

2. Management of acute episode of retinal Artery occlusion

There are number of experimental studies reporting irreversible damage to the inner retinal tissue 90 to 100 minutes, following the obstruction of central retinal artery. However, there is concensus that any patient of CRAO reporting with in 24 hours of the acute episode of aterial obstruction needs to be subjected to the following aggressive measures in an attempt to restore blood circulation which may be successful in select number of patients only.

- *Digital ocular massage* to dislodge the embolus to more peripheral vessel.
- *Anterior chamber paracentesis* which suddenly lower the IOP may also help in dislodging the embolus.

- *Medical vasodilators* like cabogen (95% oxygen and 5% carbon dioxide) may cause vasodilation of retinal vessels. In the absence of this, rebreathing into a paper bag may be considered in the office. Sublingual nitroglycerin, calcium channel blockers have been used to improve retinal circulation however, without much visual improvement.
- *Fibrinolytic therapy.* Since less than 16% of CRAO are due to platelet fibrin type of embolus therefore, the decision to institute fibrinolytic therapy having doubtful visual recovery and with potential systemic complications should be made carefully.
- *Surgical treatment* like vitrectomy with cannulation of CRA has also been proposed. Laser photodisruption of embolus has been reported in select patients to cause the passage of embolus through arterial tree with improvement in visual outcome. However, no randomized trial data have confirmed the efficacy of any of these treatments.
- *If giant cell arteritis is established* by clinical and laboratory investigations high dose steroid therapy should be initiated early in order to avoid CRAO in the other eye.

3. Management of sequelae

Neovascular glaucoma is reported in 2–16% of these eyes. The treatment consists of laser or cryotherapy of retina, topical antiglaucoma drugs, glaucoma valve implants and cyclodestructive procedures as is with any other form of NVG.

CLINICAL TRIAL IN CRAO

Eagle study conducted in CRAO is depicted in Table 17.1.

Study	No. of patients	Year	Intervention	Outcome	Recommendation	Period
Eagle study (CRAO)	82	2007	Intra-arterial fibrinolysis with TPA vs observation in patients with non-arteritic CRAO	Equal improvement in VA in both groups but up to 37% patients had worse outcomes with fibrinolysis	Due to higher number of adverse effects, fibrinolysis is not recommended for CRAO	5 years

Table 17.1 *Eagle study of CRAO*

OPHTHALMIC ARTERY OCCLUSION

Ophthalmic artery is the first intracranial branch of the internal carotid artery and the CRA is the first branch of ophthalmic artery as it enters the orbit.

Etiopathogenesis

The ophthalmic artery occlusion has the same etiopathogenesis and similar to that of CRAO.

Clinical features

Essentially, clinical features of ophthalmic artery occlusion are similar to that of CRAO; however:
- *Visual loss* in the former is more profound since both choroidal and retinal circulation are blocked.
- *RAPD* is present.
- *Classic fundus picture* is that of an acutely infarcted retina with extensive retinal whitening without any cherry red spot (Fig. 17.6).

Investigations

- *FFA* shows absent or markedly delayed choroidal flush and delayed filling of retinal circulation.
- ERG can also help in differentiating the two conditions. In ophthalmic artery occlusion both a and b waves are absent while in CRAO b wave is absent and a wave is present.

Prognosis

Visual prognosis is poor in ophthalmic artery occlusion. Ultimately, the blockage leads to optic atrophy, attenuation of retinal artery and venules and retinal pigment epithelial abnormalities because of ischemia of RPE.

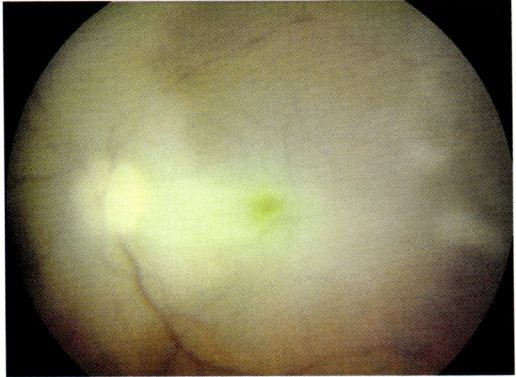

Fig. 17.6 *Left fundus photo of a case of ophthalmic artery occlusion showing presence of thread like vessels, generalized retinal whitening with absence of cherry red spot*

BIBLIOGRAPHY

1. Atebara NH, Brwon GC, Cater J, et al. Efficacy of anterior chamber paracentesis and carbogen in treating acute nonarteritic CRAO. Ophthalmology 1995;102:2029–35.
2. Beatty S, AuEong AK: Local intra-arterial fibrinolysis for acute occlusion of CRA: a meta analysis of published data Br. J. Ophthalmol 2000; 84:914–6.
3. Glacet-Bernard A, Bayani N, Chretien P, et al. APLA in retinal vascular occlusions. A prospective study of 75 patients. Arch. Ophthalmol 1994;112:790–5.
4. Greiner K, Hafner G, Dick B, et al. Retinal vascular occlusion and deficiencies in the protein C pathway. Am J Ophthalmol 1999;128:69–74.
5. Greven CM, Weaver RG, Owen J, Slusher MM. Protein S deficiency and B/L BRAO. Ophthalmology 1991;98:33–34.
6. Hayreh SS, Zimmerman B. Central retinal artery occlusion: visual outcome Am J Ophthalmol 2005;140:376–91.
7. Klein R, Klein BEK, Moss SE, et al. Retinal emboli and cardiovascular disease. The Beaver Dam Eye Study. Arch Ophthalmol 2003; 121:1446–51.
8. Kuritzky S. Nitroglycerin to treat acute loss of vision. N Engl J Med 1990;323:1428.
9. Pianka P, Almog Y, Man O, et al. Hyperhomocystinemia in patients with nonarteritic AION, CRAO, CRVO. Ophthalmology 2000;107:1588–92.
10. Ros MA, Magaragal LE, Uram M. Branch retinal-artery obstruction: a review of 201 eyes. Ann Ophthalmol 1989;21:103–4.
11. Rumelt S, Brown GC. Update on treatment of retinal arterial occlusions. Curr Opin Ophthalmol 2003;14:139–41.
12. Schumacher M, Schmitt D, Jurklies B, Gall C, Wanke I, Schmoor C, et al. Central retinal artery occlusion: local intra-arterial fibrinolysis versus conservative treatment, a multi-center randomized trial. Ophthalmology 2010;117:1367–75.
13. Sharma S. The systemic evaluation of acute retinal artery occlusion. Curr Opin Ophthalmol 1998:9:1–5.
14. Tayyanipour R, Pulido JS, Postel EA, et al. Arterial vascular occlusion associated with factor V Leiden gene mutation. Retina 1998; 18:376–7.

18 DIABETIC RETINOPATHY

Subina Narang, Panchmi Gupta

EPIDEMIOLOGY
- Introduction
- Incidence

PATHOGENESIS
- Signature pathologies
- Hematological and biochemical changes
- Angiogenic factors

CLINICAL PROFILE
Classification
- Nonproliferative diabetic retinopathy
- Proliferative diabetic retinopathy
- Clinically significant macular oedema
- OCT based classification of CSME

MANAGEMENT
- Indication of FFA and OCT
- Treatment of diabetic macular edema
- Treatment of proliferative diabetic retinopathy
- Management of cataract in presence of DR
- Follow-up

CLINICAL TRIALS IN DIABETIC RETINOPATHY
- Diabetic retinopathy study
- Early diabetic retinopathy study
- Diabetic control and complication trial

EPIDEMIOLOGY

INTRODUCTION

Diabetic retinopathy (DR) is one of the leading causes of blindness in people aged 20–64 years. Diabetes mellitus (DM), according to the current definition from the World Health Organization, is typically diagnosed if a patient has two readings of fasting plasma glucose ≥ 7.0 mmol/L (126 mg/dl) and glycosylated haemoglobin (HbA_{1c}) $\geq 6.5\%$. Its causes are not fully understood, but genetic background, obesity, and sedentary lifestyle all confer increased risk of developing diabetes. There is increase in number of diabetics due to changing life style.

INCIDENCE

- In the year 2000 the number of people with diabetes was 171 million and it is expected to be over 350 million by year 2030.
- The global population is projected to increase by 64% between the years 1995 and 2025 while the prevalence of diabetes mellitus is expected to rise by more than 120%.
- India is the world capital of diabetes with 31 million diabetics in the year 2000 and the figure is projected to be 79 million by the year 2030.
- Wisconsin epidemiological study (WES) of diabetic retinopathy strongly suggested association of the incidence of diabetic retinopathy to the duration of disease.
- At the time of diagnosis no patient of type 1 DM and 3–4% patients of type II diabetes mellitus have diabetic retinopathy.
- After 20 years of diabetes mellitus, 99% patients of type I and 60% patients of type II DM have diabetic retinopathy and of these 3.6% of type I (86% due to retinopathy) and 1.6% of type II DM (1/3rd due to diabetic retinopathy) are legally blind.
- The ten year incidence of clinically significant macular edema (CSME) is 20.1% in type I diabetes and 25.4% in older onset on insulin and 13.9% in older onset not on insulin.

PATHOGENESIS

DM is a microvascular disease and the primary targets are kidneys, nerves and retina. Other organs like heart, central nervous system and peripheral vessels may also be affected by macroangiopathic complications of diabetes.

Signature pathologies in DR are:
- Leukostasis
- Vascular leakage due to breakdown of blood retinal barrier
- Histologic changes.

Hematological and biochemical changes

The major factor is hyperglycemia which stimulates various hematological and biochemical changes, which include:
- Abnormality in serum and blood viscosity
- Increased platelet adhesiveness
- Increased erythrocyte aggregation
- Defective fibrinolysis
- Abnormal serum lipids
- Abnormal levels of growth hormone
- Increased intracameral adhesion molecule-1 (ICAM1) and neutrophilic expression of CD18 mediated leucocyte adhesions
- Upregulation of VEGF which further increases ICAM-1 level expression leading to increased leukostasis.

Hyperglycemia also leads to non-enzymatic glycation and **advanced glycation end products** leading to disruption of extracellular matrix protein interaction. There is also **increased polyol pathway** leading to accumulation of sorbitol and galactilol which in turn leads to basement membrane thickening. Due to all the above factors there are **structural alterations** like pericyte degeneration, basement membrane thickening, endothelial damage, leucocyte mediated retinal cell apoptosis (special type of cell death in which cell plays active role in its own death-cell suicide), capillary acellularity (basement membrane tubes devoid of any visible endothelial cells or pericytes) and ultimately decompensation leading to leakage.

Characterisation of molecular and cellular processes involved in the vascular growth and hyperpermeability has lead to recognition of angiogenic growth factor and vascular permeability factor which play pivotal role in microvascular complications of diabetic retinopathy. There are various proangiogenic factors and in healthy adult equilibrium is kept under control by antiangiogenic factors.

Proangiogenic factors are VEGF, platelet derived growth factor (PDGF), hepatocyte growth factor (HGF), erythropoietin, leptin, angiogenin, insulin growth factor 1 and 2, ICAM1, onco feto fibronectin endothelin 1, angiopoietin 1, angiotenin 2, angiotensin convertin enzyme, C4 factor, TNF-α, TNF-β.

Anti-angiogenic factors are endostatin, angiostatin, pigment epithelial derived factor (PEDF), thrombospondin 1, platelet factor 4.

The above factors are found in high levels in vitreous and regulate the neovessel growth and fibrosis. The high glucose mediated oxidative stress has effect on VEGF expression and action. There is also activation of protein kinase C and cytokines which leads to increase in angiogenic factors leading to neovascularisation and retinal edema.

Diabetic retina also has oxidative stress leading to increased oxygen free radicals which increases apoptosis of retinal capillary cells. There is **failure of autoregulation** of retinal circulation. Hyperglycemia leads to release of factors leading to vasodilatation. Prolonged vasodilatation further leads to pericyte loss, basement membrane thickening and endothelial cell proliferation. Hyperperfusion leads to stress damage of vessel wall adding to vicious cycle of vasodilatation which leads to macular edema by Starling forces.

To understand retinal neovascularisation we must understand that there is astrocyte precursor meshwork which exists from disc to periphery and forms template for glial fibers of new vessels. The precursors of astrocytes secrete VEGF along with the neovessel growth with aid of PDGF synthesized by retinal ganglion cells. With VEGF and angiopoietin-2 neovessels are formed.

Thus, in diabetic retinopathy changes may result from both the direct effect of hyperglycemia, advanced glycation end-products, and hyperlipidemia on vascular endothelial cells and the indirect effect of these metabolites

through induction of growth factors and these alter the tight junction complexes leading to increased endothelial permeability and with angiopoietin-2 neovessels are formed.

CLINICAL PROFILE

CLASSIFICATION OF DIABETIC RETINOPATHY

Diabetic retinopathy is classified as nonproliferative, which is early stage, and proliferative, which is advanced stage of diabetic retinopathy. Nonproliferative diabetic retinopathy (NPDR) could further be classified as mild, moderate and severe NPDR. The classical finding seen in NPDR is presence of microaneurysms which are outpouchings of retinal capillaries in inner nuclear layer (INL) seen as red dots. Microaneurysms more than 30 μm are visualized ophthalmoscopically. These are the first findings of diabetic retinopathy. We also see areas of capillary nonperfusion (CNP) which are more marked on fundus fluorescein angiography (FFA). 70% of microaneurysms disappear in first 3 months but new ones appear. If the control is good there will be overall decrease in microaneurysms. So microaneurysms are one of the ways to detect progression of diabetic retinopathy.

The other clinical findings in NPDR include hard exudates, soft exudates (cotton wool spots), intraretinal microvascular anomalies (IRMAs), dot blot hemorrhages, superficial hemorrhages and macular edema. Hard exudates are extracellular lipid deposition in outer plexiform layer (OPL). These are absorbed over months to years. Nerve fiber layer (NFL) infarcts are visible as soft exudates due to axoplasmic flow stasis. These appear on FFA as areas of capillary nonperfusion (CNP) surrounded by microaneurysms. These take 3–17 months to resolve. Intraretinal microvascular anomalies (IRMAs) are dilated capillary vascular segments in areas of capillary nonperfusion which serve as shunt vessels, do not leak as much as neovascularisation on FFA. These are areas of CNP and are suggestive of collateral channels due to hypoxia.

Arteriolar abnormal dilatation and beading or loop formation of retinal vessels also occurs suggesting progression of disease. Superficial

and dot blot hemorrhages are seen in NFL, OPL, INL. Macular edema is the most common cause of moderate visual loss in diabetics. Retinal edema appears as cystoid spaces or spongiform thickness, etc (discussed later).

Diabetic retinopathy can be clinically staged as:

NONPROLIFERATIVE DIABETIC RETINOPATHY

Nonproliferative diabetic retinopathy can be classified as (Fig. 18.1A to C):

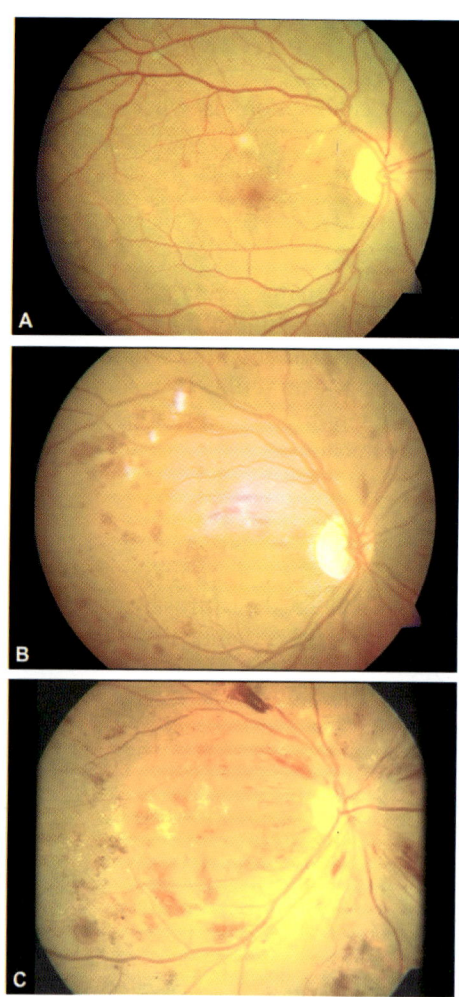

Fig. 18.1 *(A) Fundus photograph showing microaneurysms, hard exudates consistent with mild NPDR; (B) Fundus photograph showing microaneurysms, hard exudates, soft exudates, superficial and deep hemorrhages consistent with moderate NPDR; and (C) Fundus photograph showing hemorrhages in all 4 quadrants, hard exudates and soft exudates, superficial and deep hemorrhages and IRMA consistent with severe NPDR*

- *Mild NPDR:* Few microaneurysms
- *Moderate NPDR:* Few microaneurysms and hemorrhages in all quadrants, cotton wool spots and venous changes may also be seen
- *Severe NPDR:* 4 quadrants retinal hemorrhages
  - 2 quadrants venous beading
  - 1 quadrant IRMA
- *Very severe NPDR:* Any 2 or more of the above

PROLIFERATIVE DIABETIC RETINOPATHY

- High risk characters: Neovascularisation (NVD) >1/4-1/3 (DA) (Fig. 18.2)
  - NVD with preretinal bleed/vitreous hemorrhage
  - Neovascularisation elsewhere (NVE) >1/2 DA with preretinal bleed/vitreous hemorrhage.

CLINICALLY SIGNIFICANT MACULAR EDEMA
(Fig. 18.3A to C)

- Thickening of the retina at or within 500 microns of the center of the macula
- Hard exudates at or within 500 microns of the center of the macula, if associated with thickening of the adjacent retina
- Retinal thickening at least one disc area or larger, with any part within 1 disc diameter of the macular center.

This is the most common cause of moderate visual loss in diabetic retinopathy.

CSME can be focal or diffuse with or without hard exudates. FFA demonstrates break down of blood retinal barrier (BRB) and further

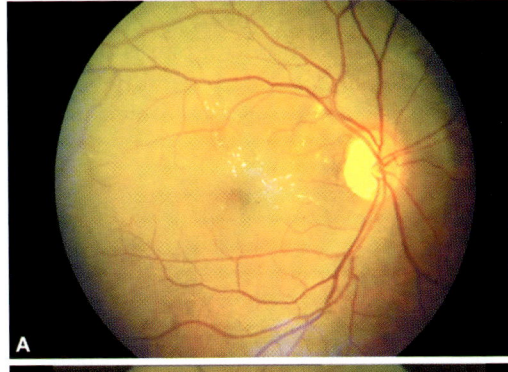

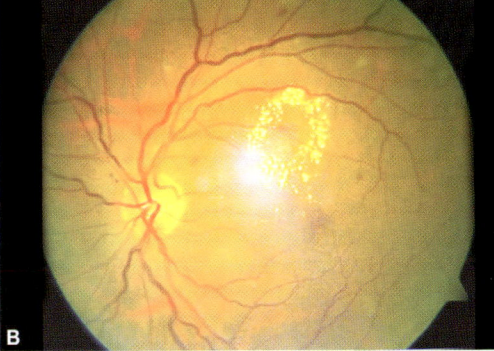

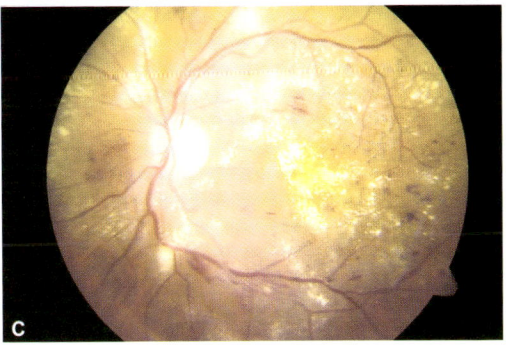

Fig. 18.3 *Fundus photograph of CSME (A) showing hard exudates and thickening involving the center of macula; (B) showing hard exudates in center with adjacent thickening; and (C) showing retinal thickening more than 1 DD a part of which is within 1 DD from center*

identifies treatable lesions. In **focal CSME** microaneurysms are the main leaking lesions. It clinically appears as focal areas of macular thickening surrounded by ring of hard exudates which are plasma lipoproteins that leak from microaneurysms. In **diffuse macular edema** FFA shows leakage from widespread capillary abnormalities, dilated capillary bed and there are areas of capillary nonperfusion (Fig. 18.4). Clinically, it may not be associated with hard

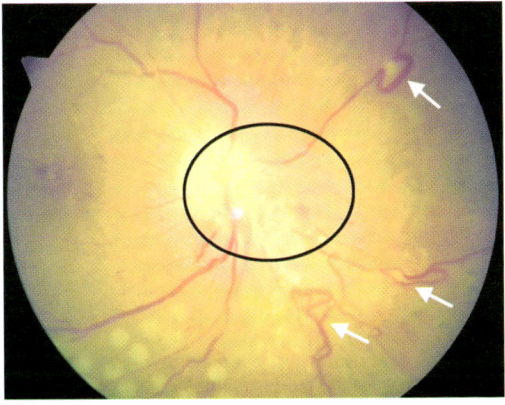

Fig.18.2 *Fundus picture showing NVD 1/3rd DD nasally (circle), venous loops (arrows) consistent with PDR*

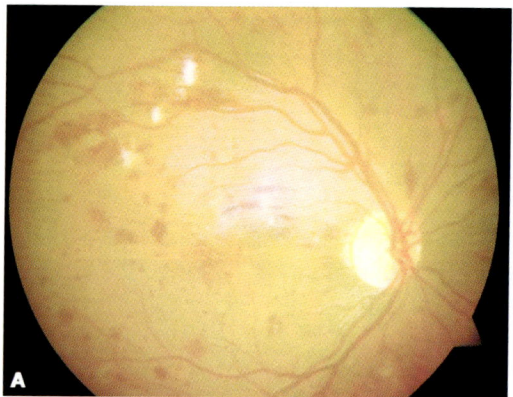

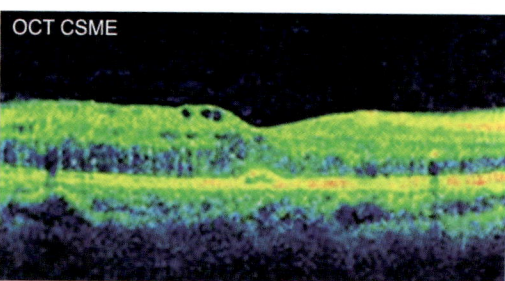

Fig. 18.5 *OCT of a diabetic patient showing clinically significant macular edema—fluid accumulation in outer plexiform layer and cystic spaces in inner retinal layers*

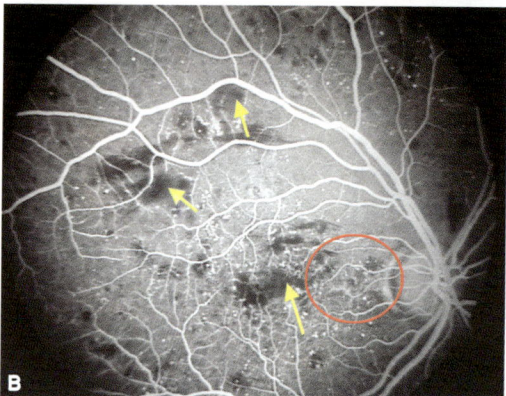

Fig. 18.4 **(A)** *Fundus photograph showing CSME; and* **(B)** *Fluorescein angiogram of the same patient showing treatable lesions hyperfluorescent dots—microaneurysms, dilated capillary bed (circle), and capillary nonperfusion areas (arrows)*

exudates as diffuse break down of inner BRB allows passage of smaller molecules and not lipoproteins.

Optical Coherence Tomography based Classification of DME

The macular thickening can be quantified on Optical Coherence Tomography (OCT) and the OCT picture helps us to decide treatment protocol for the patient (Fig. 18.5).

Five distinct forms of CSME can be appreciated on optical coherence tomography (OCT) (Fig. 18.6A to E).

1. *Sponge-like retina* due to diffuse leakage, the macular edema is between outer plexiform layer (OPL) and outer nuclear layer (ONL).

2. *Cystoid macular edema.* The edematous retina has cystic spaces that are separated by hyper

reflective membrane like structure. At first it involves ONL and OPL and then it eventually involves the entire retina.

3. *Serous retinal detachment.* Hyporeflective space under neurosensory retina.

4. *Tractional macular edema.* The foveovitreal traction is clearly evident on OCT and such macula requires surgical treatment to release this traction.

5. *Taut posterior hyaloid membrane (TPHM).* This is easily identified on OCT as hyperreflective membrane on retinal surface and needs surgical treatment. This often leads to recalcitrant diabetic macular edema.

Diabetic papillopathy (Fig. 18.7) is another rare sight threatening complication of diabetic retinopathy. It is usually seen in old patients but may be seen in either form of diabetes mellitus. Nonproliferative or proliferative diabetic retinopathy as well as macular edema may also be associated with this disorder. It is a self-limiting, sometimes bilateral disease. It is characterized by optic disc swelling caused by axonal edema and vascular leakage. Occasionally, it may be accompanied by intraretinal hemorrhages and hard exudates. Diabetic papillopathy tends to be mild and is usually associated with good visual prognosis; however, there are some cases in which permanent visual impairment can develop. The pathogenesis is still not clear and it has been associated with a small cup/disc ratio and rapid reduction in glycemia. Local injections of corticosteroids as well as bevacizumab (Avastin), may be tried in these cases.

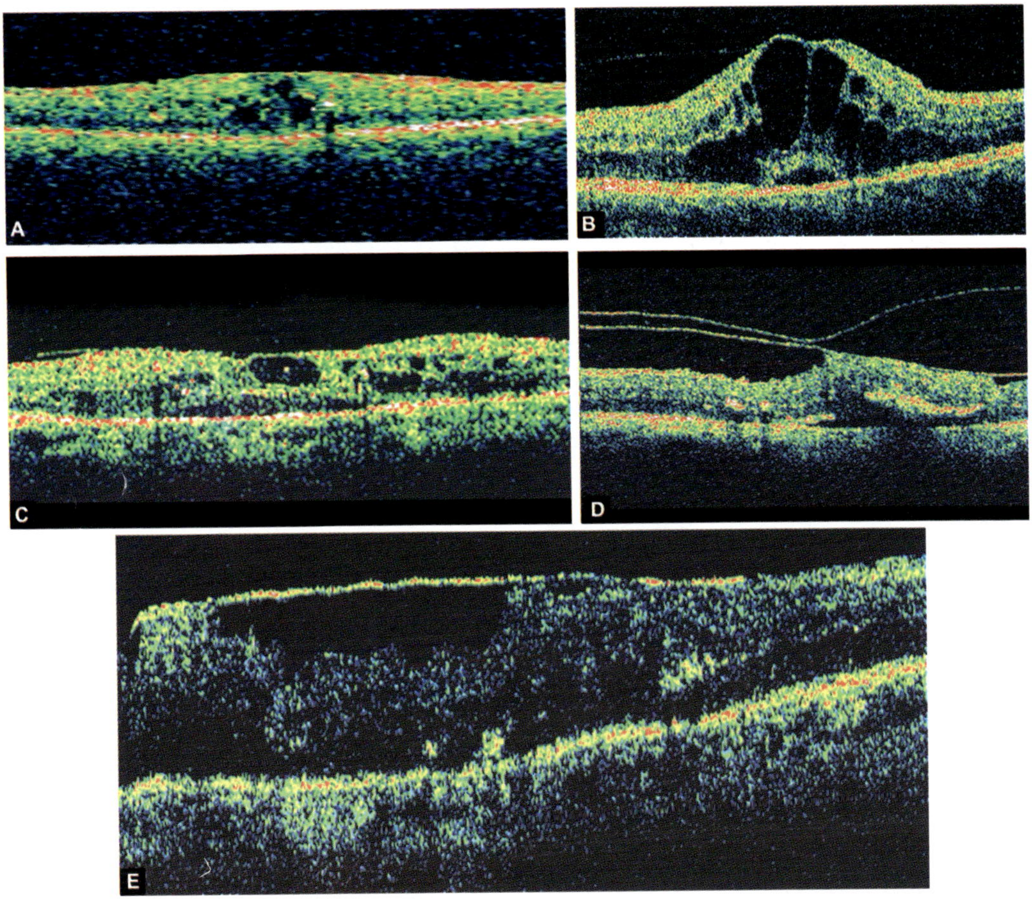

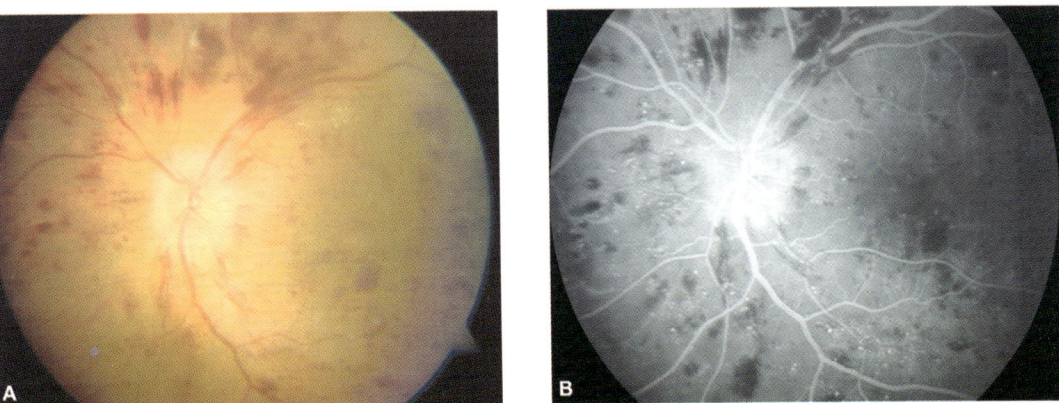

Fig. 18.6 *(A)* *Horizontal OCT scan of CSME patient showing increased foveal thickness, loss of foveal contour, spongiform pattern of retinal thickening with submacular detachment;* *(B)* *Cystoid macular edema. The edematous retina has cystic spaces that are separated by hyper reflective membrane like structure. At first it involves ONL and OPL and then it eventually involves the entire retina;* *(C)* *Horizontal OCTscan shows serous retinal detachment: hyporeflective space under neurosensory retina;* *(D)* *Vertical OCTscan shows taut posterior hyaloid membrane (TPHM) and CSME; and* *(E)* *Horizontal OCT scan of a patient with recalcitrant macular edema showing traction on macula*

Fig. 18.7 *(A)* *Fundus photograph of left eye showing severe NPDR with disc edema consistent with diabetic papillopathy; and* *(B)* *FFA shows leakage in late frames*

MANAGEMENT

The treatment of diabetic retinopathy is mainly laser. With the better understanding of pathogenesis of diabetic retinopathy the trends are shifting to pharmacotherapy and surgery in recent years. We must undertake a multidisciplinary approach in all patients with diabetes for treatment of CSME and PDR. OCT and FFA play an important role in treatment of DR.

INDICATION OF FLUORESCEIN ANGIOGRAPHY AND OCT

Indications of FFA have decreased over a period of time:
- If diffuse DME is present, we use the angiogram to identify sources of perimacular leakage and non-perfusion, to guide focal and grid laser
- To assess signs of likely macular ischemia (Fig. 18.8A and B)
- To assess amount of ischemia in severe NPDR and subtle NVE
- In selected patients with PDR, or after PRP therapy for PDR to assess response.
- Before retreatment in CSME
- In advanced cases with featureless retina, FFA could identify clinically in apparent vascularisation

The presence of cystoid macular edema and ischaemic macula are poor prognosticators of the disease.

OCT helps us to identify the type of CSME and helps in treatment planning. Surgical treatment is the only treatment for CSME with TPHM/traction. It also defines the planes which guide the surgical intervention in DR. OCT is an important part of DR workup before planning treatment.

TREATMENT OF DIABETIC MACULAR EDEMA

The treatment of CSME is guided by FFA and OCT. Clinically significant macular edema is treatable macular edema. Before treating CSME we must achieve optimal glycaemic control (target HbA_{1c} levels 7.0% or lower) and to adequately manage blood pressure (target systolic blood pressure less than 130 mm Hg) and serum lipids (target LDL cholesterol of less

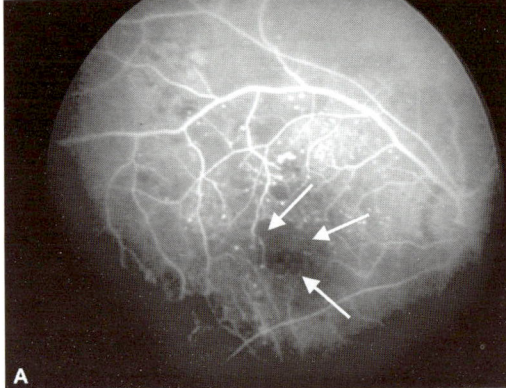
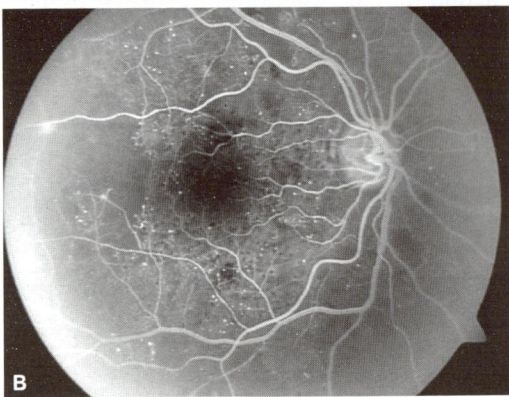

Fig. 18.8 *(A)* Fundus fluorescein angiography arteriovenous phase shows hypofluorescence due to capillary non-perfusion and *(B)* Fundus fluorescein angiography shows ischemic macula as FAZ is irregular and enlarged

than 2.5 mmol/L and a target triglycerides of less than 2.0 mmol/L) (Fig. 18.9A and B). The kidney status also needs to be assessed by 24 hour urinary proteins, blood urea, serum creatinine. The life style modification is required. Sedentary life style must be replaced by exercise, better controlled blood sugar, blood pressure, blood lipids, body mass index and smoking cessation is required.

The aim is to achieve:
- Target HbA_{1c} levels 7.0% or lower
- Target systolic blood pressure less than 130 mmHg
- Serum lipids (target LDL cholesterol of less than 2.5 mmol/L and a target triglycerides of less than 2.0 mmol/L).

Dyslipidemia may increase DR risk, particularly macular hard exudate deposition and

CSME. Consider lowering blood lipids by the use of statins to reduce DME progression or in patients with extensive hard exudates (Fig. 18.9A and B). Aspirin is safe to use in the presence of DR, at any severity level.

Randomised controlled trials, including the Early treatment of diabetic retinopathy study (ETDRS) group, established the role of focal or grid laser photocoagulation which reduces the risk of moderate vision loss (doubling of the visual angle) from CSME by at least 50% (Fig. 18.10A and B). However, CSME with TPHM or traction on OCT cannot be managed by laser. These two types of CSME are candidates for surgical treatment. With laser we treat treatable lesions which are microaneurysms, dilated capillary bed, areas of non- perfusion.

Focal laser treatment using 100 μm laser burns is applied to areas of focal leakage in focal CSME (i.e. leaking microaneurysms) sparing the central 500 μm. The threshold laser power for any retina is determined in nasal retina to get just visible burns and then the same power burns are safely applied in macular region.

Grid laser photocoagulation, using 100 μm threshold burns, is applied in a grid pattern less than one burn width apart to areas of capillary dilatation leading to diffuse leak and non-perfusion around the macula (Fig.18.11). Although treatment is ideally guided by fluorescein angiography, this may not be needed for first time treatment of focal DME but this is always required for supplement treatments to evaluate the area not treated with previous laser

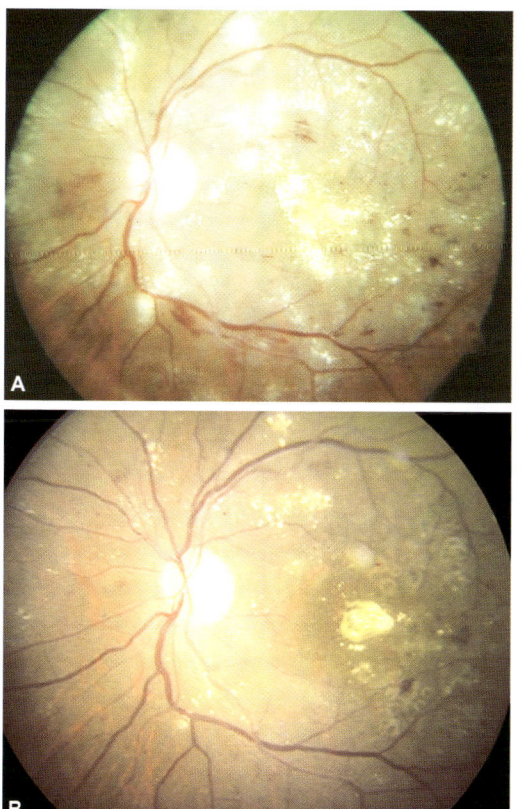

Fig. 18.9 *(A)* Fundus picture at initial visit shows massive hard exudates and thickening in center CSME. The patient was started on atorvastatin and strict metabolic control; and *(B)* There was subsequent decrease in hard exudates in subsequent 6 months

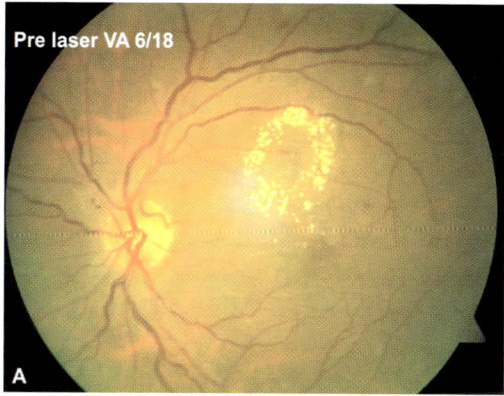

Pre laser VA 6/18

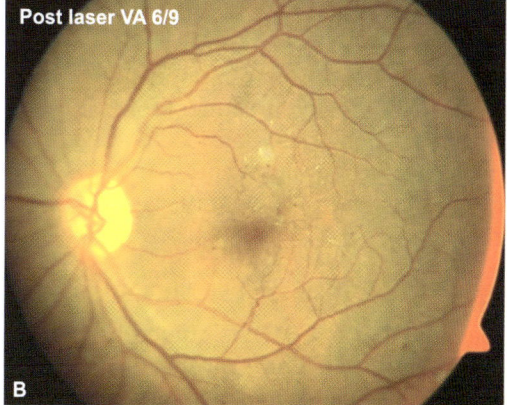

Post laser VA 6/9

Fig. 18.10 *(A)* Fundus picture showing CSME in left eye; and *(B)* Fundus picture of the same patient showing resolution of CSME after modified grid laser treatment at 6 months

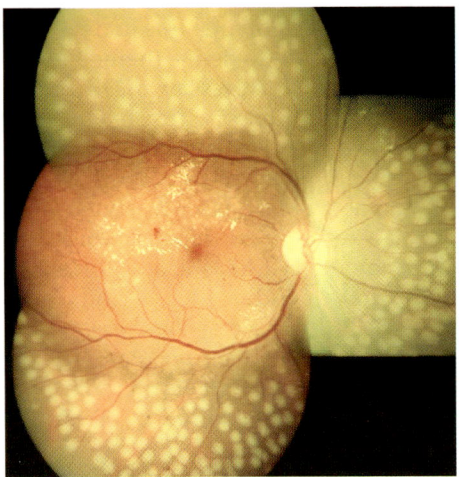

Fig. 18.11 *Modified grid laser treatment and PRP in a case of PDR with CSME*

and responsible for nonresolution of macular edema. The sparing of papillomacular bundle is not required. If the CSME does not resolve then supplement laser may be required at 3–4 months after first laser treatment. In supplement treatment, we hit the areas not treated during primary treatment and we can go up to 300 µm from center. Laser treatment is associated with minor loss in visual fields as paracentral scotoma, transient increase in macular edema and decreased vision, rarely choroidal neovascularisation, subretinal fibrosis (in case of hard exudates in center), photocoagulation scar expansion, inadvertent foveolar burns. The treatment is unlikely to be beneficial in the presence of significant macular ischmia.

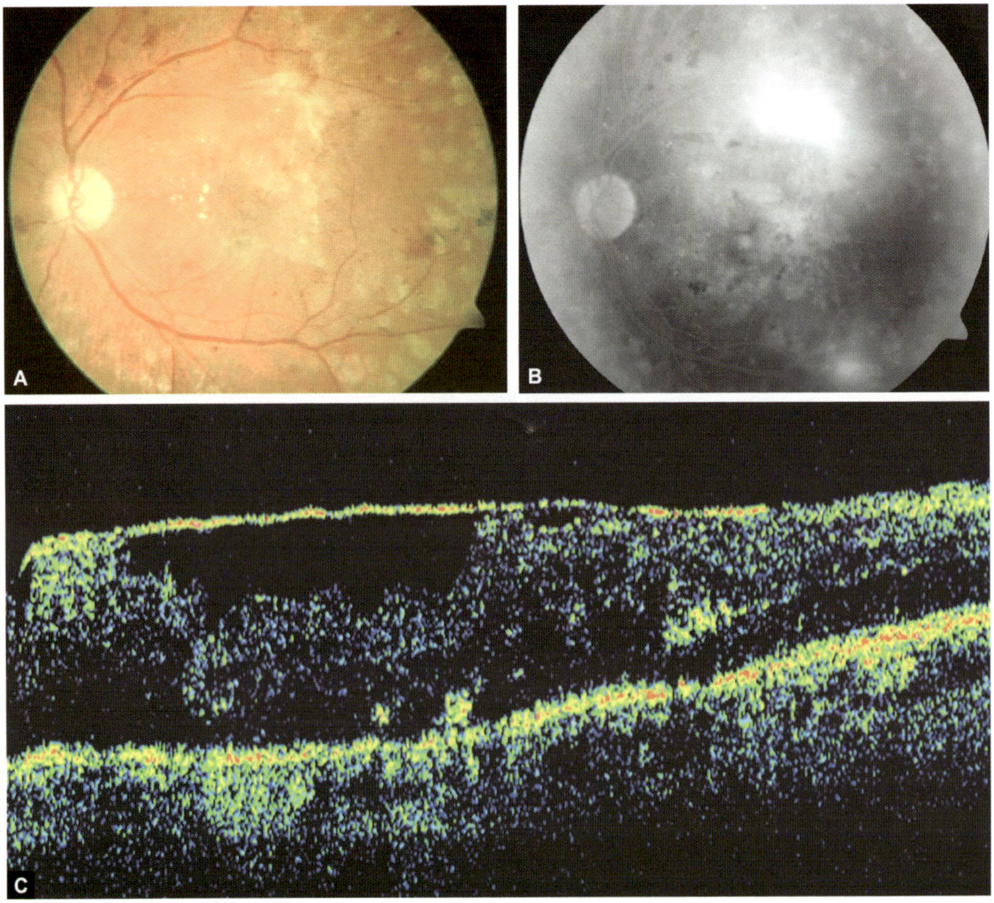

Fig. 18.12 *(A) Fundus picture of a metabolically stable NIDDM patient shows treated PDR and recalcitrant macular edema; (B) FFA shows diffuse leakage in macular area despite laser treatment; and (C) OCT vertical scan of the same patient shows traction on the macula. The patient is a candidate for PPV for posterior hyaloids removal*

Recalcitrant CSME and Pharmacotherapy

Recalcitrant macular edema (Fig. 18.12A to C) is one of the most important causes for significant visual loss in diabetic patients. In these patients the diabetic status is complicated by the presence of other systemic conditions such as hypertension, hyperlipidemias, and nephropathy. Eyes with gross retinal thickening and presence of plaques of hard exudates will respond poorly to laser photocoagulation. Presence of a thickened taut posterior hyaloid membrane exerting traction on the macula resulting in shallow macular detachment could be another cause for recalcitrant macular edema in a diabetic. Treatment modalities include laser photocoagulation, intravitreal steroid injection, pars plana vitrectomy with or without internal limiting membrane peeling or a combination of these. Laser photocoagulation targets vascular pathology and is associated with significant adverse effects due to destruction of neural tissue. VEGF plays pivotal role in development of DR, so it is valid to define therapeutic target that controls VEGF expression in DR. For CSME with serous neurosensory detachment on OCT, pharmacotherapy (anti VEGF intravitreal injections of pegaptanib, bevacizumab, ranibizumab) before laser treatment may be beneficial. Intravitreal depot steroid therapy (triamcinolone, IVTA) is useful for extensive macular hard exudate deposition, or as an adjunct to PRP. The major adverse effects of steroids are elevated intraocular pressure or posterior subcapsular cataract. The repeat injections are often required in all anti-VEGF drugs (Fig. 18.13A to C).

Recent clinical trials support anti-VEGF therapy for diffuse diabetic macular edema (DDME) which lead to significant improvement over laser therapy. Thus of now focal laser therapy is a Gold standard treatment for focal CSME while anti-VEGF drugs may have the same role in center involving DDME.

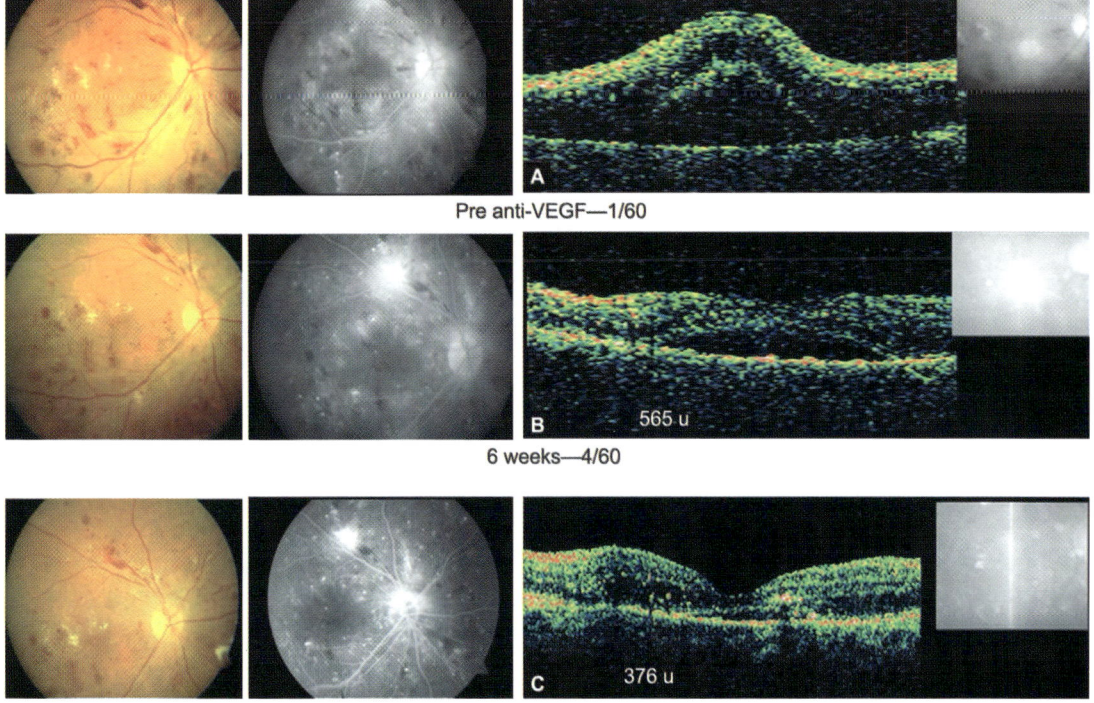

Pre anti-VEGF—1/60

565 u

6 weeks—4/60

376 u

3 months—6/60

Fig. 18.13 *(A) Fundus picture showing diffuse CSME and OCT horizontal scan shows central macular thickness of more than 500 um; (B) Same patient after single injection bevacizumab showing decrease in foveal thickness and persistence of submacular detachment; and (C) After 3 months, patient shows decrease of macular edema and restoration of foveal contour*

TREATMENT OF PROLIFERATIVE DIABETIC RETINOPATHY

PDR with HRC need urgent laser treatment in the form of panretinal photocoagulation where we do not treat the area showing traction as laser would further aggravate traction. PRP is performed using 200 to 500 μm burns placed approximately one-half burn width apart, from the posterior fundus to the equator (Fig. 18.11).

For high-risk PDR, PRP should be performed as soon as possible and usually is completed in 3 sittings. Patients should be regularly reviewed after laser treatment is completed. If high risk characteristics fail to regress or if they re-develop, supplemental laser treatment is needed at 6 weeks. Laser in PDR could be associated with reduction in more than or equal to one line in 11% patients and visual fields in 5%.

If PDR has already bled then perform laser in relatively clear area and supplement with more laser burns as the hemorrhage clears. Anti-VEGF drugs can be given to prevent rebleed till the time PRP is complete. Anti- VEGF drugs must be given with caution in presence of traction as this could be aggravated with anti-VEGF.

PDR and CSME

For eyes with both PDR and CSME, but without high-risk PDR, PRP should be delayed until focal or grid macular laser treatment is completed. However, for eyes with high-risk PDR and focal CSME, the first sitting of PRP can be performed in nasal quadrant along with focal/grid laser treatment. There is transient increase in CSME maximum retinal thickness after PRP (Fig. 18.11). Indiffuse CSME, leaser (PRP) may be combined with antiVEGF during the 1st sitting of laser.

Vitrectomy in PDR

The Diabetic Retinopathy Vitrectomy Study (DRVS) was the landmark randomized controlled trial to evaluate indications and timing of pars plana vitrectomy for the management of advanced diabetic retinopathy (DR). Complete as much PRP as possible before considering vitrectomy surgery, in order to minimise postoperative complications. The indications and rationale for vitrectomy established by the DRVS still guide therapy, but the thresholds for performing surgery are now lower, due to improved surgical results. Early vitrectomy (within 3 months) for treatment of vitreous hemorrhage secondary to DR was highly cost-effective in a cost-utility analysis using DRVS results. The benefits of early vitrectomy for non-resolving severe vitreous hemorrhage were greater for patients with type 1 diabetes mellitus and lower for type 2 diabetes mellitus.

Indications of vitrectomy

Urgent pars plana vitrectomy (within three months) should be considered for:

- Type 1 diabetes with severe vitreous hemorrhage
- In eyes considered to have very severe PDR;
- Severe PDR, not responding to aggressive, extensive PRP
- To relieve macular or other retinal traction in advanced PDR cases, in an attempt to salvage some vision (Fig. 18.14)
- Selected cases with diffuse, severe DME not responsive to other therapies, particularly if

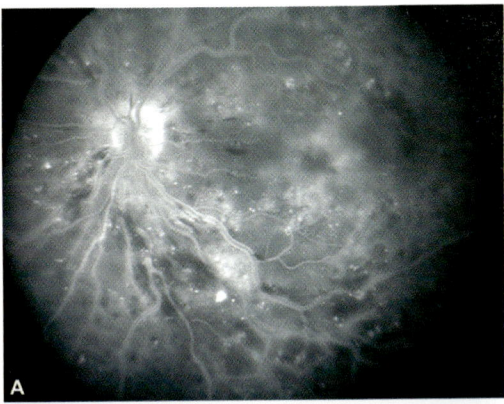

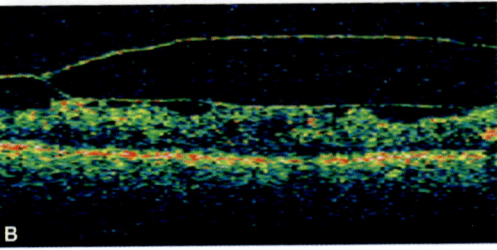

Fig. 18.14 *(A) Late arteriovenous phase FFA of recalcitrant macular edema; and (B) OCT scan of the same patient showing TPHM and vitreoschisis*

vitreomacular traction is present (Fig. 18.14A and B).

OCT has been beneficial in diagnosing the many vitreoretinal interphase changes which play major role in determining PPV in cases that were previously undiagnosed on clinical examination. Apart from diagnosing tractional forces, OCT also helps in guiding the surgery in these cases (Figs 18.4 and 18.5). The trends are shifting to combined cataract surgery with vitrectomy which results in earlier visual rehabilitation by avoiding the need for later cataract surgery. Complications from vitrectomy include recurrent vitreous hemorrhage, glaucoma, endophthalmitis, retinal detachment, rubeosis, and premature cataract. Anti-VEGF drugs before vitrectomy lowers incidence of bleed during surgery and increases the ease during surgery.

MANAGEMENT OF CATARACT IN PRESENCE OF DIABETIC RETINOPATHY

Cataract surgery may be needed to adequately assess need for laser and to permit laser treatment to be completed. Cataract surgery may also lead to substantial visual improvements in diabetic patients. The visual outcome after cataract surgery in people with diabetes depends on the severity of pre-operative DR and presence of DME. Asymmetric retinopathy progression can occur in the operated eye after cataract surgery. The presence of preoperative DME and active PDR are strong predictors of a poor visual result. DME needs to be treated before operating the patient for cataract surgery. Although modern cataract surgical techniques show consistently improved visual outcomes in diabetic patients, a systematic review of case series and clinical trials consistently demonstrated worse visual results from cataract surgery in persons with than without DR. The progression of DR after cataract surgery is correlated with diabetic control at the time of surgery and the presence of Type 2 DM and PDR at baseline. Adequate laser treatment of significant DR should be completed before cataract surgery. Where possible, adequate laser treatment of significant DR (particularly DME) should be performed before

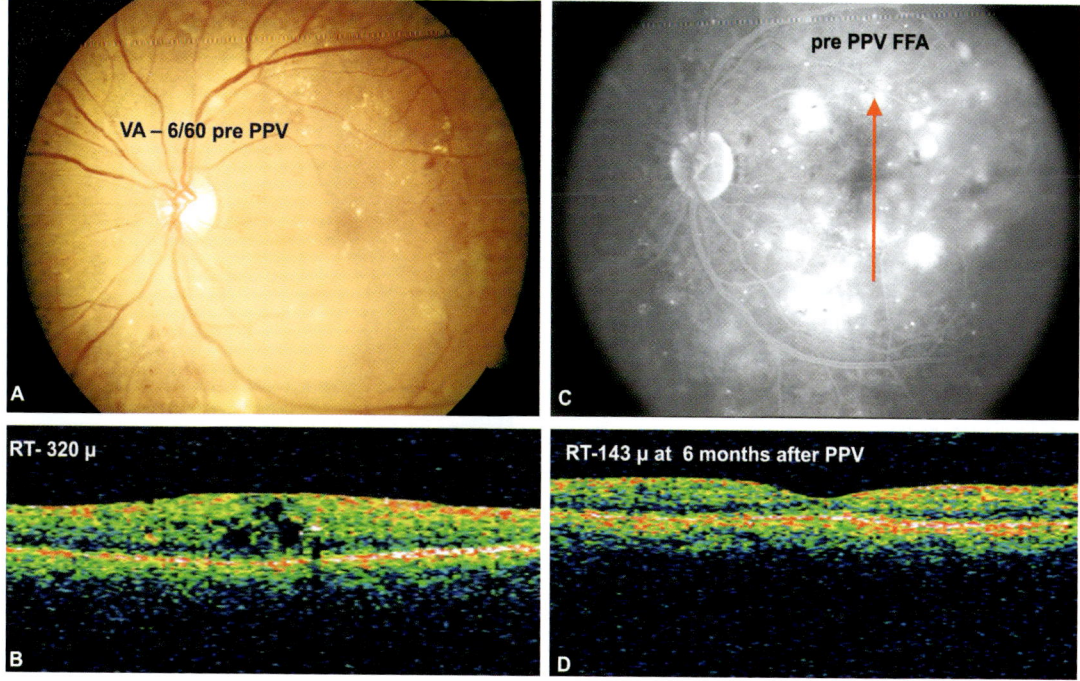

Fig. 18.15 *(A and C) Fundus picture of late phase FFA shows recalcitrant CSME and (B) OCTscan shows TPHM; (D) OCT scan of the same patient 6 months after PPV showing resolution of macular edema and restoration of foveal contour*

cataract surgery. Cataract surgery should be delayed until DR and DME signs are stabilised. Once DR is stable, consider cataract surgery to improve vision in diabetic patients. If cataract is moderate to advanced and preoperative laser not possible, cataract surgery may be done along with intravitreal anti-VEGF or steroids at the time of surgery.

FOLLOW-UP

DR increases with the duration of the disease thus timely follow-up is mandatory to preserve vision. The first examination in Type 1 DM is recommended after 5 years of diagnosis and in Type 2 DR is recommended immediately at the diagnosis. Thereafter in patients with no retinopathy one yearly follow-up is required. Risk of NPDR progression to PDR is severity dependent. Severe NPDR has 15% chance to progress to high-risk PDR. Very severe NPDR has 45% chance to develop high-risk PDR in 1 year. Complications of PDR can result in severe visual loss (SVL) if left untreated. The neovessels can bleed and progressive fibrovascular

proliferation can lead to tractional retinal detachment or combined retinal detachment if we have progressive thinning of retina and break formation along with TRD. The follow-up for moderate to severe NPDR is 6 monthly and for PDR is 3 monthly. After CSME treatment, patients needs to be followed up after 3–4 months for supplement treatment and for PDR regular follow-up 6 weekly may be done for any supplement treatment if required.

CLINICAL TRIALS IN DIABETIC RETINOPATHY

Various clinical trials in diabetic retinopathy are summarized in Table 18.1.

Common clinical trials in diabetic retinopathy include:
- Diabetic retinopathy study (DRS),
- Early treatment diabetic retinopathy study (ETDRS),
- Diabetes contrl and complications trial (DCCT).

Table 18.1 Summary of the various clinical trials in diabetic retinopathy

Study	No. of patient	Aim and year	Severity diabetic retinopathy	Intervention	Outcome	Clinical implication	Follow-up
Diabetic retinopathy study	1747	To evaluate photocoagulation for PDR 1971–1977	Severe NPDR (bilateral) or PDR (± DME)	Peripheral PRP ± Focal laser vs. observation	PRP ↓ risk of SVL by 52% at 2 years. 14% treated vs 33% of deferred treatment had SVLRR 0.42 (0.34–0.53) Eyes with "high risk" features had most benefit (57% ↓ risk SVL) **Treat if "high risk" PDR present**	Decreased VA and constriction of peripheral visual field in some eyes. Xenon effect was greater than Argon but has harmful side effects too. **Complete regression of NV in 30%, partial regression in 25% 12 months post PRP**	5 years
Early treatment Diabetic retinopathy study (ETDRS)	3711	1. When in the course of DR is it most effective to initiate PRP? 2. Is laser effective in the TX of macular edema? 3. Is ASA TX effective in altering the course of DR? 1979–1985	1. Mild to severe NPDR or early PDR (± DME in both eyes) 2. For DME with NPDR focal argon laser vs observation	One eye of each patient assigned to early PRP ± focal vs. deferral of treatment.	↓ risk of SVL or vitrectomy 4% with early photocoagulation vs 6% in deferred group. ⇓ risk of moderate visual loss by 50% over 5 years in treated group. Moderate visual gain inc from 5 to 17% in treated eyes with CSME	PRP is not indicated for mild to moderate NPDR but should be considered as retinopathy approaches the high risk stage. Grid/ focal laser treatment of treatable lesions indicated for clinically significant macular edema	5 years
Diabetes control and complications trial (DCCT)	1441	To compare intensive sugar control with conventional diabetes therapy on development and progression	IDDM patients 1. Primary intervention → no DR 2. Secondary intervention → mild to	Conventional TX consisted of 1 to 2 injections of insulin. Intensive TX consisted of three or more injections or insulin pump	Strict control of blood sugar can lead to early worsening of retinopathy. Primary intervention: Until 36 months no difference. >36 months at least **50% reduction**	For each 10% decrease in the hemoglobin A_{1c} there was a 39% decrease in the long-term risk of progression of retinopathy over the range of hemoglobin A_{1c} values. In the DCCT	6.5 years

Contd.

Table 18.1 Summary of the various clinical trials in diabetic retinopathy (Contd.)

Study	No. of patients	Aim and year	Severity diabetic retinopathy	Intervention	Outcome	Clinical implication	Follow-up
		of diabetic retinopathy	moderate DR		Mean 6 years 76% reduction of DR. Secondary intervention: >36 months 54% reduction. There was overall 47% reduction in severe DR.	there was a three-fold increase in severe hypoglycemic events and excess weight gain among patients using intensive treatment regimens	
Epidemiology of diabetes interventions and complications (EDIC) trial	95% patients of DCCT 1294–1335	-do-	-do-	Continued follow-up of patients enrolled in DCCT trial	Further progression of diabetic retinopathy during the first 4 years of the EDIC study was 66 to 77% less in the former intensive treatment group than in the former conventional treatment group. The benefit persisted even at 7 years. This benefit included an effect on severe diabetic retinopathy, including severe NPDR, PDR, CSME, and the need for focal/grid or panretinal laser photocoagulation	The change in hemoglobin A_{1c} accelerate or retard progression of diabetic retinopathy in the former intensive treatment group. Thus, it takes time for improvements in control to negate the long-lasting effects of prior prolonged hyperglycemia, and once the biological effects of prolonged improved control are manifest, the benefits are long-lasting. Furthermore, the total glycemic exposure of the patient (i.e., degree and duration) determines the degree of retinopathy observed at any one time	7 years
United Kingdom prospective diabetes study (UKPDS)	1148	Hypertension (mean BP of 160/94 mmHg) 1998	Type 2 diabetes with hypertension	Tight BP control (<150/85 mm Hg) vs less tight BP control (<180/105 mm Hg)	It ↓ risk of progression DR (≥2 ETDRS steps) by 34% and ↓ risk VA loss 3 ETDRS lines by 47%. It also ↓ risk of laser photocoagulation by 35%	Tight BP control is recommended in diabetics	8 years

Contd.

Table 18.1 *Summary of the various clinical trials in diabetic retinopathy (Contd.)*

Study	No of patient	Aim and year	Severity diabetic retinopathy	Intervention	Outcome	Clinical implication	Follow-up
Appropriate blood pressure control in diabetes trial (ABCD)	480	Hypertensive type 2 DM (mean baseline DBP >90 mm Hg) and normotensive (<140/90) type 2 DM 1996	Type 2 DM	Intensive BP control (aiming for a DBP of 75 and in normotensive 10 mm below mean DBP) vs moderate control (DBP 80–89 mmHg)	No difference in progression of DR between intensive therapy (mean BP 132/78) and CT (mean BP 138/86). In normotensives mean BP of 128/75 mm Hg ↓ progression of DR compared to conventional treatment (mean BP 137/81 mmHg)	No difference in progression of DR with nisoldipine vs enalapril	5 years
The EURODIAB Controlled Trial of Lisinopril in Insulin-dependent Diabetes Mellitus (EUCLID)	325	Normotensive and normoalbuminuric type 1 DM2009	Normotensive and normo-albuminuric type 1 DM	Lisinopril	Lisinopril ↓ progression DR (2 ETDRS steps) by 50% and ↓ progression to PDR by 80%	Lisinopril group had lower HbA$_{1c}$ levels	2 years
The diabetic retinopathy vitrectomy study (DRVS)	616	Does early vitrectomy improve long term visual outcome 1983–87	Recent severe diabetic vitreous haemorrhage reducing VA ≤5/200 at least 1 month	Early vitrectomy vs deferral of vitrectomy for 1 year with early surgery (25% vs	Early surgery ↑ recovery of VA ≥10/20 (25% vs 15% deferred group) Trend for more frequent loss of LP 19%). Greatest benefit ↑ VA ≥10/20 in type 1 DM with more severe PDR (36% vs. 12% deferred group) and proportion losing LP was similar (28% vs 26%)	Most benefit in patients with very advanced PDR. No benefit in group with less severe NV	4 years

Contd.

Table 18.1 *Summary of the various clinical trials in diabetic retinopathy (Contd.)*

Study	No. of patients	Aim and year	Severity diabetic retinopathy	Intervention	Outcome	Clinical implication	Follow-up
Diabetic retinopathy vitrectomy study	370	1983–1987	Advanced PDR with fibrovascular proliferation, and VA ≥10/200	Early vitrectomy vs conventional management	Early surgery ↑ proportion of eyes with VA ≥10/20 (44% vs 28% conventional treatment) No difference in proportion having loss of vision to light perception or less		
DRCRN (DRCR net) Diabetes retinopathy clinical research network	121 eyes	To provide short-term effect of intravitreal bevacizumab on diabetic macular edema 2011	DME and Snellen acuity equivalent ranging from 20/32 to 20/320	Five groups: focal photocoagulation at baseline, intravitreal injection of 1.25 mg bevacizumab at baseline and 6 weeks (N=22, Group B), intravitreal injection of 2.5 mg bevacizumab at baseline and 6 weeks (N = 24, Group C), intravitreal injection of 1.25 mg bevacizumab at baseline and sham injection at 6 weeks (N=22, Group D), or intravitreal injection of 1.25 mg bevacizumab at baseline and 6 weeks with photocoagulation at 3 weeks (N = 22, Group E)	Only about half of the eyes showed response to intravitreal bevacizumab (exceeding an 11% reduction in retinal thickness compared with baseline) at either the 3-week or 6-week visit. For visual acuity, with both bevacizumab doses, on average there was about one line greater improvement relative to photocoagulation throughout the 12-week	Needs phase III trial. These short-term results of the current study should not be generalized to conclude that there is a clinically meaningful benefit in treating DME with intravitreal bevacizumab	On-going

Contd.

Table 18.1 *Summary of the various clinical trials in diabetic retinopathy (Contd.)*

Study	No of patients	Aim and year	Severity diabetic retinopathy	Intervention	Outcome	Clinical implication	Follow-up
DRCR net	323	To compromise modified ErDRS to mild macular grid laser treatment (2007)	CSME with VA ≥ 20/200 OCT thickness CFT ≥ 250 to one of inner subfields ≥ 300	Modified ETDRS laser (162 eyes) vs. mild grid laser (161 eyes) (Mild grid meant wider and spaced burns throughout macula avoiding foveal region)	No significant difference in OCT central macular thickness or visual acuity (treatment ↓ CMT 88 μm in the modified ETDRS group vs CMT 49 μm in the mild macular grid laser group, p = 0.04)	The new technique causes less decrease in OCT macular thickness than conventional therapy. No change in technique is recommended	1 year
DRCR net	854	To evaluate efficacy and safety of 0.5 mg intravitreal ranibizumab plus prompt (within 1 week) or deferred laser (≥24 weeks), or 4 mg intravitreal triamcinolone plus prompt laser, in comparison with sham plus prompt laser for treatment of DME (2011)	At least one eye meeting all the following criteria: • Electronic ETDRS BCVA letter score of 78 to 24 (≈20/32 to 20/320) • Definite retinal thickening due to DME involving center of macula on clinical examination • Central subfield (stratus OCT) ≥250 μm	4 groups Group 1 – Sham + prompt laser Group 2 – Ranibizumab + prompt laser Group 3 – Ranibizumab + deferred laser Group 4 – Triamcinolone + prompt laser	• Intravitreal ranibizumab with prompt or deferred (≥24 weeks) focal/grid laser had superior VA 9 letter gain and OCT outcomes compared with focal/grid (3 letter gain) laser treatment alone • Intravitreal triamcinolone combined with focal/grid laser did not result in superior VA outcomes compared with laser alone	• Ranibizumab should be considered in patients with DME and characteristics similar to those in this clinical trial • In pseudophakic eyes, intravitreal triamcinolone with prompt focal/grid laser may be equally effective as ranibizumab at improving visual acuity and reducing retinal thickening, but is associated with an increased risk of IOP elevation	3 years
RISE and (Ranibizumab injection in	RISE 377 patients	To evaluate the efficacy and safety of monthly intravitreal ranibizumab	CSME with center involvement in type 1 and 2 DM)	RISE 127 to sham, 125 to 0.3 mg, 125 to 0.5 mg	Gained ≥15 letters • 18.1% of sham patients • 44.8% of 0.3 mg • 39.2% of 0.5 mg	Ranibizumab rapidly and sustainably improved vision, reduced the risk of further vision loss,	2 years

Contd.

Table 18.1 Summary of the various clinical trials in diabetic retinopathy (Contd.)

Study	No. of patients	Aim and year	Severity diabetic retinopathy	Intervention	Outcome	Clinical implication	Follow-up
		subjects with CSME with center involvement in type 1 and 2 DM)			ranibizumab	and improved macular edema in patients with DME, with low rates of ocular and nonocular side effects	
RIDE	RIDE 382 patients	To evaluate the efficacy and safety of monthly intravitreal ranibizumab in diabetic macular edema (DME) patients (2010)	CSME with center involvement in type 1 and 2 DM	RIDE 130 to sham, 125 to 0.3 mg, 127 to 0.5 mg	Gained ≥15 letters: • 12.3% of sham patients • 33.6% of 0.3 mg patients • 45.7% of 0.5 mg	Ranibizumab rapidly and sustainably improved vision, reduced the risk of further vision loss, and improved macular edema in patients with DME, with low rates of ocular and nonocular harm	2 years
BOLT study	80	To evaluate the efficacy and safety of intravitreal bevacizumab in diabetic macular edema (DME) patients 2012	Center-involving CSME and visual acuity of 20/40 to 20/320	Intravitreous bevacizumab vs modified early treatment diabetic retinopathy study (ETDRS) macular laser therapy (MLT)	• Bevacizumab arm had a mean gain of 8.6 letters vs a mean loss of 0.5 letters for MLT. • Forty-nine percent of patients gained 10 or more letters (P = .001) and 32% gained at least 15 letters (p =.004) for bevacizumab vs 7% and 4% for MLT • Percentage who lost fewer than 15 letters in the MLT arm was 86% vs 100% for bevacizumab (p=.03) • Mean reduction in central macular thickness was 146 μm in the bevacizumab arm vs	Improvements in BCVA and central macular thickness seen with bevacizumab at 1 year were maintained over the second year with a mean of 4 injections	2 years

Contd.

Table 18.1 *Summary of the various clinical trials in diabetic retinopathy (Contd.)*

Study	No. of patients	Aim and year	Severity diabetic retinopathy	Intervention	Outcome	Clinical implication	Follow-up
					118 μm in the MLT arm. The median number of treatments over 24 months was 13 for bevacizumab and 4 for MLT		
READ 2	126	To compare efficacy of ranibizumab monotherapy or combined with laser vs laser monotherapy in DME patients, based on mean change in BCVA from baseline to 6-month (2011)	Done with BCVA 20/40 to 20/320 and CFT ≥ 250	Patients randomized into 3 groups: Group 1 – Intravitreal Ranibizumab 0.5 mg at baseline, month 1, 3 and 5 Group 2 – Laser at baseline and again at month 3 if CFT ≥250 μm Group 3 – Ranibizumab 0.5 mg + Laser at baseline and at month 3	Ranibizumab treated patients showed greater mean BCVA improvement (+ 10.3 letters) when compared with patients treated with laser (+1.4 letters) or ranibizumab + laser (+ 8.9 letters) at month 36	Visual potential can be maintained in DME patients with less frequent ranibizumab injections, as long as edema is moderately controlled. However, maximum benefits can be achieved with more frequent administration	
READ 3 trial	152	Evaluated the use of an even higher dose of ranibizumab versus the standard 0.5 mg dose given to manage DME (2011)		152 eyes with DME were randomized to receive 0.5 mg or 2 mg of ranibizumab in three consecutive monthly doses Patients found to have a central foveal thickness >250 μm were retreated	Data from the READ 3 trial showed a mean change in BCVA from baseline to month 6 of: • +7.46 ETDRS letters in the 2-mg group • +8.69 ETDRS letters in the 0.5 mg group. No serious ocular or systemic adverse events were reported in either treatment group gain in VA at 12 months 7.8 letters	Monthly intravitreal injection of 0.5 mg or 2 mg of ranibizumab is similarly effective in managing DME The 6-month duration of this study is probably insufficient to detect differences in efficacy between the two doses	

Contd.

Table 18.1 Summary of the various clinical trials in diabetic retinopathy (Contd.)

Study	No. of patients	Aim and year	Severity diabetic retinopathy	Intervention	Outcome	Clinical implication	Follow-up
RESOLVE study	151	To evaluate safety and efficacy of Ranibizumab in Diabetic Macular Edema (confirmed by FFA, OCT, FP) (2011)	DME with center involved BCVA of 20/40–20/160 CRT ≥300 µm	Patients divided in 3 groups: Group 1 – 0.3 mg ranibizumab Group 2 – 0.5 mg ranibizumab Group 3 – Sham 3 monthly injections given after month 1, the ranibizumab dose could be doubled by increasing the injection volume from 0.05 to 0.1 ml if CRT remained >300 µm or was >225 µm and the reduction in retinal edema from the previous assessment was <50 µm	Loss of >10 letters was seen in 4.9% of study group vs 24.5% in sham treatment	Ranibizumab was well tolerated in patients with visual impairment due to DME There were no incidence of glaucoma or cataract progression	1 year
RESTORE study	345	To demonstrate superiority of ranibizumab 0.5 mg monotherapy or combined with laser over laser alone	Type 1 or 2 diabetes mellitus DME with BCVA ≥73 letter and CRT < 300 µm	3 groups Group 1 - Ranibizumab + Sham laser Group 2 - Ranibizumab + laser Group 3 - Sham injections + Laser	Ranibizumab alone (7.4 letters) and combined with laser (7.2 letters) were superior to laser (2.4 letters) monotherapy in improving mean average change in BCVA letter score from baseline to month 1 through 12 (+6.1 and +5.9 vs +0.8)	Ranibizumab is superior to laser in improving BCVA with low incidence of ocular and systemic adverse effects Patients pretreated with ranibizumab showed rapid gain in BCVA whereas laser pretreated patients showed slow gain in BCVA during extensions period	1 year

Contd.

Table 18.1 Summary of various clinical trials in diabetic retinopathy (Contd.)

Study	No. of patients	Aim and year	Severity diabetic retinopathy	Intervention	Outcome	Clinical implication	Follow-up
RESTORE extension study	240	To evaluate Two-year safety and efficacy data core study from the RESTORE 2011. Patients who completed restore study at 12 months		Patients were treated at monthly intervals until they again reached stable visual acuity	The gains in BCVA that were observed during the first 12 months were maintained at month 2 The average number of injections in the ranibizumab monotherapy arm was **3.9**, compared with **3.5** in the combined ranibizumab/laser therapy arm	Ranibizumab (Rzb) PRN re-treatment according to visual acuity stability and disease progression supports the long-term safety and efficacy of ranibizumab in patients with visual impairment due to DME	1 year
REVEAL study	396	Further corroborated the results of the RESTORE trial in DME	A scan patients with DME with BCVA 20/32 to 20/160 (2012)	3 groups Group 1 – 0.5 mg ranibizumab Group 2 – 0.5 mg ranibizumb + Laser Group 3 – Laser alone After receiving three monthly injections, the patients were treated as needed if they experienced declines in BCVA and/or DME progression, as found on OCT	As in the RESTORE trial, ranibizumab used alone and with laser therapy resulted in similar results (gains of **5.9** and **5.7** ETDRS letters, respectively). Both treatments were superior to laser therapy alone (gain of **1.4** ETDRS letters). The mean number of injections needed was **7.8** in the ranibizumab monotherapy group and **7.4** in patients given combination therapy	Ranibizumab given alone or with laser therapy offered the best outcomes with respect to best-corrected central foveal thickness	1 year

BIBLIOGRAPHY

1. Bahadir M, Ertan A, Mertoglu O. Visual acuity comparison of vitrectomy with and without internal limiting membrane removal in the treatment of diabetic macular edema. Int Ophthalmol 2005;26:3–8.
2. Chaturvedi N, Sjolie AK, Stephenson JM, et al. Effect of lisinopril on progression of retinopathy in normotensive people with type 1 diabetes. The EUCLID Study Group. EURODIAB Controlled Trial of Lisinopril in Insulin-Dependent Diabetes Mellitus. Lancet 1998;351:28–31.
3. Definition and diagnosis of diabetes mellitus and intermediate hyperglycemia: report of a WHO/IDF consultation. Geneva: World Health Organization. 2006. p. 21. ISBN 978-92-4-159493-6
4. Diabetes Control and Complications Trial Research Group. Progression of retinopathy with intensive versus conventional treatment in the Diabetes Control and Complications Trial. Ophthalmology. 1995;102:647–61.
5. Diabetes Control and Complications Trial Research Group. The effect of intensive diabetes treatment on the progression of diabetic retinopathy in insulin-dependent diabetes mellitus. The Diabetes Control and Complications Trial. Arch.Ophthalmol. 1995;113:36–51.
6. Diabetes Control and Complications Trial/Epidemiology of Diabetes Interventions and Complications Research Group. Retinopathy and nephropathy in patients with type 1 diabetes four years after a trial of intensive therapy. N Engl J Med 2000;342:381–9.
7. Diabetic Retinopathy Clinical Research Network (DRCR.net). Three-year follow-up of a randomized trial comparing focal/grid photocoagulation and intravitreal triamcinolone for diabetic macular edema. Arch Ophthalmol 2009;127:245–51.
8. Diabetic Retinopathy Clinical Research Network; Writing Committee. Rationale for the diabetic retinopathy clinical research network treatment protocol for center-involved diabetic macular edema. Ophthalmology 2011; 118:e5–14.
9. Early Treatment Diabetic Retinopathy Study Research Group. Early photocoagulation for diabetic retinopathy. ETDRS report number 9. Ophthalmology 1991;98:766–85.
10. Early Treatment Diabetic Retinopathy Study Research Group. Photocoagulation for diabetic macular edema. Early Treatment Diabetic Retinopathy Study report number 1. Arch. Ophthalmol 1985;103:1796–806.
11. Early vitrectomy for severe proliferative diabetic retinopathy in eyes with useful vision. Results of a randomized trial—Diabetic Retinopathy Vitrectomy Study Report 3. The Diabetic Retinopathy Vitrectomy Study Research Group. Ophthalmology 1988;95:1307–20.
12. Early vitrectomy for severe vitreous hemorrhage in diabetic retinopathy. Two-year results of a randomized trial. Diabetic Retinopathy Vitrectomy Study report 2. The Diabetic Retinopathy Vitrectomy Study Research Group. Arch. Ophthalmol 1985;103:1644–52.
13. Estacio RO, Jeffers BW, Gifford N, Schrier RW. Effect of blood pressure control on diabetic microvascular complications in patients with hypertension and type 2 diabetes. Diabetes Care 2000;23 Suppl 2:54–64.
14. Flynn HW (Jr.), Chew EY, Simons BD, Barton FB, Remaley NA, Ferris FL 3. Pars plana vitrectomy in the Early Treatment Diabetic Retinopathy Study. ETDRS report number 17. The Early Treatment Diabetic Retinopathy Study Research Group. Ophthalmology1992;99:1351–57.
15. Fong DS, Strauber SF, Aiello LP, et al. Comparison of the modified Early Treatment Diabetic Retinopathy Study and mild macular grid laser photocoagulation strategies for diabetic macular edema. Arch Ophthalmol 2007;125:469–80.
16. Gupta V, Gupta A, Kaur R, Narang S, Dogra MR. Efficacy of various laser wavelengths in the treatment of clinically significant macular edema in diabetics. Ophthalmic Surg Lasers. 2001;32:397–405.
17. Klein R, Klein BE, Moss SE, Cruickshanks KJ. The Wisconsin Epidemiologic Study of Diabetic Retinopathy. XV. The long-term incidence of macular edema. Ophthalmology.1995;102:7–16.
18. Matthews DR, Stratton IM, Aldington SJ, Holman RR, Kohner EM. Risks of progression of retinopathy and vision loss related to tight blood pressure control in type 2 diabetes mellitus: UKPDS 69. Arch Ophthalmol. 2004;122:1631–40.
19. Narang S, Sood S, Kaur B, Singh R, Mallik A, Kaur J. Atorvastatin in clinically-significant macular edema in diabetics with a normal lipid profile. Nepal J Ophthalmol 2012;4:23–8.
20. Nguyen QD, Brown DM, Marcus DM, et al. RISE and RIDE Research Group. Ranibizumab for diabetic macular edema: results from 2 phase III randomized trials: RISE and RIDE. Ophthalmology 2012;119:789–801.

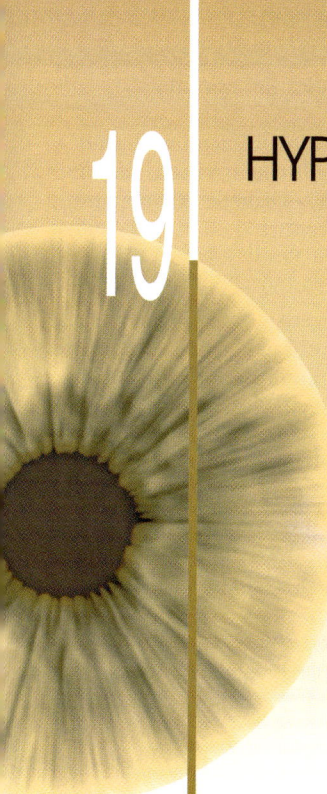

HYPERTENSIVE RETINOPATHY

Sunandan Sood, Neha Khurana

INTRODUCTION

Acute and chronic hypertensive changes may manifest in the eyes from acute changes due to malignant hypertension and chronic changes because of long-term essential hypertension respectively. High blood pressure can damage blood vessels in the retina. The higher the blood pressure and the longer it has been high, the more severe the damage is likely to be. Sometimes, the sudden rise in blood pressure can cause more severe changes in the eye.

Ocular involvement in the setting of malignant hypertension was first described by Liebreich, in 1859. Hayreh, over the course of 1970s and 1980s, elucidated pathophysiologic mechanisms for ocular involvement and described clinical findings through direct patient management observations and animal models.

EPIDEMIOLOGY

The prevalence of hypertensive retinal changes is variable and is often confounded by the presence of other retinal vascular disease, such as diabetes. In the Beaver Dam Eye Study, which evaluated hypertensive patients without coexisting, confounding vascular diseases, the overall incidence of hypertensive retinopathy was about 15% globally in fifth decaders or older. India being a developing country, has a lower prevalence of the disease. In India, community surveys have documented that between last four decades, prevalence of hypertension has increased by about 30 times among urban dwellers and by about 10 times among the rural inhabitants. The prevalence is higher in males than females till menopause and equal later. The predictive value of diagnosing systemic hypertension from ophthalmic findings on examination was only 47–53%, demonstrating that measurement of blood pressure is a more accurate means of diagnosis. Thus, it is a silent killer. It is responsible for vascular occlusions in the eye and morbid diseases like stroke and myocardial infarction systemically.

PATHOPHYSIOLOGY

Fundamentally, the ocular effects of hypertension arise from the impact on the ocular vasculature. Arteriosclerosis is an age related hardening of arterioles due to fibrosis in the tunica media layer. Atherosclerosis refers to the deposition of cholesterol beneath tunica intima of blood vessels. Both these changes are accelerated by hypertension.

The major branch arteries are about 110 μm in diameter as they cross the disc margin. They course within the nerve fiber layer and ganglion cell layer of the retina. Usually, after the first branch, the retinal arteries do not contain elastic fibers and internal elastic membrane; no nerve fibers have been found in the media or adventitia of human retinal vessels. Although the ophthalmic artery contains sympathetic nerve fiber endings, and therefore, is under the control of the autonomic nervous system, apparently no central regulation of the blood flow occurs in the retina itself.

The retinal arteries and arterioles remain in the inner retina, and only capillaries are found as deep as the inner nuclear layer. The retinal venous drainage of the retina generally follows the arterial supply. The retinal veins (mainly venules) are present in the inner retina, where they occasionally interdigitate with their associated arteries. When two vessels cross, the artery usually lies anterior to the vein, and the two vessels share a common adventitial sheath. Many more arteriovenous crossings occur temporally than nasally because the nasal vessels assume a much straighter course. The crossings are important because they represent the most common site of branch retinal vein obstructions. The retinal veins drain into the central retinal vein, which also acts as the major efferent channel. Near the disc, the retinal veins are approximately 150 μm in diameter.

Changes in the luminal diameter of the arterioles are the most important component in regulating systemic arterial blood pressure. The resistance of flow is equivalent to the fourth power of the diameter. The tight junctions of the retinal endothelium and the retinal pigment epithelium form the inner and outer blood retinal barriers. Acute hypertension causes disruption of the blood retinal barriers.

Since nervous system control of the retinal circulation does not occur, the retinal circulation must depend upon local chemical auto-regulation to maintain a constant metabolic environment. The process of autoregulation in a vascular bed maintains constant or nearly constant blood flow through a wide range of perfusion pressures. Blood flow in the retina appears to be primarily controlled by metabolic needs, especially the need for oxygen, and the accumulation of metabolic by-products such as carbon dioxide and changes in pH.

Regulation of blood flow through the choroid, as in the body in general, is under the control of the autonomic nervous system. The choroid does not show evidence of autoregulation, which may have serious consequences such as changes in IOP are not echoed by compensatory changes in the choroidal vascular pressure, and thus sudden decompression during surgery, may induce choroidal hemorrhage.

Optic nerve-head vessels exhibit intermediary characteristics with autoregulation but an incompetent blood-ocular barrier as a result of the peripapillary choroidal vessels. Because of the vascular differences between the retina, the choroid, and the optic nerve, each of these anatomic regions responds differently to hypertension. Together, however, they represent the clinical picture of the ocular response to systemic hypertension.

TREATMENT AND CLINICAL FEATURES

Most people with hypertensive retinopathy do not have symptoms until late in the disease. However, malignant hypertension may cause the symptoms which usually manifest suddenly and should be considered a medical emergency. The symptomatology may include moderate to severe headache, diplopia, dimness in vision, photopsia and scotoma in the field of vision.

CLINICAL TYPES

CHRONIC HYPERTENSIVE RETINOPATHY

Retinal vascular changes occurring from chronically elevated systemic arterial hypertension include the following:

- Arteriolosclerosis—Localized or generalized narrowing and irregularity of vessels
- Arteriovenous (AV) nicking as a result of arteriolosclerosis
- Copper wiring and silver wiring of arterioles as a result of arteriolosclerosis
- Retinal hemorrhages
- Cotton wool spots and retinal nerve fiber layer losses
- Remodelling changes due to capillary nonperfusion, such as shunt vessels and microaneurysms.

Generalized attenuation of the arterioles results from diffuse vasospasm, which occurs when a significant elevation of blood pressure has persisted for an appreciable period. Focal arteriole narrowing is closely related to control of hypertension. It occurs from spasm of local areas of the vascular musculature (Fig. 19.1).

At the arteriovenous crossing, the arteriole presses upon the vein causing hourglass constrictions on both sides of the crossing (the Gunn sign). This increases the resistance to blood flow in the veins. Thus the veins that cross at an acute angle to the vein normally may now cross by making a more obtuse angle (Salu's sign) (Fig. 19.2).

The normal light reflex of the retinal vasculature is formed by the reflection from the interface between the blood column and vessel wall. Initially, in the young age, the linear blood reflex seen over the surface of the arteriole is sharp and thin and it is predominantly because of blood column in the arteriole, since the vessel wall is by and large transparent. Subsequently, the increased thickness of the vessel walls causes the reflex to be more diffuse and less bright.

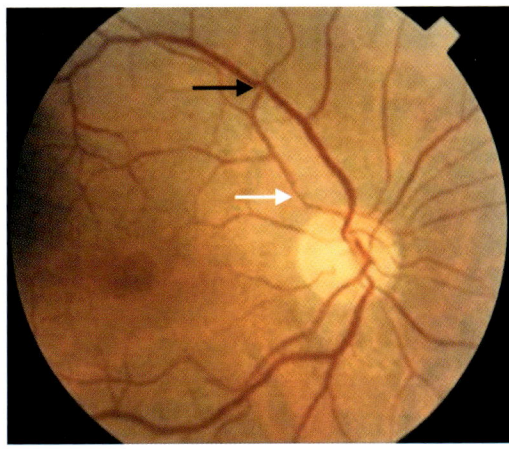

Fig 19.2 *Fundus photo showing (black arrow) narrowing of retinal vein at AV crossing (Gunn's sign) along with right angled deflection of vein (Salu's sign). White arrow shows presence of focal narrowing*

Progressive sclerosis and hyalinization causes the reflex to become red brown, known as copper wiring, and ultimately opaque white, known as silver wiring. The patency of these vessels can be confirmed on fluorescein angiography.

Superficial flame-shaped retinal hemorrhages occur at the posterior pole due to the disruption of capillaries in the retinal nerve fiber layer. These hemorrhages disappear in about 3–5 weeks.

Disruption of the blood flow dynamics lead to leaky capillaries that cause accumulation of plasma lipids in the outer plexiform layer. These refractile yellow flat lesions are called as hard exudates. Characteristic patterns like macular star and macular fan may also be seen. These are also temporary and may disappear in 3–6 weeks.

Occlusion of terminal arterioles leads to ischemic edema followed by infarction of the retinal nerve fiber layer. These fluffy, white lesions are found at the level of the nerve fiber layer and are called cotton-wool spots or soft exudates. These are located more commonly at the posterior pole and are related to the distribution of the radial peripapillary capillaries. These cotton-wool spots last approximately 3–6 weeks before fading away and leaving retinal nerve fiber (RNFL) defects in their place, clinically visible in red free illumination. Their fluorescein

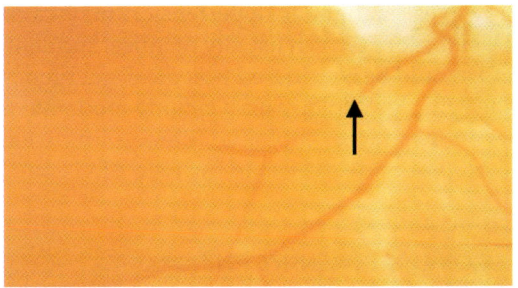

Fig 19.1 *Fundus photo shows presence of focal narrowing (black arrow) of the retinal arterioles in a case of mild hypertensive retinopathy*

angiographic appearance is hypofluorescent confirming the infarction of inner retinal layer.

ACUTE HYPERTENSIVE RETINOPATHY

The following retinal, choroidal, and optic nerve head changes are seen in malignant hypertension:

In response to sudden rise of blood pressure, there occurs a spasm of retinal arterioles and the retinal arteriolar tree instead of following a sinuous course, now has a straighter course. It appears as if the whole retinal tree is stretched. Thus, there occurs marked arteriolar narrowing.

As with chronic hypertensive retinopathy, superficial flame shaped retinal hemorrhages occur at the posterior pole due to the disruption of capillaries in the retinal nerve fiber layer. However, these hemorrhages are more in number as well as greater in severity. Even sheets of hemorrhages may be seen. These hemorrhages disappear in about 3–5 weeks provided the blood pressure is brought under control (Fig. 19.3).

First described by Hayreh, focal intraretinal periarteriolar transudates (FIPTs) are observed in malignant arterial hypertension ensuing from focal dilation of terminal retinal arterioles. Consisting of small, white, focal, oval lesions deep in the retina, they are located along the major arteriole vessels in crops and are among the earliest retinal lesions caused by malignant hypertension.

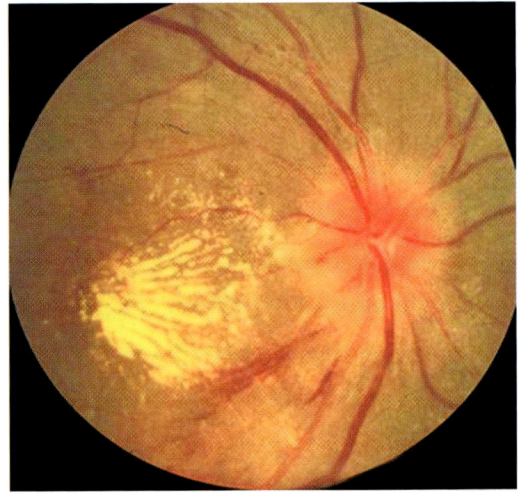

Fig 19.3 *Fundus photo of a case of malignant hypertension showing marked disc edema with dilated veins, scattered hemorrhages and hard exudates in the form of macular star*

FIPTs are related to dilation of terminal arterioles and the breakdown of autoregulatory mechanisms due to an acute, malignant increase in blood pressure. This results in the breakdown of the blood-retinal barrier, allowing transudation and accumulation of macromolecules. FIPTs are not associated with capillary obliteration and are not cotton-wool spots. They are hyperfluorescent and leak on fluorescein angiography (Fig. 19.4A and B).

Cotton-wool spots as already described are more characteristic of malignant arterial

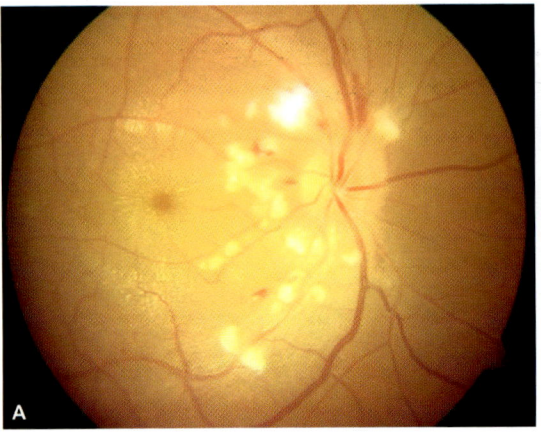

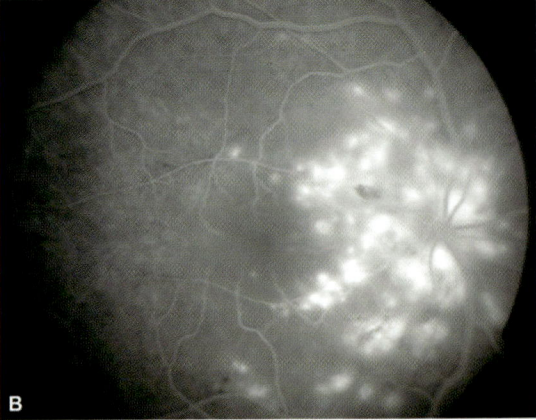

A B

Fig. 19.4 *Fundus photo of hypertensive retinopathy showing hard exudates on the macula in the form of macular star, few scattered superficial hemorrhages and focal intraretinal periarteriolar transudates (FIPTs) **(A)** which hyperfluorescence on FFA **(B)***

hypertension and may be larger in size and greater in number. They result from occlusion of terminal retinal arterioles. Capillary obliteration results in the development of microaneurysms, shunt vessels, and collaterals.

Clinical picture in acute hypertensive retinopathy resembles clinical picture in diabetic retinopathy, CRVO, hyperviscosity syndrome, neuroretinitis, and radiation retinopathy must be differentiated from these.

ACUTE HYPERTENSIVE CHOROIDOPATHY

Absence of blood ocular barrier in choriocapillaris leads to marked leakage of plasma with angiotensin II and all other vasoconstrictors into choroidal fluid. Vasoconstriction of choroidal vessels causes choroidal and RPE ischemia.

Acute ischemic changes in the choriocapillaris and overlying retinal pigment epithelium result in acute, focal retinal pigment epithelium lesions. These focal, white spots at the level of the retinal pigment epithelium are small, white, focal, oval lesions deep in the retina similar to FIPTs clinically. They can be differentiated from FIPTs by macular distribution along the major arcades. Gradually, these areas of retinal pigment epithelium clump and atrophy called as Elschnig's spots. Fluorescein angiography shows presence of window defects in the area of Elschnig's spots.

Ischemic damage to the retinal pigment epithelium leads to breakdown of the blood-retinal barrier and the accumulation of fluid beneath the retina. This leads to serous neurosensory detachment of the retina which preferentially affects the macular area.

ACUTE HYPERTENSIVE OPTIC NEUROPATHY

Initial optic disc changes include optic disc edema, hemorrhages on disc and peripapillary retina. Variable degree of disc pallor may occur late in the course. Optic nerve head is supplied by the peripapillary choroid. Vasoconstriction of peripapillary choroid leads to optic nerve head ischemia leading to edema and AION.

Thus, to summarise, following features are seen on funduscopy in malignant hypertension:
- Retinal arteriolar spasm
- Superficial retinal hemorrhages
- Cotton-wool spots and FIPTs
- Elschnig's spots
- Serous retinal detachment
- Optic disc edema.

STAGING OF HYPERTENSIVE RETINOPATHY

The original classification system for hypertensive retinopathy was conceived in 1939 by Keith and colleagues. Since that time, there have been several criticisms of the original system concerning the reproducibility and the relevance of the system to clinical practice. Two of the major schemes are presented here.

KEITH-WAGENER-BARKER CLASSIFICATION (1939)

Patients were grouped according to their ophthalmoscopic findings. As such, this was the first system to correlate retinal findings with the hypertensive disease state. Classifica-tion is as follows:
- Stage 1: Slight narrowing, sclerosis, and tortuosity of the retinal arterioles
- Stage 2: Definite narrowing, focal constriction, sclerosis, and AV nicking
- Stage 3: Retinopathy (stage 2 changes along with cotton-wool spots, hard exudates, hemorrhages) (Fig. 19.5)
- Stage 4: Papilledema (along with stage 2 and 3 changes).

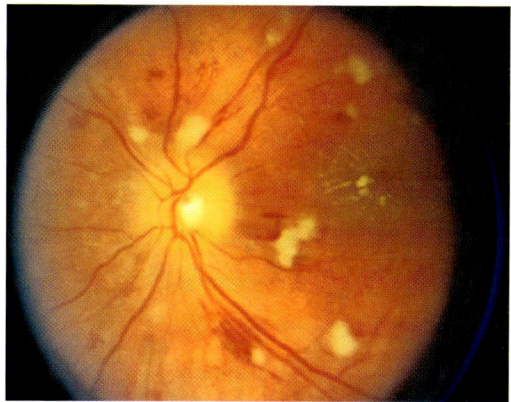

Fig 19.5 *Fundus photo shows moderate chronic hypertensive retinopathy (Keith-Wagener-Barker grade 3) with marked attenuation of arterioles and multiple scattered hemorrhages and cotton-wool spots. Macula shows presence of hard exudates*

Table 19.1 *Wong and McIntosh classification*

Retinopathy	Description	Systemic associations
Mild	One or more of the following signs: generalized arteriolar narrowing, focal arteriolar narrowing, AV nicking, arteriolar wall opacity (silver-wiring)	Weak associations with stroke, coronary heart disease and cardiovascular mortality
Moderate	Mild retinopathy with one or more of the following signs: retinal haemorrhages (blot, dot or flame-shaped), microaneurysms, cotton-wool spot, hard exudates	Strong association with stroke, congestive heart failure, renal dysfunction and cardiovascular mortality
Accelerated	Moderate retinopathy signs plus optic disk swelling, may be associated with visual loss	Associated with mortality and renal failure

SCHEIE CLASSIFICATION

In 1953, Scheie attempted to differentiate vascular changes from retinopathy changes. The former can occur without hypertension due to arteriosclerosis, however hypertension can accelerate these.

Staging of retinopathy changes is as follows:
- Stage 0—No visible retinal abnormalities
- Stage 1—Diffuse arteriolar narrowing; no focal constriction
- Stage 2—More pronounced arteriolar narrowing with focal constriction
- Stage 3—Focal and diffuse narrowing, with retinal hemorrhage
- Stage 4—Retinal edema, hard exudates, optic disc edema

Grading of the light reflex changes resulting from arteriolosclerosis is as follows:
- Grade 0—Normal
- Grade 1—Broadening of light reflex with minimal arteriolovenous compression
- Grade 2—Light reflex changes and crossing changes more prominent
- Grade 3—Copper-wire appearance; more prominent arteriolovenous compression
- Grade 4—Silver-wire appearance; severe arteriolovenous crossing changes.

WONG AND MCINTOSH CLASSIFICATION

Recently, Wong and McIntosh (2005) have introduced a new classification of hypertension into mild, moderate and accelerated hypertension and predicted the risk of systemic association (Table 19.1).

TREATMENT AND PROGNOSIS

TREATMENT

Medical care for hypertensive optic complications involves evaluation of secondary causes and appropriate medical management involving lifestyle changes and pharmacotherapy. In the presence of hypertensive optic neuropathy, a rapid reduction of blood pressure may pose a risk of worsening ischemic damage to the optic nerve. The optic nerve demonstrates autoregulation, so there is an adjustment in perfusion based on the elevated blood pressure. A precipitous reduction in blood pressure will reduce perfusion to the optic nerve and central nervous system as a result of their autoregula-tory changes, resulting in infarction of the optic nerve head, and potentially, acute ischemic neurologic lesions of the central nervous system. Surgical management is indicated to address certain secondary causes of systemic hypertension.

PROGNOSIS

The retina will generally recover if the blood pressure is controlled. However, some patients with grade 4 hypertensive retinopathy will have permanent damage to the optic nerve or macula. Patients with grade 4 (severe hypertensive retinopathy) often have propensity of heart and kidney complications of high blood pressure. They are also at higher risk for stroke.

BIBLIOGRAPHY

1. Nocturnal arterial hypotension and its role in optic nerve head and ocular ischemic disorders. Am J Ophthalmol 1994;117:603–24.

2. Systemic arterial blood pressure and the eye. Eye 1996;10:5–28.

3. Role of nocturnal arterial hypotension in optic nerve head ischemic disorders. Ophthalmologica 1999;213:76–96.

4. Beta-blocker eye drops and nocturnal arterial hypotension. Am J Ophthalmol 1999;128:301–9.

5. Role of nocturnal arterial hypotension in the development of ocular manifestations of systemic arterial hypertension. Curr Opin Ophthalmol 1999;10:474–82.

6. Hypertensive retinopathy: Introduction. Ophthalmologica 1989;198:173–7.

7. Retinal arteriolar changes in malignant arterial hypertension. Ophthalmologica 1989;198:178–96.

8. Cotton-wool spots (inner retinal ischemic spots) in malignant arterial hypertension. Ophthalmologica 1989;198:197–215.

9. Retinal lipid deposits in malignant arterial hypertension. Ophthalmologica 1989;198:216–29.

10. Macular lesions in malignant arterial hypertension. Ophthalmologica 1989;198:230–46.

11. Classification of hypertensive fundus changes and their order of appearance. Ophthalmologica 1989;198:247–60.

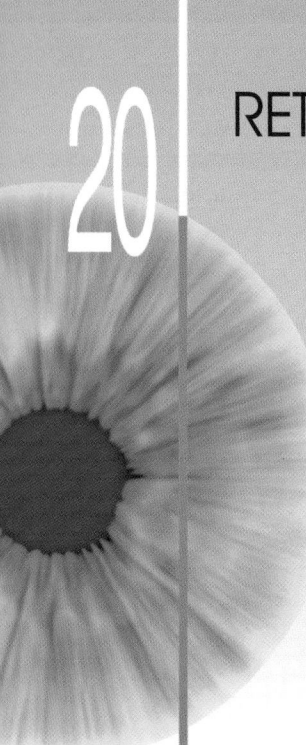

20 | RETINOPATHY OF PREMATURITY

Subina Narang

INCIDENCE, PATHOGENESIS AND RISK FACTORS

Retinopathy of prematurity (ROP) is potentially blinding disease of premature babies. Terry in 1942 first reported retrolental fibroplasia which probably represented stage V retinopathy of prematurity. There are many risk factors for the disease and among these the period of gestation (POG) and birth weight (BW) are of prime importance.

INCIDENCE OF ROP

The incidence of ROP among premature babies with gestational age of 28–29 weeks is 83%, 30–31 weeks is 60% and 32–33 weeks is 50%. For each 100 gram increase in birth weight, there is a 27% decrease in the percentage of infants who develop threshold ROP. Middle income group countries such as India and Latin America, are currently believed to be experiencing a "third epidemic" of ROP.

The incidence of ROP in India ranges from 11 to 47.7%. It has been estimated that 0.2% of childhood blindness in India is because of ROP. The number of premature deliveries in India is 10% and about 50% of these develop ROP. On follow up 15% will be needing treatment which if untreated could be blind. If we calculate the number of blind years that a baby lives the economic burden is tremendous.

PATHOGENESIS OF ROP

The vascularization of the retina starts posteriorly, around the optic nerve, at 16 weeks of gestation as spindle cells from adventitia of hyaloidal artery. These solid cords metamorphose into mature vessels and migrate in the process of angiogenesis to extend vascularization towards the ora serrata. These reach nasal ora serrata by 7–8 months and temporal ora serrata by 9 months. After birth these vessels are not fully mature in premature babies and there are two phases of development of ROP. In phase I there is hyperoxia leading to cessation of VEGF driven retinal vascular growth after premature birth. There is also vaso obliterations and capillary regression leading to

retinal ischemia. Phase II follows when hypoxia of phase I induces release of factors to stimulate vessel growth (after 34 wks POG). The oxygen-regulated factors like vasculo-endothelial growth factor (VEGF) and non-oxygen-regulated factors like insulin like growth factor-1 (IGF-1) are critical for development of ROP. The neovessels and accompanying glial cells develop contractile properties.

RISK FACTORS OF ROP

Most of our understanding of ROP is based on CRYO-ROP study, the largest multicentric trial of ROP. This included 4099 premature infants with a birth weight less than 1251 gram prospectively screened in the CRYO-ROP from 23 study centers. It included 291 babies with threshold ROP randomized into cryotherapy or observation. The most important risk factor in addition to low birth weight (LBW) and period of gestation (POG) is oxygen supplementation and the other risk factors include light, vit E deficiency, apnea, respiratory distress syndrome, asphixia, anoxia, shock, septicaemia, acidosis, patent ductus arteriosus, blood transfusions, double volume exchange transfusion, intra-ventricular hemorrhage and bronchopulmonary dysplasia, etc. CRYO-ROP study also found that younger POG, multiple births, out of nursery birth, low birth weight, white race, zone I ROP, plus disease, stage 3, greater than 6 clock hours stage 3, and iris vessel dilatation were associated with development of unfavorable macular outcome.

CLASSIFICATION AND CLINICAL FEATURES

The international classification of ROP (ICROP) gave one common language to research work in ROP in 1984. It describes the early levels of severity of ROP based on several parameters: zone, stage, extent of ROP and the presence of plus disease. Zone tells about the extent of the disease.

ZONES OF ROP

Zone of ROP (Fig. 20.1) are:

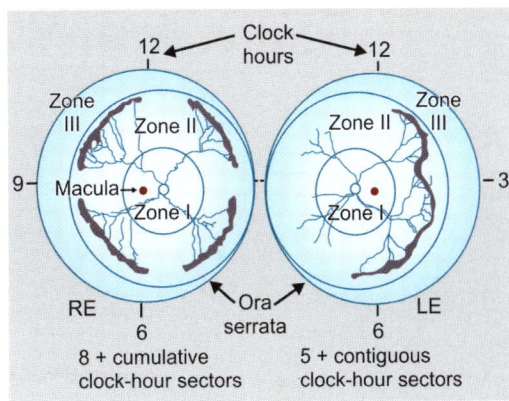

Fig. 20.1 *Line diagram showing zones of ROP*

- *Zone 1* includes disease in circle of radius twice the distance between disc and macula with disc at center.
- *Zone II* is circle outer to zone 1 with radius touching nasal ora and disc at center.
- Zone III includes the temporal crescent of retina left behind.

STAGES OF ROP

The stage of ROP defines the clinical appearance of the retina at the junction of vascularized retina and the avascular area. There are 5 stages. This classification was further modified in 2005 to include zone I aggressive posterior ROP.

- *Stage 1* ROP is demarcation line between vascular and avascular retina (Fig. 20.2)
- *Stage 2* is ridge formation when the line gets volume (Fig. 20.3).

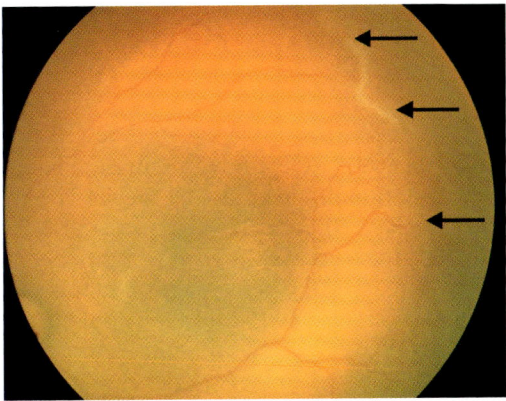

Fig. 20.2 *Fundus picture showing demarcation line (arrows) between vascular and avascular peripheral retina   stage 1 in zone II ROP (Courtesy: Prof MR Dogra)*

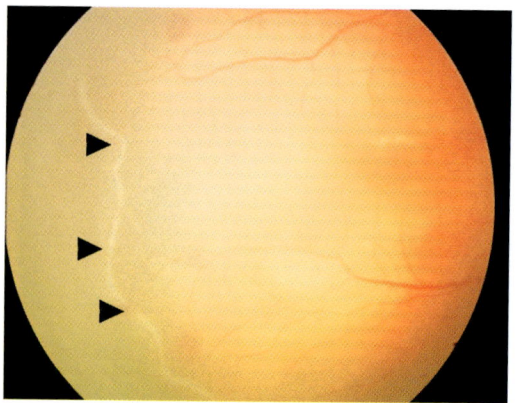

Fig. 20.3 *Fundus picture showing ridge(arrow heads) stage2 zone II ROP (Courtesy: Prof MR Dogra)*

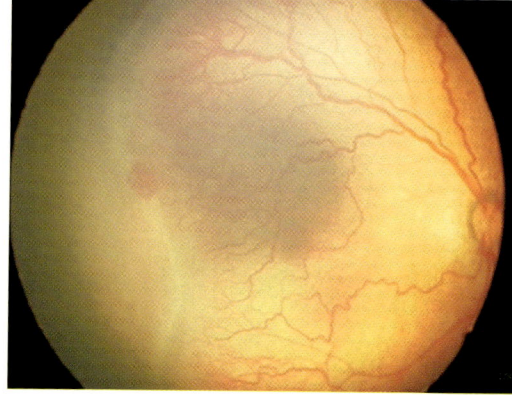

Fig. 20.5 *Fundus picture shows stage 3 zone II ROP with extraretinal proliferation (Courtesy: Prof MR Dogra)*

- *Stage 3* is extraretinal fibrovascular proliferation (Figs 20.4 and 20.5)
- *Stage 4A* is macula sparing partial retinal detachment (Fig. 20.6) and
- *Stage 4B* is partial retinal detachment involving macula (Fig. 20.7).
- *Stage 5* is total retinal detachment or retrolenticular fibroplasias (Fig. 20.8).

EXTENT OF ROP

- *The extent of ROP* refers to the number of clock hours of the highest stage.
- *Plus disease* refers to dilatation and tortuosity of the retinal arterioles and veins and is based on a standard photograph published in the CRYO-ROP. In later clinical trials, the definition of plus disease was changed to

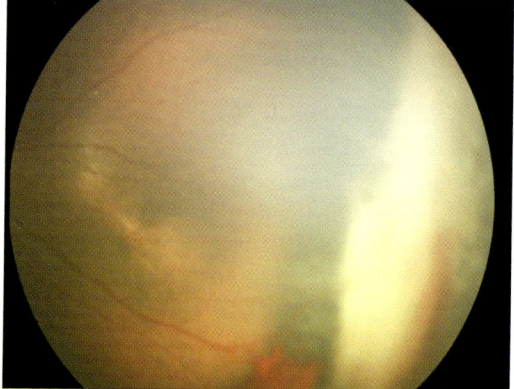

Fig. 20.6 *Fundus picture shows stage 4 A ROP, retina is lifted up in periphery (white marking) after laser treatment (Courtesy: Prof MR Dogra)*

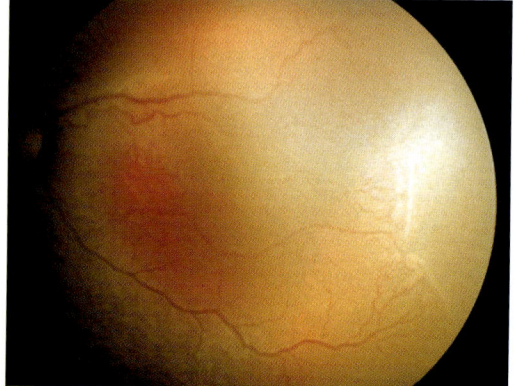

Fig. 20.4 *Fundus picture showing extraretinal proliferation on ridge stage 3 zone II ROP (Courtesy: Prof MR Dogra)*

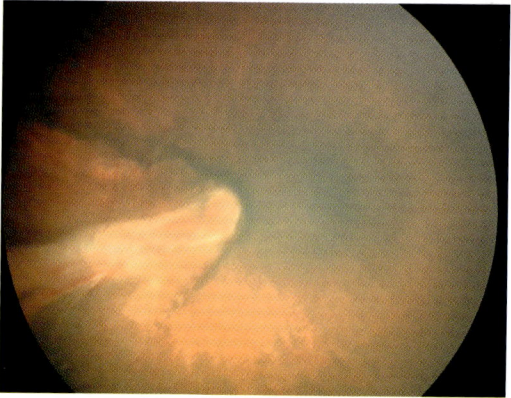

Fig. 20.7 *Fundus picture shows stage 4 B ROP (Courtesy: Prof MR Dogra)*

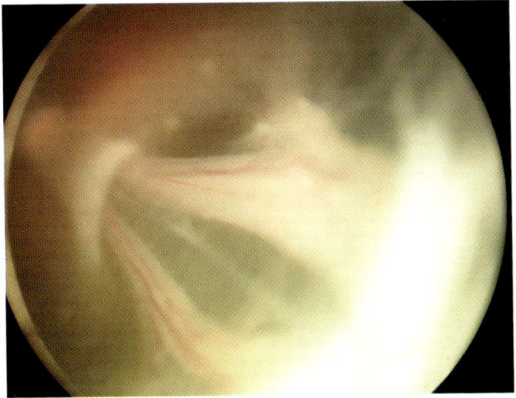

Fig. 20.8 *Fundus picture shows total retinal detachment stage 5 ROP. (Courtesy: Prof MR Dogra)*

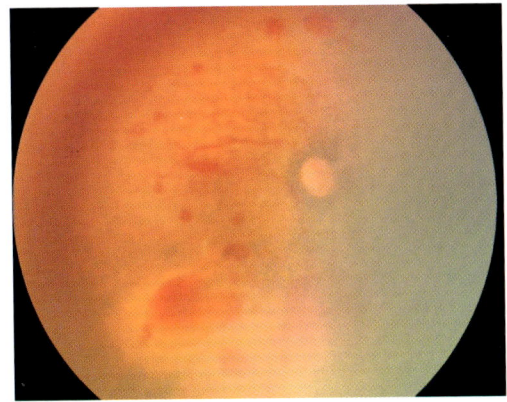

Fig. 20.10 *Fundus picture shows APROP with multiple preretinal bleeds. (Courtesy: Prof MR Dogra)*

include less severe degrees of vascular tortuosity and dilatation.

AGGRESSIVE POSTERIOR ROP

- *Aggressive posterior ROP* (AP-ROP), also called *Rush disease*, is a rapidly progressive form of ROP. In APROP, the ROP is confined to zone 1 (Figs 20.9 and 20.10) and posterior zone 2.
- *Aggressive posterior ROP may differ from zone 2 ROP* in appearance, progression, pace, treatment, and treatment response.
- *APROP is characterized by* neovascular fronds that lay flat on the retinal surface and no ridge tissue is seen in these eyes, and yet the AV shunting, which occurs within the ridge tissue in more typical ROP, is seen throughout the

posterior pole. Vessels are dilated and tortuous in a syncytial pattern.

- *APROP may progress considerably* more rapidly than ROP located in zone 2, sometimes in a matter of days without the conventional stage wise progression of ROP.

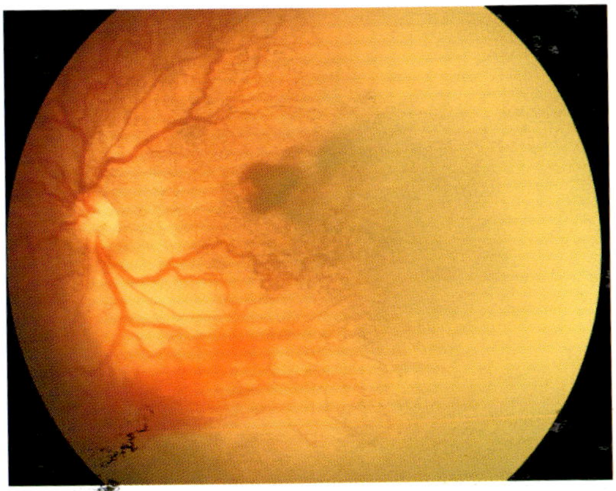

DEFINITION OF THRESHOLD DISEASE AND ITS MODIFICATION

CRYO-ROP study

- *CRYO-ROP study* defines threshold ROP when the eye has an equal chance of spontaneous regression or progression to unfavourable outcome.
- *Unfavorable outcome* is defined as presence of a macular fold, retinal detachment involving zone I, or obscuration of the posterior pole by cataract or retrolental fibroplasia.
- CRYO-ROP defines treshold ROP as presence of 5 contiguous or 8 total clock hours of stage 3 ROP in zones I or II with plus disease.
- *This however did not talk about stage 1 zone I ROP* which behaves a lot more aggressively than other zones of disease. *The zone 1 eyes had an unfavourable* outcome in high frequency (87%) in the CRYO-ROP study.

ETROP study (early treatment of ROP study)

- *ETROP study showed* that they at that time were seeing more cases of more severe zone 2 ROP than were seen during CRYO-ROP study (severe ROP accounted for 36.9% in ETROP versus 27.1% in CRYO-ROP study). The data

Fig. 20.9 *Fundus picture showing zone 1 APROP with plus disease and preretinal bleed (Courtesy: Prof MR Dogra)*

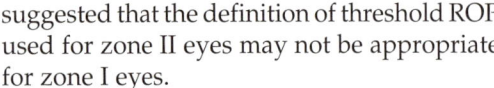

suggested that the definition of threshold ROP used for zone II eyes may not be appropriate for zone I eyes.

- ETROP study, recommends early treatment once they attained 15% risk of unfavourable outcome or more which is defined as high-risk prethreshold eyes or type1 ROP.
- *Type 2 retinopathy of prematurity signifies* the ROP disease is not severe enough to require treatment. So the child can be followed up in the routine ROP screening programme till either the disease regresses or progresses to type 1 to need treatment.

Type 1 ROP which include:
- Any eye that has any stage of ROP in zone I with plus disease
- Stage 3 ROP in zone I with or without plus disease
- Stages 2 or 3 ROP in zone II with plus disease

Type 2 ROP includes:
- Zone I, stage 1–2 without plus
- Zone II, stage 3 without plus.

SCREENING, TREATMENT, SEQUELAE AND CLINICAL TRIALS

SCREENING AND FOLLOW-UP OF ROP

Every country has its own guidelines for ROP screening. Guidelines for screening in America. Infants that should be screened for ROP include:
- All infants born weighing less than or equal to 1500 g, or less than or equal to 28 weeks gestational age
- Infants born weighing more than 1500 g but who experience an unstable course
- The first examination should be performed prior to hospital discharge, or at 4 to 6 weeks after birth, or between 31 and 33 weeks post-menstrual age (PMA) whichever is later.

Guidelines for screening in India are as follows:
- Preterm babies with birth weight of 2,000 g or less
- Gestational age of 34 or 35 weeks
- If other risk factors are present or neonato-logist feels the need of screening.

Timing of Screening

Screening in India should be at 4 weeks after birth or 32 weeks postmenstural age (PMA) whichever is earlier. We, in India, have higher birth weight criteria, based on the concern that at-risk infants may be missed since the babies with higher birth weight in developing countries develop ROP. In Asian countries the entire sequence of events occurs one to two weeks earlier. Hence the first exam is at 32 weeks PMA or 4 weeks after birth whichever is earlier. However, infants born < 28 weeks of gestation or < 1200 grams are screened by 2–3 weeks of chronological age keeping in mind the risk of APROP. As higher cutoff limit, Jalali *et al* have recommended screening babies born at ≤ 37 weeks GA and/or BW 2000 g in the presence of a high sickness score in order to prevent missing any infant with threshold ROP. Moreover, since ROP is seen in heavier and larger babies in India that have consequently a shorter window period for development of ROP earlier examinations are essential, in contrast to the West wherein threshold ROP is seen in smaller babies that have a longer window period to develop ROP. Hence, an examination carried out later would suffice in the west but would lead to missing of early stages of ROP in our country.

Retinal findings indicative of poor outcome (namely prethreshold ROP, threshold ROP, plus disease, or stage 3 disease) were seen in only 1% of infants before 31 weeks of PMA and in only 1% of infants after 46.3 weeks of PMA. Therefore, for most eyes the time window for development of serious ROP (prethreshold or worse) is between 30.9 weeks and 46.3 weeks of PMA or between 4.7 and 18.7 weeks of chronologic age.

Retinal findings indicative of minimal risk of poor outcome (namely vascularization into zone III without previous ROP or full retinal vascularization) were seen in 99% of infants by 45.9 weeks of PMA. The study investigators suggest that screening examinations be initiated at 31 weeks of PMA or at 4 weeks of chronologic age for infants born before 27 weeks of PMA and be continued until 45 weeks of PMA or progression of retinal vascularization into zone III.

Results of the ETROP place appropriate emphasis on the importance of timely identification of prethreshold ROP. In the ETROP, infants were followed on a weekly basis after developing zone II, stage 2 ROP or if they had retinal vessel immaturity with vessels ending in zone I but without ROP. Infants with low-risk prethreshold disease received follow-up fortnightly.

Telemedicine (i.e., on-site acquisition of clinical data relayed to a remote site for interpretation) overcomes many barrier to approach patients in remote areas. The trained technicians acquire digital fundus images from at-risk infants in a neonatal intensive care unit, transmit these to a regional reading center. Trained certified graders could provide timely and cost-effective input into ROP management, identifying infants requiring on-site examination or treatment.

Newer investigations like OCT have been used for ROP babies and have revealed ophthalmoscopically unapparent findings like macular edema, retinoschisis which could have bearing on their long term visual outcome.

TREATMENT OF ROP

Laser versus cryotherapy

Laser treatment has practically replaced cryotherapy now-a-days. Although the merit of cryopexy versus laser retinopexy for ROP has been debated, laser is the current standard for treating ROP (Figs 20.11 and 20.12). Cryotherapy needs to be done under general anesthesia and laser treatment may be done under topical anesthesia with pediatric support to pick up any complications of the procedure like bradycardia, apnoea, aspiration at the earliest.

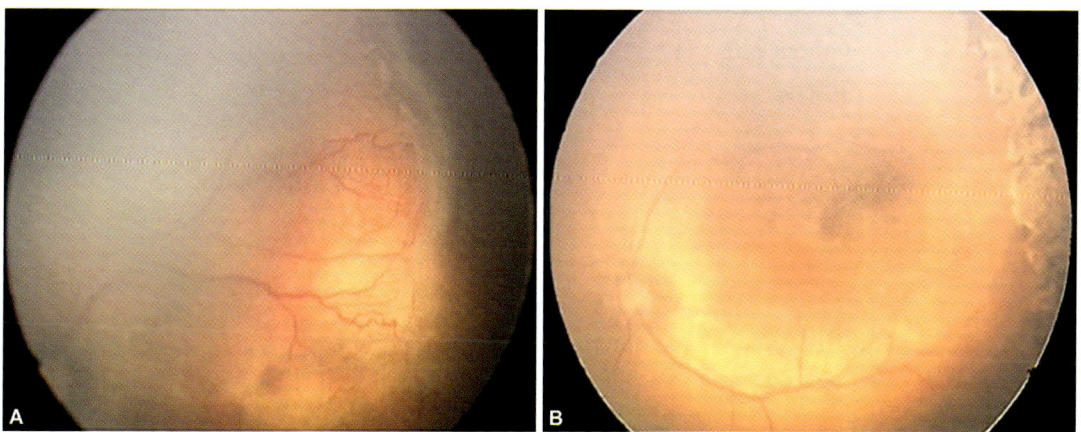

Fig. 20.11 *(A) Fundus picture showing stage 3 plus zone II ROP, (B) Fundus picture of same eye after laser showing regressed ROP (Courtesy: Prof MR Dogra)*

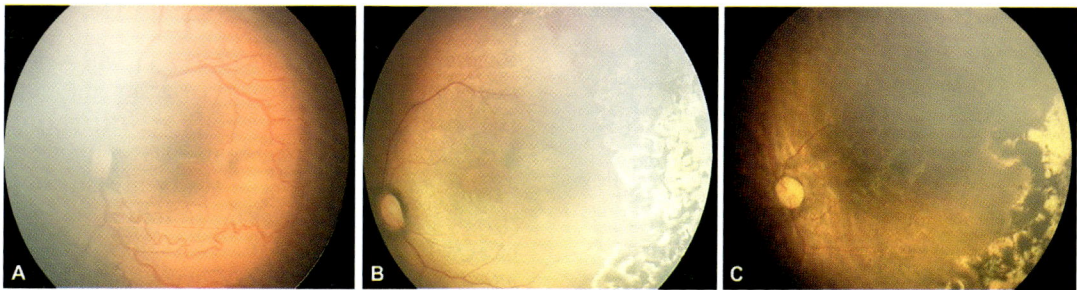

Fig. 20.12 *(A) Fundus picture of a preterm baby with POG 28 weeks and BW 900 grams developed stage 3 zone II (B and C) ROP and regressed after laser treatment (Courtesy: Prof MR Dogra)*

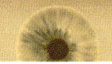
Long-term structural and functional outcomes using laser to be superior to those obtained with cryotherapy. The difference is perhaps most dramatic in eyes with posterior ROP.

Conventional laser treatment pattern is best described as nearly confluent burns placed 0.5 to 1 burn width apart.

Complications of laser treatment include anterior segment ischemia, cataract, and burns of the cornea, iris, or tunica vasculosa lentis.

Indications for using cryopexy instead of laser in the management of ROP include poor fundus visibility (vitreous hemorrhage or anterior segment problems), lack of availability of laser, and lack of treating physician's familiarity with indirect laser retinopexy.

APROP Treatment

In APROP the avascular retina beneath the flat posterior stage 3 ROP is difficult to treat at the initial laser session. Once flat stage 3 ROP regresses, the untreated avascular retina remains as a source of VEGF and can slowly continue to drive the ROP process. A second laser session may be necessary a week later, with application to the avascular retina now exposed by regression of the flat stage 3 ROP. Pharmacotherapy has been found to be effective in APROP in Beat ROP study. In zone I eyes, favourable anatomic results have been reported in 83% of eyes treated with laser, whereas cryotherapy, by contrast, provide favourable outcomes in only 25% of eyes with zone I disease.

The extent of ROP affected final anatomical outcome. For each clock hour of stage 3 ROP greater than 5 clock hours, there was a 26% increased risk of an unfavourable macular outcome. In the 5½ year report from the natural history cohort of CRYO-ROP, an unfavourable anatomic outcome occurred in 62.5% of zone I eyes compared to 44.2% of zone II eyes. In the ETROP trial, guidelines were given for early treatment which reduced unfavourable visual acuity from 19.8% in conventional group to 14.3% (p<0.05) and unfavourable structural outcome was also reduced from 15.6 to 9.0% (p<0.0001) at 9 months in type I ROP.

Pharmacotherapy

Beat ROP study, trial to establish efficacy of pharmacotherapy with anti-VEGF drugs in ROP. It concluded that Intravitreal bevacizumab monotherapy, as compared with conventional laser therapy, it showed a significant benefit for zone I stage 3+ retinopathy of prematurity. The result could not be generalized for zone II disease. The timing of intravitreal antiVEGF drugs are important. In their study the drug was injected when VEGF levels were high (32–42 weeks of PMA).

Surgical Management

ROP stage 4

ROP related retinal detachments in present day must not be managed by scleral buckling procedures.

Lens sparing vitrectomy is fairly safe surgery especially in stage 4 A. The major disadvantage of scleral buckle for stage 4A ROP are the dramatic anisometropic myopia and the second intervention required for transection or removal so that the eye may continue to grow. Partial detachments initially may look stable. However, the stability of neither partial detachment nor visual acuity is predictable on the basis of retinal appearance in infants with ROP. This holds true especially in babies with incomplete peripheral retinal ablation. Vitreoretinal surgery for stage 5 disease was associated with some structural success but not very good functional outcomes. Awareness of all tractional forces and their alleviation is important. The goal of intervention for ROP is an undistorted or minimally distorted posterior pole, total retinal reattachment, and preservation of the lens and central fixation vision.

Vitreous surgery can interrupt progression of ROP from stage 4A to stage 4B or 5 by directly addressing transvitreal traction resulting from fibrous proliferation. In experienced hands, lens-sparing vitrectomy allows primary retinal reattachment in at least 90% of eyes with stage 4A ROP.

ROP stage 5

In leucocoria in stage 5 *lens needs to be sacrificed* and the aim is to slowly open the funnel by

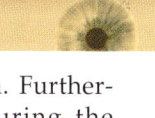

repeated surgeries without a break. There have been trials on *plasmin assisted vitrectomy* for stage 5 which would ensure complete removal of vitreous. Autologous plasmin (0.3–0.22 IU) is injected into the vitreous cavity after lensectomy.

SEQUELAE OF ROP

Residual changes following spontaneous regression of ROP. These include foveal pigmentation, posterior pole pre-retinal membrane, exudative detachment, vitreous hemorrhage and membranes, and abnormal angle of insertion of major vessels at the optic disc.

Sequelae reported after treatment include narrow temporal vascular arcade, tortuosity of posterior pole vessels, macular pigment disturbances, preretinal membranes and macular heterotopia.

Prevalence of myopia varied from 64.5–69.4% in the ETROP and CRYO-ROP studies, and that of severe myopia (more than 5 dioptres) varied from 25.5–28.3% respectively.

Strabismus in ROP from present ETROP results 30% of infants with strabismus at 6 months may show normal ocular alignment at 9 months. The ophthalmologist should be aware of greater variability in strabismus in high risk prethreshold ROP during the first year of life.

*Retinal folds and retinal detachments a*t 10 to 15 years follow up in the CRYO-ROP study group, new retinal folds were seen. Furthermore, retinal detachments obscuring the posterior pole occurred in 4.5% of treated and 7.7% of untreated eyes. An unfavourable visual outcome at 15 years was found in 49.7% of treated and 64.3% of untreated control eyes (p<0.001).

Long-term sequ elae include early nuclear sclerotic cataract, glaucoma, exudative retinopathy, and rhegmatogenous retinal detachment. These are a few of the long-term sequelae of ROP prompting the need for lifelong ophthalmic monitoring of formerly premature adults. Rhegmatogenous retinal detachments in adults with ROP may be challenging to repair because of irregular tears, atrophied peripheral retina, and abnormalities of the vitreoretinal interface, especially in areas of originally nonvascularized retina.

CLINICAL TRIALS IN ROP

Various clinical trials conducted in ROP are summarized in Table 20.1.
- Multicenter rial of cryo-therapy for retinopathy of prematurity CRYO- ROP)
- Light reduction in ROP study (LIGHT-ROP)
- Supplemental therapeutic oxygen to prevent PTh ROP (STOP-ROP)
- High oxygen percentage retinopathy of prematurity (HOPE-ROP)
- Vitamin E
- Early treatment for retinopathy of prematurity (ETROP)
- Beat ROP

Table 20.1 Summary of various clinical trials conducted in ROP

Trial	Enrollment time	Inclusion criteria	Number	Endpoint (follow up)	Rationale (hypothesis)	Outcome measures	Outcomes
Multicentre trial of cryo-therapy for retinopathy of prematurity (CRYO-ROP)	1986–1988	<1251 g birth weight; survived 28 days of life; without major ocular or systemic anomalies	Enrolled 4099 babies; 291 with Th ROP rando-mized to Cryo or observation 247 analyzed at 10 yr	Reports at 3 mo, 1 yr, 3.5 yr, 5.5 yr, 10 yr, 15 yr	Treatment of avasular zone in ThROP reduces poor visual and structural outcomes	Visual function and structural findings	31.6% cryo treated versus 51.4% observation gp had poor structural outome; 44.4% cryo treated vs 62.6% observation gp had VA <20/200 and 27.2% vs 47.9% had unfavourable structural outcomes; p<0.001
Light reduc-tion in ROP study (LIGHT-ROP)	1995–1997	<1251 g birth weight and GA<31 weeks; NICU admission within 24 hours of birth	409 enrolled; 205 wore goggles (Gog) and 204 did not (NGog)	Through regression of ROP, 6 mo follow up	Light reduction reduces ROP	Primary – any ROP; secondary Pth or ThROP (CRYO-ROP standard for defini-tion of PTh and Th ROP)	54% gog vs 58% NGog developed ROP; 15% gog vs 14%NGog developed either PTh
Supplemental therapeutic oxygen to prevent PTh ROP (STOP-ROP)	1994–1999	PTh in atleast one eye;≤94% SaO$_2$ in RA, no lethal anomalies or ocular congenital anomalies	649 enrolled; 325 given Con (to achieve 89–94% SaO$_2$), 324 given S (to achieve 96–99% SaO$_2$)	3 mo after 40 wk PMA	Oxygen supple-mentation relieves the hypoxic stimulus (for stage 3 ROP) caused through normal retinal differentiation and oxygen consumption	ThROP or worse; 3 mo F/U for structural outcome	ThROP in at least one eye in 48% Con vs 41% in S; PTh with plus disease 52% in Con vs 57% plus disease 46% in con vs 32% in S developed ThROP, p = 0.004
High oxygen percentage retinopathy of prematurity (HOPE-ROP)	1996–1999	PTh in atleast one eye and median SaO$_2$ >94%	136 HOPE ROP compared to 229 STOP-ROP infants enrolled at	Through the development of threshold ROP or regression of	Fewer HOPE-ROP infants would progress to Th ROP than STOP-	Th ROP(adverse) or regressed ROP (positive)	HOPE-ROP infants progressed less frequently (25%) to Th ROP than STOP ROP (46%) but

Contd.

Table 20.1 *Summary of various clinical trials conducted in ROP (Contd.)*

Trial	Enrollment time	Inclusion criteria	Number	Endpoint (follow up)	Rationale (hypothesis)	Outcome measures	Outcomes
			same time from same 15 hospitals	ROP	ROP infants		when race, GA, PMA at PTh, zone I disease, plus disease at PTh were controlled the difference was snot significant, p = 0.0623
Vitamin E	Meta-analysis of controlled clinical trials (n = 6;1978–1981)	≤ 1500 g birth weight	536/704 infants received vitamin E prophylaxis and 551/714 were control; all completed trial	ROP	Antioxidant vitamin E reduces oxidative damage to particularly vulnerable PUFA of retina	Any ROP; Stage 3 + ROP	39.8% receiving vitamin E compared to 43.5% control had any ROP; 2.4% of vitamin E vs 5.3% of control developed stage 3 + ROP; p<0.02
Early treatment for retinopathy of prematurity (ETROP)	2000–2002	<1251 g birth weight; PTh	Multicentre trial; enrolled 7000 in 2 years. 401 consented to be in the study. Randomized into early or con treatment	9 mo corrected age	Early treatment (laser or Cryo) of eyes with > 15% of unfavourable outcome will reduce blindness (based on model integrating risk factors to assign a risk of blindness without treatment).	BCVA at 9 mo corrected age using teller acuity cards; Favourable result >1.85 cycles/second	Unfavourable visual acuity was 19.8% in conventional group to 14.3% (p<0.05) and unfavourable structural outcome was also reduced from 15.6–9.0% (p<0.0001) at 9 mo in type I ROP and trial supported wait and watch policy for type II ROP.

Contd.

Table 20.1 *Summary of various clinical trials conducted in ROP (Contd.)*

Trial	Enrollment time	Inclusion criteria	Number	Endpoint (follow up)	Rationale (hypothesis)	Outcome measures	Outcomes
Beat ROP	2008–2010	Intravitreal bevacizumab monotherapy for zone I or zone II posterior stage 3 plus ROP.	300 eyes of 150 infants, 143 infants survived	factor inhibitors	Vascular endo-thelial growth factor inhibitors may be useful in treating ROP without any destructive ablation. Infants were randomly assigned to receive intra-vitreal bevacizumab (0.625 mg in 0.025 ml of solution) or conventional laser therapy, bilaterally.	The primary ocular outcome was recurrence of ROP in one or both eyes requiring retreatment in 54 wk PMA	ROP recurred 4% in bevacizumab group and 22% in laser treated group. A significant treatment effect was found for zone I but not for zone II ROP

BIBLIOGRAPHY

1. An international committee for the classification of Retinopathy of Prematurity. The international classification of retinopathy of prematurity revisited. Arch Ophthalmol 2005; 123:991–9.

2. Capone A, Trese MT. Lens-sparing vitreous surgery for tractional stage 4A retinopathy of prematurity retinal detachments. Ophthalmology 2001; 108:2068–70.

3. Cryotherapy for Retinopathy of Prematurity Cooperative Group. The natural outcome of premature birth and retinopathy. Arch Ophthalmol 1994; 112:903–12.

4. Cryotherapy for Retinopathy of Prematurity Cooperative Group. Multicenter trial of cryotherapy for retinopathy of prematurity. Preliminary results. Arch Ophthalmol 1988; 106:471–9.

5. Cryotherapy for Retinopathy of Prematurity Cooperative group. Multicentric trial of cryotherapy for retinopathy of prematurity: natural history ROP: ocular outcome at 5½ years in premature infants with birth weight less than 1251 g. Arch Ophthalmol 2002; 120:595–9.

6. Cryotherapy for Retinopathy of Prematurity Cooperative Group. Multicenter Trial of Cryotherapy for Retinopathy of Prematurity Ophthalmological Outcomes at 10 Years Arch Ophthalmol 2001;119:1110–18.

7. Dogra MR, Narang S, Biswas C, Gupta A, Narang A. Threshold retinopathy of prematurity: ocular changes and sequelae following cryotherapy. Indian J Ophthalmol. 2001 Jun; 49(2):97–101.

8. Dutta S, Narang S, Narang A, Dogra M, Gupta A. Risk factors of threshold retinopathy of prematurity. Indian Pediatr 2004 Jul; 41(7):665–71.

9. Early treatment for Retinopathy of Prematurity Cooperative Group: Revised indications of treatment for retinopathy of prematurity: Results of Early treatment for Retinopathy of Prematurity randomized trial. Arch Ophthalmol 2003;121:1684–94.

10. Helen A. Mintz-Hittner, Kathleen A Kennedy, MD, Alice Z Chuang. BEAT-ROP Cooperative Group. Efficacy of Intravitreal Bevacizumab for Stage 3 + Retinopathy of Prematurity N Engl J Med 2011; 364:603–15.

11. International Committee for the classification of the late stages of Retinopathy of Prematurity. An international classification of Retinopathy of Prematurity: II. The classification of retinal detachment. Arch Ophthalmology 1987;105: 906–12.

12. Maguire AM and Trese MT. Visual results of lens-sparing vitreoretinal surgery in infants. J Pediatr Ophthalmol Strabismus 1993;30:28–32.

13. Palmer EA, Hardy RJ, Dobson V, et al. Cryotherapy for Retinopathy of Prematurity Cooperative group. 15 years outcome following threshold retinopathy of prematurity final results from multicentric trial of cryotherapy for retinopathy of prematurity. Arch Ophthalmol 2005;123:311–8.

14. Repka MS, Tung B, Good WV, et al. Outcome of eyes developing retinal detachment during the ETROP study. Arch Ophthalmol 2006; 124:24–30.

15. The Committee for the Classification of Retinopathy of Prematurity. An international classification of retinopathy of prematurity. Arch Ophthalmol 1984;102:1130–34.

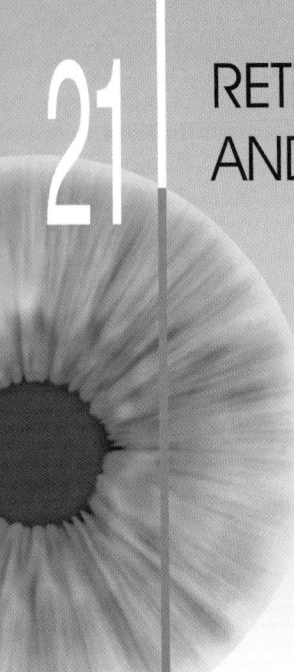

21 | RETINAL TELANGIECTASIA AND COATS' DISEASE

Sunandan Sood, Parul Chawla and Subina Narang

COATS' DISEASE

INTRODUCTION

Coats' disease is an idiopathic, ocular condition caused by a defect in the development of retinal vasculature, which is characterized by retinal telangiectasis, hemorrhage, intraretinal and subretinal exudation. It was first described in 1908 by Dr George Coats, a Scottish medical student, as a unilateral condition with retinal exudation and telangiectasis in male children. Coats originally classified disease into three groups:

i. Eyes without marked vascular disease
ii. Eyes with marked vascular disease
iii. Eyes with "large arteriovenous communications".

Groups (i) and (ii) were later grouped into exudative retinitis and group (iii) was later known as von Hippel angiomatosis retinae. Later, Leber defined a similar non-exudative retinal degeneration which was characterised by multiple retinal aneurysms rather than

telangiectasis and was termed *Lebermiliary aneurysms*. However, later on it was recognised as milder or earlier stages of Coats' disease. Subsequently, Shields et al defined Coats' disease as 'idiopathic retinal telangiectasia associated with intraretinal exudation and frequent exudative retinal detachment without signs of appreciable retinal or vitreal traction'.

Coats' disease can also be further differentiated into congenital or juvenile form (Coats' disease) and adult form in patients older than 30 years (Coats' reaction or Coats' syndrome). However, the clinical, pathologic and angiography findings are similar in both. The disease can present as early as first year of life and as late as eight decade of life. However, most of the cases (two-thirds) occur before 10 years of life. 90% of the disease is **unilateral** and 70–90% children are **boys.**

PATHOGENESIS AND CLASSIFICATION

Coats' disease is mostly a unilateral, progressive condition affecting mainly males during childhood, with the average age of diagnosis

ranging being between 8 and 16 years, although several cases have also been reported in adults. It is commonly described as 'light bulb telangiectasia' due to the large amounts of yellow exudates accompanying the disease (Fig. 21.1).

There are two pathological processes which are seen in Coats' disease. The first consists of a breakdown of the blood-retinal barrier at the endothelial level, which causing leakage of plasma into the vessel wall resulting in thickening of parts of the vessel wall, which may become necrotic and disorganized and give rise to a 'sausage-like' shape of the vessel. The second is related to the presence of abnormal pericytes and endothelial cells in retinal blood vessels, which subsequently degenerate, causing abnormal retinal vascula-ture and formation of aneurysms, as well as closure of vessels, leading to ischemia. The loss of endothelial cells and pericytes from the capillaries and the dilated telangiectatic arterioles cause leakage of a cholesterol-rich exudates, hemorrhage, cysts, edema, lymphocytic infiltration and fibrin deposition into the retina, which can lead to thickening of the retina, cystic changes or exudative retinal detachment.

Several studies assume that the condition is idiopathic whereas others suggest that there may be a genetic cause. It has recently been shown that Coats' disease could be a consequence of a mutation in the NDP gene, which results in a deficiency of norrin, a protein which is thought to be important for normal retinal vasculogenesis. Black et al reported a case of a mother with unilateral Coats' disease,

who gave birth to a son with Norrie disease, in which both had mutations in the NDP gene. Additionally, Coats' retinopathy has been associated with a variety of exudative retinopathies, as well as several conditions, including familial renal-retinal dystrophy (Senior-Loken syndrome), autosomal dominant fascioscapulohumeral muscular dystrophy (Hallermann-Streiff syndrome) and Turners syndrome.

Shields et al proposed the most recent classification system, as shown in Table 21.1. Patients can present with a range of signs, with the most common being decreased visual acuity, strabismus and leucocoria. Other signs that can be present in patients with Coats' disease are pain, heterochromia of the iris and nystagmus. Coats' disease is mainly a progressive condition, which can be asymptomatic in early stages and diagnosed during routine ophthalmologic examination.

CLINICAL FEATURES

The disease presents as strabismus, leucocoria or impaired vision (Fig. 21.1). There could be turbid fluid filling the anterior chamber. In cases the diagnosis is made on routine ophthalmoscopic examination, the characteristic findings are retinal telangiectasia and aneurysmal dilation ('light bulbs') of the retinal vasculature which may be associated with sheathing of the vessels by yellow cholesterol deposits. The majority of these vessels have been noted to be at the temporal and inferior quadrants. Fusiform aneurysms are more commonly seen rather than saccular aneurysms. At the initial stages, there may only be vascular abnormalities, but as the disease progresses, extensive intraretinal and subretinal exudation is seen (Fig. 21.2A and B). Advanced macular disease can be associated

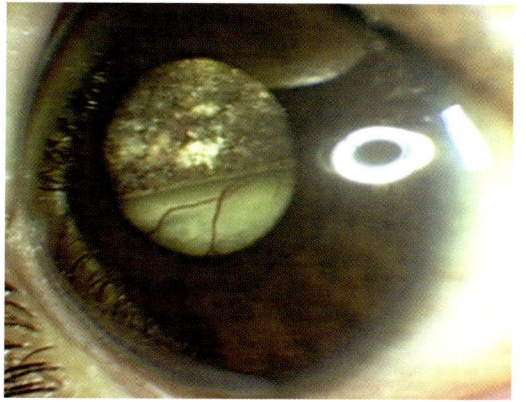

Fig. 21.1 *Coat's disease presenting as leucocoria*

Table 21.1 *Classification of Coats' disease*	
Stage	*Findings*
1	Retinal telangiectasia only.
2	Telangiectasia and exudation.
3a	Exudative subtotal retinal detachment.
3b	Exudative total retinal detachment.
4	Total retinal detachment and glaucoma.
5	Advanced end-stage disease.

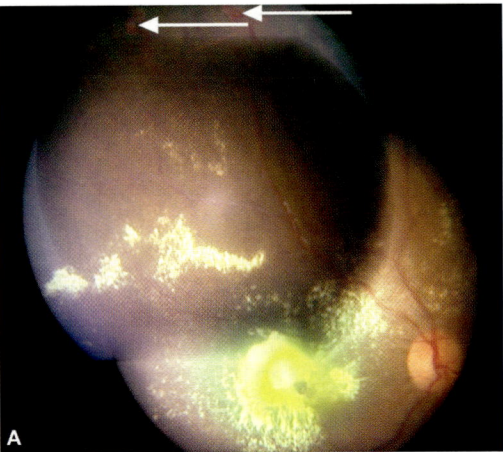

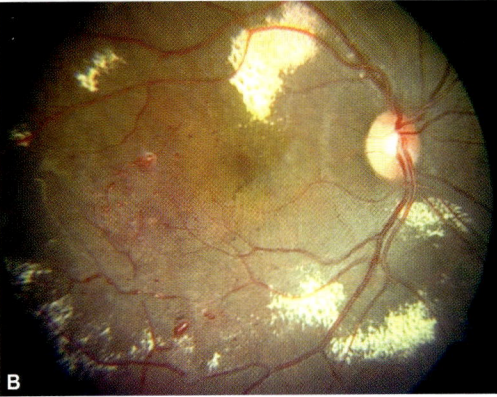

Fig. 21.2 (A) *A fundus picture showing dilated tortuous vessels (arrow) superiorly and massive macular as well as mid peripheral exudation in a young boy; and **(B)** fundus photo-graph showing retinal telangiectasia, aneurysmal dilatation and intraretinal and subretinal exudation in an adult patient of Coats' disease*

with macular fibrosis and formation of subfoveal nodules as well as macular holes. The vitreous commonly remains clear, until areas of vitreous condensation cause retinal detachment and vitreous hemorrhage. The vision may remain unaffected, till the vascular abnormalities are in the periphery, but can be affected as the exudates move towards the macular area. Macular edema can occur at the area of telangiectasia also.

DIFFERENTIAL DIAGNOSIS

In the **differential diagnosis** of Coats' disease, the most important lesion to be ruled out is **retinoblastoma.** It is considered to be the most common primary intraocular malignancy in

children, and as it could be fatal if left untreated, significant attention should be paid to its diagnosis. Mass lesion with calcification differentiates retinoblastoma from Coats' disease. Differentiation from diffuse infiltrative disease of retinoblastoma is difficult. Coats' disease misdiagnosed as retinoblastoma has also been reported to be the most common cause of wrongful enucleation. Calcification can also be seen in submacular nodule in Coats' disease or in phthisical eyes after Coats' disease. **Retinopathy of prematurity**, which causes abnormal peripheral retinal vascularisation due to peripheral avascular retina can be excluded since it is bilateral and occurs at a very early stage of life in premature infants. Additionally, we should take into account **familial exudative vitreoretinopathy** (FEVR) which has clinical features of a peripheral retinal fibrovascular mass, retrolental membranes, and exudative detachment and **persistent fetal vasculature syndrome or persistent hyper-plastic primary vitreous (PHPV)** which is characterized by retrolental fibrovascular membranes reminiscent of Norrie disease. It is observed in fullterm infants and is attributed to failure of regression of the hyaloid and vasculature. Involvement is usually unilateral but can be bilateral. Occurrence is usually sporadic but occasionally familial. In contrast to FEVR and Coats'disease, the involved eyes are often microphthalmic. **Haemangioblastoma von Hippel** (a phakomatosis involving central nervous system and viscera with a feeding arteriole and a draining venule). Retinal capillary hemangiomas seen in 50% of the patients are usually supplied by large, dilated feeder vessels, may occur in any part of the retina. Serum leakage from these vessels and hemangiomas leads to retinal exudates. Organized fibroglial bands with traction retinal detachment and vitreous hemorrhage may occur. **Incontinentia pigmenti** is a rare X-linked dominant disorder affecting the skin, hair, teeth, nails, and eyes. The eye phenotype is present in one third of affected individuals and resembles FEVR and Coats' disease. **Ocular toxocariasis**, which tend to be acquired, usually unilateral, infestation with the round-worm *Toxocaracanis*. In one form, a peripheral granulomatous mass

develops. Retinal traction may ensue, forming a retinal fold. The uveitis that can be associated with toxocariasis is not a feature of FEVR or Coats' disease.

Although, it is possible to reach a diagnosis from clinical examination alone, in the majority of cases, some form of ancillary testing is needed, including fluorescein angiography, ultrasound, computerized tomography (CT) and magnetic resonance imaging (MRI).

Fluorescein angiography plays a vital role in both diagnosis and assessment of disease progression. Telangiectasias cause early hyperfluorescence and exudation causes blocked hypofluorescence (Fig. 21.3). Moreover, in larger blood vessels, the aneurysms will be clearly visible, characteristically described as 'light bulb' dilations.

Ultrasonography can also be a useful diagnostic tool, as shown by Atta and Watson. The typical features of Coats' disease on ultrasound is subretinal opacities due to cholesterolosis present from the exudates, as

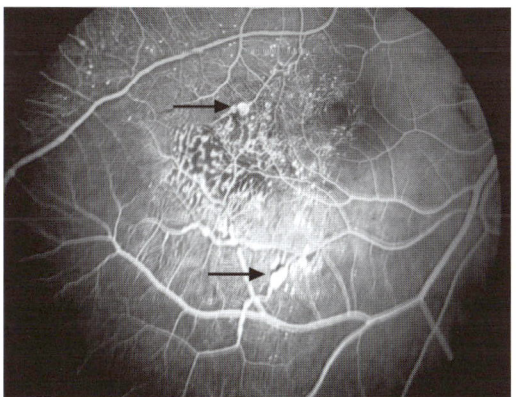

Fig. 21.3A *Fundus fluorescein angiogram showing early hyperfluorescence due to telangiectasia, 'aneurysmal dilatation seen as "light bulb" sign (arrow heads). Exudation cause blocked fluorescence*

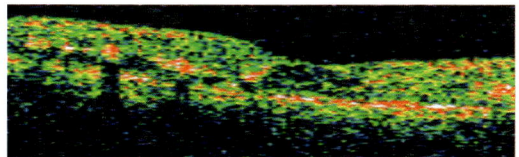

Fig. 21.3B *Prelaser OCT vertical scan shows spongiform macular thickness*

well as retinal detachment which is visualized as a linear echo. It can also be used to exclude retinoblastoma, as it allows visualization of the intraocular space and no mass lesion is seen.

CT too can be very useful to rule out retinoblastoma. Patients with retinoblastoma can present with solid tumors and calcifications, visualized with CT, whereas in Coats' disease these lesions would be absent. However, it should be noted that CT may not be useful in distinguishing cases of retinoblastoma without calcification, which can be seen in up to 46% of the retinoblastomas. On the other hand, recently cases of Coats' disease have been seen where there has been intraocular bone formation alongside the vascular and exudative retinopathy, showing a calcification in both CT and ultrasound. Moreover, in advanced Coats' disease, in up to 20% of cases, a submacular nodule may be formed and calcified. In advanced cases, CT can also show the lipid exudate as a hyperdense area within the orbit, as well as a retinal detachment but without any mass lesion.

MRI is also extremely useful in the diagnosis of advanced Coats' disease, but may have lesser utility during the initial stages of the disease. MRI is superior to CT, in ruling out retinoblastoma as the difference between subretinal exudation and a solid mass is clearer on MRI. Being more specific, the exudate in Coats' disease is hyperintense on both T1-weighted and T2-weighted MRI images, whereas in retinoblastoma, T1 weighted image will show a hyperintense mass, but T2-weighted image shows a hypointense mass. Eisenberg et al also utilized magnetic resnonance spectroscopy, which can provide biochemical information non-invasively from various body tissues. Also, the use of gadolinium contrast may also aid in the differential diagnosis of retinoblastoma as it enhances the solid tumors like retinoblastoma, which is not seen in Coats' disease.

In the majority of cases, invasive diagnostic modalities, such as **fine-needle aspiration (FNA)**, are not recommended, however, FNA can be used to confirm the diagnosis when non-invasive modalities are not diagnostic. Shields

et al emphasised that FNA is contra-indicated if there is a total retinal detachment or if there is a strong clinical suspicion of retinoblastoma.

TREATMENT

If left untreated 64% patients developed total retinal detachment and 32% developed secondary glaucoma. Spontaneous regression of telangiectasias is rarely noticed. There are several treatment modalities for Coats' disease, depending on its stage and they are briefly summarized in Table 21.2. The main aim of treatment in mild disease is ablation of the abnormal retinal vasculature, preservation of vision and prevention of disease progression to retinal detachment. For many years, the main treatment options have been laser photo-coagulation and cryotherapy, especially for mild or moderate stages of the disease. In more advanced disease, where there are extensive telangiectasias, retinal detachment and widespread exudation, laser photocoagulation and cryotherapy can still be used, although vitreoretinal surgery may be more effective and in severe cases enucleation may be necessary or simply observation depending upon the magnitude of pain.

Laser photocoagulation is useful to ablate and cauterise the retinal vasculature and can be used in mild disease with limited exudation,

corresponding to stages 1, 2 and 3a according to the Shields' classification. Argon lasers are most commonly used and often up to five sessions may be required for adequate regression of the disease (Fig. 21.4A to C). Laser is usually only effective when the retina is attached. Schefler et al. also showed that in patients with advanced disease and subtotal retinal detachment, they were able to preserve some vision with laser treatment. Until now, laser photocoagulation is thought to be the best option for early stages of Coats' disease. If thick exudation is present, laser treatment may not be particularly useful, as it may not be able to reach the vessels, and in these cases, cryotherapy is preferred.

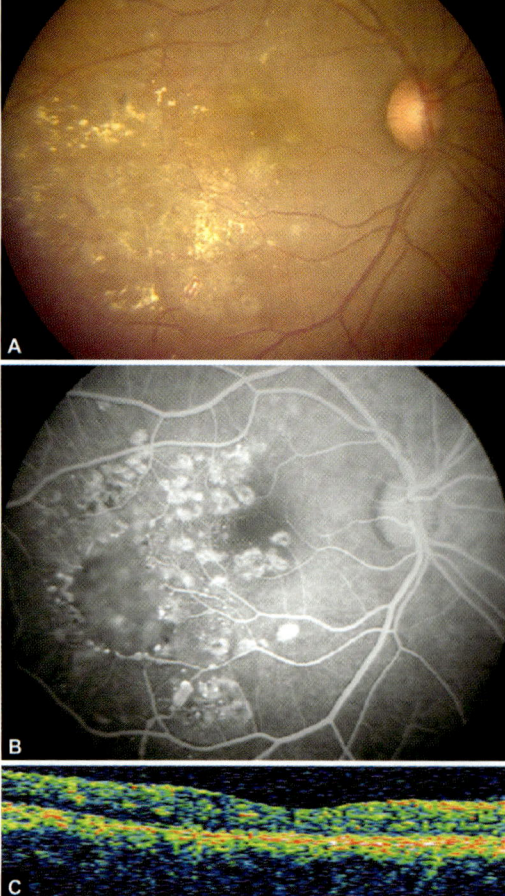

Fig. 21.4 *Laser photocoagulation in a patient of Coats' disease*

Table 21.2 *Treatment modalities according to stage of the disease*

Stage	Treatment
Mild disease (1, 2)	Laser photocoagulation/ cryotherapy
Mild disease (1, 2) without progression	Observation — no treatment
Advanced disease (3, 4)	Vitreoretinal surgery
Advanced end-stage disease (5) with painful eye	Enucleation
Advanced end-stage disease (5) with comfortable eye	Observation — no treatment
Adjuvant therapy	Intravitreal triamcino-lone
Adjuvant therapy	Anti-VEGF agents

Cryotherapy is used in Coats disease especially in patients presenting with exudative disease and retinal detachment, which corresponds to stages 1–3b of the Shields' classification. When laser photocoagulation is not possible, even being the treatment of choice for mild Coats disease, cryotherapy is utilized and believed to be more effective than laser in more advanced cases. It is used as primary treatment in up to 42% of patients. Like laser photocoagulation, it may require multiple sessions, however, if it is excessive, it may conversely lead to an increase in subretinal exudation and an increase in retinal detachment. Therefore, it is advisable to use it for only up to two quadrants at a time, with a gap of one month between treatments. Laser photocoagulation and cryotherapy are not recommended in cases of total retinal detachment.

In severe forms of Coats' disease, there is a variety of treatment options, with **vitreoretinal surgery** playing a major role in late-stage Coats' disease. Vitrectomy for eyes with Stage 3a Coats disease also may be effective for visual prognosis compared to conventional therapy, i.e., laser photocoagulation and cryotherapy, by enabling retinal attachment in the early postoperative period and by causing the foveal exudation to disappear. In the vitrectomy, posterior vitreous detachment has either occurred previously or it is induced. An intentional retinal hole is made and the subretinal fluid and exudates is drained through the hole. The abnormal vessels are coagulated by endodiathermy and/or laser photocoagula-tion. The vitreous fluid is replaced with long-lasting gas or air.

Recent reports suggest, **intravitreal triamcinolone (IVTA)** has been found to be effective in the treatment of Coats' disease as an adjuvant therapy. Othman et al showed an improvement in visual acuity, as well as absorption of subretinal fluid and macular exudates in 15 consecutive patients having been treated with intravitreal triamcinolone in combination with other treatment modalities, such as laser photocoagulation and/or cryopexy. This is in accordance with other reports which also suggest an improvement in visual acuity, a decrease in central retinal thick-

ness, resolution of exudates and no recurrence at an average 6-month follow-up, in patients treated with intravitreal triamcinolone as an adjuvant therapy. However, a very common complication is a possible development of cataract and glaucoma that could restrict its use.

The latest development in the treatment of Coat's disease has been the use of anti-vascular endothelial growth factor (**anti-VEGF**) agents. Kaul et al recommend, it as a future adjunctive treatment alongside traditional therapies, which is in accordance with the majority of other authors, as it seems to reduce macular edema and exudates, improve or even stabilize visual acuity and expedite the regression of dilated abnormal vessels. On the contrary, Ramasubramanian et al suggested that bevacizumab should be used with caution, as vitreoretinal fibrosis and, more importantly, traction retinal detachment were found in patients treated with bevacizumab in addition to standard therapy, but not in patients receiving only standard measures. It is also very impor-tant to mention that anti-VEGF agents can be used only if the diagnosis of Coats' disease is confirmed and retinoblastoma excluded as it is known that intraocular injections can cause seeding of extraocular tissue in some cases of retino-blastoma.

Enucleation may also be required in some cases of Coats' disease and is carried out in approximately 16% of patients with confirmed Coats' disease, complicated with neovascular glaucoma, pain, nausea and vomiting.

ADULT COATS' DISEASE

Coats' disease can first be diagnosed in adulthood with unilateral retinal vascular abnormalities similar to those seen in younger patients. There are a number of important differences in disease manifestation in adults, including limited area of involvement, slower apparent progression of disease, and hemorrhage near larger vascular dilatations.

In adult patients, vascular abnormalities appear in the equatorial and peripheral regions in all the patients and also in the juxtamacular region in the majority of patients. Lipid deposition and exudation, frequently massive

and diffuse in children, is localized and limited in the adults. Hemorrhage, less common in typical Coats' disease in young patients, occurred in many adult patients, with the bleeding localized to macroaneurysms. Coats' disease in adults seems to advance at a slower rate than it does in children, with the majority of patients reaching a stable final visual acuity (Fig. 21.2B).

IDIOPATHIC JUXTAFOVEAL TELANGIECTASIA

INTRODUCTION

Idiopathic juxtafoveal telangiectasia (also known as idiopathic parafoveal, perifoveal or macular telangiectasia or telangiectasis) is a term used for various disease conditions presenting with incompetence, ectasia, and/or irregular dilations of the capillary network affecting only the juxtafoveal region of one or both eyes. These entities are distinguished from more generalized retinal telangiectasia (such as in Coats' disease) or secondary juxtafoveal telangiectasia due to retinal vein occlusions, diabetes, irradiation, or carotid artery obstruction.

TERMINOLOGY AND CLASSIFICATION

The term *idiopathic juxtafoveal telangiectasia* (IJFT) was coined by Gass and Oyakawa in 1982, who gave the first classification of these entities into four groups based largely on their clinical and fluorescein angiographic (FA) features. In 1993, Gass and Blodi further updated this classification, by subdividing IJFT into three distinct groups I, II, and III (also known as groups 1, 2, and 3), with two subgroups in each (A and B), based on demographic difference or clinical severity (Table 21.3). Each main group had an independent etiology. **Group I** was **congenital** and predominantly presenting in **males** with **unilateral** telangiectasia and macular edema. **Group II** was **acquired bilateral** telangiectasia with atrophy of the fovea. **Group III** was extremely **rare** and characterized by **progressive obliteration** of the perifoveal capillary network. This classification, based on clinical examination and angiographic findings comprised additional

staging for IJFT group II into five stages. Despite its complexity, the Gass-Blodi classification is the most commonly used to date.

The most common IJFT is group IIA followed by group I and Group III is extremely rare. Hence, only group IIA and group I are discussed in detail and for the description of the other types, the readers are advised to consult reference books and suggested reading. Gass and Blodi have further described the five stages of group IIA (Table 22.4):

Yannuzzi et al. proposed a simplified classification of IJFT, which was a revision and simplification of the Gass-Blodi model. They coined the term "idiopathic macular telangiectasia" with two distinct types: Type 1 or "aneurysmal telangiectasia" equivalent to IJFT group I (A and B combined), which is the second most common form of IJFT; and type 2 or "perifoveal telangiectasia" equivalent to IJFT group IIA, the most common type of IJFT. The remaining types described by Gass and Blodi (group IIB and groups IIIA and B) were omitted from Yannuzzi's classification because of their rarity. Yannuzzi et al. also simplified the five stages of group IIA proposed by Gass and Blodi into two distinct stages which have clinical, therapeutic, and prognostic relevance: non-proliferative and proliferative stage (Table 21.4).

GROUP I: IDIOPATHIC JUXTAFOVEAL TELANGIECTASIA ("IDIOPATHIC MACULAR TELANGIECTASIA TYPE 1" OR "ANEURYSMAL TELANGIECTASIA")

CLINICAL FEATURES

This congenital or developmental form of IJFT occurs mostly in males and is typically unilateral (97% of cases). Although the onset of symptoms can occur at any age, the mean age at presentation is 40 years. On fundus examination, prominent telangiectatic retinal capillaries, with aneurysmal dilations of various sizes are a typical hallmark feature of this type of IJFT. The telangiectasia usually involve a two-disc diameter area or greater temporal to the fovea. Macular edema and lipid deposition is also a characteristic feature. No blunted right-angled venules, superficial vitreoretinal interface crystalline deposits, plaques of retinal pigment

Table 21.3 *Classification of idiopathic juxtafoveal telangiectasia*

	I–A:	I–B:	II–A:	II–B:	III–A:	III–B:
According to Gass and Blodi	*Visible and exudative*	*Visible, exudative and focal*	*Occult and non-exudative*	*Juvenile, occult and familial*	*Occlusive*	*Occlusive associated with central nervous system vasculopathy*
Frequency	Second most common	Rare	Most common	Extremely rare	Very rare	Very rare
Gender	Male (90%)	Male	Male=Female	2 siblings	Female	Male=Female
Age (mean yrs)	15–54 (40)	middle age	35–65 (56)	< 12 yrs	40–60	middle age
Congenital/acquired	Congenital	Congenital	Acquired	Acquired	Acquired	Dominant inheritance
Biomicroscopic features						
laterality	Unilateral	Unilateral	Bilateral (asymmetric)	Bilateral	Bilateral	Bilateral
Juxtafoveolar telangiectasis location	Temporal half of macula	Temporal half of macula	Temporal to fovea++++ up to entire perifovea	Temporal to fovea	Perifoveal	Perifoveal
Juxtafoveolar telangiectasis size	≥ 2DD	< 2 clock hours	≈ 1DD around foveola	Small	Variable	Variable
Visual acuity at presentation	≈ 20/40	≥ 20/25	20/20–20/300	NM	20/25–20/50	variable
Visible macular edema	+++	±	–(unless SRNV)	–	NM	NM
Loss of retinal transparency	+	±	+	+	+	NM
Easily visible microaneurysms/telangiectasis	+++	+	–	–	+	+
Yellow exudates	+	±	–(unless SRNV)	–	Minimal	Minimal
Blunted right-angled venules	–	–	+	–	–	–
Superficial crystalline deposits	–	–	+	–	–	–
Intraretinal pigment plaques/hyperplasia	–	–	+	–	–	–
Fibrous metaplasia	–	–	+	NM	–	–
Subretinal neovascularization/RCA	–	–	+ (in stage 5)	+ (OU)	–	–
Fluorescein Angiographic features						
Visible telangiectasia	+++	±	±	±	± *	+
Late intraretinal staining	+	+	+	+	+	Minimal
Capillary occlusion	Minimal	–	–	NM	+++ *	+++
Cause of vision loss	Macular oedema, exudation	No visual loss	Foveal atrophy SRNV	SRNV	Capillary occlusion and obstruction	Capillary occlusion and obstruction
Systemic associations	None	None	Possible diabetes mellitus	None	Polycythemia, hypoglycemia, gouty arthritis, ulcerative colitis, multiple myeloma, chronic lymphocytic leukemia	CNS involvement, extra macular telangiectasis

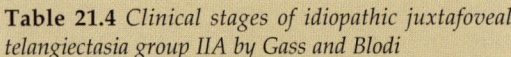

Table 21.4 *Clinical stages of idiopathic juxtafoveal telangiectasia group IIA by Gass and Blodi*

Stage 1	No biomicroscopic abnormality, no or minimal capillary dilation, mild staining of outer perifoveal retina.
Stage 2	Slight graying of perifoveolar retina, no or minimal biomicroscopically visible telangiectatic vessels, but capillary telangiectasia of outer capillary network temporally on fundus autofluorescence.
Stage 3	One or several slightly dilated and blunted retinal venules descending into outer perifovea, typically temporally.
Stage 4	Pigment hyperplasia, often surrounding right-angle venules.
Stage 5	Subretinal neovascularization, often in proximity to intraretinal pigment migration.

epithelial hyperplasia, intraretinal pigment migration or subretinal neovascularization are seen in this type of IJFT.

On fluorescein angiography (FA), the telangiectatic vessels are easily visible straddling the horizontal raphe and filling rapidly in both the superficial and deep juxtafoveolar capillary plexus. Minimal nonperfusion or capillary ischemia exists sometimes and is easily visible on FA. Central cystic or noncystic macular edema is evident angiographically as late intraretinal staining and confirmed with OCT in all cases. The OCT characteristically demonstrates increased central retinal thickness and fluid-filled spaces. In some patients, shallow detachments of the macula visible only with OCT are seen. On ultra-high resolution OCT (UHR-OCT), abnormally large intraretinal blood vessels located near the fovea and deep in the outer nuclear layer can be visualized. Müller cells bodies span the separation between the outer nuclear layer and outer plexiform layer. The outer retina (i.e., outer nuclear layer, external limiting membrane, and inner segment/outer segment junction), remains uninvolved.

Macular edema and exudation are the main cause of visual loss in these patients. Some patients retain excellent VA for years without treatment. In some cases, spontaneous resolu-tion may occur. If progressive visual loss occurs however, treatment with laser photocoagulation may be effective in reducing the exudation and improving or stabilizing vision.

In addition to the juxtafoveal vascular lesions, which are essential for the diagnosis, this group of IJFT may also develop focal vascular changes in the mid-peripheral fundus and even in the more anterior fundus. In fact Gass et al believed that this group of IJFT may be a localized form or part of the spectrum of congenital retinal telangiectasia or Coats' disease, identical to what Leber had previously described as miliary aneurysms of the retina. Similarly, Yannuzzi et al considered aneurysmal telangiectasia to be a type of Coats' disease that is found in the macula. On histopathology, the findings of IJFT I are consistent with the clinical observa-tions of dilation of capillaries, aneurysms, leakage, and minimal nonperfusion.

Gass and Blodi identified a separate subgroup of IJFT I named group IB carrying identical features described above but confined to two-clock hours or less in the juxtafoveolar areas with much better VA.

DIFFERENTIAL DIAGNOSIS

When IJFT I is suspected, it must be differen-tiated from secondary telangiectasis caused by retinal vascular diseases such as retinal venous occlusions, diabetic retinopathy, radiation retinopathy, sickle cell maculopathy, ocular ischemic syndrome/carotid artery obstruction, hypertensive retinopathy, polycythemia vera retinopathy, and a localized retinal capillary hemangioma. In addition, IJFT I should also be differentiated from dilated perifoveal capillaries with evidence of vitreous cellular infiltration secondary to acquired inflammatory disease, or from Coats' disease which is defined by extensive peripheral retinal telangiectasis, exudative retinal detachment, relatively young age of onset, and male predilection. Less commonly, macular telangiectasis has been described in association with fascio-scapulo-humeral muscular dystrophy, incontinent a pigmenti, and familial exudative vitreo-retinopathy with posterior pole involvement.

TREATMENT

Treatment options for IJFT I include laser photocoagulation, intravitreal injections of steroids, or antivascular endothelial growth factor (VEGF) agents. Photocoagulation was recommended by Gass and it still remains the mainstay of treatment. It seems to be successful in causing resolution of exudation and VA improvement or stabilization in many eyes. Photocoagulation should be used sparingly to reduce the chance of producing a symptomatic paracentral scotoma and metamorphopsia. Small burns (100–200 μm) of moderate intensity in a grid-pattern are recommended. Dilated capillaries on the edge of the capillary-free zone should always be avoided.

Intravitreal injections of triamcinolone acetonide (IVTA) have proved to be beneficial in the treatment of macular edema by means of their anti-inflammatory effect, their down-regulation of VEGF production, and the stabilization of the blood retinal barrier. However, the effect of IVTA is short-lived and complications, mainly increased intraocular pressure and cataract, limit its use.

Indocyanine green angiography-guided laser photocoagulation directed at the leaky micro-aneurysms and vessels combined with posterior sub-Tenon's injection of triamcinolone acetonide has also been reported in a limited number of patients with IJFT I with improve-ment or stabilization of vision after a mean follow-up of 10 months. Further studies are needed to validate the efficacy of this treatment modality.

Recently, intravitreal injections of anti-VEGF agents, namely bevacizumab, a humanized monoclonal antibody targeted against pro-angiogenic, circulatory VEGF, and ranibizumab, a FDA-approved monoclonal antibody frag-ment that targets all VEGF-A isoforms, have shown improved visual outcome and reduced leakage in macular edema due to diabetes and retinal venous occlusions. It is likely that patients of IJFT I with macular edema from leaky telangiectasia may benefit from intra-vitreal anti-VEGF injections, but this requires further studies.

Today, laser photocoagulation remains most effective, but the optimal treatment of IJFT I is questioned, and a larger series comparing different treatment modalities is required. The rarity of the disease however, makes it difficult to assess in a randomized controlled manner.

GROUP IIA: IDIOPATHIC JUXTAFOVEAL TELANGIECTASIA ("IDIOPATHIC MACULAR TELANGIECTASIA TYPE 2" OR "PERIFOVEAL TELANGIECTASIA")

CLINICAL FEATURES AND NATURAL HISTORY

This is the most common type of IJFT, and differs completely from IJFT I. It is acquired, not congenital. Affected patients are middle-aged or older (mean 55 years). Males and females are affected equally. This disorder is bilateral, but may be asymmetric appearing unilaterally in its early stages. Initially, the patients are asympto-matic but subsequently patients have gradual painless loss of vision. Metamorphopsia is a frequent symptom in IJFT IIA which was reported to be present in 83% of eyes with nonproliferative IJFT IIA. It has been subdivided by Gass and Blodi into five stages (Table 21.4).

In *Stage 1*, patients are generally asympto-matic. A slight loss of the retinal transparency, typically grayish appearance usually in the temporal juxtafoveal area is mostly the only finding seen. Fluorescein angiography is required for detection and shows no evidence of capillary dilation, but mild late retinal staining of the outer juxtafoveal retina surrounding a part or whole of the foveolar border but sparing the foveola itself is seen (Fig. 21.5A to H).

In *Stage 2*, patients may be asymptomatic or have minimal disturbances in central vision such as blurred vision, metamorphopsia, or paracentral positive scotoma. A slight graying of the parafoveolar retina approximately one disc diameter in size, confined temporally is seen. The foveal center is spared and may appear thinned out. The telangiectasia is minimally or not visible, hence the term "occult" as opposed to the easily visible telangiectasia of IJFT I. Superficial crystals may be seen. There is little or no thickening. FA demonstrates early staining of the thickened walls of the outer capillary network, mostly temporally, followed by diffuse late staining in the middle and outer retina (Fig. 21.6A to F).

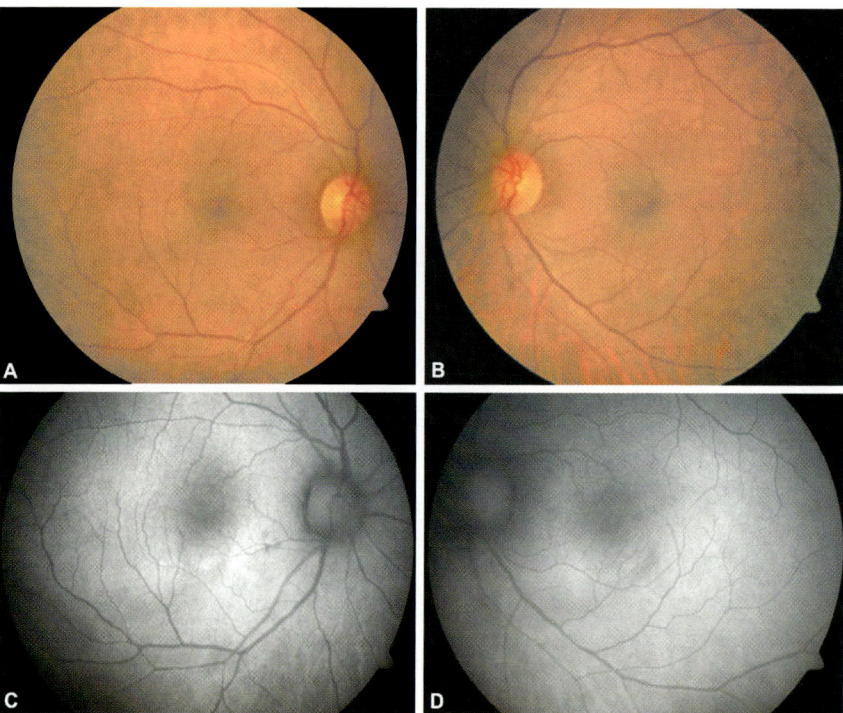

Fig. 21.5 *Fundus examination of a 64-year-old woman with blurred vision showed no biomicroscopic abnormality* **(A and B)**. *Fundus autofluorescence was normal* **(C and D)** *(Courtesy: Prof. Amod Gupta)*

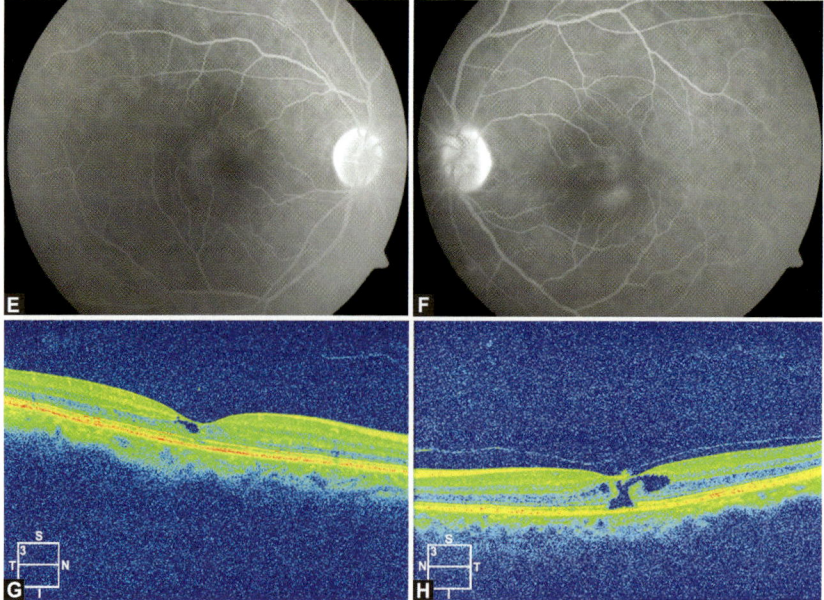

Fig. 21.5 *Fluorescein angiography showed mild staining of foveal capillaries in the late phase* **(E and F)**. *Optical coherence tomography scan through the fovea showed a hyporeflective area in the inner retinal layers in right eye* **(G)** *and all retinal layers in the left eye* **(H)** *(Courtesy: Prof. Amod Gupta)*

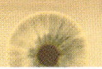

In *Stage 3*, patients may experience decreased vision, which is slow in onset and progression. Paracentral vertically oriented and slightly dilated right-angled venules draining the telangiectatic area are seen on fundus examination temporally. These vessels have

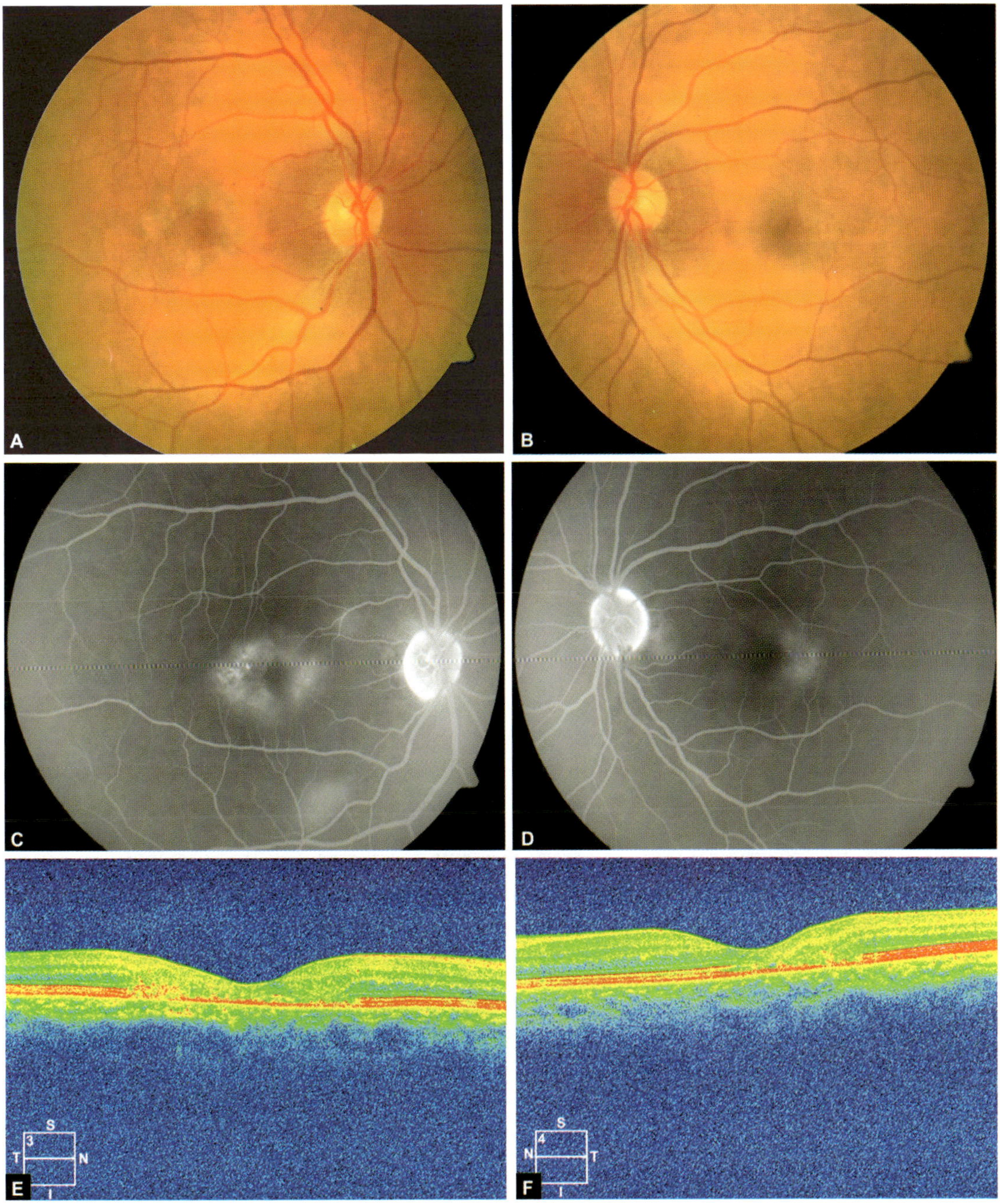

Fig. 21.6 *Fundus examination of a 50-year-old woman with decreased vision showed area of retinal greying all around the fovea in right eye* **(A)** *and temporal to fovea in the left eye* **(B)**. *Fluorescein angiography showed staining from telangiectatic vessels* **(C and D)**, *including photoreceptor-RPE complex.* **(E and F)** *Optical coherence tomography scan showed atrophy of all retinal layers in the foveal region in both eyes). (Courtesy: Prof. Amod Gupta)*

both a venule and an arteriole that in combination leads to a network of proliferating vessels in the deep retinal layers. Prominent dilation of the capillaries may be seen clinically. The foveolar depression may simulate macular hole. FA often shows unusual capillary dilation and permeability changes in the outer retina causing the retinal staining. However, there is no fluid causing ballooning or cystic spaces in the outer plexiform layer (as occurs in eyes with IJFT I) on OCT (Fig. 21.7A to H).

In *Stage 4*, as a result of RPE migration into the retina along the course of the right-angled vessels, one or more foci of black retinal

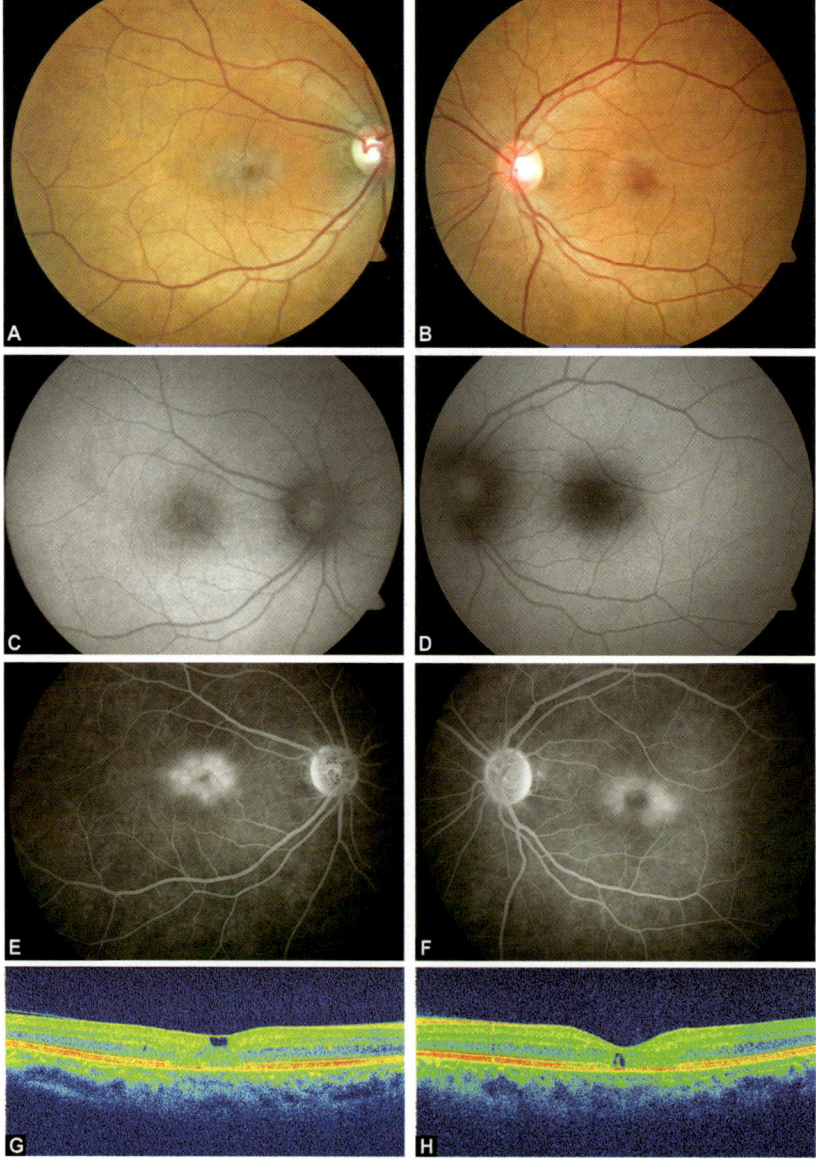

Fig. 21.7 *Fundus examination (A and B) as well as fundus autofluorescence (C and D) of a 47-year-old woman with decreased vision showed parafoveal dilated and blunted retinal venules. Fluorescein angiography showed capillary dilatation with leakage (E and F). Optical coherence tomography scan through the fovea showed a hyporeflective area in the inner retinal layers in the right eye (G) and outer retinal layers in the left eye (H), suggesting a localized loss of these layers. (Courtesy: Prof. Amod Gupta)*

pigmented epithelial hyperplasia or clumps may be seen around the parafoveolar right-angled vessels. In some cases, the pigment extends into the inner retina and forms an irregular or stellate shaped plaque enveloping the right angled-vessel (Fig. 21.8A to D).

Stage 5 is marked by subretinal neo-vascularisation (SRNV) which occurs as a result of retinal capillary remodelling, proliferation, and invasion of the outer retina which has progressively atrophied. A subretinal network, often with a retino-retinal anastomosis (RRA) or retinal-subretinal anastomosis is seen. Retino-choroidal anastomosis may also exist. The SRNV usually occurs temporally, often near the intraretinal pigment epithelial migration or unrelated to the latter. Rapid visual decline follows as the SRNV causes exudation, neuro-sensory elevation, intra and subretinal

hemorrhage, and fibrovascular proliferation. These features are evident clinically and angio-graphically. On FA, the SRNV has angiographic features similar to classic neovascularization demonstrating early lacy hyperfluorescence which increases and leaks in the late phases of the angiogram. However, it is not associated with RPE detachment and its final size is generally smaller compared to classic choroidal neovascularization in AMD and visual acuity does not deteriorate any further. The fibrovascular tissues remodelling leads to retinal vascular distortion and dragging of neighbouring venules and arterioles into the tissue itself. At any stage (Stages 2–5), tiny golden crystals may be seen near the retinal surface often anterior to the retinal vessels over the area of telangiectasis. This is an inconsistent feature (Fig. 21.9A to F).

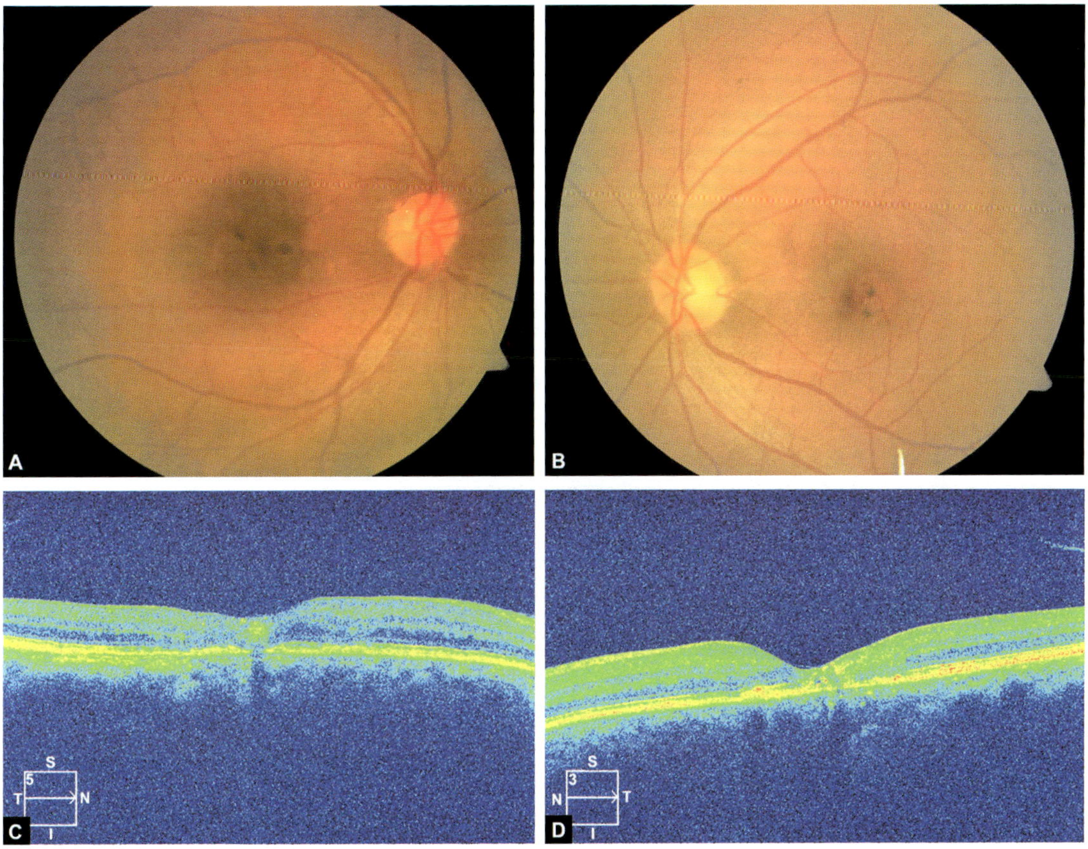

Fig. 21.8 *Fundus examination (**A and B**) of a 65-year-old man with decreased vision showed black stellate foci of RPE hyperpigmentation at the end of retinal venules. OCT through the fovea showed foveal atrophy with hyperplasia of RPE extending in the inner retinal layers (**C and D**). (Courtesy: Prof. Amod Gupta)*

Three key and distinguishing features of IJFT IIA are:

1. The absence of prominent aneurysms or hemorrhage

2. The absence of cystic macular edema or lipid exudation (unless SRNV has developed). The loss of retinal transparency and fluorescein staining are primarily caused by intracellular

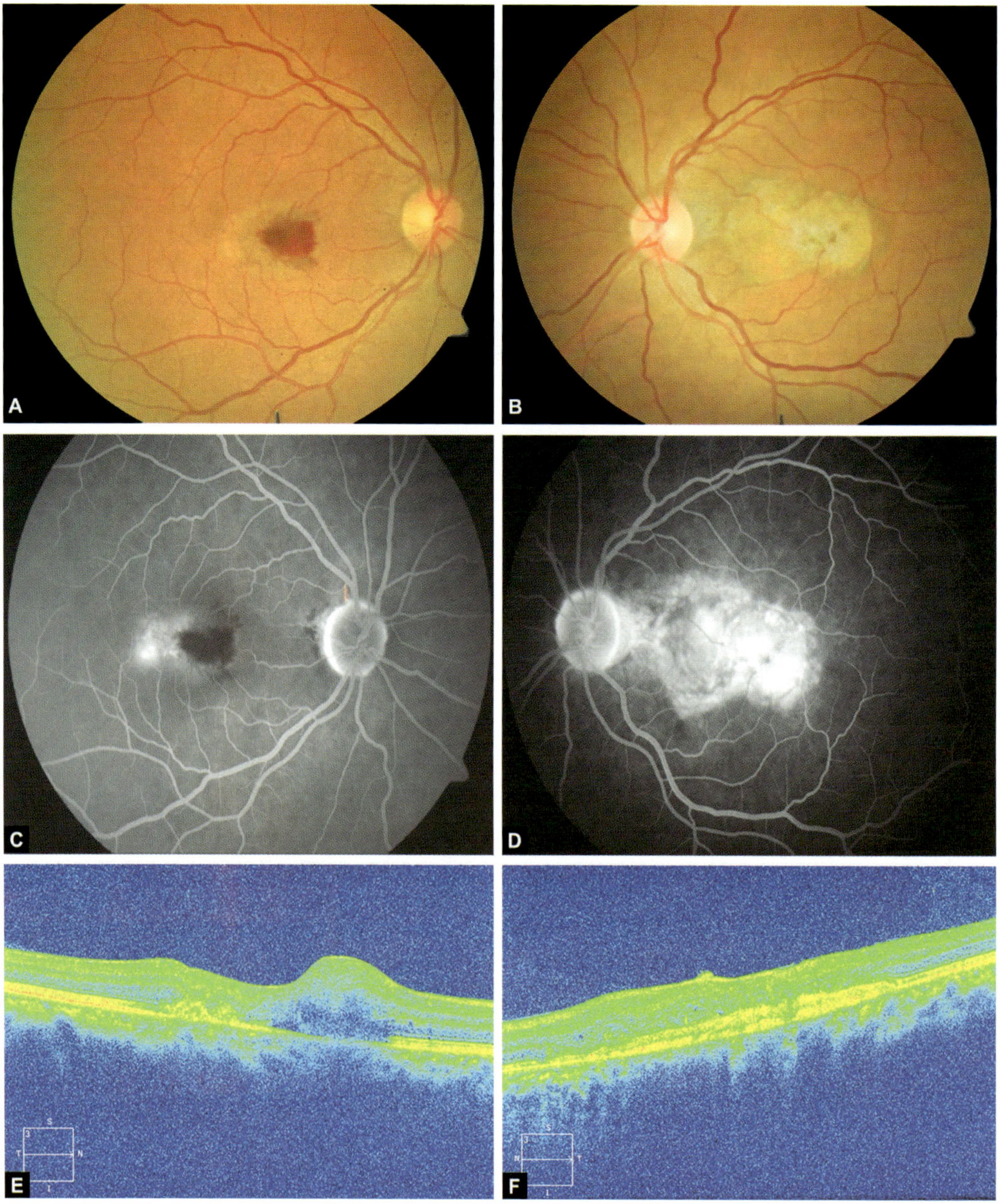

Fig. 21.9 *Fundus examination of a 64-year-old man with decreased vision showed a hemorrhage in the macula of right eye with area of retinal greying temporal to it (A) Left eye had a macular scar of an old choroidal neovascular membrane (CNVM) (B) Fluorescein angiography showed leakage temporal to haemorrhage suggesting a CNVM in the right eye (C) and window defect with staining of scar tissue in the left eye (D) OCT of right eye showed intraretinal thickening corresponding to the hemorrhage due to a CNVM temporal to it (E) and a hyperreflective complex in deep retinal layers suggesting a CNVM scar in the left eye (F) (Courtesy: Prof. Amod Gupta)*

edema (contrary to the extracellular fluid causing CME and lipid exudation in IJFT I); and

3. The presence of foveolar atrophy, best seen with OCT which can simulate a lamellar macular hole. Foveal atrophy is the primary cause of the slow progressive visual loss occurring over years in these patients (to 20/200 or worse), distinguishable from the rapid and severe visual loss that may occur with the advent of SRNV and fibrosis.

The five stages were simplified by yannuzzi et al into two distinct stages that have clinical, prognostic, and therapeutic implications: non-proliferative stage (Stages 1–4), characterized by telangiectasis and foveal atrophy without SRNV, and proliferative stage (Stage 5 of Gass and Blodi) defined by the presence of SRNV and fibrosis. The pathogenesis of subretinal proliferation is similar to the neovascular form of age-related macular degeneration known as retinal angiomatous proliferation (RAP).

The thickening of retinal capillaries due to marked proliferation of the basement membrane and narrowing of the caliber of the lumen with degeneration of pericytes, and occasionally endothelial cells, has been reported in IJFT. Intracellular and extracellular edema, especially prominent in the inner retinal layers has been observed.

IJFT IIA is the most common type of IJFT. It has been reported in monozygotic twins as well as in siblings and families.

RETINAL IMAGING

OCT in IJFT

The following OCT features have been described in IJFT IIA:

1. Central foveolar thickening is consistently absent, and intraretinal edema is either absent or minimal. Thinning and disruption of photoreceptor layer, as seen on UHR-OCT, is common, confirming that foveal atrophy is the primary cause for reduced vision. This disruption is found to correlate with VA in 63% of eyes and increases with advancing disease.

2. Cyst-like structures in the foveola and inner retinal layers are very common (50–100% of eyes with Stage 3 or higher). They are referred to as "cystoids," have variable size and are not seen clinically or on FA. Because of the consistent absence of associated cystoid macular edema or petaloid pooling on FA, these cysts are not a result of exudation, but rather due to a progressive retinal tissue loss. At the foveola, the inner lamellar cyst appears as a loss of tissue with the ILM spanning across it and draping over it. This unique feature, the ILM drape, may be specific to IJFT II. Full-thickness macular holes are uncommon in IJFT IIA but have been reported.

3. Blunting of the foveal pit is common to all stages. Foveal flattening or thinning is encountered with more advanced disease.

4. Intraretinal neovascularization near the foveola, seen as highly reflective dots in the inner and outer nuclear layers is found in 21% of eyes.

5. Central intraretinal hyper-reflective lesions that cause posterior shadowing and correspond to hyperpigmented RPE plaques are observed.

All of the changes mentioned above (foveal cyst, intraretinal RPE hyperplasia, foveal atrophy, and absence of edema) are consistent with the hypothesis of progressive retinal tissue loss, possibly due to Müller cells degeneration.

Adaptive optics imaging

In recent years, confocal reflectance imaging using the confocal scanning laser ophthalmoscope (cSLO; HRA2, Heidelberg Engineering, Heidelberg, Germany), has emerged as a very sensitive and noninvasive method for the diagnosis of IJFT IIA, monitoring its progression as well differentiating it from other conditions. Confocal blue reflectance (CBR) imaging (at 488 nm) is very helpful in the diagnosis of the early stages of IJFT IIA showing a well-defined generally oval parafoveal area of increased reflectance that corresponds to, but is slightly larger than, the area of leakage in late-phase angiography. Confocal infrared reflectance (at 820 nm), on the other hand, is helpful in monitoring progression, showing in the early stages, a uniform increased reflectance corresponding to the area of leakage on angiography, and in late stages with pigment clumping or

SRNV, a decreased reflectance in the area of leakage. Confocal reflectance imaging might not substitute for angiography, but the combination may improve the diagnostic sensitivity. Abnormalities of macular pigment distribution and Müller cell pathology have been suggested to contribute to the phenomenon of increased CBR. In fact, a central depletion of macular pigment has recently been established in patients with IJFT IIA.

FUNDUS AUTOFLUORESCENCE(FAF)

FAF imaging may provide the earliest fundus alterations in IJFT IIA, i.e., before angiographic signs are visible, making this technique useful for the diagnosis and monitoring disease progression. Recently, Wong et al examined 22 eyes with IJFT IIA with multiple imaging methods [fundus photography, FA, OCT, FAF, and microperimetry (MP)] and proposed a classification of IJFT IIA into five categories (0–4) based on the sequence of progressive changes observed (Table 21.5). Mild increases in FAF at the fovea (attributed to a loss of macular pigment) are detectable before clinical or angiographic findings are visible. As the disease progresses, foveal FAF signal becomes progressively more prominent until hyperpigmentation develops, where the FAF signal becomes mixed, showing both increased and decreased autofluorescence. This mixed FAF signal is proposed to relate to a changing composition of fluorophores in the RPE, which points to the possible involvement of the RPE in disease pathogenesis.

FLUORESCEIN ANGIOGRAPHY

The hallmark finding in IJFT IIA has been the characteristic telangiectactic capillaries on FA, again starting predominantly temporal to the fovea. Eventually, the entire parafoveal area is involved. Stereoscopic angiography has demonstrated that the deeper vasculature is involved but more superficial capillaries may also contribute to the fluorescein leakage. Traditionally, the use of FA was essential in the diagnosis of macular telangiectasia type 2. However, OCT changes, as described above, may precede the development of any angiographic findings.

Table 21.5 *Categorization of IJFT IIA eyes based on combined fundus photography, FA, FAF, OCT, and MP (Wong et al.)*

Category no.	Description
0	Normal results on all imaging methods (fellow eyes).
1	Mild increased foveal autofluorescence on FAF; no other abnormalities.
2	Mild-to-moderate increased foveal autofluorescence + funduscopic and angiographic features of IJFT IIA. No atrophic or cystic abnormalities on OCT imaging. No MP deficits.
3	Moderate to marked increased foveal autofluorescence + funduscopic and angiographic features of IJFT IIA + foveal atrophy and cysts on OCT + centrally decreased retinal sensitivity on MP.
4	Mixed patterns of increased and decreased FAF signal + clinically evident pigment clumping + central outer retinal atrophy on OCT + scotomas on MP correlating with decreased FAF signal or retinal atrophy on OCT.

Functional deficits

Since the macular abnormality in IJFT IIA is mainly located parafoveally, VA testing which is dependent on foveal function, may not represent the optimal method to evaluate macular dysfunction in these patients. Another method of evaluating function is the use of microperimetry (MP), which may help to correlate the structural changes with the functional changes. Retinal sensitivity defects appear to correlate with the outer retinal atrophy seen on OCT imaging. In areas of retinal pigment hyperplasia, there is often a dense scotoma. The use of microperimetry to correlate with changes seen on OCT may result in a reasonable outcome measurement for measuring changes over time.

IJFT IIA may lead to a sharply demarcated parafovealscotoma that correspond topographically to the angiographically and ophthalmoscopically visible alterations and to outer retinal

atrophy on OCT. These distinct parafoveal functional deficits may be present even in non-proliferative stages. Early in the course of the disease, light increment sensitivity (LIS) could be preserved despite angiographic leakage. LIS reduction then starts temporal to the fovea, progresses above and below the fovea, and involves the nasal area in later disease stages. These findings suggest that angiographic leakage precedes functional consequences, and only chronic retinal alterations may lead to a reduction of LIS. Light increment sensitivity reduction temporal to the fovea may be present despite preserved VA, but lead to the significant functional deficits and reading difficulty reported in these patients.

Wong et al. added three important observations:

1. Areas with mildly or moderately elevated FAF changes correlated with intact retinal structure on OCT and function on MP, whereas areas of significantly elevated or decreased FAF abnormalities correlated with disrupted retinal structure on OCT and decreased sensitivity on MP testing.
2. The five categories described did not follow a strict pattern of decreasing central VA. Wong noted that VA depended less on the presence of retinal atrophy, pigment migration or hypofluorescence signals per se, and more on their position relative to the foveal center. Central VA is decreased when these changes occur in the fovea, but may be preserved if they are limited to the parafovea.
3. The development of SRNV was also not limited to eyes in a single category. SRNV occurred in eyes in which there was no retinal atrophy and only mild changes in FAF signal (Category 2), as well as in eyes with advanced pigment clumping (Category 4).

Differential diagnosis

Retinal capillary telangiectasia may result from a multitude of retinal vascular inflammatory or occlusive conditions. However, IJFT IIA is quite distinct from other conditions where retinal telangiectasia is a prominent feature. Branch retinal vein occlusions can give rise to segmental capillary changes, but this can be readily distinguished since it involves an area of distribution distal to an arteriolar-venular crossing, and does not cross the horizontal raphe, unless there is already collateral formation. Radiation retinopathy usually involves a larger retinal area, and is accompanied by cotton-wool spots and preretinal neovascularization, both features that are not characteristic of mac tel type 2. Foveolar atrophy in IJFT IIA may simulate a macular hole. OCT permits the distinction. Some eyes demonstrate in the early stages a yellow foveal lesion that may be mistaken for adult vitelliform dystrophy or Best's disease. Retinal crystals may be mistaken for other causes of crystalline retinopathies, but FA readily establishes the correct diagnosis. The macular pigment plaques with SRNV may be mistaken for age-related macular degeneration, but drusen and pigment epithelial detachment are generally absent in IJFT IIA.

Treatment

When considering treatment, we must distinguish between the therapeutic attempts for nonproliferative IJFT IIA, and treatment modalities for the SRNV of the proliferative stage.

Treatment of nonproliferative IJFT IIA

Argon laser photocoagulation (ALPC), Verteporfin photodynamic therapy (PDT), Intravitreal triamcinolone acetonide(IVTA) though tried, have not proven to be effective in IJFT.

Intravitreal anti-VEGF agent, namely bevacizumab, has also been used for nonproliferative IJFT IIA and it has only a transient effect. However, the inhibition of VEGF may be useful particularly before atrophic changes occur since VEGF plays a pathophysiological role in IJFT IIA. But the small cystic changes seen on OCT remained unchanged, emphasizing that visual deterioration is caused by microcystic degeneration and progressive retinal atrophy and not by intraretinaledema, and therefore cannot be halted with intravitreal anti-VEGF injections. There seems to be no apparent visual acuity or OCT benefit to using intravitreal anti-VEGF in the absence of SRNV. Moreover, it has been suggested that VEGF plays a role in

photoreceptor differentiation, may contribute to photoreceptor survival, and may serve a role in maintaining retinal vascular homeostasis. Therefore, it cannot be ruled out that blocking VEGF may cause an acceleration of apoptosis among ganglion cells and photoreceptors in IJFT IIA and thus may harm the condition rather than benefitting it.

Treatment of proliferative IJFT IIA

Before the advent of VEGF antagonists, therapeutic options for SRNV associated with IJFT IIA included laser photocoagulation, PDT with or without IVTA, transpupillary thermotherapy (TTT), and surgical removal of the SRNV. Ablation of the SRNV by photocoagulation has been described as being able to prevent deterioration of VA only in selected cases. This treatment, however, is only feasible if the SRNV is distant enough from the fovealcenter. Prognosis for visual recovery is guarded despite the laser treatment, and treatment will result in a scotoma close to fixation.

Vascular endothelial growth factor has been implicated as the major angiogenic stimulus responsible for neovascularization in IJFT IIA. Given the risk of permanent RPE damage with PDT, coupled with the huge evidence of efficacy of VEGF antagonists in the treatment of choroidal neovascularization in various entities, the anti-VEGF approach is a reasonable treatment alternative for proliferative IJFT IIA, particularly in the presence of retinochoroidal anastomosis. Several case series in the literature investigated bevacizumab or ranibizumab for the treatment of proliferative IJFT IIA but with limited (12 months or less) follow-up. The best-corrected VA remains unchanged or improved after treatment. All eyes demonstrate decreased intraretinal leakage and decreased growth and leakage of the SRNV and decrease in central retinal thickness on OCT.

In conclusion, the preliminary results of studies suggest that intravitreal delivery of anti-VEGF therapy combined with or without PDT appears efficacious and should be considered as a treatment option for proliferative IJFT IIA. Long-term follow-up and larger series are needed to address the long-term outcomes, the needed frequency of anti-VEGF drug delivery,

and specific side effects or complications of anti-VEGF therapy in this condition.

GROUP III: IDIOPATHIC JUXTAFOVEAL RETINAL TELANGIECTASIA

This is a rare form of IJFT described by Gass characterized by progressive bilateral perifoveolar capillary obliteration, capillary telangiectasia, minimal exudation clinically and on FA and visual loss in association with systemic or cerebral familial disease. It has been omitted in the recent classification of IJFT based on its rarity.

Conclusion

Coats' disease is an idiopathic, progressive ocular entity, with retinal telangiectasia and exudates, which can cause retinal detachment. Its diagnosis can be challenging and retinoblastoma is the most important lesion that should be ruled out in the differential diagnosis. There are several treatment modalities, especially laser photocoagulation and cryotherapy for mild to moderate stages of the disease as well as vitrectomy for advanced stages. Today, anti-VEGF agents are used as adjuvant therapy to other treatment options, but clinical trials or case series with a large number of patients are limited due to the low incidence of the disease.

Idiopathic juxtafoveal telangiectasia comprises essentially three groups that are considerably different in their appearance, their presumed pathogenesis and management strategies. In group I, the unilateral telangiectasis is easily visible and vision loss is primarily a result of serous and lipid exudation in the macula. Photocoagulation is generally effective in controlling the macular edema. In group II, the most common, the bilateral capillary telangiectasis is more difficult to detect biomicroscopically, but the angiographic and OCT findings are characteristic and diagnostic. Vision loss is progressive and primarily due to retinal atrophy, not exudation. More rapid visual loss can occur with SRNV, not uncommonly. Treatment options for this group are still very limited, and have shown effectiveness only for the subretinal neovascular component. This is

primarily because the pathogenesis of this telangiectasis remains an enigma and is possibly secondary to a retinal neuronal dysfunction. New imaging modalities and functional tests, along with worldwide longitudinal studies will hopefully improve the understanding and treatment capabilities of this condition. As for group III, it is featured primarily as a perifoveolar capillary occlusive condition, and is poorly understood because of the rarity of cases reported.

BIBLIOGRAPHY

1. Bergstrom CS, Hubbard GB 3rd. Combination intravitreal triamcinolone injection and cryotherapy for exudative retinal detachments in severe Coats disease. Retina 2008;28:33–7.
2. Entezari M, Ramezani A, Safavizadeh L, Bassirnia N. Resolution of macular edema in Coats' disease with intravitreal bevacizumab. Indian J Ophthalmol 2010;58:80–2.
3. Gass JD, Blodi BA. Idiopathic juxtafoveolar retinal telangiectasis. Update of classification and follow-up study. Ophthalmology. 1993;100: 1536–46.
4. Gass JD, Oyakawa RT. Idiopathic juxtafoveolar retinal telangiectasis. Arch Ophthalmol. 1982;10:769–80.
5. Gass JD. Diagnosis and Treatment. 4 ed. Mosby: St Louis; 1997. In Stereoscopic Atlas of Macular Diseases; pp. 505–11.
6. Goel N, Kumar V, Seth A, Raina UK, Ghosh B. Role of intravitreal bevacizumab in adult onset Coats' disease. IntOphthalmol 2011;31:183–90.
7. Gupta V, Gupta A, Dogra MR, Agarwal A. Optical coherence tomography in group 2A idiopathic juxtafoveolartelangiectasis. Ophthalmic Surg Lasers Imaging 2005;36:482–6.
8. Hershberger VS, Hutchins RK, Laber PW. Photodynamic therapy with verteporfin for subretinal neovascularization secondary to bilateral idiopathic acquired juxtafoveolar telangiectasis. Ophthalmic Surg Lasers Imaging. 2003;34:318-20
9. Jones JH, Kroll AJ, Lou PL, Ryan EA. Coats' disease. Int Ophthalmol Clin 2001;41:189–98.
10. Kovach JL, Rosenfeld PJ. Bevacizumab (avastin) therapy for idiopathic macular telangiectasia type II. Retina 2009;29:27–32.
11. Lee BL. Bilateral subretinal neovascular membrane in idiopathic juxtafoveolar telangiectasis. Retina. 1996;16:344–6.
12. Li KK, Goh TY, Parsons H, Chan WM, Lam DS. Use of intravitreal triamcinolone acetonide injection in unilateral idiopathic juxtafoveal telangiectasis. Clin Experiment Ophthalmol. 2005;33:542–4.
13. Macular Telangiectasia (MacTel) Project. Invest Ophthalmol Vis Sci. 2008;49:4340–6.
14. Moon SJ, Berger AS, Tolentino MJ, Misch DM. Intravitreal bevacizumab for macular edema from idiopathic juxtafoveal retinal telangiectasis. Ophthalmic Surg Lasers Imaging 2007;38:164–6.
15. Potter PD, Shields CL, Shields JA, Flanders AE. The role of magnetic resonance imaging in children with intraocular tumors and simulating lesions. Ophthalmology 1996;103:1774–83.
16. Reichstein DA, Recchia FM. Coats disease and exudative retinopathy. Int Ophthalmol Clin 2011; 51:93–112.
17. Ridley ME, Shields JA, Brown GC, Tasman W. Coats' disease. Evaluation of management. Ophthalmology 1982;89:1381–87.
18. Schmitz-Valckenberg S, Ong EE, Rubin GS, Peto T, Tufail A, Egan CA, et al. Structural and functional changes over time in MacTel patients. Retina 2009;29:1314–20.
19. Shields CL, Uysal Y, Benevides R, Eagle RC Jr, Malloy B, Shields JA. Retinoblastoma in an eye with features of Coats' disease. J Pediatr Ophthalmol Strabismus 2006;43:313–5.
20. Shields JA, Shields CL, Honavar SG, Demirci H, Cater J. Classification and management of Coats disease: The 2000 Proctor Lecture. Am J Ophthalmol 2001;131:572–83.
21. Shields JA, Shields CL, Honavar SG, Demirci H. Clinical variations and complications of Coats disease in 150 cases: the 2000 Sanford Gifford Memorial Lecture. Am JOphthalmol 2001; 131: 561–71 and 572–83.
22. Treatment of adult Coats' disease: a case report. Korean J Ophthalmol 2010;24:374–6.
23. Wong WT, Forooghian F, Majumdar Z, Bonner RF, Cunningham D, Chew EY. Fundus auto-fluorescence in type 2 idiopathic macular telangiectasia: Correlation with optical coherence tomography and microperimetry. Am J Ophthalmol 2009;148:573–83.
24. Yannuzzi LA, Bardal AM, Freund KB, Chen KJ, Eandi CM, Blodi B. Idiopathic macular telangi-ectasia. Arch Ophthalmol. 2006;124:450–60.

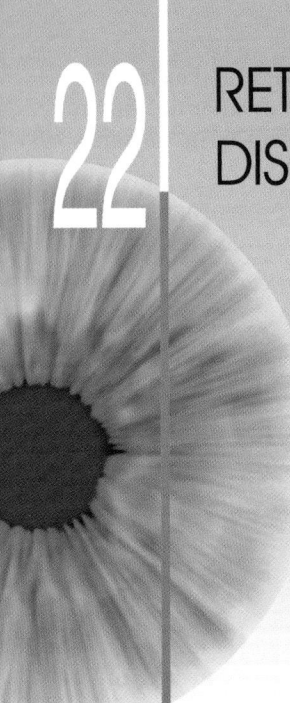

22 | RETINOPATHIES IN DISORDERS OF BLOOD

Sunandan Sood, Manisha Nada, AK Khurana, A. Khanna

INTRODUCTION

Hematological diseases include disorders of erythrocytes, leucocytes and platelets and disorders of coagulation and plasma proteins. These diseases may affect the eye either as local ocular involvement or as ophthalmic manifestations arising in the disease process. Ocular manifestations can be presenting symptom of hematological disease. Disorders of blood can produce retinopathy which may present clinically or may remain silent. Complete ocular and systemic examination is essential to diagnose these retinopathies. Treatment of the underlying disease may cure the retinopathy, however, lasers and surgical intervention are sometimes required. The common retinopathies in blood disorders can be divided broadly into two groups:

Retinopathy in non-malignant hematological disorders
• Anemic retinopathy
• Sickle cell retinopathy
• Retinal involvement in hemorrhagic disorders
• Dysproteinemic retinopathy.

Retinopathy in malignant hematological disorders
• Leukemic retinopathy
• Lymphoma (*see* page 155)
• Multiple myeloma

RETINOPATHY IN NON-MALIGNANT HEMATOLOGICAL DISORDERS

ANEMIC RETINOPATHY

GENERAL CONSIDERATIONS

Anemia is a group of disorders characterized by decrease in the number of circulating red blood cells, decrease in the amount of hemoglobin in each cell or both. Anemia can result from decreased or faulty red cell synthesis, decreased red cell life span or increased destruction. Anemia is classified according to red cell size and hemoglobin content. The morphologic classification of anemia divides the anaemias

into three broad groups on the basis of average cell size and hemoglobin content: the macrocytic anemias; the microcytic and hypochromic anemias; and the normocytic, normochromic anemias.

The most frequent cause of anemia is iron deficiency and this is microcytic hypochromic type. Pyridoxine deficiency and mild forms of thalassemia have similar morphology. Normocytic normochromic anemia is usually associated with acute blood loss where red blood cells are decreased in number. However, shortened life span can lead to normocytic normochromic anemia. Macrocytic anemia is caused by vitamin B_{12}/folic acid deficiency. Pernicious anemia is caused by the deficiency of vitamin B_{12} or folic acid deficiency or both. RBC'S are larger in size, DNA synthesis gets affected and cell nuclei mature slowly compared to cytoplasm. Production of platelets and granulocytes is also affected and this is the reason of more retinal hemorrhages in this type of anemia.

PATHOGENESIS

- Retinal changes are liable to occur when hemoglobin level falls by 50 percent and consistently present when hemoglobin level falls below 5 gm%. Retinal changes in anemia are innocuous and rarely of diagnostic importance.
- Duration and type of anemia do not influence the occurrence of retinopathy.
- Factors that have been implicated in the pathogenesis of anemic retinopathy include anoxia, venous stasis, angiospasm, increased capillary permeability and thrombocytopenia.
- Severity of the anemia, increased blood viscosity as seen in leukemic and other myeloproliferative disorders and periods of hypotension (especially following severe hemorrhage), are other contributing factors for anaemic retinopathy.

CLINICAL FEATURES

Characteristic features of retinopathy in anemia

- *Fundus background* becomes pale.
- *Retinal arterioles* appear less deeply red.

- *Retinal veins* become dilated and tortuous. This is related to severity of anemia, but may become otherwise also as in patients of thalassemia major.
- *Retinal hemorrhages* are present and these may be superficial, deep or preretinal (sub-hyaloid).
  - *Hemorrhages in superficial* (inner) capillary plexus tend to accumulate along the nerve fibers, and thus take on flame or feather shape, with fine striations and indstinct margins. These are seen within two disc diameter of the optic disc.
  - *Hemorrhages in deep* capillary plexus tend to orient vertically along the inner plexiform layers and outer plexiform layers. Only the end of column of blood is seen, which appears as dot or blot.
  - *Sub-hyaloid* hemorrhages are massive and occur just below the internal limiting membrane or between posterior vitreous face and internal limiting membrane. Such hemorrhages can be round or boat-shaped. These hemorrhages occur at posterior pole. These hemorrhages can extend into vitreous cavity also.
  - The severity of the hemorrhages is related to both the degree of the anemia and the presence of accompanying thrombocytopenia.
  - *Roth spots,* i.e white-centered hemorrhages are seen. Platelet-fibrin emboli constitute the white center.
- *Cotton-wool spots,* i.e grey or white ischemic areas are seen (Fig. 22.1).

Note. Roth spots and cotton wool spots are more common with coexisting thrombocyto-penia in aplastic anemia.

Optic neuropathy and other features include:
- Pernicious anemia may also lead to optic neuropathy with centrocaecal scotomas.
- Permanent optic atrophy follows if vitamin B_{12} supplements are not given to the patient.
- Pernicious anemia may lead to dementia, peripheral neuropathy and subacute combined degeneration of spinal cord characterised by posterior and lateral column disease.

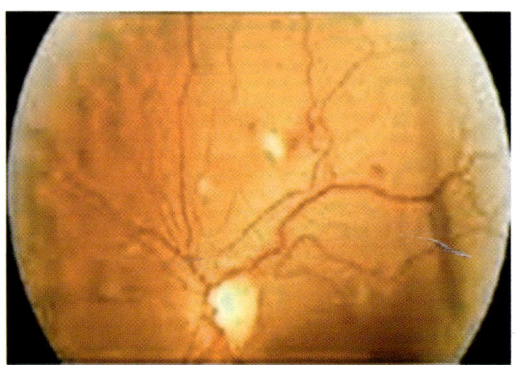

Fig. 22.1 *Venous dilatation and tortuosity, superficial hemorrhages and cotton-wool spots in anemic retinopathy*

MANAGEMENT

Treatment of anemia should be carried out by hematologist. Anaemic retinopathy is almost always reversible with the treatment of anemia. Surgical intervention may be is required if spontaneous resorption is insufficient.

SICKLE CELL RETINOPATHY

Sickle cell hemoglobinopathies (abnormal hemoglobins) lead to systemic and ocular manifestations. Sickling hemoglobinopathies are caused by the presence of one or a combination of abnormal hemoglobins in the red blood cells. The normal red blood cell hemoglobin comprises four polypeptide globin chains, each associated with a central heme ring (ferriprotoporphyrin).

The sickle cell hemoglobinopathies are characterized by a genetic error in B-chain synthesis, which results in abnormal function of the hemoglobin molecule. The imperfect globin chain induces pathological alterations in red blood cells morphology under particular conditions like ischemia and metabolic stress.

There are four common variants of sickle cell anemia which include sickle cell anemia (SS), sickle-hemoglobin C disease (SC), sickle beta thalassemia (S thal) and sickle cell trait (AS). When both parents contribute S globin chain sickle cell anemia occurs. If one parent contributes S globin chain and other contributes hemoglobin C then sickle SC trait is created. Thalassemia mutations can occur with normal hemoglobin to produce heterozygous S-Thalassemia disease. The normal hemoglobin

confers pliability to oval shaped red blood cells. Sickle hemoglobin results in red blood cells with a crescentic, elongated shape, particu-larly under conditions of hypoxia or acidosis. Due to their crescent shape, the altered red blood cells are called *sickle cells*. These patients have higher haematocrit and higher blood viscosity there by increasing the chances of vaso-occlusion in the retinal microvasculature. This causes the blood cells to stack, leading to local ischemia. A vicious circle of ischemia, red cell sickling, tissue hypoxia and necrosis gets set in motion (Fig. 22.2).

CLINICAL FEATURES

The most severe systemic symptoms are observed in sickle SS disease, while severe ocular features are most commonly noted in patients with sickle SC or sickle thalassemia (S-thal). Sickle cell anemia can involve both anterior as well as posterior segment.

Characteristic features of anterior segment involvement in sickle cell anemia are:
- *Conjunctival sickle sign:* This is characterized by linear, comma shaped or truncated seg-ments of bulbar conjunctival vessels. These abnormalities are due to flow obstruction or impedance by sickled cells. These are not pathognomic, as they may be seen rarely in patients with AIDS, chronic myeloid leukemia and other vaso-occlusive diseases.
- *Iris atrophy and neovascularisation*: These may be extensive and even pupil may become irregular. Iris neovascularisation occurs secondary to retinal detachment or major arteriole obstruction. Rarely there may be neovascular glaucoma.
- *Hyphaema*: It may cause permanent ocular damage in sickle cell patient with minimal trauma or surgery.

Charteristic features of posterior segment involvement in sickle cell disease (sickle cell retinopathy) are:
- *Vitreous hemorrhage* .
- *Salmon-colored retinal hemorrhages (Salmon patch)* occur adjacent to a retinal arteriole and are often found in the equatorial retina. The salmon hue is attributed to color changes in the hemorrhage. The initial color is bright red. These hemorrhages result from rupture of a

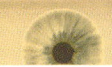

Abnormal, sickled, red blood cells
(sickle cells)

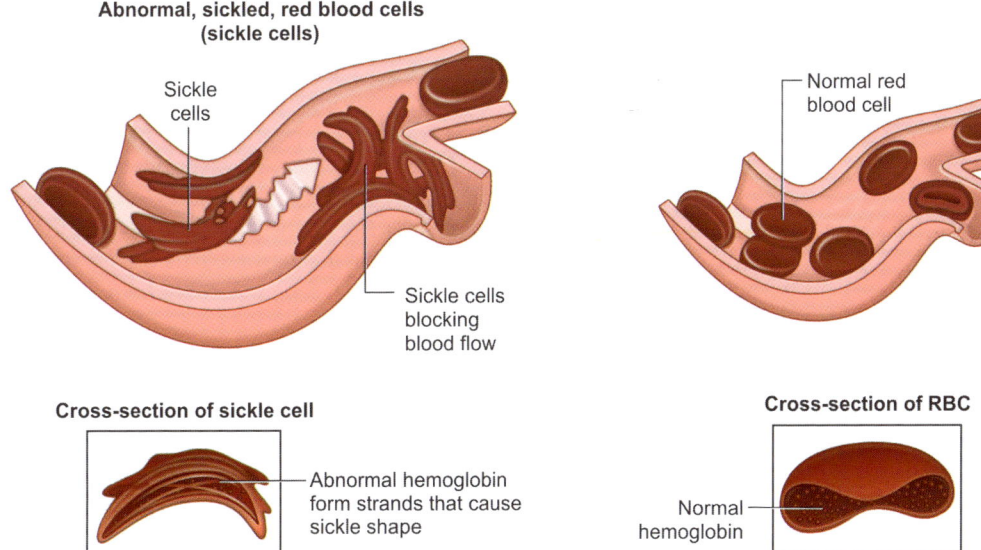

Sickle cells

Normal red blood cell

Sickle cells blocking blood flow

Cross-section of sickle cell

Abnormal hemoglobin form strands that cause sickle shape

Cross-section of RBC

Normal hemoglobin

Fig. 22.2 *Normal red blood cells and sickle cells*

medium sized retinal arteriole. They resolve, however, a schisis cavity with iridescent yellow particles in the lining of the cavity may be seen. These are macrophages who have engulfed blood breakdown products and hemoglobin.

- *Black sunburst sign:* Intra-arteriolar hemorrhages dissects into the sub-neural retinal space and disturbs the retinal pigment epithelium, a black sunburst lesion is formed. The stellate or spiculated lesions are due to retinal pigment epithelial hyperplasia and intraretinal migration. These are seen in equatorial region, hence no visual symptoms are observed (Fig. 22.3).

- *Optic disc sign*: This is a transient sign where sludging red cell within prepapillary retinal capillaries lead to dark spots or vascular lines. Unlike, some retinal vasoocclusive diseases, sickle cell retinopathy is rarely associated with optic disc neovascularisation.

- *Macular small vessel occlusions (sickling maculopathy):* The macular depression sign represents atrophy and thinning of the neural macula, resulting in oval depression of the bright central reflex. This is better appreciated with red-free illumination. This area of macular ischemia may be associated with a decrease in vision.

- *Large macular infarction* can occur with multiple retinal arteriolar occlusions. Fluorescein angiography shows increased size of foveal avascular zone.

- *Cotton-wool spots* and less commonly *retinal arterial microaneurysms* are observed.

- *Retinal arteriolar sclerosis* and *venous tortuosity* are non-specific signs.

- *Angioid streaks* have been described in association with sickle cell disease.

- *Epiretinal membranes* may be formed.

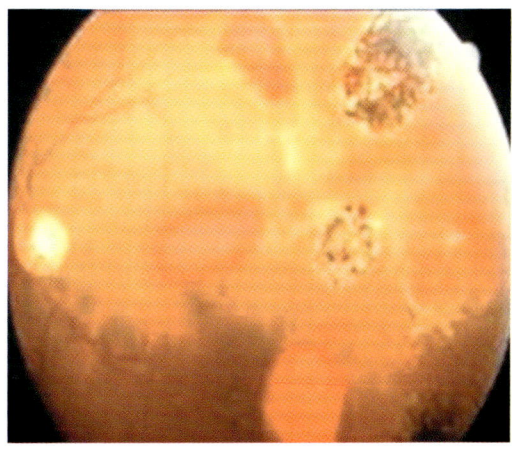

Fig. 22.3 *Salmon patches and sun-burst lesions in sickle cell retinopathy*

- *Macular holes* may be formed if traction occurs from peripheral neovascularisation.
- *Proliferative sickle retinopathy (PSR)* is the most severe ocular complication leading to severe visual disability.

It rapidly progresses in children and adolescents than adults and is more common in patients with hemoglobin SC and S-thal disease than with hemoglobin SS disease. The development of PSR is not only genotype dependent but also age dependent. It occurs earlier in hemoglobin SC than in hemoglobin SS disease. Highest risk period is 20 to 34 years in hemoglobin SC, whereas 40–50 years in hemoglobin SS disease.

Classification of proliferative sickle cell retinopathy

Goldberg has classified PSR into five stages:

Stage 1: Peripheral arteriolar occlusion: This is the earliest ophthalmoscopic abnormality that can be visualised in periphery. Venular occlusions including central as well as branch occlusions are rare.

Stage 2: Peripheral arteriolar-venular anastomosis: Neovascularisation develops at the junction of arteriolar-venular anastomosis. Fluorescein angiography reveals that no leakage occurs hence these are not true neovascularisations.

Stage 3: Neovascular proliferation: Characteristic sea-fan neovascularisation fronds form in the periphery. They have one feeder arteriole and one draining venule. However, with time more fronds develop with more and more feeding and draining vessels. Neovascularisation occurs at the junction of normal and ischemic retina. White glial tissue envelops these neovascular tufts. Fluorescein angiography shows leakage from new vessels (Fig. 22.4A and B).

Stage 4: Vitreous hemorrhage: Spontaneous hemorrhages from new vessels are more common than hemorrhages with trauma.

Stage 5: Retinal detachment: Localised retinal detachment or retinoschisis may progress posteriorly. Full thickness breaks occur and may cause rhegmatogenous retinal detachment.

- *Early detection* of neovascularisation and its treatment should be done.

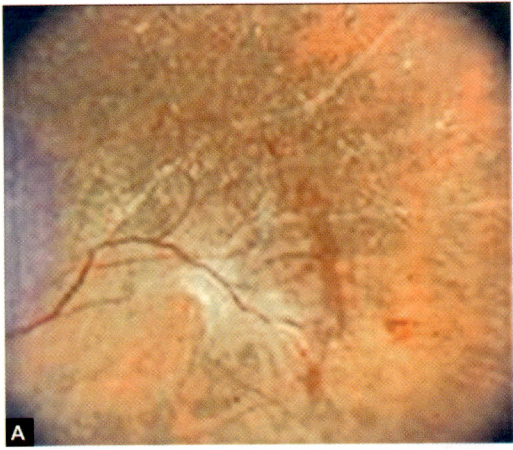
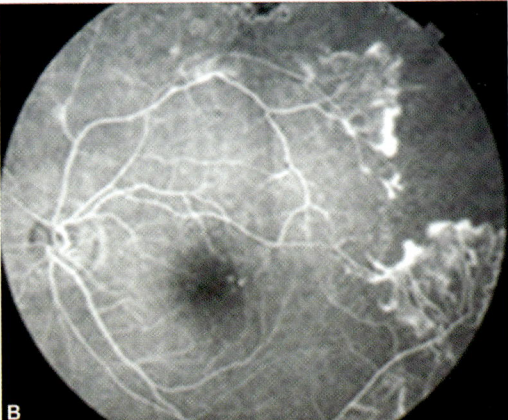

Fig. 22.4 *Fundus picture:* **(A)** *Fluorescein angiography; and* **(B)** *sea-fan neovascularisation in sickle cell retinopathy*

Treatment modalities include:
- Diathermy, cryotherapy and laser photocoagulation.
- For vitreous hemorrhages and retinal detachment scleral buckling, vitrectomy, Nd:YAG laser vitreolysis can be done.

Ocular complications which can occur with surgical procedures include: Anterior segment ischemia, intraoperative hemorrhages and secondary glaucoma. Iatrogenic retinal breaks in the ischemic and atrophic peripheral retina are easily made if peripheral dissection is attempted. Every effort should be made to maintain a low intraocular pressure during surgery as even a small elevation in IOP can result in optic nerve ischemia and retinal arterial occlusion.

RETINAL INVOLVEMENT IN HEMORRHAGIC DISORDERS

Hemorrhagic disorders comprise a heterogenous group of diseases which manifest clinically by easy bruising, spontaneous bleeding or excessive bleeding after injury. The retina is not typically involved in hemorrhagic disorders unless there is ocular trauma but thrombocytopenia is an exception (Fig. 22.5). Common hemorrhagic disorders which may cause retinopathy are as under:

1. *Disorders of platelets* e.g. idiopathic thrombocytopenic purpura (ITP), thrombotic thrombocytopenic purpura (TTP).
2. *Disorders of clotting factors*, e.g. hemophilia.
3. *Connective tissue disorders*, e.g. pseudoxanthoma elasticum.
4. *Miscellaneous disorders*, e.g. scurvy, steroid use, Kaposi's sarcoma, disseminated intravascular coagulation and bone marrow disorders.

Characteristic features of retinopathy due to hemorrhagic disorders include:
- Vitreous hemorrhage.
- Retinal hemorrhages.
- Optic disc edema, optic disc neovascularisation and optic atrophy.
- Serous macular detachment secondary to choriocapillary occlusion by platelet-fibrin thrombi.

DISSEMINATED INTRAVASCULAR COAGULOPATHY

Disseminated intravascular coagulopathy is characterized by massive activation of the coagulation cascade, microvascular thrombosis, consumption of coagulation factors and platelets, and results in bleeding. It can be the result of sepsis, massive tissue necrosis, malignancy, toxemia of pregnancy, crush injuries, or severe burns. Thrombocytopenia with prolongation of prothrombin time and activated partial thromboplastin time (aPTT) is seen. Reduced plasma fibrinogen level correlates most closely with bleeding. Low ESR, elevated levels of fibrindegradation products and schistocytes (fragmented RBCs) on peripheral smear are also seen.

Characteristic features of retinopathy in DIC
- Bilateral submacular choroidal thrombosis.
- Fibrin deposition underneath the retina often with overlying serous retinal detachments.
- There is pinpoint leakage through the RPE On fluorescein angiography. Macular involvement can result in permanent vision loss.

Treatment modalities include elimination of underlying cause, fresh whole blood, fresh frozen plasma or platelet concentrates infusion. Heparin infusion is given to stop the onging coagulation after correction of bleeding risk.

BONE MARROW DISORDERS

Bone marrow disorders that increase blood viscosity such as polycythemia vera can result in stasis retinopathy and vision loss that may be reversible once the hyperviscosity is treated. Ischemic retinopathy similar to diabetic and hypertensive retinopathy can also be seen in polycythemia vera. Clinical signs of hyperviscosity begin with a hematocrit value greater than 50%. Retinal manifestations are bilateral and more common with primary polycythemia than secondary.

Characteristic features of retinopathy in Polycythemia vera are
- Fundus shows dark dilated tortuous veins.
- The disc is hyperemic and swollen and intraretinal hemorrhages may be seen.
- There may be retinal edema and central or branch vein occlusion.
- Loss of vision due to retinal edema or vein occlusion.

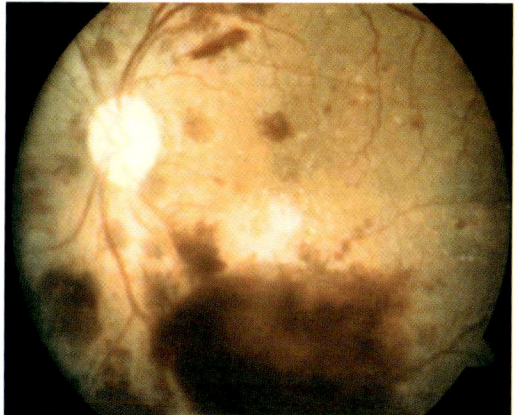

Fig. 22.5 *Retinal and subhyaloid hemorrhages in thrombotic thrombocytopenic purpura*

Treatment reverses findings unless venous occlusion has occurred.

Bone marrow disorders that result in bone marrow failure can result in thrombocytopenic or anemic retinopathy. Dyskeratosis congenita, an exceedingly rare inherited bone marrow failure syndrome, can result in retinal hemorrhages, optic atrophy, nerve fiber layer infarction, a peripheral retinal vasculopathy resulting in a Coats' like exudative retinopathy, retinal neovascularization, or retinal detachment.

DYSPROTEINEMIC RETINOPATHY

Dysproteinemic retinopathy occurs due to hyperviscosity of the serum because of dysproteinemia caused by:
- Hypergammaglobulinemia.
- Cryomacroglobulinemia.
- Waldenstrom's macroglobulinemia.
- Chronic lymhocytic leukemia with macroglobulinemia and multiple myeloma with hyperglobulinemia.

Note. Presence of retinopathy correlates with degree of associated anemia.

Characteristic features of dysproteinemic retinopathy are as follows (Fig. 22.6):
- Vitreous hemorrhage, neovascular glaucoma.
- Central or branch retinal vein occlusions may be found.
- Retinal veins are dark, dilated and tortuous.

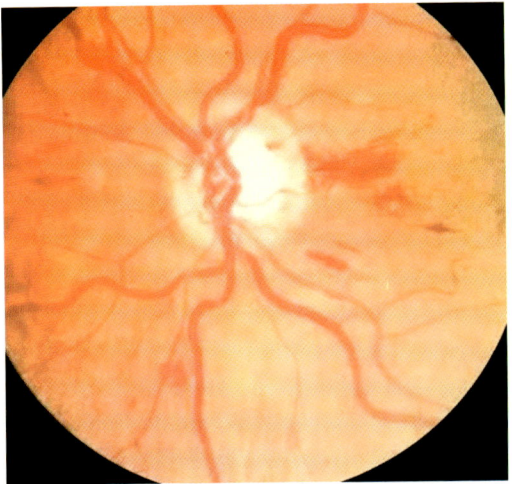

Fig. 22.6 *Dark, dilated tortuous veins and hemorrhages in dysproteinemic retinopathy*

- Intraretinal hemorrhages.
- Cotton wool spots may be seen.
- Disc hyperemia.
- Retinal hemorrhages, both superficial and deep.
- Retinal edema.
- Retinal micro-aneurysms are seen in chronic cases.
- Retinal detachment (exudative type) is seen.
- Neovascularisation of the retina or iris.

RETINOPATHY IN MALIGNANT HEMATOLOGICAL DISORDERS

LEUKAEMIC RETINOPATHY

General considerations

Leukemia refers to a group of neoplastic proliferation of leucocytes. These can be lymphocytic or myelocytic depending on the cell of origin. Ocular involvement is more frequent in acute leukemia than in chronic leukemia. Any ocular structure can get involved. *Leukemic retinopathy* was first described by Richard Liebreish in 1861. Involvement of retina can be either primary or secondary.
- Primary involvement is due to infiltration of the retina by leukemic cells.
- Secondary involvement in leukemia occurs due to associated anaemia, thrombocytopenia, hyperviscosity and opportunistic infections.

Clinical features

Characteristic features of primary involvement in leukemia are:
- *Leukemic retinal infiltrates* seen as grayish-white nodules that may be associated with surrounding hemorrhages.
- *Choroidal involvement* is rarely clinically evident but histopathological involvement is quite common. Leukemic infiltration of the choroid diminishes perfusion of choriocapillaries, resulting in pigment epithelial ischemia and subsequent breakdown of pigment epithelial barrier and pump functions. The retinal pigment epithelium shows mottled or tigroid appearance and serous retinal detachment may occur.

- *Optic nerve head* infiltration may appear as a pale grey swelling which is associated with a high frequency of CNS involvement and poor prognosis. Intraocular leukemic lesions are usually not a presenting feature of the disease but are more likely to occur during leukemic relapse.

Characteristic features of secondary involvement in leukemia are:
- *Fundus* background is pale and orange.
- *Retinal veins* are dilated and tortuous. It is the first change to be observed.
- *Retinal arterioles* become pale and narrow due to decreased RBC count and increased WBC count.
- *Roth spots,* i.e white centered hemorrhages are very common. These are either of leukemic cells or platelet-fibrin emboli.
- *Subhyaloid hemorrhages* are sometimes seen.
- *Retinal hemorrhages and cotton wool spots* are caused by vascular occlusion by leukemic cells, thrombocytopenia and stasis, hyperviscosity and anaemia.
- *Retinal vascular sheathing* — Grey-white streaks along retinal vessels.
- *Microaneurysms* (may be related to increased viscosity from elevated WBC count) and *hard yellow-white exudates* (indicative of vascular insufficiency) may sometimes be seen (Fig. 22.7).
- *HTLV-1 leukemia* has somewhat different clinical picture that includes pigmentary retinopathy, lymphoma-like picture, uveitis, and vasculitis.
- *Retinal neovascularization* is a rare finding but has been found in the periphery and on the

optic nerve in patients with leukemia. The mechanism is thought to be peripheral nonperfusion and ischemia due to increased blood viscosity. Angiogenic factors from leukemic cells may play a role in this process. Overall, secondary ophthalmic manifestations of leukemia have been found in up to 39% of patients with leukemia.

Other ocular features in leukemia are:
- Orbital infiltrations presenting as proptosis, especially in children.
- Spontaenously occurring subconjuctival hemorrhages and hyphema.
- Iris thickening, iritis and pseudohypopyon.

Multiple myeloma

It is malignancy of plasma cells producing abnormal amounts of monoclonal immunoglobulins causing pancytopenia, multiple punched out skull or vertebral lesions and hypercalcemia. The ocular manifestation can be multiple pars plana cysts, ciliochoroidal effusions, uveal plasmocytoma, retinal vasculitis, neurosensory or RPE detachments. Hyperviscosity can cause dilated tortuous veins, segmentation in vascular blood flow, cotton-wool spots, microaneurysms, intraretinal and preretinal hemorrhages, venous occlusion and optic nerve edema.

BIBLIOGRAPHY

1. Diseases of the Retina. In: AK Khurana, editor. Comprehensive Ophthalmology. 5th ed. New Delhi: New Age International Publishers/2012
2. Relationship between fundus and haematological parameters at diagnosis. Opthalmology 1989 June 96(6): 860–4
3. Retinal Vascular Disease. In: Jack J Kanski, editor, Clinical Ophthalmology: A systemic approach. 6th ed. Philadelphia: Butterworth Heinemann 2007.
4. Retinopathy associated with blood anomalies. John I. Loewenstein. In: Albert DM, Jakobiec FA (editors). Principles and Practice of Ophthalmology 2nd ed Saunders 2000.
5. Robert H Rosa JR, Richard D Cunningham. Retinopathy of Blood Dyscrasias. In: William Tasman, Edward A Jaegar, editors. Duane's Clinical Ophtha lmology, Philadelphia: Lippincott-Raven 2006.

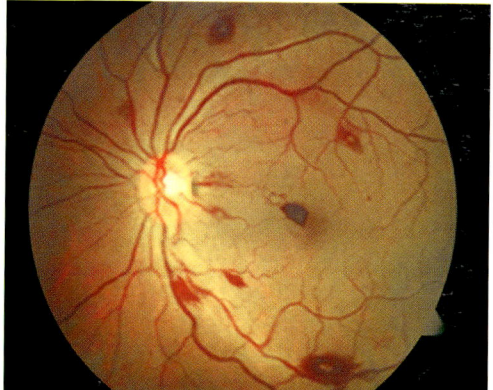

Fig. 22.7 *Superficial retinal hemorrhages, Roth spots and subhyloid hemorrhage in leukemic retinopathy*

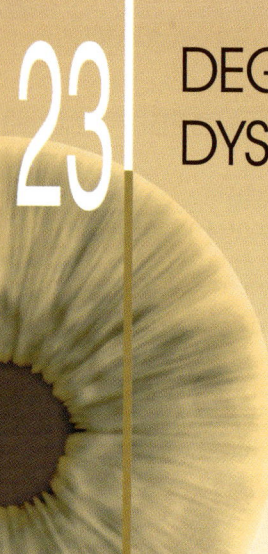

23 | DEGENERATIONS AND DYSTROPHIES OF THE RETINA

Atul Kumar, Thirumalesh, Mohan Raj

RETINITIS PIGMENTOSA
- Clinical presentation
- Variants of retinitis pigmentosa
- Conditions that resemble retinitis pigmentosa
- Epidemiology
- Genetics
- Natural course of RP
- Syndromic associations of RP
- Management

OTHER DIFFUSE RETINAL DYSTROPHIES
Cone Dystrophies
- Progressive cone-rod dystrophy
- Pericentral inverse RP
- Inner retinal dystrophies
  - X-linked juvenile retinoschisis

- **Familial foveal retinoschisis**

RETINITIS PIGMENTOSA

Retinitis pigmentosa is an inherited retinal dystrophy which leads to the loss of photoreceptors characterized by classic triad of:
- Arteriolar attenuation
- Retinal bony spicule pigmentation
- Waxy disc pallor.

The photoreceptor degeneration in retinitis pigmentosa is characterized by primary degeneration of rods with secondary degeneration of cones which explains the first symptom of nyctalopia in patients of retinitis pigmentosa.

CLINICAL PRESENTATION
Symptoms

1. *Night blindness* (nyctalopia) first symptom to appear.
2. *Visual field changes include:*
   - Patchy loss of peripheral vision.
   - Ring shape scotoma
   - Tunnel vision

Fundus examination reveals (Fig. 23.1A)

1. Pigmentary deposits in the peripheral retina resembling bony spicules.
2. Waxy disc pallor.
3. Arteriolar attenuation.
4. Tessellated fundus due to atrophy of retinal pigment epithelium.
5. Atrophy of macula with cellophane membrane formation. Cystoids macular edema shown in Fig. 23.1B.

VARIANTS OF RETINITIS PIGMENTOSA
1. Pigmental paravenous chorioretinal atrophy

Pigmental paravenous chorioretinal atrophy (PPCRA) is associated with mutation of crumbs homdos 1 (CRB 1) gene 3 (Mc Kay GJ, Clarke et al) (Fig. 23.2). It is a stable condition showing mild to moderate abnormality in ERG. EOG is significantly affected.

2. Uniocular retinitis pigmentosa

Francois and Verriest criteria for diagnosis of unilateral retinitis pigmentosa:

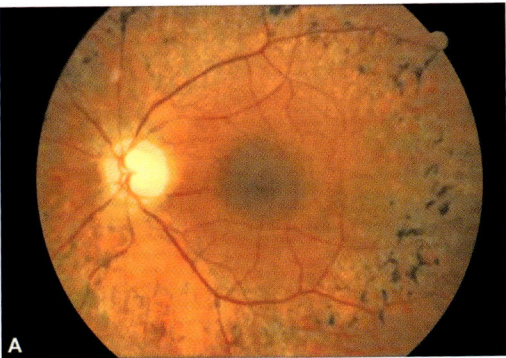

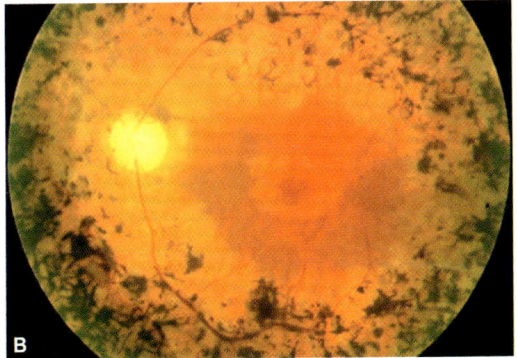

Fig. 23.1 *Classical retinitis pigmentosa without* **(A)** *and with cystoid macular oedema* **(B)**

i. Fundus picture showing typical pigmentary degeneration in involved eye.
ii. Absence of pigmentary changes or other features of retinitis pigmentosa in fellow eye with normal ERG over 5 years.
iii. Presence of symptoms of retinitis pigmentosa in affected eye.
iv. Exclusion of inflammatory causes in affected eye.

3. Central retinitis pigmentosa

It is an atypical variant where:
- Pigmentary changes particularly localized over the macula
- Central vision is defective
- Defective color and contrast sensitivity

4. Sectoral retinitis pigmentosa

Sectoral RP is characterized by fundus picture showing pigmentary changes, attenuated vessels and atrophy of RPE over one of the segments of the fundus. Visual acuity is retained but visual fields are reduced corresponding to the segment of the fundus involved. ERG shows subnormal response in these patients.

There is preferential involvement of inferonasal quadrants, and with progressive ageing, entire fundus may get involved.

5. Retinitis pigmentosa sine pigmento

In contrast to the typical retinitis pigmentosa fundus picture shows characteristic absence of pigmentary changes in the form of bony spicules. But the waxy disc pallor and varying degree of arteriolar attenuation are usually present (Fig. 23.3). Diagnosis is established by an extinguished ERG response and defective dark adaptation.

6. Retinitis punctata albescens

The fundus picture (Fig. 23.4) shows discrete yellowish white spots scattered up to the equator. The disc is usually normal but can at

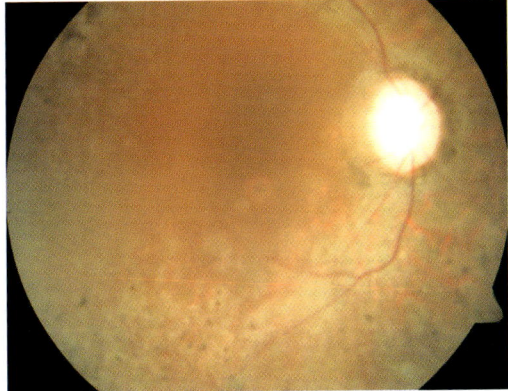

Fig. 23.2 *Pigmental paravenous chorioretinal atrophy*

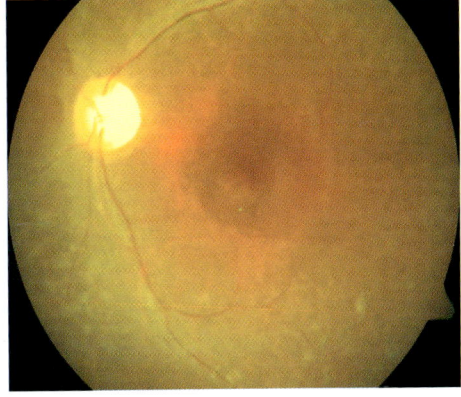

Fig. 23.3 *Retinitis pigmentosa sine pigmento*

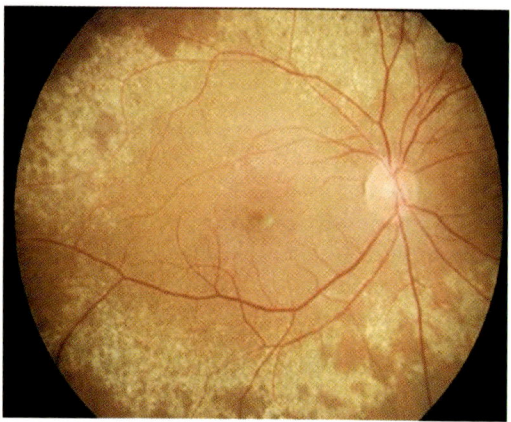

Fig. 23.4 *Retinitis punctata albescens*

times show waxy disc pallor. There is involvement of peripheral visual fields.

CONDITIONS THAT RESEMBLE RETINITIS PIGMENTOSA

Conditions that resemble retinitis pigmentosa are also known as pseudoretinitis pigmentosa and include:

1. *Drug induced pigmentary retinopathy*
   • Thioridazine
   • Chloroquine
2. *Infective*
   • Syphilis
   • Rubella
   • Measles
3. *Scarring*
   • Chronic CSR
   • Trauma
   • Uveitis (VKH syndrome)

EPIDEMIOLOGY

The incidence of retinitis pigmentosa is around 1:4000. A study by Jai Rup Singh et al over 400 families in 16 states of India has shown that the autosomal recessive form is the most common variety accounting for 75% of the cases. The X-linked inheritance pattern was least common with 1% of cases but carried the worst prognosis. 14% of the cases in the above study did not show a definite inheritance pattern.

GENETICS

More than 100 genes have been mapped and identified, the current list of these genes are available in the Ret Net site at http://www.sphuth.tmc.edu/Retnet/sum-dis.htm.

The most common genes involved are as follows:

1. *Rhodopsin gene* encoded the chromosome 3 a Pro 23. This mutation accounts for majority of AD case. Other genes are PAP 1 and PRPF 31 genes which are AD with variable points.
2. *Nonsense mutation of rhodopsin gene* is involved autosomal recessive type retinitis pigmentosa.
3. *Other genes involved* are red and green pigmentosa on chromosome X and blue pigment on chromosome.

NATURAL COURSE OF RETINIITS PIGMENTOSA

Typically retinitis pigmentosa is a chronic long lasting disease involving over several decades but in few aggressive cases it evolves very rapidly with a visual acuity of perception of hand movement close to face by second decade of life.

The natural history of the disease can be divided into 3 stages.

1. Early stage

Night blindness is the main symptom usually appearing during 1st or 2nd decade of life. There are peripheral field defects in scotopic conditions usually ignored by patient. Fundus picture to a large is extent normal. Field defects difficult to pick up as visual fields are examined under mesopic conditions not photopic conditions.

Diagnosis is difficult unless there is a family history, color vision is usually normal at this stage. ERG is the key test and shows suppression of the b wave.

2. Mid stage

Symptoms become obvious with difficulty in doing routine activities like night driving, maneuvering staircase in dark, loss of peripheral field.

Decreased color and contrast sensitivity is often present particularly to pale color.

Patient also develop photophobia in diffuse bright light described as white cloudy appearance thus allowing a very narrow range of

brightness between insufficient brightness and too bright light.

There is diminution of vision due to macular edema or foveolar atrophy. The typical fundus picture of retinitis pigmentosa becomes obvious.

The ERG is extinguished in scotopic condition and cone response is markedly diminished.

3. End stage

Patient left only with central few degree of visual field around fixation point making it extremely difficult for autonomous mobility. Near vision is reduced requiring the use of magnifying glasses.

Fundus shows wide spread pigment deposition with marked attenuation of vessels with waxy disc pallor.

Patients are more prone to cataract and open angle glaucoma.

Progression of disease shows gradual and severe loss of central vision.

SYNDROMIC ASSOCIATIONS OF RETINITIS PIGMENTOSA

Usher syndrome
- Most frequent syndromic form (14% of RP)
- Typical RP with neurosensory deafness
- Vestibular dysfunction with ataxia

Bardet-Biedl syndrome
- Less common 1:150,000
- Characterized by:
  - RP
  - Obesity
  - Mental retardation
  - Post-axial polydactyly
  - Hypogenitalism
  - Nephrogenic diabetes insipidus

Alport syndrome
- Anterior lenticonus
- Sensori-neural deafness
- Progressive renal failure with persistant nephritis and hematuria
- Diffuse leiomyomatosis of esophagus

Facial dysmorphic syndromes

Cohen syndrome
- Facial dysmorphism
  - Micrognathia
  - Short philthrum
  - Prominent incision
- Obesity, mental retardation
- Neutropenia
- Retinitis pigmentosa

Jeune syndrome
- Asphyxiating thoracic dystrophy
- Brachydactyly
- Chronic nephritis
- Retinitis pigmentosa

Cockayne syndrome
- Dwarfism
- Progeria
- Mental retardation
- RPC fine granular spot

Metabolic diseases

Methylmalonyl aciduria
- Genetic defect in metabolism of vitamin B_{12}
- Macular atrophy, salt pepper retinopathy with vascular attenuation

Abetalipoproteinemia **(Bassen-Kornzweig disease)**
- Progressive ataxia
- Steatorrhoea
- Decreased plasma lipids
- Retinitis pigmentosa resembling retinitis puntata albescens

Cystinosis
- Hypothyroidism
- Diabetes mellitus
- Renal failure
- Crystalline deposition cornea
- RP

Mycopolysaccharidoses (types I, II and III only)
- Facial dysmorphism (coarse facies)
- Mental retardation
- Skeletal changes
- RP

Refsum's disease
- Ataxia cerebellar degeneration
- Icthyosis
- Hearing loss
- Retinitis pigmentosa

Other rare metabolic syndromes
- Rhizomelic chondrodysplasia punctata
- Zellweger syndrome

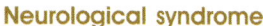
Neurological syndrome

Joubert syndrome
- Vermis hypoplasia
- Renal cysts
- Retinitis pigmentosa.

Hallevorden-Spatz disease
- Iron pigment deposition
- Basal ganglia (extra-pyramidal dysfunction)
  - Dementia
  - Dysarthria
- Flecked retinopathy.

Neuronal ceroid lipofuscinosis
- Mental retardation
- Seizure
- Ataxia
- Retinitis pigmentosa.

Kearns-Sayre syndrome
- Mitochondrial myopathy with chronic progressive external ophthalmoplegia
- Cerebral ataxia
- Cardiac conduction abnormality
- Deafness
- Diabetes mellitus
- Endocrinopathies

MANAGEMENT

Clinical work-up

Diagnosis is usually straight forward with classical fundus picture of pigmentary changes attenuation of vessels.

Also look:
- Macula for CME, epiretinal membrane, and atrophy
- Anterior segment for keratoconus and cataract
- IOP measurement to rule out glaucoma
- Look for extraocular movement, if restricted think of chronic progressive external ophthalmoplegia (Kearns-Sayre syndrome)

Evaluate systemically for:
- Hearing (Usher's, Refsum's, Kearns-Sayre)
- Neurological evaluation (neurological syndromes)
- Peripheral smear examination, lipid profile (abetalipoproteinemia)
- Renal function test (cystinosis, Joubert's syndrome)
- ECG (Kearns-Sayre syndrome)

Also examine other family members

Treatment

Currently there is no therapy that stops the evolution of pigmentary retinopathy or restore lost vision. Main strategy is to slow down the degeneration and management of complications.

I. *Slowing down degeneration*

1. Animal studies and clinical data have shown some types of RP are partly light dependent. Hence are advised to wear dark glasses out doors with lateral protection to protect against dazzling side rays.
2. High doses of vitamin A of 15,000 IU/day slightly slow down the loss of ERG amplitude. However, if at all this vitamin A supplementation is considered, a regular assay of:
   - Serum retinol
   - Serum triglycerides
   - Liver enzymes (AST, ALT, alkaline phosphatase) should be regularly done as there is a risk of hypervitaminosis.

II. *Management of complications*

1. *Cataract:* Usually presents in the mid stage of the disease as posterior subcapsular cataract. Prompt phacoemulsification with PCIOL implantation should be done.
2. *Macular edema:* Important cause for sudden drop in visual acuity. Responds well to oral carbonic anhydrase inhibitors (Acetazolamide 500 mg daily). Response with topical dorzolamide is varied. However, long-term use of azetazolamide, metazolamide lead to recalcitrant macular edema. Oral third generation synthetic glucocorticoid-deflazacort has also been tried with promising results.

III. *Future treatment*

Lot of work is going on all over the world to understand the pathophysiology and genetic basis of this disease and to establish efficient therapeutic strategies.

1. *Gene therapy.* Currently 50% of the cases of RP can be accounted to the known genes and there is a need to identify remaining genes and establish an efficient method of testing genotype of a single patient for several genes in a short time.

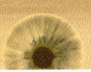

Short time efficacy demonstrated in animal studies but long term results not established. Moreover suitable vectors have not been identified.

The risks of gene therapy like neoplasia, autoimmunity in a non life-threatening disease seem overwhelming in regards to potential benefits.

Gene therapy have been achieved in animal models of RP and human trials have begun.

2. *Neuroprotection.* Neuroprotection with ciliary neurotrophic growth factor after animal studies has been tried in humans with phase I study completed with technology that used encapsulated cell with intravitreal sustained release of ciliary neurotrophic growth factor was well tolerated, with some patient report improved vision.

3. *Retinal prosthesis.* Micro photodiodes arrays which can be implanted intraocularly replacing degenerated photoreceptors stimulating the optic nerve or visual cortex have been developed.

It is yet to be established how much of functional vision will be obtained with these devices. Attempts have been made to improvise the resolution of these systems.

4. *Retinal transplantation.* Transplantation of photoreceptors under retina has also been advocated. But there are no data that show these transplanted cells form viable synaptic connections with other retinal layers. Kaplan and coworkers in 2003 transplanted vibratome-harvested adult photoreceptor cells into the sub retinal space of eight patients with advanced RP. Adult human cadaver photoreceptor sheets harvested with the excimer laser were transplanted into the recipient eyes. Patients were followed for 12 months postoperatively. The change in Best-correct visual acuity (Bailey-Lovie chart), median reading speed, contrast sensitivity, and visual fields for the operated eye were not statistically significant. The ampli tude and latency of the electroretinogram, as well as the log threshold for dark adaptation, did not change between the operated and control (unoperated) eye. Kaplan et al reported on

intraoperative or postoperative complications or clinical evidence of rejection but also observed no improvement in vision. Allogeneic adult human photo-receptor transplantation is feasible in RP but was not associated with rescue of central vision or a delay in visual loss.

5. *Pharmacotherapy.* Neuroprotection with calcium channel blocker like D-cis-diltiazem which lowers c-GMP seen in some degeneration has shown no benefits.

6. *Stem cell therapy.* It has been shown that bone marrow stem cells can differentiate into various lineages like hepatocytes, endothelial cells, epithelial cells of gut and bronchus myocardium, skeletal muscle, neural cells and retinal cells.

Several animal studies have established the vasculotropic rescue and neurotrophic rescue of intravitreally injected lineage negative, bone marrow stem cells. In a study by Tomita and co-workers, it has been shown that stem cells derived from bone marrow when injected into injured eyes can differentiate into retinal neural cells in vivo in animals models suggest that bone marrow stem cells contain more primitive stem cells than hippocampus-delivered neural stem cells and that the injection of bone marrow stem cells into eyes can potentially rescue the injured retinal tissue even in human.

A pilot study was done at the Dr Rajendra Prasad Center for Ophthalmic Sciences, AIIMS by us to assess the safety of stem cells injected intravitreal in patients with advanced retinitis pigmentosa which showed no adverse events.

Right now an efficacy trial is going on in collaboration with the stem cell facility, AIIMS. The results of analysis of first 30 patients has shown

- In 6 months follow up period, mean value of best corrected visual acuity, central macular thickness and multifocal ERG p1 wave amplitude and latency with in 2 degrees from fovea showed improvement (p value >.05).
- 56.61% showing some improvement on Goldmann visual field (Fig. 23.5A and B).

Multifocal ERG (Fig. 23.6) has been a key tool in evaluating follow up patients of retinitis pigmentosa after intravitreal stem cell injection.

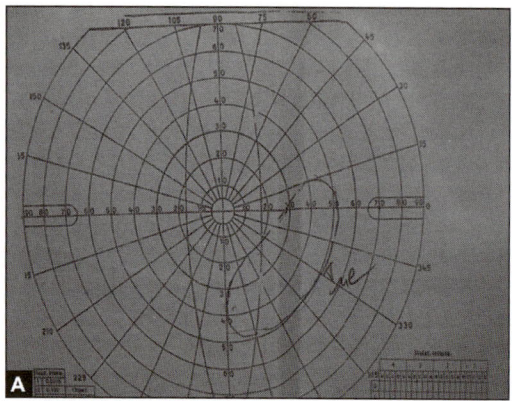

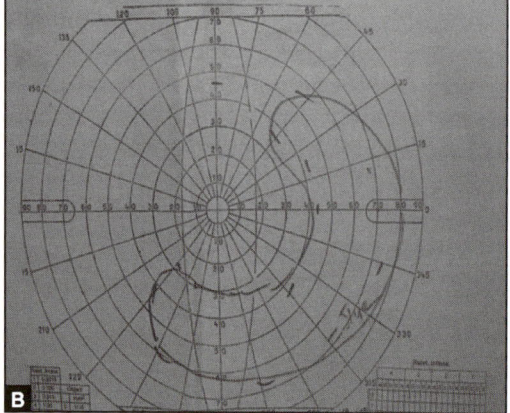

Fig. 23.5 *Goldmann visual fields.* **(A)** *Preinjection and* **(B)** *6 months following injection of stem cells*

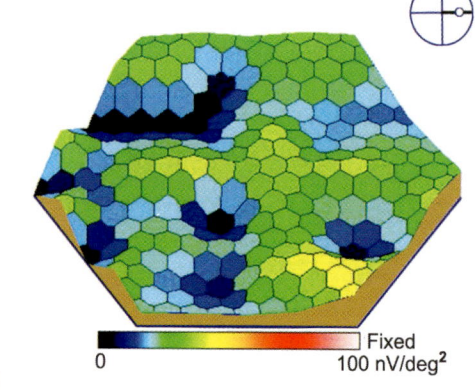

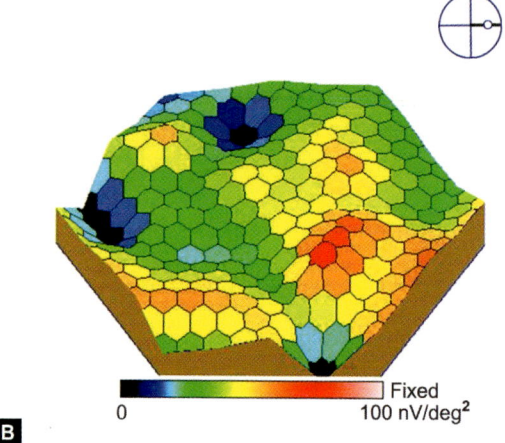

Fig. 23.6A and B *Multifocal ERG 3-D map of wave amplitudes.* **(A)** *Preinjection and* **(B)** *6 months of post-injection*

OTHER DIFFUSE RETINAL DYSTROPHIES

CONE DYSTROPHIES

INTRODUCTION

The cone dystrophies represent a heterogenous group of disorders that can be inherited as an autosomal recessive, autosomal dominant or X-linked recessive trait. The stationary cone dystrophies present as congenital disorders with various degrees of cone dysfunction but normal rod function. In contrast, the progressive cone dystrophies often present in childhood or even early adulthood. These patients often develop rod dysfunction in later life and therefore overlap in clinical features with cone-rod dystrophies.

PROGRESSIVE CONE-ROD DYSTROPHIES

Synonym: Progressive cone dystrophy.

Introduction

This dystrophy is characterized by the presence of progressive color defects and a progressive decrease in visual acuity. There is a gradual decrease in visual acuity during the first or second decades of life, followed by a gradual loss of color vision. Frequently, these patients may go undiagnosed for years and they may be mistakenly believed to have a functional disorder.

The inheritance pattern is usually autosomal dominant, although autosomal recessive and X-linked recessive inheritance pattern have been described. Even within these inheritance modes, multiple different locations of mutations have

been documented. Autosomal dominant progressive cone dystrophy has been mapped to chromosome 19q13.3, 17q12-p13, and to specific mutations of the peripherin/RDS gene on chromosome 6p. In patients with X-linked recessive progressive cone dystrophy, several loci have been mapped, including Xp21-p11.1, Xq27, and Xq28.

Histopathologic study shows a complete disappearance of the photoreceptors in the macular and paramacular regions, with associated degeneration and disappearance of the retinal pigment epithelium.

Clinical findings

Defective color vision and a decrease in visual acuity are the presenting complaints. Photophobia is extremely common, along with hameralopia. Patients may develop total achromatopsia with visual acuities in the 20/200 range.

Foveal reflex may be absent and there may be some increased granularity of the retinal pigment epithelium in the macula. There can be oval atrophy of the macular retinal pigment epithelium ("beaten bronze" atrophy), and associated choroidal atrophy. A characteristic Bulls eye maculopathy, similar to that seen in patients with chloroquine retinopathy, may also be seen.

In the early stages of the dystrophy, the optic disc, retinal vessels, and peripheral retina are usually normal (Fig. 23.7).

Fluorescein angiography demonstrates increased transmission of choroidal fluorescence in the macula during early phases of the study (Fig. 23.8), without late leakage of dye or staining. In addition, an annular pattern of hyperfluorescence is often seen in the macula, highlighting the Bulls eye pattern seen on fundus examination.

Visual field defects include central scotoma, peripheral field loss, and ring scotoma.

Electrophysiologic testing

In the early stages of the dystrophy, electrophysiologic testing reveals normal photopic and scotopic ERG responses. With progression of the disease, there is a moderate-to-marked loss of cone function, associated with a slight-to-moderate loss of rod function, markedly decreased or absent photopic responses and mildly decreased scotopic responses.

The EOG in the early stage of the dystrophy is normal. With more widespread involvement of the retina, a reduction of the light rise develops and the EOG becomes a sensitive indicator of the progress of the dystrophy. The EOG first becomes subnormal, and is then followed by the presence of a subnormal ERG.

Dark adaptation curves late in the course of the dystrophy are monophasic with slightly elevated rod thresholds.

Differential diagnosis

The differential diagnosis includes rod monochromatism, pericentral and sine pigmento

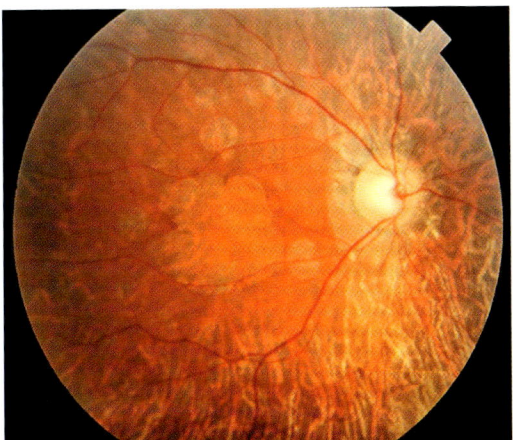

Fig. 23.7 *Progressive cone-rod dystrophy*

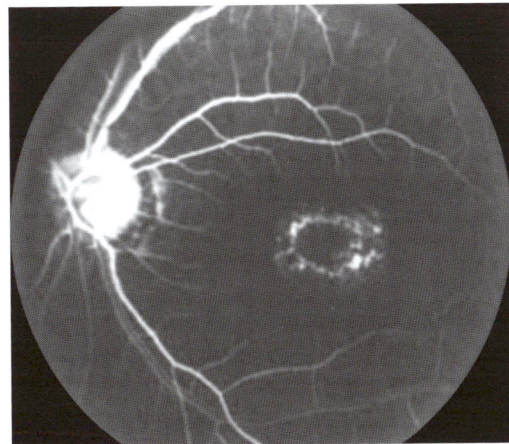

Fig. 23.8 *Fluorescein angiography showing transmission defects at the macula*

forms of retinitis pigmentosa (rod-cone dystrophy), Stargardt's disease, central areolar choroidal dystrophy, chloroquin retinopathy, and congenital optic atrophy.

PERICENTRAL (INVERSE) RETINITIS PIGMENTOSA (ROD-CONE DYSTROPHY)

Synonyms. Pericentral pigmentary retinopathy, pericentral pigmentary dystrophy, peripapillary pigmentary retinal degeneration, pericentral pigmentary degeneration.

Introduction

Pericentral retinitis pigmentosa is characterized by pigmentary disturbances similar to those occurring in classic Retinitis pigmentosa, but which occur solely in the pericentral retina with no involvement of the peripheral retina.

The disease has an autosomal recessive mode of inheritance.

Clinical Findings

Vision is usually normal in the early stage and patients are often diagnosed on routine fundus examinations in the second and third decades of life. In later stages, vision may be markedly reduced. Color vision is normal early on, but becomes defective accompanied by a progressive decrease in central vision. Nyctalopia is often present. The pigmentary changes may take the form of bone spicules or scattered black dots and are the earliest signs of the dystrophy. Because the fovea is lacking in vessels, no bone spicules are present in this region. Atrophy of the retinal pigment epithelium may also be present. Unlike retinitis pigmentosa (Fig. 23.9), the disc and retinal vessels are usually normal until late in the course of the disease.

Tritan color defects have been reported on Ishihara and Farnsworth-Munsell testing. Despite the common presenting symptom of nyctalopia, the dark adaptometry is normal or slightly delayed. FFA usually normal in early course of the disease.

Differential diagnosis

The differential diagnosis includes classic retinitis pigmentosa (rod-cone dystrophy), progressive cone-rod dystrophy, the late stage

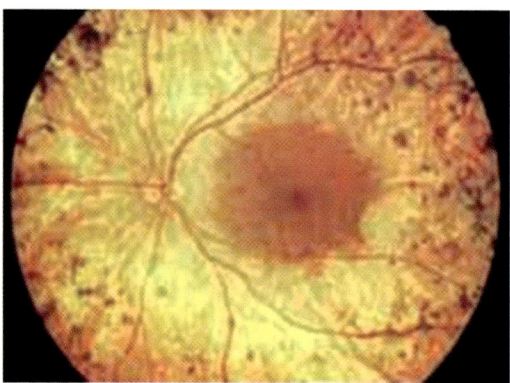

Fig. 23.9 *Pericentral retinitis pigmentosa*

of fundus flavimaculatus, and inflammatory and infectious causes of chorioretinitis. The ERG should enable one to differentiate this dystrophy from the progressive cone-rod dystrophies and classic retinitis pigmentosa (rod-cone dystrophy). The dark adaptation curve may be biphasic.

Electro-physiologic tests

Patients have normal scotopic ERG, absent or markedly subnormal photopic ERG, and a normal EOG.

INNER RETINAL DYSTROPHIES

X-linked juvenile retinoschisis

Synonyms: Congenital hereditary retinoschisis, congenital vascular veils, anterior dialysis of the young, cystic disease of the retina, inherited retinal detachment.

Introduction

Initially described by Haas in 1898, X-linked juvenile retinoschisis is an X-linked recessive condition with 100% penetrance, but varying expressivity. The pathogenesis is unknown, but histopathologic and electrophysiological studies have suggested an underlying defect in the Müller's cells.

The gene locus for this condition is located on the distal short arm of the X-chromosome localized to the p22 region. Only males are affected and female carriers have normal vision and are normal on clinical examination and electrophysiological testing.

The characteristic histopathologic feature of juvenile retinoschisis is a split between the nerve fiber and ganglion cell layers. This is to be distinguished from the split between the outer plexiform and adjacent nuclear layers seen in senile or acquired retinoschisis.

Clinical findings

There is wide variation in the presentation of the disorder. The major finding within the macula is a classic radial cystic maculopathy. Although retinal signs have been described in infants as young as 3 months, foveal schisis may be difficult to detect, leading to under diagnosis. It is characterized by the presence of radiate perifoveal microcysts located in the nerve fiber layer with radiate plications of the overlying internal limiting membrane that are seen especially well on monochromatic (red-free) photography.

Peripheral features of this disorder include peripheral schisis, vitreous changes, perivascular sheathing, dendritiform patterns, retinal dragging, subretinal exudates, pigment lines, and a generalized tapetal-like reflex (Fig. 23.10).

Vision in this disease is variable and cannot be predicted based on the fundus findings alone. On occasion, it has been shown to be normal even in the presence of a foveal schisis. Visual acuity is usually in the 20/60 range in the affected young adult and may remain stationary for many years, with gradual deterioration to about 20/100 by the sixth decade. Most affected patients are legally blind by the seventh decade.

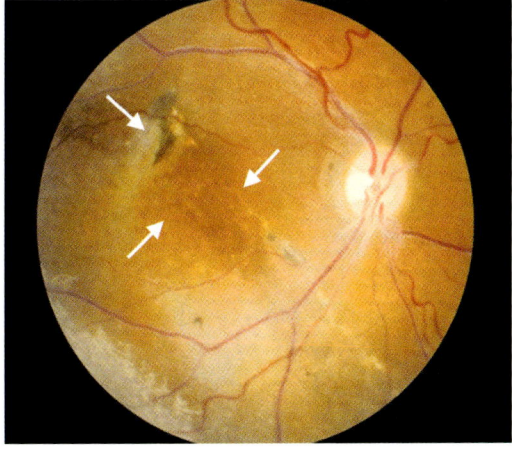

Fig. 23.10 *X-linked juvenile retinoschisis*

Laser photocoagulation, cryopexy, and scleral buckling have been used with varying degrees of success to treat peripheral schisis that is rapidly advancing and threatening the posterior pole. The incidence of retinal detachment has varied from 0% to more than 20%. For these patients, scleral buckling may be used to treat retinal detachment that may arise in areas of peripheral retinoschisis with inner and outer layer holes.

Ancillary tests

Although OCT show hyporeflective cystoid spaces but the posterior pole most often appears normal on fluorescein angiography and this may be helpful in the clinical differentiation of this entity from cystoid macular edema.

Color testing using the Farnsworth-Munsell 100-hue test shows a tritan defect. Later, a progressive deutan defect is found, correlating well with the visual acuity. Absolute visual field defects corresponding to zones of peripheral retinoschisis are present, as are relative central scotomas.

Electrophysiologic tests

In X-linked retinoschisis, the electroretinogram (ERG) is often abnormal. Both the photopic and scotopic b-wave, which arise from the bipolar cell layer, are usually reduced, whereas the a-wave, which arises from the inner segments of the photoreceptors, is intact, suggesting an inner retinal localization for these diseases. A demonstrated decrease in amplitude over several years indicates progressive disease, with non-recordable ERG responses in advanced disease.

The electro-oculogram (EOG) is normal in mild cases, but may become subnormal in advanced cases.

Dark adaptometry shows normal-to-sub-normal cone and rod segments.

Differential diagnosis

X-linked juvenile retinoschisis must be differentiated from Goldmann-Favre disease and the other forms of inherited juvenile retinoschisis described in the next section, senile or acquired retinoschisis, cystoid macular edema, idiopathic macular hole formation, Wagner's disease.

FAMILIAL FOVEAL RETINOSCHISIS

It is an autosomal recessive condition.

Fundus. Findings are similar to Juvenile Retinoschisis but fundus changes are limited to the fovea. The pathology is identical to that seen in the early stages of X-linked retinoschisis.

- *Fluorescein angiography* reveals a barely discernible area of hyperfluorescence within the fovea .
- *Visual fields* show a relative central scotoma.
- *Electrophysiologic testing* (ERG and EOG) is normal.
- *Dark adaptometry* show normal-to-subnormal cone and rod segments, and color testing reveals a mild tritan defect. The complete natural history of this disorder has not yet been elucidated.

BIBLIOGRAPHY

1. Berson EL. Rosner B, Sandberg MA, et al. A Randomized Trial of Vitamin A and Vitamin E Supplementation for Retinitis Pigmentosa Arch Ophthalmol 1993; 111: 761–72.
2. Berson EL. Retinitis Pigmentosa and allied diseases: Electrophysiologic findings; Trans Am Acad journal of Ophtalmol and Otorhinolaryngology 1976;91:659–66.
3. Bush RA, et al. Encapsulated cell-based intraocular delivery of ciliary neurotrophic factor in normal rabbit: dose-dependent effects on ERG and retinal histology. Invest. Ophthalmol. Vis. Sci. 2004;45:2420–30.
4. C. Giusti, R Forte, EM. Vingolo, Deflazacort treatment of cystoid macular edema in patients affected by Retinitis Pigmentosa: European Review for Medical and Pharmacological Sciences; 2002;6:1–8.
5. Clinical Genetic Analysis of Retinitis Pigmentosa in Indian Population, Subhabrata Chakrabartia, Virinder Kaur Sarhadia, Daljit Singh; IJHG 2001;1(2):133–37

6. Cox SN, Hay E, Bird AC Treatment of chronic macular edema with acetazolamide. Arch Ophthal 1988;106:1190–5.
7. Fetkenhour CL, Chromokos E, Weinstein J, et al. cystoid macular edema in retinitis pigmentosa: Trans Am Acad journal of Ophtalmol and Otorhinolaryngology 1977;83:515–21.
8. Gareth J. McKay, Stephen Clarke, Jason A. Davis et al; Investigative Ophthalmology & Visual Science, January 2005, Vol. 46, No. 1; 32–328.
9. Hamel C. Retinitis Pigmentosa; Orphanet encyclopedia July 2003.
10. Kaplan HJ, Tezel TH, Berger AS, Wolf ML, Del Priore LV. Human Photoreceptor Transplantation in Retinitis Pigmentosa: A Safety Study. Arch Ophthalmol; 1997;115:1168–72.
11. Minoni Tomitaa, Yasuthi Adachia C, Harunito Yamadate Kany, et al. bone marrow derived stem cells can differentiate into retinal cells in injure rat retina. Stem Cells 2002;20:279–83.
12. Otain A, Kindes K, Ewalk K, et al. Bone marrow derived stem cells target retinal astrocytes and can promote and inhibit retinal angiogenesis. Nat Med 2002;21:857–64.
13. Otami A, Dorell MI, Kinder K. Neurotrophic rescue of retinal degeneration by intravitreally injected adult bone marrow delivered lineage negative hematopoiectic stem cells. J Clin Invest 2001;114:765–774.
14. Pawlyk BS, Li T, Scimeca MS, et al. absence of photoreceptor rescue with D-cis-ditiazem in rd mouse. Invest Ophthalmol Vis Sci 2002;a3:1912–5.
15. Sieving, Caruso, Tao w, et al. Ciliary neurotrophic factor (CNTF) for human retinal degeneration: Phase I trial of CNTF delivered by encapsulated cell intraocular implants Proc Nat Acad Sci USA 2006;103:3896–901.
16. Travis GH, et al. The human retinal d egeneration slow (RDS) gene: chromosome assignment and structure of the mRNA. Genomics. 1991.
17. Wang M, Lang TT, Tso MOM, Nash MI. (1997); expression of mutant opsin gene increases susceptibility of retina to light damage. Vis Neurosci 1997;14:55–62.
18. Weilland JD, Humayun MS. A Biometric Retinal Stimulating Array; IEEE Eng Med Biol Mag. 2005;24:14–21.

24 DISORDERS OF MACULA

Atul Kumar, Anusha K, Bhavin Shah

24.1 MACULAR DYSTROPHIES

STARGARDT'S DISEASE

INTRODUCTION

Originally described by Stargardt in 1909, Stargardt's disease is a bilaterally symmetric, autosomal recessively inherited condition that is characterized by a progressive loss of central vision. The locus is identical to that described in fundus flavimaculatus, the short arm chromosome 1.

Synonym of Stargardt's is juvenile macular degeneration.

CLINICAL FINDINGS

The appearance of the fundus (Fig. 24.1.1) and the decrease in acuity may not always parallel each other, the macula is generally involved first, usually between the ages of 6 and 20.

Parafoveal and mid peripheral yellow-white flecks may occur late in the disease, representing

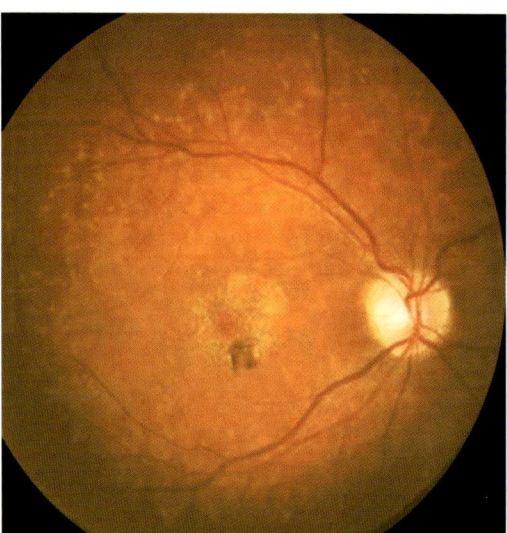

Fig. 24.1.1 *Stargardt's disease*

the large degree of heterogeneity between Stargardt's disease and fundus flavimaculatus. When the periphery is involved, it may demonstrate the presence of round, granular black spots of increased pigmentation with surrounding depigmented areas. As the atrophic process extends deeper, the choroid becomes exposed and, in the later stages, the geographic atrophy within the posterior pole may resemble that seen in central areolar choroidal dystrophy. Meanwhile, the peripheral retina may develop an appearance simulating retinitis pigmentosa (rod-cone dystrophy) with bone spicule pigmentation and irregular zones of pigment atrophy.

Visual acuity usually diminishes to the 20/200 level or worse if peripheral involvement is extensive. Central scotomas are present, while peripheral fields remain little affected until late in the course of the disease.

The classic dark or silent choroid is a diagnostic angiographic finding that has been postulated as a secondary effect of blockage of the choroidal fluorescence from the accumulation of lipofuscin. Fluorescein angiography may also show expected pigment epithelial and choroidal transmission defects also described in fundus flavimaculatus.

An acquired red-green dyschromatopsia may be characteristic in these patients with color testing.

ELECTROPHYSIOLOGIC TESTS

Both the Electroretinogram and the Electro-oculogram are normal with purely central involvement, but they are often abnormal with more diffuse involvement extending into the periphery. Visual-evoked responses are often subnormal, even with good vision and minimal fundus changes and may be helpful in establishing an early diagnosis.

Histopathologic studies reveal a complete disappearance of the visual elements in the macula. However, it is uncertain whether this represents a primary defect in the photoreceptors themselves or it is secondary to a defect in the retinal pigment epithelium. It is probable that the defects in the photoreceptors are secondary to the retinal pigment epithelium abnormalities.

FUNDUS FLAVIMACULATUS

INTRODUCTION

Although described as two separate entities, it is now believed that, apart from their ophthalmoscopic appearance, there is no clear distinction between fundus flavimaculatus and Stargardt's disease. They are most common causes for macular diseases in children.

Fundus flavimaculatus is an autosomal-recessive dystrophy now localized to the short arm chromosome 1p . It is usually diagnosed before the third and fourth decades of life and affects both genders equally. It may be discovered on routine ophthalmoscopic examination, or the patient may present with a slowly progressive decrease in vision secondary to macular involvement. Histopathologic examination of an eye with fundus flavimaculatus has demonstrated that the yellow flecks are dense accumulations of periodic acid-Schiff (PAS)-positive lipofuscin-like material within engorged RPE cells.

CLINICAL FINDINGS

The bilaterally symmetric fundus picture (Fig. 24.1.2A) is characterized by the presence of multiple Angulated or fishtail-shaped (pisciform) yellow-white lesions confined to the retinal pigment epithelium of the posterior pole. The size, shape, and confluence of the yellow flecks vary considerably, and new clusters may appear periodically as old ones fade. The optic

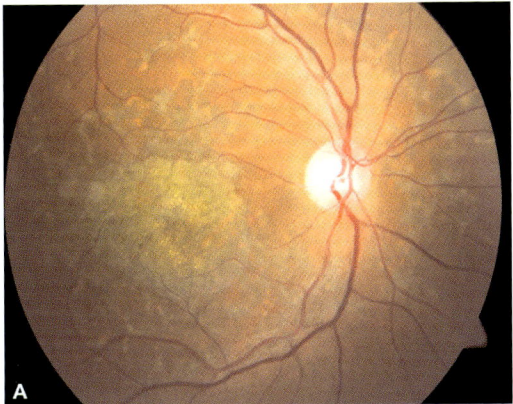

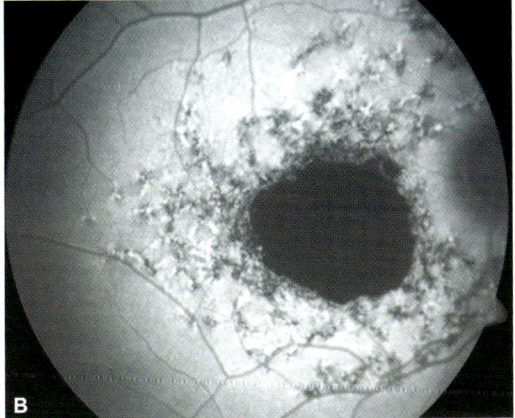

Fig. 24.1.2 *(A) Fish-tail shaped discrete macular flecks; (B) Autofluorescence picture of fundus flavimaculatus*

disc, retinal vessels, and periphery are normal in the early stage of the disease.

In the typical case, there are no atrophic macular lesions and flecks may be present within the posterior pole without significant accompanying visual loss.

Fundus exam shows fish-tail shaped discrete macular flecks (Fig. 24.1.2A) while fluorescein angiography reveals generalized decrease in choroidal fluorescence, dark choroidal flecks due to intact RPE and hyperfluorescence along areas of RPE atrophy. Autofluorescence (Fig. 24.1.2B) shows hypofluorescence due to RPE degeneration, while surrounding flecks loaded with lipofuschin appear hyper-flourescent (Fig 24.1.2B).

ELECTROPHYSIOLOGIC TESTS

The ERG may be normal and show mild abnormalities, but it is never nonrecordable as

is the case with the diffuse tapetoretinal dystrophies. The EOG is usually subnormal, suggesting a widespread defect in the retinal pigment epithelium.

DIFFERENTIAL DIAGNOSIS

The differential diagnosis of fundus flavi-maculatus includes familial drusen, fundus albipunctatus, and fleck retina of Kandori.

AUTOSOMAL DOMINANT FUNDUS FLAVIMACULATUS

Synonyms: Dominant progressive foveal dystrophy, Dominant Stargardt's disease.

This dystrophy presents a picture similar to that just described for Stargardt's disease with retinal flecks occasionally being present. It has, in fact, been called a dominant form of Stargardt's disease.

Dominant progressive foveal dystrophy is much less common than autosomal recessive Stargardt's disease; mapping of the autosomal dominant form was located at chromosome 6q and chromosome 13q.

Patients may present at a later age with decreased vision and/or decreased color discrimination. Peripheral retinal involvement is usually less extensive, the course of the disease is usually less progressive, and any accompanying macular changes may be more subtle.

Central scotomas may accompany the decrease in vision. Dark adaptometry and the ERG are normal. The EOG, however, may be abnormal. These findings tend to place the primary level of involvement as that of the retinal pigment epithelium and photoreceptors.

VITELLIFORM DYSTROPHY

Synonyms: Best's disease, vitelliruptive macular dystrophy, polymorphic macular degeneration of Braley, central exudative detachment of the retina, hereditary macular pseudocysts.

INTRODUCTION

The age of onset ranges from 3 to 15 years and may vary widely and the condition may not be detected until much later in life.

CLINICAL FINDINGS

The visual acuity may be surprisingly good, despite the apparently severe macular disturbance, and often remains relatively stable for many years. Despite relatively good visual acuity testing, patients have noted visual field defects. Progressive severe visual loss is unusual and is often associated with the development of atrophic macular changes or fibrous scarring. Hyperopia, esotropia, and strabismic amblyopia are commonly encountered in this disorder.

The disease progresses in a sequential pattern through various stages:

Stage 0: The macula may be relatively normal in appearance with a mild degree of foveal hypoplasia and an abnormal EOG.

Stage I: A speckled fine pigmentary disturbance in the macula is seen. Typical vitelliform or egg-yolk lesion composed of a round, homogeneous, opaque yellow lesion with discrete margins measuring approximately 1 disc diameter in size is present.

Stage II: This lesion (Stage I) may degenerate, leading to a scrambled-egg appearance (Fig. 24.1.3).

Stage III: The yellow material within the vitelliform cyst develops a fluid level, resulting in the appearance of a pseudohypopyon.

Stage IV: Represents advanced disease with an atrophic macular pigment epithelium (stage IVa), fibrous scarring (stage IVb), or subretinal neovascularization (stage IVc).

Fluorescein angiography (Fig. 24.1.4) demonstrates hypofluorescence of the vitelliform lesion due to blockage of dye transmission by the yellow deposition material. When this material partially or completely disappears, hyperfluorescence due to RPE transmission defects and staining may be seen.

Visual fields show relative central scotoma early in the disease, with denser scotoma being noted after degeneration and organization of the macular lesions.

ELECTROPHYSIOLOGIC TESTS

The a-waves and b-waves of the ERG are normal and it is the EOG that demonstrates the most important electrophysiologic findings.

The EOG is markedly depressed, a finding that may precede any ophthalmoscopic or clinical evidence of abnormality. This indicates that the degenerative process is not confined to the macula, but probably includes more widespread involvement of the retinal pigment epithelium, Bruch's membrane, or the potential space between these two layers.

Dark adaptometry is normal, while color defects proportional to the degree of visual loss may be noted.

DIFFERENTIAL DIAGNOSIS

The differential diagnosis of macular vitelliform lesions includes pattern dystrophies, Stargardt's disease, age-related macular degeneration,

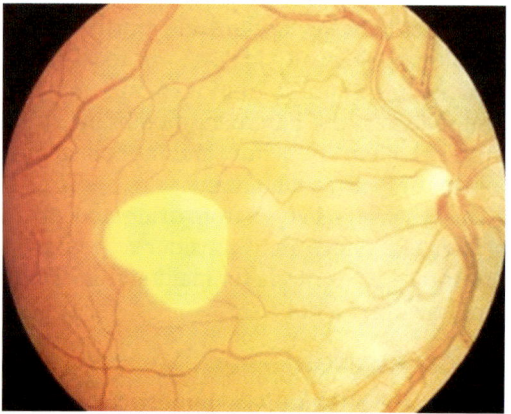

Fig. 24.1.3 *Vitelliform dystrophy Stage II*

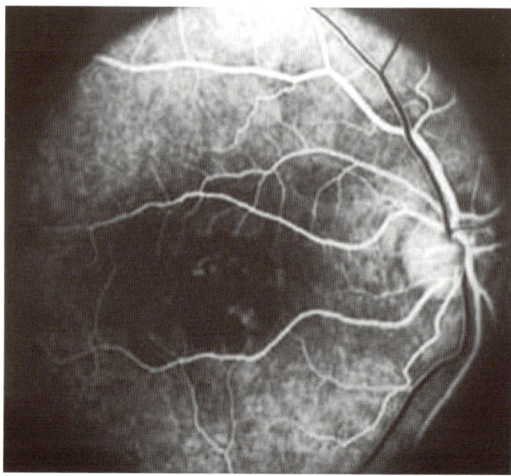

Fig. 24.1.4 *FFA early phase Stage II vitelliform dystrophy*

foveomacular vitelliform dystrophy: adult type (adult-onset foveomacular pigment epithelial dystrophy [AOFPED]), confluent drusen, and acquired RPE detachments.

FOVEOMACULAR VITELLIFORM DYSTROPHY: ADULT TYPE

Synonyms: Peculiar foveomacular dystrophy of Gass, AOFPED, pseudovitelliform macular degeneration, adult vitelliform macular degeneration.

INTRODUCTION

This autosomal dominant condition was first described by Gass in 1974 and the gene has been localized to GPT1 locus on the short arm of chromosome 16.

The histopathologic description of this dystrophy demonstrated focal loss of the photoreceptors and atrophy of the retinal pigment epithelium within the fovea.

CLINICAL FINDINGS

Visual acuity is usually better than 20/80 despite the obvious ophthalmoscopic and fluorescein angiographic changes, a mild degree of slowly progressive deterioration may occur.
Ophthalmoscopic appearance of this dystrophy consists of bilaterally symmetric, round or oval, slightly elevated, yellow subretinal lesions measuring one-third disc diameter in size with a central pigmented spot within the fovea of each eye. In addition, small paracentral, discrete yellow lesions resembling drusen may be seen at the level of the retinal pigment epithelium in some patients. Subretinal neovascularization and perifoveal capillary leakage have been reported, but are rare entities.
Fluorescein angiography during the early stage of the disease demonstrates either a hypofluorescent lesion or, more typically, a small irregular ring of hyperfluorescence surrounding a central hypofluorescent spot, a finding called the corona sign (Fig. 24.1.5).
Color testing demonstrates a mild tritan defect
Visual fields may reveal a small central scotoma.

ELECTROPHYSIOLOGIC TESTS

The ERG is normal and EOG is normal to subnormal. A reduction in the EOG Arden ratio below 1.8 is seen in majority of the eyes.

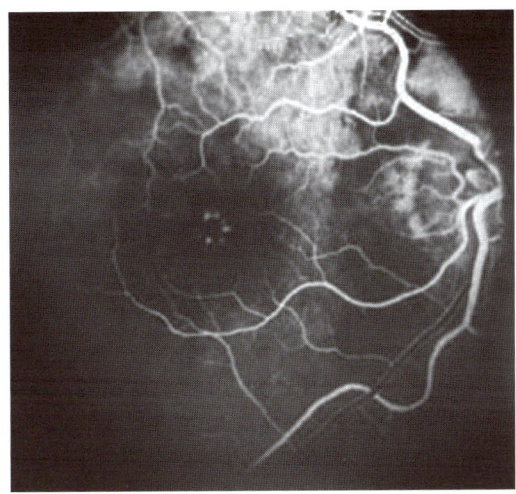

Fig. 24.1.5 *Foveomacular dystrophy FFA a-v phase*

DIFFERENTIAL DIAGNOSIS

The differential diagnosis includes age-related macular degeneration, Best's vitelliform dystrophy, and adult vitelliform macular degeneration

FAMILIAL DRUSEN

Synonyms: Dominant drusen of Bruch's membrane, Doyne's honeycomb choroiditis, Hutchinson-Tay central guttate choroiditis, Holthouse-Batten superficial choroiditis, Malattia-leventinese, Sorsby's macular dystrophy.

INTRODUCTION

It is an autosomal dominant dystrophy which is isolated to Chromosome 2p16-p21, with the onset often between the third and fourth decades.

Histopathologically, drusen are focal collections of eosinophilic homogeneous material lying between the basement membrane of the retinal pigment epithelium and the collagenous portion of Bruch's membrane.

This disease is distinct from drusen occurring in later life, which they consider to be part of senescence. The criteria for making this distinction, however, is not clear.

CLINICAL FINDINGS

Drusen are bilaterally symmetric, multiple, deep, yellow lesions of various sizes and

configurations (Fig. 24.1.6). Early in life, they may be relatively difficult to detect on ophthalmoscopy, although they can be seen with slit-lamp retroillumination as semi-translucent depositions. As the pigment epithelium overlying the deposits becomes thinned, the drusen turns yellow and are more easily detected. Drusen change in size, shape, distribution, and consistency over years, with some drusen eventually becoming calcified and demonstrating a crystalline appearance ophthalmoscopically, while others may disappear and leave behind small areas of geographic atrophy of the overlying pigment epithelium. These lesions are characteristically seen on the nasal side of the disc as well.

INVESTIGATIONS

Fluorescein angiography reveals RPE transmission defects corresponding to the areas of drusen deposition and thinning of the overlying retinal pigment epithelium. The fluorescent areas usually remain constant in size, reach peak fluorescence within the first minute following dye injection, and rapidly begin to fade along with the background choroidal fluorescence. In some instances, however, the lesions continue to show fluorescence even after the background choroidal fluorescence has faded, indicating fluorescein dye staining of the deposition material itself. In addition, fluorescein angiography often reveals the presence of more drusen than are apparent on fundus examination alone.

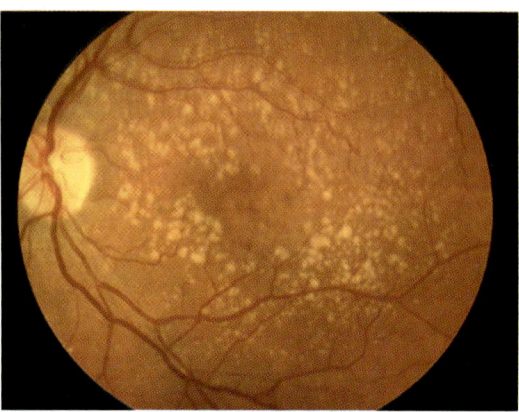

Fig. 24.1.6 *Familial dominant drusen*

Dark adaptation, color testing, and *visual field* studies are usually normal.

Electrophysiologic tests

The ERG is generally normal, while the EOG may be subnormal, especially in advanced cases, indicating a more widespread defect than would be revealed based on ophthalmoscopy or angiography.

DIFFERENTIAL DIAGNOSIS

The differential diagnosis includes age-related macular degeneration, fundus flavimaculatus, retinitis punctata albescens and Best's vitelliform dystrophy with multifocal vitelliform lesions (polymorphic macular degeneration of Braley).

CENTRAL AREOLAR PIGMENT EPITHELIAL DYSTROPHY

Synonyms: North Carolina macular dystrophy, Lefler-Wadsworth-Sidbury dystrophy.

INTRODUCTION

Central areolar pigment epithelium (CAPE) dystrophy is an autosomal dominant disorder with a high degree of penetrance and variable expressivity. The North Carolina Macular dystrophy locus (MCDR1) has been mapped to 6q14–q16.2.

Characteristics of this dystrophy include onset in the first decade, lack of visual symptoms, normal visual acuity, and a nonprogressive course.

CLINICAL FINDINGS

The fundus lesions of CAPE dystrophy consist of an RPE disturbance within the fovea which may progress to become confluent zone of RPE atrophy (Fig. 24.1.7).

Fluorescein angiography reveals RPE transmission defects corresponding to the punctate and confluent lesions within the fovea. Occasionally, when the disorder is complicated by subretinal neovascular membrane formation, subretinal hemorrhage, retinal edema, dye leakage, and fluorescein pooling may be seen within the macula.

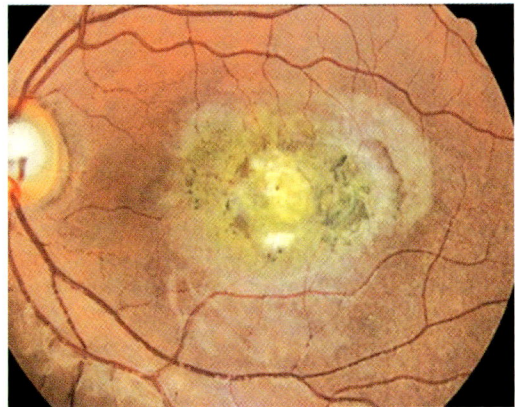

Fig. 24.1.7 *CAPE dystrophy*

ELECTROPHYSIOLOGIC TESTS

ERG and EOG studies performed on patients with CAPE dystrophy are normal.

The results of dark adaptometry and color testing are normal. The normality of these results helps to distinguish this entity from most other macular dystrophies.

DIFFERENTIAL DIAGNOSIS

The differential diagnosis includes dominant progressive foveal dystrophy (dominant Stargardt's), familial drusen, central areolar choroidal dystrophy, and congenital macular colobomas.

NORTH CAROLINA MACULAR DYSTROPHY

Synonyms: Lefler-Wadsworth-Sidbury dystrophy, CAPE dystrophy.

INTRODUCTION

It is an autosomal dominant foveal dystrophy.

CLINICAL FINDINGS

The dystrophy develops during the first year of life, and the foveal lesions were thought to progress throughout childhood to reach their final stage by late puberty. The final visual acuity is also reached by late puberty. Ophthalmoscopically, the macular changes can be divided into three stages:

Stage 1. Scattered drusen and pigment dispersion within the fovea. Visual acuity is usually 20/20, and central or paracentral scotomas are not present.

Stage 2. Confluent drusen with or without pigment clumping within the central macula. RPE atrophy and partial choroidal atrophy may be seen. The visual acuity is usually in the 20/50 range, and small central or paracentral scotomas may be present (Fig. 24.1.8).

Stage 3. Choroidal atrophy. Total RPE and choriocapillary atrophy of the fovea, parafovea, or entire macula may develop.

Visual acuity is usually in the 20/50 to 20/200 range and large central or paracentral scotomas are present. The foveal lesion is always moderately severe before any decrease in visual acuity occurs. Thereafter, the decrease in visual acuity closely parallels the severity of the foveal lesion. Likewise, the size and development of central scotomas correspond closely to the stage and size of the foveal lesions. There is no known therapy for this dystrophy.

ANCILLARY TESTS

Stage 1. Fluorescein angiography reveals transmission defects within the fovea corresponding to the drusen.

Stage 2. Fluorescein angiography shows a more confluent pattern of transmission defects with no evidence of dye leakage or pooling.

Stage 3. Angiography demonstrates diffuse transmission defects secondary to total RPE and choriocapillary atrophy.

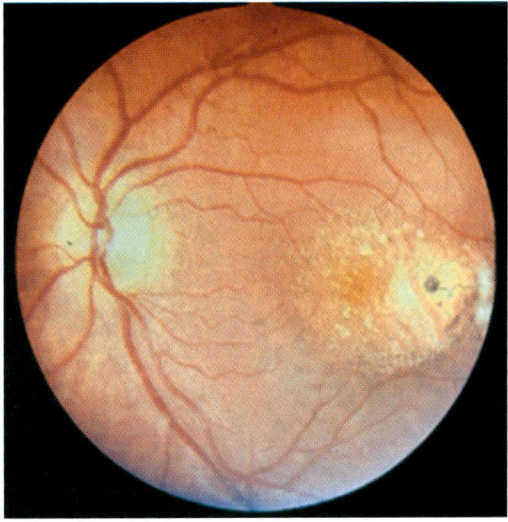

Fig. 24.1.8 *North carolina macular dystrophy*

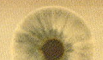

ELECTROPHYSIOLOGIC TESTING

The ERG and EOG are normal, as are dark adaptometry and color vision testing.

DIFFERENTIAL DIAGNOSIS

The differential diagnosis includes dominant progressive foveal dystrophy (dominant Stargardt's), familial drusen, central areolar choroidal dystrophy, and congenital macular colobomas.

DOMINANT SLOWLY PROGRESSIVE MACULAR DYSTROPHY OF SINGERMAN-BERKOW-PATZ

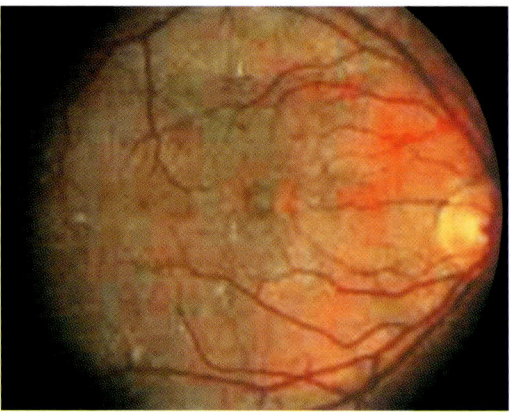

Fig. 24.1.10 *Slowly progressive macular dystrophy type 2*

This dystrophy manifests itself in the fifth to sixth decades, and patients are generally asymptomatic or show a slight decrease in central vision in the 20/25 to 20/40 range.

Younger patients demonstrate only a subtle degree of pigment epithelial mottling within the fovea.

Older patients have macular lesions that can be divided into one of two types:

Type 1 lesions consist of an ovoid RPE defect measuring less than 1 disc diameter in size with a central spot of grayish yellow deposition material and no associated flecks or spots within the posterior pole (Fig. 24.1.9).

Type 2 lesions are similar to type 1 lesion but are associated within definite flecks in the posterior pole (Fig. 24.1.10).

Fluorescein angiography demonstrates an ovoid area of hyperflourescence and late staining corresponding to the RPE defect surrounding a central hypofluorescent spot related to the grayish yellow deposition material (Fig. 24.1.11).

ELECTROPHYSIOLOGIC TESTS

The ERG usually reveals normal-to-subnormal photopic and scotopic responses.

The EOG is usually normal

Color vision testing is normal.

Visual field studies demonstrate para central scotoma and a generalized field constriction.

DOMINANT CYSTOID MACULAR DYSTROPHY

INTRODUCTION

It is an autosomal recessive condition and the gene has been localized to chromosome 7p.

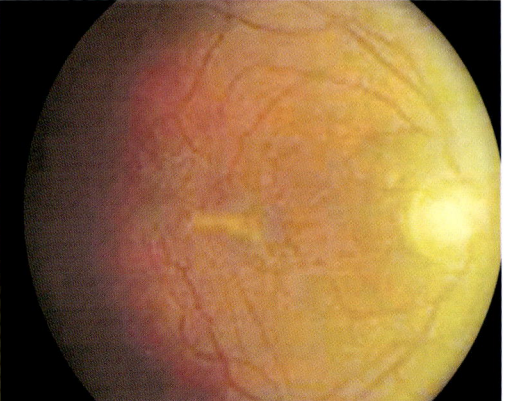

Fig. 24.1.9 *Slowly progressive macular dystrophy type 1*

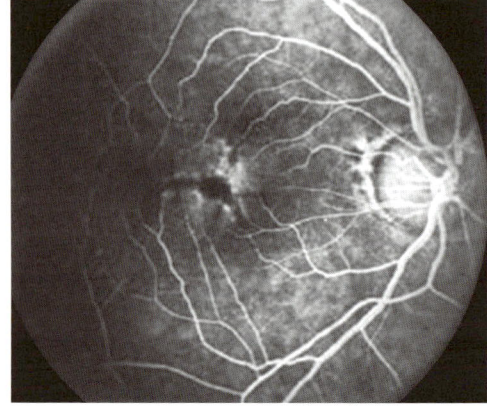

Fig. 24.1.11 *FFA appearance of slowly progressive macular dystrophy*

CLINICAL FINDINGS

Dominant cystoid macular edema is characteristically seen in the first and second decades with a prolonged course of macular cystoid change and progressive loss of central vision.

Hyperopia from +2.00 to +10.00 D is seen along with hypopigmentation within the central macula. Macular atrophy is a fairly prominent finding late in the course of the disease. Subsequently, vision may be reduced to finger counting range and a relative-to-absolute central scotoma may be present.

Fluorescein angiography reveals leakage from perifoveal capillaries with dye pooling in a cystoid pattern. Later in the disease, transmission defects are seen in areas of RPE atrophy. In some cases, fluorescein leakage from optic disc capillaries has also been noted.

Color testing in some patients often demonstrated blue yellow defects which is likely to be secondary to macular edema and in chronic cases red green deficiencies secondary to photoreceptor damage.

ELECTROPHYSIOLOGIC STUDIES

- **ERG** is normal in all patients.
- **EOG** and results of dark adaptometry, however, are subnormal in most, but not all, patients. The subnormal EOG would indicate widespread dysfunction of the retinal pigment epithelium.

DIFFERENTIAL DIAGNOSIS

The condition should be differentiated from retinitis pigmentosa with cystoid macular edema, and dystrophies characterized by the presence of foveal retinoschisis (which may be mistaken for cystoid macular edema) such as X-linked juvenile retinoschisis and familial foveal retinoschisis. In these conditions, OCT shows cystoid space but no leakage on FFA. Cystoid macular edema is seen after ophthalmic surgeries, pars planitis, and other ocular inflammatory disorders.

FENESTRATED SHEEN MACULAR DYSTROPHY

INTRODUCTION

Fenestrated sheen macular dystrophy is an autosomal dominant condition with high penetrance.

CLINICAL FINDINGS

Fenestrated sheen macular dystrophy is a slowly progressive disease presenting in childhood. In the early stages, small, red demarcated lesions can be seen within the deep neurosensory retina. It is characterized by the presence of yellowish refractile sheen with red fenestrations within the macula. The sheen is also present within the foveal avascular zone and may be related to the macular luteal pigment. The fenestrations appear to be tiny windows within the sheen that allow increased visualization of the underlying pigment epithelium. The changes within the sensory retina are slowly progressive and are eventually accompanied by changes of the retinal pigment epithelium. By the third decade, an annular zone of hypopigmentation of the retinal pigment epithelium appears around the area of sheen and progressively enlarges to form a bull's-eye macular lesion.

Visual acuity usually remains normal throughout, although paracentral scotomas develop by the sixth decade of life. The prognosis for maintenance of central vision is excellent and despite the ophthalmoscopically evident macular changes, central visual acuity remains normal.

The fluorescein angiographic features (Fig. 24.1.12) of this dystrophy are dependent on chronicity of the disorder. Younger patients have essentially normal studies. Older patients

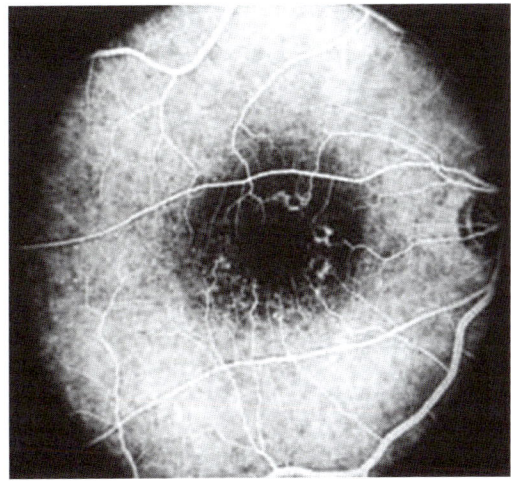

Fig. 24.1.12 *Fenestrated sheen macular dystrophy*

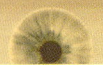

demonstrate multiple punctate window defects in an annular zone ringed by an area of slightly subnormal choroidal fluorescence due to increased pigmentation of the retinal pigment epithelium

ELECTROPHYSIOLOGIC TESTS

Retinal function studies correlate with age. Younger patients have normal ERGs and EOGs and a mild red-green color defect.

Older patients have subnormal photopic ERGs and normal-to-subnormal EOGs.

DIFFERENTIAL DIAGNOSIS

Acute macular neuroretinopathy, Stargardt's disease, progressive cone-rod dystrophy, benign concentric annular macular dystrophy, central areolar pigment epithelial dystrophy, and central areolar choroidal dystrophy.

BUTTERFLY-SHAPED PIGMENT DYSTROPHY OF THE FOVEA

INTRODUCTION

Deutman and associates in the Netherlands first described this autosomal dominant dystrophy with a peculiar pigmentary pattern in the central macula in 1970.

CLINICAL FINDINGS

This disorder manifests itself in the second to fifth decades and is accompanied by normal or only slightly decreased vision in the 20/20 to 20/25 range. The characteristic feature (Fig. 24.1.13) of this dystrophy is the presence of a bilaterally symmetric reticular pattern of pigmentation (the so-called butterfly-shape) within the central macula which is best seen with fluorescein angiography.

Fluorescein angiography demonstrates a reticular hypofluorescent pattern corresponding to the areas of hyperpigmentation with no obvious hyperfluorescence or dye leakage (Fig. 24.1.14).

Dark adaptometry and **color testing** are normal, while **visual field** studies may reveal a relative central scotoma with normal peri-pheral fields.

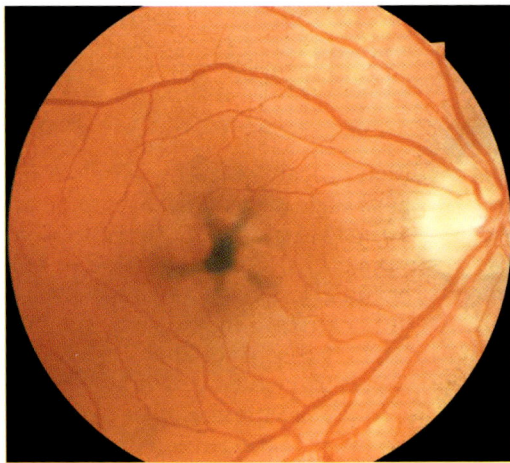

Fig. 24.1.13 *Pigment dystrophy of the fovea*

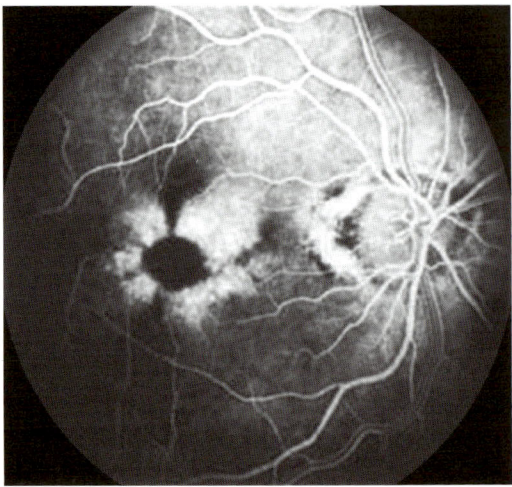

Fig. 24.1.14 *FFA appearance of pigment dystrophy of the fovea*

ELECTROPHYSIOLOGIC STUDIES

The ERG is normal, while the EOG demonstrates subnormal-to-abnormal values, suggesting a more widespread disturbance of the retinal pigment epithelium than visualised ophthalmoscopically.

SJÖGREN'S RETICULAR DYSTROPHY OF THE RETINAL PIGMENT EPITHELIUM

INTRODUCTION

In 1950, Sjögren reported a rare dystrophy which has an autosomal recessive mode of inheritance,

distinguishing it from the autosomal dominant pattern dystrophies of the retinal pigment epithelium just discussed.

CLINICAL FINDINGS

This condition probably manifests itself at first decade. At this stage, patients are asymptomatic and have normal visual acuities. However, some loss of vision may occur later in the disease process. The initial lesion is a dark pigment spot within the central macula measuring approximately 1 disc diameter in size (Fig. 24.1.15). A hyperpigmented network first forms around the central accumulation of pigmented granules with a gradual extension of the pattern toward the midperiphery up to around 5-7 disc diameters.

Fluorescein angiography demonstrates a netlike hypofluorescent pattern corresponding to the reticular pattern of increased pigmentation with hyperfluorescence of the meshes of the network. No leakage or staining is observed in the later phases of the fluorescein angiogram (Fig. 24.1.16).

Dark adaptometry is normal-to-abnormal, while color testing and visual field studies are normal.

ELECTROPHYSIOLOGIC TESTS

The ERG is normal, while the EOG is normal-to-subnormal, suggesting the presence of diffuse involvement at the level of the retinal pigment epithelium.

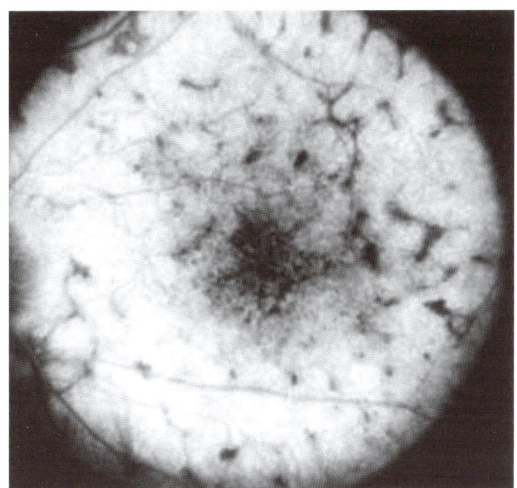

Fig. 24.1.16 *FFA of pattern dystrophies of the retinal pigment epithelium*

DIFFERENTIAL DIAGNOSIS

The differential diagnosis includes the dominant reticular dystrophies of Werner-Benedikt and of Kingham-Fenzl-Willerson-Aaberg, macro reticular dystrophy, fundus flavimaculatus, senile reticular peripheral degeneration, and the other pattern dystrophies of the retinal pigment epithelium.

PIGMENT EPITHELIAL DYSTROPHY OF NOBLE-CARR-SIEGAL

INTRODUCTION

In 1977, Noble and his colleagues studied a family exhibiting hereditary syndrome of myopia, nystagmus, and an RPE dystrophy. This disorder has an autosomal dominant pattern of inheritance with complete penetrance and variable expressivity and is believed to occur early in life, perhaps even being present at birth.

CLINICAL FINDINGS

Several features that characterize this entity include decreased central vision in the 20/40 to hand motions range, pendular nystagmus, and a moderate-to-severe degree of myopia. Changes in the retinal pigment epithelium range from a mild pigmentary disturbance with irregularity or loss of the foveal reflex to an advanced derangement that involved loss of the retinal pigment epithelium and chorio-capillaris

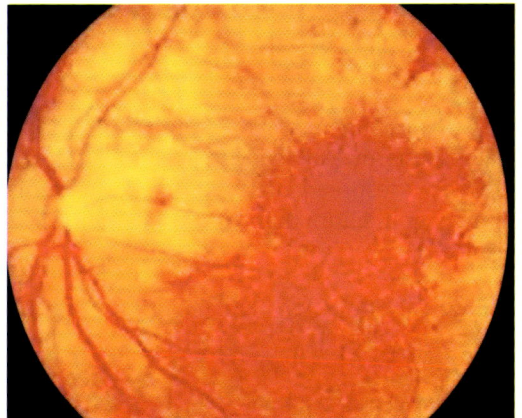

Fig. 24.1.15 *Pattern dystrophies of the retinal pigment epithelium*

with increased visibility of the choroidal vasculature and pigment clumping noted both focally within the posterior pole and diffusely throughout the retina. This dystrophy is stationary or slowly progressive.

Fluorescein angiography demonstrates an irregular pattern of hypofluorescence corresponding to areas of increased pigmentation, and hyperfluorescence related to zones of RPE atrophy.

ELECTROPHYSIOLOGIC TESTS

ERG abnormalities were always present in the reported cases and ranged from a moderate decrease in scotopic b-wave amplitudes to a nonrecordable response. A direct relationship between the retinal changes and electrophysiologic results was noted, patients with greater losses in their scotopic b-wave amplitudes showed more extensive fundus lesions.

The EOG was normal, and visual field studies demonstrated a central scotoma when the posterior pole alone was involved.

BENIGN CONCENTRIC ANNULAR MACULAR DYSTROPHY

INTRODUCTION

In 1974, Deutman described this autosomal dominant macular dystrophy with an onset in the second decade. The characteristic lesion was a bull's-eye macular lesion consisting of a ringlike zone of atrophic retinal pigment epithelium surrounding an intact central fovea.

CLINICAL FINDINGS

Decreased visual acuity, varying degrees of peripheral pigmentary disruption are described, and ranged from a subtle granular change to obvious bone spicule pigmentary changes. Varying degrees of retinal arteriolar attenuation, waxy optic disc pallor, and peripapillary atrophy were also noted

Fluorescein angiography demonstrates a pattern of hyperfluorescence corresponding to the area of RPE atrophy with hypofluorescence of the central intact zone. Scattered areas of extramacular hyperfluorescence secondary to RPE transmission defects may also be seen.

Dark adaptometry reveals normal-to-abnormal cone and rod segments.

Color vision testing shows an acquired tritan defect.

Visual field charting reveals ring scotoma with varying degrees of peripheral contraction.

ELECTROPHYSIOLOGIC TESTS

The ERG is initially normal to subnormal. Most individuals eventually develop subnormal scotopic and photopic responses, with early involvement of the photopic system.

The EOG is normal in less severely affected individuals, and is subnormal-to-markedly abnormal in severely affected patients. This dystrophy may be due to a primary abnormality of the retinal pigment epithelium with secondary nonselective dysfunction of the photoreceptors, or it may represent a mild benign variant of the progressive cone-rod dystrophies.

CENTRAL AREOLAR CHOROIDAL DYSTROPHY

Synonyms. Central areolar choroidal sclerosis, central areolar choroidal atrophy.

INTRODUCTION

Central areolar choroidal dystrophy is an autosomal dominant disorder, as was first reported by Sorsby and Crick, and later confirmed by others. Hoyng et al described an autosomal dominant form caused by a mutation in codon 142 in the peripherin/RDS gene while Lotery et al localized the gene to chromosome 17p. An autosomal recessive pattern of inheritance has also been demonstrated in some families.

CLINICAL FINDINGS

The onset of symptoms usually occurs in the second decade, with the initial symptom being a mild-to-moderate decrease in central vision depending on the location of the changes within the macula. This may be followed by a progressive decrease in visual acuity.

The earliest fundus changes seen in patients with central areolar choroidal dystrophy consist of a mild degree of nonspecific granularity within the fovea. It is only after many years does

the pathognomonic round or oval zone of neurosensory, RPE, and choriocapillary atrophy appear within the posterior pole. When this occurs, the underlying choroid becomes much more clearly visualized, with the larger choroidal vessels appearing yellowish white simulating the appearance of heavily sheathed, fine red lines (Fig. 24.1.17).

Fluorescein angiography of the early lesions may show faint areas of hyperfluorescence within the fovea corresponding to RPE transmission defects. Lesions seen later in the course of the dystrophy demonstrate findings consistent with a sharply demarcated zone of chorioretinal atrophy with no choroidal fluorescence in the early phases of the study.

Color vision testing reveals the presence of moderate protan-deutan defects.

Visual field studies demonstrate large central scotomas in those patients manifesting zones of RPE and choriocapillary atrophy within the central macula.

ELECTROPHYSIOLOGIC STUDIES

The ERG may demonstrate normal-to-slightly subnormal photopic responses and normal scotopic responses

The EOG may reveal normal-to-slightly subnormal results.

Multifocal electroretinogram has shown localized areas of depressed retinal function despite normal full-field electroretinograms.

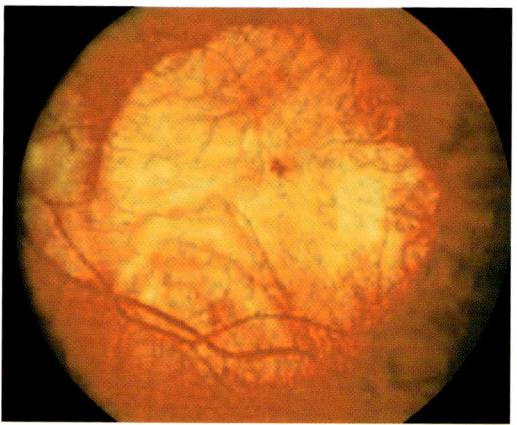

Fig. 24.1.17 *Central areolar choroidal dystrophy*

DIFFERENTIAL DIAGNOSIS

The differential diagnosis includes CAPE dystrophy, dominant progressive foveal dystrophy (dominant Stargardt's), North Carolina macular dystrophy, Best's disease, and age-related macular degeneration with geographic atrophy within the central macula.

INNER RETINAL AND VITREO RETINAL DYSTROPHIES

X-LINKED JUVENILE RETINOSCHISIS

Synonyms: Congenital hereditary retinoschisis, congenital vascular veils, anterior dialysis of the young, cystic disease of the retina, inherited retinal detachment

INTRODUCTION

Initially described by Haas in 1898, X-linked juvenile retinoschisis is an X-linked recessive condition with 100% penetrance, but varying expressivity. The pathogenesis is unknown, but histopathologic and electrophysiological studies have suggested an underlying defect in the Müller's cells.

The gene locus for this condition is located on the distal short arm of the X chromosome localized to the p22 region. Only males are affected and female carriers have normal vision and are normal on clinical examination and electrophysiological testing

The characteristic histopathologic feature of juvenile retinoschisis is a split between the nerve fiber and ganglion cell layers. This is to be distinguished from the split between the outer plexiform and adjacent nuclear layers seen in senile or acquired retinoschisis.

CLINICAL FINDINGS

There is wide variation in the presentation of the disorder. The major finding within the macula is a classic radial cystic maculopathy. Although retinal signs have been described in infants as young as 3 months, foveal schisis may be difficult to detect, leading to under-diagnosis. It is characterized by the presence of radiate perifoveal microcysts located in the nerve fiber layer with radiate plications of the overlying internal limiting membrane that are seen

especially well on monochromatic (red-free) photography.

Peripheral features of this disorder include peripheral schisis, vitreous changes, perivascular sheathing, dendritiform patterns, retinal dragging, subretinal exudates, pigment lines, and a generalized tapetal-like reflex (Fig. 24.1.18).

Vision in this disease is variable and cannot be predicted based on the fundus findings alone. On occasion, it has been shown to be normal even in the presence of a foveal schisis. Visual acuity is usually in the 20/60 range in the affected young adult and may remain stationary for many years, with gradual deterioration to about 20/100 by the sixth decade. Most affected patients are legally blind by the seventh decade.

Laser photocoagulation, cryopexy, and scleral buckling have been used with varying degrees of success to treat peripheral schisis that is rapidly advancing and threatening the posterior pole. The incidence of retinal detachment has varied from 0% to more than 20%. For these patients, scleral buckling may be used to treat retinal detachment that may arise in areas of peripheral retinoschisis with inner and outer layer holes.

ANCILLARY TESTS

The posterior pole most often appears normal on fluorescein angiography and this may be helpful in the clinical differentiation of this entity from cystoid macular edema.

Color testing using the Farnsworth-Munsell 100-hue test shows a tritan defect. Later, a progressive deutan defect is found, correlating well with the visual acuity. Absolute visual field defects corresponding to zones of peripheral retinoschisis are present, as are relative central scotomas.

ELECTROPHYSIOLOGIC TESTS

In X-linked retinoschisis, the electroretinogram (ERG) is often abnormal. Both the photopic and scotopic b-wave, which arise from the bipolar cell layer, are usually reduced, whereas the a-wave, which arises from the inner segments of the photoreceptors, is intact, suggesting an inner retinal localization for these diseases. A demonstrated decrease in amplitude over several years indicates progressive disease, with nonrecordable ERG responses in advanced disease.

The electro-oculogram (EOG) is normal in mild cases, but may become subnormal in advanced cases.

Dark adaptometry shows normal-to-subnormal cone and rod segments.

DIFFERENTIAL DIAGNOSIS

X-linked juvenile retinoschisis must be differentiated from Goldmann-Favre disease and the other forms of inherited juvenile retinoschisis described in the next section, senile or acquired retinoschisis, cystoid macular edema, idiopathic macular hole formation, Wagner's disease, Stickler disease.

FAMILIAL FOVEAL RETINOSCHISIS

It is an autosomal recessive condition.

Findings are similar to juvenile retinoschisis but fundus changes are limited to the fovea. The pathology is identical to that seen in the early stages of X-linked retinoschisis.

Fluorescein angiography revealed a barely discernible area of hyperfluorescence within the fovea. Visual fields show a relative central scotoma.

Electrophysiologic testing (ERG and EOG) is normal.

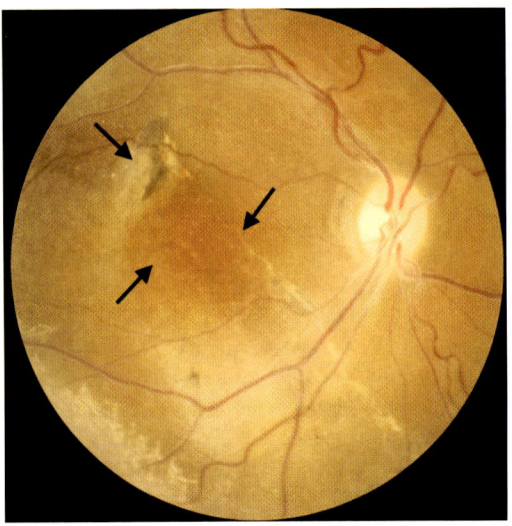

Fig. 24.1.18 *X-linked juvenile retinoschisis*

Dark adaptometry show normal-to-subnormal cone and rod segments, and color testing reveals a mild tritan defect. The complete natural history of this disorder has not yet been elucidated.

BIBLIOGRAPHY

1. Aaberg TM. Stargardt's disease and fundus flavimaculatus: evaluation of morphologic progression and intra-familial co-existence. Trans Am Ophthalmol Soc, 1986; 84:453
2. Burgess DB, Olk RJ, Uniat LM. Macular disease resembling adult foveomacular vitelliform dystrophy in older adults. Ophthalmology, 1987; 94:362
3. Cardillo Piccolino F, Singirian M. Pattern dystrophy of the retinal pigment epithelium with vitelliform macular lesion: evolution in ten years. Int Ophthalmol, 1988; 11:207
4. Carr RE. Central areolar choroidal dystrophy. Arch Ophthalmol, 1965; 73:32
5. Cavender JC. Fundus flavimaculatus: variable fundus findings in a dominant pedigree. Invest Ophthalmol Vis Sci, 1978; 17(Suppl 2):204
6. Constantaras AA, Dobbie JG, Choromakis EA, et al. Juvenile sex-linked recessive retinoschisis in a black family. Am J Ophthalmol, 1972; 74:1166
7. Curry HF, Moorman LT. Fluorescein photography of vitelliform macular degeneration. Arch Ophthalmol, 1968; 79:705
8. Daily MJ, Mets MB. Fenestrated sheen macular dystrophy. Arch Ophthalmol, 1984; 102:855
9. Deutman AF, Van Blommenstein JDA, Henkes HE, et al. Butterfly-shaped pigment dystrophy of the fovea. Arch Ophthalmol, 1970; 83:558
10. Deutman AF. Benign concentric annular macular dystrophy. Am J Ophthalmol, 1974; 78:384
11. Falls HF. A classification and clinical description of hereditary macular lesions. Trans Am Acad Ophthalmol Otolaryngol, 1966; 70:1034
12. Ferrell RE, Hittner HM, Antoszyk JH. Linkage of atypical vitelliform macular dystrophy (VMD-1) to the soluble glutamate pyruvate transaminase (GPT1) locus. Am J Hum Genet, 1983; 35:78
13. Fishman GA. Inherited macular dystrophies: a clinical overview. Aust NZ J Ophthalmol, 1990 18:123
14. Gass JDM. A clinicopathologic study of a peculiar foveomacular dystrophy. Trans Am Ophthalmol Soc, 1974; 72:139
15. Goodman G, Ripps H, Siegel IM. Cone dysfunction syndromes. Arch Ophthalmol, 1963; 70:214
16. Heon E, Piguet B, Munier F, et al. Linkage of autosomal dominant radial drusen (malattia leventinese) to chromosome 2p16-21. Arch Ophthalmol, 1996; 114:193
17. Hittner HM, Ferrel RE, Borda RP, et al. Atypical vitelliform macular dystrophy in a 5-generation family. Br J Ophthalmol, 1984; 68:199
18. Hoyng CB, Heutink P, Testers L, et al. Autosomal dominant central areolar choroidal dystrophy caused by a mutation in codon 142 in the peripherin/RDS gene. Am J Ophthalmol, 1996; June; 121(6); 623–9
19. Kremer H, Pinchers A, van den Helm B, et al. Localization of the gene for dominant cystoid macular dystrophy on chromosome 7. Hum Mol Genet, 1994; 2:299
20. Krill AE, Deutman AF. Dominant macular degenerations: the cone dystrophies. Am J Ophthalmol, 1972; 73:352
21. Lotery AJ, Ennis KT, Silvestri G, Nicholl S, et al: Localization of a gene for central areolar chroidal dystrophy to chromosome 17p. Hum Mol Genet, 1996; 5:705
22. Meire F, Bergan AA, De Rouck A, et al. X-linked to progressive cone dystrophy: localization of the gene locus to Xp21-p11.1 by linkage anyalysis. Br J Ophthalmol, 1994; 78:103
23. Merin S. Inherited macular disease. In Inherited Eye Diseases: Diagnosis and Clinical Management. New York: Dekker, 1991:137–175.
24. Mosarella MA. Gene mapping of ocular disease. Surv Ophthalmol, 1992; 36:285
25. Noble KG, Carr RE, Siegel IM. Pigment epithelial dystrophy. Am J Ophthalmol, 1977; 83:751
26. Noble KG: Central areolar choroidal dystrophy. Am J Ophthalmol, 1977; 84:310
27. Okun E, Cibis PA. The role of photocoagulation in the management of retinoschisis. Arch Ophthalmol, 1964; 72:309
28. Pearce WG. Hereditary macular dystrophy: a clinical and genetic study of two specific forms. Can J Ophthalmol, 1975; 10:319
29. Pinckers A, Deutman AF. X-linked cone dystrophy. Int Ophthalmol, 1987; 10:241
30. Ruddock KH: Psychophytsics of inherited color vision deficiencies. In: Foster D, Ed. Inherited and Acquired Color Vision Deficiencies. Basingstoke: Macmillan Press, 1991; 88:114

24.2 MACULAR HOLE

A macular hole is a full-thickness defect of the neurosensory retina involving the anatomical fovea. Idiopathic full-thickness macular holes are an important cause of central visual loss; these lesions are twice as common in females as in males and three-quarters of affected individuals are in their sixth decade. The prevalence of macular hole increases with each decade it is 0.1% in fourth decade and increases up to 0.8% by seventh decade.

PATHOGENESIS

The pathogenesis of idiopathic full-thickness macular holes is not well understood. Macular holes are commonly idiopathic in etiology, although trauma and high myopia are implicated in a minority of cases.

On the basis of clinical observations, ocular imaging, histological studies, and the results of vitrectomy surgery, the mechanism underlying idiopathic macular hole is widely believed to involve tangential as well as antero-posterior traction exerted by the posterior vitreous cortex on the neurosensory retina at the fovea. Evidence of the role of posterior vitreous attachment in the development of macular holes includes its association with an increased risk of macular hole development in the fellow eyes of individuals with unilateral macular holes and with the subsequent enlargement of established holes.

Tangential traction may be the result of contraction of the prefoveal vitreous cortex following invasion and proliferation of Muller cells. Antero-posterior traction may occur from dynamic tractional forces on an abnormally persistent vitreo-foveal attachment following perifoveal vitreous separation.

The role of antero-posterior vitreo-foveal traction is supported by optical coherence tomography (OCT) studies that clearly identify perifoveal posterior hyaloid separation with persistent adherence of the posterior hyaloid to the center of the fovea.

A cone-shaped, zone of Muller cells, the 'Muller cell cone' forms the central and inner part of the fovea centralis and appears to confer structural support, serving as a plug to bind together the foveolar photoreceptor cells.

Vitreo-foveal traction may result in dis-insertion of the Muller cell cone from underlying foveolar photoreceptor cells and in the formation of a foveal schisis or "cyst".

A dehiscence develops in the roof of the foveal cyst that may extend by centric expansion, or more commonly in a pericentric fashion, to form a crescentic hole that progresses to a horse-shoe tear. Complete avulsion of the cyst roof results in a fully detached operculum that is suspended on the posterior vitreous cortex in the prefoveal plane. Opercula primarily comprise vitreous cortex and glial elements with a variable amount of foveal tissue that includes photoreceptor cells in 40% of cases. The photoreceptor layer, which is no longer anchored by the Muller cell cone at the foveola, undergoes passive centrifugal retraction to form a full-thickness retinal dehiscence with centrifugal displacement of xanthophyll. The edge of the hole becomes progressively elevated and a cuff of subretinal fluid develops. In the event of vitreo-foveal separation during the development of the macular hole, the relief of traction may result in regression of a cyst, but spontaneous closure of an established full-thickness macular hole is relatively uncommon.

Full-thickness macular holes may also occur in association with high myopia, following posterior segment surgery such as pneumatic retinopexy, and following ocular trauma. Traumatic macular holes typically result from blunt injury, but have also been reported following laser injury and lightning strike.

CLINICAL STAGING

Macular hole formation typically evolves through a series of four major stages that were first described according to their biomicroscopic features by Gass.

Stage 1 ('impending') macular hole is loss of the normal foveal depression, associated with the development of a yellow spot (stage 1a) or ring

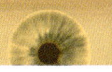

(stage 1b) in the center of the fovea, changes that reflect the intraretinal schisis that progresses into an intraretinal cyst. A foveal dehiscence may be masked on biomicroscopy (stage 1-b, occult hole) by semi-opaque contracted prefoveolar vitreous cortex bridging the yellow ring.

Stage 2 is a small full-thickness hole (≤ 200 μm), typically with a pericentric configuration, associated with persistent vitreo-foveal attachment.

Stage 3 is a larger full-thickness hole (250–400 μm) with a rim of elevated retina and separation of the posterior hyaloid from the macula. A fully detached operculum on the posterior hyaloid may be evident on biomicroscopy.

Stage 4 is a full-thickness hole (≥ 450 μm) with complete posterior vitreous separation from the optic disc, typically demonstrated by the presence of a Weiss ring (Fig. 24.2.1).

NATURAL HISTORY OF MACULAR HOLES

An estimated 40% of stage 1 (impending) macular holes progress to full-thickness holes, but up to 50% resolve spontaneously. Stage 2 macular holes typically enlarge, with progression to stage 3 in at least 75% of cases and spontaneous closure has been reported in no

more than 15–21%. Stage 3 holes progress to stage 4 in approximately 30% of cases over 3 years. Full-thickness holes tend to enlarge modestly; by 25% during the first 12 months and by 29% at 24 months, associated with deterioration in mean visual acuity from 6/36 to 6/60. Spontaneous closure of stage 3 and stage 4 holes is rare, occurring in no more than 6% of cases.

While macular holes frequently stabilize at stage 3, they may resolve spontaneously with associated improvement in visual acuity at any stage during the course of their progression. Spontaneous regression occurs in association with vitreo-foveal separation and is more likely during the early stages than during the later stages of macular hole evolution; it has been suggested that holes relieved of traction at an early stage may be more amenable to glial repair. Spontaneous resolution of small full-thickness macular holes following trauma in young patients is not uncommon and can be associated with good visual recovery (Table 24.2.1).

SIGNS AND SYMPTOMS

Stage 1 and stage 2 macular holes are asymptomatic and are identified only on routine eye examination.

Table 24.2.1 *Symptoms signs and natural history of macular holes*				
	Stage 1	*Stage 2*	*Stage 3*	*Stage 4*
Symptoms	Asymptomatic, or mild meta-morphopsia	Metamorphopsia and loss of central vision	Metamorphopsia and loss of central vision	Metamorphopsia and loss of central vision
Visual acuity	20/20–20/60	20/40–20/100	20/60–20/200	20/60–20/400
Biomicroscopy	Loss of foveal depression Yellow spot (1a) or yellow ring (1b)	Full-thickness retinal defect Typically ≤200 μm in diameter	Full-thickness retinal defect Typically 250–400 μm in diameter	Full-thickness retinal defect Typically ≥450 μm in diameter
			Operculum may be evident	Operculum may be evident
Posterior vitreous	Attached to fovea and optic disc	Attached to fovea and optic disc	Typically detached from fovea, but attached to optic disc	Detached from both fovea and optic disc
Natural history	50% regress 40% progress 10% stabilize	15–21% regress 75% progress	5% regress 30% progress	20% enlarge

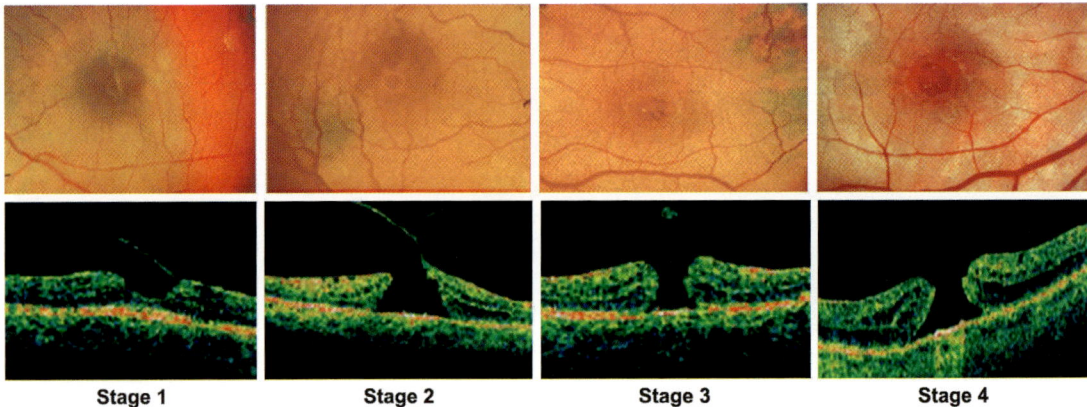

| Stage 1 | Stage 2 | Stage 3 | Stage 4 |

Fig. 24.2.1 *Fundus photograph and OCT finding of different stages of macular holes*

Stage 3 and 4 features are depicted in Table 24.2.1 and Fig. 24.2.1

- *Typical presenting features* are progressive blurring of central vision and metamorphopsia, classically with micropsia and pincushion distortion, and occasionally a pericentral positive scotoma.
- *Visual acuity* may be relatively well preserved in stage 1 holes (6/6–6/24), but deteriorates with progression to stage 2 (6/12–6/36), and further to stage 3 (6/18–6/60).

Biomicroscopic examination
- The diagnosis of full-thickness macular is clinically made by biomicroscopic examination.
- The features of a full-thickness macular hole comprise a circular defect of the neurosensory retina, the edges of which are typically elevated by a cuff of subretinal fluid. Small yellow spots of xanthophyll pigment may be seen in the retinal pigment epithelium at the base of a full-thickness macular hole.

Differential diagnosis of a full-thickness macular hole includes a pseudo-hole in an epiretinal membrane and a lamellar hole associated with arrested macular hole development or cystoids macular edema.

INVESTIGATIONS

Watzke-Allen slit beam test can be a valuable sign if the diagnosis is uncertain. In the Watzke-Allen test, a narrow vertical slit beam is projected across the fovea. The diagnosis of full-thickness macular hole is supported if the slit beam is perceived by the patient to be discontinuous (Watzke-Allen positive).

Laser aiming beam test is performed in a similar way. The diagnosis of macular hole is supported if the patient is unable to perceive a 50 μm laser aiming beam projected within the lesion, but is able to do so when the beam is projected onto adjacent normal retina.

OCT: Optical Coherence Tomography

Optical coherence tomography (OCT) is novel non-invasive, non-contact imaging technique capable of producing cross-sectional images of ocular tissue *in vivo* of high resolution (10 μm) which has now become a mandatory and investigation of choice because it not only establishes the diagnosis but also provides important prognostic clue with reference to surgical outcomes.

OCT is useful in the diagnosis of full-thickness macular holes, especially where there is uncertainty on biomicroscopy, and is able to distinguish full-thickness macular holes from partial thickness holes, macular pseudoholes, and cysts.

OCT is also useful for defining the stage of macular hole development and providing a quantitative measure of hole size (which can be used to calculate the hole form factor (a+b/c >0.8 and macular hole index: height/base >0.5 has good closure rate (Fig. 24.2.2)).

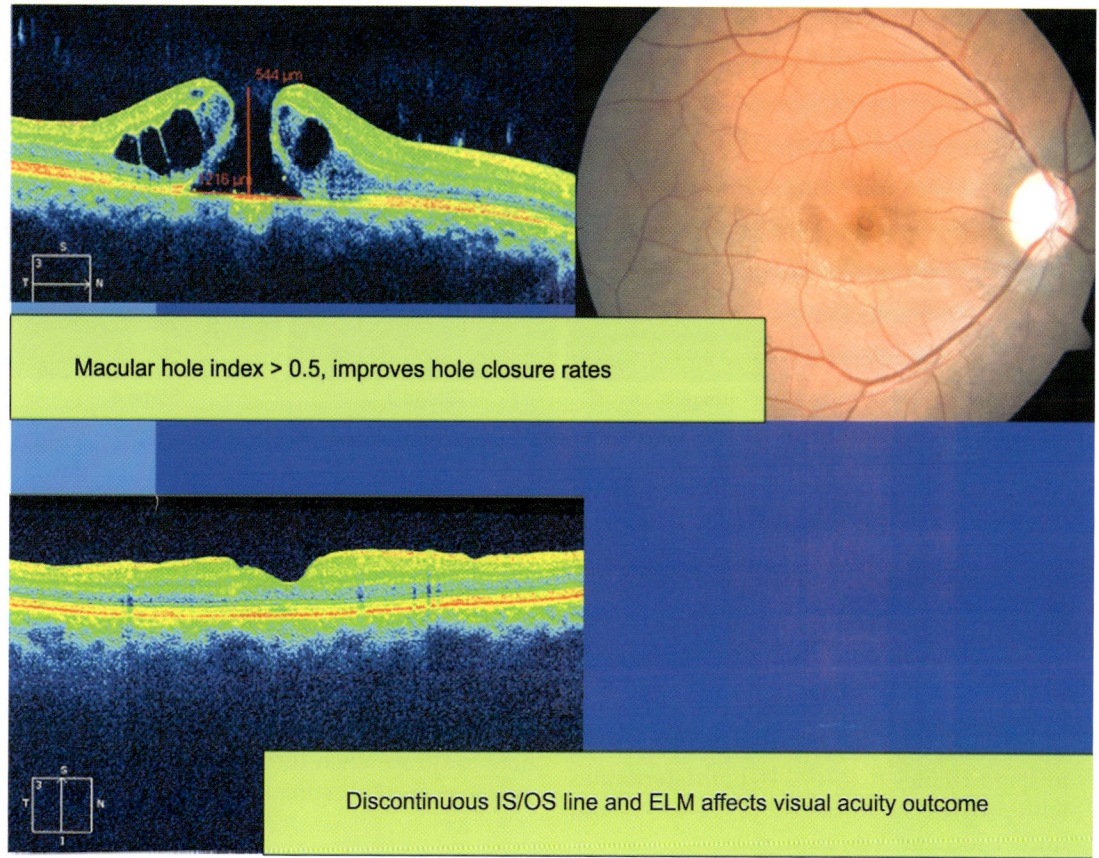

Macular hole index > 0.5, improves hole closure rates

Discontinuous IS/OS line and ELM affects visual acuity outcome

Fig. 24.2.2 *Fundus photograph and OCT picture of stage IV MH depicting macular hole index*

Diameter Hole Index (DHI): Ratio of minimum diameter of MH to base diameter, it is an Indicator of extent of tangential traction.

Tractional Hole Index (THI): Ratio of maximal height of MH to minimum diameter. It is a indicator of antero-posterior traction and retinal hydration. Patients with higher THI values (1.41) and low DHI values (< 0.50) had best post-op VA recovery.

OCT has been used to evaluate the vitreo-retinal interface in the fellow eyes of individuals with macular holes and enables the detection of subtle separations of the posterior hyaloid from the retina that are not evident clinically.

Other clinical investigation

Other clinical investigations which can help in diagnosing macular hole are FFA and auto fluorescence.

SURGICAL MANAGEMENT OF MACULAR HOLE

See Chapter 32.

PROGNOSIS FOLLOWING MACULAR HOLE SURGERY

Visual recovery following surgical closure of macular holes may be gradual. Although substantial improvement in visual acuity occurs soon after cataract extraction as cataract is known to commonly occur following macular hole surgery, further improvement may be observed for up to 2 years. Visual recovery is inversely correlated with vision in the fellow eye, tending to be greater where vision in the fellow eye is subnormal. Bilateral visual function improves in a significant proportion of patients after macular hole surgery, particularly where vision in the fellow eye is subnormal. Successful closure improves stereo-acuity and has a bene-

ficial effect on patients' subjective perception of visual function, but the effect of macular hole surgery on patients' quality of life has yet to be fully evaluated. The outcome of macular hole surgery is dependent on the stage of the hole and the duration of symptoms, but is not dependent on the age of the patient. Anatomic and visual outcomes are inversely correlated to the stage of the hole and are greatest following surgery for small stage 2 holes. The closure rate in patients undergoing surgery within 1 year of onset is 94.0%, and in those waiting 1 year or more it is 47.4%. However, in our study, we found even chronic macular holes improved vision after surgery with a closure rate of up to 94%. Although the best functional results are obtained if surgery is performed within 6 months of the onset of symptoms, visual improvement may be achieved in patients who have been symptomatic for much longer. Surgery for macular holes secondary to trauma can result in closure rates comparable to those of idiopathic holes, but high myopia or the presence of a localized macular detachment are associated with a relatively poor prognosis. Following failure of primary surgery to close macular holes, further surgery involving rigorous dissection of epiretinal membranes, with or without ILM peeling, and long-acting gas tamponade can result in anatomical closure and improvement in visual acuity. Alternatively, in eyes with unclosed macular holes following vitrectomy with ILM peeling, additional gas injection during the early postoperative period can result in successful closure. In the MMHS, eyes in which hole closure was achieved after a second procedure attained slightly poorer Log-MAR and Snellen acuities than eyes in which closure had been achieved after a single procedure, but achieved similar near acuities.

BIBLIOGRAPHY

1. Al-Abdulla NA, Thompson JT, Sjaarda RN. Results of macular hole surgery with and without epiretinal dissection or internal limiting membrane removal. Ophthalmology 2004; 111(1):142–49.
2. Ando F, Sasano K, Ohba N, Hirose H, Yasui O. Anatomic and visual outcomes after indocya-nine green-assisted peeling of the retinal internal limiting membrane in idiopathic macular hole surgery. Am J Ophthalmol 2004; 137(4):609–14.
3. Ando F, Sasano K, Suzuki F, Ohba N. Indocya-nine green-assisted ILM peeling in macular hole surgery revisited. Am J Ophthalmol 2004; 138(5):886–7.
4. Apostolopoulos MN, Koutsandrea CN, Moschos MN, Alonistiotis DA, Papaspyrou AE, Mallias JA, et al. Evaluation of successful macular hole surgery by optical coherence tomography and multifocal electro retinography. Am J Ophthalmol 2002; 134(5):667–74.
5. Aycock PD, Bunce C, Xing W, Thomas D, Poon W, Gazzard G, et al. Outcomes of macular hole surgery: implications for surgical management and clinical governance Eye 2005; 19(8):879–84.
6. Azzolini C, Patelli F, Brancato R. Correlation between optical coherence tomography data and biomicroscopic interpretation of idiopathic macular hole. Am J Ophthalmol 2001; 132(3):348–55.
7. Banker AS, Freeman WR, Azen SP, Lai MY. A multicentered clinical study of serum as adjuvant therapy for surgical treatment of macular holes. Vitrectomy for Macular Hole Study Group. Arch Ophthalmol 1999; 117(11): 1499–502.
8. Banker AS, Freeman WR, Kim JW, Munguia D, Azen SP. Vision-threatening complications of surgery for full-thickness macular holes. Vitrectomy for Macular Hole Study Group. Ophthalmology 1997; 104(9):1442–52; discussion 1452–53.
9. Brooks HL Jr. Macular hole surgery with and without internal limiting membrane peeling. Ophthalmology 2000; 107(10):1939–48; discussion 48-49.
10. Chen CJ. Glaucoma after macular hole surgery. Ophthalmology 1998; 105(1):94–99; discussion 99–100.
11. Comparative evaluation of anatomical and functional outcomes using brilliant blue G versus triamcinolone assisted ILM peeling in macular hole surgery in Indian population Atul Kumar, Varun Gogia, Vinit M. Shah and Tapas C. Nag. Graefe's Archive for Clinical and exp ophthalmology. Volume 1/1854 –2011.
12. Da Mata AP, Burk SE, Foster RE, Riemann CD, Petersen MR, Nehemy MB, et al. Long-term follow-up of indocyanine green-assisted peeling of the retinal internal limiting membrane during vitrectomy surgery for idiopathic macular hole repair. Ophthalmology 2004; 111(12):2246–2253.

13. Da Mata AP, Burk SE, Riemann CD, Rosa RHJr, Snyder ME, Petersen MR, et al. Indocyanine green-assisted peeling of the retinal internal limiting membrane during vitrectomy surgery for macular hole repair. Ophthalmology 2001; 108(7):1187–1192.

14. De Bustros S. Vitrectomy for prevention of macular holes. Results of a randomized multi-center clinical trial. Vitrectomy for Prevention of Macular Hole Study Group. Ophthalmology 1994; 101(6):1055–59; discussion 60.

15. Engelbrecht NE, Freeman J, Sternberg P Jr, Aaberg TM Sr, Aaberg TM Jr, Martin DF, et al. Retinal pigment epithelial changes after macular hole surgery with indocyanine green-assisted internal limiting membrane peeling. Am J Ophthalmol 2002; 133(1):89-94.

16. Evans JR, Schwartz SD, McHugh JD, Thamby-Rajah Y, Hodgson SA, Wormald RP, et al. Systemic risk factors for idiopathic macular holes: a case control study. Eye 1998; 12(Pt 2):256–59.

17. Ezra E, Aylward WG, Gregor ZJ. Membranec-tomy and autologous serum for the retreatment of full-thickness macular holes. Arch Ophthalmol 1997; 115(10):1276–80.

18. Ezra E, Gregor ZJ. Surgery for idiopathic full thickness macular hole: two-year results of a randomized clinical trial comparing natural history, vitrectomy, and vitrectomy plus autologous serum: Morfields Macular Hole Study Group Report no.1. Arch Ophthalmol 2004; 122(2):224–36.

19. Ezra E, Munro PM, Charteris DG, Aylward WG, Luthert PJ, Gregor ZJ. Macular hole opercula. Ultrastructural features and clinico-pathological correlation. Arch Ophthalmol 1997; 115(11):1381–87.

20. Ezra E, Wells JA, Gray RH, Kinsella FM, Orr GM, Grego J, et al. Incidence of idiopathic full-thickness macular holes in fellow eyes. A 5-year prospective natural history study. Ophthalmo-logy 1998; 105(2):353–9.

21. Ezra E. Idiopathic full thickness macular hole: natural history and pathogenesis. Br J Ophthalmol 2001; 85(1):102–8.

22. Foulquier S, Glacet-Bernard A, Sterkers M, Soubrane G, Coscas G. [Study of internal limiting membrane peeling in stage–3 and –4 idiopathic macular hole surgery]. J Fr Ophtalmol. 2002; 25(10):1026–31.

23. FreemanWR, AzenSP, KimJW, el-HaigW, Mishell DR III, Bailey I. Vitrectomy for the treatment of full-thickness stage 3 or 4 macular holes. Results of a multicentered randomized clinical trial. The Vitrectomy for Treatment of Macular Hole Study Group. Arch Ophthalmol 1997; 115(1):11–21.

24. Gandorfer A, Haritoglou C, Kampik A. Retinal damage from indocyanine green in experimental macular surgery. Invest Ophthalmol Vis Sci. 2003; 44(1):316–23.

25. Gass CA, Haritoglou C, Messmer EM, Schaum-berger M, Kampik A. Peripheral visual field defects after macular hole surgery: a complica-tion with decreasing incidence. Br J Ophthalmol 2001; 85(5):549–51.

26. Gass CA, Haritoglou C, Schaumberger M, Kampik A. Functional outcome of macular hole surgery with and without indocyanine green assisted peeling of the internal limiting membrane. Graefes Arch Clin Exp Ophthalmol 2003; 241(9):716–720.

27. Gass JD. Idiopathic senile macular hole. Its early in stages and pathogenesis. Arch Ophthalmol 1988; 106(5):629–39.

28. Gass JD. Muller cell cone, an over looked part of the anatomy of the fovea centralis: hypotheses concerning its role in the pathogenesis of macular hole and foveo macular retinoschisis. Arch Ophthalmol 1999; 117(6):821–823.

29. Gass JD. Reappraisal of biomicroscopic classifi-cation of stages of development of a macular hole. Am J Ophthalmol 1995; 119(6):752–9.

30. Gaudric A, Haouchine B, Massin P, Paques M, Blain P, Erginay A. Macular hole formation: new data provided by optical coherence tomography. Arch Ophthalmol 1999; 117(6):744–51.

31. Glaser BM, Michels RG, Kuppermann BD, Sjaarda RN, Pena RA. Transforming growth factor-beta 2 for the treatment of full-thickness macular holes. A prospective randomized study. Ophthalmology 1992; 99(7):1162–72; discussion 73.

32. Goldbaum MH, McCuen BW, Hanneken AM, Burgess SK, Chen HH. Silicone oil tamponade to seal macular holes without position restrictions. Ophthalmology 1998; 105(11):2140–7; discussion 2147–8.

33. Haritoglou C, Gandorfer A, Gass CA, Schaum-berger M, Ulbig MW, Kampik A. Indocyanine green-assisted peeling of the internal limiting membrane in macular hole surgery affects visual outcome: a clinicopathologic correlation. Am J Ophthalmol 2002;134(6):836–841.

34. Haritoglou C, Gass CA, Schaumberger M, Gandorfer A, Ulbig MW, Kampik A. Long-term follow-up after macular hole surgery with internal limiting membrane peeling. Am J Ophthalmol 2002;134(5):661–666.

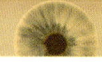

24.3 AGE-RELATED MACULAR DEGENERATION

INTRODUCTION

Age-related macular degeneration (AMD), also known as age-related maculopathy (ARM), is the leading cause of blindness in the Western world. It is also the leading cause of irreversible central vision loss in whites over 50 years of age in the United States. The disease affects approximately eight million people in the United States; its advanced form affects more than 1.75 million people. The prevalence and progression of AMD increases with age, from a prevalence of 1.6% in the age group 52 to 64 years to 28% in the age group 74 to 85 years. In the Blue Mountain Study, the prevalence of early AMD was reported to increase from 1.3% in the age group 49 to 54 years to 28.0% for those over 80 years of age; the prevalence of late ARM, on the other hand, increased from 0.1% in the age-group 49 to 54 years to 7.1% in the age group 75 to 86 years. The population older than 65 years is the fastest growing segment of our society and the prevalence of AMD is predicted to increase dramatically in the next decade. Though dry AMD is the most common form of AMD, wet AMD is responsible for 90% of the cases of visual loss. There is a pressing need for new therapies to either prevent AMD or treat the exudative AMD.

PATHOPHYSIOLOGY OF AMD

Pathologic changes in age-related macular degeneration (AMD) occur in the various structures in the posterior pole, such as the outer retina, the retinal pigment epithelium (RPE), Bruch's membrane and the choriocapillaries. Early lesions of AMD are located either between the RPE and its basement membrane [e.g. basal laminar deposits (BlamD)] or between the basement membrane of the RPE and the remainder of Bruch's membrane [e.g. basal linear deposits (BlinD)]. Focal and diffuse deposition between the RPE and Bruch's membrane is called drusen. Alterations of RPE such as hypopigmentation, depigmentation or atrophy as well as attenuation of photoreceptor

cells are also observed. This form of macular degeneration is known as dry AMD (non-exudative AMD), whereas choroidal neovascularization (CNV) is the main feature of wet AMD (exudative AMD), which ultimately results in a disciform scar in end stage AMD.

CHANGES IN NON-EXUDATIVE (DRY) AMD

1. *Changes of Bruch's Membrane:* Bruch's membrane increases in thickness with age with deposition of calcium salts in the elastic tissue. Focal thinning and disruption of Bruch's membrane is also found associated with an increased cellular activity. This may suggest an inflammatory etiology.

2. *Changes of retinal pigment epithelium:* RPE cells with AMD have cytoplasmic "lipofuscin granules, as the result of incompletely digested photoreceptor outer segments. Another clinical finding called non-geographic RPE atrophy is related to moderate RPE hypopigmentation and atrophy in areas overlying diffuse BlamD and BlinD. Hypopigmentation, attenuation or atrophy of the RPE may also be accompanied by soft drusen, RPE detachment and geographic atropy.

3. *Changes of choriocapillaries:* The choriocapillaris in eyes with AMD is usually thinned and sclerosed.

4. *Changes of neurosensory retina:* Aging changes of the neurosensory retina occur in Muller cells and axons of ganglion cells. While rods gradually disappear with aging even without evidence of overt RPE disease, cones only begin to degenerate by advanced stages of non-exudative AMD. Red-green cones seem to be more resistant than blue cones to aging and may also increase in size in AMD. The greatest photoreceptor cell loss is located in the parafovea and may finally result in disappearance of all photoreceptors in the presence of geographic atrophy or disciform degeneration.

Basal deposits

Accumulation of waste material between the RPE and Bruch's membrane is termed "basal

deposit", one of the earliest pathologic features of AMD.

1. ***Basal laminar deposit:*** BlamD is composed of granular material with much wide-spaced collagen located between the plasma and basement membranes of the RPE. Studies have shown that BlamD is composed of collagen (type IV), laminin, glycoproteins, glycosamino-glycans (chondroitin, heparinsulfate), carbo-hydrates (N acetylgalactosamine), cholesterol (unesterified, esterified), and apolipoproteins B and E.

2. ***Basal linear deposit:*** BlinD is located external to the RPE basement membrane (e.g. in the inner collagenous zone of Bruch's membrane. Electron microscopy shows that BlinD is primarily composed of an electron dense, lipid-rich material with coated and non-coated vesicles and granules that result in diffuse thickening of the inner aspect of Bruch's membrane. BlinD appears to be a more specific marker than BlamD for AMD, particularly for progression to late stage disease, whereas the amount of BlamD seems to be a more reliable indicator of the degree of RPE atrophy and photoreceptor degeneration.

Drusen

Drusen are important features of AMD, which can be ophthalmoscopically observed as small yellowish white lesions located deep to the retina in the posterior pole (Fig. 24.3.1)

1. ***Nodular (hard) drusen:*** Nodular (hard) drusen are smooth surfaced, dome-shaped structures between the RPE and Bruch's membrane. They consist of hyaline material and stain positively with periodic acid-Schiff. The RPE overlying the drusen is often attenuated and hypopigmented.

2. ***Soft drusen:*** Cleavage in BlamD and BlinD may occur with the formation of a localized detachment (soft drusen). Soft drusen may become confluent with diameters larger than 63 µm, and are then termed "large drusen." Soft drusen formation may result in a diffuse thickening of the inner aspect of Bruch's membrane with separation of the overlying RPE basement membrane from the remaining Bruch's membrane. The hydrophobic space between these types of soft drusen and Bruch's membrane is a potential space for CNV. The overlying RPE may be attenuated, diminished or atrophic. In late stages, geographic atrophy may occur.

3. ***Diffuse drusen:*** Diffuse drusen is a diffuse thickening of the inner aspect of Bruch's mem-brane. This term also includes basal laminar (cuticular) drusen, which are characterized by an internal nodularity.

Geographic atrophy

Geographic atrophy, which is characterized by the areas of well demarcated atrophy of RPE, represents the classic clinical picture of end-stage non-exudative AMD (Fig. 24.3.2). Although

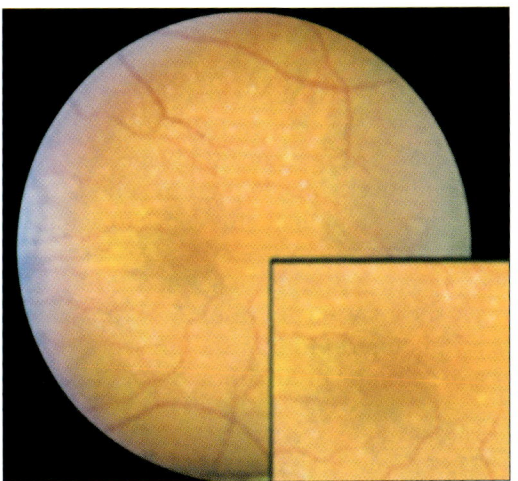

Fig. 24.3.1 *Clinical photograph of drusen*

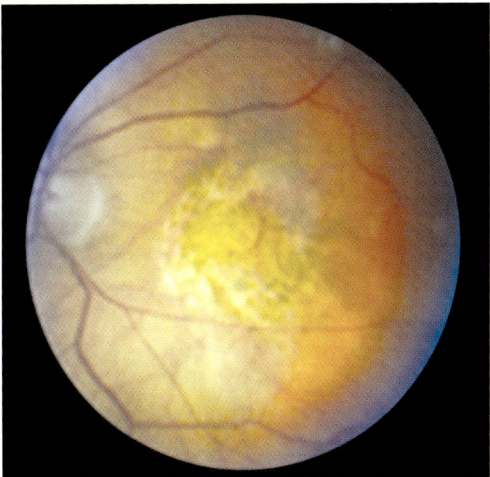

Fig. 24.3.2 *Clinical photograph of geographic atrophy*

drusen are apparently central direct factors for initiation of RPE cell loss, they may disappear over time, especially when geographic atrophy occurs. Histological studies have shown that the loss of RPE is usually accompanied by a gradual degeneration of the outer layers of the neurosensory retina (photoreceptors, outer nuclear layer, external limiting membrane), marked atrophy and sclerosis of the choriocapillaris, without breaks in Bruch's membrane.

CHANGES IN EXUDATIVE (WET) AMD

Choroidal neovascularization

The hallmark of exudative (wet type) AMD is the development of CNV. CNV represents new blood vessel formation typically from the choroid. Such changes in Bruch's membrane as calcification and focal breaks correlate with the presence of exudative AMD. Decreased thickness and disruption of the elastic lamina of Bruch's membrane in the macula may also be a prerequisite for invasion of CNV into the space underneath the RPE. Vascular channels supplied by the choroid begin as a capillary-like structure and evolve into arterioles and venules. Most of the vessels arise from the choroid, although a retinal vessel contribution has been observed in about 6% of CNV in AMD. These choroidal vessels traverse the defects in the Bruch's membrane and grow into the plane between the RPE and Bruch's membrane (sub-RPE CNV: type 1 growth pattern), between the retina and RPE (subretinal CNV: type 2 growth pattern), or in the combination of both patterns (combined growth pattern) (Fig. 24.3.3).

1. Subretinal Pigment Epithelium CNV (Type 1 Growth Pattern)

In type 1 pattern, CNV originates with multiple ingrowth sites, ranging from 1 to 12, from the choriocapillaris. After breaking through Bruch's membrane, CNV tufts extend laterally and merge in a horizontal fashion under the RPE. This is facilitated by a natural cleavage plane in the space between BlamD and Bruch's membrane that has accumulated lipids with aging. Patients with type 1 CNV have relatively intact retina and few visual symptoms. This growth pattern likely corresponds to the "occult" type of angiographic appearance of

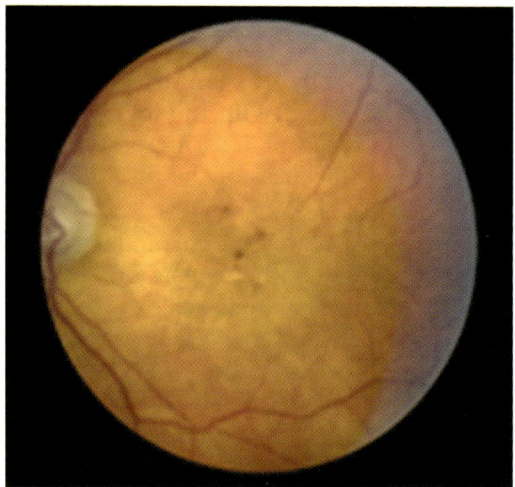

Fig. 24.3.3 *Clinical photograph of CNV*

CNV. Secondary changes can be noted in the surrounding retina such as serous or hemorrhagic detachment of the RPE and overlying retina, RPE tears, and lipid exudation follows.

2. Subretinal CNV (Type 2 Growth Pattern)

The type 2 (subretinal) growth pattern demonstrates single or few ingrowth sites with a focal defect in Bruch's membrane. There is a reflected layer of RPE on the outer surface of the CNV and little or no RPE on its inner surface. Since there is no support from the RPE, the overlying outer layers of retina become atrophic. Angiographically, type II CNV membranes leak under the RPE and in the outer retina. This growth pattern correlates with the "classic" angiographic appearance.

3. Combined Growth Pattern CNV

There are many theoretical variations leading to a combined pattern of CNV growth. A progression from the type 1 to the type 2 growth pattern as well as temporal development of the type 2 growth prior to the type 1 growth have been discussed (Fig. 24.3.10). These growth patterns correspond to angiographic "minimally classic" and "predominantly classic" appearances.

Disciform scar

Disciform scar represents the end-stage of the exudative form of AMD. Disciform scars are usually vascularized, but predominantly

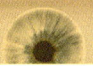

composed of fibrotic scar tissue. The vascular supply is provided from the choroid (96%), retina (2.5%) or both (0.6%). A disciform scar is generally associated with the loss of neural tissue. Photoreceptor loss increases as the diameter and thickness of the disciform scar increases (Fig. 24.3.4).

Over the past few years our understanding of the molecular pathogenesis of CNV has improved. It is clear that VEGF is a critical stimulus and antagonism of VEGF has led to the first treatment that improves vision in a substantial number of patients with neovascular AMD.

IMMUNE RESPONSE IN AMD

1. *Innate immunity:* Activation by retinal or choroidal injury or infection
2. *Antigen specific immunity:* Normal activation by foreign antigens, Aberrant activation in AMD by molecular mimicry, antigen desequestration, neoantigen formation, or antigen trapping
3. *Amplification mechanisms:* Complement, cytokines, oxidants, others
4. *Immune cells:* Monocytes/macrophages, DC, mast cells, lymphocytes

Innate immunity, antigen-specific immunity, and amplification cascades may contribute to AMD.

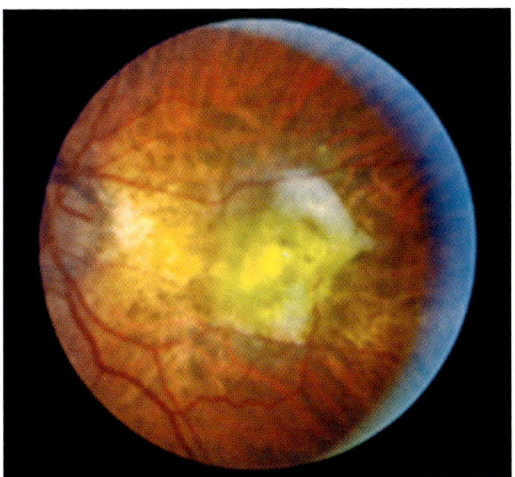

Fig. 24.3.4 *Clinical photograph of disciform scar*

GENETICS OF AMD

Linkage mapping, which searches for chromosomal regions that cosegregate with the AMD disease trait, and multicandidate gene screening have implicated multiple genetic loci in almost every chromosome, including 1q25–31, 2q14.3, 2q31.2-2q32.3, 2p21, 3p13, 4q32, 4p16, 5p, 5q34, 6q25.3, 6q14, 8, 9p24, 9q31, 9q33, 10q26, 12q13, 12q23, 14q13, 15q21, 16p12, 17q25, 18p11, 19p, 20q13, 22q, and X. Recent case-association studies have identified allelic variations of several genes thought to be major risk loci for AMD. These are CFH, BF/C2, PLEKHA1, LOC387715 and HTRA1. The etiology of AMD is multifactorial, involving the presence of multiple disease loci as well as environmental factors.

RISK FACTORS FOR AMD

1. *Age:* Age is the strongest risk factor associated with AMD. The prevalence, incidence, and progression of all forms of AMD rise steeply with advancing age. There is a consistent finding across multiple population-based studies of an increase in prevalence of late AMD with age, from near absence at age 50 years to about 2% prevalence at age 70, and about 6% at age 80
2. *Gender:* In the Blue Mountains Eye Study, there was consistent, although not statistically significant, sex differences in prevalence for most lesions of AMD, with women having higher rates for late AMD and soft indistinct drusen than men, but not retinal pigmentary abnormalities, which were slightly more frequent in men.
3. *Race:* Several studies have suggested that AMD is more prevalent among whites than blacks.
4. *Heredity:* Plays an important role in AMD. Chromosome and genes related to AMD are highlighted in genetics of AMD.
5. *Ocular factors:*
   a. *Macular pigment optical density:* Macular pigments, lutein and zeaxanthin have a protective role against AMD.
   b. *Cataract surgery:* In the Blue Mountains Eye Study, a higher prevalence of late AMD in eyes with past cataract surgery (6.3%) than in phakic eyes (1.3%) was observed.

c. *Iris color:* A number of studies have reported an increased risk of AMD in people with blue or light iris color compared with those with darker iris pigmentation.

d. *Refractive error:* Several case-control studies have found an association between AMD and refractive error, with hyperopic eyes at greater risk of AMD.

6. **Systemic risk factors** includes:

a. *Cardiovascular disease and smoking:* A number of inflammatory biomarkers which are known to be associated with cardiovascular disease have now been found to be independently associated with the progression of AMD. These include C-reactive protein and interleukin 6.

b. *Hypertension*

c. *Increased serum lipids* and increased dietary fat intake

d. *Diabetes*

e. *Chlamydiae pneumonia* infection

7. **Sunlight exposure:** It has also been blamed to be one of the risk factor for AMD.

8. **Risk factors for progression to choroidal neovascularization:** Presence of five or more drusen, focal hyperpigmentation, systemic hypertension, one or more large drusen or confluent drusen, caucasians, and smoking.

CLINICAL FEATURES OF AMD

The clinical hallmarks of non-exudative AMD are soft drusen, localized deposits noted between the basement membrane of the retinal pigment epithelium (RPE) and the Bruch's membrane, associated RPE pigmentary changes, and mild loss in visual acuity (VA). The advanced form of non-exudative AMD, termed geographic atrophy (GA), is characterized by outer retinal and RPE atrophy with loss of choriocapillaris. The presence of subretinal fluid, subretinal hemorrhage, RPE detachment, a subretinal greenish-greyish membrane, or hard exudates indicates choroidal neo-vascularization (CNV), which heralds the onset of exudative macular degeneration. Fluorescein angiography delineates the exact location (subfoveal, juxtafoveal, or extrafoveal), the size, and the pattern of leakage (classic vs. occult). Loss of central vision is usually due to RPE

atrophy or GA in non-exudative AMD and due to subretinal fluid or subretinal hemorrhage in exudative AMD. Early-stage AMD (or early ARM) is defined as the presence of soft drusen (63 µm) alone, RPE depigmentation alone, or a combination of distinct/indistinct drusen with pigment irregularities. Latest age AMD (or late ARM) is defined as pure GA (both central and noncentral), signs of exudative macular degeneration, or a combination of both.

TYPES OF DRUSEN

Different types of drusen are noted in the retina: (i) hard, (ii) soft, (iii) crystalline, and (iv) cuticular or basal laminar.

1. **Hard drusen:** Hard drusen are discrete, small, yellow, nodular hyaline deposits in the sub-RPE space, between the basement membrane of RPE and the inner collagenous layer of Bruch's membrane. These drusen are smaller than 50 µm in diameter. Focal densifications of Bruch's membrane, termed microdrusen, may precede the formation of hard drusen. These are structurally different from basal linear deposit. Hard drusen are common in young people and do not lead to macular degeneration. Small, hard, distinct drusen were found in the macula of 94% of the Beaver Dam Eye Study population. These were not noted to increase in number with age. If present in excessive number, however, they may predispose to RPE atrophy. Hard drusen act as window defects on fluorescein angiogram with early hyperfluorecence and fading of fluorescence in late frames

2. **Soft drusen:** Soft drusen are clinically noted as pale yellow lesions with poorly defined edges (Fig. 24.3.1). They can also represent focal accentuations of basal linear deposits. They also represent localized accumulation of basal laminar deposits in an eye with diffuse basal laminar deposits. They gradually enlarge and may coalesce, termed confluent drusen, to form multiple irregular areas of localized RPE detachments. With time, soft drusen can become crystalline in nature.

3. **Crystalline drusen** are discrete calcific refractile drusen (Fig. 24.3.4). These are dehydrated soft drusen that predispose to GA (Fig. 24.3.2). Soft drusen are classified by size into small, medium, and large. A small soft drusen is 63 mm wide,

intermediate is between 63 and 128 μm and large is more than 128 μm. (The width of the retinal vein off the optic nerve head is 128 μm.) The risk of progression from non-exudative to exudative AMD increases with the size and the total area of the drusen. Clinical and histological studies have shown that soft drusen precede macular degeneration. They lead to secondary Bruch's membrane thickening and RPE atrophy with subsequent photoreceptor loss. This promotes the development of choroidal neovascular membrane. On fluorescein angiography, soft drusen show early hypofluorescence followed by hyperfluorescence with no late leakage.

4. *Basal laminar drusen:* Basal laminar or cuticular drusen are tiny, white deposits found between the plasma membrane of RPE and its basement membrane. Such drusen are mainly composed of collagen, laminin, membrane-bound vesicles, and fibronectin. The deposits tend to accumulate over the thickened Bruch's membrane, suggesting that they may be a local response to altered filtration at these sites. Basal laminar drusen are typically very numerous, distributed in a bilaterally symmetrical pattern, and are most prominent in the posterior poles. These unusual drusen are often seen in association with other typical hard, soft, or semisolid drusen. VA is typically minimally affected despite the large number of these drusen. They tend to occur in younger individuals and in normal eyes and do not predispose to macular degeneration. On fluorescein angiography, the basal laminar drusen hyperfluoresce early and give an appearance of "starry night."

GEOGRAPHIC ATROPHY

Soft drusen can lead to RPE atrophy, with resultant overlying photoreceptor atrophy and vision loss. When the vision falls below or equal to 20/30, the disease process is termed nonexudative or dry macular degeneration. Subretinal fluid, subretinal hemorrhage, RPE detachment, hard exudates, and subretinal fibrosis, all signs of exudative maculopathy, are absent in dry macular degeneration. GA is an advanced form of dry macular degeneration. This involves RPE atrophy with subjacent choriocapillaris and small choroidal vessel atrophy. This condition progresses slowly over years and often spares the center of the foveal avascular zone until late in the course of the disease. Non-exudative AMD is the most common form of AMD, accounting for 80% to 90% of cases overall. Focal hyperpigmentation along with the presence of greater than five soft, large, and confluent drusen is associated with the increased risk of progression of RPE atrophy and choroidal atrophy. These eyes have a higher incidence of developing CNV. The five-year risk of eyes with bilateral soft drusen and good VA to develop CNV is 0.2% to 18%. This risk increases to 7 to 87% if the fellow eye has CNV.

The AREDS research study group has described a simplified clinical scale to define risk categories for a five-year risk of developing advanced AMD in eyes without advanced AMD at baseline, or the risk in the unaffected fellow eye when advanced AMD is present in one eye at baseline. It is a five-step scale (0–4) that predicts an approximate five-year risk of developing advanced AMD in at least one eye as follows: 0 factor, 0.5%; 1 factor, 3%; 2 factors, 12%; 3 factors, 25%; and 4 factors, 50%. The scale sums retinal risk factors in both eyes. The risk factors are the presence of one or more large drusen (125 μm width of a retinal vein at the disk margin) and pigment stippling; each characteristic gets one point for each eye. Advanced AMD in one eye at baseline is given two scores. The presence of intermediate drusen (63–28 μm) in both eyes is given one score. The AREDS trial also noted that the drusen area was stronger and a more consistent predictor of progression to advanced AMD than the drusen size. However, for practical clinical purposes, the drusen number and type was used for calculating the severity score.

MONITORING DRY AMD

Patients with intermediate drusen (O63 μm) or those with exudative AMD in fellow eyes are recommended to take high-dose vitamins as per the AREDS study. Amsler grid testing is a sensitive indicator of progression of the disease process. Patients are encouraged to seek medical help if visual distortion, metamorphopsia, loss of central vision, or any new symptoms occur.

These herald the growth of choroidal neo-vascular membranes. The early detection of the choroidal neovascular membranes may facilitate early treatment.

NEOVASCULAR AMD

Symptoms

Symptomatic patients with exudative AMD typically present complaining of sudden onset decreased visual acuity, metamorphopsia, and central or paracentral scotomas. Patients who are at risk for CNV should be periodically screened for development of CNV and should be encouraged to self monitor their vision daily. Monitoring options include using an Amsler grid or the preferential hyperacuity perimeter (PHP).

Amsler's grid: The Amsler grid is a useful test for detecting the early visual symptoms of exudative AMD in patients with high risk AMD. Each box on the grid represents one degree of visual field. Thus, the Amsler grid tests the central 10 degrees of visual field beyond fixation. The patient is asked to fixate on the central black dot and to note whether surrounding lines are wavy, missing or obscured by scotomas (dark areas). If these findings are present, the patient should be instructed to seek attention urgently with his or her ophthalmologist as it is likely that the cause is neovascular AMD. There are limits to Amsler grid testing which includes the cortical completion phenomenon, crowding phenomenon and lack of forced fixation. A newly developed computer-automated, three dimensional, threshold, Amsler grid visual field test has been shown to be useful in earlier detection of AMD.

Potential hyperacuity perimeter: The PHP is based upon the concept of vernier (hyperacuity) acuity, the ability to detect a subtle mis-alignment of an object. The threshold of vernier acuity is three to six seconds of arc in the fovea-10 fold smaller than to resolve an object clearly on the fovea. When photoreceptors are misaligned because of edema, CNV and or RPE elevation, the brain is able to detect the misalignment. The PHP is useful even in patients with media opacities due to its resistance to retinal image degradation. The central 14 degrees are tested in about five minutes. Patients are shown a series of linear dots with an area of artificial distortion. The artificial distortion is progressively made smaller. If a patient has CNV, the CNV results in a true area of distortion of the dots. When their distortion is larger than the artificial distortion, the patient preferentially chooses that area. A computerized map of these areas is created.

Clinical signs

The major clinical features of active exudative AMD include subretinal fluid, subretinal hemorrhage, sub-RPE fluid, sub-RPE hemorrhage, RPE pigment alterations and hard exudates. Chronic exudative AMD is characterized mainly by the presence of subretinal fibrosis with or without the other features of active exudation. These features may appear clinically as any one or any combination of the following: a serous or a hemorrhagic PED (Fig 24.3.5A), grayish subretinal membrane, area of subretinal fluid, area of RPE alteration, subretinal hemorrhage, or hard exudates (Fig. 24.3.5B). The late manifestation of exudative AMD is a disciform scar or geographic atrophy (Fig. 24.3.4), with or without subretinal fluid or subretinal blood. Spontaneous involution of CNV may manifest as any of the above findings with RPE alterations and or scar formation.

Stereoscopic fundus examination is the best method for examining a patient with suspected CNV. A fundus contact or non-contact lens in conjunction with slit lamp biomicroscopy should be utilized for the exam. During the exam, it is helpful to have the patient look directly at the thin slit lamp beam and to ask the patient whether the beam appears distorted. Elevation of the RPE or retina (due to underlying CNV) causes the patient to perceive distortion of the slit beam.

OCT has been an extremely useful tool in the detection and management of CNV in AMD patients. The OCT resolution may be 3 to 5 μm for high resolution OCT and 10 μm for the third generation OCT machine. Microscopic areas of subretinal fluid and areas of elevation can be detected on OCT imaging of the macular area

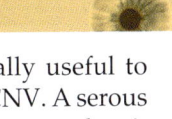

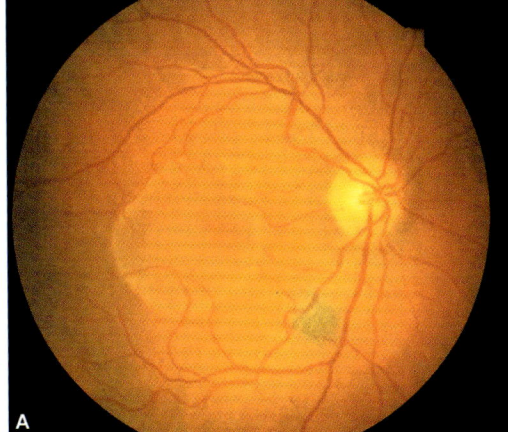

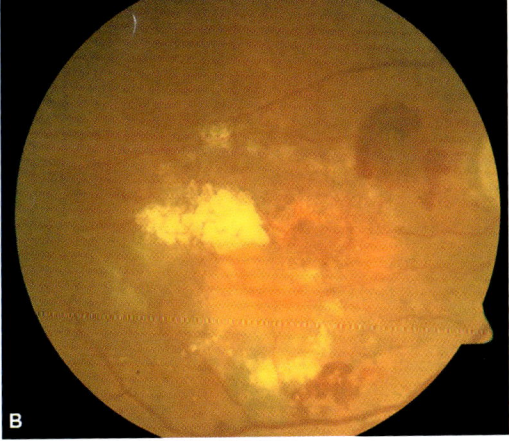

Fig. 24.3.5 *(A) ARMD with serous PED; and (B) CNV with hard exudates and heme*

of AMD patients. Areas of CNV appear as RPE thickening with or without intraretinal cysts and subretinal fluid. PEDs are clearly seen on the OCT (Fig. 24.3.8). OCT has been used in the recent anti-angiogenesis clinical trials as another measurement of treatment outcome. Successful treatment of PEDs and CNVMs has been shown to result in normalization of the OCT appearance. Recurrence of the CNV can appear as slight areas of elevation of the RPE, neurosensory retina or presence of cystic retinal change.

Pigment epithelial detachment: The borders of a PED are usually sharply demarcated (Fig. 24.3.5A). Clinically, hemorrhage or hard exudates may or may not be present depending upon the presence or absence of associated CNV. A fluorescein angiogram or indocyanine

green (ICG) angiogram is clinically useful to detect the presence of associated CNV. A serous PED shows early hyperfluorescence and uniform fluorescence on the late frames of the angiogram (Fig. 24.3.7).

The dye pools in the PED on the late phase. The borders remain sharp and the area does not increase in size. On ICG angiography, the PED is hypofluorescent. Whereas a serous PED will show uniform filling of the PED, a vascularized PED shows irregular filling, notching of the PED or irregular margins on the FA. On the OCT, the RPE elevation is readily seen. If there is CNV present with the PED, occult CNV will frequently show associated subretinal fluid, hard exudate, or subretinal blood. The fluorescein angiogram typically demonstrates irregular filling of the PED and the PED borders may be blurred in the area of the CNV. Leakage on the late frames of the FA is commonly noted. ICG angiography has been shown to be helpful in this regard. The association of CNV with PED increases the chance for visual acuity loss.

The risk of an RPE tear/rip occurring in this setting is a real concern in these eyes. An RPE tear is readily identifiable as a sharply-demarcated area of bare choroid with a straight, linear edge. This straight, linear edge corresponds to the location of the associated retracted, scrolled RPE. The fluorescein angiogram shows blocked fluorescence in the area of scrolled RPE and hyperfluorescence in the area without RPE. The natural history of PEDs includes RPE tears, but treatment of CNV with PEDs has also been temporarily associated with RPE tears.

Choroidal neovascularisation: The macular photocoagulation study (MPS) group has defined the various forms and components of CNV. The entire complex of components termed a "CNV lesion" includes the CNV itself, blood, elevated blocked fluorescence (due to a pigment or scar that obscures the neovascular borders), and any serous detachment of the RPE. The classic clinical description of a choroidal neovascular membrane is that of a dirty gray-colored membrane. There is associated subretinal fluid and there may or may not be subretinal blood and lipid. The fluorescein angiogram is a key test in the evaluation of patients with CNV.

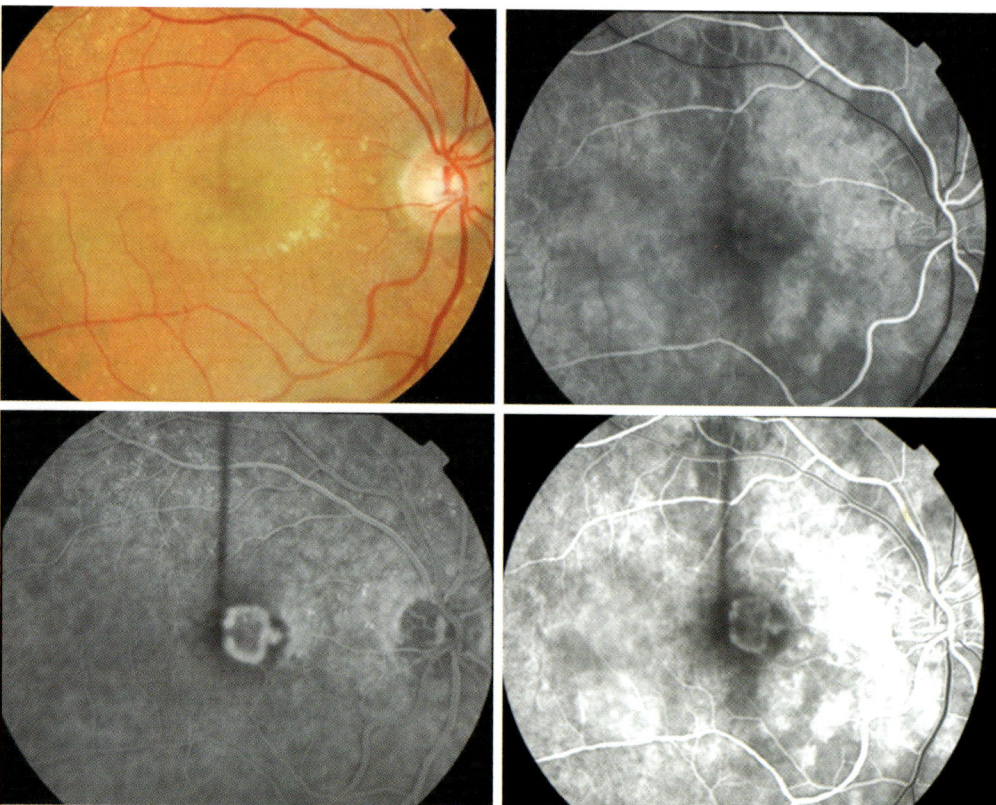

Fig. 24.3.6 *Clinical photograph and FFA of a patient with classic CNV. FFA shows the lacy membrane in the early phases with late leakage*

Classic CNV: The MPS group characterized classic CNV as only occasionally showing a lacy pattern of hyperfluorescence in the early fluorescein phases (Fig. 24.3.6). In the later frames of the angiogram, the boundaries of the CNV are obscured by progressive pooling of dye in the subneurosensory space. With the advent of photodynamic therapy (PDT), the term "predominantly classic" was coined. A predominantly classic lesion is one in which the lesion is more than 50% classic CNV in composition.

Occult CNV: It has been classified as either fibrovascular PED (FVPED) or late leakage of undetermined source (LLUS). These types of occult CNVs are differentiated on the basis of the fluorescein angiogram.

FVPEDs show early hyperfluorescence with irregular elevation of the RPE. These areas are

not as bright or as discrete as the classic CNV seen on the transit phases.

Within one to two minutes, an area of stippled hyperfluorescence is present. By ten minutes, there is persistent fluorescein staining or leakage within the subneurosensory detachment. The borders of the occult CNV may be either well-demarcated or poorly demarcated. Late leakage is present, although it is not as intense as that seen in classic CNV.

There is subretinal fluid overlying the entire lesion in addition to the sub retinal pigment epithelium (PED) fluid. Grayish area on the superonasal edge of the PED corresponds to the CNV (Fig. 24.3.7A). The corresponding fluorescein angiogram from the late transit phase shows a notch of the PED superonasally. The corresponding fluorescein angiogram from the late phase shows fluorescein dye leakage in

the area corresponding to the CNV. The adjacent PED shows sharp edges in the areas not involving the CNV.

LLUS in contrast does not show early hyperfluorescence. LLUS appears as speckled hyperfluorescence with pooling of dye in the overlying neurosensory space; choroidal leakage is apparent between two and five minutes after fluorescein injection. The boundaries of this type of occult CNV are never well-demarcated. In fact, the later frames show hyperfluorescent leakage in an area that showed no hyperfluorescence on the early frames (Fig. 24.3.7B). Lastly, there is a slow-filling form of classic CNV in which hyperfluorescence is not seen until two minutes. However, in this form of CNV, the late frames of leakage and pooling of the dye in the subneurosensory space correspond with the area seen at two minutes. Using ICG angiography, occult CNVs can be further classified into those with hot spots, plaques, combination of these two types, retinal-choroidal anastomosis and polypoidal-type CNV. ICG angiography is also useful for evaluating eyes with subretinal hemorrhage for the presence of CNV.

Disciform scar: A disciform scar shows an area of subretinal fibrosis or subRPE fibrosis. Dull, white fibrous tissue is seen and may accompany the CNV lesion or replace it over time. Areas of retinal pigment epithelial atrophy may or may not be present. FA may show leakage associated with the scar if active CNV is present. The fibrotic scar may otherwise show only staining of the fibrotic tissue.

ROLE OF OCT IN AMD

1. OCT can help characterize retinal pathology, even when this information is difficult to discern on clinical examination or angiography. It is possible to define the location of choroidal neovascular membranes above or below the RPE (Fig. 24.3.8).
2. Solid fibrous tissue can be differentiated from subretinal fluid when these findings may be angiographically equivocal.
3. Other features of AMD, including cystoid macular edema (CME), drusenoid RPE detachments and RPE tears can be imaged by OCT.
4. Optical coherence is useful for quantitative assessment of retinal thickness and subretinal fluid when associated with choroidal neovascularization (CNV).

A characteristic appearance of CNV has also been described, consisting of thickening and fragmentation of the reflective layer corresponding to the RPE and choriocapillaris. The extent and location of subretinal fluid associated with CNV can be used to assess whether the pathology is subfoveal, as long as there is preservation of some foveal architecture. As noted on clinical examination and FA, CME is frequently associated with CNV in wet AMD. However, the presence of CME may be difficult to definitively diagnose through those modalities alone.

In addition to imaging subretinal fluid, OCT is effective in identifying intraretinal edema, compared to both clinical stereoscopic images and FA. The appearance of CME on OCT images

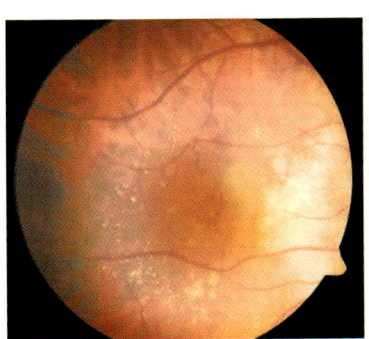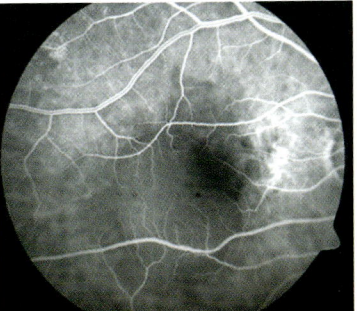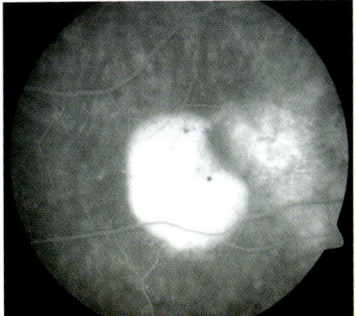

Fig. 24.3.7A *Pigment epithelial detachment (PED) with associated CNV*

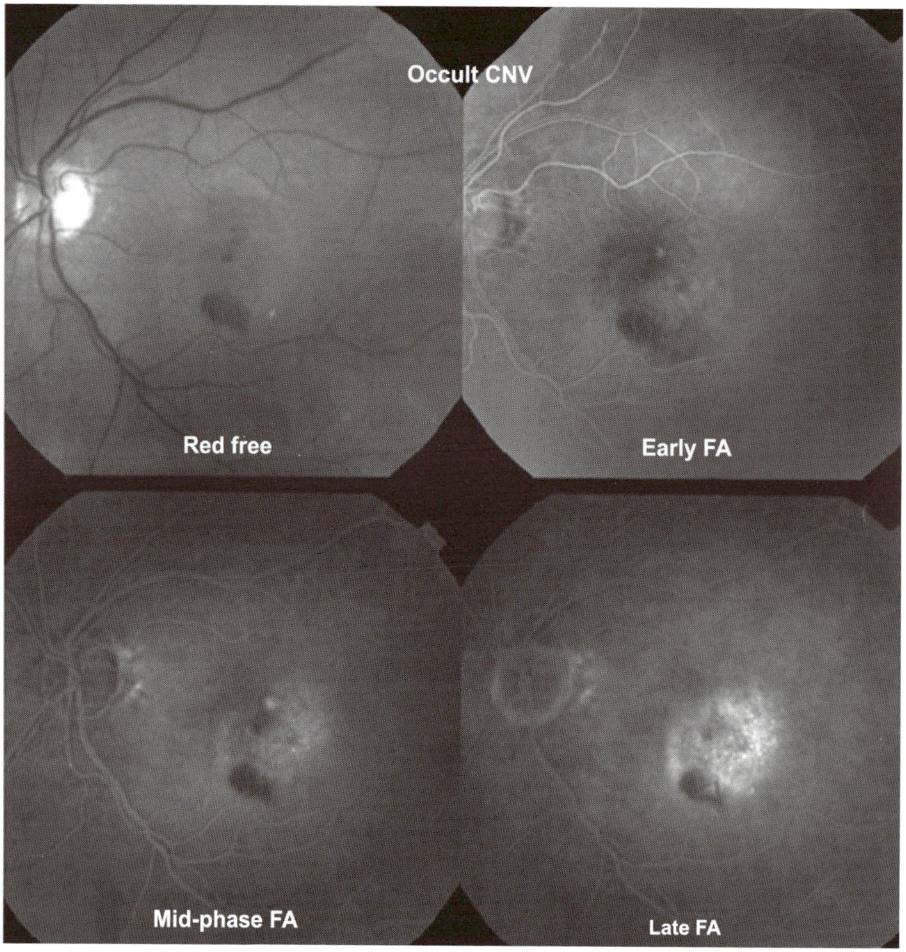

Occult CNV

Red free

Early FA

Mid-phase FA

Late FA

Fig. 24.3.7B *FFA of an occult CNV showing stippled hyperfluorescence in the late phases*

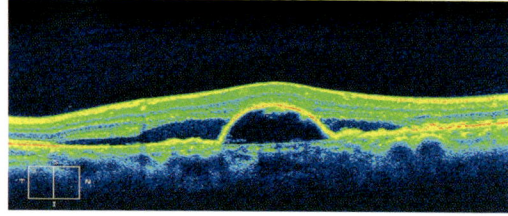

Fig. 24.3.8 *OCT image of an occult CNV*

is seen as hyporeflective, dark spaces within retinal tissue. Its presence is important clinically, since CME as seen on OCT scan in wet AMD correlates with decreased visual acuity. RPE detachments and sub-RPE neo-vascularization has been associated with occult CNV in AMD as defined histopathologically.

IDIOPATHIC POLYPOIDAL CHOROIDAL VASCULOPATHY OR POLYPOIDAL CHOROIDAL VASCULOPATHY (PCV)

Idiopathic polypoidal choroidal vasculopathy (PCV) has recently been classified as a form of CNV that may occur in elderly patients. A recent study by Yannuzzi and colleagues determined the frequency and nature of PCV in patients suspected of harboring exudative AMD. In their prospective study of 167 newly diagnosed patients with exudative AMD, CNV was diagnosed in 154 (92.2%) and PCV in 13 (7.8%). Nonwhite race (23.1%), absence of drusen (16.7% had drusen) and peripapillary location were felt to distinguish between PCV and AMD. Since then, it is now recognized that PCV occurs

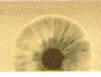

in all races. PEDs are commonly seen in PCV. Investigation of choice is ICG and the polyps are picked up as an outpouching of the choroidal vasculature (Fig. 24.3.9). In the absence of subretinal bleed, these can also be picked up on FFA (Fig. 24.3.10).

RETINAL ANGIOMATOUS PROLIFERATION (RAP)

One other distinct type of neovascular AMD is retinal angiomatous proliferation (RAP). This entity is characterized by an anomalous retinal vascular complex which is most commonly associated with retinal and subretinal neo-vascularization (Fig. 24.3.11). It has been described predominantly in elderly Caucasians and is often seen bilaterally. While its natural history is not fully understood, it is thought to progress ultimately to a disciform scar. Prior to the recognition of this entity, it was often misdiagnosed as occult CNV.

A three-stage classification system of RAP has been proposed by Yannuzzi and colleagues to describe the various clinical presentations and to theorize on the disease's natural history.

Stage I, a nodular mass of intraretinal neo-vascularization is seen and originates from the deep capillary plexus in the paramacular area. There is usually one or more associated retinal vessels which either perfuse or drain the vascular complex. Intraretinal hemorrhages and intraretinal edema are often present. FA typically shows a focal area of staining corres-ponding to the intraretinal neovascularization. Surrounding leakage is present and often misinterpreted as occult CNV. ICG angiography can aid in the diagnosis by identifying the neovascularization as a focal "hot spot" and

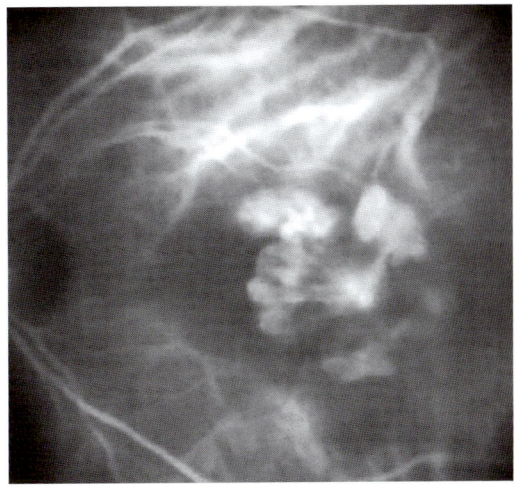

Fig. 24.3.9 *Polyps picked up on ICG*

intraretinal cystic spaces as focal hyper-fluorescent areas.

Stage II, subretinal neovascularization, involves both retinal and subretinal vascular prolifera-tion. The neovascularization occurs in a tangen-tial direction with minimal horizontal extension. Other common signs include increased intra-retinal edema, neurosensory retinal detachment, serous PED, and preretinal and subretinal hemorrhages. In many cases, a clear retinal-retinal anastomosis can be seen. FA often shows a diffuse area of leakage which is, again, often misinterpreted as occult CNV.

Stage III of RAP is defined by the Stage II findings plus the clear presence of CNV. This is most often documented by the presence of a FVPED or a predisciform scar. Occasionally, the presence of a retinal-choroidal anastomosis helps confirm the staging.

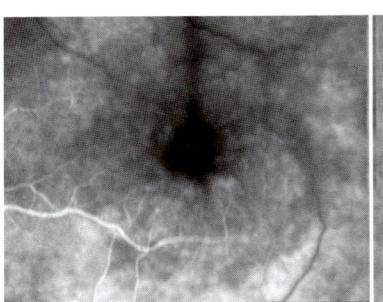
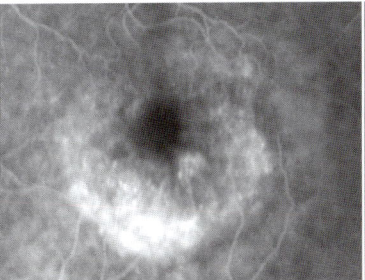
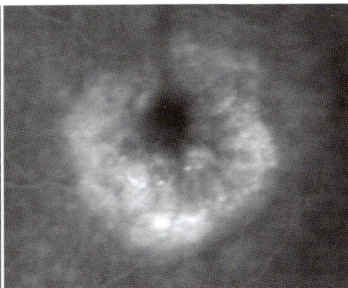

Fig. 24.3.10 *PCV on FFA*

occlusion occurs following PDT and is marked by the release of vasoactive molecules, vasoconstriction, blood cell aggregation, endothelial cell damage, blood flow stasis, and hemorrhage. Verteporfin at 6 mg/m^2 was infused intravenously for 10 minutes. Then, a diode laser was used to activate the dye (689–nm diode laser, 50 J/cm^2, 600 mW/cm^2, 83–second duration, spot size 1000 μm larger than greatest linear diameter of the CNV lesion) 15 minutes after the start of infusion. PDT has traditionally focused on the treatment of cancer, but the potential for selective destruction of diseased vessels, while sparing normal overlying tissues, coupled with promising clinical efficacy, resulted in its use for the treatment of age-related macular degeneration (AMD), particularly subfoveal choroidal neovascularization (CNV).

VERTEPORFIN TRIALS

Treatment of age-related macular degeneration with photodynamic therapy trial (TAP study)

Eligible AMD patients had subfoveal CNV whose greatest linear dimension was up to 5400 μm and best-corrected visual acuity ranged from 20/40 to 20/200. Subgroup analysis demonstrated the greatest benefit (67% vs. 39% losing less than 15 letters of visual acuity, p<0.001) for those eyes with predominantly classic CNV (greater than 50% of the entire lesion being classic CNV at baseline before treatment).

Verteporfin in photodynamic therapy (VIP) study

In this study, patients with pathologic myopia, occult CNV, and classic CNV were evaluated. Eyes with new or recurrent CNV, and AMD with the following criteria were included:
- Classic CNV with visual acuity better than 20/40.
- Occult CNV with evidence of blood or deterioration within the last 3 months defined either visually as the loss of ≥ 5 letters or anatomic as ≥ 10% increase in the greatest linear diameter of the lesion.

For the subgroup of occult-only CNV, the PDT group was less likely than placebo to lose 15 and

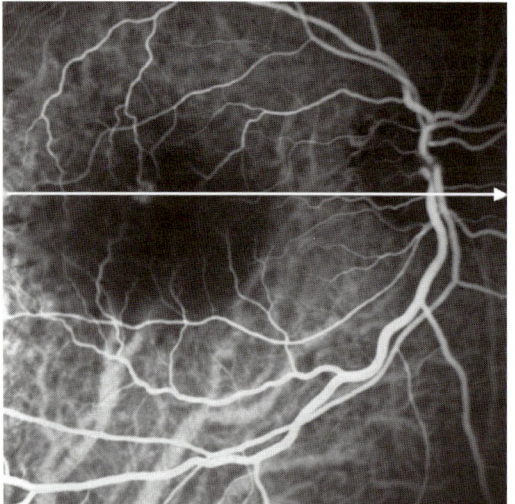
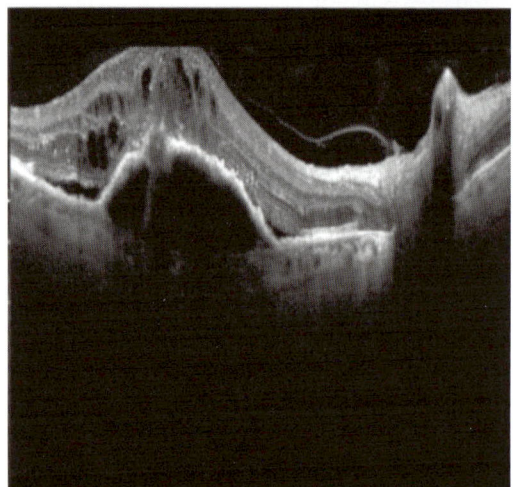

Fig. 24.3.11 *RAP lesion on FFA and the corresponding SL-OCT image demonstrating the level of the lesion*

TREATMENT OF WET AMD

Photodynamic therapy (PDT) is a therapeutic modality that entails the administration of a photosensitizer with its subsequent accumulation in the target tissue and then its activation by non-thermal monochromatic light corresponding to the sensitizers absorption profile. Uptake of the dye is facilitated by the increased expression of low-density lipoprotein receptors on tumor cells and neovascular endothelial cells. Powerful oxidizing agents such as cytotoxic singlet oxygen and free radicals are produced causing irreversible cellular damage. Vascular

30 ETDRS letters at the 24-month follow-up. For the subgroup of patients with a visual acuity score of less than 65 ETDRS letters (Vision less than 20/50) or lesion size less than or equal to four disc areas, verteporfin PDT-treated patients were less likely than placebo to lose 15 and 30 ETDRS letters at the 24-month follow up.

The TAP and VIP trial data were combined and analyzed in a series of reports. The most significant data to be gleaned from these reports was that baseline lesion size was the most important predictor of visual acuity following verteporfin PDT, regardless of lesion composition. Size was a significant factor for patients with predominantly classic lesions greater than one disc area, minimally classic lesions less than four disc areas, and occult-only lesions less than five disc areas.

Verteporfin PDT has been approved by the FDA for eyes with predominantly classic CNV as well as for eyes with pathologic myopia and ocular histoplasmosis.

ANTI-VEGF TREATMENT

Aptamers: pegaptanib sodium (macugen)

The first anti-VEGF therapy to undergo clinical testing was a VEGF aptamer. Approved by the Food and Drug Administration (FDA) in 2004, Pegaptanib was the first anti-VEGF agent with proven efficacy for the treatment of CNV secondary to age-related macular degeneration (AMD). Pegaptanib is an aptamer a short single-stranded oligonucleotide sequence that functions as a high affinity inhibitor of a specific protein target. Pegaptanib is a 28-base RNA oligonucleotide that is covalently linked to two 20 kD polyethylene glycol moieties to extend the half-life. Pegaptanib selectively binds to the heparin-binding domain of VEGF165 and larger isoforms, preventing ligand-receptor binding. The smaller VEGF isoforms and proteolytic fragments are therefore not inhibited by pegaptanib.

Safety and efficacy of pegaptanib for the treatment of neovascular AMD was established through the VEGF inhibition study in ocular neovascularization (VISION) study. VISION consisted of two phase III prospective, multi-center, randomized, controlled, double-masked trials comparing intravitreal injections of pegaptanib with sham injections. Patients (1186

total) were randomized to receive pegaptanib (at a dose of 0.3, 1.0, or 3.0 mg) or sham injection (usual care), every six weeks for a total of 54 weeks. The primary end point of the study was the number of patients losing less than 15 letters of early treatment diabetic retinopathy study (ETDRS) visual acuity at 54 weeks. Patients with all CNV lesion subtypes with sizes up to and including 12 disc areas in size were included. In the pooled analysis, efficacy was demonstrated for all three doses, without a dose-response relationship. Seventy per cent of pegaptanib-treated patients lost less than 15 letters, compared with 55% of usual care patients. More pegaptanib-treated patients maintained or gained visual acuity (33%) at 54 weeks than usual care patients (23%). In addition, the usual care group was twice as likely to experience severe vision loss (>30 letters) during the study period than pegaptanib-treated patients. However, only 6% of pegaptanib-treated patients in the study gained > 15 letters at 54 weeks (compared with 2% of usual care controls), and as a group, the pegaptanib-treated patients lost an average of eight letters over the study period (compared with 15 letters in the usual care group).

Further research

1. **VERITAS study:** A phase III prospective, multicenter, randomized, double-masked trial comparing PDT combined with one of two doses of intravitreal triamcinolone (1 mg, 4 mg) versus PDT combined with 0.3 mg of intravitreal pegaptanib.
2. Sustained release preparations to reduce the frequency of intra vitreal injections.

Monoclonal Antibodies: Ranibizumab (Lucentis)

In June 2006, ranibizumab (Lucentis-Genentech, South San Francisco, California, USA) became the second VEGF inhibitor approved by the FDA for use in the treatment of CNV secondary to AMD. Ranibizumab is a humanized, affinity-maturated Fab fragment of a murine mono-clonal antibody directed against human VEGF-A. Ranibizumab is a potent, non-selective inhibitor of all VEGF-A isoforms and bioactive proteolytic products. Ranibizumab was specifi-

cally designed as a molecule smaller than its parent full-size precursor anti-VEGF antibody, because it was felt that the full-sized antibody was unable to cross the inner retina and choroid.

Efficacy and safety of ranibizumab has thus far been established through two large prospective, multicenter, randomized, double-masked, controlled clinical trials: Minimally classic/occult trial of anti-VEGF antibody ranibizumab in the treatment of neovascular age-related macular degeneration (MARINA) and anti-VEGF antibody for the treatment of predominantly classic CNV in AMD (ANCHOR).

The MARINA trial was limited to patients with subfoveal occult or minimally classic CNV, either primary or recurrent, with evidence of recent disease progression. In MARINA, 716 patients were randomized 1:1:1 to receive monthly intravitreal injections of ranibizumab (either 0.3 or 0.5 mg) or sham injections. The primary outcome measure was the proportion of patients losing less than 15 ETDRS letters at 12 months. 94.5% of patients assigned to the 0.3 mg group and 94.6% of patients assigned to the 0.5 mg ranibizumab treatment arms, compared with 62.2% in the sham-treatment arm, met this endpoint. More eyes gained 15 or more letters of visual acuity by month 12 in the ranibizumab treatment arms than the control arms: 24.8% in the 0.3 mg group, 33.8% in the 0.5 mg group, 5.0% in the sham-treated group. Mean visual acuity increased by 6.5 letters in the 0.3 mg group and 7.2 letters in the 0.5 mg group at 12 months. In contrast, mean visual acuity dropped by 10.4 letters in the sham-treated group. In general, vision gains were maintained throughout year two of the MARINA trial in ranibizumab-treated patients, whereas vision continued to decline in the sham treated patients; mean loss was 14.9 letters in the sham group.

The ANCHOR trial has likewise demonstrated efficacy of ranibizumab for the treatment of predominantly classic CNV lesions secondary to AMD. ANCHOR was designed as a head-to-head comparison between ranibizumab and PDT with verteporfin (Visudyne), which was then the standard of care for subfoveal CNV. 423 patients were randomized 1:1:1 to receive

monthly intravitreal injections with ranibizumab 0.3 mg and sham PDT, ranibizumab 0.5 mg with sham PDT or monthly sham injections plus active verteporfin PDT. The primary end point was the number of patients losing fewer than 15 letters of baseline visual acuity at 12 months. This end point was achieved in 94.3% of the patients receiving 0.3 mg ranibizumab and 96.4% of patients receiving 0.5 mg ranibizumab versus 64.3% of the verteporfin group.

The percentage of patients experiencing an improvement over baseline visual acuity of at least 15 letters was 35.7% and 40.3% respectively, in the ranibizumab treated patients, versus only 5.6% in the verteporfin treated patients. Mean visual acuity increased by 8.5 letters in the 0.3 mg ranibizumab group and 11.3 letters in the 0.5 mg ranibizumab group at 12 months. In contrast, mean visual acuity dropped by 9.5 letters in the verteporfin PDT group at 12 months.

The PIER study is a phase IIIb, prospective, multicenter, randomized, double-masked, controlled study of 184 patients with predominantly classic or occult CNV randomized to receive ranibizumab or sham injections monthly for the first three months, followed by once every three months for a total of 24 months. The purpose of PIER is to help determine the optimal dosing schedule for ranibizumab. The one year results of the PIER study showed that 83% (0.3 mg) and 90% (0.5 mg) of ranibizumab-treated eyes lost less than 15 letters of visual acuity, compared to 49% of sham eyes. However, the percentage of eyes improving 15 or more letters was only 12% (0.3 mg) and 13% (0.5 mg) in ranibizumab-treated eyes, compared with 10% of sham eyes.

Prospective optical coherence tomography (PRONTO) imaging of patients with neovascular AMD treated with intraocular ranibizumab is a two-year, single site, open-label, uncontrolled study of 40 patients designed to evaluate the durability of response of ranibizumab and whether optical coherence tomography (OCT) can be used to guide treatment of neovascular AMD. As in the PIER study, patients receive monthly injections of ranibizumab for the first three months. There-

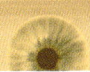

after, re-treatment with ranibizumab is performed if one of the following changes were observed between visits: a loss of 5 letters in vision in conjunction with fluid on OCT, increase in OCT central retinal thickness of at least 100 μm, new onset classic CNV, new macular hemorrhage, or persistent macular fluid detected by OCT at least 1 month after the previous injection of ranibizumab. At 12 months, mean visual acuity improved by 9.3 letters (p < 0.001) and the mean OCT central retinal thickness decreased by 178 mm. Visual acuity improved 15 or more letters in 35% of patients. These visual acuity and OCT outcomes were achieved with an average of 5.6 injec-tions over 12 months. Once a fluid-free macula was achieved, the mean injection-free interval was 4.5 months before another reinjection was necessary. PRONTO outcomes suggest that OCT can be useful for guiding re-treatment with intravitreal ranibizumab in neovascular AMD.

Monoclonal antibodies: **Bevacizumab (Avastin Genentech, South San Francisco, California, USA)** is a full-length humanized murine monoclonal antibody directed against human VEGF-A. It was FDA approved in 2004 for the intravenous treatment of metastatic colorectal cancer. Several retrospective, uncontrolled, open label case series have been published regarding the use of intravitreal bevacizumab as an off label drug for the treatment of CNV secondary to AMD.

One important aspect in which ranibizumab and bevacizumab may differ is their pharmacokinetics. Because of its larger molecular weight, it is assumed that bevacizumab has a significantly longer half-life in the vitreous, and possibly systemically as well. A longer half-life may allow for less frequent injections to achieve the same biologic effect. The half life of ranibizumab, as seen in animal studies, in the vitreous is 3 days as compared to 4.3 days in case of bevacizumab.

Bevacizumab comes in preservative-free 100 mg vials, containing 4 cc of a 25 mg/cc solution, intended for one-time use only for treatment of a single cancer patient. A single vial can theoretically be aliquoted out to provide up to eighty individual 0.05 cc intravitreal doses in 1 cc tuberculin syringes. The pharmacy should confirm the dose and sterility, provide proper storage instructions, and mark all aliquots with an expiration date. Although bevacizumab is a very stable drug with a shelf-life of many months, compounded aliquots will usually have an expiration date due to sterility concerns.

Combination therapy with PDT

The RhuFab V2 ocular treatment combining the use of VISUDYN to evaluate safety; (FOCUS) study is a two-year, phase I/II, multicenter, randomized, single-masked, controlled study of 162 patients with predominantly classic CNV. FOCUS compared the safety and efficacy of intravitreal rani-bizumab (0.5 mg) combined with verteporfin PDT versus verteporfin PDT alone (combined with sham injection). Patients received monthly ranibizumab (0.5 mg) (nZ106) or sham (nZ56) injections. The PDT was perfor-med seven days before initial ranibizumab or sham treatment and then quarterly as needed. The primary outcome measure was the propor-tion of patients who lost fewer than 15 letters from baseline at 12 months. At 12 months, 90.5% of the ranibizumab treated patients and 67.9% of the control patients lost fewer than 15 letters (p0.001). In addition, the FOCUS study showed that despite a history of prior PDT therapy, a significant proportion of these patients were able to gain visual acuity when treated with ranibizumab and PDT.

siRNAs

Double stranded RNA binds to a protein complex called *dicer*, which cleaves it into multiple smaller fragments. A second protein complex called RNA induced silencing complex (RISC) then binds these RNA fragments and eliminates one of the strands. The remaining strand stays bound to RISC, and serves as a probe that recognizes the corresponding messenger RNA transcript in the cell. When the RISC complex finds a complementary messenger RNA transcript, the transcript is cleaved and degraded, thus silencing that gene's expression.

Bevasiranib/Cand5 is a siRNA inhibitor of VEGF, which is given as an intravitreal injection. A phase I, open-label, dose escalation study of 15 patients revealed no serious ocular or syste-mic adverse effects at a dose up to 3.0 mg.

Receptor tyrosine kinase inhibitors

Non-RNA inhibitors of VEGF receptor tyrosine kinase activity have been identified, and their anti-angiogenic properties are being investigated for use in the treatment of systemic malignancy, as well as CNV. One advantage of this class of drugs over those discussed thus far in this chapter is the possibility of an oral route of administration, thereby avoiding the ocular complications associated with frequent intravitreal injections.

One promising compound is PTK787, which is a non-selective inhibitor of all known VEGF receptors. A multicenter phase I trial of PTK787/Vatalanib in patients with AMD is the ADVANCE study. Patients with all CNV lesion types will receive PDT with Visudyne at baseline, and will be randomized to receive concurrent treatment with either 500 or 1000 mg of oral PTK787/Vatalanib or placebo, once daily for three months. ADVANCE is designed to assess the safety and efficacy of the drug.

AG-013958 (Pfizer, San Diego, California, USA) is a selective VEGFR and PDGFR inhibitor that is currently in phase I/II testing. The route of administration being examined is subtenon injection. Preliminary results of 21 patients with subfoveal CNV indicated that adverse events were mild.

ADVANCES IN THE TREATMENT OF WET AGE-RELATED MACULAR DEGENERATION

Research has continued to evolve since the advent of antivascular endothelial growth factor (VEGF) treatment for AMD. Several studies have been conducted to assess the efficacy of combination therapy with anti-VEGFs, as well as investigative approaches to treatment, and the risk of side effects.

CATT Results: avastin and lucentis equivalent for AMD

NEI launched CATT in 2008 to compare lucentis and avastin for the treatment of wet AMD. The study has now reported results for 1,185 patients treated at 43 clinical centers in the United States. Patients were randomly assigned and treated with one of four regimens for a year. They received lucentis monthly or PRN, PRN (Prorenata means as and when required) or avastin monthly or PRN. Enrollment criteria required that study participants had active disease.

Patients in the monthly dosing groups received an initial treatment and then had an injection every 28 days. Patients in the PRN groups received an initial treatment and were then examined every 28 days to determine medical need for additional treatment. PRN groups received subsequent treatment when there were signs of disease activity, such as fluid in the retina. Ophthalmologists involved in patient care did not know which study drug a patient was getting, to make sure that the data was not affected by how anyone felt about the treatment.

Change in visual acuity served as the primary outcome measure for CATT. Thus far, visual acuity improvement was virtually identical (within one letter difference on an eye chart) for either drug when given monthly. In addition, no difference was found in the percentage of patients who had an important gain or loss in visual function. Also, when each drug was given on a PRN schedule, there also was no difference (within one letter) between drugs. PRN dosing required four to five fewer injections per year than monthly treatment. In addition to the primary finding of equivalence between lucentis and avastin for visual acuity, CATT also demonstrates that PRN dosing is a viable treatment option for either of these drugs. Serious adverse events (primarily hospitalizations) occurred at a 24% rate for patients receiving Avastin and a 19% rate for patients receiving lucentis. The number of deaths, heart attacks, and strokes were low and similar for both drugs during the study. CATT was not capable of determining whether there is an association between a particular adverse event and treatment. Differences in serious adverse event rates require further study. Investigators in the CATT study will continue to follow patients through a second year of treatment. These additional data will provide information on longer-term effects of the drugs on vision and safety.

COMBINATION THERAPY: DENALI, MONT BLANC, MOUNT EVEREST

A randomized, double-blinded prospective study evaluating the efficacy of photodynamic therapy (PDT) and intravitreal triamcinolone versus triple therapy consisting of PDT, triamcinolone, and 0.5 mg intravitreal ranibizumab in 15 patients with subfoveal choroidal neovascularization (CNV) secondary to AMD was conducted in Mexico. Group 1 (n = 7) received PDT followed by 4 mg triamcinolone (n = 7) and group 2 (n = 8) received triple therapy. At 6 months, 5 of 7 patients (71.4%) from group 1 and all the patients from group 2 had lost fewer than 15 letters (P < .001). Three patients (37.5%) from group 2 had an improve-ment of 3 lines or more. Only visual acuity had a statistically significant effect (P = .006) on outcome. The median number of treatments in both groups was 1. Both groups had significant and similar increases in IOP (25–28%) and cataract progression (12.5–14.2%). There were no cases of endophthalmitis nor were there any cardiac or cerebrovascular accidents. The authors concluded that the combination of PDT, triamcinolone, and intravitreal ranibizumab is a safe and efficacious treatment option for neovascular AMD. These findings lend support to the work of Augustin, who presented a promising case series using triple therapy with PDT, dexamethasone, and bevacizumab.

VEGF TRAP

A new experimental antiangiogenic drug, called VEGF Trap-Eye (aflibercept ophthalmic solution) is being tested for its ability to being benefits over current therapies. VEGF Trap is a fusion protein of key domains from human VEGF Receptors 1 and 2 with a human IgG Fc portion. VEGF Trap-Eye is a protein that binds to and inactivates a growth factor called VEGF (vascular endothelial growth factor) that stimulate blood vessel growth in AMD. Inhibiting these blood vessels reduces vision loss. Two phase 3 clinical trials, called **VIEW 1** and **VIEW 2,** have been conducted to examine the benefits of VEGF Trap-Eye. The results indicate that this new drug is just as effective as a standard therapy, but requires fewer injections into the eyes. In VIEW 1 and VIEW 2, at least 95% of patients who received the experimental medication maintained their vision during the 52-week follow-up period. Maintenance of vision was defined as losing fewer than three lines (equivalent to 15 letters) on the early treatment diabetic retinopathy study (ETDRS) eye chart. VEGF Trap-Eye is also in clinical development for the treatment of central retinal vein occlusion (CRVO), another major cause of blindness, and diabetic macular edema (DME).

ADVANCES IN THE TREATMENT OF DRY AMD

Brimonidine intravitreal implant in patients with geographic atrophy due to age-related macular degeneration (AMD)

This is a randomized, double-masked, dose-response, sham-controlled evaluation of the safety and efficacy of brimonidine tartarate intravitreal implant in patients with geographic atrophy from age-related macular degeneration. It is hypothesized that the implant may promote the release of neuroprotective factors that may slow the progression of retinal degenerative disease.

AREDS1

AREDS1 was designed as both a study of the clinical course of age-related lens opacity and AMD as well as a randomized, controlled trial of high-dose antioxidants and zinc to reduce progression of eye diseases common in the elderly. Participants with AMD were defined as:

- *Category 1:* Early AMD. Having few small drusen (<63 μm)
- *Category 2:* Mild AMD, having small drusen (<63 μm) and few intermediate drusen (≤63 μm and <125 μm);
- *Category 3:* Intermediate AMD, having extensive intermediate drusen or large drusen (≥125 μm); or
- *Category 4:* Advanced AMD in one eye, either geographic atrophy in the center or neovascular AMD (Fig. 24.3.12A to C).

Participants were randomized in a factorial design to receive either antioxidant vitamins, zinc, antioxidants and zinc, or placebo.

The formulations included:
- vitamin C (500 mg);
- vitamin E (400 International Units [IU]);

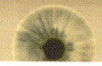

- beta-carotene (15 mg);
- zinc (80 mg of zinc oxide); and
- copper (2 mg of cupric oxide).

The results of AREDS demonstrated a statistically significant benefit for the combination of high-dose antioxidant vitamins and zinc in providing a moderate reduction in the risk of developing advanced AMD over a median of 6.3 years of follow-up in persons at high risk. Specifically, the risk for progression was reduced by 25% for the entire study population (Categories 2-4) and 34% for the population of patients with Categories 3 or 4 AMD. The overall risk for moderate vision loss (decrease of 15 or more letters on the logarithmic chart compared with baseline) was reduced by 19% at 5 years.

The beneficial effects of the AREDS-type supplements were demonstrated to persist at 4 years follow up. It was therefore recommended that persons with intermediate AMD or AREDS Category 3 (bilateral large drusen) or those with advanced AMD (neovascular AMD or geographic atrophy) in one eye consider taking the AREDS-type formulation to prevent the development of advanced AMD. For persons with early AMD, however, the AREDS-type supplements did not prevent progression from Category 2 to Category 3. The risk of developing advanced AMD was also exceedingly low, making it unlikely that persons with less severe AMD than Category 3 disease will benefit from the use of AREDS-type supplements.

Adverse effects: Beta-carotene: It was demonstrated to increase the risk for lung cancer and its associated mortality in smokers. Beta-carotene also increased the yellowing of the skin but this was of no health consequence. Currently, the AREDS formulation is not recommended for smokers.

Zinc. A potential for an increase in genitourinary hospitalizations (e.g. unspecified urinary tract infection and prostatic hyperplasia in men and stress incontinence in women) was more frequent in participants randomly assigned to the zinc arms compared with those not assigned to zinc (7.5% vs. 4.9%; P = .001)

Age-related eye disease study 2 (AREDS2): results awaited

Objectives

1. To evaluate the effect of the two dietary xanthophylls (10 mg lutein and 2 mg zeaxanthin that accumulate in macula and two omega-3 long-chain polyunsaturated fatty acids (LCPUFAs), docosahexaenoic acid and eicosapentaenoic acid (350 mg DHA and 650 mg E PA as 2 soft-gel capsules), on progression to advanced age-related macular degeneration (AMD) and/or moderate vision loss in people at moderate to high risk for progression.
2. To evaluate the effects of eliminating beta-carotene from the original AREDS formulation on the development and progression of AMD.
3. To evaluate the effects of reducing zinc in the original AREDS formulation on the development and progression of AMD.
4. To contribute data for validation of the photographic AMD scales developed from the age-related eye disease study.

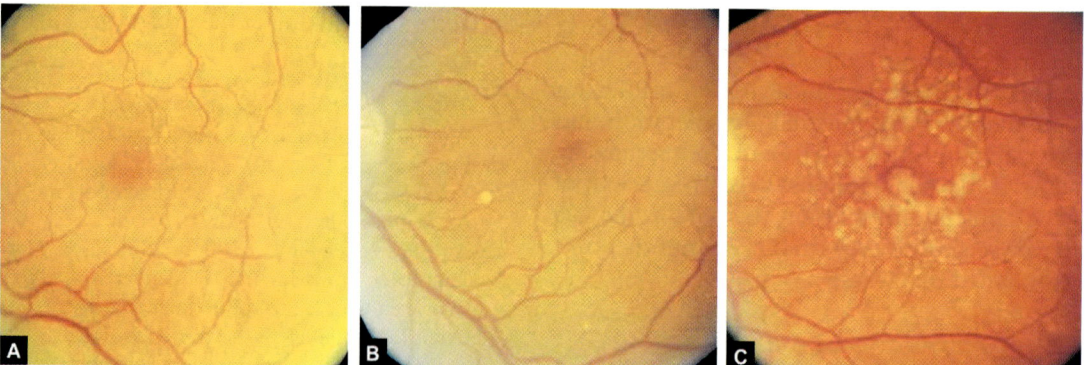

Fig. 24.3.12 *Category of participants in AREDS I study,* **(A)** *Category 2,* **(B)** *Category 3, and* **(C)** *Category 4*

Conclusions of AREDS–2 Study

1. Addition of omega-3 fatty acids or lutein and zeaxanthin to original AREDS formulation is not recommended, as it does not offer any added benefit.
2. Reduction of the dose of zinc from AREDS 1 formulation had no effect on prevention of advanced AMD. Side effects were also same in both groups.
3. Elimination of β-carotene from AREDS 1 formulation is recommended, as it increases rates of lung cancer in both smokers and non-smokers.
4. Patients with low dietary levels of lutein and zeaxanthin, may benefit from addition of these carotenoids to AREDS 1 formulation.
5. Addition of lutein and zeaxanthin to AREDS 1 formulation may decrease rates of cataract progression in patients with low dietary levels of the same.

Fenretinide in dry AMD

This drug is an oral vitamin A binding protein antagonist and is being studied in patients with geographic atrophy (GA). It halts the accumulation of retinol (vitamin A) toxins through affinity for retinol-binding protein. One of the hallmarks of dry macular degenera-tion is the accumulation of cellular "debris". The debris is also called "lipofuscin". In a healthy eye, lipofuscin is reabsorbed and does not cause problems. In dry AMD, it shows up as drusen, those small deposits of proteins that appear on the retina. The debris is also present in the geographic atrophy that is the advanced form of dry macular degeneration. The hope is that fenretinide will block the process that creates this lipofuscin and have a positive effect on drusen and geographic atrophy.

This is a Phase II clinical trial of a PILL for patients with dry macular degeneration and geographic atrophy (GA). One year interim data showed that fenretinide slowed the growth of geographic atrophy lesions by 45% in the 300 mg dose. Follow-up at the 24-month point maintained this result.

CNTF in dry AMD

Ciliary neurotrophic factor (CNTF) is a protein that effects cellular function and is classified as a "neuroprotective" agent. It means, it stops cell death and may rescue the photoreceptors, even if they are already on their way to dying. One year results of a clinical trial involving CNTF for geographic atrophy in dry AMD were recently released. The eyes receiving the high-dose showed a change in the total macular volume and an increase in retinal thickness. This was tied to maintaining vision, which occured in 96.3% of these patients, versus 75% of the sham and low-dose patients. The device, made by Neurotech Pharmaceuticals, is called the NT-501 Implant.

Copaxone (glatiramer acetate)

This small phase 1 clinical trial of 30 people with dry AMD involves a weekly vaccination with the drug Copaxone. This is NOT an injection in the eye.

Macular degeneration, Alzheimer's disease and multiple sclerosis have some things in common, including inflammation and the formation of deposits. In Alzheimers, the deposits are plaque in the brain; in AMD, the deposits are drusen in the retina. Copaxone is being investigated as a treatment for all three diseases. It is already used to treat multiple sclerosis and has been proven safe in that treatment.

The intention of the study is to see if copaxone will reduce the drusen in dry AMD. Earlier studies showed that eyes treated with copaxone showed a reduction in drusen area of over 53% after 12 weeks. This is compared to patients without treatment those eyes showed an average 25% increase in the total area of drusen over 6 months. None of the untreated eyes showed any shrinking of the drusen area at all.

BIBLIOGRAPHY

1. Age-Related Eye Disease Study Research Group. Potential public health impact of Age-Related Eye Disease Study results: AREDS report no. 11. Arch Ophthalmol 2003; 121:1621–4.
2. American Academy of Ophthalmology. New Therapies for Macular Degeneration, 2005. (www.aao.org/newsroom/facts/amd.cfm)
3. Evans J, Wormald R. Is the incidence of registrable age related macular degeneration increasing? Br J Ophthalmol 1996; 80:9–14.

4. Eye Diseases Prevalence Research Group. Prevalence of age-related macular degeneration in the United States. Arch Ophthalmol 2004; 122:564–72.

5. Kahn HA, Leibowitz HM, Ganley JP, et al. The Framingham Eye Study. I. Outline and major prevalence findings. Am J Epidemiol 1977; 106:17–32.

6. Leibowitz HM, Krueger DE, Maunder LR, et al. The Framingham Eye Study monograph: an ophthalmological and epidemiological study of cataract, glaucoma, diabetic retinopathy, macular degeneration, and visual acuity in a general population of 2631 adults, 1973–1975. Surv Ophthalmol 1980; 24 (Suppl.):335–610.

7. Thylefors B. A global initiative for the elimination of avoidable blindness. Am J Ophthalmol 1998; 125:90–3.

Pathophysiology of AMD

1. Ambati J, Ambati BK, Yoo SH, et al. Age-related macular degeneration: etiology, pathogenesis, and therapeutic strategies. Surv Ophthalmol 2003; 48:257–93.

2. Bressler NM, Silva JC, Bressler SB, et al. Clinicopathologic correlation of drusen and retinal pigment abnormalities in age-related macular degeneration. Retina 1994; 14:130–42.

3. Chong NHV, Keonin J, Luthert PJ, et al. Decreased thickness and integrity of the macular elastic layer of Bruch's membrane correspond to the distribution of lesions associated with age-related macular degeneration. Am J Pathol 2005; 16:241–51.

4. Curcio CA, Medeiros NE, Millican LC. Photoreceptor loss in age-related macular degeneration. Invest Ophthalmol Vis Sci 1996; 37:1236–49.

5. Curcio CA, Millican CL, Allen KA, et al. Aging of the human photoreceptor mosaic: evidence for selective vulnerability of rods in the central retina. Invest Ophthalmol Vis Sci 1993; 34:3278–96.

6. Curcio CA, Millican CL. Basal linear deposit and large drusen are specific for early age-related maculopathy. Arch Ophthalmol 1999; 117:329–39.

7. Eisner A, Klien ML, Zilis JD, et al. Visual function and the subsequent development of exudative age-related macular degeneration. Invest Ophthalmol Vis Sci 1992; 33:3091–102.

8. Green WR, Enger C. Age-related macular degeneration histopathologic studies: the 1992 Lorenz E. Zimmerman. Lecture. Ophthalmology 1993; 100:1519–39.

9. Green WR, Key SN. Senile macular degeneration: a histopathologic study. Trans Am Ophthalmol Soc 1977;75:180–254.

10. Green WR, McDonnell PH, Yeo JH. Pathologic features of senile macular degeneration. Ophthalmology 1985; 92:615–27.

11. Green WR. Histopathology of age-related macular degeneration. Mol Vis 1999; 5:27–36.

12. Grossniklaus HE, Gass JDM. Clinicopathologic correlation of surgically excised type 1 and type 2 submacular choroidal neovascular membranes. Am J Ophthalmol 1998; 126:59–69.

13. Grossniklaus HE, Green WR. Choroidal neovascularization. Am J Ophthalmol 2004; 137:496–503.

14. Hogan M, Alvarado J. Studies on the human macula: IV. Aging changes in Bruch's membrane. Arch Ophthalmol 1967; 77:410–20.

15. Kliffen M, Van der Schaft TL, Mooy CM, et al. Morphologic changes in age-related maculopathy. Microsc Res Tech 1997; 36:106–22.

16. LaFaut BA, Bartz-Schmidt KU, van den Broecke C, et al. Clinicopathologic correlation in exudative age-related macular degeneration: histological differentiation between classic and occult neovascularization. Br J Ophthalmol 2000; 84:239–43.

17. Löffler KU, Lee WR. Basal linear deposits in the human macula. Graefes Arch Clin Exp Ophthalmol 1986; 224:493–501.

18. Malek G, Li C-M, Guidry C, et al. Apolipoprotein B in cholesterol-containing drusen and basal deposits of human eyes with age-related maculopathy. Am J Pathol 2003; 162:413–25.

19. Penfold PL, Killingsworth MC, Sarks SH. Senile macular degeneration. Invest Ophthalmol Vis Sci 1986; 27:364–71.

20. Ramrattan RS, van der Schaft TL, Mooy CM, et al. Morphometric analysis of Bruch's membrane, the choriocapillaris and the choroid in aging. Invest Ophthalmol Vis Sci 1994; 35:2857–64.

21. Sarks JP, Sarks SH, Killingsworth MC. Evolution of geographic atrophy of the retinal pigment epithelium. Eye 1988; 2:552–77.

22. Sarks SH. Ageing and degeneration in macular region: a clinicopathological study. Br J Ophthalmol 1976; 60:324–41.

23. Schneider S, Greven CM, Green WR. Photocoagulation of well-defined choroidal neovascularization in age-related macular degeneration: clinicopathologic correlation. Retina 1998; 18:242–50.

24. Spraul CW, Grossniklaus HE. Characteristics of drusen and Bruch's membrane in post-mortem

eyes with age-related macular degeneration. Arch Ophthalmol 1997; 115:267–73.

25. van der Schaft TL, de Bruijn WC, Mooy CM, et al. Histologic features of the early stages of age-related macular degeneration: a statistical analysis. Ophthalmology 1992; 99:278–86.

Immunology in AMD

1. Khodr B, Khalil Z. Modulation of inflammation by reactive oxygen species: implications for aging and tissue repair. Free Radic Biol Med 2001; 30:1–8.
2. Mullins RF, Russell SR, Anderson DH, Hageman GS. Drusen associated with aging and age-related macular degeneration contain proteins common to extracellular deposits associated with atherosclerosis, elastosis, amyloidosis, and dense deposit disease. Faseb J 2000; 14:835–46.

Genetics in AMD

1. Klein ML, Mauldin WM, Stoumbos VD. Heredity and agerelated macular degeneration. Observations in monozygotic twins. Arch Ophthalmol 1994; 112(7):932–7.
2. Klein R, Klein BEK, Linton LKP. Prevalence of age-related maculopathy: the Beaver Dam Eye Study. Ophthalmology 1992; 99(6):933–43.
3. Meyers SM, Zachary AA. Monozygotic twins with agerelated macular degeneration. Arch Ophthalmol 1988; 106(5):651–3.

Risk factors for AMD

1. Krishnaiah S, Das T, Nirmalan PK, et al. Risk factors for age-related macular degeneration: findings from the Andhra Pradesh Eye Disease Study in South India. Invest Ophthalmol Vis Sci 2005; 46(12):4442–9.
2. Klein R, Klein BEK, Jensen SC, Meuer SM. The five-year incidence and progression of age-related maculopathy: the Beaver Dam Eye Study. Ophthalmology 1997; 104(1):7–21.
3. Seddon JM, George S, Rosner B, Rifai N. Progression of age-related macular degeneration prospective assessment of C-reactive protein, interleukin 6, and other cardiovascular bio-markers. Arch Ophthalmol 2005; 123(6):774–82.
4. Wang JJ, Mitchell P, Cumming RG, Lim R. Cataract and age-related maculopathy: the Blue Mountains Eye Study. Ophthalmic Epidemiol 1999; 6(4):317–26.

Clinical features of AMD

1. Ambati J, Ambati BK, Yoo SH, Lanchulev S, Adamis AP. Age-related macular degeneration: etiology, pathogenesis, and therapeutic strategies. Surv Ophthalmol 2003; 48(3):257–93.
2. Klein R, Klein BE, Linton KL. Prevalence of age-related maculopathy. The Beaver Dam Eye Study. Ophthalmology 1992; 99:933–43.
3. Spraul CW, Grossniklaus HE. Characteristics of drusen and Bruch's membrane in postmortem eyes with agerelated macular degeneration. Arch Ophthalmol 1997; 115:267–73.
4. Green WR, Enger C. Age-related macular degeneration histopathologic studies. The 1992 Lorenz E. Zimmerman Lecture. Ophthalmology 1993; 100:12519–35.
5. Sarks SH. Ageing and degeneration in the macular region: a clinicopathologic study. Br J Ophthalmol 1976; 60: 324–421.
6. Sarks SH, Arnold JJ, Killingsworth MC, Sarks JP. Early drusen formation in the normal and ageing eye and their relation to age-related maculopathy: a clinicopathological study. Br J Ophthalmol 1999; 83:358–68.
7. Sarks SH. Drusen patterns predisposing to geographic atrophy of the retinal pigment epithelium. Aust J Ophthalmol 1982; 10:91–7.
8. Bressler NM, Silva JC, Bressler SB, et al. Clinico-pathologic correlation of drusen and retinal pigment epithelial abnormalities in age-related macular degeneration. Retina 1994;14:130–42.
9. Gass JD. Stereoscopic Atlas of Macular Diseases: Diseases and Treatment. Vol 1. Louis: CV Mosby, 1987.
10. Age-Related Eye Disease Study Research Group. A simplified severity scale for age-related macular degeneration: AREDS Report No. 18. Arch Ophthalmol 2005; 123:1570–4.
11. Bressler SB, Maguire MG, Bressler NM, Fine SL, The Macular Photocoagulation Study Group. Relationship of drusen and abnormalities of the retinal pigment epithelium to the prognosis of neovascular macular degeneration. Arch Ophthalmol 1990; 108:1442–7.
12. Bressler NM, Bressler SB, Seddon JM, Gragoudas ES, Jacobson LP. Drusen characteristics in patients with exudative vs non-exudative age-related macular degeneration. Retina 1988; 8:109–14.
13. Holz FG, Wolfensberger TJ, Piguet B, et al. Bilateral macular drusen in age-related macular degeneration. Prognosis and risk factors. Ophthalmology 1994; 101:1522–8.
14. Gass JD. Drusen and disciform macular detachment and degeneration. Trans Am Ophthalmol Soc 1972; 70:409–36.
15. Sarks SH. Council lecture. Drusen and their relationship to senile macular degeneration. Aust J Ophthalmol 1980; 8:117–30.

16. Kahn HA, Leibowitz HM, Ganley JP, et al. The Framingham Eye Study. II. Association of ophthalmic pathology with single variables previously measured in the Framingham Heart Study. Am J Epidemiol 1977; 106:33–41.

17. Sunness JS, Rubin GS, Applegate CA, et al. Visual function abnormalities and prognosis in eyes with age-related geographic atrophy of the macula and good visual acuity. Ophthalmology 1997; 104:1677–91.

18. Bressler NM, Bressler SB, Gragoudas ES. Clinical characteristics of choroidal neovascular membranes. Arch Ophthalmol 1987; 105:209–13.

19. Bressler NM, Bressler SB, Fine SL. Age-related macular degeneration. Surv Ophthalmol 1988; 32:375–413.

20. Goldstein M, Loewenstein A, Barak A, et al. Results of a multicenter clinical trial to evaluate the preferential hyperacuity perimeter for detection of age-related macular degeneration. Retina 2005; 25:296-303.

21. Loewenstein A, Malach R, Goldstein M, et al. Replacing the Amsler grid: a new method for monitoring patients with age-related macular degeneration. Ophthalmology 2003; 110:966–70.

22. Fine AM, Elman MJ, Ebert JE, Prestia PA, Starr JS, Fine SL. Earliest symptoms caused by neovascular membranes in the macula. Arch Ophthalmol 1986; 104:513-4.

23. Nazemi PP, Fink W, Lim JI, Sadun AA. Electronic Amsler grid scotomas of age-related macular degeneration detected and characterized by means of a novel three dimensional computer-automated visual field test. Retina 2005; 25:446–53.

24. Srinivasan VJ, Wojtkowski M, Witkin AJ, et al. High definition and 3-dimensional imaging of macular pathologies with high-speed ultrahigh-resolution optical coherence tomography. Ophthalmology 2006; 113:2054–65.

25. Lim JI, Aaberg TM, Sr., Capone A, Jr., Sternberg P, Jr. Indocyanine green angiography-guided photocoagulation of choroidal neovascularization associated with retinal pigment epithelial detachment. Am J Ophthalmol 1997; 123:524–32.

26. Elman MJ, Fine SL, Murphy RP, Patz A, Auer C. The natural history of serous retinal pigment epithelium detachment in patients with age-related macular degeneration. Ophthalmology 1986; 93:224–30.

27. Dhalla MS, Blinder KJ, Tewari A, Hariprasad SM, Apte RS. Retinal pigment epithelial tear following intravitreal pegaptanib sodium. Am J Ophthalmol 2006; 141(4):752–4.

28. Macular Photocoagulation Study Group. Subfoveal neovascular lesions in age-related macular degeneration: guidelines for evaluation and treatment in the macular photocoagulation study. Arch Ophthalmol 1991; 109:1242–57.

29. Lafaut BA, Leys AM, Snyders B, Rasquin F, DeLaey JJ. Polypoidal choroidal vasculopathy in Caucasians. Graefes Arch Clin Exp Ophthalmol 2000; 238:752–9.

30. Latfaut BA, Aisenbrey S, Broeck CV, Bartz-Schmidt KU. Clinicopathological correlation of deep retinal vascular anomalous complex in age-related macular degeneration. Br J Ophthalmol 2000; 84:1269–74.

31. Yannuzzi LA, Negrao S, Iida T, et al. Retinal angiomatous proliferation in age-related macular degeneration. Retina 2001; 21:416–34.

Treatment of wet AMD

1. Arnold JJ, Blinder KJ, Bressler NM, et al. Acute severe visual acuity decrease after photodynamic therapy with verteporfin: case reports from randomized clinical trials- TAP and VIP Report No. 3. Am J Ophthalmol 2004; 137(4):683–96.

2. Azab M, Benchabourne M, Blinder KJ, et al. Verteporfin therapy of subfoveal choroidal neovascularization in age related macular degeneration: meta-analysis of 2-year safety results in three randomized clinical trials: treatment of age-related macular degeneration with photodynamic therapy and verteporfin in photodynamic therapy study. Report No. 4. Retina 2004; 24(1):1–12.

3. Barbazetto I, Burdan A, Bressler NM, et al. Photodynamic therapy of subfoveal choroidal neovascularization with verteporfin: fluorescein angiographic guidelines for evaluation and treatment-TAP and VIP Report No. 2. Arch Ophthalmol 2003; 121(9):1253–68.

4. Blinder KJ, Bradley S, Bressler NM, et al. Effect of lesion size, visual acuity, and lesion composition on visual acuity change with and without verteporfin therapy for choroidal neovascularization secondary to age-related macular degeneration: TAP and VIP Report No. 1. Am J Ophthalmol 2003; 136(3):407–18.

5. Brown DM, Kaiser PK, Michels M, et al. Ranibizumab versus verteporfin for neovascular age-related macular degeneration. N Engl J Med 2006; 355:1432–44.

6. Dougherty TJ, Gomer CJ, Hender BW, et al. Photodynamic therapy. J Natl Cancer Inst 1998; 90(12):889–905.

7. Fung AE, Lalwani GA, Rosenfeld PJ, et al. An OCT guided, variable dosing regimen with intravitreal ranibizumab (Lucentis) for Neovascular age-related macular degeneration. Am J Ophthalmol.

8. Gragoudas ES, Adamis AP, Cunningham ET, Jr., et al. Pegaptanib for neovascular age-related macular degeneration. N Engl J Med 2004; 351:2805–16.

9. Heier JS, Boyer DS, Ciulla TA, et al. Ranibizumab combined with verteporfin photodynamic therapy in neovascular age-related macular degeneration: year 1 results of the FOCUS study. Arch Ophthalmol 2006; 124:1532-42.

10. Henderson BW, Dougherty TJ. How does photodynamic therapy work? Photochem Photobiol 1992; 55(1):145–57.

11. Joondeph BC, Szczesny P, Sforzolini B. Abstract of Papers, Combined Meeting of Club Jules Gonin and The Retina Society, Cape Town, South Africa, October 15–20, 2006.

12. Ng EW, Shima DT, Calias P, et al. Pegaptanib, a targeted anti-VEGF aptamer for ocular vascular disease. Nat Rev Drug Discov 2006; 5:123–32.

13. Regillo CD, Brown DM, Abraham H, Kaiser PK, Mieler WF. Randomized, double-masked, sham-controlled trial of ranibizumab for neovascular age-related macular degeneration: PIER study year 1. Am J Ophthalmol 2007.

14. Reich SJ, Fosnot J, Kuroki A, et al. Small interfering RNA (siRNA) targeting VEGF effectively inhibits ocular neovascularization in a mouse model. Mol Vis 2003; 9:210–6.

15. Rosenfeld PJ, Brown DM, Heier JS, et al. Ranibizumab for neovascular age-related macular degeneration. N Engl J Med 2006; 355:1419–31.

16. Wood JM, Bold G, Buchdunger E, et al. PTK787/ZK 222584, a novel and potent inhibitor of vascular endothelial growth factor receptor tyrosine kinases, impairs vascular endothelial growth factor-induced responses and tumor growth after oral administration. Cancer Res 2000; 60: 2178–89.

24.4 CENTRAL SEROUS CHORIORETINOPATHY

INTRODUCTION

Central serous chorioretinopathy (CSCR) is one of the several chorioretinal disorders characterized by idiopathic serous detachment of the neurosensory retina and/or retinal pigment epithelium (RPE) at the posterior pole of the fundus. Described first by Albrecht von Graefe in 1866 as recurrent central retinitis characterized by recurrent serous macular detachment, this disorder has been variously termed central serous retinopathy by Bennet and idiopathic central serous choroidopathy by Gass. Using fluorescein angiography, Maumenee showed that the detachment of the macula resulted from a leak at the level of the retinal pigment epithelium.

EPIDEMIOLOGY

The epidemiology of CSC has not been reviewed systematically. CSC mostly affects healthy males between 25 and 55 years of age. The disorder is more common in males compared to females with the ratio varying from 3:1 in some studies to 6:1 in others. The peak age of prevalence is around 45 years though it may be higher in females and in patients with chronic CSC. CSC has been reported to be more severe in Asians and Hispanics and relatively rare in African-Americans. Other reported risk factors include hyperopia or emmetropia, stress, Type A personality, hypertension and chronic use of corticosteroids or psychotropic medications, pregnancy and oral contraceptives.

PATHOPHYSIOLOGY

Several theories have been proposed to explain the pathogenesis of CSC based on the information of the physiology known at that point in time; though each has its own deficiencies. Broadly, the following hypotheses have been proposed to explain the presence of fluid in the subretinal space in CSC.

a. A break in the integrity of the RPE causing the subretinal accumulation of fluid in CSC had been proposed based on the fluorescein angiographic finding of leakage at the level of RPE in patients with CSC.

b. RPE dysfunction theory: According to this theory, what appeared to be RPE leaks on fluorescein angiography were actually areas where the dye had diffused into the sub-retinal space

c. Alteration of RPE polarity: This theory proposes that a focus of RPE cells lose their normal polarity and pump fluid in the reverse direction thereby causing neuro-sensory detachment.

d. Choroidal vascular hyperpermeability: This theory correlates the clinical findings in CSC with indocyanine green angiography findings. It proposes that sympathomimetics and corticosteroids alter the choroidal vascular permeability either directly or indirectly by affecting its autoregulation. This, in turn, increases the tissue hydrostatic pressure in the choroid causing PED, disruption of RPE barrier and abnormal egress of fluid under the neurosensory retina leading to CSC.

CLINICO-INVESTIGATIVE PROFILE

CLINICAL PRESENTATIONS

Based on the clinical presentation, CSC can be classified into three types:

i. *The first* and the most common type is the typical or classic variant characterized by acute localized detachment of the retina with mild to moderate loss of visual acuity associated with one or few leaks on fluorescein angiography.

ii. *The second presentation* of CSC, associated with chronic corticosteroid usage, is termed as diffuse retinal pigment epitheliopathy, decompensated RPE or chronic CSC and has widespread alteration of RPE pigmentation due to chronic accumulation of shallow subretinal fluid.

iii. *A third* less common form of CSC seen more frequently after organ transplantation and in patients of Asian descent is associated with inferior bullous retinal detachment with shifting fluid. CSC may be active in which accumulation

of serous fluid between the photoreceptor layer and the RPE causes a neurosensory detachment in combination with unifocal or multifocal RPE abnormalities; or inactive in which the neurosensory detachment resolves but residual RPE abnormalities are present which may mimic several other conditions posing diagnostic challenges.

Symptoms

The most common presenting symptoms of CSC are decreased and distorted vision. The visual acuity is usually lowered to 20/30 to 20/60 and may be partially corrected with a low plus lens. Patients with severe or recurrent disease often have visual acuities as low as 20/200. Other symptoms include metamorphopsia, micropsia, altered color vision, and a central dimness in vision that may have a grey or purple cast. Bilateral involvement has been reported in up to 40% cases and may be more frequent in older patients. Patients with an inferior bullous detachment may complain of a corresponding superior field defect.

Ocular Findings

Acute classic CSC usually presents as a solitary, localized neurosensory detachment at the posterior pole. Biomicroscopic examination reveals a blister of clear fluid elevating the macula with the base of the CSC ringed by light reflexes where the sloping edge of the retina reflects light back to the observer (Fig. 24.4.1). serous retinal pigment epithelial detachments

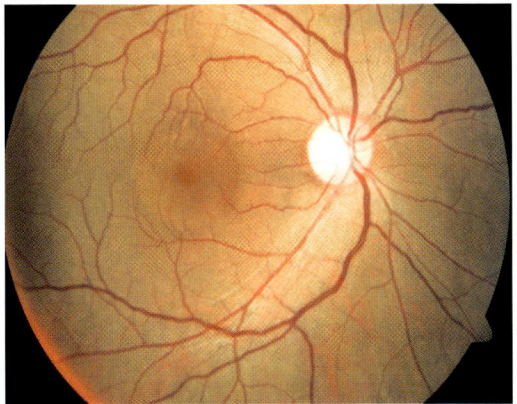

Fig. 24.4.1 *Clinical appearance of central serous chorio-retinopathy*

(RPEDs) seen as smooth, circumscribed, orange colored elevations with darker rims, may be found in association with classic CSC; though these may also be seen in association with occult choroidal neovascular membranes (CNVMs) or polypoidal choroidal vasculopathy (PCV).

Chronic CSC or DRPE on the other hand presents as relatively broad and shallow areas of neuosensory detachment with thinning or even cystoid changes within the retina. These are often accompanied by RPE alterations including atrophy or loss of pigmentation, focal areas of hyperpigmentation or RPE hyperplasia to the point of formation of bony spicules. In addition, tracks of fluid descending inferiorly up to the equator may also be seen.

The third form of CSC, more commonly reported in Japanese patients and in patients who have undergone organ transplantation, is associated with inferior bullous retinal detachments. These patients show larger and more numerous areas of choroidal hyperpermeability on ICG angiography.

In addition, patients with all forms of CSC may show subretinal deposits. These may be either subretinal fibrin or lipids. In addition, patients in whom the disease has lasted for a few months also show small, white dots on the outer retinal surface which probably represent macrophages with phagocytised outer segments.

INVESTIGATIONS

Fundus fluorescein angiography

Fundus fluorescein angiography (FFA) in patients with acute classic CSC show one or more leaks at the level of the RPE. In a minority of cases (10%), the dye rises up under the neurosensory detachment as a "smoke-stack" leak (Fig. 24.4.2); probably representing the increasing protein concentration under the detachment. A more commonly seen pattern is a blot like leak (Fig. 24.4.3) that increases in size during the angiographic evaluation. Focal leaks in CSC are more common nasally than temporally and superiorly than inferiorly. The FFA picture in chronic CSC or DRPE shows areas of granular hyperfluorescence (due to RPE atrophy) with subtle, indistinct leaks and inferiorly descending atrophic RPE tracks. Other

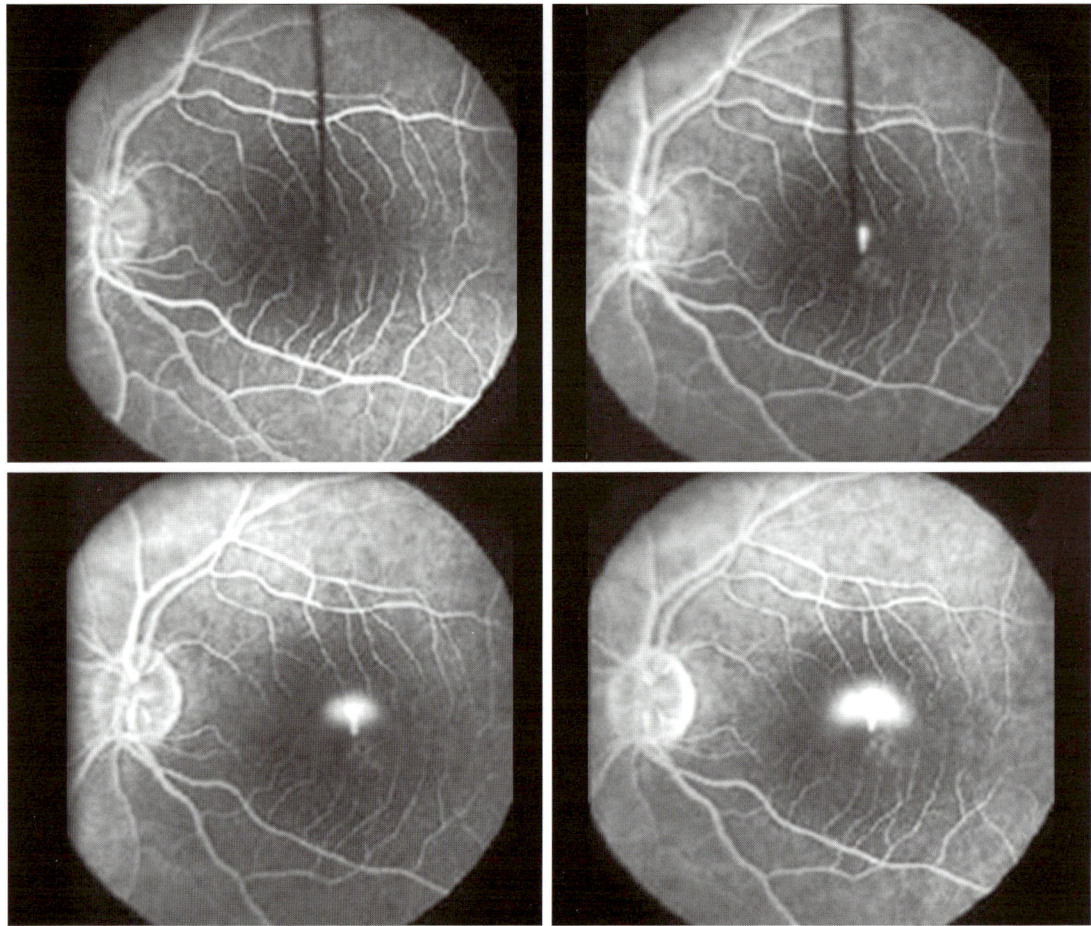

Fig. 24.4.2 *Smoke stack pattern on FFA*

findings include capillary telangiectasias, capillary nonperfusion and secondary neovascularisation in chronic detachments.

Indocyanine green (ICG) angiography

ICG in patients with classic CSC shows patchy areas of choroidal hyperpermeability typically in the mid phases of the angiogram and appears to involve the inner choroid. With time, as the dye diffuses into the outer choroid, characteristic hyperfluorescent patches with silhouetting of the larger choroidal vessels are seen in the late phases of ICG. Other reported abnormalities include delay in the filling of choroidal arteries and choriocapillaris and venous dilatation. Patients with chronic CSC or DRPE also show similar abnormalities on ICG

except the number and area of hyperpermeability are greater in DRPE.

Optical Coherence Tomography (OCT)

OCT is an excellent, non-invasive imaging modality for the diagnosis and for following the resolution of subretinal fluid in CSC. It can pick up subtle fluid accumulation beneath the sensory retina and the RPE not detectable clinically or on FFA. Recently, spectral domain OCT has been used to study ultrastructural abnormalities including external limiting membrane (ELM) and photoreceptor inner segment outer segment junction (IS-OS junction) discontinuities in patients with active and inactive CSC. These studies may provide further insight into the microstructural abnormalities in

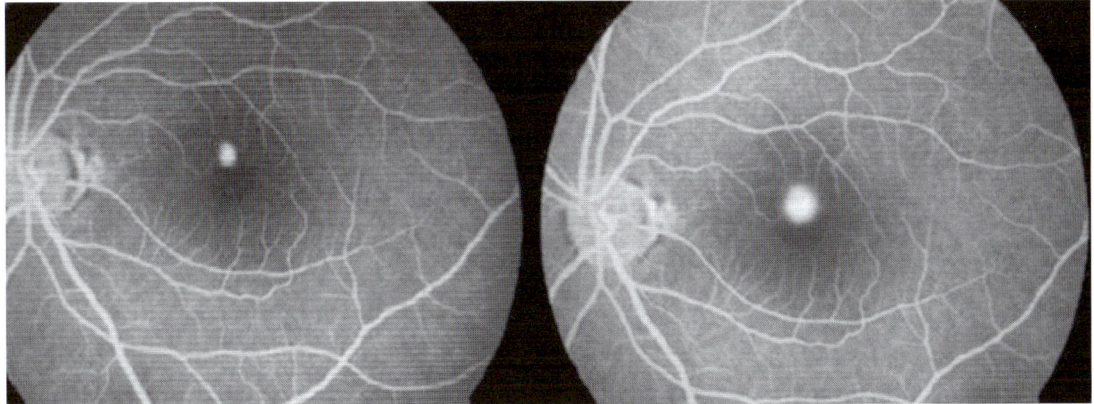

Fig. 24.4.3 *Ink blot pattern on FFA*

patients with CSC and correlation with visual acuity outcomes following resolution.

Fundus autofluorescence

Fundus autofluorescence shows hypofluore-scence that correlates well with the area of focal leakage on FFA in patients with active CSC and also shows pigment mottling in areas of RPE disturbance. In addition, central macular auto-fluorescence correlates with the central RPE atrophy and lower levels may be associated with poorer vision.

DIFFERENTIAL DIAGNOSIS

Young healthy males presenting with acute classic CSC rarely possess a diagnostic dilemma. However, the presence of subretinal fluid in an older patient requires the ophthalmologist to consider a differential diagnosis of CNV asso-ciated with age related macular degeneration, optic nerve pits with serous macular detach-ment, polypoidal choroidal vasculopathy and Vogt-Koyanagi-Harada syndrome. Whereas CSC is usually associated with a pin point leak on FFA relative to a large area of subretinal fluid, the area of leakage on FFA in CNV and PCV usually corresponds to the area of sub-retinal fluid. ICG also helps to differentiate the entities from CSC due to their characteristic appearances. Optic nerve pits are often visible on OCT and show a contiguous track of fluid with the schisis cavity or subretinal fluid. Vogt-Koyanagi-Harada syndrome may show additional signs of granulomatous intraocular inflammation, associated optic disc staining on FFA, and thickening of the choroid on ultra-sound in addition to the characteristic extra-ocular findings associated with this syndrome.

NATURAL COURSE

While a large majority of patients with acute classic CSC resolve spontaneously and experience complete restoration of vision; some patients may notice a slight permanent decrease in their visual acuity, brightness or color vision in their affected eye or a slight distortion of their central vision. On the other hand, a few patients regain only a part of their vision following resolution of their neurosensory detachment owing to photoreceptor damage, atrophy, RPE pigmentary abnormalities or subretinal fibrosis. In general, patients with chronic CSC or those with associa-ted bullous detachments have a poorer visual prognosis.

Recurrence is not uncommon and is reported to occur in about 40–50% cases. Some of these patients go on to have recurrent focal leaks while others progress inexorably to chronic CSC or DRPE. Secondary CNV may occur especially in older patients and must be suspected in cases with persistent subretinal fluid associated with blood or lipid.

TREATMENT

The current treatment approaches for CSC can be broadly divided into observation, medical, photocoagulation therapy and photodynamic therapy. Corticosteroids have long been descri-

bed as an exacerbating or precipitating factor in CSCR. The ophthalmologist should carefully question a patient with CSCR to determine any recent corticosteroid use. Affected individuals may have forgotten previous intra-articular corticosteroid injections or may not realize that their inhaler, nose spray or skin cream contains corticosteroids.

Though several drugs have been advocated targeting different steps in the pathophysiology of CSC, none have been confirmed to be of benefit by a randomized controlled trial. Diet modification, antihistamines, carbonic anhydrase inhibitors, beta blockers, non-steroidal antiinflammatory drugs, anti-VEGF agents and several others have been reported to aid the resolution of CSC in uncontrolled studies. Acetazolamide has been suggested to hasten the resolution of subretinal fluid. Corticosteroids are contraindicated and have no therapeutic role in CSCR. Scattered case reports also describe use of intravitreal avastin, but unsubstantiated.

The goal of focal laser photocoagulation is to reduce the leakage of fluid through the RPE and cause resolution of CSC. Though laser photocoagulation shortens the duration of macular detachment in patients with classic CSC, it does not alter the final visual outcome compared to untreated eyes and may not reduce the rate of recurrence as well. Moreover, the timing of laser photocoagulation is also debatable. As a result, laser photocoagulation is usually reserved for eyes in which the serous macular detachment persists for more than 4 months, the site of leakage on the FFA is > 375 µ from the foveal center, there is a history of permanent visual deficit from CSC in the fellow eye, there are signs of chronicity such as cystic changes in the retina or widespread RPE abnormalities or the occupational needs of the patient require prompt restoration of visual acuity. The usual settings for laser photo-coagulation include a spot size of 200 µ, power of 100 mw and duration of 100 ms. The site of leakage on the FFA and a small surrounding region of normal RPE are treated. As a small percentage of patients may develop CNV, it is essential to follow up the patients every 2 weeks for the first few visits following photocoagulation.

The use of photodynamic therapy with verteporphin has been investigated in patients with chronic CSC or DRPE. These cases present a therapeutic challenge owing to the diffuse nature of the disease process. Application of grid laser photocoagulation to a small area of diffuse leakage decreased the subretinal fluid but did not improve the visual outcome. In such cases PDT with verteporphin may be helpful in resolution of the subretinal fluid. The treatment spot for PDT is aimed at treating areas of choroidal hyperpermeability on ICG. Small retrospective series have reported encouraging results using standard fluence ($600\ mW/m^2$) or reduced fluence ($300\ mW/m^2$). It may be prudent to avoid direct treatment of the central fovea to avoid unwanted side effects of foveal atrophy with PDT. In addition, PDT may also be useful in patients with acute classic CSC in whom the site of leak on FFA is closer than 375 µ in which case laser photocoagulation may be contraindicated.

However, randomized controlled trials with a larger sample size may be needed to clearly define the role of early photocoagulation and photodynamic therapy in patients with CSC.

BIBLIOGRAPHY

1. Battaglia Parodi M, Da Pozzo S, Ravalico G. Photodynamic therapy in chronic central serous chorioretinopathy. Retina 2003; 23:235–237.
2. Bennett G. Central serous retinopathy. Br J Ophthalmol 1955; 39:605–18.
3. Brancato R, Scialdone A, Pece A, Coscas G, Binaghi M. Eight-year follow-up of central serous chorioretinopathy with and without laser treatment. Graefes Arch Clin Exp Ophthalmol 1987; 225:166–8.
4. Cardillo Piccolino F, Eandi CM, Ventre L, et al. Photodynamic therapy for chronic central serous chorioretinopathy. Retina 2003; 23:752–63.
5. Eandi CM, Ober M, Iranmanesh R, Peirett E, Yannuzzi LA. Acute central serous chorioretinopathy and fundus autofluorescence. Retina 2005; 25:989–93.
6. Ficker L, Vafidis G, While A, Leaver P. Long-term follow-up of a prospective trial of argon laser photocoagulation in the treatment of central serous retinopathy. Br J Ophthalmol 1988;72:829-34.

7. Gackle HC, Lang GE, Freissler KA, Lang GK. Central serous chorioretinopathy. Clinical, fluorescein angiography and demographic aspects. Ophthalmology 1998; 95:529–533.

8. Gass JDM Pathogenesis of disciform detachment of the neuroepithelium. II. Idiopathic central serous choroidopathy. Am J Ophthalmol. 1967; 63:587–615.

9. Gass JDM. Bullous retinal detachment: an unusual manifestation of idiopathic central serous choroidopathy. Am J Ophthalmol 1973; 75:810.

10. Gilbert CM, Owens SL, Smith PD, Fine SL. Long-term follow-up of central serous chorioretinopathy. Br J Ophthalmol 2004; 68:815–20.

11. Gilbert CM, Owens SL, Smith PD, Fine SL. Long-term follow-up of central serous chorioretinopathy. Br J Ophthalmol 1984; 68:815–20.

12. Haimovici R, Koh S, Gagnon DR. Risk factors for central serous chorioretinopathy: a case-control study. Ophthalmology 2004; 111:244–49.

13. Ie D,Yannuzzi LA, Spaide RF, et al. Subretinal exudative depostis in central serous chorioretinopathy. Br J Ophthalmol 1993; 77:349–53.

14. Karadimas P, Bouzas EA. Glucocorticoid use represents a risk factor for central serous chorioretinopathy: a prospective, case-control study. Graefes Arch Clin Exp Ophthalmol 2004; 242:800–2.

15. Marmor MF. New hypotheses on the pathogenesis and treatment of serous retinal detachment. Graefes Arch Clin Exp Ophthalmol 1988;226:548–52.

16. Matsunaga H, Nangoh K, Uyama M, Nanbu H, Fujiseki Y, Takahashi K. Occurrence of choroidal neovascularization following photocoagulation treatment for central serous retinopathy. Nippon Ganka Gakkai Zasshi 1995; 99:460–8.

17. Maumenee AE Symposium: Macular diseases, clinical manifestations. Trans Am Acad Ophthalmol Otolaryngol 1965; 69:605–13.

18. Ojima Y, Hangai M, Sasahara M, et al. Three-dimensional imaging of the foveal photoreceptor layer in central serous chorioretinopathy using high-speed optical coherence tomography. Ophthalmology 2007; 114:2197–207.

19. Okushiba U, Takeda M. Study of choroidal vascular lesions in central serous chorioretinopathy using indocyanine green angiography. Nippon Ganka Gakkai Zasshi 1997; 101:74–82.

20. Prunte C, Flammer J. Choroidal capillary and venous congestion in central serous chorioretinopathy. Am J Ophthalmol 1996; 121:26–34.

21. Spaide RF, Campeas L, Haas A, et al. Central serous chorioretinopathy in younger and older adults. Ophthalmology 1996; 103:2070–80.

22. Spaide RF, Hall L, Haas A, et al. Indocyanine green videoangiography of central serous chorioretinopathy in older adults. Retina 1996; 16:78–80.

23. Spitznas M, Huke J. Number, shape, and topography of leakage points in acute type I central serous retinopathy. Graefes Arch Clin Exp Ophthalmol 1987; 225:438–40.

24. Spitznas M. Pathogenesis of central serous retinopathy: a new working hypothesis. Graefes Arch Clin Exp Ophthalmol 1986; 224:321 4.

25. von Graefe A Ueber centrale recidivierende Retinitis. Graefes Arch Clin Exp Ophthalmol. 1866; 12:211

26. Wang M, Sander B, Lund-Andersen H, Larsen M. Detection of shallow detachments in central serous chorioretinopathy. Acta Ophthalmol Scand 1999; 77: 402–5.

27. Yannuzzi LA, Shakin JL, Fisher YL, Altomonte MA. Peripheral retinal detachments and retinal pigment epithelial atrophic tracts secondary to central serous pigment epitheliopathy. Ophthalmology 1984; 91:1554–72.

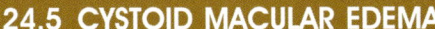
24.5 CYSTOID MACULAR EDEMA

ETIOPATHOGENESIS

INTRODUCTION

Cystoid macular edema (CME) represents a common pathologic sequelae of the retina occuring in a variety of pathological conditions such as intraocular inflammation, central or branch retinal vein occlusion, diabetic retinopathy and most commonly following cataract extraction. Histological studies show that radially orientated cystoid spaces consisting of ophthalmoscopically clear fluid are often clinically detectable in the macula area. These cysts seem to be areas of retina in which the cells have been displaced (Henle's layer).

PATHOGENESIS

The exact pathogenesis of CME remains uncertain. CME develops when excess fluid accumulates within the macular retina. This is thought to occur following disruption of the inner blood-retinal barrier (BRB). Fluorescein angiography in the normal eye demonstrates the intact barrier as the dye stays within blood vessels and does not leak into the retinal tissues. In particular, the avascular zone at the macula remains dark with no egress of dye. When the BRB is damaged, fluid accumulates within the retina both intra- and extracellularly.

Extracellular fluid accumulation disturbs cell function and retinal architecture. Müller cells are thought to play an important role in acting as metabolic pumps which keep the macula dehydrated. However, intracellular fluid accumulation in the Müller cells may also occur in CME and further reduce macular retinal function. Vitreous traction may also play a part as demonstrated by the findings of Hirokawa and colleagues (1985) who showed that uveitic eyes with complete vitreous detachment tend to have fewer macular changes than those eyes without complete vitreous detachment. In eyes with uveitis, damage to the integrity of the BRB results in leakage of dye during fluorescein angiography which accumulates in the macular area, often with a characteristic petalloid appearance.

Numerous different T-cell cytokines have been detected in both the intraocular fluids of inflamed eyes and the biopsies of involved ocular tissue and it is thought that cytokines such as interferon-γ, interleukin-2, interleukin-10, and tumor necrosis factor-α are key players in the generation of intraocular inflammation.

Macular edema and consequent loss of vision are the most frequent and serious complications of pars planitis. Persistent macular edema for more than 6–9 months leads to chronic macular changes, with permanent impairment of central vision; the degree of impairment reflects the severity of the changes. The presence of the pars plana exudates or membrane is more often, but not invariably, associated with more severe vitreous inflammation and CME.

Cystoid macular edema following cataract surgery was initially reported by Irvine in 1953 and is known as the Irvine-Gass syndrome. Approximately 20% of the patients who undergo uncomplicated phacoemulsification or extracapsular extraction develop angiographically proven CME. However, a clinically significant decrease in visual acuity is seen only in about 1% of these eyes. If cataract extraction is complicated by posterior capsule rupture and vitreous loss, severe iris trauma or vitreous traction at the wound, there is a significantly higher incidence (up to 20%) of clinically apparent CME, which is unrelated to the presence of AC-IOL. Clinically significant CME usually occurs within 3–12 weeks postoperatively, but in some instances its onset may be delayed for months or many years after surgery. Spontaneous resolution of the CME with subsequent visual improvement may occur within 3–12 months in 80% of the patients. Cataract surgery in diabetic patients may result in a dramatic acceleration of pre-existing diabetic macular edema leading to poor functional visual outcome. This can be prevented provided the severity of the retinopathy is recognized preoperatively and treated appropriately with prompt laser photocoagulation

either before surgery, if there is adequate fundal view, or shortly afterward.

Diabetic macular edema (DME) is one of the most common causes of vision loss in patients with diabetes. The severity may range from mild and asymptomatic to profound loss of vision. DME is a general term defined as retinal thickening within two disc diameters of the foveal center; it can be either focal or diffuse in distribution. Focal edema is often associated with circinate rings of hard exudates (lipoprotein deposits) resulting from leakage from microaneurysms. Diffuse edema represents more extensive breakdown of the BRB, with leakage from both microaneurysms and retinal capillaries. Cystic changes may appear within the macula, representing focal coalescence of exudative fluid.

Retinal vein obstructions represent another common retinal vascular cause of CME. In patients with central retinal vein occlusion or a tributary branch occlusion involving the macula, CME is a major cause of visual loss. This edema, if severe or chronic (>8 months), causes permanent diminution of vision secondary to disruption of the microscopic intraretinal connections and to the intracellular damage suffered by the visual elements.

Trauma anterior uveitis, drugs like prostaglandin analouges eye drops and pilo carpine eye drops, hypotony and raised intraocular pressure and post surgical are the other causes.

CLINICO-INVESTIGATIVE PROFILE

CLINICAL PRESENTATION

Slit lamp examination with contact or noncontact lens makes it possible to detect retinal thickening, localized or extending to the posterior pole. The use of a narrow slit beam is useful in detecting cystoid spaces.

Tests may be grouped into three categories according to whether one is analyzing the underlying pathogenesis, the effect of the macular edema on the retina, or its impact on visual function.

DIAGNOSTIC METHODS

Tests detecting disturbances in the blood-retinal barrier

Macular edema may result from the breakdown of the BRB. This may occur at the level of the retinal pigment epithelium or the capillary endothelial cells. Various methods of investigation are utilized to detect disruption of the BRB in order to determine the presence and the extent of macular edema.

The fundus fluorescein angiogram is clinically the most widely available and useful test. The amount of fluorescein leakage depends on the dysfunction of the retinal vascular endothelium. Although there is a significant correlation between visual acuity and the area covered by these cystoid changes, there is no relation between visual acuity and distance of cysts from the foveal avascular zone (Fig. 24.5.1). FFA shows typical patelloid hyperfluorescence.

Tests detecting retinal tissue thickness

Assessment of retinal thickness can be useful in the treatment and follow-up of macular edema. Retinal thickness at the posterior pole can be assessed by several methods. Because slit-lamp biomicroscopy and stereoscopic fundus photography are to some extent subjective, new imaging techniques for objective measure-ment of retinal thickness have been introduced to clinical use. The two most commonly used techniques are the OCT and the retinal thickness analyzer (RTA).

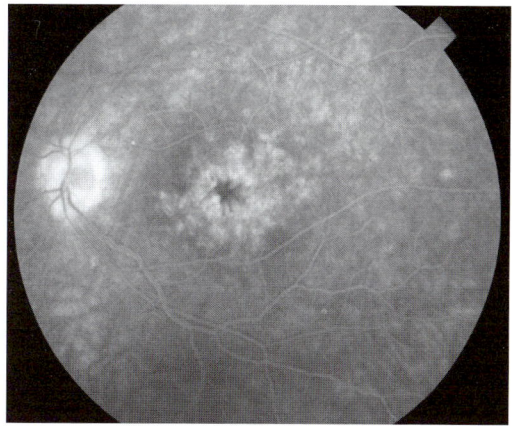

Fig. 24.5.1 *Shows petalloid fluorescein pattern suggesting gross CME*

Optical coherence tomography is a non-invasive device that obtains cross-sectional, high-resolution images of the retina and thus may detect retinal thickening (Huang et al 1991). Microstructural features are determined by measuring the 'echo' time it takes for the light to reflect from the different structures at varying distances, analogous to A-scan ultrasonography. As the OCT operates with a near-infrared wavelength (about 840 nm), the examination is of minimal discomfort for the patient (Ripandelli et al 1998). Optical coherence tomography examination is possibly indicated in the early detection and follow-up of patients with macular edema (Hee et al 1998). It has been shown to produce highly reproducible measurements and it is as effective at detecting macular edema as fluorescein angiography, but is superior at demonstrating axial distribu-tion of the fluid. The typical OCT picture shows large cystic spaces in the macula having CME (Fig. 24.5.2).

The RTA (retinal thickness analyser) is a rapid screening instrument that generates a detailed map of retinal thickness.

Tests assessing retinal function

Macular edema may potentially affect macular function as far as visual acuity and contrast sensitivity are concerned. Tests assessing macular function may be used indirectly to detect the effects of macular edema and during follow up treatment. Contrast sensitivity charts and electroretinography are both clinical and experimental tools. Contrast sensitivity has been documented as suffering specific changes in

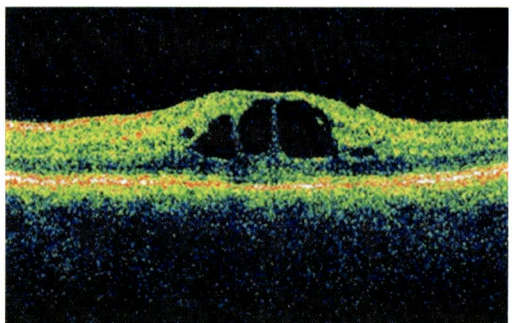

Fig. 24.5.2 *OCT shows large cystic spaces in the retina having CME*

CME as well as other localized and generalized retinal disorders.

Electroretinography (ERG) may also be utilized to follow up the treatment of macular edema. The focal electroretinogram (ERG) is the response evoked by the foveal cones of the retina to a brief flash of light focused on the fovea. The foveal ERG provides objective information on the presence or absence of organic disease at the macula. A very important development in the ERG-field in recent years is the multifocal-ERG recording system. This system allows assessment of ERG activity in small areas of retinal dysfunction.

MANAGEMENT

I. MEDICAL

The challenge concerning the management of macular edema arises in the chronic and persistent case, for which a stepwise therapeutic approach is optimal. The clinician must always be alert to the possible side effects of the many effective, but potentially toxic, pharmaceutical agents used to treat this entity. Additionally, surgical management should be considered for unremitting cases of CME.

1. Nonsteroidal anti-inflammatory drugs

In aphakic or pseudophakic CME, the occurrence of intraocular inflammation with synthesis of prostaglandins results in disruption of the tight junctions of the perifoveal retinal capillaries. Nonsteroidal anti-inflammatory drugs (NSAIDs) are useful as they inhibit the enzyme cyclooxygenase, which is required for the production of the prostaglandins as a degradation product of arachidonic acid.

2. Carbonic anhydrase inhibitors

Medical treatment of CME with carbonic anhydrase inhibitors (CAIs) has been known for over a decade. Carbonic anhydrase inhibitors may alter the polarity of the ionic transport systems in the retinal pigment epithelium through the inhibition of carbonic anhydrase and γ-glutamyl transferase. As a result there is increased fluid transport across the retinal

pigment epithelium from the sub-retinal space to the choroid with reduction of the edema. Carbonic anhydrase inhibitors have also been shown to have other direct effects both on retinal and retinal pigment epithelial cell function by inducing an acidification of the sub-retinal space, a decrease of the standing potential as well as an increase in retinal adhesiveness.

3. Steroids

Steroids also inhibit the production of prosta-glandins, but at a higher level in the biochemical pathway, by inhibiting the enzyme phospho-lipase A2, which catalyses the conversion of membrane lipids to arachidonic acid. By this process, steroids inhibit the forma-tion of both prostaglandins and leukotrienes (Abe et al 1999). Locally their vasoconstrictive properties decrease intracellular and extra-cellular edema, suppress macrophage activity, and decrease lymphokine production. Corticosteroids may be administered topically, by periocular injection, orally and parenterally. Topical corticosteroids penetrate the corneal epithelium and reach the anterior chamber. The anti-inflammatory properties of topical corticosteroids can be potentially helpful in treating CME caused by chronic iritis or iridocyclitis. Intravitreal injection of triamcinolone acetonide has become a popular treatment, subsequently, a number of corticosteroid-based intravitreal implants have been developed to provide a sustained release of drug and make repeated intravitreal injections unnecessary. A promising treatment modality for patients poorly controlled or intolerant to repeated periocular corticosteroid injections, systemic corticosteroids, or steroid sparing immuno supressive agents has been suggested with the introduction of intraocular steroid-sustained drug delivery devices. There are currently four corticosteroid-based intravitreal implants under development. These include the dexamethasone biodegradable implant (Posurdex®, Allergan, Irvine, CA), the helical triamcinolone acetonide implant 2(I-vation™ TA, SurModics, Eden Prairie, MN), the fluocinolone acetonide implant (Retisert®, Bausch and Lomb, Rochester, NY), and the fluocinolone acetonide — based implant that is injectable (Medidur™, pSivida, Boston, MA/

Alimera Sciences, Alpharetta, GA). Triam-cinolone acetonide has been reported to be effective in the management of macular edema because it suppresses inflammation, reduces extravasation of fluid from leaking blood vessels, inhibits fibrovascular proliferation, and downregulates production of VEGF. Triamcino-lone can be administered by several routes, including intravitreal depot injection, periocular injection, posterior subtenon injection, and intravitreal implant. After depot injection, corticosteroid action peaks at 1 week, with residual activity persisting for 3 to 6 months. Intravitreal injection of triamcinolone is associated with significant adverse events, including elevated intraocular pressure in up to half of injected eyes and cataract formation, as well as injection-related complications such as endophthalmitis and retinal detachment.

II. *LASER PHOTOCOAGULATION*

Photocoagulation is a therapeutic technique using a strong light source to coagulate tissue. Laser lesions in experimental animals show a temporary breakdown of the BRB and a sub-sequent repair, as the retinal pigment epithe-lium cells adjacent to the burns proliferate and slide to replace the necrotic cells. The new retinal pigment epithelium cells produce tight junctions within several weeks, which restore the integrity of the retinal pigment epithelium barrier. An alternative hypothesis states that the grid laser by destroying photoreceptors reduces the oxygen consumption of the outer retina and allows oxygen to diffuse from the choroid to the inner retina, where it raises the oxygen tension and relieves hypoxia. This increased oxygen tension causes retinal arteriolar constriction and increased resistance in the arterioles, leading to reduced hydrostatic pressure in the capillaries and venules.

III. *VITRECTOMY*

Diabetic macular edema. Vitrectomy can be useful in eyes with DME if there is evidence of vitreomacular traction. There is a higher rate of posterior vitreous detachment in eyes without DME than in diabetic eyes with DME. In one published series, vitrectomy resulted in a 61 to

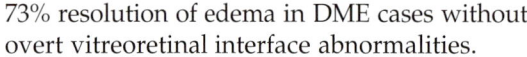

73% resolution of edema in DME cases without overt vitreoretinal interface abnormalities.

Aphakic/pseudophakic CME. The vitrectomy-aphakic-cystoid macular edema study, a prospective, multicenter study of patients with chronic aphakic CME, showed significant improvement in visual acuity following vitrectomy.

IV. ANTI-VEGF TREATMENT

Inhibition of VEGF has become a topic of interest in recent years in the area of age-related macular degeneration. The properties of VEGF, and the consequences of its inhibition, also suggest a role for this approach in the management of DME.

In the pathophysiologic cascade leading to DME, chronic hyperglycemia leads to oxidative damage to endothelial cells as well as to an inflammatory response. The ensuing ischemia results in overexpression of a number of growth factors, including not only VEGF but also insulin-like growth factor-1, angiopoietin-1 and -2, stromal-derived factor-1, fibroblast growth factor-2, and tumor necrosis factor (Grant et al 2004). Synergistically, these growth factors mediate angiogenesis, protease production, endothelial cell proliferation, migration, and tube formation. Tumor necrosis factor-α (TNF-α) and VEGF play a role in the early stages of angiogenesis, with TNF-α promoting leukocyte adhesion and VEGF promoting leukostasis, resulting in ischemia.

Blockade of all involved growth factors will likely be necessary to completely suppress the detrimental effects of ischemia, but even isolated blockade of VEGF may have beneficial effects on DME. VEGF increases vascular permeability by relaxing endothelial cell junctions, which increases permeability and leakage. Inhibition of VEGF blocks this effect to some extent, as demonstrated in several recent clinical trials and case series involving the anti-VEGF molecules pegaptanib, ranibizumab, and bevacizumab. Pegaptanib sodium (Macugen®, Eyetech Pharmaceuticals, Melville, NY/Pfizer, New York, NY) is an anti-VEGF aptamer, a small piece of RNA that self-folds into a shape that binds to and blocks the effects of VEGF165, one

isoform of the VEGF family of molecules. The drug is approved by the FDA for the treatment of age-related macular degeneration, and it has recently been studied in a phase II trial for DME. In that study, 172 subjects with DME were randomized to receive a series of 3 intravitreal injections of pegaptanib (at entry and every 6 weeks) in 1 of 3 doses, or a sham injection, and were followed for 36 weeks. Additional injections or photocoagulation were permitted every 6 weeks through the end of the study. A total of 52% of patients in the 0.3-mg and sham groups had baseline visual acuity of <58 letters; the remaining 48% had baseline visual acuity of ≥58 letters. At the 36-week mark, mean visual acuity had improved to 20/50 in the pegaptanib 0.3-mg group (the dose that was approved by the FDA) versus only 20/63 in the sham group (P = 0.04). Mean central retinal thickness decreased by 68 µm in the 0.3-mg group, whereas it increased by 4 µm in the sham group (P = 0.02). In addition, photocoagulation was required in 25% of the 0.3-mg group compared with 48% of the sham group (P = 0.04). The injections were well tolerated, with a single case of endophthalmitis reported (1/652 injections, 0.15%).

Ranibizumab (Lucentis™, Genentech, San Francisco, CA) is an antibody fragment that also binds and blocks the effects of VEGF. Unlike pegaptanib, ranibizumab binds and inhibits all isoforms of VEGF. Ranibizumab is also approved by the FDA for the treatment of age-related macular degeneration. A small, single-site, open-label trial was conducted in which 10 patients with DME were treated with a series of 3 monthly injections of 1 of 2 doses of ranibizumab (0.3 or 0.5 mg; the FDA approved the latter for macular degeneration) and then followed for 2 years. Recently published data from this study indicate that at 3 months, 4 patients gained 15 or more letters of vision, 5 patients gained 10 or more letters, and 8 patients gained at least 1 letter. Mean central retinal thickness was reduced by 45 µm in the 0.3-mg group and by 198 µm in the FDA-approved 0.5-mg group.

Bevacizumab (Avastin®, Genentech, San Francisco, CA) is the full antibody from which

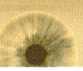

ranibizumab is derived. This anti-VEGF molecule is FDA approved for systemic treatment of metastatic colon cancer, but not for any ophthalmic indications. Its use in conditions such as age-related macular degeneration, diabetic retinopathy, and DME is currently off-label.

A small, retrospective review of 16 eyes of 15 patients with macular edema secondary to central retinal vein occlusion recently reported the short-term anatomic and visual acuity outcomes after treatment with intravitreal bevacizumab (Iturralde et al 2006). Subjects received at least one injection of bevacizumab 1.25 mg, with repeat injections at 1 month at the investigator's discretion, with a mean of 2.8 injections per eye. One month after the initial injection, mean central macular thickness measured by OCT decreased from 887 to 372 μm (P < 0.001). Mean visual acuity improved from the pretreatment baseline of 20/600 to 20/200 at 1 month (P = 0.001) and to 20/138 at 3 months (P < 0.001). In all, 14 of the 16 eyes demonstrated a halving of the visual angle, and no adverse events were noted. In a recent study, Moschos and Moschos (2008) showed that 3 months after the intravitreal use of bevacizumab, the electrical activity of the fovea and perifovea increased significantly. Anti-VEGF therapy for DME shows promise in preliminary studies. Larger studies are ongoing. VEGF inhibition may represent an important component of DME therapy in the future. Improvements in drug delivery will be necessary in order to avoid repeated intravitreal injections and the cumulative risk of endophthalmitis associated with this route of administration.

BIBLIOGRAPHY

1. Aiello LP, Pierce EA, Foley ED, et al. Suppression of retinal neovascularization in vivo by inhibition of vascular endothelial growth factor (VEGF) using soluble VEGF-receptor chimeric proteins. Proc Natl Acad Sci USA 1995; 92:10457–61.

2. Androudi S, Letko E, Meniconi M, et al. Safety and efficacy of intravitreal triamcinolone acetonide for uveitic macular edema. Ocul Immunol Inflamm 2005; 13:205–12.

3. Argon laser photocoagulation for macular edema in branch vein occlusion. The Branch Vein Occlusion Study Group. Am J Ophthalmol 1984; 98:271–82.

4. Bergman M, Laatikainen L. Cystoid macular edema after complicated cataract surgery and implantation of an anterior chamber lens. Acta Ophthalmol (Copenh) 1994; 72:178–80.

5. Bergman M, Laatikainen L. Cystoid macular edema after complicated cataract surgery and implantation of an anterior chamber lens. Acta Ophthalmol (Copenh) 1994; 72:178–80.

6. Bonnet S. Repercussions of cataract surgery on the development of cystoid macular edema in the diabetic patient. Bull Soc Belge Ophtalmol 1995; 256:127–9.

7. Bonnet S. Repercussions of cataract surgery on the development of cystoid macular edema in the diabetic patient. Bull Soc Belge Ophtalmol 1995; 256:127–9.

8. Burnett J, Tessler H, Isenberg S, et al. Double-masked trial of fenoprofen sodium: treatment of chronic aphakic cystoid macular edema. Ophthalmic Surg 1983; 14:150–2.

9. Chun DW, Heier JS, Topping TM, et al. A pilot study of multiple intravitreal injections of ranibizumab in patients with center-involving clinically significant diabetic macular edema. Ophthalmology 2006; 113:1706–12.

10. Cox SN, Hay E, Bird AC, et al. Treatment of chronic macular edema with acetazolamide. Arch Ophthalmol. 1988; 106:1190–5.

11. Cox SN, Hay E, Bird AC, et al. Treatment of chronic macular edema with acetazolamide. Arch Ophthalmol 1988; 106:1190–5.

12. Cunningham ET, Jr, Adamis AP, Altaweel M, et al. A phase II randomized double-masked trial of pegaptanib, an anti-vascular endothelial growth factor aptamer, for diabetic macular edema. Ophthalmology 2005; 112:1747–57.

13. Dowler JG, Sehmi KS, Hykin PG, et al. The natural history of macular edema after cataract surgery in diabetes. Ophthalmology 1999; 106:663–8.

14. Dowler JG, Sehmi KS, Hykin PG, et al. The natural history of macular edema after cataract surgery in diabetes. Ophthalmology 1999; 106:663–8.

15. Federman JL, Annesley WH, Jr, Sarin LK, et al. Vitrectomy and cystoid macular edema. Ophthalmology. 1980; 87:622.

16. Finkelstein D. Ischemic macular edema. Recognition and favourable natural history in branch vein occlusion. Arch Ophthalmol 1992; 110:1427–34.

17. Finkelstein D. Ischemic macular edema. Recognition and favourable natural history in

branch vein occlusion. Arch Ophthalmol 1992; 110:1427–34.

18. Flach AJ. Topical nonsteroidal anti-inflammatory drugs in ophthalmology. Int Ophthalmol Clin 2002; 42:1–11.

19. Flach AJ. Topical nonsteroidal anti-inflammatory drugs in ophthalmology. Int Ophthalmol Clin 2002; 42:1–11.

20. Fung WE. Vitrectomy for chronic aphakic cystoid macular edema. Results of a national, collaborative, prospective, randomized investigation. Ophthalmology 1985; 92:1102–11.

21. Guex-Crosier Y. The pathogenesis and clinical presentation of macular edema in inflammatory diseases. Doc Ophthalmol 1999; 97:297–309.

22. Guex-Crosier Y. The pathogenesis and clinical presentation of macular edema in inflammatory diseases. Doc Ophthalmol 1999; 97:297–309.

23. Henderly DE, Genstler AJ, Rao NA, et al. Pars planitis. Trans Ophthalmol Soc UK. 1986; 105(Pt 2):227–32.

24. Henderly DE, Genstler AJ, Rao NA, et al. Pars planitis. Trans Ophthalmol Soc UK 1986; 105(Pt 2):227–32.

25. Irvine AR. A newly defined vitreous syndrome following cataract surgery: interpreted according to recent concepts of the structure of the vitreous. Am J Ophthalmol 1953; 36:599–619.

26. Irvine AR. A newly defined vitreous syndrome following cataract surgery: interpreted according to recent concepts of the structure of the vitreous. Am J Ophthalmol 1953; 36:599–619.

27. Jaffe NS, Luscombe SM, Clayman HM, et al. A fluorescein angiographic study of cystoid macular edema. Am J Ophthalmol 1981; 92:775–7.

28. Jaffe NS, Luscombe SM, Clayman HM, et al. A fluorescein angiographic study of cystoid macular edema. Am J Ophthalmol 1981; 92:775–7.

29. Katzen LE, Fleischman JA, Trokel S, et al. YAG laser treatment of cystoid macular edema. Am J Ophthalmol 1983; 95:589–92.

30. Kylstra JA, Brown JC, Jaffe GJ, et al. The importance of fluorescein angiography in planning laser treatment of diabetic macular edema. Ophthalmology 1999; 106:2068–73.

31. Kylstra JA, Brown JC, Jaffe GJ, et al. The importance of fluorescein angiography in planning laser treatment of diabetic macular edema. Ophthalmology 1999; 106:2068–73.

32. Loewenstein A, Goldstein M. Intravitreal triamcinolone acetonide for diabetic macular edema. Isr Med Assoc J 2006; 8:426–7.

33. Loewenstein A, Goldstein M. Intravitreal triamcinolone acetonide for diabetic macula edema. Isr Med Assoc J 2006; 8:426–7.

34. Methods in optical coherence tomography studies of diabetic macular edema. Ophthalmology 2008; 115:1366–71.

35. Miyake Y, Miyake K, Shiroyama N, et al. Classification of aphakic cystoid macular edema with focal macular electroretinograms. Am J Ophthalmol 1993; 116:576–83.

36. Miyake Y, Miyake K, Shiroyama N, et al. Classification of aphakic cystoid macular edema with focal macular electroretinograms. Am J Ophthalmol 1993; 116:576–83.

37. Nasrallah FP, Jalkh AE, Van Coppenolle F, et al. The role of the vitreous in diabetic macular edema. Ophthalmol 1988; 95:1335–9.

38. Oshima Y, Emi K, Yamanishi S, et al. Quantitative assessment of macular thickness in normal subjects and patients with diabetic retinopathy by scanning retinal thickness analyzer. Br J Ophthalmol 1999; 83:54–61.

39. Oshima Y, Emi K, Yamanishi S, et al. Quantitative assessment of macular thickness in normal subjects and patients with diabetic retinopathy by scanning retinal thickness analyzer. Br J Ophthalmol 1999; 83:54–61.

40. Peterson M, Yoshizumi MO, Hepler R, et al. Topical indomethacin in the treatment of chronic cystoid macular edema. Graefes Arch Clin Exp Ophthalmol 1992; 230:401–5.

41. Peterson M, Yoshizumi MO, Hepler R, et al. Topical indomethacin in the treatment of chronic cystoid macular edema. Graefes Arch Clin Exp Ophthalmol 1992; 230:401–5.

42. Recchia FM, Ruby AJ, Carvalho-Recchia CA, et al. Pars plana vitrectomy with removal of the internal limiting membrane in the treatment of persistent diabetic macular edema. Am J Ophthalmol 2005; 139:447–54.

43. Wakefield D, Lloyd A. The role of cytokines in the pathogenesis of inflammatory eye disease. Cytokine 1992; 4:1–5.

44. Wakefield D, Lloyd A. The role of cytokines in the pathogenesis of inflammatory eye disease. Cytokine 1992; 4:1–5.

24.6 EPIRETINAL MEMBRANE

ETIOPATHOGENESIS

Gass proposed two mechanisms for the development of ERM.

- *The first mechanism* involves dehiscence in the inner limiting membrane (ILM) caused by vitreous separation from the macular surface, which allows retinal glial cells entry onto the retinal surface that then proliferate and contract.
- *A second proposed mechanism* of ERM formation involves contraction of vitreous cortical remnants and proliferation of hyalocytes on inner retinal surface after a PVD. The cortical remnants may act as a scaffold for cellular elements composing the membrane.

CLINICO-INVESTIGATIVE PROFILE

Various types of cells may gain access to the internal surface of the retina and proliferate to form fibrocellular tissue, which forms thin membrane sheets that cover the retinal surface. Numerous and overlapping terms have been used to describe such proliferative membranes: ERM, premacular membrane, preretinal macular fibrosis, surface wrinkling retinopathy, cellophane maculopathy and macular pucker. ERM can be secondary to many ocular conditions such as ocular inflammatory disease, retinal vascular disease, rhegmatogenous retinal detachment and accidental or surgical trauma, particularly after retinal cryotherapy or photocoagulation. ERM may also be idiopathic.

CLINICAL FEATURES

Patients associated with ERM may be asymptomatic in most cases. If retinal distortion occurs, patients may recognize variable degrees of vision loss, metamorphosia and micropsia. The clinical features vary, depending on the severity of the membrane, membrane thickness, membrane location and degree of contraction. In more advanced cases, distinct retinal findings can be seen, retinal striae radiating from the center of the ERM, retinal vessels straightened towards the membrane center, or tortuosity of retinal vessels (Fig. 24.6.1) and dilated retinal

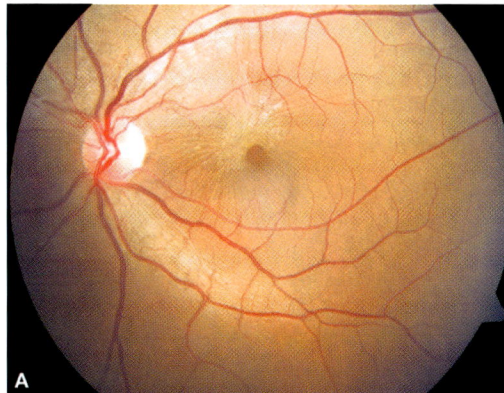

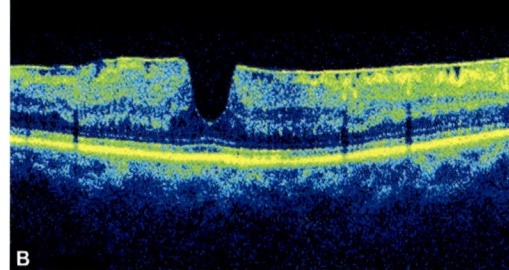

Fig. 24.6.1 *(A)* Showing retinal striae and psuedomacular hole; and *(B)* OCT of the same patient confirms the psuedomacular hole and ERM

veins. Pseudomacularholes or lamellar holes (Fig. 24.6.2) may also be associated with ERMs and may simulate full thickness macular holes.

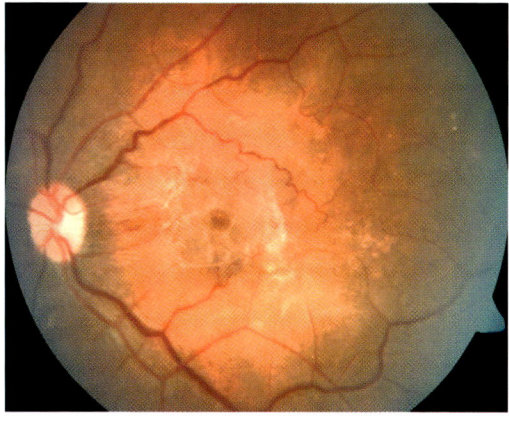

Fig. 24.6.2 *ERM with pseudomacular hole*

Slit lamp biomicroscopy with a contact lens evaluation

Slit lamp biomicroscopy with a contact lens evaluation has traditionally, been considered the best method for the evaluation of an ERM. It remains the most important diagnostic tool in such cases.

Fluorescein angiography

Fluorescein angiography is also a useful tool in the diagnosis of ERM. Anatomical features of retinal distortion may be better seen on FA. Fluorescein leakage and macular edema (Fig. 24.6.3) secondary to ERM induced traction-causing vascular leakage may also be assessed. FA may also help to distinguish between a full thickness macular hole and a pseudohole because transmitted fluorescence is not usually present in a pseudohole. Another important role of FA would be to detect the presence of other retinal pathologies, such as choroidal neo-vascular membranes.

Optical coherence tomography

Optical coherence tomography may be helpful in evaluating patients with ERM. OCT provides good visualization of the vitreoretinal interface and may show membrane over the retinal surface. It also helps in assessment of macular edema, cystoid changes (Fig. 24.6.4) if any, can also be assesed. It may also differentiate a pseudomacular hole (Fig. 24.6.5) from full thickness hole. OCT plays an important role in preoperative and postoperative evaluation of

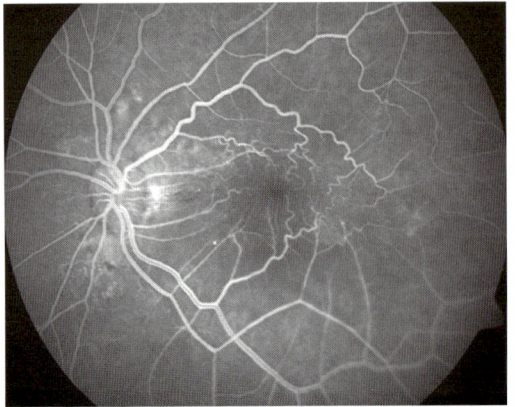

Fig. 24.6.3 *FFA showing vascular tortuosity with dye* leak in same patient as in Fig. 24.6.2

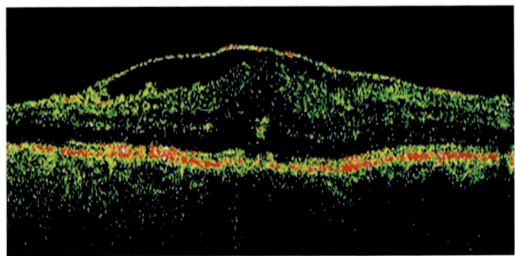

Fig. 24.6.4 *OCT: ERM with cystoid edema*

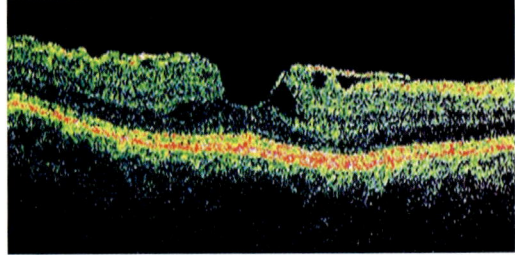

Fig. 24.6.5 *ERM with pseudomacular hole as seen on OCT*

surgery for ERMs by assessment of thickness and extent of the ERM on line scans.

CLASSIFICATION OF ERM

A commonly used method of classification of ERM proposed by Gass, is based on **severity of retinal distortion:**
- **Grade 0:** Cellophane maculopathy
- **Grade 1:** Crinkled cellophane maculopathy
- **Grade 2:** Macular pucker

Yet another classification is based on biomicroscopy findings.

FOOS classification based on histology and etiology is defined as given in Table 24.6.1.

MANAGEMENT

Most idiopathic ERMs remain stable both anatomically and visually over time. Surgical intervention with pars plana vitrectomy and epiretinal membrane peeling is indicated only if vision is markedly reduced and distortion is symptomatic. Favorable prognostic factors for visual improvement are good preoperative vision and short duration of symptoms preoperatively.

SURGICAL TECHNIQUE

The preferred vitrectomy technique is 23 or 25 age gauge trans-conjunctival sutureless

Type	Predominant histological features	Etiology	Mechanism	Biological mediators
Simple	ILM, laminocytes	PVD, laminocyte migration and activation	Surface tension on retina Disruption to the ILM	GNF, GFRα, RET1
Tissue repair	ILM, laminocytes, RPE cells, fibroblasts macrophages	Retinal tear, trauma, infection, and blunt injury	Cytokine-driven tissue rapair process	NF-xB pathway, TGF β, IL6, PDGF
Neovascular	Capillaries and acellular stromal tissue	PDR, radiotherapy, and vasoformative tumors	Hypoxia and neo-vasular cytokines	VEGF, HIFα ANG1

Table 24.6.1 *FOOS classification of ERM*

vitrectomy. After the placement of the infusion cannula using, the other two ports are also made 160-180 degrees apart.

• *A core vitrectomy* is performed, followed by posterior vitreous separation or PVD induction (triamcinolone assisted for optimum results). Following this , the membrane can be peeled off without any staining agent or stained with trypan blue dye (0.15%), brilliant blue G dye which stains the ILM and causus a negative staining effect for effective ERM peel can be also attempted. Using membrane peeling or ILM forceps (Fig. 24.6.6). After the ERM peeling the ILM is also peeled (Double peel) so as to prevent the recurrence of ERM formation.

• *Peripheral vitrectomy* is now completed under wide angle viewing system. Once complete the peripheral retina is inspected for any breaks. Air fluid exchange is done and for

short term tamponade either it is left under air or a 20% isoexpansile mixture of SF6 used. The cannulae are removed, and slight conjunctival massage is done at the minimal gauge opening site. Subconjunctival antibiotics are injected away from the sites of sclerotomies. The postoperative care includes a broad spectrum antibiotics, topical steroids for a short period and a cycloplegic.

VISUAL OUTCOMES

The usual visual outcome is gain of two or more lines of visual acuity.

Although visual acuity usually recovers within two months, metamorphopsia usually takes up to a year to resolve.

BIBLIOGRAPHY

1. Applah AP. Secondary causes of premacular fibrosis: Ophthalmology 1989; 96:389–92
2. Capone A Jr. Macular surface disorders. Focal points: Clinical modules for Ophthalmologists. San Francisco: American Academy of Ophthalmology 1996, module 4.
3. Jofnson MW.Tractional cystoid macular edema: a subtle variant of vitreomacular traction syndrome. Am J Ophthalmol 2005; 140:184–192
4. Johnson MW. Epiretinal membrane. In: Yanoof M, Duker J, Eds. Opthalmology, 2nd ed. St Louis: Mosby 2004; 947–950
5. Martinez et al. Differentiating macular holes from macular Pseudoholes. Am J ophthalmology 1994; 762–67
6. Wise GN. Clinical features of idiopathic pre-retinal macular fibrosis: Am J Ophthamol 1975; 79:349.

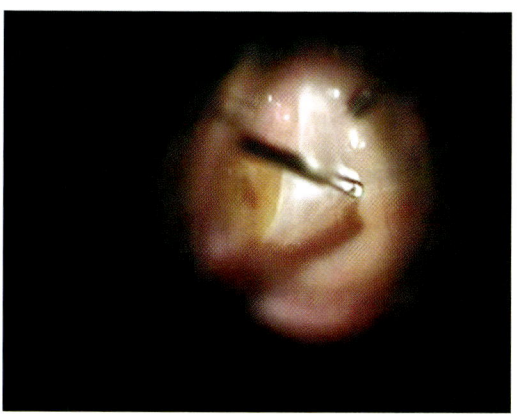

Fig. 24.6.6 *Epimacular membrane being peeled*

24.7 TOXIC MACULOPATHIES

Several medications and other exogenous substances can cause potential toxicity to the macula. Some of the main substances that can cause maculopathy include:
- Chloroquine maculopathy
- Quinine ocular toxicity
- Phenothiazines maculopathy
- Tamoxifen maculopathy
- Canthaxanthin maculopathy
- Talc maculopathy

CHLOROQUINE MACULOPATHY

Chloroquine (Nivaquine, Avlocor) and Hydroxychloroquine (Plaquenil) are used in treating malaria and rheumatological disorders (i.e. rheumatoid arthritis, lupus). Excess of 300 gm cumulative oral dose (250 mg/day for 3 years) significantly increases risk of maculopathy. Hydroxychloroquine has less maculopathy risk than chloroquine, and as such is typically the preferred medication to prescribe. Chloroquine associated ocular side effects can be divided to three categories; (1) accommodation abnormality, which is the most common; (2) corneal deposition, and (3) pre and true-retinopathy. The accommodation defect, corneal deposition, and pre-retinopathy are in general completely reversible with drug discontinuation. On the other hand, "Bull's eye maculopathy" is a major concern as it has irreversible damage.

Levels of chloroquine maculopathy from antimalarials are directly related to duration and dose are described as follows.
- *Premaculopathy:* Scotoma to red target between 4–9 degrees.
- *Established maculopathy:* 20/30 to 20/40 BCVA, faint halo of RPE pallor (Fig. 24.7.1A).
- *Bull's eye maculopathy:* 20/60 to 20/80 BCVA, dark ring surrounds halo (Fig. 24.7.1B).
- *Severe maculopathy:* 20/120 to 20/200 BCVA, pseudohole and atrophy.
- *End-stage:* Legally blind, large RPE atrophy, pigment clumps.

Antimalarials tend to concentrate in melanin-containing structures such as the RPE and choroid. Corneal deposits also can occur, but are relatively benign. The maculopathy, however, is potentially serious.

Pre-treatment baseline retinal evaluation is recommended, and should include:
- Visual acuities
- Amsler grid
- Color vision
- Visual fields (10–2, macular threshold)
- Dilated retinal examination
- Fundus photos
- Electroretinography

Post-treatment retinal evaluations utilizing the tests above should be performed minimum annually if no signs or symptoms are noted.

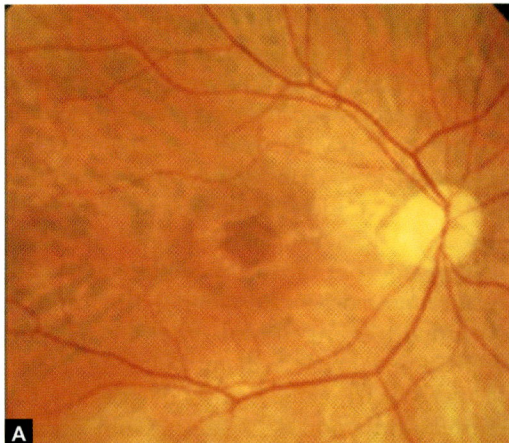

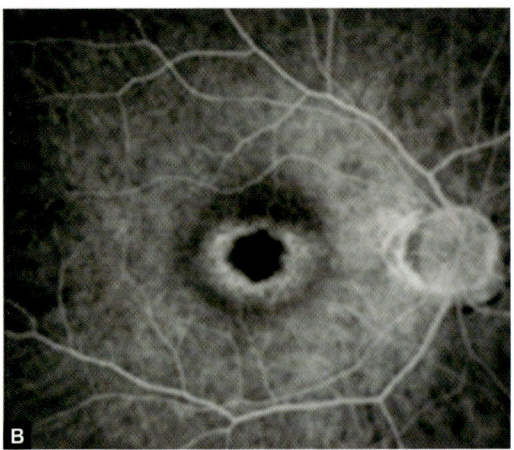

Fig. 24.7.1 *(A) Fundus photograph showing Bull's eye maculopathy; and (B) FFA picture of the same patient*

Home Amsler grids should be provided for daily monitoring of the central vision in each eye.

QUININE OCULAR TOXICITY

Quinine is an antimalarial alkaloid compound that also reduces nocturnal muscle cramps. An overdose of quinine may cause cinchonism, an ocular complex which has the following findings:
- Visual acuity loss (can also occur with normal dose)
- Fixed and dilated pupils
- Retinal edema (unknown mechanism)
- Attenuated arterioles
- Constricted visual fields
- Optic atrophy (Fig. 24.7.2)

PHENOTHIAZINE MACULOPATHY

Thioridazine (Melleril) and chlorpromazine (Largactil) are each used in treating schizophrenia and related psychoses. Chlorpromazine is also used as sedative. A normal dose of thioridazine is 150 to 600 mg/day, while chlorpromazine is 75 to 300 mg/day. Greater than 800 mg/day of thioridazine for a few weeks can cause retinotoxicity, while greater than 2400 mg/day chlorpromazine over many weeks can cause retinotoxicity. This retinopathy presents as pigment changes that create a 'salt and pepper' appearance to the macula (Fig. 24.7.3). Macular toxicity usually causes decreased visual acuities and poor dark adaptation. Coarse granular macular pigmentation usually appears first, which may not progress if cessation of the

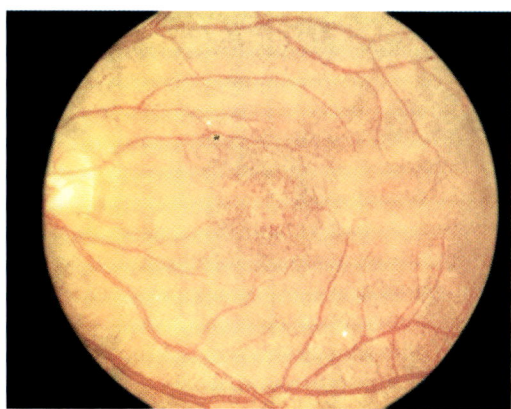

Fig. 24.7.3 *Salt and pepper maculopathy in phenothiazine toxicity*

drug occurs. Later, geographic RPE/choriocapillaris atrophy with hyperpigmented clumps and plaques may occur with continued drug use.

TAMOXIFEN MACULOPATHY

Tamoxifen (Nolvadex, Emblon, Noltam, Tamofen) is an anti-estrogen used to treat breast carcinoma. It has few systemic side-effects at a traditional normal dose of 20 to 40 mg/day. Current dosages prescribed today may be even less, reducing the prevalence of side-effects. Vortex keratopathy and optic neuritis can rarely occur, which usually is reversible on cessation of therapy. Retinotoxicity presents as multiple superficial yellow crystalline ring-like deposits at the macula, that can cause visual acuity loss (Fig. 24.7.4).

CANTHAXANTHIN MACULOPATHY

Canthaxanthin is an oral agent that enhances sun tanning. Prolonged use over time can cause maculopathy. This appears as tiny glistening yellow dots arranged in a donut-shaped ring around both maculae. These deposits appear in the superficial retina (ganglion cell layer), and generally benign (Fig. 24.7.5).

TALC MACULOPATHY

Talc maculopathy appears as multiple tiny, yellow-white, glistening particles scattered throughout posterior poles of both eyes

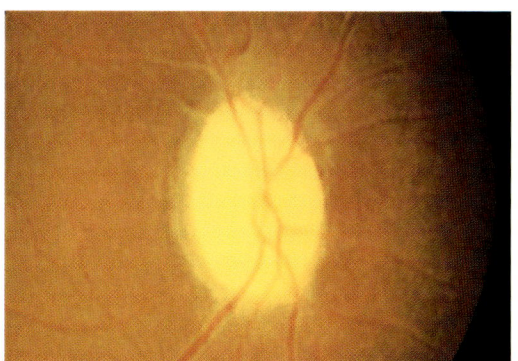

Fig. 24.7.2 *Quinine toxicity: Disc pallor with arteriolar attenuation*

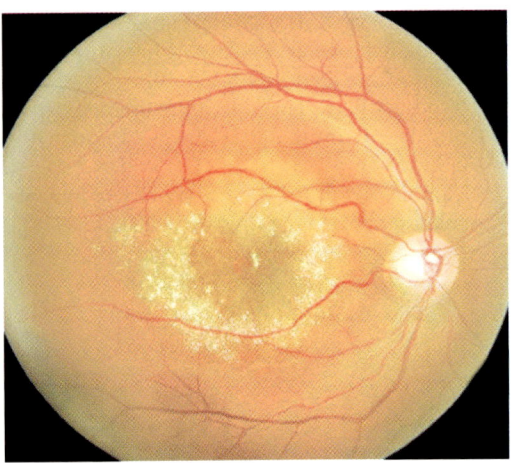

Fig. 24.7.4 *Crystalline retinopathy involving the peri-foveal region in tamoxifen toxicity*

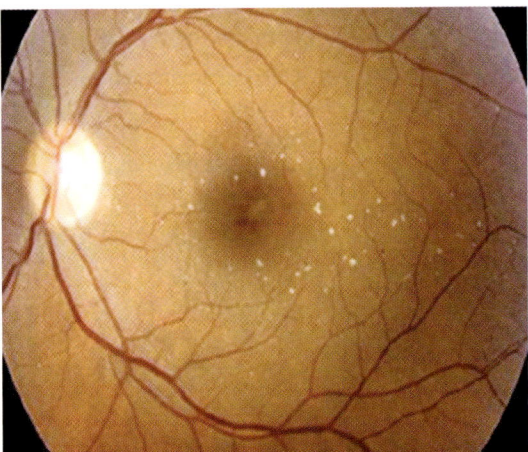

Fig. 24.7.6 *Talc maculopathy secondary to cocaine abuse*

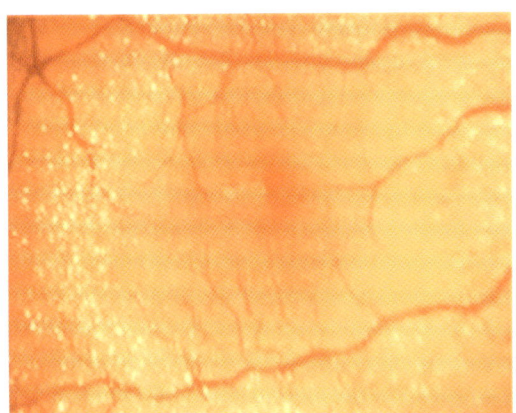

Fig. 24.7.5 *Crystalline deposits in canthaxanthine maculopathy*

(Fig. 24.7.6). The talc is more numerous in the capillary bed and small arterioles of perimacular area. Some patients can get macular edema, venous engorgement, punctate and flame hemorrhages, and arterial occlusion associated with the talc emboli. Talc retinal granulomas and neovascularization can also rarely occur.

Cases of associated paramacular scarring on certain patients who have injected cocaine or Ritalin over several years have been noted. Talc has a more destructive association with substance abuse. Drug abusers typically crush tablets of cocaine, methylphenidate (Ritalin) or other narcotic in water, boil the suspension, and filter it before injecting it. Injection is typically by intravenous, subcutaneous, and/or intramuscular routes of administration. Talc particles enter the circulation and embolize in various tissues. Most parts of bloodstream including the retina will be infused with the talc deposits over a long period of time of injections.

The extent of talc corresponds with amount and duration of drug abuse. It is routinely found if the person has injected the equivalent of over 12,000 tablets. Most patients have no visual symptoms, and the visual acuities are usually normal. However, blur and/or blind spots in visual fields can occur. 'Microtalc retinopathy' is a variant of talc retinopathy, involving finer deposits. This type of retinopathy may be associated with nerve fiber layer (NFL) defects and 'glaucoma-like' visual field loss.

Talc maculopathy observation usually involves careful questioning of the patient's medicinal and social drug history. Ocular talc indicates excess lung involvement, whereby lung function may be compromised. Drug abuse counseling and possibly a pulmonary consultation may be needed. Annual retinal evaluations with fundus photography and threshold VF testing are recommended. If there are glaucoma risk factors along with visual field loss, ocular hypotensive medications may be indicated.

BIBLIOGRAPHY

1. Fraunfelder FW. Corneal toxicity from ocular and systemic medications. Cornea 2006; 25:1133–8.
2. Fraser Bell S, Capon M. Talc Retinopathy. Clin Exp Ophthalmol 2002; 30:432–3.
3. Miriam M Rolf. Clinical implications of tamoxifen ocular toxicity. Clinical Eye and Vision Care 1998; 10(3):135–40.
4. Rynes RI, Bernstein HN. Ophthalmologic safety profile of antimalarial drugs. Lupus 1993; 2(Suppl 1): S17–9.
5. Yam JC, Kwok AK. Ocular toxicity of hydroxy-chloroquine. Hong Kong Med J 2006;12:294–304.

24.8 PHOTORETINITIS

INTRODUCTION

Photoretinitis or light induced photochemical damage to the retina may occur with or without the use of exogenous photosensitizers. An example of photochemical injury using exogenous photsensitizer is photosensitized Verteporfin which is used to sclerose CNV in Photodynamic therapy. Photochemical retinal damage that occurs without exogenous photosensitizers is also termed as photic retinopathy. The retinal phototoxicity depends on the duration, intensity and the spectrum of the light exposure.

PROTECTIVE MECHANISMS IN THE NORMAL EYE

Optical radiation includes visible light between 400 to 700 nm and ultraviolet (UV) radiation at lower wavelengths. The human cornea absorbs UV radiation below 300 nm protecting the retina from its harmful effects. The cornea is transparent between 300 and 400 nm but the crystalline lens protects the retina by absorbing most of this radiation. Shadowing by the eyebrow, corneal reflection of light rays that are not incident perpendicular to its surface (Fresnal's Law) and aversion, squint and blink responses are some of the other protective mechanisms against Photoretinitis. In addition, the human retina is rich in superoxide dismutase, glutathione, catalase, Vitamins E and C, lutein and zeaxanthin and macular xanthophylls, all of which protect the retina from photochemical damage by acting as free radical scavangers.

CLASSIFICATION OF PHOTIC RETINOPATHY

The UV-blue type of retinal phototoxicity is also termed Type 2 or Ham-type photic retinopathy. As the crystalline lens blocks the UV and shorter wavelength visible light, this type of photic retinopathy peaks at 440 nm, requires light exposures less than 12 hours and primarily affects the RPE. It is probably responsible for solar and operating microscope injuries.

The blue-green type of photic retinopathy is also termed white light, type 2 or Noell-type of photic retinopathy. It requires prolonged light exposures more than 12 hours, primarily affects the neural retina and RPE, and may be responsible for reduced blue color contrast vision in long time users of older argon-green photocoagulators.

Chief forms of photoretinitis in clinical practice include acute solar exposure, welder's maculopathy and operating microscope maculopathy.

Acute solar exposure

The retinal image of the sun at its zenith is about 160 µ in size, far smaller than the foveolar diameter of 350 µ. Most cases of solar maculopathy are due to retinal phototoxicity rather than retinal photocoagulation. This is because the threshold for retinal photocoagula-tion is a temperature rise of about 10°C which is more than the temperature rise of about 4°C observed with solar exposure at noon time with a 3 mm pupil. Solar eclipses are particularly dangerous because of possible pupil dilatation.

The typical lesion of solar retinopathy is a yellowish foveolar lesion which usually fades over a few weeks but may sometimes result in foveolar distortion or hole formation. Fluorescein angiography is usually normal; but may reveal a few RPE transmission defects in some cases. Visual acuity usually returns to the 20/20 to the 20/40 range over a 6 month period. The predilection for foveal involvement may be due to the Henle-layer facilitated fibre-optic transmission which may increase the foveal irradiance by channeling blue light photons from the perifoveal region to the fovea.

Partial solar eclipse, annular eclipse and partial phases of total eclipse are more dangerous than total phase of an eclipse. The safest and most inexpensive method of "sun-gazing" during an eclipse is the projection method in which the pin-hole or a similar small opening is used to cast the image of the sun on a screen placed half a meter or more away. Specially designed filters that have a layer of aluminium, chromium or silver deposited on their surface are also safe for solar viewing. Recently,

aluminium mylars which can be cut to adapt to any kind of viewing device have also become available. As developed color films pack silver, these are not safe for solar viewing.

Welder's maculopathy

Though photokeratitis is a common welding injury, welder's maculopathy is quite rare. It has the same ophthalmoscopic appearance and clinical course as solar retinopathy. Visible light from the welding arc in the spectrum of 400–440 nm may be sufficient to cause photic retinopathy. Moreover, crystalline lens transmittance in younger individuals is higher; thus a small fraction of UV-B radiation in the 300–310 nm window may also penetrate the cornea and lens to cause retinal damage.

Operating microscope maculopathy

Typical operating microscope injuries are oval shaped, 0.5 to 2 disc diameters in size, oriented parallel to the long filament of the microscope's bulb and more common in the inferior macula due to the microscope tilt and illumination positioning. Photosensitizing systemic medications such as chloroquine, benzodiazepines, allopurinol and furosemide as also systemic diseases like diabetes and hypertension increase the risk of injury. Theoretically, use of infra-red blocking filters reduces the thermal enhancement of retinopathy while the use of blue-blocking filters may reduce the risk of acute retinal phototoxicity; however, some blue light may be useful for tissue visualization during surgery.

BIBLIOGRAPHY

1. Boettner EA, Walter JR. Transmission of the ocular media. Invest Ophthalmol 1962; 1:304–10.
2. Boulton M, Rozanowska M, Rozanowski B. J Photochem Photobiol B 2001; 64:144–61.
3. Broad RD, Olsen KF, Ball SF, et al. The site of operating microscope light-induced injury on human retina. Am J Ophthalmol 1989; 107: 390–7.
4. Feeney L, Berman ER. Oxygen toxicity: damage by free radicals. Invest Ophthalmol 1976; 15: 789–92.
5. Gass JDM. Stereoscopic Atlas of macular diseases, 3rd ed. St. Louis: Mosby-Year book; 1987.
6. Ham WT, Muller HA, Ruffolo LL Jr, et al. Basic mechanisms underlying the production of photochemical lesions in mammalian retina. Curr Eye Res 1984; 3:165–74.
7. Ham WT, Muller HA, Sliney DH. Retinal sensitivity to damage from short wavelength light. Nature 1976; 260:153–5.
8. Keates RH, Armstrong PF. Use of short wavelength filter in an operating microscope Ophthalm Surg 1985; 16:40–41.
9. Kirshfeld K. Carotenoid pigments: their possible role in protecting against photoxidation in eyes and photoreceptor cells. Proc R Soc Lond B Biol Sci 1982; 216:71–85.
10. Li S, Lam TT, Fu J et al. Systemic hypertension exaggerates retinal photic injury. Arch Ophthalmol 1985; 103:28-30.
11. Macfaul PA. Visual prognosis after solar retinopathy. Br J Ophthalmol 1969; 53:534–51.
12. Mainster MA. Henle fibers may direct light towards the center of the fovea. Lasers Light Ophthalmol 1988; 2:79–86.
13. Manzouri B, Egan CA, Hykin PG. Phototoxic maculopathy following uneventful cataract surgery in predisposed patient. Br J Ophthalmol 2002; 86:705–6.
14. Mellerio J. Light effects on the retina. In: Albert DM, Jakobeic FA, Eds. Principles and practice of Ophthalmology. Philadelphia: WB Saunders 1994; 1326–45.
15. Michels M, Sternberg P Jr. Operating microscope-induced retinal phototoxicity: pathophysiology, clinical manifestations and prevention. Surv Ophthalmol 1990; 34:237–52.
16. NASA RP 1383 Eye safety during solar eclipses
17. Sliney DH, Wolbarsht ML. Safety with lasers and other optical sources: a comprehensive handbook. New York: Plenum Press; 1980:1035.
18. Sliney DH. Defining biologic exposures to light. In: Cronly-Dillon J, Rosen ES, Marshal J, Eds. Hazards of light. New York: Pergamon Press; 1986.
19. Sliney DH. Eye protective techniques for bright light. Ophthalmology 1983; 90:937–44.
20. Stampr DA, Lund DA, Molchany JW, et al. Human pupil and eyelid response to intense laser light: implications for protection. Percept Motor Skills 2002; 95:775–82.

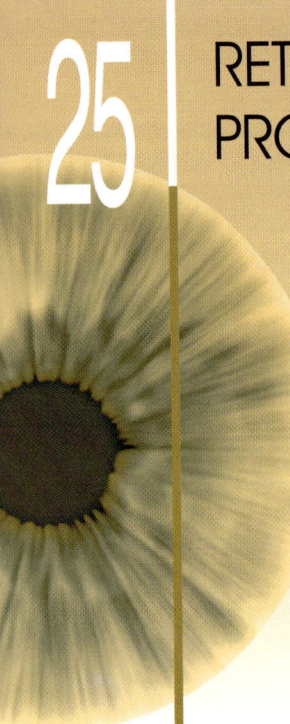

25

RETINAL DETACHMENT AND PROLIFERATIVE VITREORETINOPATHY

Sunandan Sood, Rajiv Gupta and Parul Chawla

GENERAL CONSIDERATIONS

The term retinal detachment (RD) is a misnomer since it is not the retina which detaches from choroid but it is the separation of neurosensory retina from retinal pigment epithelium (RPE). However, the old term die hard therefore this separation continues to be called as retinal detachment. There is an embryological fact behind this vulnerability of retinal separation since a potential space exist between the neurosensory retina and retinal pigment epithelium (RPE) embryologically as these two layers develop from the invaginated optic vesicle. Despite the existence of potential space between two layers, it is hard to separate them in normal circumstances. There are certain anatomical and physiological factors which lend to bind the two layers together.

FACTORS FOR NORMAL RETINAL ADHESION

1. Fluid is driven passively from vitreous to choroid by both intraocular pressure (IOP) and the osmotic pressure of the extracellular fluid in the choroid and the latter is less than IOP. This outward movement of fluid acts to push the retina against RPE.

2. The locaction of Na^+K^+ ATPase mediated metabolic pump of the RPE which actively pump fluid from subretinal space to choroid at a very high rate thus keeping the subretinal space dry.

3. Formed vitreous supports the retina from inside. It is known to plug the break and thus

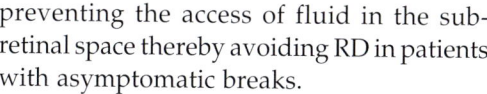

preventing the access of fluid in the sub-retinal space thereby avoiding RD in patients with asymptomatic breaks.

4. Intact retina without any break is as important as the abovesaid formed vitreous in safeguarding against detachment. Infact formation of break in the retina is a precursor for RD.

5. Although anatomic bridges do not exist between retina and RPE but the current evidence indicates that the matrix material between the two layers serves as a "glue" in the adhesive process. In addition interdigitations of photoreceptor outer segments and RPE microvilli probably also serves to hold the two issues together.

CLASSIFICATION

Depending upon the underlying pathological mechanism retinal detachment has been classified as under:
- Rhegmatogenous retinal detachment
- Tractional retinal detachment
- Exudative retinal detachment

1. *Rhegmatogenous retinal detachment.* Rhegma means break and in rhegmatogenous RD which occurs as a result of full thickness retinal break, liquefied vitreous after passing through the retinal break enters the potential subretinal space, thereby dissecting the retina into two layers, i.e. neurosensory retina and RPE thus causing retinal detachment. It is the most common type of RD seen in 90% of cases.

2. *Tractional retinal detachment* is next common and as the name suggest it is caused by vitreo-retinal fibroproliferative membranes that mechanically pull the retina away from RPE. In some cases the progressive traction may tear the retina resulting in combined tractional and rhegmatogenous detachment. This type of RD is characteristically seen in proliferative diabetic retinopathy.

3. *Exudative retinal detachment* is caused by retinal or choroidal conditions that disturbs RPE or outer retinal barrier such as tumor or inflammation resulting in accumulation of fluid in the subretinal space without traction or full-thickness retinal breaks. A pathognomic finding associated with this detachment is the presence of shifting fluid which leads to variation in the location of RD as the patient is examined in different postures.

RHEGMATOGENOUS RETINAL DETACHMENT

As already mentioned it is the most common type of RD and arises from one or more full thickness retinal breaks. In retinal detachment the normal forces maintain the neurosensory retinal attachment to the RPE as discussed above are overwhelmed by the opposing forces causing RD.

The opposing forces causing RD are: (1) the existence of liquefied vitreous gel; (2) the tractional forces that can precipitate a retinal break; (3) the presence of a retinal break that will allow the passage of liquefied vitreous into the subretinal space. All the factors need to be present to cause rhegmatogenous RD. In the absence of any of the factors, it is unlikely that retina will detach, i.e. if hole is there in the absence of liquefied vitreous or tractional forces, the RD will not occur. This is also the reason of finding asymptomatic breaks in 5 to 10% of the population without any apparent detachment.

PATHOGENESIS

- Changes in vitreous
- Peripheral retinal degeneration predisposed to retinal detachment.
- Developmental variations predisposed to retinal detachment
- High risk factors of retinal detachment.

1. Changes in vitreous

In adulthood the formed vitreous is in gel form. It consists of collagen fibrillar network intertwined with the molecules of hyaluronic acid. With age there occurs fragmentation of collagen fibers and leaking of hyaluronic acid leading to liquefaction of vitreous (synchisis) and collapse of fibrillar frame work of vitreous gel (syneresis). Initially there are small pockets of liquefied vitreous which coalesce to form larger pockets. This is followed by a defect in the dense posterior cortical vitreous through which liquefied vitreous pass into subhyaloid space leading to the separation of posterior

hyaloid from the internal limiting membrane producing a true posterior vitreous detachment (PVD). PVD is found in 27% of patients aged 60–69 years and in 63% of patients after 70 years. The factors leading to early PVD are pathological myopia, trauma, inflammation and cataract extraction.

PVD can be diagnosed by 90D slit lamp examination by finding a circular weiss ring which is the attachment of vitreous on optic nerve head. In 90% of cases the PVD is eventless, however, in the rest it might be complicated. In the process of separation if abnormal vitreo-retinal adhesions are encountered as in lattice/snail track degeneration it may lead to tractional horse shoe shaped break formation with convexity towards disc. In case retinal vessels is also involved in the process of PVD, break formation may be associated with vitreous hemorrhage. Thus a patient nearing 60 years presenting with rapid onset of floaters and flashes (photopsiae) warrants 90D slit lamp and indirect ophthalmoscopic examination after dilating pupil in order to arrive at the diagnosis of PVD and to rule out retinal break formation (Figs 25.1 and 25.2).

2. Peripheral retinal degeneration predisposed to retinal detachment

There are number of peripheral retinal degenerations some of them are predisposed and other are not predisposed to retinal detachment. The ones which are not predisposing to RD are peripheral cystoid degeneration, pavingstone

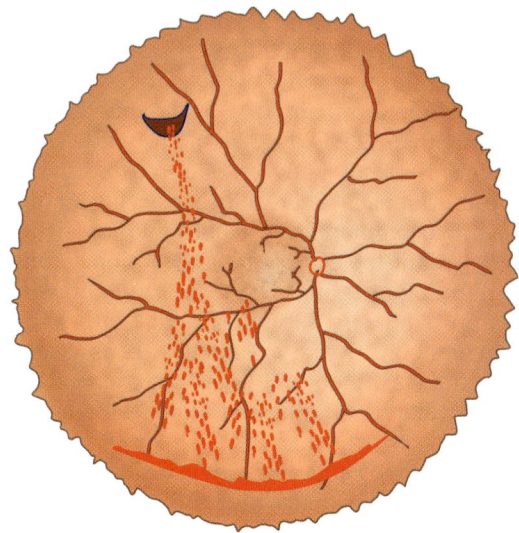

Fig. 25.2 *Diagrammatic representation of PVD, retinal break formation and vitreous hemorrhage*

degeneration and pigmentary degeneration of retina. The peripheral degeneration which are predisposed to RD are:
• Lattice degeneration
• Snail tract degeneration
• Retinoschisis
• White without pressure and white with pressure.

i. Lattice degeneration

It is most commonly recognized vitreoretinal abnormality of the peripheral fundus known to predispose to rehegmatogenous retinal detachment. Approximately 30–40% of patients with retinal detachment have lattice degeneration. It is otherwise seen in 7–8% of general population. The condition is bilateral in 42 to 45% of cases with no sex and racial predilection. Patients with lattice degeneration have myopia more frequently than the general population. It is more commonly located in the temporal than the nasal fundus and superiorly rather than inferiorly.

Lattice lesions are sharply outlined, round or oval mostly circumferentially but may be radially oriented, commonly located between equator and the posterior border of the vitreous base. Characteristic feature is an arborsing network of white lines which represent occluded or sheathed retinal blood vessels and

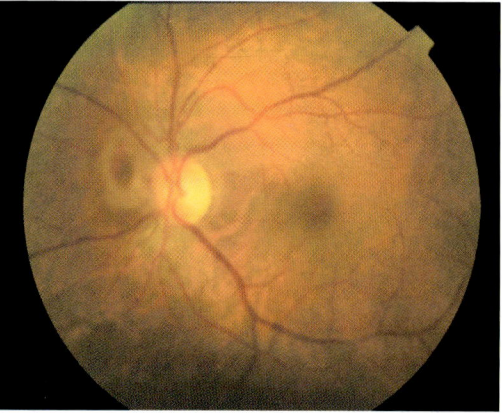

Fig. 25.1 *Weiss ring strongly suggestive of PVD*

these lines are seen in 17% of patients. The term lattice is derived from the interlacing pattern of these white lines only. The patches vary in length from a fraction of a disc diameter (DD) to more than 12 DD (Fig. 25.3). The width of the patches is mostly between one-fourth of DD to two-thirds of DD. There may be varying amount of retinal pigmentation, yellow-white surface flecks, reddish patches within the lesion because of thinning of retina. The former two are seen in approximately 80% of patients with lattice degeneration. The lattice patches are associated with liquefaction of overlying vitreous gel and firm vitreoretinal adhesion along the edges of the lesion which can be visualized by indirect ophthalmoscoy and scleral depression. Vitreous traction on these areas after PVD often leads to retinal break formation along the posterior edge of the lesions resulting into RD which is typically seen in high myopes of more than 50 years. In addition round atrophic holes are seen in lattice patches in about 16–18% of patients with lattice degeneration. Most of the round holes are solitary, although multiple holes may be present with in a lattice lesion.

ii. Snail track degeneration

It is a variation of lattice degeneration in which there are sharply demarcated shiny wet looking bands which are due to multiple tiny, yellowish-white flecks that appear to lie on the inner surface of retina giving the peripheral retina a white frost like appearance. These flecks have been observed in up to 80% of snail track lesions although extent varies considerably. These lesions are usually longer than lattice with or without overlying vitreous liquefaction or vitreoretinal adhesion, thus tractional breaks seldom occur however, atrophic round holes within the snail track may be present (Fig. 25.4).

iii. Degenerative retinoschisis

It is splitting (schisis) of neurosensory retina. It is of two types:
- Typical retinoschisis
- Reticular retinoschisis

In typical retinoschisis which is more common of the two the splitting occurs at the level of outer plexiform layer whereas in reticular type it occurs at the level of nerve fiber layer. The typical retinoschisis is the extension of the process of peripheral cystoid degeneration towards the posterior pole. It is found in 4–22% of the normal population older than 40 years. Men and women are equally affected and it frequently involves both eyes.

Inferotemporal quadrant (82%) is most commonly involved followed by supero-temporal (72%) and thereafter both nasal quadrants (32%) which are equally affected. In the early stage retinoschisis is seen as flat smooth, retinal elevation which is best appreciated by binocular indirect ophthalmo-scope when it is viewed tangentialy using scleral depression. The elevated inner layer of retinoschisis always contain blood vessels, some of which may appear white in periphery as if occluded. The inner layer is interspersed with small, shiny yellow-white dots resembling snow

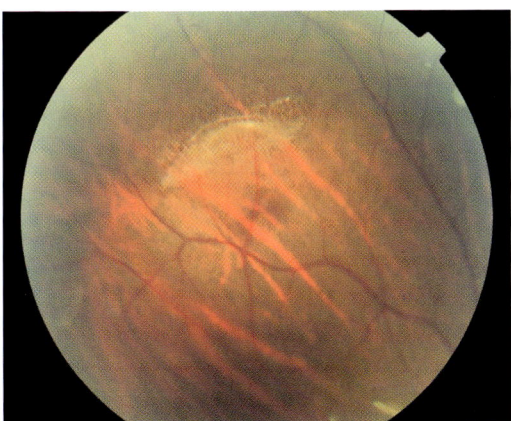

Fig. 25.3 *Patch of lattice degeneration*

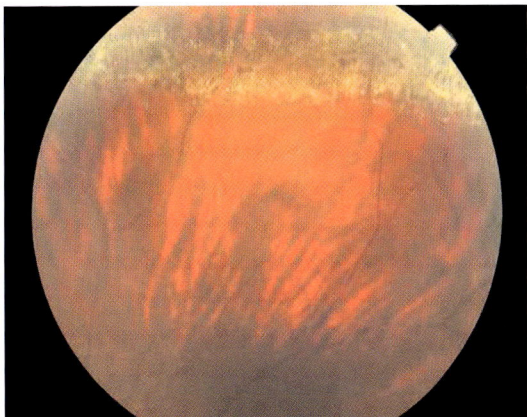

Fig. 25.4 *Patch of snail track degeneration*

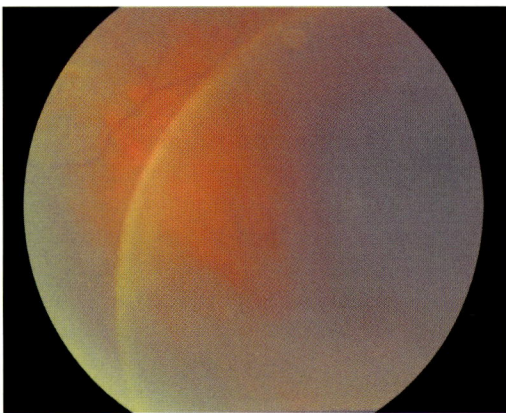

Fig. 25.5 *Flat, smooth retinal elevation suggestive of retinoschisis*

flakes which are the remanants of the foot steps of the pillars of the Müller cells (Fig. 25.5).

Retinoschisis in most cases remain stationary however in some cases it may progress posteriorly circumferentially and towards the vitreous cavity thereby increasing in height. In advanced stage the retinoschisis appears as large, fixed, almost transparent dome shaped elevation. The surface of the dome is smooth and does not undulate. The outer layer of retinoschisis often has multiple reddish round spots which resemble clusters of fish or frog eggs the same is demonstrated by white with pressure sign on indirect ophthalmoscopy with scleral depression. The breaks are found in both the layers, the outer layer breaks tend to be single and larger whereas those in inner layer are less frequent and small.

Retinal detachment develops occasionally as a complication in patients with breaks in both the layers. Inner layer breaks alone do not cause retinal detachment, however, a break or breaks in the outer layer alone or in both layers may lead to retinal detachment. It is important to differentiate retinoschisis from retinal detachment. The possible features which may differentiate the two are given in Table 25.1. The reticular retinoschisis is discussed at p-348.

iv. White without pressure and white with pressure

It refers to geographic areas of relative whiteness of peripheral retina when seen by indirect ophthalmoscopy without scleral depression. Earlier the same features when seen with scleral depression used to be called white with pressure. However, keeping blanching of choroids by indentation and possibility of optical phenomenon in mind, it is very difficult to diagnose white with pressure. Hence, it is no longer considered significant clinical sign and white without pressure (WWP) remains to be an important peripheral retinal degeneration predisposed to retinal detachment.

White without pressure areas are circumferentially oriented. The posterior boundaries are scalloped irregular and sharply defined rarely extending beyond equator where as anterior limits are less precise (Fig. 25.6). There may be small island of normal colored retina in white area which may be mistaken for retinal break. It is more frequently seen in temporal quadrants particularly in inferotemporal quadrant. It is present in about 30% of otherwise normal eyes and is bilateral in approximately 20% patients. It is about 10 times more common in blacks than white. Patients younger than 40 years and in myopic eyes WWP is observed more frequently. The presence of WWP does not

Features	Retinal detachment	Retinoschisis
1. Clinically	Undualating folds	Dome shaped elevated, smooth
2. Mobility	Mobile	Fixed
3. Transparency	Translucent	Transparent
4. Extent	From ora to disc	From ora to equator usually
5. Break	Must	May or may not be there
6. Reaction to photocoagulation	Absent	Whitening, usually present
7. Field defect	Sloping border	Sharp border
8. USG with scleral depression	Becomes shallow	No change

Table 25.1 *Difference between retinal detachment and retinoschisis*

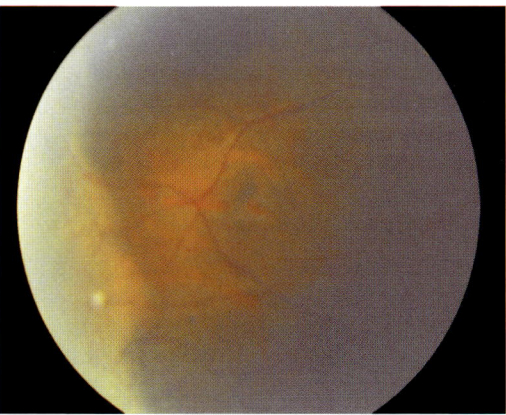

Fig. 25.6 *Circumferentially oriented whitish patch with scalloped posterior border suggestive of white without pressure*

appear to predispose to retinal detachment with possible exception of giant retinal tear (GRT) where in the fellow eye the significance has been attached to its presence since WWP is noted in 40% of fellow eyes of cases of GRT (Fig. 25.7). Hence, prophylactic 360° barrage laser has been recommended in the fellow eye with WWP.

3. Developmental variations predisposing to retinal detachment

These include:
• Enclosed oral bays
• Meridional folds and complexes

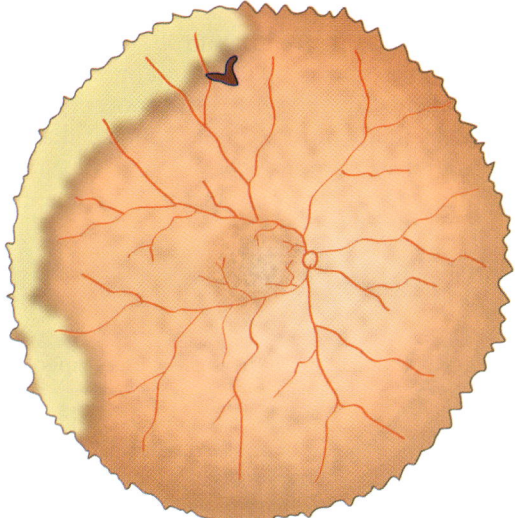

Fig. 25.7 *HST along the posterior border of WWP in the fellow eye of a patient of GRT*

• Cystic retinal tufts
• Zonular traction tufts.

i. Enclosed oral bays

These result from coalescence of adjacent denatate processes to form a ring. These were found in 3% of eyes in large autopsy series. These are seen in nasal meridian where dentate processes are more prominent (Fig. 25.8).

These are of clinical importance since they can mimic retinal holes and because they are associated with the development of retinal breaks.

The appearance of enclosed oral bays differ from retinal breaks in two aspects. These are brown in color rather than red and the surface with in the lesion is granular instead of smooth. The relationship between enclosed oral bays and retinal breaks have been reported to be 17% and the break is posterior to the enclosed oral bay. All these breaks are associated with PVD.

The retinal breaks occur probably due to the local posterior extension of the vitreous base in the area of enclosed oral bays which causes focal traction behind the enclosed oral bays in the process of vitreous detachment, thus causing break.

ii. Meridional folds and complexes

Meridional folds and complexes are common developmental variations at the ora and are found in 20% and 12% of eyes respectively.

Meridional folds are oblong radially oriented areas of thickened retinal tissue. 80% of meridional folds arise from denate process. In fact they are prominent dentate processes only

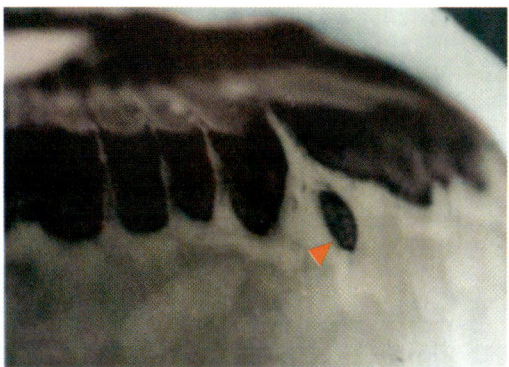

Fig. 25.8 *Enclosed oral bays*

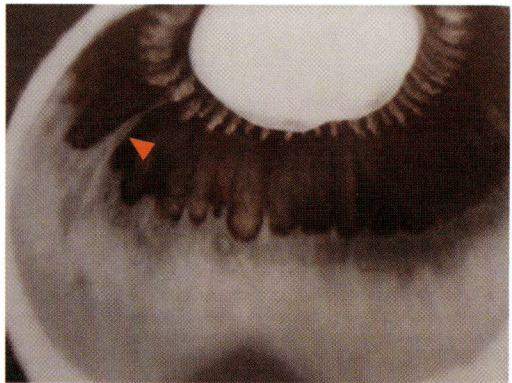

Fig. 25.9 *Meridional complex*

and are usually located in the superonasal quadrant (Fig. 25.9).

When a prominent dentate process (meridional fold) align with a cilliary process afront in the same meridian, it is called as meridional complex and are again located superonasally.

The importance of meridional folds and complexes as precursors of RD has not been confirmed. However, if RD occurs in an eye with meridional folds, retinal break may be located at the posterior end of these lesions.

iii. Cystic retinal tufts

They are noduar projections of retinal tissue that are typically surrounded by cystic retinal degeneration.

On indirect ophthalmoscopy they appear as a discrete, sharply circumscribed opaque white lesions frequently with pigment alteration at their bases and vitreous may be attached to their surface (Fig. 25.10).

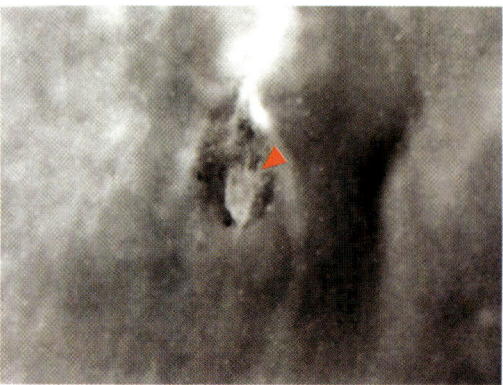

Fig. 25.10 *Cystic retinal tuft*

These occur in 5% adults and are unilateral in 95%. 80% of these tufts occur in the equatorial region and are usually not present with in the vitreous base.

These are commonly associated with retinal breaks which may be flap tears, horse shoe tears or breaks with operculum. In a clinical study of 200 consecutive primary retinal detachment cystic retinal tufts were associated with pathogenically important break in 6.5% eyes. However, 7 to 10% of RDs are said to be because of breaks related to cystic retinal tufts.

iv. Zonular-traction tufts

These are anterior projections of the retina attached to one or more thickened zonular fibers. They are usually single and unilateral, located within the vitreous base in the nasal quadrant. They differ from other tufts by their large size, anterior angulation and closed proximity to ora serrata.

Although zonular-traction tufts are important cause of small flap tears but these are insignificant because they lie within the vitreous base and hardly ever responsible for retinal detachment, however, sometimes these are regarded as important in the production of aphakic retinal detachment.

4. High risk factors of retinal detachment
- Myopia
- Cataract extraction
- Trauma
- Family history of retinal detachment
- Retinal detachment in the other eye.

i. Myopia

A strong statistical relation has been established between axial myopia and rhegmetogenous RD and more than 35% of all rhegmetogenous retinal detachments occur in myopic eyes. The incidence of retinal detachment is directly related to degree of myopia. The lifetime incidence of retinal detachment among myopic patients is said to be 0.7 to 6% compared to the incidence of 0.06% in emetropic patients. It is because of early liquefaction of vitreous leading to PVD and association of myopia with lattice degeneration and snail track degeneration.

ii. Cataract extraction

It is a major risk factor of retinal detachment since more than 40% of retinal detachment occur in aphakic and pseudophakic eyes. The incidence of retinal detachment is 2–5% after ICCE, 0–3.6% after ECCE and 0.8 to 2% after phacoemulsification. The incidence may rise to 20% in patients with vitreous loss and posterior capsular rent. YAG capsulotomy also leads to three-fold increase in the incidence of retinal detachment. It is all because of vitreous disturbaneces, i.e. leakage of hyaluronic acid and precipitation of synchisis and syneresis of vitreous leading to PVD and formation of break in the retina thereby causing retinal detachment.

iii. Trauma

In children and in young adults closed globe injury is a leading cause of retinal detachment and studies have shown that up to third of retinal detachments may be attributed to trauma. Retinal dialysis is the most common type of break found (75%) in traumatic retinal detachments which is frequently located superonasally as a countercoup lesion with direct force of blunt trauma coming from inferotemporal quadrant. Detachment after penetrating injuries are usually characterized by the presence of transvitreal fibroproliferative membranes.

iv. Family History

The two most common hereditary ocular conditions associated with retinal detachment are axial myopia and lattice degeneration. The importance of these two conditions have been discussed earlier and these are present in both familial and non-familial cases of retinal detachment. The inheritance of myopia is uncertain, however, it is usually autosomal dominant in lattice degeneration. In addition the most important distinctive familial vitreoretinal condition associated with retinal detachment is Stickler's vitreoretinal dystrophy. The main features are that the vitreous cavity is optically empty, patches of lattice degeneration, high myopia and progressive cataract at young age. Other noticeable hereditary systemic disorders associated with retinal detachment include Marfan's syndrome and homocystinemia. Lastly bilateral infertemporal dialyses at a younger age without any history of trauma and associated retinal detachment is also seen in certain familial cases. Thus the family history is very important in patients of retinal detachment particularly in younger age group.

v. Retinal detachment in the other eye

It is a well known fact that in case one eye has suffered from retinal detachment then the chances of development of retinal detachment in the other eye is 8–10%. Therefore, it is important to examine the other eye by indirect ophthalmoscopy so that prophylactic laser application is carried out to seal the breaks if any in order to prevent retinal detachment.

PERIPHERAL RETINAL DEGENERATIONS NOT PREDISPOSED TO RD

1. Peripheral cystoid degeneration
2. Paving stone degeneration
3. Pigmentary degeneration of retina

1. PERIPHERAL CYSTOID DEGENERATION

The pathogenesis of peripheral cystoid degeneration is unknown. It occurs in the outer plexiform layer of neurosensory retina which is the junction of the dual blood supply of retina. However, it is suggested that degenerative retinoschisis is preceded by peripheral cystoid degeneration. It is said to be of two types:

• Typical
• Reticular

Clinical Features

Typical peripheral cystoid degeneration

It is said to be present in all patients 8 years or older and both the sexes are equally affected. Cystoid degeneration begins at ora serrata and the extent and severity is known to progress both circumferentially and posteriorly with increasing age, however, it is symmetrical in the two eyes. Initially microcysts form and these coalesce to form macrocysts around 0.15 mm in diameter. These areas of involvement increase in size and later the cystoid degeneration has a circumferential band like distribution around the eye which tend to be more extensive temporally than nasally and superiorly than inferiorly (Fig. 25.11).

Ophthalmoscopically typical peripheral cystoid degeneration has characteristic stippled pattern and honeycomb appearance close to ora serrata. The affected retina is 1½ to 3 times thicker than the normal adjacent retina.

It is not associated with any pathologic lesions or anatomic variation other than retinoschisis. It is not predisposed to RD.

Reticular peripheral cystoid degeneration

It is less common and in one series was found in 18% patients and was bilateral in about 40% patients. The age and sex distribution is the same as in typical form.

The development of small spaces microscopically occur at the level of nerve fiber layer with the loss of ganglion cells and these are bounded by inner plexiform layer and internal limiting membrane (ILM).

Ophthalmoscopically it is characterised by a prominent linear or reticular pattern corresponding to the pattern of retinal vessels. The involved areas have fine stippled appearance and angular borders and are often demarcated posteriorly by retinal blood vessels. The second characteristic is gray appearance deep to the retinal vessels, which partly obscures RPE. However, it is mostly difficult to clinically differentiate between reticular and typical form of peripheral cystoid degeneration.

2. PAVING STONE DEGENERATION

It occurs at the level of RPE and was first described by Donders in 1855. It was also known as cobble stone degeneration but Mayer-Schwickerath in 1960 introduced the term

paving stone which is preferred to cobble stone since the later are elevated.

The incidence of paving stone degeneration is about 17 to 20% and is bilateral in about 40%. Once bilateral it is symmetrical in two eyes.

It has the tendency for increased prevalence in patients above 40 years and in one study 35% of patients above 80 years exhibited these changes.

Paving stone degeneration has predilection for eyes with long axial length. Thus bilateral paving stone degeneration was reported in 57% of myopic patients.

Choroidal vascular insufficiency is believed to be responsible for the development of paving stone degeneration because retinal changes in histopathological examination are limited to the area supplied by choriocapillaris. It leads to loss of RPE and outer retinal layers. There is no change in the vitreous gel overlying areas of paving stone degeneration.

Ophthalmoscopically it has a typical appearance with areas of apparent loss of the RPE. The lesions are located in the periphery and are pale, flat and sharply demarcated. The lesions are separated from ora by a band of intact RPE. The visible large vessels of the choroid are normal in appearance. The small lesions are circular while the large lesions have scalloped margins probably due to confluence of smaller lesions and the margins have increased pigmentation (Fig. 25.12).

It is not predisposed to the development of RD or primary retinal breaks.

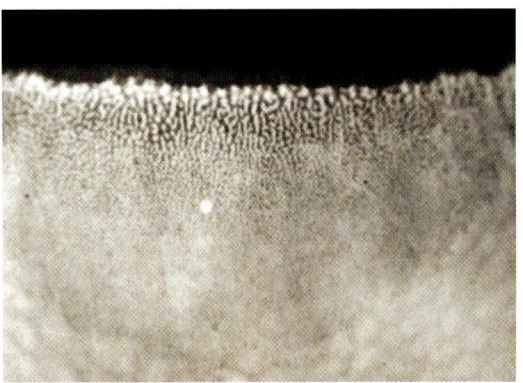

Fig. 25.11 *Peripheral cystoid degeneration*

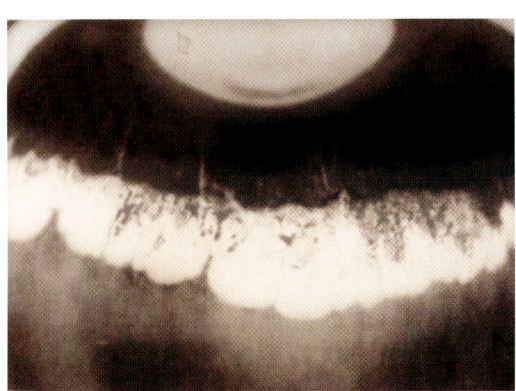

Fig. 25.12 *Paving stone degeneration*

3. PIGMENTARY DEGENERATION OF RETINA

Pigmentary degeneration of retina is characterized by variations in amount of pigmentation in the middle and far periphery of retina. This may vary from a diffuse dark appearance to discrete focal areas of clumping of the peripheral retina. The posterior margin of abnormal pigmentary zone may extend several disc diameters posterior to equator and is usually relatively indistinct.

It is strongly age related and related to axial length of the eyeball. The changes are usually bilateral and both sexes are equally affected.

Its pathogenesis is unknown but probably a reaction of the choriocapillaris and RPE to the elongation of globe and aging.

It is probably not related to retinal breaks and RD.

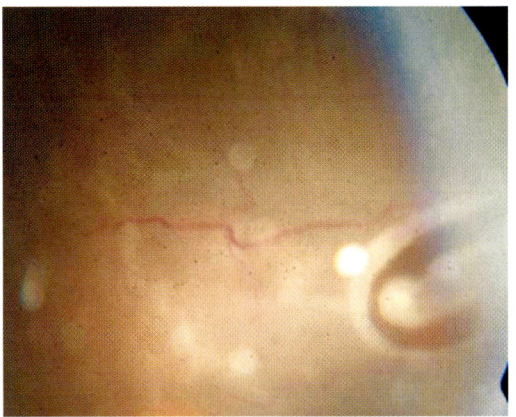

Fig. 25.13 *Horse-shoe break in the superotemporal quadrant*

RETINAL BREAKS

These are precursors of the occurrence of rhegmatogenous retinal detachment. Retinal break is a full thickness defect in the neuro-sensory retina. There are three types of retinal breaks depending upon the pathogenesis:

- Tears
- Holes
- Dialysis

1. **Tear** is caused by vitreoretinal traction. It is of following type:

 i. *Horseshoe tear (HST):* It occurs because of the vitreo-retinal adhesion which tears away the retina behind the vitreous base in the process of posterior vitreous detachment. The convexity of the horse shoe tear is always towards the disc (Fig. 25.13).

 ii. *Operculated tears:* In this the flap of the tear is completely torn away from the retina and the operculum remains attached to the detached vitreous gel (Fig. 25.14).

 iii. *Giant retinal tears (GRT):* It is circumferential retinal break of 90 degree or more in expense. In horse shoe tear the vitreoretinal adhesion is localized whereas it is more wide spread in GRT. The posterior edge of the tear is free from vitreous that is why it gets inverted, however, the anterior edge of the tear remain attached to the vitreous gel (Fig. 25.15).

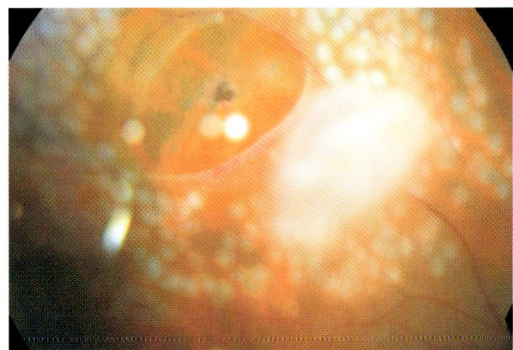

Fig. 25.14 *Lasered operculated break*

2. **Hole.** It is caused by arophy and degeneration and vitreoretinal traction has no role to play. These are round or oval in shape and mostly associated with lattice and snail track peripheral retinal degeneration (Fig. 25.16).

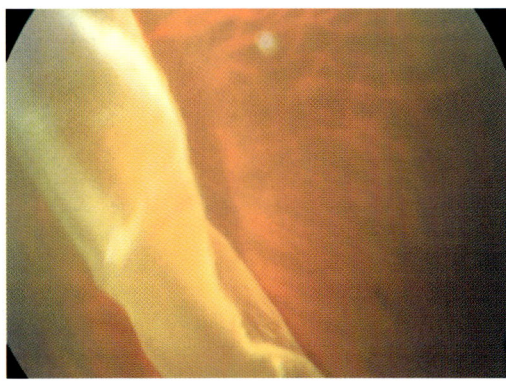

Fig. 25.15 *Grant retinal tear (GRT) with inverted flap*

3. **Dialysis.** It is full thickness disinsertion of the retina at the ora serrata and is often, but not always associated with blunt trauma to the globe. In this the vitreous gel remain attached to the posterior margin preventing it from curling on itself (Fig. 25.17).

Retinal breaks are found most frequently in superotemporal quadrant (60%) followed by superonasal (25%), then inferotemporal (15%) and least commonly in inferonasal (10%) quadrant.

CLINICAL FEATURES AND EXAMINATION

CLINICAL FEATURES

Symptoms

These are denoted by four Fs, i.e. flashes, floaters, field defects and failing vision. Flashes of light and floaters are the symptoms which may precede the retinal detachment. These are actually the symptoms of acute posterior vitreous detachment (PVD) following its synchisis and synresis.

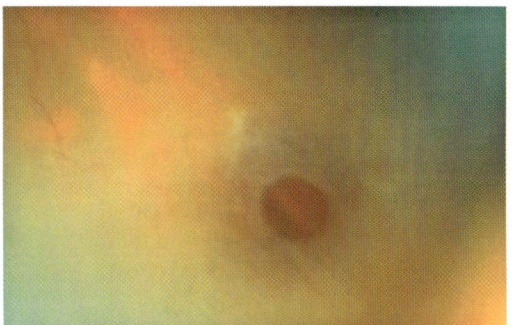

Fig. 25.16 *Round atrophic hole in the peripheral retina*

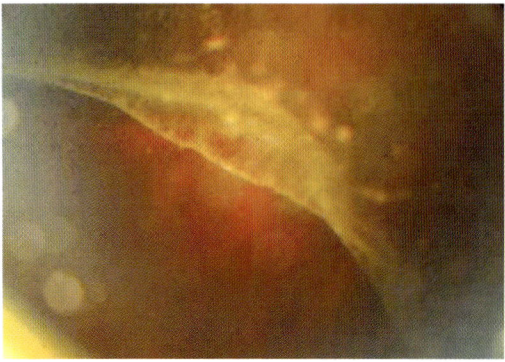

Fig. 25.17 *Retinal dialysis*

a. Flashes. It is called as photopsiae which means the subjective sensation of flash of light. It is caused by the mechanical irritation of retina because of vitreoretinal traction at the site of adhesion which the patient may experience in the process of separation of posterior hyaloid from internal limiting membrane. It is better seen in dim light and is induced by the eye movements. The cessation of flash means either the PVD has negotiated the adhesion and posterior vitreous detachment has been completed or the flap of retina has got separated from retina (operculum) and traction has been released resulting into a break in the retina.

b. Floaters. These are the black spot seen in the field of vision. These are because of moving vitreous opacities casting their shadow on the retina and thus perceived as dark spot (entopic phenomenon). The vitreous opacities are of the following types:

i. *Cobwebs:* are perceived because of conden-sation of collagen fibrillar network of vitreous due to is collapse (synresis).

ii. *Weiss ring* is the detached attachment of the cortical vitreous on the optic nerve head seen as single annular floater. Its presence is a surest sign of PVD, however, its absence does not ensure posterior hyaloid attachment.

iii. *Sudden shower of minute red colored or dark floaters* are experienced when the retinal tear involves the retinal vessels in the process of PVD leading to small and sparse vitreous hemorrhage.

c. Fielf defect. It is appreciated by the patient as a dark veil or curtain interrupting the field of vision. The appearance of the dark veil will depend upon the quadrant from where the retinal detachment is initiating. Since mostly it starts from superior quadrant so the dark veil is seen inferiorly as a lower field defect. The progress of the detachment will be seen as increase in the size of field defect till such time total field inclusive of central vision is knocked out.

d. Failing vision. Retinal detachment is a well known cause of rapid painless loss of vision which occurs when the detachment process involves the macula.

SIGNS

Can be divided as anterior or posterior segment signs.

Anterior segment signs

- Leucocoria-white pupillary reflex may denote retinal detachment.
- Marcus gun pupil (RAPD) is present in the affected eye if there is an extensive detachment.
- Low intraocular pressure is due to backward flow of the aqueous in the vitreous cavity and then through the retinal break into the subretinal space.
- Tobacco dust means pigment cells may be seen in the anterior vitreous on slit lamp examination.
- Iritis may be seen in old retinal detachment due to the irritation of uvea from the metabolic product of detached retina. Thus retinal detachment masquerading as iritis may be missed on cursory examination by a novice.

Posterior segment signs

Retinal detachment can be best diagnosed and examined by indirect ophthalmoscopy in case the media is clear and diagnosed by B scan ultrasound in hazy media. The clinical signs will vary depending upon the duration of retinal detachment. The conspicuous features of the following types of retinal detachment are discussed as under:

- Fresh retinal detachment
- Old retinal detachment
- Inferior retinal detachment
- Aphakic/pseudophakic retinal detachment
- Traumatic retinal detachment.

a. Fresh retinal detachment

The detached retina appears greyish-white, it is convex in configuration and is having corrugated folds, the choroidal pattern is lost, the vessles are reflexless and darker and it is difficult to differentiate between artery and vein. The mobility of retina is good and it is not difficult to bring sclera-choroid close to retina by depressor indirect ophthalmoscopy. The edges of breaks are flat (Fig. 25.18).

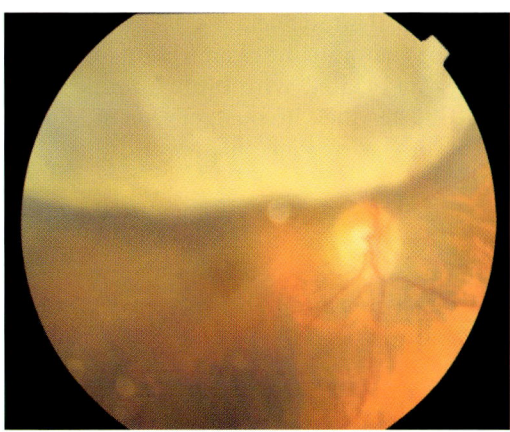

Fig. 25.18 *Fresh retinal detachment*

b. Old/long-standing retinal detachment

The retina with time become more fixed and less mobile. The PVR changes sets in, the margins of breaks become everted, the star folds appear in the inferior quadrants followed by superior quadrants. Intraretinal cysts may appear which may disappear after retinal reattachment. The retina which was greyish-white initially may become transparent because of atrophic changes (Fig. 25.19).

c. Inferior retinal detachment

These detachments occur because of presence of breaks inferiorly. The subretinal fluid collects and rises gradually and it leave behind high water marks (demarcation lines) caused by proliferation of RPE cells at the junction of flat and detached retina. These are called chronic retinal detachments because of relatively slow course and the patient visits ophthalmologist once the macula is detached. These are not bullous as in retinal detachments with superior breaks, but are relatively shallow retinal detachments. Since these are long-standing, therefore, may be having intraretinal cysts (Fig. 25.20).

d. Aphakic/pseudophakic retinal detachment

The breaks in these detachments are relatively small in the far periphery just posterior to vitreous base. The detachment is more extensive than phakic eyes and involve macula more

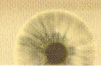

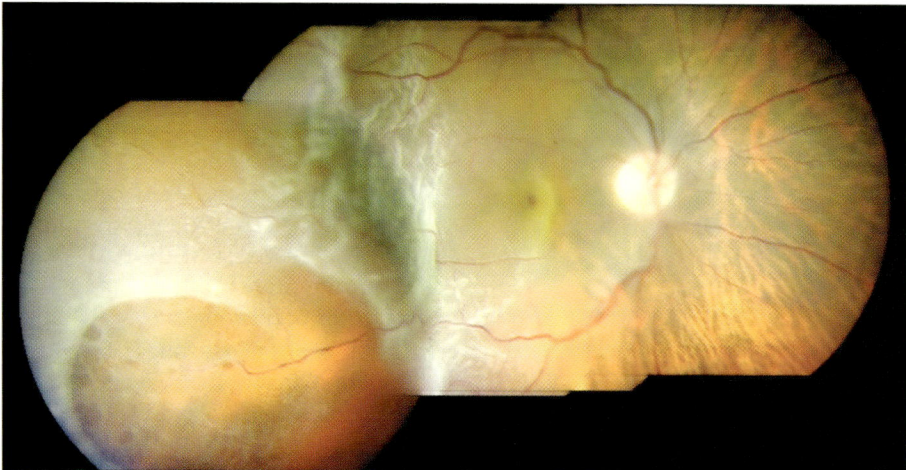

Fig. 25.19 *Long-standing RD with fixed folds*

frequently. The signs of proliferative vitreo-retinopathy are also more common (Fig. 25.21).

e. Traumatic retinal detachment

These detachments characteristically occur after blunt trauma, with direct injury in the infero-temporal quadrant and counter coup effect in the superonasal quadrant. The patients involved mostly are male young adults less than 40 years. Oral dialysis account for three-fourth of the cases in the superonasal quadrant. Retinal detachment usually do not follow blunt trauma immediately since the vitreous is gel, however, it may manifest 4 weeks to within 2 years of trauma after liquefaction of vitreous. Traumatic detachments are mostly associated with vitreous hemorrhage inferiorly (Fig. 25.22).

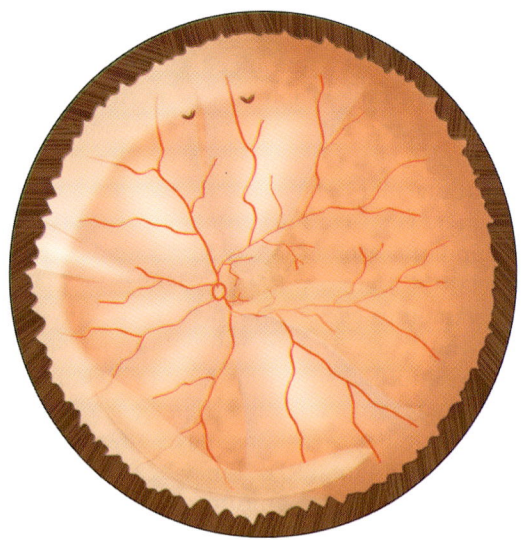

Fig. 25.21 *Aphakic RD with small breaks at the posterior edge of vitreous base*

EXAMINATION OF A CASE OF RETINAL DETACHMENT

• Exact record of best corrected visual acuity of each eye is made. Retinoscopy is carried out to assess the refractive status of the patient, e.g. aphakia or myopia or otherwise. Low level of visual acuity < 1/60 is carefully recorded, i.e. finger counting 1 meter, half meter, close to face, hand movements close to face, followed by accurate projection of light and

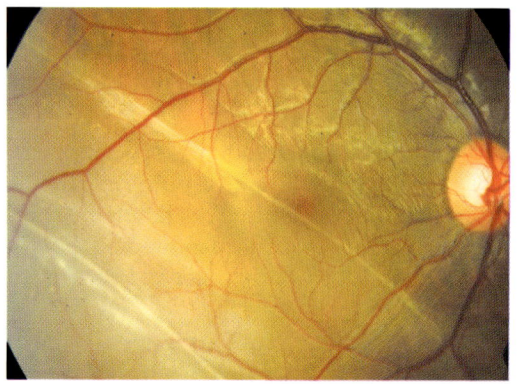

Fig. 25.20 *Inferior RD with high projection marks*

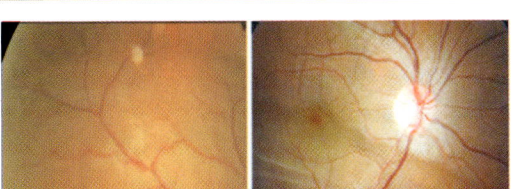

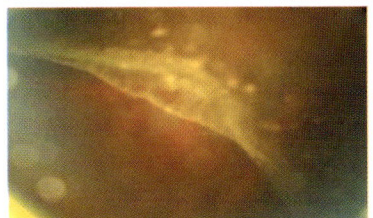

Inferotemporal dialysis with RD

Fig. 25.22 *Traumatic RD with inferotemporal retinal dialysis*

lastly perception of light. Negative perception of light is contraindication for surgery. In a patient of RD if the macula is attached but threatened the vision may be normal. This is an emergency situation warranting admission, complete bed rest with binocular bandage so that macular detachment is arrested and the patient is posted for urgent surgery.

- Pupillary reactions are carefully evaluated. A relative afferent pupillary defect (RAPD) is common in eyes with extensive RD. In eyes with RAPD the visual prognosis after successful RD surgery is guarded because of marked permanent retinal damage. In subtotal RDs pupillary reactions may be normal and in fresh and total RDs it may be sluggish and illsustained. The amount of preoperative dilatation will indicate the anticipated size of pupil during surgery.
- Sclera is examined to detect ectasia, staphyloma in high myopes because thinning of sclera may influence choice of surgery.

a. Slit lamp examination

It includes examination of anterior segment, anterior vitreous gel and record of IOP by applantation tonometry.

- Clarity of cornea is noted which may influence the visibility during surgery.
- Anterior chamber is examined for flare and cells which may indicate chronic uveitis often seen in chronic RDs. Assessment of AC depth

is made since application of a buckle in shallow AC might cause further shallowing and precipitation of an attack of secondary narrow angle closure glaucoma by shifting iris lens diaphragm forward. Preoperative gonioscopy may help and laser iridotomy can be considered in indiated cases. In addition gonioscopy can also help in ruling out NVA and NVI (rubeosis iridis particularly in cases of proliferative retinopathies of diabetes and vascular occlusion, etc.

- Intra ocular pressure as measured by applanation tonometry is expected to be lower than fellow eye in patients of RD. It may be elevated in patients of RD with OAG or in post-traumatic RDs. Gonioscopy is again important in eyes with RD and raised IOP.
- After dilating pupil crystalline lens is evaluated. Any subluxation may point towards Marfan's syndrome, homocystinuria or trauma. Transparency of the lens is assessed, in case it interferes with the examination of retina, phacoemulsification is carried out before or in combination with parsplana vitrectomy (PPV).
- In aphakic eyes the anterior hyaloid face is examined for performing paracentasis during the surgery. If it is intact paracentasis may be performed, in case it is ruptured and vitreous is in AC then paracentass during the scleral buckling procedure is avoided lest vitreous should incarcerate in the paracentasis site causig later complications. For similar reason pseudophakic eyes with intact posterior capsule or pseudophakic eyes with central posterior capsular rent, however, plugged with the optic of an IOL may be safely subjected to paracentasis. It should be avoided in pseudophakic eyes where vitreous is presenting into AC from the peripheral portion of optic of an IOL.
- Iris supported IOLs required special precautions before dilatation of pupil and before injecting the gas. During dilatation the haptic might dislocate and after gas injection the optic might touch the central corea and damage the endothelium.
- Examination of anterior vitreous gel is performed, there is a dictum which states that if there is pigment cells in the anterior vitreous

without the signs of uveitis and without the history of trauma, RD must be ruled out (Fig. 25.23). However, presence of larger gray or pigmented clumps of cells with the vitreous gel suggest beginning of proliferative vitreoretinopathy (PVR).

- The mobility of vitreous is assessed by having the patient look up and down and then instantaneously stopping the movement. Normally vitreous moves freely and posterior surface of vitreous is seen indicating PVD, and most obvious movements lasts for 3–5 seconds. Marked reduction of mobility of vitreous is suggestive of PVR in patients of RD.

b. Vitreoretinal examination by binocular indirect ophthalmoscope

- It is performed by binocular indirect ophthalmoscopy aided by scleral indentation. This may be supplemented by 90D biomicroscopic examination to evaluate macula and posterior vitreous gel. The modern head mounted binocular indirect ophthalmoscope was invented by Charles Schepens in 1947. It provides a stereoscopic view of the fundus with considerable depth and with 20D aspheric condensing lens one can have real, inverted, laterally reversed and 3X magnified view of about 37 to 40 degree wide field of retina. With the decrease in dioptric power of condensing lens the working distance, magnification and depth of focus increases but the field of view decreases and vice versa.

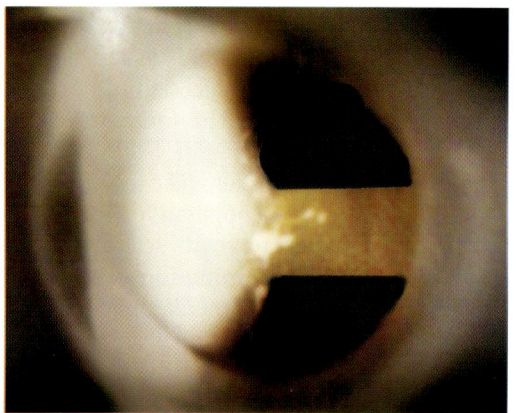

Fig. 25.23 *Slit lamp photograph in diffuse light showing pigmented cellular clumps in the anterior vitreous gel*

Since the image of the fudus is vertically inverted and laterally reversed therefore the observer learns through experience to mentally transpose the image into the true anatomic relations in the patient's eye. Learning this technique and interpretation of the images seen require hours of practice and considerable experience.

- It is always advisable for the trainee to learn the indirect ophthalmoscopy under the guidance of an expert which is likely to cut short the learning curve.
- The crux is that there are four components in conduit pipe, i.e. observer's eye, indirect ophthalmoscope, condensing lens and patient's eye; all these have to be perfectly aligned for seeing the sharp and clear image of the retina. In case any one component is not aligned the image will disppapear. Mastering the alignment of these four components is the art of indirect ophthalmoscopy (Fig. 25.24).

Procedure

- The pupils are dilated with 0.8% tropicamide and 5.0% phenylepherine.
- The patient is lying supine in a semi dark room on an examination table.
- The observer places the indirect ophthalmoscope on his head and inter pupillary distance is adjusted after switching on the equipment. The illuminatin of the beam is adjusted initially to moderate intensity so that the glare to the patient is minimized. The beam is aligned so that it is located in the center of the viewing frame (Fig. 25.25).
- The patient is instructed to keep both the eyes open at all the time and his gaze is directed towards his thumb in the desired direction.
- The condensing lens is taken in one hand with the flat surface facing the patient and this surface should be kept parallel to the plane of iris of the patient all throughout the examination.
- The other hand of the observer may be used in keeping the lids of the patient apart.
- First of all the central area, i.e. disc, macula and surrounding area just anterior to equator is examined when the patient is asked to see straight towards the ceiling.

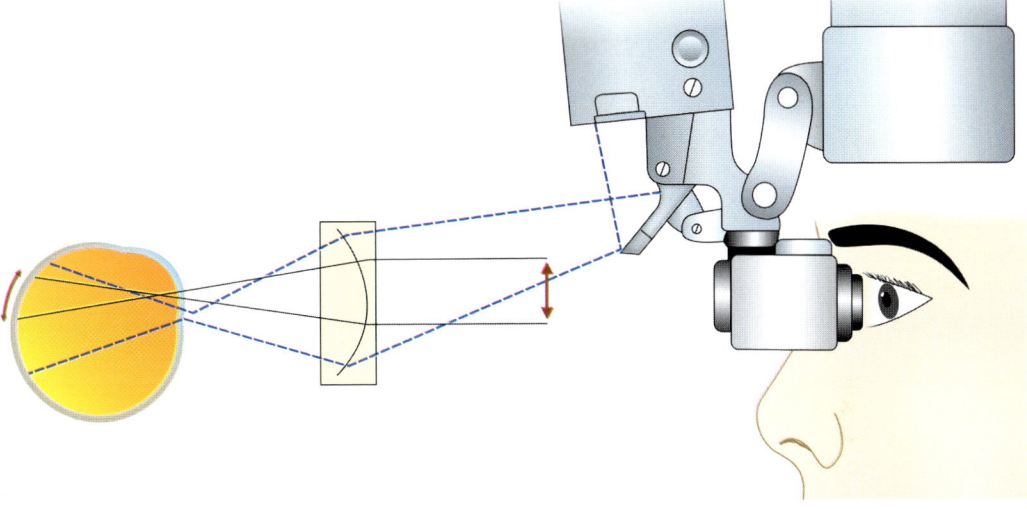

Fig. 25.24 *Diagrammatic representation of four components of indirect ophthalmoscopy consisting of patient eye, 20D lens, indirect ophthalmoscopy and observer's eye*

- The condensing lens is moved in anterior posterior direction to bring the image into focus and titled slightly to displace troublesome reflexes out of viewing axis in order to have sharp view of the retina.
- The anterior retina up to ora can be seen by asking the patient to see away from the observer without scleral indentation only in high myopes and aphakes with wide dilatation of pupil.
- In rest of the cases the peripheral retina anterior to equator upto ora serrata can only be seen by scleral indentation by thimble depressor. It also permits kinetic evaluation of the retina as the observer can move the depressor from anterior to posterior and sideways which enhances the contrast and can thus differentiate between retinal hemorrhage and retinal break.
- The thimble depressor is placed on the eyelid at the peripheral margin of the tarsus and gently pushed against the sclera. This indents sclera, thereby permitting the visualization of the peripheral retina, which is not normally visible in phakic eye. The force applied is tangential to the surface of sclera not perpendicular since the latter will cause pain and render the patient uncooperative (Fig. 25.26).
- Indirect ophthalmocopy with scleral indentation also permits examination of the peripheral fundus through media opacities such as mild to moderate cataract and vitreous hemorrhage because of its bright illumination.
- In preparing the fundus drawing the fundus chart is kept on the chest of the patient upside down. The boundaries of the retinal detachment

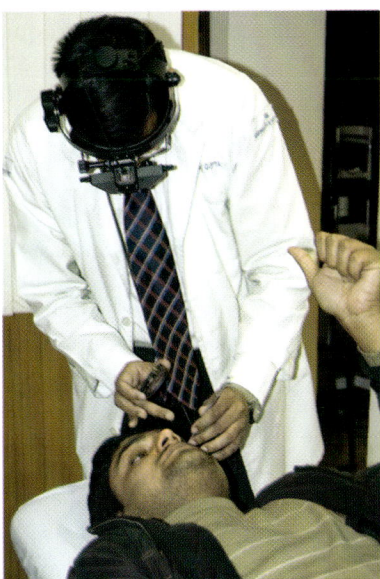

Fig. 25.25 *IDO procedure*

around the optic nerve head are recorded first and special care is taken to determine whether macula is involved or not. Now as per the topography of RD and Lincoff's rule the probable sites are explored for the localization of break.

- The starting of the examination from the superior retina is simplified because of uprolling of the eyeball caused by stimulus of bright light (Bell's phenomenon). In the meantime the eye gets adapted to bright light and then the inferior retina is examined which can be assisted by gazing of the patient towards the thumb with the fellow eye.
- Thus it is convenient to begin in the 12 o'clock meridian and proceed clockwise. Since the chart is kept up side down, the observer stationed at 6 o'clock and examining at 12 o'clock can record all the findings in the clock hour wherever he is positioned.
- In this way all retinal breaks suspicious breaks, areas of retinal thinning, and zones of abnormal vitreoretinal adhesion, including the lattice degeneration are recorded in the clock hour wherever the observer is positioned. The pigment or hemorrhagic spots in the peripheral fundus are carefully recorded since these assist in the localization of breaks which are mostly in their vicinity.
- The other features of RD like (a) the height of the RD (b) the presence of demarcation lines, intraretinal cysts and fixed retinal folds (c) areas of epiretinal membrane formation are recorded on the chart and/or written notes are made.

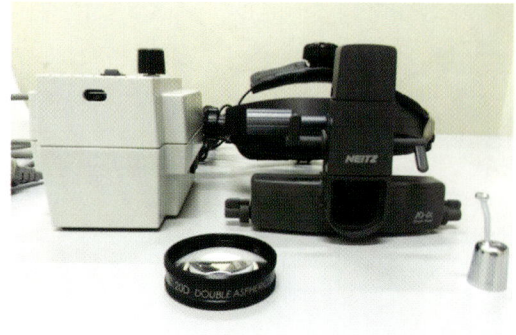

Fig. 25.26 *Indirect ophthalmoscope, thimble depressor and 20D aspheric lens*

- After completing the examination the fundus chart is brought back to its normal erect position and is interpreted as depicted.
- The fellow eye is examined in the same fashion as the eye with detachment and a fundus drawing of the fellow eye is also made if any abnormality is seen.

Localization of retinal break

It is the most important routine preoperative ocular part of the workout of the patient of retinal detachment. It is preferably be done by indirect ophthalmoscopy although in the past it used to be practiced by Goldman three mirror examination also. The later procedure is reserved these days in case the break is not found and sometime to confirm the doubtful finds as seen by indirect ophthalmoscopy. The modern indirect ophthalmoscope invented by Charles Schepens opened a new chapter in the preoperative localization of the retinal breaks. However, it was Lincoff who after examining hundreds of retinal detachments defined a rule known as Lincoff's rule by which one can ascertain the possible site of retinal break by examining the topography of retinal detachment.

The topography of the retinal detachment is of great value in predicting the location of retina breaks (Lincoff's rule — Fig. 25.27).

- If a detachment involves one upper quadrant or both upper and lower quadrants on one side of the vertical meridian, the primary break is likely to be there near the superior edge of the detachment. It is usually with in 1½ clock hours of the more superior margin of the detachment.
- If the detachment is total and high then it is caused by a primary break 1 clock hour from the vertical meridian, i.e. 11 o'clock to 1 o'clock hour.
- If the detachment is involving both the lower quadrants, and the level on both sides is equal then it is due to retinal break at 6 o'Clock.
- If the detachment is inferior involving both the lower quadrants, however level is higher on one side than the other, then the primary break is 1 clock hour on the side of 6 o'clock where the level is higher.

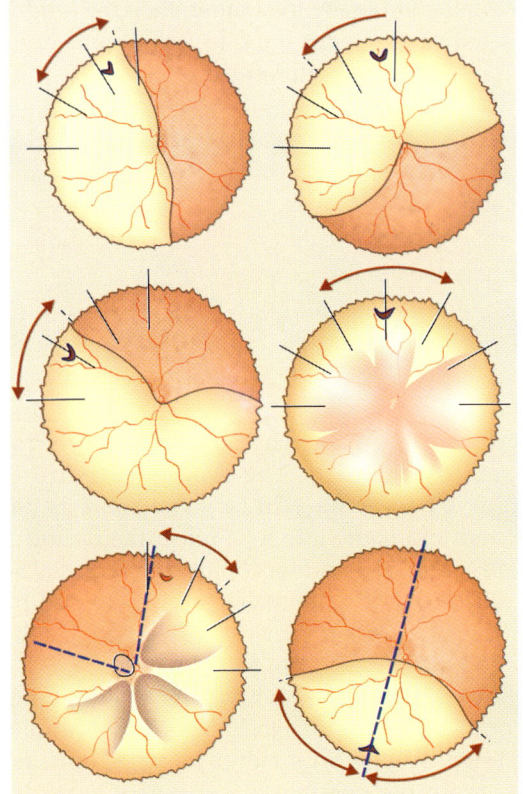

Fig. 25.27 *Localization of break depending upon the topography of retina as per Lincoff's rule (for detail see text)*

the middle circle correspond to the ora serrata and the outermost circle depicts pars plana. Vortex vein ampullae are slightly posterior to the equator. The location of 3 and 9 o'clock meridians are indicated by long posterior cilliary arteries and nerves. There is globally accepted color coding of fundus drawing chart which is shown in Fig. 25.28, Table 25.2 and Fig. 4.19, p-62.

Important clues to localise and identify breaks

Although the topography of the retinal detachment as discussed above points towards primary break still sometimes it is not possible to localize the break by indirect ophthalmoscopy. Either one can examine the detachment by Goldmann three mirror lens or one can be guided by the following clues:

- The recognition of lattice degeneration in the detached retina is important since it might have atrophic holes.
- Look for a operculum in the vitreous, the break is close to the operculum.
- Look for spots of pigment or blood, breaks are usually seen in closed proximity.
- The retinal break is usually within 1½ clock hours of the superior edge of the detachment.
- During indirect ophthalmoscopy and scleral depression look for tiny flaps elevated above

- If the detachment involves both lower quadrants and it is bullous then the primary break is above the horizontal meridian.
- If there is subtotal retinal detachment with a superior wedge of attached retina then the primary break is located near its highest border.

In all the retinal detachments there is one break which is responsible for it and is called as primary break. In 50% of retinal detachments there is more than one break and when two are there, they are usually within 90° of each other. The second break known as secondary break is not a culprit break and is present as a result of the process of their genesis. However, it is equally important to localize and to treat secondary breaks failing which retina is not going to settle.

Fundus drawing chart

It has three circles and 12 clock hour meridians. The innermost circle correspond to the equator,

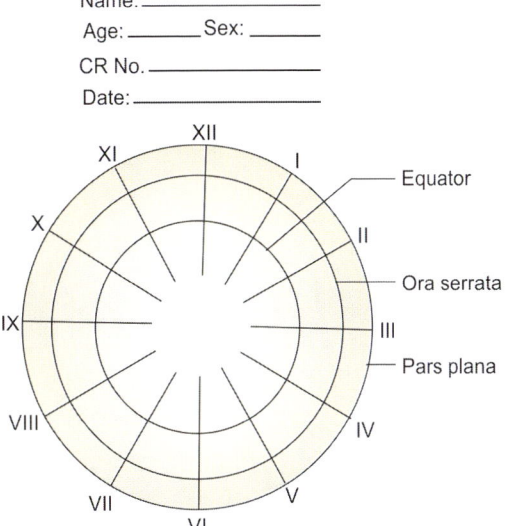

Fig. 25.28 *Fundus chart having three circles. Inner circle represent equator, middle represent ora serrata, outer represent pars plana. There are 12 clock hours*

Table 25.2 *Color codes for fundus drawing chart*

Color	Retinal findings
Red	Attached retina, retinal arteries and all types of hemorrhages.
Blue	Detached retina, retinal veins and retinal folds.
Red surrounded by blue	Retinal breaks.
Cross-hatched blue	Lattice degeneration in detached retina.
Hashed blue	Retinoschisis.
Green	Opacities in media including vitreous hemorrhage.
Black	Retinal pigmentation and choroidal pigmentation seen through attached retina.
Cross-hatched black	Lattice degeneration in attached retina.
Brown	Choroidal pigmentation seen through detached retina.
White	Normal attached retina.
Yellow	Active chorioretinitis, retinal edema, recent treatment with laser, cryo or diathermy.
Purple	Flat NV.
Orange	Elevated NV.

the plane of retina which might indicate break (s) concealed underneath. Such tiny flap tears are most likely to occur in a circumferential line corresponding to the anterior limit of PVD. This line of mild vitreous traction is often visible with sclera depression with in the area of detachment where the retina is mobile, whereas it is usually not seen in attached retina.

c. Vitreoretinal examination by fundus biomicroscope and Goldmann three mirror lens

Vitreoretinal examination can also be carried out by fundus biomicroscopy with Goldmann three mirror lens or by a double aspheric 90D lens. Out of these the former has the advantage of examining the entire fundus and the later can discern only up to equator. With both lenses the disc and macula can be evaluated stereoscopically under high magnification. However, the main clinical uses of fundus biomicroscopy are:

i. Search for small retinal breaks at a site suggested by topography of RD which are not detected by indirect ophthalmoscopy.

ii. Confirm the suspicious breaks or to dertermine whether the areas of thin retina are actually full thickness breaks.

iii. Study the vitreoretinal anatomy in eyes having complex RDs with PVR.

- Goldmann three mirror contact lens best suits for this purpose. It require a coupling material, e.g. 2% methylcellulose for fixing it on the cornea of the patient after topical anesthesia. It has central contact lens and three mirrors incorporated in it (Fig. 25.29).
- Central part provides a 30° upright view of posterior pole.
- Equatorial mirror (largest and oblong shaped 73°); by this retina from 30° to equator can be examined.
- Peripheral mirror (medium sized and square shaped 67°; by this retina from equator to ora serrata can be visualized.
- Gonioscopy mirror (smallest and dome shaped); by this extreme retinal periphery and pars plana can be seen.

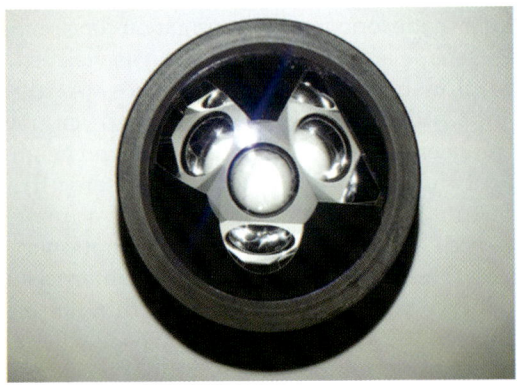

Fig. 25.29 *Goldmann three mirror contact lens*

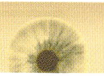

- The mirror is positioned opposite the area of the fundus to be examined, i.e. to examine 12 o'clock the mirror is positioned at 6 o'clock.
- When viewing the vertical meridian, the image is seen upside down but not laterally reversed in contrast to indirect ophthalmoscopy. However, when viewing the horizontal meridian, the image is laterally reversed.
- For having a comprehensive view of the 360° of the retina both oblong shaped and square shaped (large and medium sized) mirrors are used and patient is asked to rotate the eye in different directions. The patient when asked to see towards the mirror more posterior regions are visualized, when eye is rotated away from the mirror more anterior areas are visualied.
- With Goldmann three mirror lens, a combination of high magnification provided by slit lamp, the variable angulation and width of slit beam not only help in the identification of small subtle retinal breaks but can also differentiate between areas of thin retina and full thickness breaks. The identified tiny retinal break should be marked with laser which stays for 24 to 48 hours. This aids in its identification intraoperatively when indirect ophthalmoscopy is used.

ROLE OF ULTRASONOGRAPHY

Indirect ophthalmoloscopy is indispensable for diagnosis and management of retinal detachment with clear media, however, in hazy media it is not easily possible to assess posterior segment. Thus in patients with hazy media it is the B scan ultraosonography by which the retinal status can be assessed. Ultrasonography can provide topographic information concerning size, shape and quality of a lesion as well as its relationship to other structures. A high amptitude echo in the vitreous cavity, equivalent to choroidal and scleral echo height, indicates RD on A scan. On B scan ultrasonography, the detached retina has a funnel-shaped configuration attached to the optic nerve head (Fig. 25.30). It is important to interpret at reduced gain setting which will differentiate between RD and vitreous hemorrhage wherein the high amptitude echo of retinal tissue will persist and those of vitreous hemorrhage will

disappear. It is equally important to differentiate between RD and PVD. Typically moderately echogenic posterior hyaloid membrane once completely detached is free from optic nerve head, whereas RD will alway be attached to optic nerve head. A thickened and partial PVD may be difficult to differentiate from RD however, a detached retina often has a characteristic undulating motion after abrupt eye movement, whereas vitreous membranes usually show more brisk motion but with more restricted excursion (kinetic ultrasonography).

EXUDATIVE AND TRACTIONAL RETINAL DETACHMENT

EXUDATIVE RETINAL DETACHMENT

The mechanisms by which the neurosensory retina remain attached to the retinal pigment epithelium (RPE) has been discussed in detail earlier (p-403)

Clinical and experimental evidence has shown that fluid movement from the vitreous across the retina into the choriocapillaris carried out

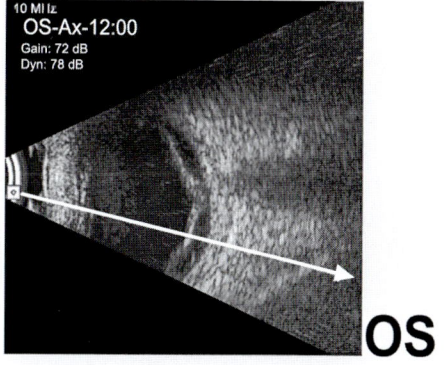

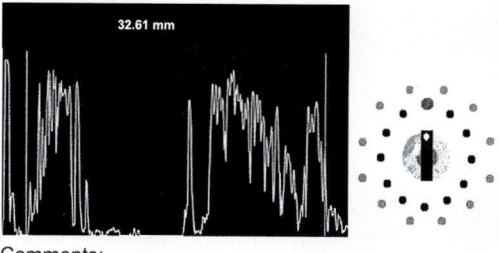

Comments:

Fig. 25.30 *A scan and B scan ultrasonography showing RD in a patient with cataract*

by the RPE pump plays a major role in keeping the retina attached. Where as the anatomic adhesion and mechanical support provided by formed vitreous contribute a small part in this regard. Thus the lesions which lead to RPE pump failure (outer retinal barrier) will cause non-rhegmatogenous or exudative retinal detachment.

CAUSES

Although there are number of conditions which are responsible for it but the following are most commonly seen in the clinical practice when retinal tears are not detected and shifting subretinal fluid is present.

Idiopathic
- Coats' disease.
- Idiopathic central serous chorioretinopathy (ICSC).
- Uveal effusion syndrome.

Congenital
- Dominant familial exudative vitreoretinopathy.

Post Surgical
- Panretinal photocoagulation.

Inflammatory
- Scleritis (posterior)
- Orbital cellulitis.

Autoimmune
- Vogt Koyanagi Harda's disease (VKH)
- Sympathetic ophthalmia.

Vascular
- Pregnancy induced hypertension (PIH)
- Hypertensive retinopathy.

Neoplstic
- Retinoblastoma.
- Choriodal malignant melanoma.
- Choriodal metastasis
- Choriodal hemangioma.

CLINICAL FEATURES AND DIAGNOSIS

Most commonly patient complain of decreased vision, but the symptoms may vary from meta-morphosia to light perception. Anterior segment should be carefully assessed for relative afferent

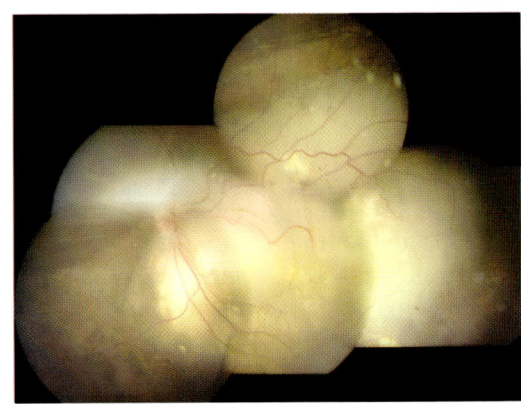

Fig. 25.31 *Exudative RD with shifting fluid in a patient of VKH*

pupillary conduction defect (RAPD), anterior chamber reaction, episcleral injection associated with scleritis.

On indirect ophthalmoscopic examination of posterior segment reveals, absence of retinal breaks, smooth (no folds) bullous retinal detach-ment with shifting subretinal fluid. When the patient is upright the bullous RD shifts inferiorly and when the patient is supine the fluid shifts posteriorly to the most dependent location (Fig. 25.31).

Apart from its utility in the hazy media ultrasonography is useful in assessing the choriodal thickening in VKH and scleral thickening in scleritis. In addition it can pick up nature, location and size of any intraocular tumors.

CT scan is indicated to rule out intraocular/ extraocular pathology like retinoblastoma in a child (calcification) or orbital pseudotumor, etc.

The management will vary with the condition causing it. The conditions like VKH and sympa-thetic ophthalmia and scleritis can be treated by corticosteroids; PIH and Hypertensive retino-pathy grade IV can be treated by termination of pregnancy and antihypertensive drugs. ICSC may be treated by photocoagulation. The treatment of intraocular tumors have been dealt at appropriate section.

TRACTIONAL RETINAL DETACHMENT (TRD)

As the term suggest, this type of RD is because of the vitreoretinal traction bands developing as a result of the underlying ocular/systemic

disease thus leading to tractional retinal detachment.

CAUSES

Most common conditions causing this type of RD are as under:

- Proliferative diabetic retinopathy (PDR).
- Retinopathy of prematurity (ROP).
- Penetrating posterior segment trauma.
- Proliferative retinopathies like CRVO/BRVO and vasculitis in their late stages.

The pathogenesis of TRD has been discussed appropriately at the respective section of their discriptions. However, it is understandable that TRD occurs because of progressive contraction of fibrovascular membranes formed over areas of vitreoretinal adhesion.

The vitreoretinal traction is largely of three types. **Tangential traction** is because of the contraction of the epiretinal fibrovascular membranes resulting into puckering of retina and distortion of the vessels. **Anteroposterior traction** is caused by the contraction of membranes extending from posterior retina to the vitreous base anteriorly. The third is **Bridging traction** (table top) which is the result of contraction of membranes usually spaning across the vascular arcades or from one part of posterior retina to another thus pulling the two involved points together causing thereby TRD.

Clinical features: These have largely been covered in the defferntial diagnosis of rhegmatogenous RD. The usual features of flashes floaters and progressive curtain of darkness as seen in rhegmatogenous RD are absent since TRD occurs due to insidious traction of membranes and is not associated with acute PVD. Again because of the same reason the visual field defect progress very slowly which may remain stationary for months and sometimes for years. The condition is usually bilateral however, one eye may be involved earlier than the other. The RD has a concave configuration and the breaks are absent unless it becomes combined (rhegmatogenous and tractional) RD due to the occurance of tractional breaks in the retina. The mobility of retina is restricted and RD hardly ever extends to ora serrata. The RD is shallow and there is no shifting of fluid. The highest elevation of

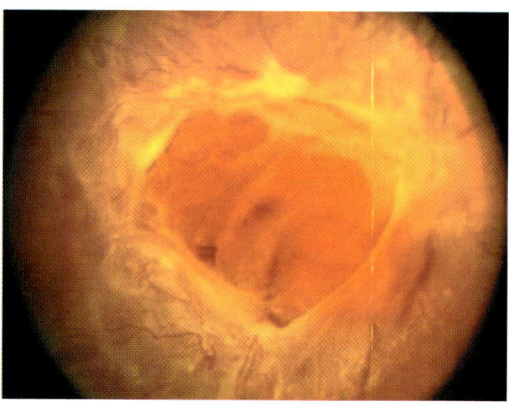

Fig. 25.32 *Traction RD in a patient of PDR*

RD occurs at the site of vitreoretinal traction (Fig. 25.32).

The treatment of the condition involves the cutting, peeling and segmentation of causative membranes, thereby releasing the traction which allows the retina to fall back to its bed by vitreoretinal surgery.

DIFFERENTIAL DIAGNOSIS, MANAGEMENT AND PROPHYLAXIS

DIFFERENTIAL DIAGNOSIS OF RHEGMATOGENOUS RD

Rhegmatogenous RD need to be differentiated from followng condition:

- Retinoschisis
- Tractional retinal detachment
- Exudative retinal detachment
- Choroidal detachment

Differential diagnosis of rhegmatogenous retinal detachment and retinoschisis has been discussed on (p-407)

Differential diagnosis of various types of RDs is given in Table 25.3.

Differentiation of rhegmatogenous RD from choroidal detachment

The differences are given in Table 25.4.

MANAGEMENT OF RHEGMATOGENOUS RETINAL DETACHMENT

Retinal detachment (RD) is managed only surgically, there is no available drug therapy of

Table 25.3 *Differences between rhegmatogenous, tractional and exudative detachment*

	Rhegmatogenous	Tractional	Exudative
1. Symptom	Floaters and flashes	Absent	Absent
2. Visual Field defect	Develops fast	Develops slowly may remain static for months	Develops fast
3. Laterality	U/L other eye may be involved later	U/L other eye may be involved later	Involves both eyes simultaneously
4. PVD	Usually follows PVD which is complete	Not associated with PVD, which is incomplete	Not associated with PVD
5. Break	Always present	Absent	Absent
6. RPE pump	Intact	Not affected	Occurs due to RPE pump failure
7. Configuration	Convex, bullous, corrugated folds	Concave	Convex but surface is smooth, no folds
8. Mobility of retina	Mobile in fresh case restricted in old case	Restricted	Mobile
9. Extent	Extends to ora	Seldom extends	Extends to ora
10. PVR	Present in due course of time	Absent	Absent
11. SRF shift	No shift	Shallous and no shift	Shift with posture
12. Treatment	Surgical	Surgical	No surgery, treat underlying cause

Table 25.4 *Differences between rhegmatogenous RD and choroidal detachment*

	Rhegmatogenous RD	Choroidal detachment
1. Symptoms	Flashes and floaters positive	Absent
2. Visual field defect	Develops fast	Absent unless it is very extensive, i.e. kissing choroidals
3. AC and IOP	Normal AC, IOP is low	Shallow AC, IOP very low
4. Break	Present	Absent
5. Configuration	Greyish white, corrugated retinal fold, mostly mobile	Convex, dome shaped brownish, smooth and not mobile
6. Extent	From disc to ora	Mostly anterior to equator, it usually extends beyond ora
7. Treatment	Surgical	Mostly there is spontaneous resolution

the condition so far. It is managed by the following three surgical procedures:

1. Scleral buckling
2. Pneumatic retinoplexy
3. Primary vitrectomy in RD

Following are the management **principles** of retinal detachment in scleral buckling:

1. Localization of all the retinal breaks by indirect ophthalmoscopy.
2. Treat all the retinal breaks by cryotherapy.
3. Bring treated retinal break close to the sclerochoroid so that adhesion forms and break seals. This is done by:
   a. Drainage of subretinal fluid (SRF).
   b. Application of episcleral buckle to make it permanent.

1. SCLERAL BUCKLING

Surgical steps

These are discussed briefly here for details see (p-542). The steps of scleral buckling also

referred to as retinal detachment (RD) surgery are as follows:

Anesthesia: RD surgery is generally performed under local peribulbar anesthesia except in children and very anxious or un-cooperative adults where it can be performed under general anesthesia.

Preparation of surgical field: A drop of 5% povidone iodine is put into the conjunctival sac. The lid margin is scrubbed with povidone iodine and periocular skin is cleaned and painted with the same. A contact time of 3 minutes is given for iodine to act. The surface is then dried with a sterile guage and an adhesive drape is applied to isolate surgical field from eye lashes, periocular skin and adjoining areas.

Conjunctival peritomy: A 360° limbal incision is given with conjunctival scissors to cut conjunctiva and Tenon's capsule in a single layer and two radial cuts are given at 3 and 9 o'clock meridian. Tenon capsule is then separated from underlying sclera in each quadrant by opening tenotomy scissors between Tenon's capsule and sclera (Fig. 25.33A).

Bridling of recti muscles: The recti muscles are then engaged one by one by passing a muscle hook underneath these. The connections to Tenon's capsule are separated by stripping the muscle with a cotton bud. A traction suture preferably a one zero silk is placed around each rectus muscle which will help in rotation of globe during surgery (Fig. 25.33B).

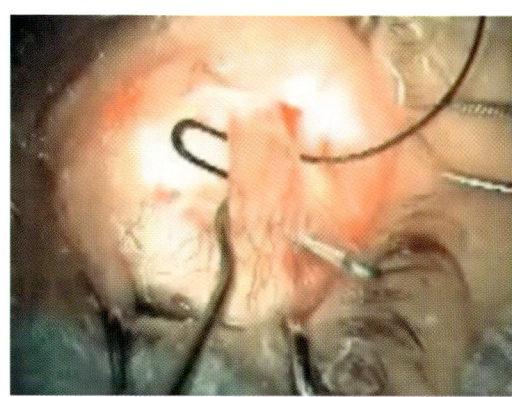

Fig. 25.33B *Bridling of recti muscles*

Localization of retinal breaks: This is an important step of the surgery. All the retinal holes as seen during preoperative period are localized using a localizer. The indentation marks created by the localizer are enhanced with a marker pen. Small tears or breaks can be marked with a single mark on the posterior edge. Large tears require localization of both anterior and posterior edges. In case of multiple tears in a quadrant circumferential extent is also to be marked (Fig. 25.33C).

Cryotherapy: The role of cryotherapy is to create adhesion between RPE and neurosensory retina. Cryo is done by applying a 2.5 mm cryo probe to the area of retinal breaks (Fig. 25.33D). The tip of cryo probe cools down to –89°C on pressing the foot switch of the equipment due to expansion of high pressure nitrous oxide at the tip of the probe. The aim of treatment is to

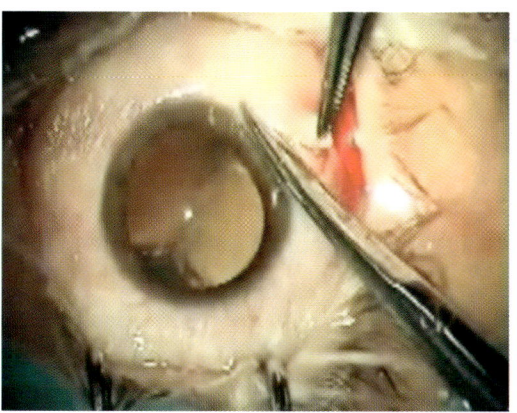

Fig. 25.33A *360° conjunctival peritomy*

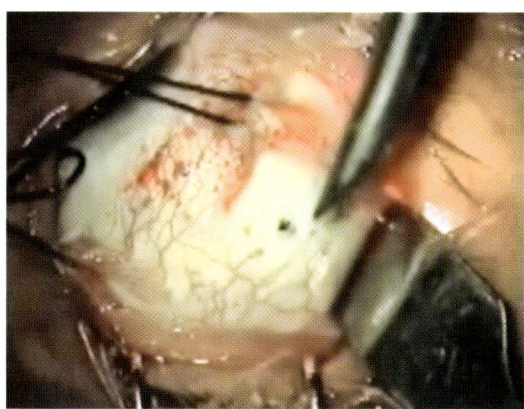

Fig. 25.33C *Localization of retinal break*

sourround the retinal break with contiguous treatment. The end point of cryo application is retinal whitening. Cryotherapy initially reduces adhesive force between RPE and sensory retina for about a week and then adhesive forces start to operate leading to cellular connections between the two layers. Disadvantage of cryotherapy is dispersion of viable retinal pigmented epithelial cells into vitreous cavity and subretinal space leading to proliferative vitreoretinopathy (PVR) in some cases. Thus latter may cause macular pucker or recurrence of RD.

Buckling: Scleral buckling was devised by Ernst Custodis in 1953. Explants are made of solid silicone rubber or silicone sponges. Most commonly used technique in RD surgery involves fixing a 2.5 mm encircling band (code 240). All around the globe and suturing a wide (7 mm or 9 mm) solid silicone tire piece (code 277, or 287) in the area of retinal breaks (Fig. 25.33E). Solid silicone tire is made up of cross-linked polydimethyl siloxane. Tires have a groove in them to accommodate encircling band in that quadrant. For posterior tears, silicone sponges can be placed in radial configuration. Explants are sutured to sclera with partial thickness scleral sutures. A 5-0 nonabsorbble suture such as polyester or nylon is used for this purpose. Sutures are placed a minimum of 2 mm more than the width of silicone explant planned for a particular location. The posterior edge of the tear should be well supported on the explant and the

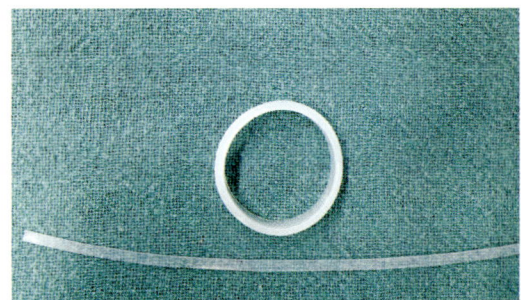

Fig. 25.33E *Showing 240 band and 277 tire*

buckling effect should extend for at least 30 degrees on either side of the tear and extend anteriorly to ora serrate. Two mattress sutures are placed normally over the explant in each quadrant. The encircling 2.5 mm solid silicone band is secured to the sclera with a single mattress suture in each quadrant. Alternatively it can be passed through scleral tunnels. The ends of the band can be secured with silicone sleeve or non-absorbable suture. Buckle height is adjusted by tightening the sutures over the explants as well as tightening the encircling band (Fig. 25.33 F and G).

Subretinal fluid drainage: Drainage of subretinal fluid (SRF) is considered in most cases of RD surgery. Drainage of SRF decreases intraocular volume so that buckle can be accommodated without raising IOP and it also allows area of retinal tear to fall back on the elevated buckle thereby facilitating closure of the retinal break. The selection of drainage site is affected by several factors:

i. SRF should be drained in an area where there is adequate fluid and it is safe to enter the subretinal space.

ii. Wherever possible, it is preferable to drain just above or below the horizontal meridian, preferably nasally. These location avoid injury to vortex veins. If these sites are not available, SRF can be drained close to vertical recti on either side. For SRF drainage, we perform a radial sclerotomy so as to reach bare choroid and then give a puncture nick in the choroid with a 30G needle tip. Subretinal hemorrhage and retinal incarceration are potential complications of SRF drainage. Towards the end of SRF drainage, the egress of SRF slows down and

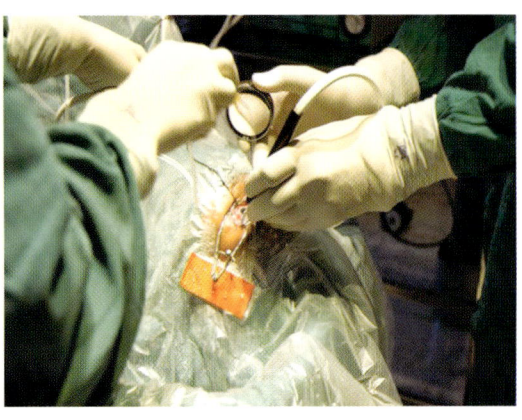

Fig. 25.33D *Application of cryotherapy*

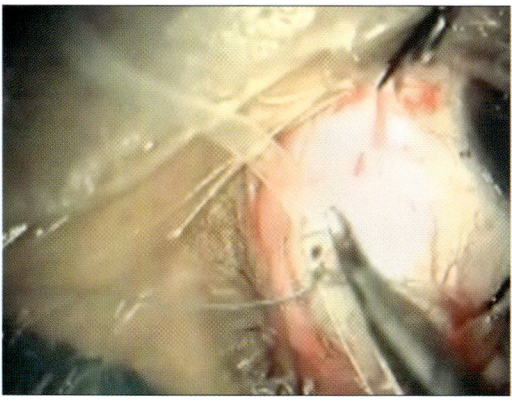

Fig. 25.33F *Fixing of 240 band*

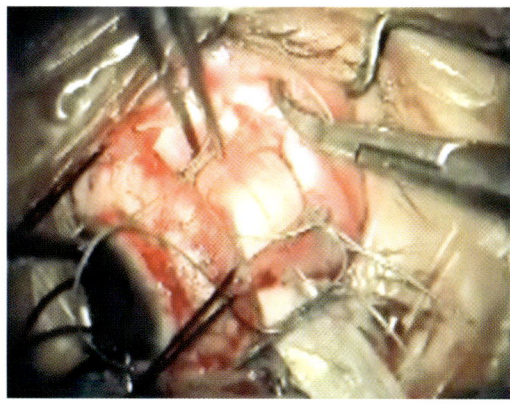

Fig. 25.33H *SRF drainage*

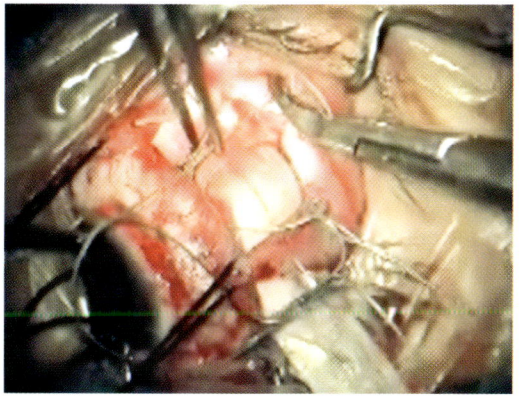

Fig. 25.33G *Fixing of 277 tire*

pigment particles are seen in SRF. Total drainage of SRF may not be necessary in all cases (Fig. 25.33H).

Buckle adjustments: After drainage of SRF, the sutures over the explant are tightened and secured with temporary ties. The ends of encircling band are also tightened and secured with temporary suture tie. Indirect ophthalmoscopy is done at this stage to assess status of retina, position of retinal breaks over the explant and perfusion of central retinal artery. Any adjustment in the height of buckle material can be done at this stage if required. Once surgeon is satisfied with the outcome, temporary ties are converted into permanent knots.

Closure All suture knots are rotated to posterior edge of buckle. Conjunctiva and Tenon's layers

are stitched together in a single layer with a running 7–0 vicryl suture. A subconjunctival antibiotic-steroid injection is given at the end of surgery (Fig. 25.33I).

Result of surgery is shown in Fig. 25.33 J and K.

Complications

Many complications can occur in intraoperative and postoperative period.

A. Intraoperative complications

1. *Corneal clouding:* It is caused by epithelial edema from increased intraocular pressure which may occur during scleral depression. If extensive, debridement of epithelium can be done to improve visualization.

2. *Miosis:* Miosis can occur during surgery either due to excessive cryotherapy induced inflammation or hypotomy caused by SRF drainage. If severe, 0.2 ml of 1:10,000 epinephrine can be injected intracamerally.

3. *Scleral perforation:* Scleral perforation can occur during suture placement in sclera. If perforation has caused retinal break, the area should be cryoed and covered with scleral buckle.

4. *Drainage complications:* A dry tap can occur if there is incomplete perforation of choroid. In that case, a deeper puncture can be given. Retinal break or incarceration can occur if the needle strikes the retina in a case of shallow SRF.

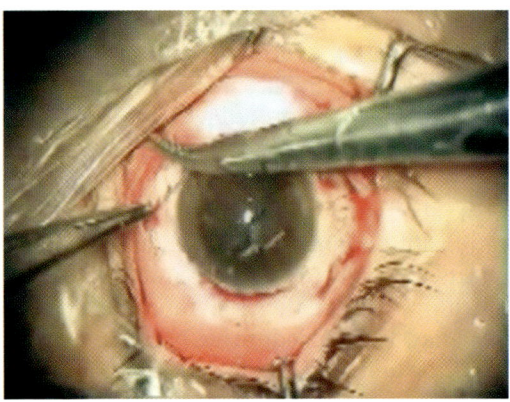

Fig. 25.33I *Closure of conjunctiva*

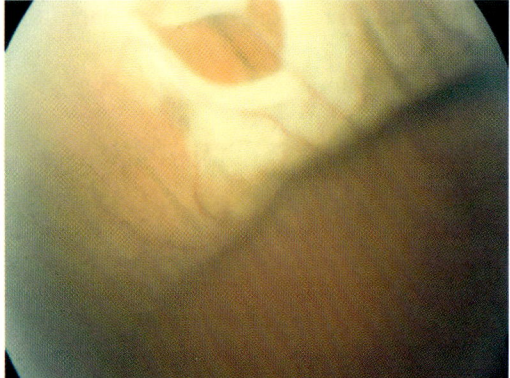

Fig. 25.33J *Buckle effect as seen by indirect ophthalmo-scopy after the surgery in a case with settled RD*

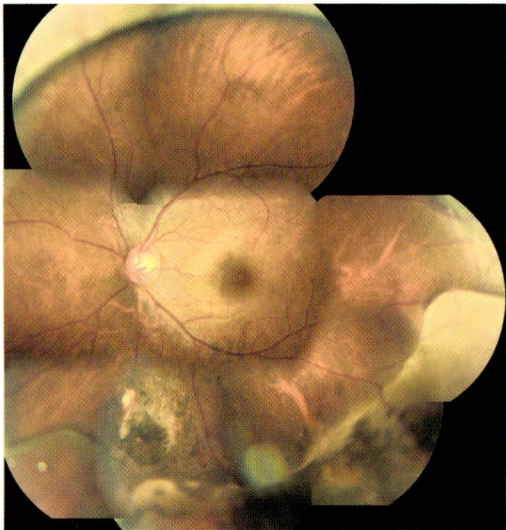

Fig. 25.33K *Attached retina after buckling procedure*

This area again should be cryoed and supported with a buckle.

Choroidal hemorrhage is the most feared complication of SRF drainage. If this occurs, the blood enters into subretinal space may gravitate unto fovea. To minimize bleeding, the draining site may be indented for a few minutes with a cotton bud and the eye may be rotated to place the drainage site as inferior as possible. Incases of large amount of subretinal hemorrhage under fovea, pars plana vitrectomy surgery with internal drainage of blood may be required.

B. Postoperative complications

They may occur from early to late postoperative period.

1. *Glaucoma:* Angle closure glaucoma may occur manifested by increased IOP, corneal edema and shallowing of peripheral angle. It occurs due to shallow detachment of ciliary body secondary to serous fluid in supra-choroidal space. It results in anterior displacement of ciliary body and angle closure. Initial management consists of medical therapy. Laser iridotomy can be done in failed cases.

2. *Anterior segment ischemia:* It is characterized by stromal edema, fibrinous anterior chamber reaction elevated intraocular pressure and occasionally a shallow anterior chamber. Late changes include iris atrophy and cataract. Mild cases may respond to topical and systemic steroids. In severe cases it may be necessary to release the knot of encircling band. Anterior segment ischemic is caused by venous obstruction by the encircling band.

3. *Infection and extrusion:* Buckle materials act as foreign bodies and are at risk of infection and extrusion. This may occur a few weeks to a few year after surgery. Signs of buckle infection include pain, purulent discharge, conjunctival congesion, granuloma formation, subconjunctival hemorrhage, tenderness and buckle exposure or partial extrusion. Topical and systemic antibiotics rarely resolve infection and the curative treatment involves removal of all buckle materials and sutures (Fig. 25.34).

4. *Choroidal detachment:* Collection of serous fluid in the suprachoroidal space is called choroidal detachement. In RD surgery, it is primarily caused by vortex vein obstruction.

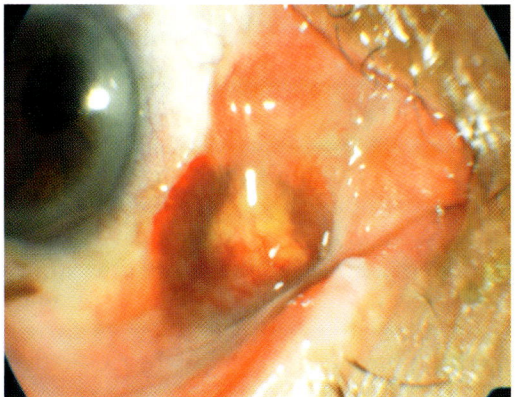

Fig. 25.34 *Postoperative complication of buckle infection*

Drainage of subretinal fluid is another factors leading to hypotony and choroidal detachment. Choroidal detachment usually appears 2 to 4 days after surgery and resolve readily with systemic steroids given for 2–3 weeks. Massive choroidals may require surgical drainage (Fig. 25.35).

5. *Proliferative viteoretinopathy:* See p-432.

II. PNEUMATIC RETINOPEXY

Scleral buckling (SB) is the most favoured surgical technique for retinal detachment with PVR up to C1 with a success rate of about 75 to 80%. However, this surgery involves hospita-lization, tissue trauma, some known complica-tions and higher cost. Pneumatic retinopexy is considered in indicated cases in order to minimize these problems.

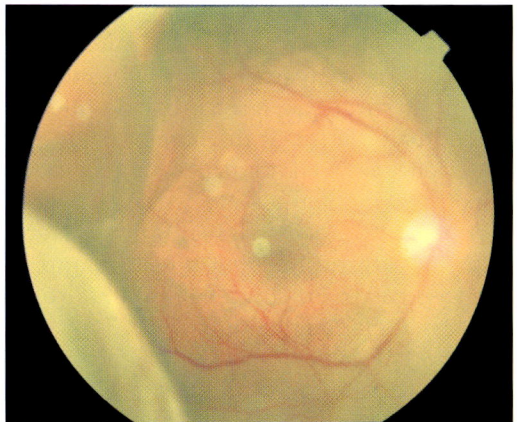

Fig. 25.35 *Choroidal detachment after buckling procedure*

In contrast to SB it is an outpatient procedure and consists of an intravitreal gas injection (C3F8/SF6) with transconjunctival cryopexy or laser photocoagulation, followed by appropriate head positioning.

It is indicated for cases with superior single break above the horizontal meridian without significant vitreoretinal traction and PVR. The results are said to be comparable to scleral buckling and morbidity is less and visual results are better. This procedure has been popularized by Hilton and Grizzard in 1986.

Case selection

Following cases are usually excluded:

i. Breaks larger than one clock hour or multiple breaks.

ii. Breaks in inferior four clock hours.

iii. Presence of PVR grade C or D.

iv. Physical disability or mental incompetence precluding maintenance of the required head positioning.

v. Severe or uncontrolled glaucoma.

vi. Cloudy media precluding full assessment of retina.

Procedure

Under topical anesthesia the break is cryoed, the conjunctival culde sac is sterilized with betadine solution. Paracentasis is performed. 0.4 to 0.6 ml SF6 gas (undiluted) is injected in one bolus. Ocular massage is carried out and if the need be second paracentasis is performed so that the IOP is with in range. Head position-ing is instructed depending upon the site of break. Antibiotic drops are instilled and eye is patched for few hours. Postoperatively the patient is examined on first or second, fifth and fourteenth postoperative day and periodically thereafter. The gas bubble absorbs by 14th day and patient can resume work after that, however, he is advised not to fly during this period otherwise rise of IOP can bother him.

The success rate is about 80% and in failed cases scleral buckling can be performed. Failed pneumatic retinopexy requiring scleral buckling does not adversely affect the final visual out-come, compared with scleral buckling alone.

Complications

a. Formation of new breaks and missed breaks occur in about 13–14%.
b. PVR is the other major complication and the incidence is close to 4%.
c. Subretinal gas is usually a preventable complication. While injecting precaution should be taken to inject in a bolus and avoid fish egging.

III. PRIMARY VITRECTOMY IN RD

Sofar primary vitrectomies have been perfor-med only for complicated cases of RD as under:
  i. RD with PVR C2, C3 and D grade.
 ii. RD with giant retinal tear.
iii. RD with multiple breaks.
 iv. RD with posterior breaks.
  v. Failed scleral buckle.
 vi. Combined tractional and rhegmatogenous RD.
vii. RD with nonclearing vitreous hemorrhage.

However, with better expertise, improvised equipment and instruments and introduction of wide angle viewing system, the indications of primary vitrectomy have broadened to even less complicated cases where routine scleral buckling technique so far was being employed.

The rationale of primary vitrectomy is that it can take care of vitreoretinal traction by near complete removal of vitreous, thus it allows the retina to settle. PPV is followed by fluid air exchange and subsequently air is exchanged with 20% SF6 or 15% C3F8 gas after lasering all the breaks.

The placement of an encircling 240 band depends upon the preference of the individual surgeon. Some expert surgeons who can remove the entire vitreous even from its base find the encircling band redundant whereas the other conservative surgeons find it useful to offset any residual vitreoretinal traction. However, sofar 240 encircling band application is still an open debate.

Complications

Most frequent intraoperative complications of primary vitrectomy are iatrogenic retinal breaks (6%) and iatrogenic lens damage (3%). In addition the development of a nuclear cataract is already a known late complication of PPV. The other posterior segment complications are macular pucker (0–18%), CME (17%). Needless to mention that there can be rarer complications like endophthalmitis and CRA occlusion asso-ciated with raised IOP due to gas temponade.

Success rate

It is comparable in primary vitrectomy versus scleral buckling (80%). However, visual results are better in primary vitrectomy group.

Nevertheless keeping iatrogenic complica-tions of primary vitrectomy in mind there is general concensus that primary vitrectomy in regular cases where buckling is an option should be reserved for aphakic, pseudophakic detachments or in phakic detachments of elderly age group.

PROPHYLAXIS OF RETINAL DETACHMENT

FACTOR TO BE CONSIDERED

In the absence of prospective, randomized long term clinical trials for prevention of RD, there is hardly any concensus of protocol of prophylaxis. However, frequently followed guidelines in the selection of the patients for prophylactic therapy depend upon the following factors:
• Risk factor of RD
• Precursors of RD
• Characteristics of breaks.

A. Risk Factor of RD

1. Pathological myopia.
2. Aphakia and pseudophakia.
3. Patient with family history of RD.
4. Patient with h/o RD in the other eye.
5. Patients undergoing YAG capsulotomy.
6. Patients with prior ocular trauma.
7. Patients with systemic disease like Marfan's, Stickler and Ehlers-Danlos syndromes.
8. Patients with CMV retinitis and acute retinal necrosis.

B. Precursors of RD

Peripheral retinal degenerations like lattice, snailtrack, white without pressure, retinoschisis and cystic retinal tufts are the lesions which predispose the eye to RD.

C. Characteristics of break

i. Traction tears like horse shoe breaks, tiny flap tears and operculated breaks are more prone to cause RD than atrophic small round holes since the former are associated with dynamic vitreoretinal traction.

ii. Larger breaks are more dangerous than small ones.

iii. Breaks located in superior quadrants are more likely to progress to RD than breaks in the inferior quadrants, obviously because of the effect of gravity. Equatorial breaks are more dangerous than breaks near ora since the latter are supported by vitreous base.

iv. Symptoms associated with break are flashes and floaters and the presence of these symptoms imply that these are possibly tractional tears, e.g. horse-shoe, operculated breaks and tiny flap tears. Thus a symptomatic break needs urgent attention since it may end up in RD.

GUIDELINES FOR PROPHYLAXIS

- Symptomatic breaks with or without high risk factors, with or without precursors of RD require immediate prophylactic treatment. The urgency of treatment is even more, if it is a horse-shoe tears, located in superior quadrant, the size is larger and is associated with cuff of subretinal fluid around it.

- The findings of an operculated symptomatic break also demands treatment, however, if it becomes asymptomatic after the separation of operculum (no more causing traction) it may be followed up since the possibility of causation of RD is quite low.

- Atrophic round holes in the presence of signs and symptoms of acute PVD should undergo prophylactic treatment.

- Asymptomatic breaks with either high risk factors or with precursors of RD must be treated particularly if these are tractional and located superiorly.

- Asymptomatic breaks which are atrophic and round in shape, without high risk factors and without precursors of RD, located near ora may be followed up with the caution that the patient should report back in case he develops symptoms. Location of the breaks near ora is safe since vitreous base support these holes.

- Break of any type, size and location in the fellow eye of a patient of RD must receive prophylactic treatment. The treatment is all the more imperative if the fellow eye happens to be aphakic or pseudophakic since these eyes are prone to have RD (14 to 40%).

- Fellow eye of patient of RD undergoing cataract extraction must receive prophylactic therapy if on indirect ophthalmoscopy symptomatic or asymptomatic break is found.

- Fellow eye of patient of RD with giant retinal ear must receive 360° barrage laser particularly if vitreous is liquefied and there is white without pressure lesion.

- Small inner layer holes in retinoschisis carry an extremely low risk of RD since there is no communication between vitreous cavity and subretinal space. However, both layer breaks may warrant prophylaxis.

- In the absence of risk factors and breaks neither lattice nor snail track degeneration require prophylactic treatment.

- The prophylactic treatment can be carried out by both laser therapy or cryopexy, however, for posterior breaks laser is preferred and for anterior breaks cryotherapy is preferred.

PROLIFERATIVE VITREORETINOPATHY

INTRODUCTION

Proliferative vitreoretinopathy (PVR) is a clinical syndrome associated with growth and contraction of cellular membranes within vitreous cavity and on both the surfaces of retina after rhegmatogenous retinal detachment (RD). It is a natural process of healing and bringing back the retina to its bed but it misfires and instead produces spectrum of changes in the retina starting from subtle retinal wrinkling, rolled out edges of the retinal breaks, fixed star folds, rigid retinal detachment, retinal shortening and advanced periretinal proliferation. It is the most common cause of recurrent RD that is estimated to be 5–11% after successful RD surgery which occur due to contraction of these membranes, thereby reopening the breaks or creating new breaks. In addition PVR can occur after severe penetrating trauma of posterior segment of the eye, after which the risk of PVR is estimated at 25%.

PATHOPHYSIOLOGY

- The vitreous compartment normally is devoid of cells with the exception of a few hyalocytes. It is protected from outside invasion by intact internal limiting membrane of the retina and from cytokines and chemoattractants by the intact blood retinal barriers.

- The occurrence of retinal break is the beginning of cascade of events in the process of PVR. It brings subretinal space in direct contact with vitreous compartment. There occurs proliferation and migration of viable retinal pigment epithelial cells (RPE) through the break into the vitreous cavity. In addition to RPE cells, glial cells and inflammatory cell also follow. They multiply and grow along both over and under surface of retina and within the vitreous gel.

- These cells have contractile property thereby exerting traction directly on the retina or through the vitreous gel leading to more new retinal breaks and retinal traction. Traction is the key feature in the pathogenesis of PVR which may vary substantially in location extent and severity.

- Breakdown of the blood retinal barrier is another key feature associated with PVR which occur simultaneously with RD. This causes increased cytokine release, influx of inflammatory cells and chemoattractant proteins and resultant inflammation.

- PVR most frequently occurs in the inferior retina which is believed to be a result of gravity whereby RPE and inflammatory cells liberated into vitreous cavity via retinal breaks settle on the inferior retina.

- Macular pucker seen after successful RD surgery can be considered as a mild form of PVR.

- Intraoperative use of cryo, laser and trauma associated with scleral buckling procedure all leads to intraocular inflammation and breakdown of blood-retinal barrier. The breakdown of blood-retinal barrier and mobilization of viable RPE cells are caused less by laser therapy than by crypoapplication. Thus laser induces less PVR changes as compared to cryotherapy.

RISK FACTORS FOR DEVELOPMENT OF PVR

PVR either develops in untreated rhegmatogenous RD or in eyes with recent repair of rhegmatogenous RD. However, there are some RDs which are more prone to have PVR changes than the other types of RDs. The risk factors are as under:

1. Eyes with large retinal breaks or giant retinal tears. Large breaks allow more migration of viable RPE cells.

2. Vitreous hemorrhage associated with RD appear to stimulate more PVR changes.

3. RDs larger then 2 quadrants are more prone to PVR.

4. Eyes with chronic rhegmatogenous RDs often spontaneously develop PVR.

5. Patients with uveitis or increased inflammation from trauma are at increased risk of having PVR.

6. RD surgery with use of cryo itself appears to hasten PVR changes and the risk is greatest about 2 month after RD repair.

7. Postoperative choroidal detachment may predispose the eye to developing PVR.

8. Excess cryotherapy of large retinal breaks because of release of more viable RPE cells and breakdown of blood retinal barrier produce an environment favorable to the development of PVR.

9. RDs associated with systemic diseases such as Diabetes, Jansen syndrome, Stickler syndrome, Marfan syndrome and familial exudative vitreoretinopathy are more prone to have PVR.

DIAGNOSIS OF PVR

- The diagnosis of PVR in the presence of rhegmatogenous RD is made by indirect ophthalmoscopy and slit lamp biomicroscopy with +78D or +90D lens or a corneal contact lens.

- Early signs of PVR are subtle and include dispersion of cells in the vitreous and on the retinal surface (Fig. 25.23). The latter proliferate to form localized fibrocellular membranes appearing as whitish opacification with small wrinkles and subsequently fixed folds of the retina.

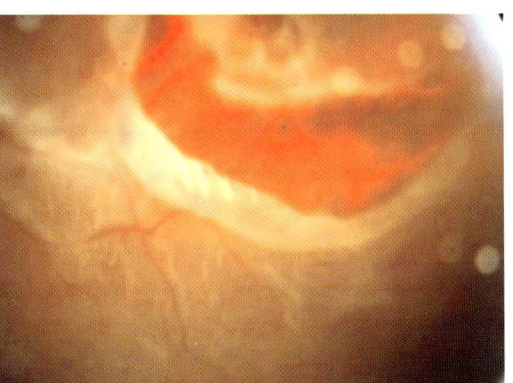

Fig. 25.36 *Horse shoe break with rolled out edges (PVR grade B)*

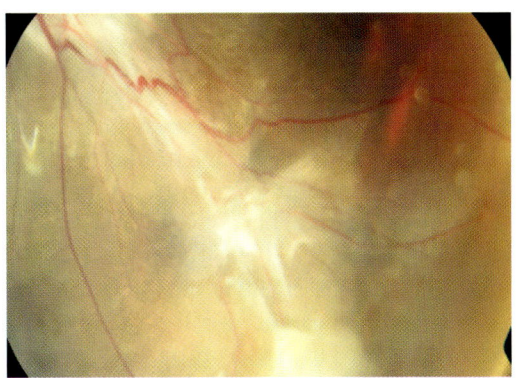

Fig. 25.37 *Startfold of the retina in one quadrant (PVR grade C1)*

- Involvement of the edge of the retinal break can lead to localized contraction and a rolled posterior edge (Fig. 25.36).
- More extensive PVR has fixed retinal folds initially in the inferior quadrants and fine membranes bridging the folds leading to the decreased mobility of the detached retina (Fig. 25.37).
- Advanced PVR results in the formation of a funnel shaped retinal detachment with contracted equatorial membranes. In some cases anterior traction at the vitreous base draws retina forward towards the ciliary body or detaches ora serrata (Fig. 25.38 to 25.40).
- In eyes with opaque media, B scan ultrasonography shows high intensity echo with a 'V' shape funnel attached to the optic nerve head and retinal stiffness during ocular movements (Kinetic ultrasonography) are strongly suggestive of a retinal detachment with PVR.

CLASSIFICATION OF PVR

The first and the most commonly used classification system remains the one that was published by the Retina Society Terminology Committee in 1983. It is popular probably because of its simplicity. It classifies the appearance of PVR on the basis of clinical signs and geographic distribution into four grades (Table 25.5 and Figs 25.36 to 25.40).

Drawbacks

- It ignores the anteroposterior locations of epiretinal proliferation and hence the importance of anterior traction in PVR.
- It is also a static classification that says nothing about the degree of cellular proliferative activity at the time of the grading.

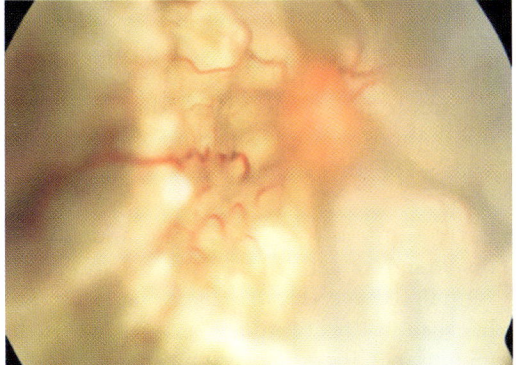

Fig. 25.38 *Open funnel RD depicting PVR grade D1*

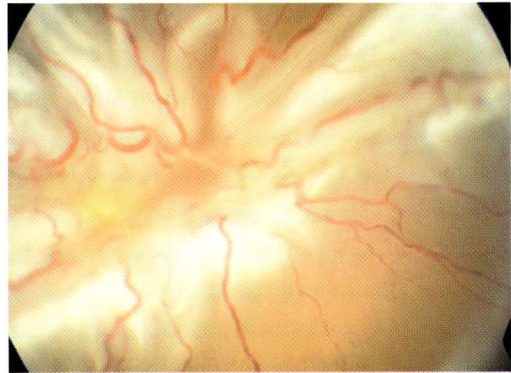

Fig. 25.39 *Narrow funnel RD depicting PVR grade D2, disc visible*

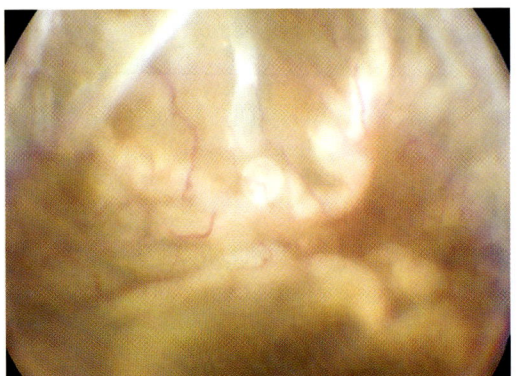

Fig. 25.40 *Closed funnel RD, disc not visible depicting PVR grade D3*

The revised classification of PVR of 1991 took into account more detailed information about the location, extent and severity of PVR and hence is more useful especially for clinical trials (Tables 25.6 and 25.7). Further modifications of the classification of PVR (1989) onwards were proposed as part of the multicenter controlled trial of silicone oil (SO) as an adjunct treatment for PVR but it was found to be more complex and less reproducible between different examiners than the more simplified Retina Society classification (1983) (Tables 25.8 and 25.9). *Thus Retina Society classification still remains the most popular in grading PVR* since it correlated well with prognosis demonstrating a trend towards poorer outcome with increasing severity from stages C3 through D3 PVR.

TREATMENT

Surgery is the mainstay of treatment of PVR. Surgical principles are as under:

1. Belt-buckle (240 band) to support the vitreous base up to PVR grade C, however, high buckle encirclage may be considered (277 tire) with extensive PVR grade D.
2. Complete or near complete vitrectomy.
3. Removal of membranes to relieve traction on retina.
4. Localization and treatment of breaks and supporting them with segmental buckle.
5. Intraocular tamponade either by long acting gas or silicone oil.

Basic operative steps in treating eyes with PVR

It is obvious that for treating patients of rhegmatogenous RD with PVR grade C1 and higher grade both scleral suckling as well as pars plana vitrectomy (PPV) is required. Till recently 20G PPV was being performed, but with advancement in technology, availability of superior instrumentation and better vitrectomy machines having sensitive control of fluidics and higher cut rate, the 23G sutureless PPV is becoming surgical technique of choice. In addition vitrectomy for PVR should be performed under operating microscope preferably using wide angle viewing system since it helps in complete removal of vitreous and fibrocellular membranes (Fig. 25.41)

Table 25.5 *Retina society PVR classification (1983)*	
Grade (stage)	*Characteristics*
A	Vitreous haze, vitreous pigment clumps
B	Wrinkling of the inner retinal surface, rolled edge of retinal break, retinal stiffness, vessel tortuosity
C	Full-thickness retinal folds in
C–1	One quadrant
C–2	Two quadrants
C–3	Three quadrants
D	Fixed retinal folds in four quadrants
D–1	Wide funnel shape
D–2	Narrow funnel shape (anterior end of funnel visible by indirect ophthalmoscopy with 20 diopter lens)
D–3	Closed funnel (optic nerve head not visible)

Table 25.6 *Updated proliferative vitreoretinopathy grade classification (1991)*

Grade	Feature
A	Vitreous haze, vitreous pigment clumps, pigment clusters on inferior retina.
B	Wrinkling of the inner retinal surface, retinal stiffness, vessel tortuosity, rolled and irregular edge of retinal break, decreased mobility of vitreous.
CP 1–12	Posterior to equator, focal, diffuse or circumferential full-thickness folds, *subretinal strands.
CA 1–12	Anterior to equator, focal, diffuse, or circumferential full-thickness folds, *subretinal strands, *anterior displacement, *condensed vitreous strands.

*Expressed in the total number of clock-hours involved

Table 25.7 *Updated proliferative vitreoretinopathy contraction type classification (1991)*

Type	Location (in relation to equator)	Features
Focal	Posterior	Starfold posterior to vitreous base
Diffuse	Posterior	Confluent star folds posterior to vitreous base; optic disc may not be visible
Subretinal	Posterior/anterior	Proliferation under the retina; annular strand near disc; linear strands; motheaten-appearing sheets
Circumferential	Anterior	Contraction along posterior edge of vitreous base with central displacement of the retina; peripheral retina stretched; posterior retina in radial folds
Anterior	Anterior	Vitreous base pulled anteriorly by proliferative tissue; peripheral retinal trough; displacement ciliary processes may be stretched, may be covered by membrane; iris may be retracted

Table 25.8 *Silicone study classifications system for proliferative vitreoretinopathy*

Grade	Clinical signs
A	Vitreous haze, vitreous pigment clumps.
B	Inner retinal wrinkling, rolled edge of retinal breaks.
CP	

P1: 1 quadrant (1–3 clock hr)
   P2: 2 quadrant (4–6 clock hr)
   P3: 3 quadrant (7–9 clock hr)
   P4: 4 quadrant (10–12 clock hr)
	Starfolds and/or diffuse contraction and/or subretinal membrane in posterior retina.

CA	

A1: 1 quadrant (1–3 clock hr)
   A2: 2 quadrant (4–6 clock hr)
   A3: 3 quadrant (7–9 clock hr)
   A4: 4 quadrant (10–12 clock hr)
	Circumferential and/or perpendicular and/or anterior traction in anterior retina

1. Conjunctiva is opened by creating 360° peritomy (Fig. 25.33A).
2. 4–0 black silk stay sutures are looped to bridle all the four recti (Fig. 25.33B).
3. The location of retinal breaks and extent of epiretinal proliferation (PVR) is noted by indirect ophthalmoscopy (Fig. 25.33C).
4. Depending upon the severity of PVR either 240 belt-buckle or buckle encirclage by silicone tire (277/287) is fixed at the equator

Table 25.9. *Silicone study classification of contraction type in proliferative vitreoretinopathy*

Type number	Contraction type	Location of PVR	Summary of clinical signs
1.	Focal	Posterior	Starfold
2.	Diffuse	Posterior	Confluent irregular retinal folds in posterior retina; remainder of retina drawn posterior; optic disk may not be visible
3.	Subretinal	Posterior	"Napkin ring" around disc, "clothes line" elevation of retina
4.	Circumferential	Anterior	Irregular retinal folds in the anterior retina; series of radial folds more posteriorly; peripheral retina within vitreous base stretched inward
5.	Perpendicular	Anterior	Smooth circumferential fold of retina at insertion of posterior hyaloid
6.	Anterior	Anterior	Circumferential fold of retina at insertion of pulled forward; trough of peripheral retina anteriorly; cilliary processes stretched with possible hypotony; iris retracted

by applying four sutures in the four quadrants which is technically easier before the actual vitrectomy (Fig. 25.33F and G). Tire has the additional advantage of supporting

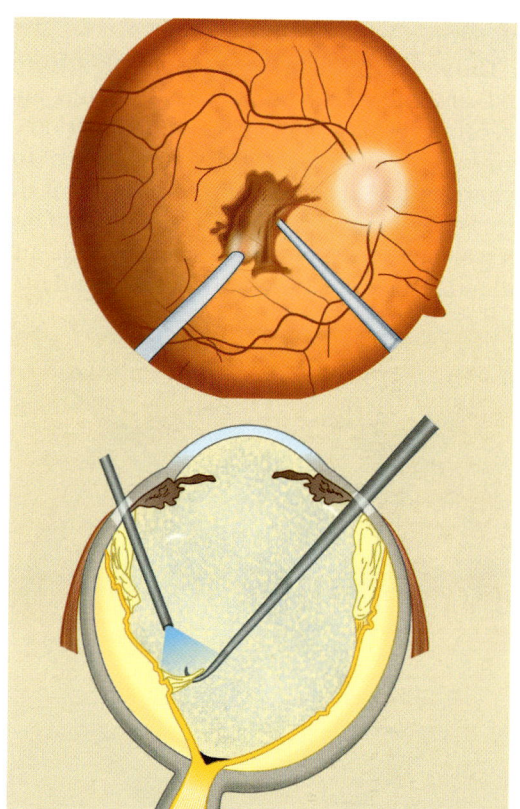

Fig. 25.41 *Diagrammatic representation of peeling of membrane during PPV*

peripheral breaks. Some surgeons prefer to thread the buckle around the equator of the eye before vitrectomy but do not tie the sutures until later in the surgical procedure which is mostly before air-silicone oil exchange.

5. Then the vitrectomy infusion cannula is sutured to the sclera and its entry into vitreous cavity is confirmed. Additional sclerotomy sites are made for fiberoptic light pipe and the vitreous cutter at 10 and 2 o'clock position 3.5 to 4 mm behind the limbus.

6. Lensectomy is performed if the lens is too opaque to allow visualization of retina and epiretinal membranes.

7. Virectomy is then performed with removal of the central and posterior vitreous. Almost all eyes with PVR have posterior vitreous detachment (PVD). Peripheral vitreous is then removed, care being taken not to create any iatrogenic retinal break.

8. Posterior epiretinal membranes are removed first followed by stabilization of retina with perfluorocarbon liquid (PFCL). Subsequently anterior membranes are peeled off with a pick, forceps or both (Fig. 25.41).

9. Location of breaks are noted and any traction around these is relieved and are marked with diathermy which make their identification easier after fluid-air exchange.

10. Once retina is relieved of all anterior and posterior traction, PFCL is removed and then

fluid-air exchange is performed preferably through a posterior supranasal retinotomy or a pre-existing break (Fig. 25.42).

11. Laser photocoagulation is then applied around all the retinal breaks and around retinotomy by endolaser probe.

12. The scleral buckle is tied to create moderate to high buckle effect depending upon the severity of PVR.

13. Air is exchanged with either long acting gas such as 15% perfluoropropane (C3 F8) or with 1000 centistoke (CS) silicone oil. In case air silicone oil exchange is decided and it is an aphakic eye, then iridectomy at 6 o'clock (Ando's iridectomy) is performed with vitreous cutter in order to avoid post-operative rise of intraocular pressure (IOP). In severe cases of PVR, 5000 CS silicone oil may be used. IOP is monitored manually by palpating the cornea.

14. Sclerotomies are closed with sutures in case of 20G PPV. However, the sclerostomies are self sealing in 23G vitrectomy, nevertheless the sealing must be ensured. Not to use subconjunctival injection in case of 23G vitrectomy which may interfere with the sealing of sclerotomies.

Intraocular tamponade

As mentioned above there are two choices of intraocular tamponade in eyes with PVR. The one is long acting gas in a nonexpansile mixture of 15 to 20% (C3F8) and the other is silicone oil. However, in general when tamponade is required for <4 weeks C3F8 is used and when >4 weeks of tamponade is desired silicone oil (SO) is used. Nevertheless many surgeons prefer SO to gas because it results in less postoperative inflammation, quicker rehabilitation and few reoperations. The use of heavier than water fluorinated 5000 centistokes SO versus 1000 centistokes SO can also improve inferior retinal tamponade especially in severe cases of PVR, and it is increasingly being used.

Silicone oil is associated with poor post-operative vision because of markedly different refractive index and owing to configuration of its anterior surface in aphakic, phakic and pseudophakic eyes. In aphakic eye its convex anterior surface acts as plus lens making the eye myopic while in phakic and pseudophakic eyes the anterior surface of the SO is concave acting as a minus lens and thus makes the eye hyperopic.

The wound-healing sequence of PVR matures like any other scar tissue over 3 months and therefore, SO is left in for at least that period of time. The eye is carefully monitored for recurrent traction and retinal breaks but if the eye is quiet and all peripheral retinal pathology is well supported by a high scleral buckle and all retinal breaks are closed, silicone liquid may

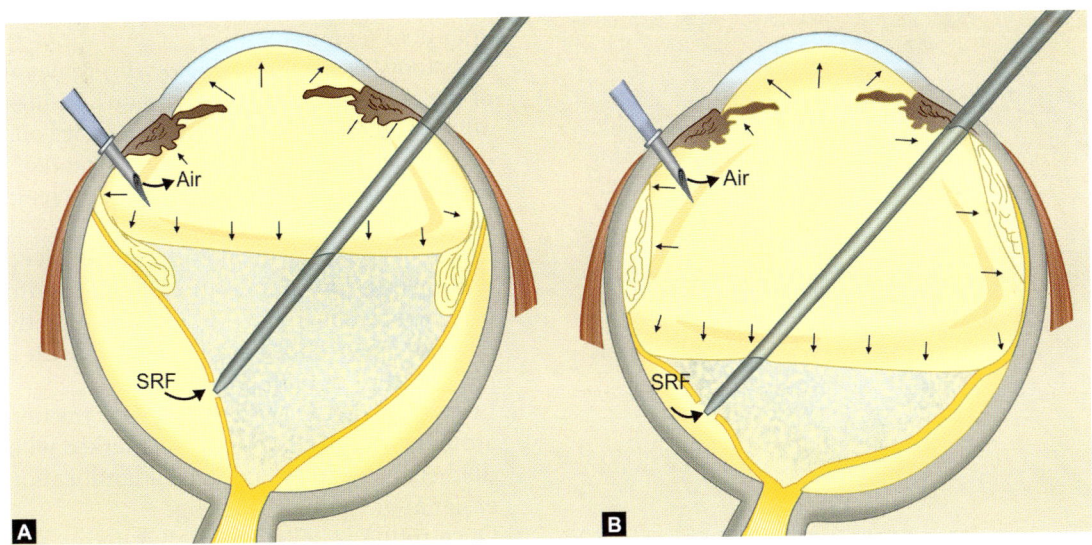

Fig. 25.42 *Fluid air exchange through supranasal retinotomy*

be removed after approximately 3 months. 360° barrage laser posterior to the encircling buckle may decrease the risk of retinal redetachment after silicone oil removal which have been reported to be as high as 20%.

Advantages and disadvantages of perfluoropropane gas versus silicone oil tamponade for proliferative vitreoretinopathy

Perfluoropropane Gas

Advantages
- Absorbs spontaneously, giving temporary tamponade to retina.
- Can control duration of tamponade from intermediate to long duration by adjusting concentration of C3F8 with air.
- Visual rehabilitation occurs more rapidly in eyes with PVR treated with gas.
- Relatively few long-term complications associated with use.

Disadvantages
- Does not last long enough to provide tamponade needed for eyes with epiretinal reproliferation 6–8 weeks after surgery.
- Air travel prohibited until bubble gets absorbed.
- Cataract formation if prone positioning not maintained.
- Some short-term complications, such as elevated intraocular pressure.
- Hypotony more likely postoperatively.

Silicone Oil

Advantages
- Provides extended tamponade for months or years, allowing surgeon to determine if and when to remove silicone oil.
- The best tamponade for eyes with numerous retinal tears or large retinectomies.
- Better in achieving partial retinal reattachment in eyes with residual traction or reproliferation
- No restrictions on air travel.
- Better tamponade for eyes with hypotony.

Disadvantages
- Does not prevent reproliferation in inferior retina.
- Visual acuity slow to improve and causes substantial changes in refraction.

- Corneal toxicity.
- Cataract formation in phakic eyes.
- Silicone oil emulsification.
- Elevated intraocular pressure.
- Must be removed by a second surgical procedure to achieve best acuity.

Postoperative management

The patient should be instructed to remain in prone position for at least the first 24 hours after gas or SO exchange to allow the retinal pigment epithelium to pump out any remaining subretinal fluid and to facilitate initial adhesion at the sites of photocoagulation or cryotherapy. Many surgeons insist on prone positioning for a much longer duration, up to 7–10 days, especially if there are inferior retinal breaks. A rise in intraocular pressure is very frequent and hence should be monitored regularly. Patients should avoid sleeping on their back as this allows the light SO to move forward away from the retinal surface and possibly into the anterior chamber. Shallowing of the anterior chamber may also occur. Corticosteroid, mydriatic and cycloplegic drops are usually used four times a day for 3–4 weeks and the patient may in addition require anti-glaucoma drops and acetazolamide tablets for postopera-tive ocular hypertension. If orbital swelling and pain occur in the absence of a high intraocular pressure, oral prednisolone should also be given in addition to the routine analgesics.

Complications
- Intraoperative
- Early postoperative
- Late postoperative

A. Intraoperative complications
1. The most common complication of PVR surgery is the creation of iatrogenic retinal breaks during dissection. A careful dissection can avoid these. More important is to recognize these breaks, relieve all the tractions and treat these breaks with endolaser after fluid air exchange.
2. Intraoperative bleeding may occur during dissection of dense membranes and during creation of a retinotomy and this is controlled by raising the infusion pressure temporarily and by using endodiathermy.

3. The view may also become obscured by intraoperative corneal edema, pupillary constriction, or lens clouding. The corneal epithelium can be scraped clearing the view. The pupil can be redilated either with 1:10000 epinephrine in the vitrectomy infusion fluid, iris hooks can be used, or rarely iridectomy/sphincterotomy using the vitreous cutter can be done. Rarely, lens clouding during the operation would necessitate a 20G fragmatome lensectomy via pars plana. More often a layer of blood or cellular debris forms on the anterior or posterior surface of lens which can be removed by painting the posterior surface with methyl cellulose and anterior chamber paracentesis.

4. During surgery air or heavy fluid perfluoro-carbons or SO may pass through a retinal break and then subretinally. Passage of air into subretinal space indicates residual traction which must be relieved. This may require further dissection and large retinotomy.

5. Choroidal hemorrhagic detachment may occur intraoperatively by accidental rupture of a choroidal vessel when placing scleral sutures or spontaneously in a susceptible eye if prolonged hypotony occurs. This is treated by the temporary injection of heavy liquid perfluorocarbon in the vitreous followed by external drainage of blood through a radial sclerotomy. Sometimes a choroidal detachment cannot be drained during the surgery and requires a repeat visit to the operation theatre a few days later.

6. Serous choroidal detachment may occur but is usually due to a malpositioned infusion cannula under the retina or in the supra-choroidal space. This is managed by transferring the infusion to another port and ensuring the entry of the infusion cannula in the vitreous cavity.

B. Early postoperative complications

1. Elevated intraocular pressure is the most commonly, occurring early postoperative complication. A rise to about 25 mmHg is treated conservatively with ocular anti-hypertensive drops and oral acetazolamide.

If higher than this, it is often due to angle closure with a forward shift of the iris diaphragm or overfill of the eye with gas or SO. In aphakic eyes filled with silicone, a pressure rise may be due to an incomplete inferior iridectomy. An overfill of intraocular gas can be readily dealt with as an office procedure with removal of around 0.2 cc through the pars plana with a 30G needle and syringe. Removal of SO is more difficult and requires a trip back to the operating room. Rarely it is because of tight belt-buckle which needs to be loosened.

2. Postoperative inflammation is common following extensive vitreoretinal surgery and fibrin may occlude the pupil or cover the posterior surface of the intraocular lens. This is treated with intensive topical and some-times systemic steroids.

3. Incomplete fill of gas can occur due to mixing errors or leakage through a sclerotomy site. It may be topped up or if the subretinal fluid persists, can be replaced with SO.

4. An incomplete fill of SO with associated fluid inferiorly may require reoperation with top-up of the oil and internal drainage of the residual fluid or possibly supplementation with an injection of heavy silicone liquid.

5. A persistent corneal epithelial defect particularly after the epithelium has been removed from a cloudy cornea during surgery may require extended patching and antibiotic ointment.

6. Endophthalmitis is very rare but since this is a prolonged operation with insertion of multiple instruments, it must always be considered a possibility. The standard injection of intravitreal antibiotics is complicated by the presence of intravitreal gas or silicone which prevent the intravitreal antibiotics from diffusing freely in the vitreous. This could be removed and prescribed antibiotics injected in the vitreous.

C. Late postoperative complications

1. Between one-fourth to one-half of eyes undergoing PVR surgery develop recurrent retinal detachment mostly because of reopening of an existing break or formation of new break.

2. Perisilicone oil proliferation occurs inferiorly because of meniscus of vitreous fluid between the inferior meniscus of SO and retinal surface. This occurs because SO is lighter and floats in the vitreous cavity in the incompletely filled eye. Vitreous fluid being rich in mitogens stimulate severe proliferation inferiorly. This leads to recurrent RD requiring repeat vitreous surgery. It is minimized by complete fill of vitreous cavity with SO.

3. Emulsification of SO into fine bubbles is common, especially with the lower-viscosity (1000 CS) material and particularly if it has been mixed with inflammatory proteins or blood and in eyes that are aphakic with an incomplete fill where there is a constant fluid/oil surface interaction. This can block the angle and lead to late secondary glaucoma. SO in the anterior chamber can also damage corneal endothelial function and eventually lead to bullous keratopathy. Emulsified SO is seen as milky white material in the Juperior part of anterior chamber with sharp horizontal lower level termed as reverse hypopyon (hyperoleon) (Fig. 25.43).

4. Cataract is universal in phakic eyes following vitrectomy and extended silicone tamponade. Phacoemulsification of cataract and intracapsular lens implantation can be done and the silicone oil can be removed at the same sitting.

5. Rubeosis of the iris is occasionally seen following surgery but is uncommon unless the patient already has coexisting diabetic retinopathy. It is more likely where there is recurrent persisting retinal detachment and intraocular inflammation. This can be managed by injecting a vascular endothelial growth factor blocker.

6. Late cystoid macular edema with or without preretinal membranes or epiretinal membranes can occur after vitrectomy and can be managed by topical steroid and nonsteroidal drops, intravitreal triamcinolone injection or internal limiting membrane peeling.

7. The scleral buckle may erode through the conjunctiva and lead to chronic low-grade infection.

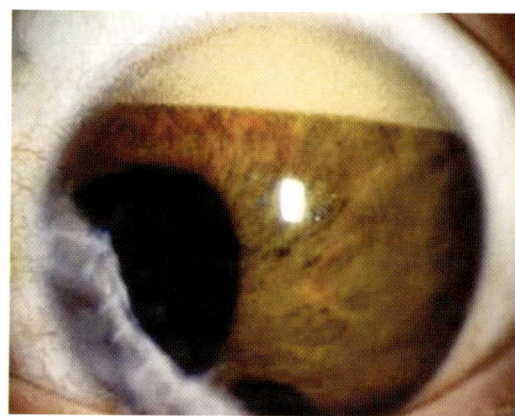

Fig. 25.43 *Emulsified silicone oil in AC seen as reverse hypopyon*

8. Scarring around the muscles due to the buckle may lead to squint and double vision.
9. Sympathetic ophthalmia is considered as a rare complication.

Adjunctive medical therapy for PVR

- A number of pharmacologic agents have been tried in an effort to inhibit proliferation that leads to PVR.
- Intravitreal and sub-Tenon's injection of long-acting triamcinolone have been investigated. This can decrease the inflammatory cascade and hence diminish the stimulus to cellular proliferation and contraction. Intravitreal triamcinolone acetonide is the most favored agent of those studied and it is increasingly being used as an adjunct during surgery to delaminate the vitreous and membranes that may not be visible with the usual operative systems of illumination. Hopefully, a beneficial dose persists even after vitreous replacement or else triamcinolone can also be injected into the SO for slow release. However, it will require periodic monitoring of IOP.
- Antiproliferative agents such as 5-fluorouracil and daunomycin have been evaluated but unfortunately the therapeutic window between inhibition of fibroblastic tissue proliferation and toxicity to the surrounding neuronal cells has not been sufficient enough to demonstrate a clinical benefit in humans.
- The many factors involved in the pathogenesis of PVR, for example, platelet-derived growth factor and connective tissue growth factor, will

probably one day provide a suitable target for a more specific intervention in the process. Genetic variations in patients with PVR, for example, an association with the gene linked to tumor necrosis factor are starting to emerge. Hopefully, clinical trials to block specific biologics using humanized antibodies, RNA interference, or gene therapy will emerge and suitable pharmacotherapy may replace the present day surgical therapy of PVR. Hence, currently the role of pharmacotherapy in the treatment of PVR is limited.

Results of surgery for PVR

Untreated, PVR inevitably leads to severe loss of vision, hypotony, and sometimes phthisis bulbi. The anatomical success, which is defined as retinal reattachment for at least 6 months, has progressively improved over the last 40 years, along with the steady improvement in instrumentation and surgical techniques. A scleral buckle without vitrectomy successfully reattached up to 50% of milder cases 30 years ago, while at present, with all the surgical techniques at our disposal, up to 90% of all cases of PVR can be anatomically reattached. However, many eyes need more than one operation because of continuing cellular proliferation and retinal traction.

Functional success defined as improved visual acuity is more difficult to achieve, as any macula detached for more than a few days is unlikely to recover more than 10–20% of central vision. In the multicenter and largely controlled silicone study, now more than 20 years old, about half the eyes overall, whether with gas or SO, obtained 5/200 vision or better. If the process was not so severe that SO was able to be removed, eyes after removal of oil were 19 times more likely to experience a visual acuity improvement of ≥3 lines. However, removal of SO resulted in recurrent retinal detachment in 19% of eyes and this was twice the risk of retinal detachment in eyes in which the SO was not removed. The visual results were relatively stable in those eyes that obtained retinal reattachment and were followed up to 6 years after surgery. Visual results were better in those that required only one surgery. There was no statistically significant difference in the anatomical reattachment rate or visual acuity between 14% perfluoropropane gas tamponade or SO after long-term follow-up of up to 6 years.

BIBLIOGRAPHY

1. Asaria RH, Kon CH, Bunce C, et al. Adjuvant 5-fluorouracil and heparin prevents proliferative vitreoretinopathy: Results from a randomized, double-blind, controlled clinical trial. Ophthalmology 2001; 108: 1179–83.
2. Byer NE. Long-term natural history of lattice degeneration of the retina Ophthalmology 1989; 96: 1396–1402.
3. Byer NE; Perspectives on the management of the complications of senile retinoschisis eye 2002; 16: 358.
4. Campochiaro PA. Pathogenic mechanisms in proliferative vitreoretinopathy. Arch Ophthalmol 1997; 115: 237–41.
5. Charteris DG, Sethi CS, Lewis GP, et al. Proliferative vitreoretinopathy-developments in adjunctive treatment and retinal pathology. Eye (Lond) 2002; 16: 369–74.
6. Coll GE, Chang S, Sun J, et al. Perfluorocarbon liquid in the management of retinal detachment with proliferative vitreoretinopathy. Ophthalmology 1995; 102: 630–8; discussion 638–639.
7. Daniel AB, Eugene SL. Pneumatic retinopexy. In: Ryan SJ, Hinton DR, Schachat AP, Wilkinson CP, (eds) Retina Vol 3, 4th ed. Philadelphia: Elsevier/Mosby: 2006: 2036–71.
8. George AW, Thoms MA. Technique of scleral buckling. In Ryan SJ, Hinton DR, Schachat AP, Wilkinson CP (eds) Retina Vol 3, 4th ed. Philadelphia: Elseier/Mosby: 2006:2021–35.
9. Glasgow BJ, Foos RY, Yoshizumi MD. Degenerative diseases of the peripheral retina. In: Tasman W, Jaeger EA (eds). Duane's Clinical Ophthalmology Vol 3, Philadelphia: Lippincott; 1994; 26: 1–30.
10. Green WR, Sebag J, Vitreoretinal interface. In: Ryan SJ, Hinton DR, Schachat AP, Wilkinson CP, (eds). Retina Vol 3, 4th ed. Philadelphia: Elsevier/Mosby: 2006: 1921–89.
11. Heinrich H, Bernd K. Primary vitrectmy in rhegmatogenous RD. In Ryan SJ, Hinton DR, Schachat AP, Wilkinson CP, (eds). Retina Vol 3, 4th ed. Philadelphia:Elsevier/Mosby: 2006: 2072–85.
12. Kean T. Oh, Mary EH, Maurice B. Landers III. Pathogenic mechanisms of retinal detachment. In: Ryan SJ, Hinton DR Schachat AP, Wilkinson CP (eds). Retina Vol 3, 4th ed. Philadephia: Elsevier/Mosby: 2006: 2013–20.

13. Lean J, Azen SP, Lopez PF, et al. The prognostic utility of the Silicone Study Classification System. Silicone Study Report 9. Silicone Study Group. Arch Ophthalmol 1996; 114: 286–92.

14. Lean J, et al. Classification of PVR used in the Silicon study. The Silicon Study Group. Ophthalmology 1989; 96: 765–71.

15. Lewis H, Aaberg TM, Abrams GW. Causes of failure after initial vitreoretinal surgery for severe proliferative vitreoretinopathy. Am J Ophthalmol 1991; 111: 8–14.

16. Lois N, Wong D.Pseudophakic retinal detachment. Surv Ophthalmol 2003; 48: 467.

17. Machemer R, Aaberg TM, Freeman HM, et al. An updated classification of retinal detachment with proliferative vitreoretinopathy. Am J Ophthalmol 1991; 112: 159–65.

18. Machemer R. Pathogenesis and classification of massive periretinal proliferation. Br J Ophthalmol 1978; 62: 737–47.

19. Peripheral retinal degenerations and the risk of retinal detachment. Am J Ophthalmol 2003; 136; 135.

20. Regillo CD, Benson WE. Retinal Detachment and management, 3rd ed. Philadelphia: Lippincott Williams and Wilkins; 1998: 60–6.

21. Sakamoto T, Kimura H, Scuric Z, et al. Inhibition of experimental proliferative vitreoretinopathy by retroviral vector-mediated transfer of suicide gene. Can proliferative vitreoretinopathy be a target of gene therapy? Ophthalmology 1995; 102: 1417–24.

22. Scott JD. Treatment of massive vitreous retraction. Trans Ophthalmol Soc U K 1975; 95: 429–32.

23. Sharma T, Gopal L, Shanmugam MP, et al. Retinal detachment in Marfan syndrome: Clinical characteristics and surgical outcome. Retina 2002; 22: 423.

24. Silicone Study Group. Vitrectomy with silicone oil or perfluoropropane gas in eyes with severe proliferative vitreoretinopathy: results of a randomized clinical trial. Silicone Study Report 2. Arch Ophthalmol 1992; 110: 780–92.

25. Singh AK, Glaser BM, Lemor M, et al. Gravity-dependent distribution of retinal pigment epithelial cells dispersed into the vitreous cavity. Retina 1986; 6: 77–80

26. Sun JK, Young LHY. Retinal detachment. In: Albert DM, Miller JW, Azar DT, Blodi BA, (eds). Albert and Jakobiec's Principles and Practice of Ophthalmology. Philadelphia: Saunders: 2008: Chap. 182.

27. The classification of retinal detachment with proliferative vitreoretinopathy. Ophthalmology 1983; 90: 121–5.

28. Van Meurs JC, Bolt BJ, Mertens DA, et al. Rubeosis of the iris in proliferative vitreo-retinopathy. Retina 1996; 16: 292–5.

29. Wiedemann P, Sorgente N, Bekhor C, et al. Daunomycin in the treatment of experimental proliferative vitreoretinopathy. Effective doses in vitro and in vivo. Invest Ophthalmol Vis Sci 1985; 26: 719–25.

30. Williams GA, Aaberg TM Jr. Technique of scleral buckling. In: Ryan SJ, Hinton DR, Schachat AP, Wilkinson CP, (eds) Retina, Vol 3, 4th ed. Philadelphia: Elsevier/Mosby 2006: 2035–70.

26 | TUMORS AND CYSTS OF THE RETINA

Vikas Khetan, Parul Chawla, G Suguneshwari, Sandhya Hegde, Sunandan Sood

TUMORS OF THE RETINA

CLASSIFICATION

Retinal tumors can arise from various tissues and cells of the retina. They can be classified as:

i. Tumors arising from retinocytes (retino-blastomas and retinomas)

ii. Tumors associated with the retinal vasculature (retinal hemangioblastomas and retinal arteriovenous [AV] communications)

iii. Tumors arising from retinal glial cells (retinal astrocytic hamartomas and astrocytomas)

iv. Intraocular lymphoid tumors and leukemias (primary retinal lymphoma)

v. Tumors that metastasize to the retina via its blood supply (retinal/vitreoretinal metastases from primary tumors located elsewhere)

vi. Tumors that are associated with the retinal pigment epithelium (RPE).

   a. Congenital anomalies, such as the simple and combined hamartomas, the congenital hypertrophy of the RPE (that can also be associated with hyperplasia)

   b. True neoplasia of the RPE, such as adenomas and adenocarcinomas.

vii. Phakomatosis-neuro-oculocutaneous syndromes (systemic hamartomatoses).

TUMORS ARISING FROM RETINOCYTES

A. RETINOBLASTOMA

Retinoblastoma is the most common intraocular malignancy in children, with an incidence ranging from 1 in 15,000 to 1 in 18,000 live births. It is second only to uveal melanoma in the

frequency of occurrence of malignant intraocular tumors. There is no racial or gender predisposition in the incidence of retinoblastoma. Retinoblastoma is bilateral in about 25 to 35% of the cases. The mean age at diagnosis is 18 months, with unilateral cases being diagnosed at around 24 months and bilateral cases before 12 months.

HISTORY OF RETINOBLASTOMA

Pawius first described retinoblastoma in 1597. In 1809, Wardrop referred to the tumor as fungus hematodes and suggested enucleation as the main mode of treatment. Initially it was thought to be derived from the glial cells and was called a glioma of the retina by Virchow (1864). Flexner (1891) and Wintersteiner (1897) believed it to be a neuroepithelioma because of the presence of rosettes. Later, there was a consensus and it was opined that the tumor originated from the retinoblasts and the American Ophthalmological Society accepted the term retinoblastoma in 1926 officially.

Retinoblastoma was associated with almost certain death in 100% cases just over a century ago. Early tumor diagnosis aided by indirect ophthalmoscopy and meticulous enucleation technique contributed to an improved survival from 5% in 1896 to 81% in 1967. Advances in external beam radiotherapy also provided an excellent alternative to enucleation and resulted in eye salvage in majority of the cases. Localised therapeutic measures such as cryotherapy, photocoagulation and plaque brachytherapy allowed targeted treatment of smaller tumors. Introduction of ultrasonography, computed tomography, and magnetic resonance imaging contributed in increasing the diagnostic accuracy and early detection of extraocular retinoblastoma.

The recent advances such as identification of genetic mutations, replacement of external beam radiotherapy by chemoreduction as the primary management modality, use of chemoreduction to minimize the size of regression scar, identification of histopathologic high-risk factors following enucleation, provision of adjuvant therapy to reduce the incidence of systemic metastasis and aggressive multimodal therapy in the management of orbital retinoblastoma have contributed to improved outcome in terms of better survival, improved eye salvage and potential for optimal visual recovery.

GENETICS OF RETINOBLASTOMA

Among the newly diagnosed cases of retinoblastoma, only 6% are familial while 94% are sporadic. Bilateral retinoblastomas involve germinal mutations in all cases. Approximately 15% of unilateral sporadic retinoblastoma is caused by germinal mutations affecting only one eye while the 85% are sporadic. In 1971, Knudson proposed the two hit hypothesis. He said that, two chromosomal mutations are needed for retinoblastoma to develop. In hereditary retinoblastoma, the initial hit is a germinal mutation, which is inherited and is found in all the cells. The second hit develops in the somatic retinal cells leading to the development of retinoblastoma. Therefore, hereditary cases are predisposed to the development of non-ocular tumors such as osteosarcoma. In unilateral sporadic retinoblastoma, both the hits occur during the development of the retina and are somatic mutations. Therefore, there is no risk of second non-ocular tumors.

Genetic counselling is an important aspect in the management of retinoblastoma. In patients with a positive family history, 40% of the siblings would be at risk of developing retinoblastoma and 40% of the offspring of the affected patient may develop retinoblastoma. In patients with no family history of retinoblastoma, if the affected child has unilateral retinoblastoma, 1% of the siblings are at risk and 8% of the offspring may develop retinoblastoma. In cases of bilateral retinoblastoma with no positive family history, 6% of the siblings and 40% of the offspring have a chance of developing retinoblastoma.

Apart from genetic counseling, the current trend is to identify the mutation and compute specifc antenatal risk. Knowledge of the full range of mutations can aid in the designing of screening tests for individuals at risk.

HISTOPATHOLOGY OF RETINOBLASTOMA

It is a fast growing tumor. Mostly its proliferation surpasses its blood supply, thus there are viable

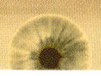

tumor tissue alternating with necrotic tissue, latter undergo calcification which is pathognomonic of retinoblastoma in a child less than 18–24 months of age.

Under magnification, basophilic areas of tumor are seen along with eosinophilic areas of necrosis and more basophilic areas of calcification within the tumor. Poorly differentiated tumors consist of small to medium sized round cells with large hyperchromatic nuclei and scanty cytoplasm with mitotic figures. Well differentiated tumors show the presence of rosettes and fleurettes. These are of various types:

a. Flexner-Wintersteiner rosettes consist of columnar cells ar ranged around a central lumen. These are highly characteristic of retinoblastoma, however, they and are also seen in medulloepithelioma.

b. Homer Wright rosettes consist of cells arranged around a central neurofibrillary tangle. This is also found in neuroblastomas, medulloblastomas and medulloepitheliomas.

c. Pseudorosette refers to the arrangement of tumor cells around blood vessels. They are signs of poor differentiation.

d. Fleurettes are eosinophilic structures composed of tumor cells with pear-shaped eosinophilic processes projecting through a fenestrated membrane.

Rosettes and fleurettes indicate that the tumor cells show photoreceptor differentiation. In addition, basophilic deposits (precipitated DNA released after tumor necrosis) can be found in the walls of the lumen of blood vessels.

CLINICAL MANIFESTATIONS OF RETINOBLASTOMA

Leucocoria is the most common presenting feature of retinoblastoma, followed by strabismus, painful blind eye due to glaucoma and loss of vision. Table 26.1 lists the common presenting signs and symptoms of retinoblastoma. The clinical presentation of retinoblastoma depends on the stage of the disease. Early lesions are likely to be missed, unless an indirect ophthalmoscopy is performed. The tumor appears as a translucent or a white fluffy retinal mass.

The child may present with strabismus or with reduced visual acuity, if the tumor involves the macula. Moderately advanced lesions usually present with leucocoria due to the reflection of light by the white mass in the fundus (Table 26.1).

Table 26.1 *Common presenting features of retinoblastoma*

Leucocoria	56%
Strabismus	20%
Red painful eye	7%
Poor vision	5%
Asymptomatic	3%
Orbital cellulitis	3%
Unilateral mydriasis	2%
Heterochromia iridis	1%
Hyphema	1%

As the tumor grows further, three patterns are usually seen:

- Endophytic, in which the tumor grows into the vitreous cavity. A yellow white mass progressively fills the entire vitreous cavity and vitreous seeds occur. The retinal vessels are not seen on the tumor surface.
- Exophytic, in which the tumor grows towards the subretinal space. Retinal detachment usually occurs and retinal vessels are seen over the tumor.
- Diffuse infiltrating tumor, in which the tumor diffusely involves the retina causing just a placoid thickness of the retina and not a mass. This is generally seen in older children and mostly there is a delay in the diagnosis.

Advanced tumors manifest with proptosis secondary to optic nerve extension or orbital extension and systemic metastasis. Retinoblastoma can spread through the optic nerve relatively easily especially once the lamina cribrosa is breached. Orbital extension may present with proptosis and is most likely to occur at the site of the scleral emissary veins. Infact in Indian scenario this is one of the common presenting feature since the diagnosis is delayed because of lack of awareness and non-availability of ophthalmologists in the far flung and remote areas (Table 26.2). Systemic metastasis usually occurs to the brain, skull, distant bones and the lymph nodes.

Table 26.2 *Comparison of demographic and presenting features of retinoblastoma in asian and caucasian population*

	Indian study	Studies from North America and Europe
Median age at presentation (unilateral retinoblastoma)	30 months	24 months
(Bilateral retinoblastoma)	24 months	13 months
Sex (Male:Female)	1.6:1	1:1
Laterality, %	70 unilateral	70 unilateral
Most common symptom	Leukocoria	Leukocoria
Buphthalmia and proptosis, %	31.3	1–2
Stage of disease %		
Intraocular	60	90
Locally advanced/ metastatic disease	35	10

DIAGNOSIS OF RETINOBLASTOMA

A thorough clinical evaluation, aided by B-scan ultrasonography helps in the diagnosis. Computed tomography and magnetic resonance imaging are generally reserved for cases with atypical manifestations and where extraocular or intracranial tumor extension is suspected.

a. A child with suspected retinoblastoma necessarily needs complete ophthalmic evaluation including a dilated fundus examination under anesthesia. The intraocular pressure is measured and the anterior segment is examined for neovascularization, pseudohypopyon, hyphema, and signs of inflammation.

b. Bilateral fundus examination with 360 degree scleral depression is essential. Direct visualization of the tumor by an indirect ophthalmoscope is diagnostic of retinoblastoma in over 90% of cases. RetCam is a wide-angle fundus camera, useful in accurately documenting retinoblastoma and monitoring response to the therapy.

c. Ultrasonography B-scan shows a rounded or irregular intraocular mass with high internal reflectivity representing typical intralesional calcification.

d. Magnetic resonance imaging is specifically indicated if optic nerve invasion or intracranial extension is suspected. It also help in detecting associated pinealoblastoma.

e. Computed tomography helps in the diagnosis of an extraocular extension. It is absolutely contraindicated in infants. It is rarely done nowadays due to the risk of irradiation and second tumor.

f. Retinoblastoma shows minimally dilated feeding vessels in the arterial phase, blotchy hyperfluorescence in the venous phase and late staining on fluorescein angiography.

In cases in which there is clear evidence of tumor outside the eye, the full metastatic workup should be pursued. Studies should include a bone scan in addition to a search for tumor cells in the CSF and bone marrow. Positron emmission tomography (PET) may be of great help in this regard. Aspiration from more than one site may be of value because bone marrow involvement can be uneven. The aspirates are typically taken from the iliac crest in young children.

CLASSIFICATION OF RETINOBLASTOMA

An ideal classification system for retinoblastoma should include two components: grouping and staging. Grouping is used for prognosticating organ salvage while staging prognosticates survival.

The Reese-Ellsworth classification (Table 26.3) was introduced to prognosticate patients treated with methods other than enucleation. This classification was devised prior to the widespread use of indirect ophthalmoscopy and focal measures of management of retinoblastoma and mainly pertained to eye salvage with external beam radiotherapy. Although the Essen classification addressed some of the shortcomings of Reese Ellsworth classification, it is considered too complex. Further, none of the older systems of classification prognosticated chemoreduction, the current favored method of retinoblastoma management.

The new International Classification of Intraocular Retinoblastoma (ICIOR) correlates tumor grading with the outcome of newer therapeutic modalities. The new International Staging system is the first such for retino-

Table 26.3 *Reese-Ellsworth classification of retinoblastoma*

Group I
a. Solitary tumor, less than 4 disc diameters in size, at or behind the equator
b. Multiple tumors, none over 4 disc diameters in size, all at or behind the equator

Group II
a. Solitary tumor, 4 to 10 disc diameters in size, at or behind the equator
b. Multiple tumors, 4 to 10 disc diameters in size, behind the equator

Group III
a. Any lesion anterior to the equator
b. Solitary tumors larger than 10 disc diameters behind the equator

Group IV
a. Multiple tumors, some larger than 10 disc diameters
b. Any lesion extending anterior to the ora seratta

Group V
a. Massive tumors involving over half the retina
b. Vitreous seeding

Table 26.4 *International classification for intraocular retinoblastoma (ICIOR)*

Group A—Very low risk
Small discrete intraretinal tumors away from the foveola and disc
• All tumors are ≤3 mm in greatest dimension, confined to the retina
• All tumors are located further than 3 mm from the foveola and 1.5 mm from the optic disc (Fig. 26.1)

Group B—Low risk
All remaining discrete retinal tumors without seeding
• All tumors confined to the retina not in group A
• Any tumor size and location with no vitreous or subretinal seeding (Fig. 26.2)

Group C—Moderate risk
Discrete local disease with minimal focal subretinal or vitreous seeding
• Tumor(s) must be discrete
• Subretinal fluid, present or past, without gross seeding, involving up to one quadrant of retina
• Local subretinal seeding, present or past up to less than 5 mm from the tumor
• Focal fine vitreous seeding close to discrete tumor (Fig. 26.3)

Group D—High risk
Diffuse disease with significant vitreous and/or subretinal seeding
• Tumor(s) may be massive or diffuse
• Subretinal fluid, present or past up to total retinal detachment
• Diffuse subretinal seeding, may include subretinal plaques or tumor nodules
• Diffuse or massive vitreous disease may include "greasy" seeds or avascular tumor masses (Fig. 26.4)

Group E—Very high risk
Presence of any one or more of these poor prognosis features
• Tumor touching the lens
• Neovascular glaucoma
• Tumor anterior to anterior vitreous face involving ciliary body or anterior segment
• Diffuse infiltrating retinoblastoma
• Opaque media from hemorrhage
• Tumor necrosis with aseptic orbital cellulitis
• Phthisis bulbi (Fig. 26.5)

blastoma and incorporates five distinct stages. Staging is based on the collective information gathered by the clinical evaluation, imaging, systemic survey and histopathology.

The International Classification System (Table 26.4) is based both on the natural history of retinoblastoma and on the likelihood of salvaging the eye when systemic chemotherapy is used.

DIFFERENTIAL DIAGNOSIS

There are several pediatric ocular conditions that can cause leukocoria and should be considered in the differential diagnosis of retinoblastoma. The conditions that most commonly present a diagnostic challenge include retinopathy of prematurity (ROP), persistent fetal vasculature (PFV), Coats' disease, toxocariasis, and medulloepithelioma (Table 26.5).

MANAGEMENT OF RETINOBLASTOMA

The primary goal of management of retino-blastoma is to save life. Salvage of the organ (eye) and function (vision) are the secondary and tertiary goals respectively. The management

of retinoblastoma needs a multidisciplinary team approach including an ocular oncologist, pediatric oncologist, radiation oncologist,

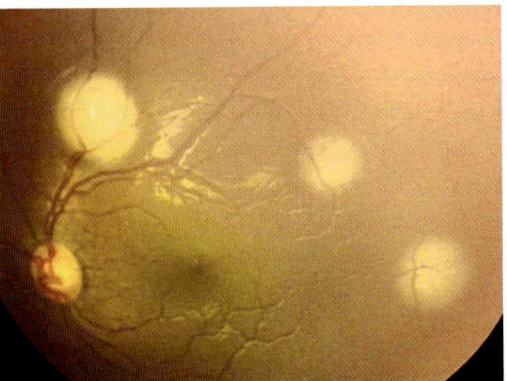

- 3 mm or smaller tumors confined to the retina
- Located further than 3 mm from the fovea and 1.5 mm from the optic disc

Fig. 26.1 *Group A intraocular retinoblastoma*

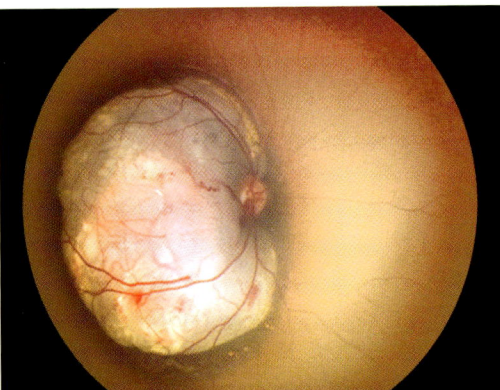

- All tumors confined to retina not in Group A
- Any tumor with associated subretinal fluid less than 5 mm from the tumor with no vitreous or subretinal seedings

Fig. 26.2 *Group B intraocular retinoblastoma*

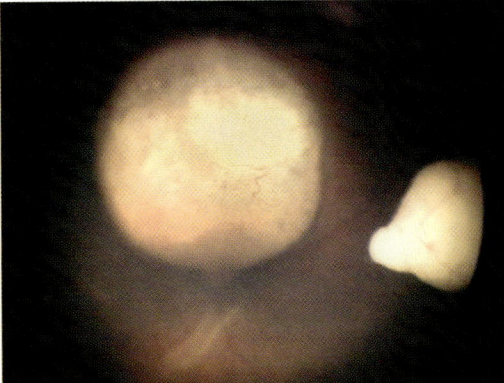

- Discrete tumors
- Less than quarter of retina with subretinal fluid
- Local subretinal seeding, less than 5 mm from the tumor
- Local fine vitreous seeding close to discrete tumor

Fig. 26.3 *Group C intraocular retinoblastoma*

radiation physicist, genetist and an ophthalmic oncopathologist. The management strategy depends on the stage of the disease – intraocular retinoblastoma, retinoblastoma with high-risk characteristics, orbital retino blastoma and metastatic retinoblastoma. Management of retinoblastoma is highly individualized and is based on several considerations-age at presentation, laterality, tumor location, tumor staging, visual prognosis, systemic condition, family and societal perception, and, to a certain extent, the overall prognosis and cost-effectiveness of treatment in a given economic situation.

A. MANAGEMENT OF INTRAOCULAR RETINOBLASTOMA

A majority of children with retinoblastoma manifest at the stage when the tumor is confined to the eye. About 90–95% of children in developed countries and 60–70% in the developing countries present with intraocular retino-blastoma. Diagnosis of retinoblastoma at this stage and appropriate management are crucial for life, eye and possible vision salvage.

There are several methods to manage intraocular retinoblastoma — focal (cryotherapy, laser photocoagulation, transpupillary thermo-therapy, transcleral thermotherapy, plaque brachytherapy), local (external beam radio-therapy, enucleation), and systemic (chemo-therapy). While primary focal measures are mainly used for small tumors, local and systemic modalities are used to treat advanced retinoblastoma.

Focal Therapy

A. Cryotherapy

Cryotherapy is performed for small equatorial and peripheral retinal tumors measuring up to 4 mm in basal diameter and 2 mm in thickness. Triple freeze thaw cryotherapy is applied at 46 weeks intervals until the complete tumor

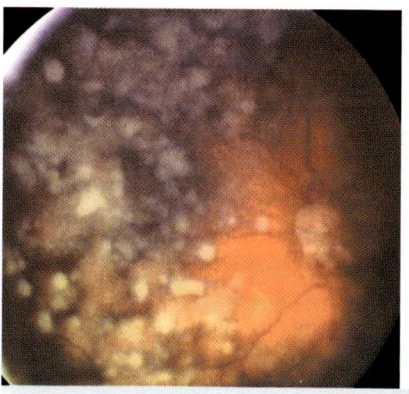
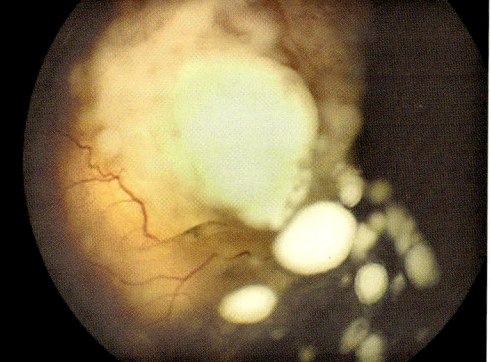

- Tumor may be massive or diffuse
- Subretinal fluid without subretinal seedings, causing total RD
- Diffuse subretinal seeding—may include subretinal plaques or tumor nodules
- Diffuse or massive vitreous disease—may include "greasy" seeds or avascular tumor masses

Fig. 26.4 *Group D intraocular retinoblastoma*

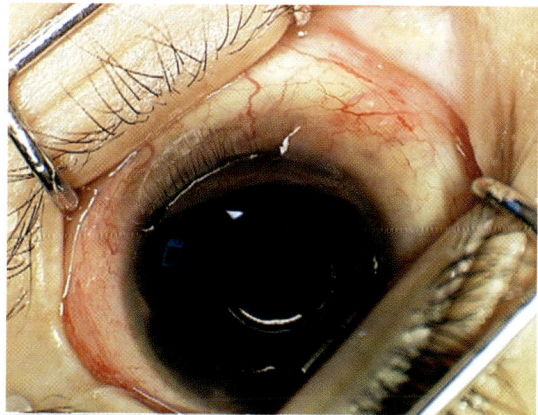
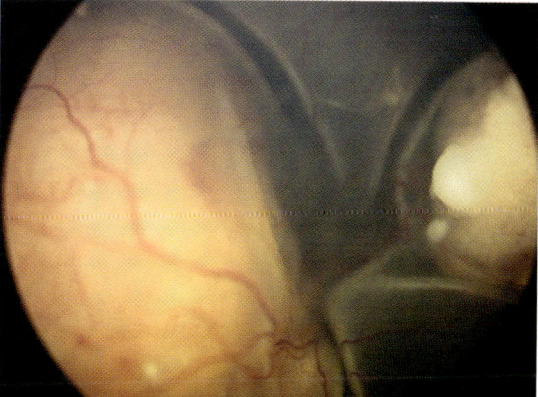

- Tumor touching the lens
- Neovascular glaucoma
- Tumor anterior to the anterior vitreous face involving ciliary body or anterior segment

- Diffuse infiltrating RB
- Opaque media from hemorrhage
- Tumor necrosis with aseptic orbital cellulitis
- Phthisis bulbi

Fig. 26.5 *Group E intraocular retinoblastoma*

regresses. Cryotherapy produces a scar much larger than the tumor. Complications of cryotherapy include transient serous retinal detachment, retinal tear and rhegmatogenous retinal detachment. Cryotherapy administered 2–3 hours prior to chemotherapy can increase the delivery of chemotherapeutic agents across the blood retinal barrier and thus has additive effect.

B. Laser Photocoagulation

Laser photocoagulation is used for small posterior tumors 4 mm in basal diameter and 2 mm in thickness. The treatment is used to delimit the tumor and coagulate the blood supply to the tumor by surrounding it with two rows of overlapping laser burns. Complications include transient serous retinal detachment, retinal vascular occlusion, retinal hole, retinal

			Table 26.5 Differential diagnosis of retinoblastoma		
Condition	Age of presentation	Risk factors	Laterality	Axial length	USG
1. Retinoblastoma	90% <3 years old	Family history	Unilateral/ bilateral	Normal	Intraretinal/ subretinal mass with calcification
2. ROP	Days to months after birth	Prematurity; oxygen supplementation	Bilateral	Short	RD with retinal bands
3. PFV	Days to weeks after birth	——	**Unilateral**	Short	Vitreous band from lens to optic nerve
4. Coats' disease	4–10 years of age	Male gender	Unilateral	Normal	Exudative RD Subretinal hyperechoic particles
5. Toxocariasis	Variable	Contact with dogs	Unilateral	Normal	Peripheral mass, vitreoretinal band, traction RD
6. Medullo-epithelioma	First decade of life	——	Unilateral	Normal	Ciliary body mass with cyst

traction, and pre-retinal fibrosis. It is less often used now with the advent of thermotherapy. In fact, laser photocoagulation is contraindicated while the patient is on active chemoreduction protocol.

C. Thermotherapy

In thermotherapy, focused heat generated by infrared radiation is applied to tissues at subphotocoagulation levels to induce tumor necrosis. A slow and sustained temperature range of 40° to 60°C within the tumor is achieved, thus sparing damage to the retinal vessels. Transpupillary thermotherapy (TTT) using infrared radiation from a semiconductor diode laser delivered with a 1300-micron large spot indirect ophthalmoscope delivery system has become a usual protocol. It can also be applied transpupillary through an operating microscope or by the trans-scleral route with a diopexy probe. The tumor is heated until it turns a subtle gray. Thermotherapy provides satisfactory control for small tumors — 4 mm in basal diameter and 2 mm in thickness. Complete tumor regression can be achieved in over 85% of tumors using 3–4 sessions of thermo-

therapy. The common complications are focal iris atrophy, focal paraxial lens opacity, retinal traction and serous retinal detachment. The major application of thermotherapy is as an adjunct to chemoreduction. The application of heat amplifies the cytotoxic effect of platinum analogues. This additive combination with chemoreduction protocol is termed chemo-thermotherapy.

D. Plaque Brachytherapy

Plaque brachytherapy involves placement of a radioactive implant on the sclera corresponding to the base of the tumor to trans-sclerally irradiate the tumor. Commonly used radioactive materials include Ruthenium 106 and Iodine 125. The advantages of plaque brachytherapy are focal delivery of radiation with minimal damage to the surrounding normal tissues, minimal periorbital tissue damage, absence of cosmetic deformity because of retarded bone growth in the field of irradiation as occurs with external beam radiotherapy, reduced risk of second malignant neoplasm and shorter duration of treatment.

Plaque brachytherapy is indicated in tumors less than 16 mm in basal diameter and less than 10 mm thickness. It could be the primary or secondary modality of management. Primary plaque brachytherapy is usually now performed only in situations where chemotherapy is contraindicated. It is most useful as secondary treatment in eyes that fail to respond to chemoreduction and external beam radiotherapy or for tumor recurrences.

Plaque brachytherapy requires precise tumor localization and measurement of its basal dimensions. The tumor thickness is measured by ultrasonography. The data is used for dosimetry on a three-dimensional computerized tumor modeling system. The plaque design is chosen depending on the basal tumor dimensions, its location, and configuration. The dose to the tumor apex ranges from 4000–5000 cGy. The plaque is sutured to the sclera after confirming tumor centration and is left in situ for generally 36 to 72 hours. The results of plaque brachytherapy are gratifying with about 90% tumor control. The common complications are radiation papillopathy and radiation retinopathy. In tumors near optic nerve-notched plaques are recommended.

Local Therapy

A. External Beam Radiotherapy

External beam radiotherapy was the preferred form of management of moderately advanced retinoblastoma earlier. However, with the invention of newer chemotherapy protocols, external beam radiotherapy is being used less often. Presently it is indicated in eyes where primary chemotherapy and focal therapy has failed, or rarely when chemotherapy is contraindicated.

The major side effects with external beam radiotherapy are the orbital growth stunting, dry eye, cataract, radiation retinopathy and optic neuropathy. External beam radiotherapy can induce second malignant neoplasm especially in patients with the hereditary form of retinoblastoma. There is a 30% chance of developing another malignancy by the age of 30 years in such patients if they are given external beam radiotherapy compared to a less than 6% chance in those who do not receive external beam radiotherapy. The risk of second malignant neoplasm is more in children under 12 months of age.

B. Enucleation

Enucleation is a common method of managing advanced retinoblastoma. Just about 3 to 4 decades ago, a majority of the patients with unilateral retinoblastoma and the worse eye in bilateral retinoblastoma underwent primary enucleation. A major reduction in the frequency of enucleation has occurred in the late last century. Concurrently, there has been an increase in the use of alternative eye and vision conserving methods of treatment.

Primary enucleation continues to be the treatment of choice for advanced intraocular retinoblastoma with neovascularization of iris, secondary glaucoma, anterior chamber tumor invasion, tumors occupying >75% of the vitreous volume, necrotic tumors with secondary orbital inflammation, and tumors associated with hyphema or vitreous hemorrhage where the tumor characteristics cannot be visualized, especially when only one eye is involved.

There are specific considerations while enucleating an eye with retinoblastoma (Table 26.6). Minimum-manipulation surgical technique should be essentially done. It is important not to accidentally perforate the eye. The sclera is thin at the site of muscle insertions and the rectus muscles have to be hooked delicately. It is important to obtain a long optic nerve stump, ideally more than 15 mm, but never less than 10 mm. The end of the stump is subjected to histopathological evaluation in order to rule out intracranial spread which is important to plan the management.

Table 26.6 *Special considerations for enucleation in retinoblastoma*

a. Minimal manipulation
b. Avoid perforation of the eye
c. Harvest long (>15 mm) optic nerve stump
d. Inspect the enucleated eye for macroscopic extra-ocular extension and optic nerve involvement
e. Harvest fresh tissue for genetic studies
f. Avoid biointegrated implant if postoperative radiotherapy is necessary

i. *Certain steps can be taken to obtain about 15 mm long optic nerve stump in all cases of advanced retinoblastoma.* Gentle traction can be applied by the traction sutures applied to recti muscle stumps prior to transecting the optic nerve. As an alternative to the traction sutures, medial or lateral rectus muscle stumps may be kept long and traction exerted with an artery clamp. A 15-degree curved and blunt-tipped tenotomy scissors is introduced from the lateral aspect (or a straight scissors from the medial aspect) and the optic nerve is palpated with the closed tip of the scissors while maintaining gentle traction on the eyeball. The scissors is moved posteriorly to touch the orbital apex while "strumming" the optic nerve. The scissors is lifted by 3 or 4 millimeters off the orbital apex (to preserve the contents of the superior orbital fissure), the blades of the scissors are opened to engage the optic nerve, and the nerve is transected with one bold cut. This maneuver generally provides at least 15 mm long optic nerve stump. Enucleation spoon and heavy enucleation scissors limit space for maneuverability and may result in a shorter optic nerve stump. In addition, one should be careful not to accidentally perforate the eye during enucleation. The enucleated eyeball is inspected for optic nerve or extraocular extension of tumor.

ii. *Eyes manifesting tumor necrosis with aseptic orbital cellulitis pose specific problem.* Imaging should be done in these patients to rule out extraocular extension. Enucleation is best performed when the inflammation is resolved. A brief course of preoperative oral and topical steroids help control inflammation. Patients with retinoblastoma presenting as phthisis bulbi need imaging to exclude extraocular and optic nerve extension. Phthisis generally results following spontaneous tumor necrosis and an episode of aseptic intraocular and orbital inflammation. Enucleation in these cases is often complicated by excessive peribulbar fibrosis and intraoperative bleeding.

iii. *Placement of an orbital implant* following enucleation for retinoblastoma is the current practice. The orbital implant promotes orbital growth, provides better cosmesis and enhances motility of prosthesis. The implants could be non-integrated (polymethyl methacrylate or silicon) or bio-integrated (hydroxyapatite or porous polyethylene). Placement of a biointegrated implant is generally avoided if postoperative adjuvant radiotherapy is considered necessary. Although most implants structurally tolerate radiotherapy well, implant vascularization may be compromised by radiotherapy thus increasing the risk of implant exposure. Use of myoconjunctival technique and custom ocular prosthesis have optimized prosthesis motility.

SYSTEMIC CHEMOTHERAPY

a. Chemoreduction

Chemoreduction, is defined as the process of reduction in the tumor volume with chemotherapy, and has become an essential part of the current management of retinoblastoma. Chemotherapy alone is however not curative and must be associated with intensive local therapy. Chemoreduction coupled with focal therapy can minimize the need for enucleation or external beam radiotherapy without signifcant systemic toxicity.

Chemoreduction in addition with focal therapy is now extensively used in the primary management of retinoblastoma. There are different protocols in chemotherapy. The commonly used drugs are vincristine, etoposide and carboplatin, for 6 cycles. Standard dose chemoreduction is provided in ICIOR groups A-C. In high dose chemoreduction, the dose of etoposide and carboplatin is increased. This is indicated in ICIOR groups D tumors (Table 26.7).

Table 26.7 *Chemoreduction regimen and doses for intraocular retinoblastoma*

Day 1: Vincristine + Etoposide + Carboplatin
Day 2: Etoposide
Standard dose (3 weekly, 6 cycles): Vincristine 1.5 mg/m^2 (0.05 mg/kg for children <36 months of age and maximum dose <2 mg), Etoposide 150 mg/m^2 (5 mg/kg for children <36 months of age), Carboplatin 560 mg/m^2 (18.6 mg/kg for children <36 months of age)
High-dose (3 weekly, 6–12 cycles): Vincristine 0.025 mg/kg, Etoposide 12 mg/kg, Carboplatin 28 mg/kg

With chemoreduction and sequential local therapy, it is now possible to salvage many eyes and maximize residual vision. Chemoreduction is most successful for tumors without associated subretinal fuid or vitreous seeding. Risk factors for tumor, subretinal seed and vitreous seed recurrence, and failure of chemoreduction leading to external beam radiotherapy and/or enucleation have been identifed. Chemoreduction offers satisfactory tumor control for Reese-Ellsworth groups I–IV eyes, with treatment failure necessitating additional external beam radiotherapy in only 10% and enucleation in 15% at 5-year follow-up. Patients with Reese-Ellsworth group V eyes require external beam radiotherapy in 47% and enucleation in 53% at 5 years. Chemoreduction is an option for some selected eyes with unilateral retinoblastoma.

It is important to be aware of the adverse effects and interactions of chemotherapeutic agents, which include myelosuppression, febrile episodes, neurotoxicity and non-specifc gastrointestinal toxicity. Chemotherapy should be given only under the supervision of an experienced pediatric oncologist.

b. *Periocular chemotherapy.* Carboplatin delivered deep posterior subtenon has been demonstrated to be efficacious in the management of Reese-Ellsworth Group VB retinoblastoma with vitreous seeds because it can penetrate the sclera and achieve effective concentrations in the vitreous cavity. This modality is currently under trial. Early studies have shown that periocular chemotherapy achieves 70% eye salvage in patients with retinoblastoma with diffuse vitreous seeds.

c. Intra-arterial Chemotherapy (IA)

Primary systemic intravenous (IV) chemotherapy for intraocular retinoblastoma administers a large volume of medication to the entire body to treat a relatively small organ.

In the 1980s, Kaneko at the National Cancer Institute in Tokyo, Japan developed a new method to administer ocular chemotherapy – he described it as selective ophthalmic arterial infusion (SOAI). With this approach, developed primarily to avoid enucleation, a balloon catheter was inserted in the femoral artery, past the internal carotid and guided just past the origin of the ophthalmic artery. The balloon was then inflated and melphalan injected into the arterial vasculature. Often adjuvant treatments were also administered but more than half of treated eyes were preserved.

In 2008, Abramson and colleagues modified this technique with direct insertion of the cannula just at the ostea of the artery. A trial of ten patients with Group V retinoblastoma salvaged seven eyes that would have otherwise been enucleated. While the initial series used melphalan additional follow-up reports have infused other agents including carboplatin and topotecan with good results. The technique has been used successfully in unilateral and bilateral cases, as a primary and salvage approach. Following up electroretinogram (ERG) data suggests improved ERG findings in some very advanced cases.

The technique is technically challenging, requiring significant expertise. It has been likened to surgery. Many practitioners have raised concerns regarding the potential systemic and CNS risks with this approach including death and stroke; especially in the context of unilateral disease, where enucleation is generally curative with low risk for morbidity and mortality. More trials will be necessary to assess whether it will be widely adopted by the ocular oncology community and whether it will replace primary systemic intravenous chemotherapy.

Bilateral RB are best managed with intravenous chemotherapy but unilateral RB should be managed with intra-arterial chemotherapy to limit the side effects. Intravitreal chemotherapy is reserved for recurrent vitreous seeds.

Management of High risk Retinoblastoma

Systemic metastasis is the main cause for mortality in patients with retinoblastoma. Although the life prognosis of patients with retinoblastoma has dramatically improved in the last three decades, with a reported survival of more than 90% in developed countries, mortality is still as high as 50% in the developing nations. Reduction in the rate of systemic metastasis by identification of high-risk factors and appropriate adjuvant therapy may help improve survival.

High-risk factors

None of the clinical high-risk factors seem to strongly correlate with mortality. Recent studies have evaluated the role of histopathologic high-risk factors which have been identified following enucleation. The identification of frequency and significance of high-risk histopathologic factors that can reliably predict metastasis is vital for patient selection for adjuvant therapy. Massive choroidal infiltration, retrolaminar optic nerve invasion, invasion of the optic nerve to transection, scleral infiltration, and extrascleral extension are the risk factors that are predictive of metastasis (Table 26.8).

Table 26.8 *Histopathologic high-risk factors predictive of metastasis*

1. Anterior chamber seeding
2. Iris infiltration
3. Ciliary body infiltration
4. Massive choroidal infiltration
5. Invasion of the optic nerve lamina cribrosa
6. Retrolaminar optic nerve invasion
7. Invasion of optic nerve transection
8. Scleral infiltration
9. Extrascleral extension

The reported occurrence of anterior chamber seeding (7%), massive choroidal infiltration (12–23%), invasion of optic nerve lamina cribrosa (6–7%), retrolaminar optic nerve invasion (6–12%), invasion of optic nerve transection (1–25%), scleral infiltration (1–8%), and extrascleral extension (2–13%), widely vary even in developed countries. Vemuganti and associates have reported that 21% of the 76 eyes enucleated for advanced retinoblastoma in India had anterior chamber seeding, 54% had massive choroidal infiltration, 46% had optic nerve invasion at or beyond the lamina cribrosa and 7% had scleral infiltration or extrascleral extension. It is apparent that the incidence of histopathologic risk factors is strikingly high in developing countries compared to the developed countries.

Adjuvant therapy

Studies on the efficacy of adjuvant therapy to minimize the risk of metastasis have provided no firm recommendation. A recent study with a long-term follow-up provides useful information. It included a subset of patients with unilateral sporadic retinoblastoma who underwent primary enucleation. The study used specific predetermined histopathologic characteristics for patient selection. A minimum follow-up of 1 year was allowed to include metastatic events that generally occur at a mean of 9 months following enucleation. The incidence of metastasis was 4% in those who received adjuvant therapy compared to 24% in those who did not. The study found that administration of adjuvant therapy significantly reduced the risk of metastasis in patients with high-risk histopathologic characteristics.

Six cycles of a combination of carboplatin, etoposide and vincristine (identical to the protocol used for chemoreduction of intraocular retinoblastoma) in patients with histopathologic high-risk characteristics are given. All patients with extension of retinoblastoma up to the level of optic nerve transection, scleral infiltration, and extrascleral extension are given high dose chemotherapy for 12 cycles and fractionated 4500 to 5000 cGy orbital external beam radiotherapy.

VARIANTS OF RETINOBLASTOMA

a. Atypical retinoblastoma

Misdiagnosis can be caused by atypical manifestations of retinoblastoma (i.e. tumors growing along the surface of the retina, tumors presenting at an older age, tumors presenting with unusual features such as pseudo-hypopyon, hyphema, or vitreous hemorrhage, or tumors presenting as benign variants (retinoma or retinocytoma). The risk of death is higher with atypical manifestations, partially because of the associated delay in establishing the correct diagnosis. Retinoblastoma may be misdiagnosed as inflammation. Diffuse infiltrating retinoblastoma may closely resemble uveitis and lead to delayed diagnosis. The tumor may manifest as pseudohypopyon, iris lesions, granulomatous uveitis, indolent endophthalmitis and, perhaps the most misleading presentation, aseptic orbital cellulitis. These children are often admitted for IV antibiotic therapy because of presumed septic orbital

cellulitis who in fact had an aseptic orbital cellulitis from necrotic intraocular retinoblastoma. Often, in such cases, the lids are swollen shut from the toxic inflammation making examination of the inside of the eye difficult. No child should be admitted for this therapy without an ophthalmologist doing a fundus examination.

Retinoblastoma has been reported in a microphthalmic eye and can appear in the same eye as persistent hyperplastic primary vitreous (PHPV) or optic nerve hypoplasia. Snowball opacities in the anterior chamber or in the vitreous have been described as the presenting sign of advanced, delayed-onset retinoblastoma.

b. Retinoma (retinocytoma)

A benign form of retinoblastoma, initially described by Gallie et al. as a "retinoma" grows only to a certain size. The original description was of a lesion with pigmentary changes closely resembling a focal regressed or treated intraocular retinoblastoma. The same lesion was referred to as "retinocytoma" by Margo et al., Aaby et al. showed histologically, that, this is a benign variant of retinoblastoma and not a regressed retinoblastoma. They described a 5-year-old male initially found to have a gray translucent mass containing calcified nodules and surrounded by retinal pigment clumping and atrophy. The eye was enucleated and the tumor was found to be composed of benign-appearing cells in a bed of well-vascularized ground substance with calcific foci. There were no mitoses, cellular pleomorphism, nuclear atypia, rosettes, or other characteristics of malignancy. There was no peripheral necrosis or signs of tumor regression. It is now likely that the typical post-treatment regression appearance described as features of retinoma or retinocytoma are, in fact, the result of slow involutionary changes that occur with time in this benign variant of intraocular retinoblastoma.

It has been observed that what appear to be early stage retinomas in young patients age ≤2 years who may or may not have typical retinoblastoma lesions in the same or the other eye. The early stage "presumed" retinoma appears gray and translucent much like the lesion described by Aaby and colleagues. However this "early retinoma" does not stain or leak intensely during fluorescein angiography and some, at least, do not decrease in size with either systemic chemotherapy or external beam radiotherapy.

The retinoma or retinocytoma has benign histopathologic features but retains the ability to undergo malignant transformation into a rapidly growing retinoblastoma in exactly the same way that a choroidal nevus undergoes malignant transformation to a choroidal melanoma. The possibility for malignant transformation underscores the need for close follow-up of these patients. But the simple presence of vitreous seeding with a retinoma need not imply that malignant transformation has taken place.

c. Diffuse infiltrating retinoblastoma

In the rare and atypical form of retinoblastoma, infiltrating retinoblastoma, no mass forms. Instead, the tumor expands by diffusely infiltrating the retina. In this form of atypical retinoblastoma calcification is rare. As a result, neither ocular ultrasound nor CT scanning may be helpful in making this diagnosis. Both imaging methods reveal diffusely thickened retina. In the case of diffuse infiltrating retinoblastoma MRI may provide useful information.

The diffusely infiltrating retinoblastoma is a frequent cause of misdiagnosis. The eye is often red and may present with a pseu-dohypopyon, nodules on the surface of the iris or in the anterior chamber, and/or endothelial tumor nodules resembling keratic precipitates. The vitreous is frequently hazy, and exudates may cover the peripheral retina. The retina may appear gray, infiltrated, and thickened. This disease has usually been described unilaterally only, and prognosis after enucleation is good. This type of retinoblastoma can also present with a hyphema. An anterior variant has been noted where the only tumor focus was in the anterior retina. Enucleation is the treatment of choice in the management of these cases. Since the lesion grows within and destroys the sensory retina, little is gained by attempts to salvage the eye.

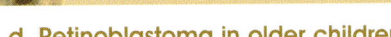
d. Retinoblastoma in older children

Almost 90% of all cases of retinoblastoma in the USA are diagnosed before the patient is 5 years old. However, newly diagnosed cases have been reported at ages 7 years, 9/10 years, 11 years, 12 years, 15 years, and in adults. The persistence of a rare embryonal retinal cell has been proposed as one explanation for this rare onset of retinoblastoma at an advanced age. An alternative explanation is that a retinoma or retinocytoma that occurs early in life may be unrecognized until it undergoes malignant transformation.

The clinically important aspect of retinoblastoma presenting in older children is that misdiagnosis is common. The possibility of retinoblastoma in children should be considered in who have unexplained vitreous hemorrhage or have signs that suggest, but are not typical for, endophthalmitis, even if they are older than 5 years of age.

e. Iatrogenic extraocular extension of tumor

Rarely, a child is referred with retinoblastoma growing out of a surgical wound. In most of these cases the underlying clinical problem of retinoblastoma lies unrecognized and intraocular surgery is performed for glaucoma, hyphema, vitreous hemorrhage, uveitis or presumed endophthalmitis. Any gross extraocular extension of intraocular retinoblastoma at the time of diagnosis should be treated with multidrug systemic chemotherapy before any surgery except for biopsy, if necessary. **The temptation to perform excisional biopsy should be resisted.** The tumor will melt away within 2–3 months following initiation of systemic chemotherapy even if the original tumor is very large.

f. Trilateral retinoblastoma (primitive neural ectodermal tumors, pinealoma)

The presence of intracranial tumor in the region of the pineal gland in association with retinoblastoma was first recognized by Jakobiec et al. in 1977. The term trilateral retinoblastoma was coined to describe the rare occurrence of a midline intracranial tumor in the presence of bilateral retinoblastoma. Originally called pinealoblastoma, typical, small, round cells with minimal cytoplasm in this region are now regarded as one of the group of primitive neural

ectodermal tumors (PNETs). The tumor that occurs in the region of the pineal gland in patients with heritable retinoblastoma is identical in histologic characteristics with the PNET (medulloblastoma) found in the posterior fossa, except that the PNET in the pineal region is characteristically more vascular than that in the posterior fossa. The pineal PNET in patients with heritable retinoblastoma occurs in approximately 2–3% of patients who carry the gene and are predisposed to the development of retinoblastoma. Most of these patients have bilateral disease. Clinical signs of pineal tumors include fever, vomiting, meningeal irritation, seizures, headaches, bilateral papilledema, and hydrocephalus. Diagnosis of PNETs may precede, appear concurrently with, or follow the diagnosis of retinoblastoma. The mean diagnosis of the midline PNET is 23 months. The diagnosis of heritable RB-associated PNET is usually made on CT scan with a demonstration of an enhancing, partially calcified suprasellar or sellar mass. Hydrocephalus may be present. The mass may extend from the sella to the foramen of Monro (located in the posterior portion of the third ventricle). Discovery of rosette formation during histology studies is helpful in the diagnosis of retinoblastoma-associated pineal PNET. These tumors apparently share antigens with retino-blastoma. The argument that these tumors arise in vestigial photoreceptors is supported by the fact that these tumors can show all the evidence of photoreceptor differentiation, fleurettes, and Flexner–Wintersteiner rosettes that is seen in retinoblastoma.

Until fairly recently, treatment of these tumors had been uniformly unsuccessful, with no survivors. Median survival after diagnosis of PNET is around 8 months. Vincristine and cyclophosphamide appeared to have some temporary beneficial effect. Survival of aggressive PNETs is rare.

The use of MRI as a screen for a midline lesion of PNET is a debatable subject. Presymptomatic detection of this lesion may result in longer survival. MRI scan of the brain is usually done every 6 months for 3 years in patients diagnosed with bilateral retinoblastoma before 6 months of age.

FOLLOW-UP SCHEDULE

The usual protocol is to schedule the first examination 3–6 weeks after the initial therapy. In cases where chemoreduction therapy has been administered, the examination should be done every 3 weeks with each cycle of chemotherapy. Patients under focal therapy are evaluated and treated every 4–8 weeks until complete tumor regression. Following tumor regression, subsequent examination should be 3 monthly for the first year, 6 monthly for three years or until the child attains 6 years of age, and yearly thereafter (Table 26.9).

PROGNOSIS

The overall survival rate from retinoblastoma in developed countries results from a mixture of causes of death. In the first 4 years of life, most of the deaths will be from metastatic retinoblastoma. Later deaths are increasingly likely to be the result of genetically predisposed second primary tumors such as osteosarcoma or fibrosarcoma. Thus, the overall survival rate will differ depending upon the time period examined. Abramson and colleagues reported that 86%, of bilateral retinoblastoma patients survive 15 years. By 5 years after diagnosis more children die of second malignant neoplasms than from retinoblastoma.

RETINAL VASCULAR TUMORS

'Retinal vascular tumors' includes both true neoplastic entities such as hemangioblastomas and cavernous hemangiomas, but also congenital AV communications. Hemangioblastomas can be encountered as solitary entities independent of any systemic disorder, but also in conjunction with the von Hippel-Lindau (VHL) syndrome,

which is a hereditary multi-tumor syndrome. Finally, retinal vasoproliferative tumors share some common features of hemangiomas and retinal glial tumors and can be either sporadic or secondary to other ocular pathology, such as uveitis and retinitis pigmentosa (Fig. 26.6).

RETINAL HEMANGIOBLASTOMA

Retinal hemangioblastoma is a benign vascular retinal tumor, which is also known as capillary retinal angioma, capillary retinal hemangioma or, in cases of multiple occurrence in an individual patient, retinal angiomatosis. In 1911 Eugen von Hippel coined the term 'angiomatosis retinae' when describing the vascular nature of the lesion. Fuchs, Wood and Collins gave earlier reports describing partial aspects of these tumors. Collins was the first to describe the hereditary nature of the disease.

Retinal hemangioblastoma may occur sporadically as a solitary tumor or associated with VHL syndrome. The frequency of **sporadic retinal hemangioblastoma** has been estimated at one in 110,000 individuals. More often it appears **in association with VHL disease**, which is an autosomal-dominant multi-tumor syndrome (Fig. 26.7). Besides retinal hemangioblastoma, further classical lesions of VHL include CNS hemangioblastoma, pheochromocytoma, pancreatic and renal cysts and renal carcinoma. VHL disease is caused by a mutation of the *VHL* gene (3p25–26). The *VHL* gene product is supposed to act as a tumor suppressor and is also involved in the cellular response to changes of intracellular oxygen levels, as well as in regulation of vascular growth.

GENETICS

Till date, more than 1500 different causative mutations of the *VHL* gene have been described, with a predominance of missense mutations. A correlation of retinal angioma phenotype and the localization of a missense mutation in the *VHL* gene has been described. A mutation in the α-domain of the *VHL* gene had a higher risk of forming juxtapapillary angiomas, whereas β-domain mutations correlated with the formation of peripheral angiomas. Since molecular genetic testing for a mutation of the *VHL* gene is informative in virtually all affected families, it

Table 26.9 *Classic regression patterns*	
Type 1	A concession of tumor to a lumpy calcified mass cottage cheese appearance
Type 2	Change in character of the tumor from a solid-looking, pink, vascular, opaque tumor to a grayish less vascular transcent tissue fish-flesh appearance
Type 3	A combination of types 1 and 2
Type 4	Total loss of tumor, retina and choroid leaving bare sclera

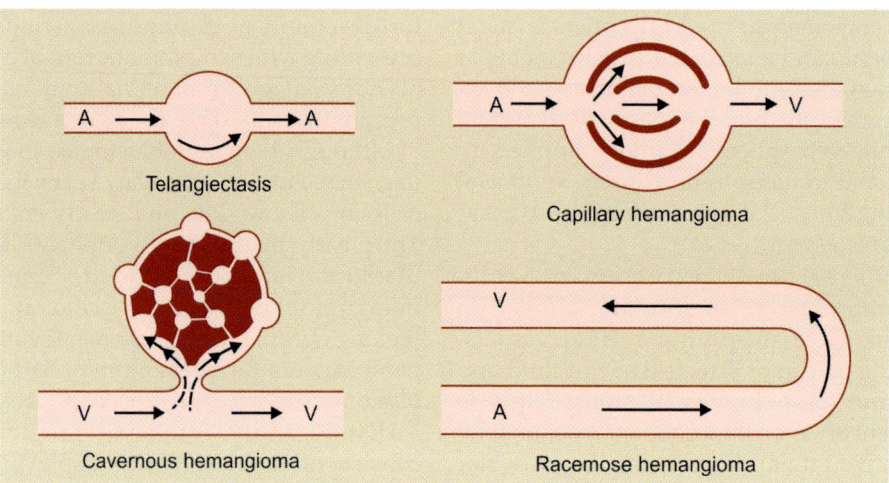

Fig. 26.6 *Schematic diagram showing the difference between retinal telangiectasis (Coats' disease), capillary hemangioma, cavernous hemangioma, and recemose hemangioma . Telangiectasis is merely a dilated vessel. Capillary hemangioma is a large arteriovenous shunt with rapid flow. Cavernous hemangioma is represented as a group of dilated vessels away from the main flow of blood. Racemose hemangioma represents an arteriovenous shunt with large vessels and rapid flow without capillary bed*

is essential for establishing the diagnosis. In the case of retinal hemangioblastoma, genetic testing for a *VHL* gene mutation, including pre- and post-test genetic counseling, is mandatory. In the case of a positive result, clinical screening for further VHL lesions should be performed. In addition, screening for further affected family members is recommended.

SCREENING PROTOCOL

Detailed recommendations for screening in individuals affected by VHL, depending on the

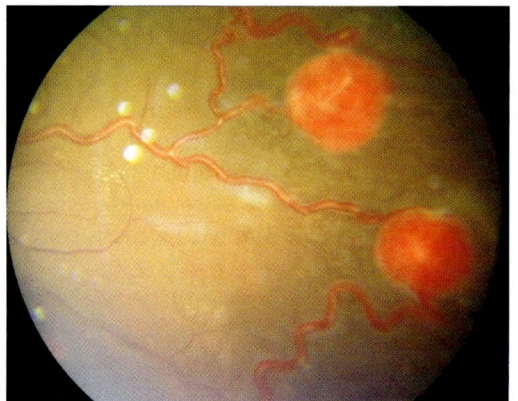

Fig. 26.7 *Fundus picture of the left eye reveals two orange-red retinal tumors in the temporal mid-periphery associated with a dilated, tortuous feeder arteriole, and draining vein*

patient's age, have been suggested. In brief, molecular genetic screening is recommended at any age. A retinal exam should be performed annually from age 1, every 6 months from age 11 to 19 years and annually again from 20 years of age. Screening for CNS lesions start at age 11 years and should be performed every 1–2 years. An annual ultrasound and a CT scan or MRI every other year for abdominal lesions should be performed. Screening should be performed throughout a patient's lifetime. However, lack of adherence to these protocols owing to pretest anxiety has been demonstrated to impede the success of these programs.

CLINICAL FEATURES

Clinically both sporadic and syndromal retinal hemangioblastoma show the same characteristics regarding age of presentation, morphology and symptoms. However, in the case of underlying VHL disease, retinal angioma is often multifocal and bilateral. In the majority of VHL patients it is the first sign of the disease to appear. It predominantly occurs in the third decade of life, but a person of any age from early childhood onwards, can be affected. The prevalence of retinal hemangioblastoma has been calculated to be 70% at age 60 years. Moreover, in the case

of retinal angiomatosis in a VHL patient bilateral involvement can be expected in all patients at age 56 years. Commonly, retinal hemangioblastoma occurs in the mid-periphery of the retina as an orangered spherical tumor, supplied by enlarged and tortuous feeder vessels. Peripheral retinal angioma is diagnosed by its typical funduscopic aspect.

Early stages, however, present as hardly visible microangiomas showing almost no enlargement of supplying retinal vessels. Depending on tumor size, leakage of fluid and lipids from the hemangioblastoma leads to impairment of vision by secondary maculopathy or exudative retinal detachment. The vascular nature of the hemangioblastoma, as well as fluid leakage from the tumor, can be visualized by fluorescein angiography. Late stages of retinal angiomatosis with large and/or multiple angiomas may be complicated by tractional epiretinal membranes, retinal detachment and vitreous hemorrhage, resulting in severe impairment of vision. Hemangioblastomas associated with the optic disc are present in 8–17% of eyes with retinal angiomatosis. The ophthalmoscopic aspect of juxtapapillary hemangioblastoma is less typical than that of peripheral hemangioblastoma. In contrast to peripheral hemangioblastomas, the borders of juxtapapillary hemangioblastomas are often irregular and less well demarcated and growth pattern is variable. They may grow into the subretinal space, intraretinally, or into the vitreous cavity. **Juxtapapillary hemangioblastoma must be differentiated** from lesions located at the optic disc as they have a similar ophthalmoscopic appearance to juxtapapillary choroidal hemangioma, amelanotic choroidal melanoma or choroidal neovascular membranes. **Fluorescein angiography** can be helpful in establishing the diagnosis. Owing to the close anatomical relation to the macula, fluid exudation, even from small juxtapapillary hemangioblastoma, may lead to a severe impairment of vision.

Clinically, patients affected by retinal hemangioblastoma present with a painless loss of visual acuity or visual field or both. In advanced cases retinal angiomatosis may lead to a painful secondary glaucoma. Since the risk for development of blindness is high in eyes presenting with symptomatic retinal hemangioblastoma, diagnosis of retinal angiomatosis in a presymptomatic stage is advantageous.

Although hemangioblastomas may remain unchanged in size over many years, the majority of lesions show slow and steady enlargement. Thus, early treatment of peripheral hemangioblastoma is recommended. Since retinal hemangioblastomas can occur at any age, lifelong ophthalmoscopic screening of the *VHL* gene carriers for presymptomatic hemangioblastoma, starting at preschool age, is mandatory.

Histologically, retinal hemangioblastoma consists of large capillaries displaying normal endothelium, basement membrane and pericytes with astrocytes containing large lipid-filled vacuoles separating the vascular channels.

MANAGEMENT

A. *Basic therapy for small peripheral retinal hemangioblastoma* is laser photocoagulation. Larger lesions may be treated by cryotherapy or radiotherapy employing ruthenium-106-plaques or proton beam irradiation. In addition, photodynamic therapy with verteporfin may be an option. Treatment of larger lesions can result in exudative or tractive retinal detachment. This complication is described to occur less frequently in plaque therapy compared with cryotherapy. In advanced cases, additional vitreoretinal surgery may be indicated. It may either be used for the treatment of secondary complications, such as angioma-associated epiretinal membrane or retinal detachment, but also for endolaser coagulation or primary resection of retinal angiomas. Prognosis in these cases can be influenced by complications such as angioma recurrence, secondary glaucoma or retinal detachment and is in general limited by these complications.

B. *Treatment of juxtapapillary retinal hemangioblastoma* is difficult, because destruction of nerve fibers or parts of the optic disc by whichever treatment modality may lead to large and persistent visual field scotomas. If juxtapapillary hemangioblastoma is asymptomatic, in contrast to the

management of peripheral hemangio-blastoma, observation is the strategy of choice. In symptomatic juxtapapillary hemangioblastoma, laser coagulation, external beam irradiation using photons or protons, vitrectomy employing photocoagulaion or cryocoagulation, and standard photodynamic therapy have all been used. However, results of treatment in these cases are variable.

C. *A modified photodynamic therapy technique* has been applied for juxtapapillary choroidal hemangiomas with success, which could also be considered for some cases of retinal hemangioblastomas associated with the optic disc. With this technique, treatment is performed in a 'paint-brush fashion', by moving the spot with constant speed eccentrically around the lesion's center over the entire tumor surface. The overall exposure time is increased from 83 to 125s. Under visual control this allows a complete and confluent photodynamic therapy of the whole tumor surface without overlapping and/or missing areas or treating the optic disc.

RETINAL CAVERNOUS HEMANGIOMA

Retinal cavernous hemangioma is a benign retinal vascular tumor that is composed of clusters of aneurysmatic dilated retinal vessels, with variable degrees of accompanying retinal gliosis and fibrosis. These lesions can be associated with similar CNS vascular anomalies, as well as cutaneous vascular malformations. Most retinal cavernous hemangiomas do not produce any retinal exudation, are not progressive and do not require any treatment.

RACEMOSE HEMANGIOMA (WYBURN-MASON SYNDROME)

The term racemose hemangioma describes the occurrence of retinal AV communications without interposed capillaries. This term is partly a misnomer, since the occurrence of hemangiomas, for example, true retinal neoplasms, is not characteristic of these lesions. If combined with vascular CNS malformations it is called Wyburn-Mason syndrome. Bonnet et al. gave an earlier description in the French ophthalmic literature, thus the term Bonnet-Dechaume-Blanc syndrome is also used in some countries.

Racemose hemangioma is rare and there are no reliable numbers describing the clinical frequency of this condition. Racemose hemangiomas are supposed to be congenital malformations remaining stationary; however, a hereditary factor predisposing to these lesions was not described.

The typical clinical aspect of the racemose hemangioma is a single or multiple direct AV communication emerging from the optic disc and extending to the posterior pole or the mid-periphery. Depending on the extent of the communication and the intravascular blood flow, the aspect of affected vessels may vary from only mild enlargement to massive dilatation, resembling feeder vessels of large retinal hemangioblastomas. However, unlike true hemangioblastomas, fluid leakage from affected vessels is often absent. Visual impairment is dependent on size and location of the lesion. It may be absent in small lesions sparing the macula but can be severe in large lesions showing widespread AV communications. Rarely, it may be complicated by vitreous or subretinal hemorrhage, retinal branch occlusion or secondary neovascular glaucoma. When followed for a very long time, AV retinal communications can show very slow progression with enhanced retinal vessel dilatation and also spontaneous regression without any treatment (Fig. 26.8).

Archer et al. proposed a **classification** for AV communications of the retina. These included:
- Grade I, retinal AV communication with interposition of an abnormal capillary plexus between major vessels.
- Grade II, single or multiple direct AV communication without capillary bed.
- Grade III, extensive and complex AV communication without capillary bed, generally with visual loss and CNS lesions.

The diagnosis is formed by the typical funduscopic appearance, and in the case of a massive and complex presentation, fluorescein angiography can be helpful to exclude the presence of a true vascular tumor. There is no

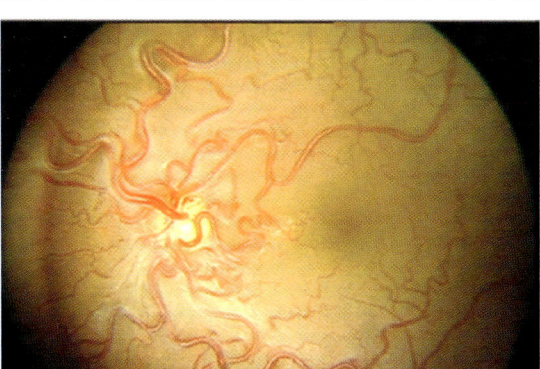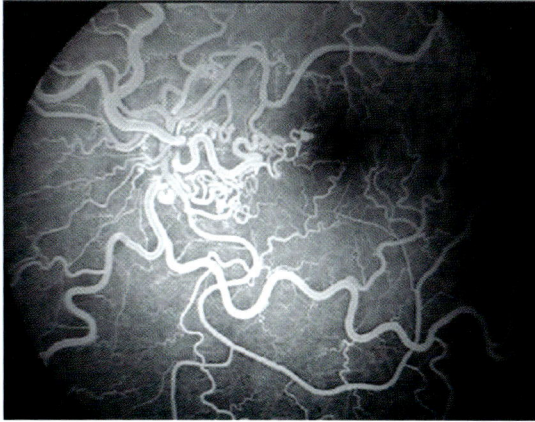

Fig. 26.8 *Racemose hemangioma in Wyburn-Mason syndrome showing the arterial side of the complex arising from the disc*

specific treatment for racemose hemangioma and clinical management of these lesions is restricted to the secondary complications.

Retinal racemose hemangioma may be combined with ipsilateral AV malformation of the CNS located in the midbrain. This can cause spontaneous intracranial hemorrhage, leading to various neurological complications. The proportion of patients with racemose hemangioma harboring a CNS AV malformation has not been determined. Considering the potentially lethal complication of CNS manifestation, however, in **every patient presenting with a racemose hemangioma, a neurological assessment should be suggested.**

RETINAL VASOPROLIFERATIVE TUMORS

Retinal vasoproliferative tumors are relatively rare, benign vascular tumors of the retinal periphery mainly occurring in patients in the fifth and sixth decade of life. They are usually unilateral and solitary, but there are rare exceptions. Retinal vasoproliferative tumors are not known to be associated with any systemic disease, but every fourth case can be associated with other intraocular, inflammatory, ischemic or vasoproliferative pathology, such as uveitis, retinitis pigmentosa, retinopathy of prematurity, sickle cell retinopathy or long-standing retinal detachment. Familiar bilateral cases have also been described.

Retinal vasoproliferative tumors most commonly occur in the inferior and/or temporal quadrant of the retinal periphery and present as yellow-orange-red-colored, well-vascularized, nonpigmented retinal lesions, almost always having a marked yellow halo composed of intra- or subretinal deposition of lipid exudates. The amount of these exudates is an indirect measure of the activity of the vasoproliferative lesions, which usually do not have very prominent feeding retinal vessels as opposed to retinal capillary hemangioblastomas. Histologically they are mainly composed of proliferating glial cells and a telangiectatic capillary network.

The main **differential diagnoses** include retinal hemangioblastoma, Coats' disease, peripheral exudative hemorrhagic chorioretinopathy, or amelanotic tumors of the retinal fundus. Peripheral fluorescein angiography can be helpful to identify the telangiectatic intrinsic vessels, but usually simple funduscopy is sufficient to diagnose these lesions. The marked lipid exudates, which usually impose first, and the lack of prominent feeder vessels, are distinct features of these tumors. In cases where a clear distinction between a retinal capillary hemangioblastomas is not possible, genetic testing to rule out VHL syndrome is recommended.

Retinal vasoproliferative tumors usually become symptomatic owing to the secondary cystoid macular edema and/or epiretinal gliosis and treatment is dependent on the symptomatology and the progressive nature of the vasoproliferative lesions. In the case of cystoid macular edema or progressive intraretinal lipid

deposition, treatment is recommended. It consists of photocoagulation or transpupillary thermotherapy in smaller vasoproliferative lesions and cryocoagulation, photodynamic therapy or brachytherapy in larger lesions (3 mm thickness). In the case of epiretinal gliosis or secondary macular pucker, additional vitrectomy is recommended.

RETINAL ASTROCYTIC HAMARTOMA (RETINAL ASTROCYTOMA)

Retinal astrocytic hamartoma or retinal astrocytomas are benign, acquired, retinal or papillary neoplasias, which are often found in association with the tuberous sclerosis complex (TSC; Bourneville-Pringle disease). They can also be associated with neurofibromatosis type 1 (NF-1), and can even rarely be found independently to any systemic diseases. Retinal astrocytic hamartomas are rarely progressive lesions. They are almost always asymptomatic, and are detected either on routine or screening fundus examinations in patients with TSC or NF-1. When associated with TSC, multifocal lesions are not uncommon.

Retinal astrocytic hamartomas are usually located in the inner layers of the retina or the optic disc, obscuring the retinal vessels. They have a milky gray–white appearance, depending on their amount of calcification. They are composed of spindle-shaped or even pleomorphic retinal astrocytes and can have various amounts of calcification. Detection of small noncalcified astrocytic hamartomas can be challenging, especially in fairly pigmented individuals. On fluorescein angiography, they produce early a relative blockade, through which the retinal vessels can be obscured in the larger lesions. The intrinsic tumor vascularization is highlighted in the middle and late phases of the angiogram.

Treatment is almost never required, with the rare exception of growing lesions, where photodynamic therapy can be effective. On rare occasions retinal astrocytomas can show progressive growth and have associated features such as vitreous seeds, vitreous hemorrhage and exudative retinal detachment, which can simulate retinoblastoma or choroidal melanoma.

RETINAL LYMPHOMA (PRIMARY INTRAOCULAR LYMPHOMA)

Retinal lymphomas are part of the intraocular manifestation of lymphomas, which can be located either in the retina or in the uvea, and can be further subclassified in primary and secondary manifestations. In the case of retinal lymphomas, these can present as isolated intraretinal lesions, infiltrating various parts of the Bruch's membrane–RPE–neuroretinal complex, as well as isolated vitreous infiltrates or, in the case of vitreoretinal lymphomas, as a combination of these. Retinal lymphoma commonly has a gray-yellowish coloration and when infiltrating under the RPE they often acquire a 'leopard fur' appearance due to RPE clumping and atrophy. Retinal lymphomas can present as 'masquerade syndromes', mimicking vitreoretinal or choroidal inflammatory diseases, such as infectious or autoimmune vitritis, retinopathies, chorioretinopathies and/or choriocapillaropathies (Fig. 26.9A to D).

Typical differential diagnoses include autoimmune vitreoretinopathies, white-dot syndromes, viral retinopathies and vitreochoroidal metastases, among others. It usually manifests in people over 60 years of age, but can also occasionally be diagnosed in immunocompromised younger patients.

Diagnosis is challenging and requires, besides systemic and neurological examinations, a variety of serological tests to rule out some of the previously mentioned entities. However, a vitreoretinal, and sometimes an additional choroidal, biopsy may establish the diagnosis. A total of 60–90% of cases are bilateral, but usually present initially as unilateral disease, with often very subtle asymptomatic manifestation in the fellow eye. The majority of vitreoretinal lymphomas are clinically aggressive and will eventually be associated with CNS lymphomas (in ~70% of cases), and therefore, regular neurological screening is recommended to detect early CNS manifestation.

RETINAL/VITREORETINAL METASTASIS

Intraocular metastasis was historically considered a rare finding; however, it is more recently

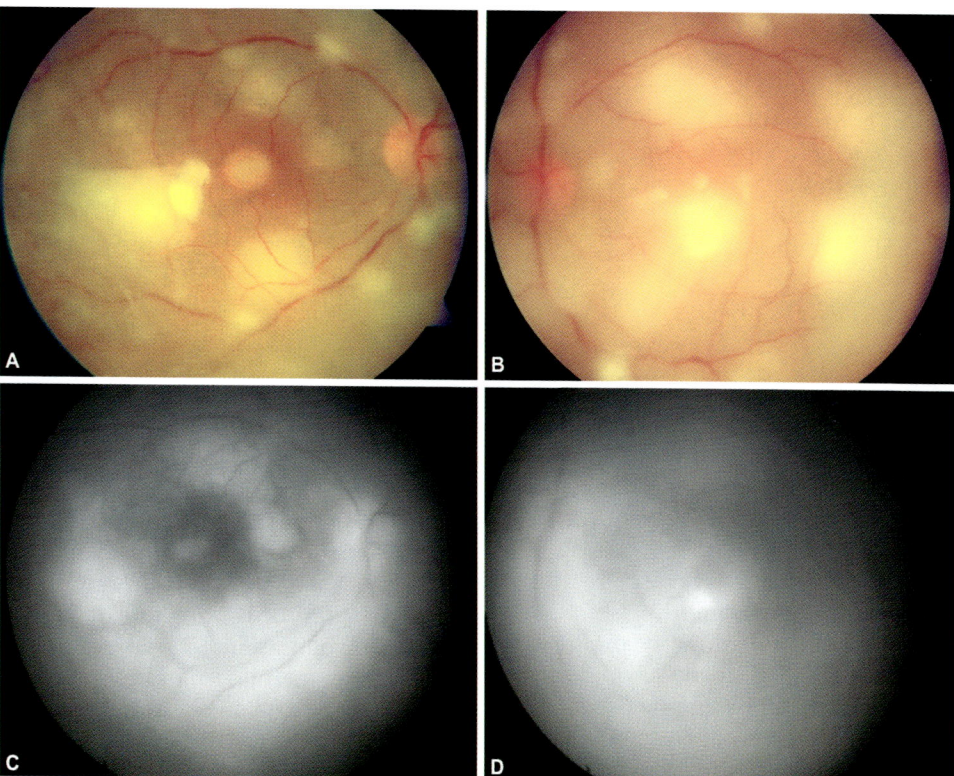

Fig. 26.9 *A 65-year-old woman had diminished vision in both eyes since 6 months. Both eyes had light perception. On examination, both eyes anterior segments were unremarkable. Posterior segment examination of both eyes showed significant vitreous cells, with creamy yellowish subretinal lesions all over the fundus (A and B). Fluorescein angiography showed diffuse leakage from retinal vessels (C and D). MRI whole body was normal. Cytology and immunohistochemistry of vitreous fluid and cerebrospinal fluid revealed B cell non-Hodgkin's lymphoma.(Coutesy: Prof. Amod Gupta).*

recognized as the most common intraocular tumor. In the majority of cases, it is located in the posterior choroid. The most common primary tumor is breast cancer, in approximately 50% of cases, followed by lung cancer. However, metastatic cancer to the retina or vitreous is a very rare entity and only a limited number of case reports exist describing this condition. In contrast to choroidal metastasis, the majority of retinal metastases reported concern metastatic cutaneous melanoma. Lung cancer is second, and breast cancer is only a rare source of these lesions.

The most common symptom of retinal metastasis is decreased or blurred vision, followed by floaters. Clinical signs depend on location and size of the lesion, and on the extent of associated secondary changes. Commonly,

retinal metastasis presents as yellow-white intraretinal patches with or without perivascular infiltration. In addition, intraretinal hemorrhage and subretinal exudates may be present. In contrast to choroidal metastasis, retinal metastasis may present with vitreous cellular infiltration. In the case of retinal metastasis due to cutaneous melanoma, vitreous infiltrates present as large, globular pigmented vitreous opacities. By contrast, vitreous infiltration from metastatic carcinoma is unpigmented. Secondary glaucoma caused by obstruction of the anterior chamber angle by clusters of tumor cells has been described as an additional complication of retinal metastasis.

Differential diagnosis comprises retinal infiltration from choroidal metastasis, infectious retinitis of various origin and vaso-occlusive

retinal disorders with exudation. Conditions causing vitreous floaters or opacities, such as uveitis, amyloidosis or intraocular lymphoma, also have to be considered.

In the case of retinal metastasis, patients commonly have a known history of cancer and nonocular metastasis. Thus, as in cases of choroidal metastasis, a systemic work-up for metastatic cancer should be performed. Fluorescein angiography may be helpful to differentiate retinal metastasis from vaso-occlusive disorders. Vitreous or retinal biopsy, either performed by vitrectomy or by fine-needle aspiration biopsy, may be helpful in establishing the diagnosis, but requires an experienced cytopathologist for an evaluation of the specimens obtained.

Choroidal metastasis is effectively treated by external beam radiotherapy. In the case of retinal metastases, the response to external beam radiotherapy has also been reported in single cases, but visual improvement was limited owing to macular involvement. However, systemic chemotherapy seems not to be effective in controlling retinal metastasis from cutaneous melanoma.

TUMORS OF THE RPE

SIMPLE HAMARTOMA OF THE RPE

Congenital simple hamartoma of the RPE, also described as congenital focal hyperplasia of the RPE (in contrast to congenital hypertrophy of the RPE) has typical clinical features consisting of intraretinal heavy pigmentation, a small size of approximately half disc diameter, macular/parafoveal location and often a small extension into the vitreoretinal interface. These findings are usually sufficient to differentiate it from malignant conditions. The disorder seems to be nonprogressive, but associated epiretinal traction may develop and surgical intervention is rarely effective. Optical coherence tomography has been quite helpful in determining the exact anatomical location of the hyperplastic RPE cells, which are most frequently located within the retina, having their apex at the vitreoretinal interface.

COMBINED HAMARTOMA OF THE RETINA AND THE RPE

Combined hamartoma of the retina and the RPE is believed to be a nonhereditary, congenital lesion, although it has been associated with neurofibromatosis (NF-2) and, in some cases, has been reported with NF-1. Combined hamartoma of the retina and the RPE is most commonly diagnosed in school-aged children, owing to reduced visual acuity. These lesions are usually unilateral, located close to or even involving the optic disc and are not progressive, although there are rare exceptions in all of these characteristics. The lesions have intermingled intra and subretinal components, and consist of the proliferation of retinal glial cells and RPE cells, having lost the normal retinal architecture. The lesions involve the retinal vasculature, which shows straightening of the larger, more superficial retinal vessels and marked tortuosity of the smaller vessels in the deeper layers of the tumor. The tumors commonly involve the macula and the optic disc, producing retinal distortion and foveal ectopia, as well as epiretinal gliosis. Preretinal and choroidal neovascularization, in association with combined hamartoma of the retina and the RPE, has also been described (Fig. 26.10A and B).

Pars plana vitrectomy with membrane peeling has been proposed to be helpful in restoring visual acuity in some cases, although in the majority of cases visual acuity improvement cannot be anticipated owing to the associated amblyopia, since these lesions are either congenital or have developed very early in childhood. On the rare occasion where an enlarging parafoveal combined hamartoma is threatening the fovea, photodynamic laser treatment has been proposed with encouraging results.

CONGENITAL HYPERTROPHY OF THE RPE (CHRPE)

Congenital hypertrophy of the RPE (CHRPE) is a relatively common finding in routine fundus examinations. These lesions are thought to be congenital, although are most commonly diagnosed in the fifth decade of life. They are asymptomatic and located in the mid-to-outer fundus periphery. CHRPE are flat lesions,

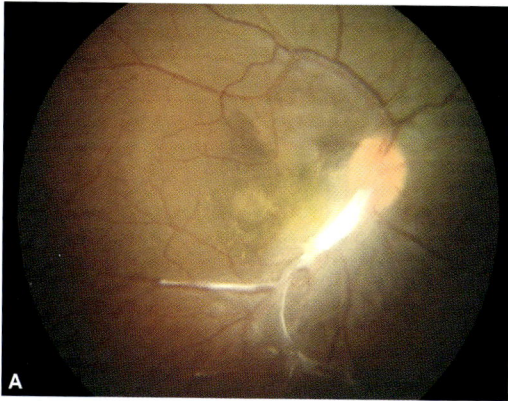

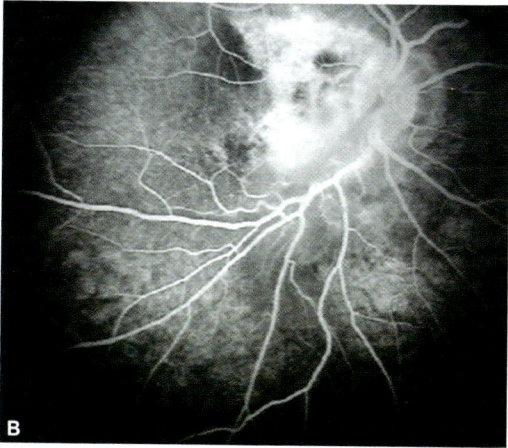

Fig. 26.10 *(A) Fundus picture of right eye showing variably pigmented macular RPE with a surrounding area of more orange appearing RPE. The temporal arcades are distorted and displaced towards the center of the fovea. There is an epiretinal membrane over the nasal portion of the fovea, extending inferiorly consistent with diagnosis of combined hamartoma; and (B) Late phase angiogram shows area of blocked fluorescence and hyperfluorescence surrounding it*

consisting most commonly of a hypertrophic heavily pigmented RPE monolayer and cannot be detected by ultrasound examination. Typically, CHRPE are well demarcated, heavily pigmented lesions at the level of the RPE and are surrounded by a thin depigmented halo, which itself is also often surrounded by a discrete, irregular, less-heavily pigmented halo (double halo pattern) (Fig. 26.11). During their evolution, CHRPE lesions can develop depigmented lacunae and present, eventually, as completely depigmented sharply demarcated lesions.

CHRPE does not need any treatment and occasional observation can be advised for documentation of progression, which can be very slow, or for observation of the development of any hyperplastic changes with secondary alterations of the vitreoretinal interface. The typical pigmented or depigmented CHRPE lesions are not associated with familial adenomatous polyposis (FAP) and bowel cancer, in contrast to RPE hamartomas, which can be associated with both FAP and Gardner syndrome. RPE hamartomas associated with FAP and/or Gardner syndrome are usually oval shaped, have irregular depigmented margins and are composed of hypertophic and hyperplastic RPE cells.

RPE–NEOPLASIA (EPITHELIOMA, ADENOMA AND ADENOCARCINOMA)

Retinal pigment epithelium–neoplasia is a very rare finding that has been described both in its benign and malignant variants. These lesions are usually deeply pigmented, although amelanotic variants have been described. Once these lesions invade the overlying retina, they develop dilated retinal feeding vessels, as well as progressive lipid exudation and exudative retinal elevations similar to retinal hemangio-blastomas. These neoplasms can develop within CHRPE lesions or hyperplastic chorioretinal scars. The aforementioned characteristics help to differentiate them from choroidal melanomas; however, in the case of atypical amelanotic lesions, the diagnosis can only be established by means of chorioretinal biopsy. Treatment will be in case of slowly growing adenomas close observation, whereas in the case of aggressive adenocarcinomas, eye-salvaging local excision, radiotherapy or enucleation will be used.

PHAKOMATOSES OF RETINA

Phakomatoses (Greek word phacomata or birth mark) are a group of complex multisystem disorders defined as neuro-oculocutaneous syndromes with multiple tumors or tumor like lesions in different organs of the body. van der Hoeve described the term Phakomatoses in 1923. Three syndromes which perfectly fits the definitional criteria and are consistently

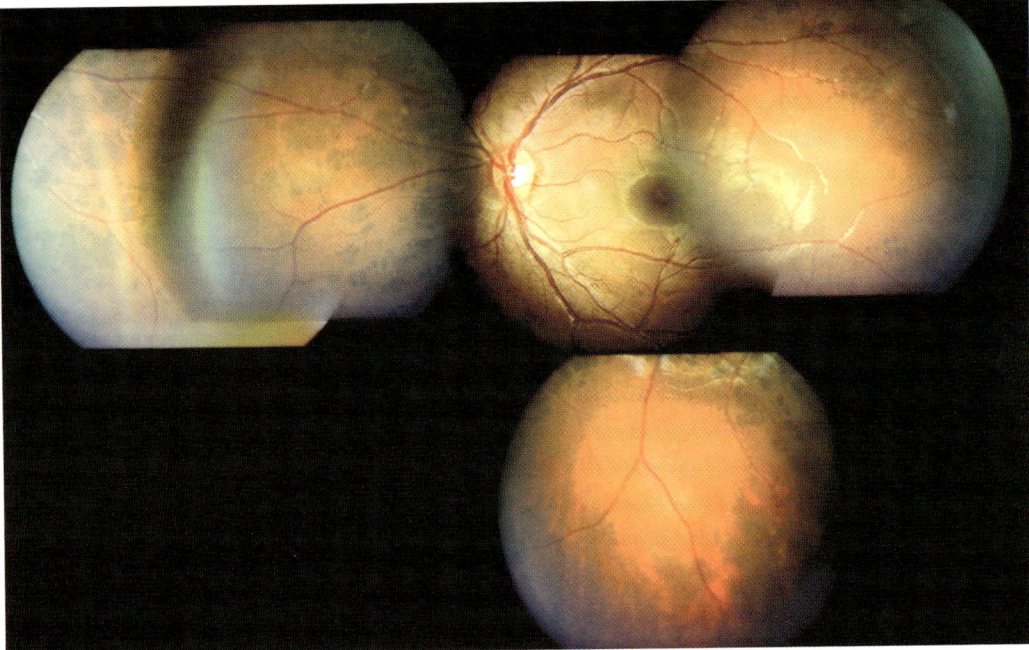

Fig. 26.11 *Multiple areas of grouped congenital hypertrophy of the retinal pigment epithelium (CHRPE) which are commonly called "bear tracks"*

classified as Phakomatoses by most authors are Neurofibromatosis (NF), Tuberous sclerosis (TS), and von Hippel-Lindau syndrome (VHLS). Two other syndromes though not conforming to the definition but still are grouped by authors as Phakomatoses are Sturge-Weber syndrome (SWS) and Wyburn-Mason syndrome (WMS).

A. NEUROFIBROMATOSIS

Neurofibromatosis is the most common type of Phakomatosis having 2 distinct inherited autosomal dominant varities: 1) Classical Neurofibromatosis (NF-1), 2) Central acoustic Neurofibromatosis (NF-2).

Classical Neurofibromatosis (NF-1)

Classical Neurofibromatosis (von Recklinghausen's disease) is the most commonest type occurring 1 in 3500 persons. Men and women are affected in similar frequency. NF-1 is inherited in an autosomal dominant manner and results from mutations in NF-1 gene on chromosome 17q11, a tumor suppressor gene. Lisch Nodules of the iris is the presenting feature of NF-1. Neurofibromatosis is a hamartomatous proliferation of neural crest derived tissues.

Clinical Features

- Ophthalmic manifestations
- Pulsatile exophthalmos
- Eyelid neurofibroma (nodular/plexiform)
- Conjunctival and sclera neurofibroma
- Prominent corneal nerves
- Congenital glaucoma
- Lisch nodules—melanocytic hamartomas of the iris
- Retinal capillary hemangiomas
- Retinal astrocytomas
- Combined retinal and retinal pigment epithelial hamartomas
- Choroidal hamartomas
- Optic nerve glioma—pilocytic hamartomas of the anterior visual pathway.

Systemic manifestations

- Café au lait spots
- Axillary freckles
- Inguinal freckles
- CNS neurofibromas

- Cutaneous neurofibromas
- Subcutaneous neurofibromas
- Scoliosis
- Learning disability
- Hypertension

Diagnostic Criteria for Neurofibromatosis Type 1 (NF1)

The criteria are met in an individual if any two or more of the features listed below are present.

- Six or more café au lait macules over 5 mm in greatest diameter in prepubertal individuals and over 15 mm in greatest diameter in postpubertal individuals
- Two or more neurofibromas of any type or one plexiform neurofibroma
- Freckling in the axillary or inguinal regions (Crowe´s sign)
- Optic nerve glioma
- Two or more Lisch nodules (iris hamartomas)
- A distinctive osseous lesion such as sphenoid dysplasia or thinning of long bone cortex with or without pseudoarthrosis
- A first-degree relative (parent, sibling, or offspring) with NF-1 by the above criteria.

Central Acoustic Neurofibromatosis (NF-2)

Central acoustic Neurofibromatosis is less common than NF-1 affecting 1 in 35,000 people and is characterized by bilateral vestibular schwannomas. NF-2 is inherited in an autosomal dominant manner with complete penetrance and results from mutations in Merlin (cytoskeletal protein encoded in chromosome 22q12) a tumor suppressor gene. Bilateral vestibular schwannomas are the diagnostic feature of NF-2. The mean age of presentation of vestibular schwannomas is less than 25 years and never beyond 55 years.

Clinical features

Ophthalmic manifestations

- Posterior subcapsular cataract
- Epiretinal membrane
- Uveal melanoma
- Optic nerve glioma
- Combined retinal and retinal pigment epithelial hamartomas

Systemic manifestations

- Sensory neural deafness with or without tinnitus
- Seizures
- Vertigo
- Numbness
- Spinal schwannomas
- Intracranial meningiomas
- Spinal epndymomas

Diagnostic criteria for Neurofibromatosis Type 2 (NF2)

Bilateral masses of the eighth cranial nerve seen with appropriate imaging techniques (e.g., CT or MRI) or a first-degree with NF 2 and either:
a. Unilateral mass of the eighth cranial nerve, or
b. Two of the following:
  - Neurofibroma
  - Meningioma
  - Glioma
  - Schwannoma
  - Juvenile posterior subcapsular cataract.

Management

Investigations

Computed tomography (CT) or magnetic resonance imaging (MRI) of the brain and spinal cord: Imaging studies should address the presence of vestibular schwannomas.

Treatment

- *Eyelid neurofibroma:* Surgical debulking done for mechanical ptosis or cosmetic deformity. Due to infiltrative nature of this lesion complete exision is not possible and has higher chance of recurrence
- *Optic nerve glioma:* Orbitotomy
- *Bilateral acoustic neuroma:* Stereotactic radiotherapy.

B. TUBEROUS SCLEROSIS COMPLEX

Desire Magloire Bourneville in 1880 suggested the terminology tuberous sclerosis on the basis of his observations of multiple potato (tubers) like lesions in the brain. It is a multiorgan disease. Incidence of tuberous sclerosis is 1 in 5800, of which two-thirds of cases occur sporadically. Two tumor suppressor genes have been identified in pathogenesis of tuberous

sclerosis: TSC 1 is found in chromosome 9q34 and TSC 2 in chromosome 16p13. TSC 1 and TSC 2 genes encode the proteins hamartin and tuberin. No gender predilection found in tuberous sclerosis. In 1908 Vogt defined the syndrome by describing the classic triad of angiofibromas, epilepsy and mental retardation. Epilepsy being the most common presenting feature described as infantile spasms (Salaam spasms). Facial angiofibromas distributed in the malar area in a butterfly fashion involving the chin called adenoma sebaceum. Ocular findings are a useful factor in the diagnosis of tuberous sclerosis in children presenting with infantile spasms. About 50% of TSC patients have mild to profound mental retardation. Ash leaf spots (Hypomelanotic macules) are the earliest cutaneous manifestation presenting at birth detectable by Wood's ultraviolet light. Shagreen patches are fibromatous infiltration of eyelids and lumbar region.

Clinical features

Ophthalmic manifestations

Angiofibromas of eyelids

Retinal hamartoma (astrocytoma)

Type 1	Type 2	Type 3
Flat	Elevated	Transitional
Smooth	Multinodular	lesion between
Noncalcified	Calcified	Type 1/Type 2
Grey,	Opaque like	
semitransparent	mulberries	

- Subretinal fluid
- Lipid exudates
- Serous retinal detachment
- Vitreous hemorrhage
- Punched out chorioretinal hypopigmentation
- Coloboma of iris, lens and choroids
- Strabismus
- Papilledema
- Sector iris depigmentation

Systemic manifestations

- Infantile spasms
- Adenoma sebaceum
- Ash leaf spots (hypomelanotic macules)
- Shagreen patches

- Subungual fibromas
- Angiomyolipoma of kidney
- Renal cyst
- Benign cardiac rhabdomyoma
- Pulmonary fibrosis
- Subpleural cysts
- Visceral hamartomas involving lung, kidney and heart.

Revised diagnostic criteria for tuberous sclerosis complex

Major features	Minor features
Facial angiofibromas or forehead plaque	Multiple randomly distributed pits in dental enamel
Non-traumatic ungual or periungual fibroma	Hamartomatous rectal polyps
	Bone cysts
Hypomelanotic macules (more than three)	Cerebral white matter migration lines
Shagreen patch (connective tissue nevus)	Gingival fibromas
	Non-renal hamartoma
Multiple retinal nodular hamartomas	Retinal achromic patch
Cortical tuber	"Confetti" skin lesions
Subependymal nodule	Multiple renal cysts
Subependymal giant cell astrocytoma	
Cardiac rhabdomyoma, single or multiple	
Lymphangiomyomatosis	
Renal angiomyolipoma	

Definite TSC: Either 2 major features or 1 major feature with 2 minor features
Probable TSC: One major feature and one minor feature
Possible TSC: Either 1 major feature or 2 or more minor features

Differential diagnosis

- Retinoblastoma
- Choroiditis secondary to toxocara and toxoplasma
- Optic disc drusen
- Coat's disease
- Myelinated nerve fibers

Investigations

- *Wood's ultraviolet light:* For detection of ash leaf spots.

- *EEG:* Abnormal hypsarrhythmic pattern with later dimunition to irregular multifocal slow waves and spikes
- *X-ray/CT scan/MRI brain:* CNS circumscribed calcifications involving periventricular/basal ganglia
- *Ultrasonography:* Califications are picked up as hyperechoic areas
- *FFA:* Autofluorescence noted in type 2 and type 3 retinal hamartoma
  – *Arterial phase:* Early filling of dilated vessels within the lesion
  – *Venous phase:* Dilated capillary loops and microaneurysms are visible.

Treatment

Genetic counseling: Adults with adenoma sebaceum, shagreen patches and ash leaf spots should be counseled about 1 in 2 risks of having child with tuberous sclerosis.
- Laser photocoagulation
- Photodynamic therapy
- Vitrectomy for hamartoma's complicated by vitreous hemorrhage.

C. STURGE-WEBER SYNDROME

Sturge-Weber syndrome (SWS) is a dermato-oculoneural syndrome. Sturge in 1879 described a syndrome characterized by facial hemangioma, ipsilateral buphthalmos, and contralateral seizures while Weber in 1922 described cortical calcification the radiological feature of leptomeningeal hemangioma causing hemiplegia. SWS is a triad of leptomeningeal hemangioma, choroidal hemangioma and cutaneous hemangioma. In the absence of CNS involvement from the triad then the diagnosis of only port wine stain should be made. SWS is the only phakomatoses that is not inherited. SWS has an estimated incidence of 1 in 50,000 live births. Men and women are equally affected.

Clinical features

Ophthalmic manifestations

1. Glaucoma — most commonest presentation.
2. *Diffuse choroidal hemangioma.* Usually unilateral and ipsilateral to the nevus flammeus. It is a diffuse angiomatosis of the choroid. These are observed in eyes where nevus flammeus involves upper eyelid. The description given

to the fundus is " tomato ketchup" (Fig. 26.12A and B).
3. Exudative retinal detachment—the commonest cause for vision loss.
4. Telangiectasia of conjunctiva and episclera.

Systemic manifestations

Leptomeningeal hemangiomatosis – seizures, developmental delay, behavioral problems.

Cutaneous hemangioma or nevus flammeus or port wine stain—this is a flat to moderately thick zone of dilated telangiectatic cutaneous capillaries lined by a single layer of endothelial cells in the dermis. The lesion is usually unilateral and involves the region of face innervated by V1 and V2 distribution of trigeminal nerve. Bilateral port wine stain has a higher likelihood of being associated with SWS. Only 10% of nevus flammeus is associated with SWS.

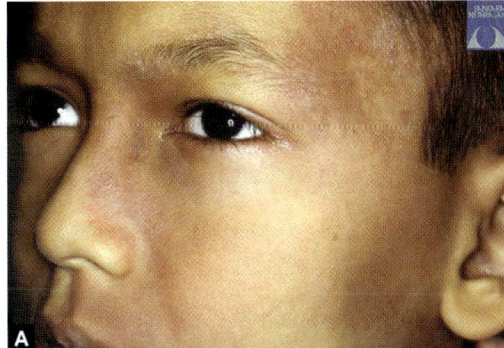

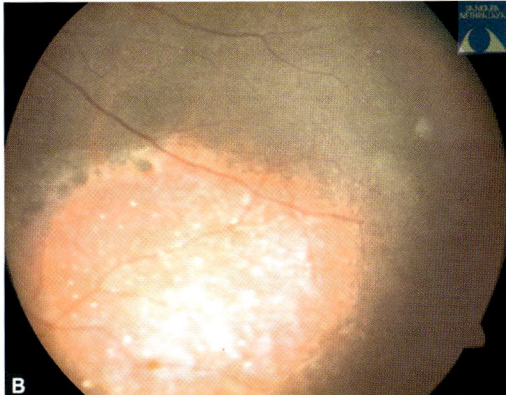

Fig. 26.12 *(A)* Left facial hemangioma (forehead); and *(B)* choroidal hemangioma on the ipsilateral side suggestive of Sturge-Weber syndrome

Investigations

- MRI (contrast enhanced)—cerebral atrophy and leptomeningeal malformations
- CT scan—intracranial calcifications

Treatment

1. *Small circumscribed choroidal hemangiomas*—Transpupillary thermotherapy, argon laser photocoagulation, plaque brachytherapy and low dose proton beam irradiation for posterior pole or sub foveal circumscribed choroidal hemangiomas.
2. *Diffuse choroidal hemangioma*—external beam radiotherapy or photodynamic therapy.
3. *Glaucoma*—medical therapy with antiglaucoma medications are effective only in certain cases. Majority of them require combined trabeculotomy with trabeculectomy or drainage implants.
4. *Seizures*—controlled with medications but intractable cases would require surgical resection of the leptomeningeal agiomatosis with the underlying cortex.
5. *Nevus flammeus*—dermatological laser therapy.
6. *Follow-up*—SWS do not have recognized propensity to develop benign or malignant neoplasms. Early deaths are reported in profound mental retardation and intractable seizures.

D. VON HIPPEL-LINDAU DISEASE

von Hippel-Lindau (VHL) disease is a multisystem disorder with a predilection for CNS and retina. Eugen von Hippel coined the term angiomatosis retinae and Arvid Lindau established the relationship between cerebellar and retinal hemangioblastomas while it was Melmon and Rosen who established the clinical spectrum of VHL disease. Affected individuals develop lesions such as CNS hemangioblastomas. Retinal hemangiomas or visceral manifestations such as renal carcinoma, pheochromocytoma and neuroendocrine tumors. Retinal capillary hemangioma is the earliest manifestation of VHL. The inheritance pattern is autosomal dominant with the VHL gene identified on chromosome 3p25–26. VHL gene encodes amino acid protein that targets hypoxia inducible factors for degradation. In the absence of pVHL

there is excessive production of vascular endothelial growth factor. The incidence of VHL disease is approximately 1 in 40,000 live births. Men and women are affected equally. Median age of detection is 20–25 years (Fig. 26.13A and B).

Clinical features

Ophthalmic manifestations

Retinal angiomas

Vail's classification of staging of retinal angiomas:

- *Stage I:* Early stage with dilation of feeding artery and draining vein and angioma formation
- *Stage II:* Development of hemorrhages and exudation
- *Stage III:* Massive exudation and retinal detachment
- *Stage IV:* Uveitis, absolute glaucoma, and loss of the eye.

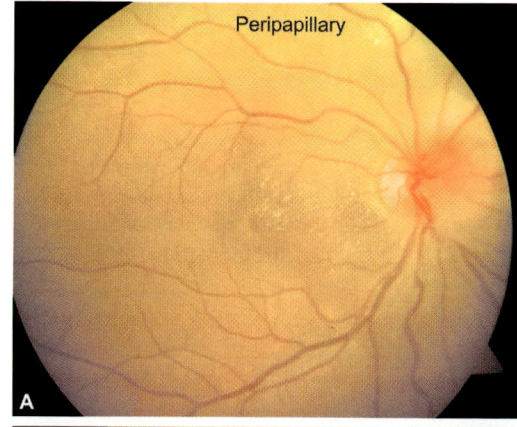

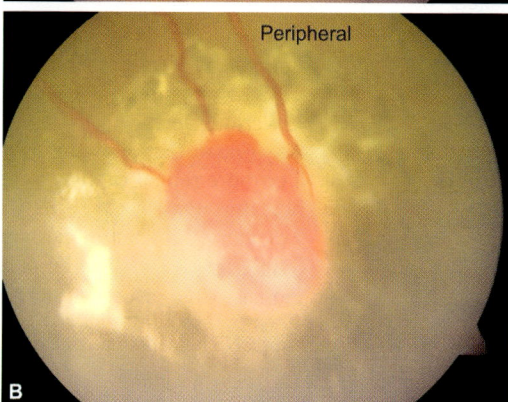

Fig. 26.13 *(A)* Capillary hemangioma on the nasal side of optic disc; and *(B)* peripheral retinal capillary hemangioma in case of VHL

*Various systems used to classify
retinal capillary hemangioma*

Basis	Classification
Retinal distribution	Peripheral
	Juxtapapillary
Morphology	Endophytic
	Sessile
	Exophytic
Effects on the retina	Exudative
	Vitreoretinal
Systemic features	Without VHL disease
	With VHL disease

Systemic manifestations

*Clinical characteristics of genotype phenotype
classifications in VHL*

Type 1	Retinal hemangioblastomas
	CNS hemangioblastomas
	Renal cell carcinoma
	Pancreatic neoplasms and cysts
Type 2A	Pheochromocytoma
	Retinal hemangioblastomas
	CNS hemangioblastomas
Type 2B	Pheochromocytoma
	Retinal hemangioblastomas
	CNS hemangioblastomas
	Renal cell carcinoma
	Pancreatic neoplasms and cysts
Type 2C	Pheochromocytoma only

Diagnostic criteria for von Hippel-lindau disease

Family history*	Required features
Positive	Any one of the following
	Retinal capillary hemangioma
	CNS hemangioma
	Visceral lesion**
Negative	Any one of the following
	2 or more retinal capillary hemangioma
	2 or more CNS hemangiomas
	Single retinal or CNS hemangioma with a visceral lesion**

*Family history of retinal or CNS hemangioma or visceral
lesion

**Visceral lesions include: Rrenal cysts, renal Ca, pheochro-
mocytoma, pancreatic cysts, islet cell tumors, epididymal
cystadenomas, endolymphatic sac tumor, adnexal papillary
cystadenoma of probable mesonephric origin

Differential diagnosis

- Coats' disease
- Racemose hemangioma
- Retinal cavernous hemangioma
- Retinal macroaneurysm
- Vasoproliferative tumor
- Retinal pigment epithelial adenoma
- Uveal melanoma with retinal invasion
- Unilateral papilledema
- Juxtapapillary choroiditis

Investigations

*Screening protocols for patients
with or at risk for VHL disease*

Test	National Institute of Health guidelines
Urinary catecholamines	Every year (age 2+)
Ophthalmoscopy	Every year (age 1+)
Fluorescein angiography	Not routine
Enhanced MRI of brain and spine	Every 2 years (age 11–60 years)
	Every 3–5 years (age 61+)
Abdominal ultrasonography	Every year (age 11–20+)
Abdominal CT	Every 1–2 years (age 21+)

Treatment

- *Observation:* Angiomas <500 microns without any exudation or subretinal fluid can be observed
- *Laser photocoagulation:* Most effective for tumors up to 1.5 mm in diameter
- *Transpupillary thermotherapy*
- *Protoporphyrin derivative therapy*
- *Photodynamic therapy* (PDT) is an effective treatment for juxtapapillary and peripheral angiomas
- *Cryotherapy:* Tumors >3 mm diameter, located between equator and ora
- *Plaque radiotherapy:* Tumors >4–5 mm
- *External beam radiotherapy*
- *Proton beam radiotherapy*
- *Pars plana vitrectomy/scleral buckling*: Retinal detachment
- *Enucleation:* Phthisis bulbi, neovascular glaucoma and painful blind eye.

E. WYBURN-MASON SYNDROME

Wyburn-Mason syndrome (WMS), also known as the Bonnet-Dechaume-Blanc syndrome, is a rare nonhereditary phakomatosis characterized by congenital ipsilateral retinal, brain (usually midbrain), and less frequently, facial angiomas. Bonnet et al first noted the combination of retinal and intracranial arteriovenous malformations (AVMs) in 1937. The condition results from a disturbance in the embryologic development of the vascular mesoderm. The retinal lesion consists of a markedly dilated and tortuous arteriole contiguous with a similar vein involving the optic disc and retina. Recognition of the association between the retinal and intracranial lesions is important because it may allow early identification of intracranial AVMs. Men and women are affected equally (Fig. 26.8).

Clinical features

Ophthalmic manifestations

Racemose hemangioma of the retinal vessels
- Group 1—abnormal capillary plexus between the major vessels
- Group 2—direct AV communication without interposition of capillary and arteriolar elements
- Group 3—extensive complex AV communication. Associated with visual loss

No exudation, Retinal detachment, vessels do not leak in fluorescein angiogram.

Systemic manifestations

- Ipsilateral midbrain hemangioma CNS features—spontaneous intracranial bleeds— neurologic symptoms, seizures and stroke.
- Skin manifestations are rare.

Investigations

Fluorescein angiography typically shows a rapid transit of dye through the lesion without leakage.

MRI and MRA of ipsilateral orbit and brain.

Treatment

- If retinal lesions are stable, no treatment is required
- *Persistent vitreous hemorrhage*—vitrectomy is the treatment of choice.

CYSTS OF THE RETINA

I. CYSTICERCOSIS

Subretinal cysticercosis is an uncommon ocular finding. It is caused by the human ingestion of the eggs of Taenia solium (pork tapeworm). Systemic dissemination may lead to bumps on the skin and symptoms of headaches, seizures, coma and even death, secondary to increased intracranial pressure.

Ocular Signs and Symptoms

Cysticerci can be found in any part of the eye or its adnexa. Possible locations include the anterior chamber, vitreous cavity, optic nerve head, subconjunctival space and recti muscles, lids, lacrimal gland, lens, and, most commonly, subretinal space. Bilateral involvement has also been reported. The larvae enter the subretinal space via the central retinal artery or posterior ciliary arteries.

Once inside the choroid, the infection causes atrophic changes in the overlying retinal pigment epithelium as the cyst develops. Enlargement of the cysticercus into the subretinal space often produces a secondary exudative detachment and focal chorioretinitis. The death of the parasite may lead to the release of large amounts of toxins, which, in turn, can produce a severe, fulminating intraocular inflammation leading to endophthalmitis. The inflammation accompanying the intraocular cysticercosis is more closely related to the host immune response than the cysticercus itself. This may explain the inefficacy of antihelminthic drugs used against the ocular disease. The vision of eyes with ocular cysticercosis can be well-preserved unless the parasite is localized in the macular area, an associated retinal detachment is present, or the intraocular inflammation is severe.

Intraocular cysticercosis may be asymptomatic in the early stages when the parasite is minute. As the parasite increases in size, it can cause gradual, painless, and progressive loss of vision. When found in the eye, the cysticercosis embryo is most commonly located beneath the retina at the posterior pole. It may migrate from one area of the fundus to another beneath the retina, or it may penetrate the retina and enter the vitreous

cavity. Over a period of many months, the parasite grows into a large cystic structure. Its funduscopic appearance can lead to the misdiagnosis of choroidal tumor, serous detachment of the retinal pigment epithelium, Valsalva retinopathy, or other parasitic infections. Recognition of the white head, or scolex, that is often invaginated and moving within the cystic body may permit accurate clinical diagnosis (Figs 26.14 A and B). Untreated subretinal cysticercosis can lead to severe ocular damage. This has been reported in about 80% of cases when cysts have not been removed.

Oral antihelminthic drugs have been used mainly to treat the central nervous system and skin presentations, whereas their uses against intraocular cysticercosis has met with limited success. Transcleral and transretinal approaches may be used to surgically remove the cyst when indicated.

II. CYSTS ASSOCIATED WITH RETINAL DETACHMENT

Retinal 'cysts' may be single or multiple, ranging from two-to-ten disc diameters in size and occur in 1–3% of the eyes with long-standing retinal detachment. Once the retina reattaches, the intraretinal cysts disappear in a few weeks. Improved nourishment of the retina gradually reverses the process responsible for cystic degeneration with eventual collapse of the cyst.

Hager and North have reported that macrocysts (medium-sized isolated cysts) are almost always seen in long-standing retinal detachments (usually greater than three months duration). They are found in about 3% of the eyes undergoing retinal detachment surgery. (Fig. 26.15) Macrocysts are believed to result from secondary degenerative changes in the retina. Retinal macrocysts are fluid-filled cavities, that is not very different from the subretinal fluid. Occasionally, there may be blood within the cyst. Drainage of the cyst is not indicated, as most cysts spontaneously resolve upon retinal reattachment and improved nutrition of the retina.

Pischel classified retinal cysts into small (up to 1 mm in size), medium or isolated (four to

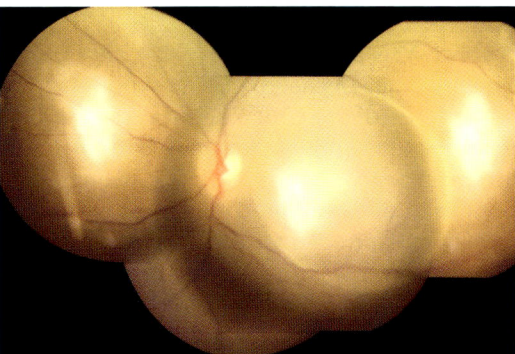

Fig. 26.14A *Subretinal cysticercosis in macular area*

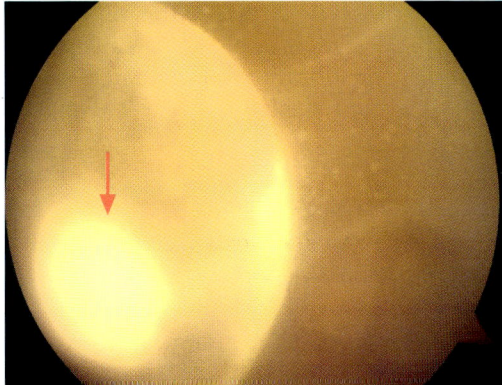

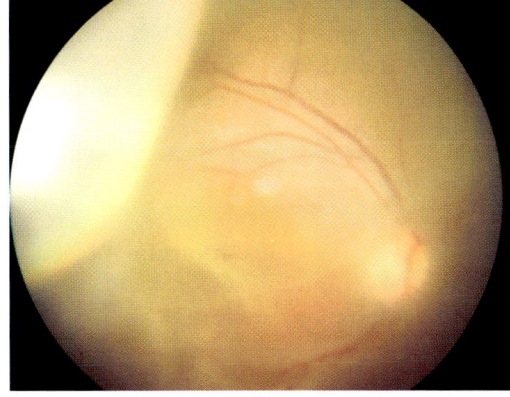

Fig. 26.14B *Motile intravitreous cystic structure without any vitreous inflammation showing refractile scolex in the cyst (arrow)*

eight disc diameters), giant (eight to ten disc diameters or more), and large cysts (retinoschisis) occupying 25% of the fundus.

Keith proposed classifying the lesions into retinal cysts and retinoschisis. He described cyst formation following retinal detachment and

doubted the causation of retinal disinsertion by the pre-existing retinal cyst.

Zimmerman and Spencer reported two unusual cases, which were diagnosed as malignant melanoma of the choroid and treated with enucleation, to be retinoschisis, which gave rise to a clinical picture of the tumor.

Ruiz reported enucleation of a blind eye with long-standing retinal detachment diagnosed clinically as malignant melanoma, which on histopathological examination turned out to be a macrocyst of the retina with organized hemorrhage.

Marcus and Aaberg, published a case series of seven patients, with retinal cysts associated with traumatic retinal detachment. In four of the seven eyes, the cysts were drained as they were felt to mechanically prevent closure of the retinal break. Hemorrhagic retinal cysts have also been described pathologically in eyes enucleated for advanced Coats' disease. The pathogenesis of a retinal cyst has been attributed to cystoid degeneration in the detached retina. In a series of seven eyes with intraretinal macrocysts associated with retinal detachment, reported by Marcus and Aaberg, none of the patients had a hemorrhagic cyst. A pathological study of one eye demonstrated that retinal macrocysts originated from the outer plexiform layer.

Although four of the seven cases in their series required drainage of the macrocysts to flatten the retinal break, we did not have to do so in our patient.

Differential diagnosis of retinal macrocysts

Macrocysts need to be differentiated from retinoschisis. In a macrocyst, there is no typical predilection for the inferotemporal quadrant, hyperopia or bilaterality, no vascular sheathing, glistening white spots, or retinal holes are seen, as in retinoschisis.

Clinically, and especially in eyes with opaque media, they may be confused with malignant melanoma, circumscribed choroidal hemangioma, subretinal abscess or posterior scleritis. The characteristic ultrasound features of each entity may help differentiate one from the other.

Malignant melanoma appears as a dome-shaped mass with a collar-stud appearance and a secondary retinal detachment away from the summit of the tumor mass. It has high surface reflectivity and low-to-moderate internal reflectivity. Acoustic hollowing with angle kappa may be seen. Choroidal excavation may also be noted. It may have extrascleral extension. In our patient, the ultrasound showed the origin of the cyst from within the retina and not the

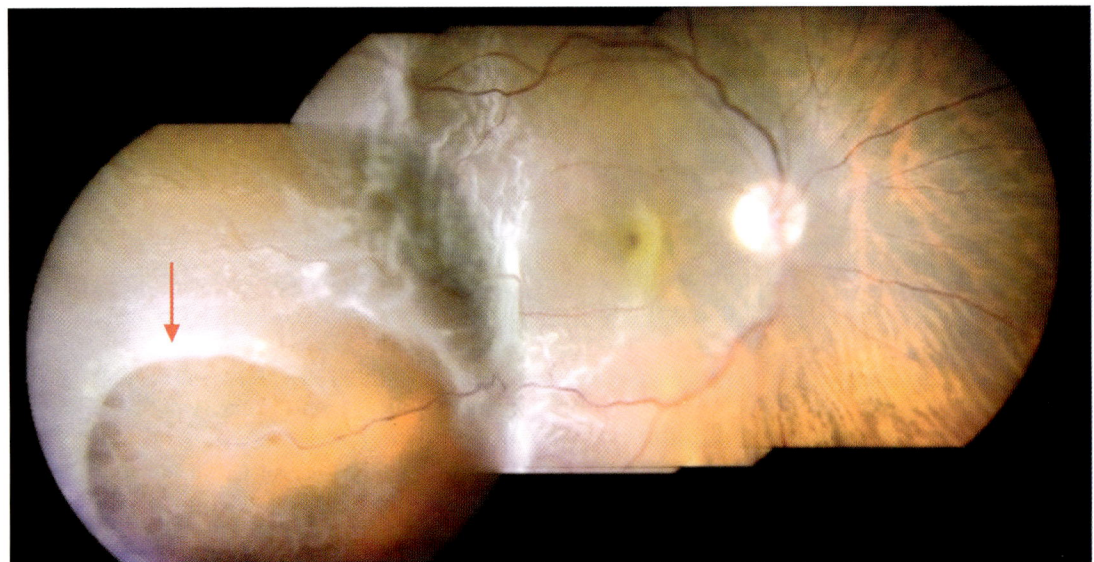

Fig. 26.15 *Fundus picture of a old long-standing retinal detachment having intravitreal cyst in the inferotemporal quadrant*

choroid. Splitting of the retina into two layers was noticeable with internal echogenic contents attributable to altered hemorrhage.

A circumscribed choroidal hemangioma appears as a relatively non-homogenous choroidal mass lesion with high surface reflectivity and moderate-to-high internal reflectivity. It may be associated with secondary retinal detachment.

A sub-retinal abscess typically appears as a well-defined, dome-shaped, elevated mass lesion, with high surface reflectivity and moderate-to-high internal reflectivity. A localized hypoechoic area of subtenon space widening is noted, adjacent to the lesion.

Posterior scleritis typically appears as a lesion with high surface reflectivity, with a regular, high internal reflective structure at the scleral level and may be associated with a localized increase in the sub-Tenon's space.

SUMMARY

There has been a dramatic change in the overall management of retinoblastoma in the last decade. Specific genetic protocols have been able to make prenatal diagnosis of retinoblastoma. Early diagnosis and advancements in focal therapy have resulted in improved eye and vision salvage. Chemoreduction has become the standard of care for the management of moderately advanced intraocular retinoblastoma. Periocular chemotherapy is now an additional useful tool in salvaging eyes with vitreous seeds. Enucleation continues to be the preferred primary treatment approach in unilateral advanced retinoblastoma. Postenucelation protocol, including identification of histopathologic high risk characteristics and provision of adjuvant therapy has resulted in substantial reduction in the incidence of systemic metastasis. The vexing orbital retinoblastoma now seems to have a cure finally with the aggressive multi modal approach. Future holds promise for further advancement in focal therapy and targeted drug delivery.

Early detection of retinal neoplasias is essential for establishing adequate diagnostic and therapeutic strategies for a variety of systemic disorders, with which they can be associated. Retinal hemangioblastomas should be treated according to their stage either by laser photocoagulation, laser hyperthermia, photodynamic therapy, radiation treatment or surgery. Adequate molecular genetic testing for the presence or absence of von Hippel-Lindau disease is important to facilitate adequate patient counseling. Novel antiangiogenic treatment methods can be integrated in these therapeutic strategies; however, the exact indications need yet to be established. Treatment of intraocular lymphomas can be local and focused on the intraocular component, but is dependent on systemic involvement and based on recommendations of general lymphoma treatment strategies. The same applies to retinal and vitreous metastases. Tumors of the RPE in general do not need any treatment, with the rare exception of RPE-carcinomas that are treated in most cases by local radiotherapy.

Better understanding of the genetic background of the systemic diseases, with which retinal neoplasia can be associated might help to develop more effective, and may be even causative, treatment methods in the future. The development of various anti-VEGF strategies in age-related macular degeneration might help to transfer therapeutic modalities in primary treatment of 'vasoactive' retinal tumors, such as retinal hemangioblastomas, retinal vasoproliferative tumors or the sequels of their primary treatment, such as exudative maculopathy/retinopathy or radiation maculopathy in the case of primary irradiation treatment.

BIBLIOGRAPHY

1. Aracena T, Roca FP. Macular and peripheral subretinal cysticercosis. Ann Ophthalmol 1981; 13:1265–7.

2. Arnold AC, Hepler RS, Yee RW, et al. Solitary retinal astrocytoma. Surv. Ophthalmol. 1985; 30(3):173–81.

3. Arun D. Singh, Carol L. Shields and Jerry A. Shields, von Hippel-Lindau Disease. Survey of ophthalmology 2001;46:117–42.

4. Augsburger JJ, Shields JA, Goldberg RE. Classification and management of hereditary

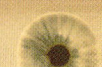

retinal angiomas. Int. Ophthalmol 4(1–2), 93–106 (1981).

5. Chan CC, Wallace DJ. Intraocular lymphoma: update on diagnosis and management. Cancer Control 2004;11(5):285–95.

6. Finger PT, McCormick SA, Davidian M, Walsh JB. Adenocarcinoma of the retinal pigment epithelium: a diagnostic and therapeutic challenge. Graefes Arch. Clin. Exp. Ophthalmol 1996;(Suppl. 1)234:S22–7.

7. Hagler WS, North AW. Intraretinal macrocyst and retinal detachment. Trans Am Acad Ophthalmol Otolaryngol 1967;71:442–54.

8. Heimann H, Bornfeld N, Vij O, et al. Vasoproliferative tumors of the retina. Br. J. Ophthalmol 2000;84(10):1162–9.

9. Honavar SG, Rajeev B. Needle Tract Tumor Cell Seeding Following Fine Nee dle Aspiration Biopsy for Retinoblastoma. Investigative Ophthalmology and Visual Science 1998;39:S 658.

10. Honavar SG, Shields CL, Shields JA, Demirci H, Naduvilath TJ. Intraocular surgery after treatment of retinoblastoma.Arch Ophthalmol 2001;119:1613–21.

11. Honavar SG, Singh AD, Shields CL, Demirci H, Smith AF, Shields JA. Postenucleation prophylactic chemotherapy in high-risk retinoblastoma. Arch Ophthalmol 2002;120:923–31.

12. Honavar SG, Singh AD, Shields CL, Meadows A, Shields JA. Does adjuvant chemotherapy prevent metastasis in high-risk retinoblastoma? Investigative Ophthalmology and Visual Science 2000; 41(S):790.

13. Honavar SG, Singh AD. Management of advanced retinoblastoma. Ophthalmol Clin North Am. 2005;18:65–73.

14. James J. Augsburger, Richard E. Goldberg, Jerry A. Changing Appearance of Retinal Arteriovenous Malformation. von Graefes Arch Klin Exp Ophthalmol 1980:215:65–70.

15. Keith CG. Retinal cyst and retinoschisis. Br J Ophthalmol 1966;50:617–28.

16. Knudson AG: Mutation and cancer: Statistical study of retinoblastoma. Proc Natl Acad Sci, USA 1971;68:820–3.

17. Kobrin JL, Blodi FC, Weingeist TA. Ocular and orbital manifestations of neurofibromatosis. Surv Ophthalmol 1979 Jul-Aug; 24(1):45–51.

18. Leys AM, van Eyck LM, Nuttin BJ, et al. Metastatic carcinoma to the retina. Clinicopathologic findings in two cases.Arch. Ophthalmol 1990; 108(10):1448–52.

19. Lopez JM, Guerrero P. Congenital simple hamartoma of the retinal pigment epithelium: optical coherence tomography and angiography features. Retina;2006;26(6):704–6.

20. Malik RK, Friedman HS, Djang WT, et al. Treatment of trilateral retinoblastoma with vincristine and cyclophosphamide. Am J Ophthalmol 1986;102:650–6.

21. McCaffery S, Wieland MR, O'Brien JM, et al. Atypical retinoblastoma presentations: a challenge for the treating ophthalmologist. Arch Ophthalmol 2002;120:1222–5.

22. Meyer JH, Witschel H. Bilateral combined hamartoma of the retina and the retinal pigment epithelium. Br. J. Ophthalmol 1996;80(6):577–8.

23. Murthy R, Honavar SG, Naik MN, Reddy VA. Retinoblastoma. In: Dutta LC, ed. Modern Ophthalmology New Delhi, India, Jaypee Brothers; 2004:849–59.

24. Neumann HP, Lips CJ, Hsia YE, Zbar B. von Hippel-Lindau syndrome. Brain Pathol, 1995; 5(2):181–3.

25. Patel U, Gupta SC. Wyburn-Mason syndrome. A case report and review of the literature. Neuroradiology 1990;31(6):544–6.

26. Riccardi VM. Neurofibromatosis: past, present, and future. N Engl J Med 1991;324:283–5.

27. Robert Williams, David Taylor, Tuberous Sclerosis. Survey of ophthalmology 1985;30:143–54.

28. Sara J. Haug, Jay M. Stewart. International ophthalmology clinics. Retinal manifestation of the phakomatosis: 2012;52:1.

29. Shields CL, De Potter P, Himelstein BP, Shields JA, Meadows AT, Maris JM. Chemoreduction in the initial management of intraocular retinoblastoma. Arch Ophthalmol 1996; 114:1330–8.

30. Shields CL, Honavar S, Shields JA, Demirci H, Meadows AT. Vitrectomy in eyes with unsuspected retinoblastoma. Ophthalmology 2000;107:2250–5.

31. Shields CL, Honavar SG, Meadows AT, Shields JA, Demirci H, Naduvilath TJ. Chemoreduction for unilateral retinoblastoma.Arch Ophthalmol 2002;120:1653–8.

32. Shields CL, Honavar SG, Meadows AT, Shields JA, Demirci H, Singh A, Friedman DL, Naduvilath TJ. Chemoreduction plus focal therapy for retinoblastoma: factors predictive of need for treatment with external beam radio therapy or enucleation. Am J Ophthalmol 2002;133:657–64.

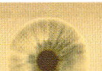

33. Shields CL, Honavar SG, Shields JA, Demirci H, Meadows AT, Naduvilath TJ. Factors predictive of recurrence of retinal tumors, vitreous seeds, and subretinal seeds following chemoreduction for retinoblastoma. Arch Ophthalmol 2002;120: 460–4.

34. Shields CL, Mashayekhi A, Ho T, et al. Solitary congenital hypertrophy of the retinal pigment epithelium: clinical features and frequency of enlargement in 330 patients. Ophthalmology 2003;110(10):1968–76.

35. Shields CL, Santos MC, Diniz W, et al. Thermo-therapy for retinoblastoma. Arch Ophthalmol 1999;117:885–93.

36. Shields CL, Shields JA, Baez K, Cater JR, De Potter P. Optic nerve invasion of retinoblastoma. Metastatic potential and clinical risk factors. Cancer 1994;73:692–8.

37. Shields CL, Shields JA, Baez KA, et a. Choroidal invasion of retinoblastoma: Metastatic potential and clinical risk factors. Br J Ophthalmol 1993; 77:54–8.

38. Shields CL, Shields JA, Cater J, et al. Plaque radiotherapy for retinoblastoma, long-term tumor control and treatment complications in 208 tumors. Ophthalmology 2001;108: 2116–21.

39. Shields CL, Shields JA. Basic understanding of current classification and management of retinoblastoma. Curr Opin Ophthalmol 2006;17: 228–34.

40. Shields JA, Shields CL, Sivalingam V. Decreasing frequency of enucleation in patients with retinoblastoma. Am J Ophthalmol 1989; 108: 185–8.

41. Shields JA, Shields CL. Intraocular tumors — A text and Atlas. Philadelphia, PA, USA, WB Saunders Company, 1992.

42. Singh AD, Shields CL, Shields JA. Prognostic factors in retinoblastoma. J Pediatr Ophthalmol Strab 2000;37:134–41.

43. Sullivan TJ, Clarke MP, Morin JD. The ocular manifestations of the Sturge-Weber syndrome. J Pediatr Ophthalmol Strabismus 1992:29: 349–56.

44. van der Hoeve J. The Doyne Memorial Lecture: Eye symptoms in phakomatoses. Trans Ophthalmol Soc, UK 1932;52:380–401.

45. Vemuganti G, Honavar SG, John R. Clinico-pathological profile of retinoblastoma in Asian Indians. Invest Ophthalmol Vis Sci 2000; 41(S):790.

46. Webb DW, Clarke A, Fryer A, Osborne JP. Cutaneous features of the tuberous sclerosis: a population study. Br J Ophthalmology 1996;9: 402–5.

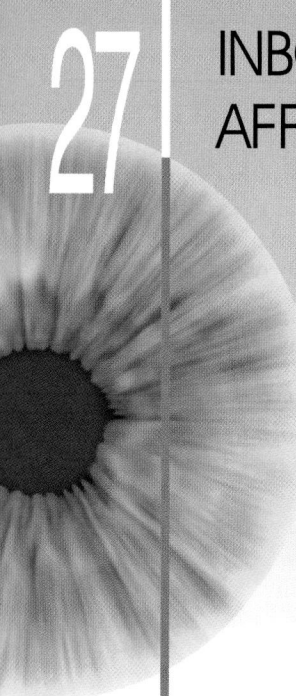

27 INBORN METABOLIC DISORDERS AFFECTING RETINA

Sunandan Sood, Paul Chawla

GENERAL CONSIDERATIONS
- Introduction
- Pathogenesis

DISORDERS OF AMINO ACID METABOLISM
- Albinism
- Cystinosis
- Homocystinuria
- Hyperornithinemia

ABNORMALITIES IN VITAMIN METABOLISM
- Congenital methylmalonic aciduria with homocystinuria

LYSOSOMAL STORAGE DISORDERS
- Mucopolysaccharidosis

DISORDERS OF LYSOSOMAL ENZYME PHOSPHORYLATION
- Mucolipidosis I, II, III, IV

DISORDERS OF GLYCOPROTEIN DEGRADATION AND STRUCTURE
- Fucosidosis
- Sialidosis I, II

DISORDERS OF LIPID METABOLISM
- Niemann-Pick disease
- Fabry's disease
- Gaucher's disease
- Metachromatic leukodystrophy
- Krabbe's disease
- Austin disease
- Farber Lipogranulomatosis

GANGLIOSIDOSIS
- Generalised gangliosidosis
- Galactosialidosis
- GM2 gangliosidoses

DISORDERS OF CARBOHYDRATE METABOLISM
- von Gierke's disease

LIPOPROTEIN AND LIPID DISORDERS
- Bassen-Kornzweig syndrome
- Refsum's disease

MISCELLANEOUS CONDITIONS
- Menke's disease
- Neuronal ceroid lipofuscinoses

GENERAL CONSIDERATIONS

INTRODUCTION

The term inherited metabolic disorders (IMDs) was coined by Archibald Garrod in 1902 when his paper on alkaptonuria was published. He recognised that some human disorders were due to enzyme deficiencies and genetic abnormalities. These observations were ignored and fell into obscurity for about 70 years and it was only in 1970 that Barton Childs reemphasized these. Henceforth, there are numerous IMDs reported in the literature. However, as per one recent study in Indian population, the incidence of IMDs is 0.1%.

IMD constitute a heterogeneous group of disorders which affect the metabolic pathways and have an underlying genetic defect. They are caused by a genetic inability to produce the full complement of a given functioning protein in its normal configuration. IMDs are fast becoming recognised where early diagnosis and appropriate treatment interventions are essential to reduce the morbidity and mortality rates amongst newborns. Early diagnosis is crucial for three reasons. First, IMDs are rapidly progressive and can cause irreversible damage early in the course of the disease. Second, the treatment can often be effective, if started early and hence the long-term outcome may also be improved. Lastly, correct early diagnosis helps in genetic counselling of the parents.

PATHOGENESIS

The eye is the fourth most common system affected by genetic diseases. More than 200 loci for genetic diseases of the eye have been mapped till date. Hereditary eye abnormalities can either manifest as primarily isolated disorders in which disease process is confined to the eye or as part of a systemic disease. The

age of onset of ocular abnormalities in metabolic disease is variable, but onset often begins in childhood, infancy, or right from birth. Although there is an extensive understanding of most of IMDs at metabolic, biochemical and molecular levels but their exact pathogenesis remains obscure. The mechanism by which these IMDs contribute to ocular defects remains to be elucidated. The various mechanisms involved could be due to direct toxic effects of abnormal metabolic products, accumulation of normal metabolites by errors of synthetic pathways, or by deficient energy metabolism. Single gene defects result in abnormalities in the anabolism or catabolism of proteins, carbohydrates, or fats. Most of them are due to a defect in an enzyme or transport protein, which results in a block in a metabolic pathway (Fig. 27.1).

IMDS INVOLVING THE RETINA

There are over 400 known inherited diseases in which the retina is majorly involved in the disease process. These can be classified into disorders of various metabolisms.

A. DISORDERS OF AMINO ACID METABOLISM

Disorders of amino acid metabolism include:

1. Albinism
2. Cystinosis
3. Homocystinuria
4. Hyperornithinemia (Gyrate atrophy)

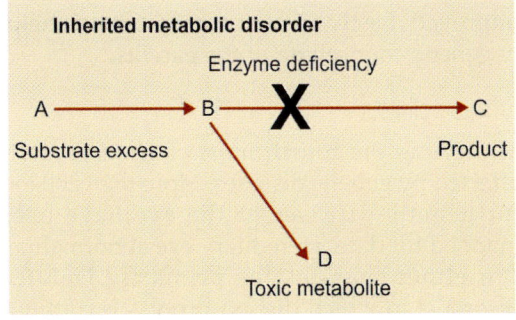

Fig. 27.1 *Garrod's hypothesis*

1. ALBINISM

Albinism consists of a heterogeneous group of hypomelanotic disorders based on heritable metabolic defects of the melanin pigment system. In this disorder either the eyes alone (ocular albinism) or the eyes, skin and hair (oculocutaneous albinism) may be affected. The latter may be either tyrosinase-positive or tyrosinase-negative.

i. Tyrosinase-negative (complete) albinos are incapable of synthesizing melanin and have white hair and very pale skin throughout life with lack of melanin pigment in all ocular structures. Inheritance is usually autosomal recessive (AR).

Visual acuity is usually <6/60 due to foveal hypoplasia. Nystagmus is typically pendular and horizontal. It usually increases in bright illumination and tends to lessen in severity with age. The iris is diaphanous and translucent, giving rise to a 'pink-eyed' appearance. *The fundus lacks pigment and shows conspicuously large choroidal vessels. There is also foveal hypoplasia with absence of the foveal pit and lack of vessels forming the perimacular arcades.* The optic chiasm has fewer uncrossed nerve fibers than normal so that the majority of fibers from each eye cross to the contralateral hemisphere. This can be demonstrated by visual evoked potential which shows predominance in the response to monocular stimulation. Other features commonly seen include refractive errors of various types, positive angle kappa, squint and absence of stereopsis.

ii. Tyrosinase-positive (incomplete) albinos synthesize variable amounts of melanin. The hair may be white, yellow or red and darkens with age. Skin color is very pale at birth but usually darkens by 2 years of age. Inheritance is usually AR with at least two gene loci. Visual acuity is usually impaired due to foveal hypoplasia. Iris may be blue or dark-brown with variable translucency. *Fundus shows variable hypopigmentation.* Associated systemic syndromes include the Chediak-Higashi syndrome (CHS), Hermansky-Pudlak syndrome (HPS) and the Waardenburg syndrome.

iii. In ocular albinism involvement is predominantly ocular with normal skin and hair

although occasionally hypopigmented skin macules may be seen. Inheritance is usually XL and occasionally AR with multiple gene loci identified. Female carriers are asymptomatic although they may show partial iris translucency, macular stippling and mid-peripheral scattered areas of depigmentation and granularity.

Diagnosis

Laboratory work-up includes hair bulb assays help to indicate the status of tyrosinase activity. The most definitive test in determining the albinism type is genetic sequence analysis. Genetic sequence analysis can be used to determine if a fetus has albinism. Amniocentesis at 16–18 weeks could be performed to obtain a sample for analysis. If HPS is suspected, bleeding time, platelet aggregation, and platelet electron microscopy is necessary. If CHS is suspected, a hematologist should evaluate polymorphonuclear leukocyte function.

Treatment

- **Low-vision aids:** Young children may simply need glasses, while older children may require bifocals. Occasionally, telescopic lenses mounted on glasses (bioptics) are prescribed for close-up work and distance vision. Tinted glasses may be used to reduce photophobia. Some patients do not like tinted lenses; they may benefit from wearing a cap or visor when outdoors.
- For the treatment of strabismus, it is preferred to start eye-patching of infants at 6 months of age. Some cases of strabismus may improve with refraction.
- Nitisinone, which is approved by the US Food and Drug Administration (FDA) for treating hereditary tyrosinemia type 1, elevates plasma tyrosine levels and increases eye and hair pigmentation. Nitisinone may soon be a potential treatment for people with ocular albinism.

2. CYSTINOSIS

The primary biochemical defect is a defective carrier mediated transport of the amino acid cystine across the lysosomal membrane. The clinical feature common to the three phenotypes of cystinosis is the pathognomonic deposition of cystine crystals in the cornea and conjunctiva. Severe photophobia often is the only presenting visual symptom. The symptoms result from the diffraction of light by the corneal crystals. Crystal deposits decrease with cysteamine eye drop therapy. The fusiform crystals initially involve the anterior portion of the central cornea but occupy the full thickness of the peripheral cornea by 1 year of age decreased tearing and painful corneal erosions occur. Corneal thickness is increased. The conjunctiva has a ground-glass appearance. Birefringent, hexagonal, polychromatic, polymorphic, rectangular, or rhomboidal crystals can be seen with the biomicroscope. The iris contains an abundance of polymorphous crystals. Clinically, these can be seen as glistening dots on the surface of the iris. Thickened iris stroma and posterior synechiae may occur. The entire uvea has polymorphic crystalline deposits, most heavily in the choroid. Pupillary block glaucoma has been reported. The crystals also deposit in sclera. *The retinal findings consist of generalized depigmentation that may assume a patchy pattern.* The pigmentary disturbance tends to be peripheral at first but progresses with age. Macular abnormalities have been observed. Intracellular crystals also have been observed within the retinal pigment epithelial cells on electron microscopy. The ERG is abnormal.

The **diagnosis** is confirmed by the demonstration of elevated cystine content in polymorphonuclear leukocytes, cultured fibroblasts, or conjunctival tissue. The ocular findings of cystinosis are sufficiently unique and characteristic to form the basis for a diagnosis of this disease. Cystinosis can be diagnosed *in utero* by cystine measurements in amniocytes or chorionic villi.

The **therapy** of cystinosis includes the use of cysteamine drops to chelate the cystine deposits from the cornea. More recently, treatment with oral phosphocysteamine was found to be useful in reducing the systemic storage of cystine.

3. HOMOCYSTINURIA

Homocystinuria is caused by a deficiency of the enzyme cystathionine β-synthase (CBS), which controls the synthesis of cystathionine, an intermediate in the degradation of homocysteine to cysteine. The block in this bio-

chemical pathway causes the accumulation of homocysteine and methionine, with increased concentrations of these amino acids in blood and urine. Normal levels of plasma homo-cysteine range from 2.2 to 13.2 µmol/L.

The principal **clinical features** of homo-cystinuria involve the eye, skeletal, nervous, and vascular systems. Diffuse osteoporosis, genu valgum, kyphoscoliosis, and pectus excavatum often are present. Mental retardation and seizures occur in approximately one half of homocystinuric patients. Thromboembolic episodes of uncertain etiology and involving both arteries and veins frequently occur. Hence, premature deaths from myocardial infarctions, pulmonary emboli, and cerebrovascular accidents are not unusual. Patients characteristically are lightly pigmented, with blond hair and blue eyes. They have a body habitus that resembles that of patients with Marfan syndrome.

Frequent **ocular features** of homocystinuria include myopia, strabismus, and retinal detachment. Less frequent are cataracts, *peripheral retinal degeneration, optic atrophy, and central retinal vascular occlusion.* Inferonasal lens dislocation or even complete dislocation into the vitreous cavity also has been observed. The subluxated lens in the anterior chamber may initially cause only myopia and mild visual impairment. The most common primary defect is fraying and disruption of the zonular fibers that anchor the lens to the ciliary body. However, pupillary-block glaucoma or complete dislocation into the anterior chamber occurs in a significant number of patients and requires emergent treatment. The glaucoma is treated by dilation of the pupil, allowing the lens to fall back behind the iris; the patient then is placed on miotic agents, and a peripheral iridectomy is performed. Lens extraction becomes necessary if the lens dislocates frequently into the anterior chamber or if there is lenticulocorneal touch leading to corneal edema.

The **diagnosis** of homocystinuria is established using amino acid—electrophoresis and chromatography of urine and plasma. There is accumulation of homocysteine and methionine, with increased concentrations of these amino acids in blood and urine. Homocystinuria is one of the few metabolic errors for which **therapy** is available. Amelioration of the characteristic biochemical abnormalities has been achieved by the use of low methionine, by cystine and betaine supplemented diets for patients not responsive to pyridoxine administration, and by supplementation of pyridoxine (vitamin B_6) for pyridoxine-responsive patients. In countries in which neonatal screening is mandatory, initiation of dietary therapy at birth leads to the prevention of mental retardation and of lens subluxation. Surgeons must bear in mind that general anesthesia is particularly hazardous in patients with homocystinuria because of frequent intra- and postoperative thrombo-embolic episodes. Good hydration and the preoperative use of antiplatelet adhesion medications should be contemplated before surgery. Deferring lens extraction until it can be done using local anesthetic is advisable.

4. HYPERORNITHINEMIA (GYRATE ATROPHY OF THE CHOROID AND RETINA)

It is a rare autosomal recessive disorder chara-cterised by progressive metabolic, retinal, and choroidal degeneration due to photoreceptor degeneration caused by the deficiency of the pyridoxal phosphate-dependent, mitochondrial enzyme ornithine d-aminotransferase, which has been mapped to chromosome 10q26. Extreme hyperornithinemia is universally seen in this disease. All the body fluids (whole blood, plasma, cerebrospinal fluid (CSF), aqueous humour, and urine) have been found to contain 10–20 times the normal levels (400–1400 mM) of ornithine. As a result, excessive ornithine build-up causes retinal thinning.

Systemic features include mild muscle weakness may occur due to tubular aggregates in type 2 muscle fibers, which can be visualized with electron microscopy and may lead to loss of these fibers and muscle wasting. Fine, straight hairs have also been observed with patches of alopecia. Slow wave background changes on EEG have been described in almost one-third of patients and peripheral neuropathy is also seen sometimes. Hearing loss has been described as well. *Ocular features include night blindness, myopia, and multiple round islands of peripheral chorioretinal degeneration which*

often appear in the first decade of life, some-times as early as five years of age. Night blindness often begins in late childhood. *The atrophic areas slowly progress to the posterior pole and may eventually affect central vision.* Both eyes are usually symmetrically affected. All patients have myopia, some with refractive errors ranging up to –20D. Fluorescein angio-graphy shows hyperfluorescent at the edges of the peripheral atrophy. A zone of pigmentary changes can be seen between normal and atrophic areas. The electroretinogram may show reduced rod and cone responses with rods affected more than cones in early phases. Dark-adapted ERG documents elevated rod thresholds. Swollen mitochondria have been described in photoreceptors, corneal epithelium, and in the nonpigmented ciliary epithelium. Macular edema is commonly present and posterior subcapsular cataracts requiring surgery are common.

Currently, gyrate atrophy can be treated with amino acid tablets and a very low protein diet with limited fruits and vegetables. The defective gene replacement therapy is also under clinical trials.

B. ABNORMALITIES IN VITAMIN METABOLISM

CONGENITAL METHYLMALONIC ACIDURIA WITH HOMOCYSTINURIA

It is inherited in an autosomal recessive fashion and results from an abnormality of cobalamin metabolism. Patients with methylmalonic aciduria with homocystinuria (cobalamin E and G mutants) present with failure to thrive, seizures, megaloblastic anemia, hemolysis, poor feeding, and lethargy in the first 2 months of life. Neurologic manifestations are prominent. Most have hematologic abnor-malities. Biochemical abnormalities include methyl-malonic aciduria, homocystinuria, hypome-thioninemia, and cystathioninuria. A large number of patients present with nystagmus, wandering eye movements, or abnormal lid movements. Lens dislocation, as in isolated homocystinuria, does not occur. *Retinal degeneration which may be most marked in the posterior pole or which may take the form of salt-and-pepper pigmentary changes in the fundus periphery is seen.* The ERG is subnormal. Ocular histopathologic studies show photoreceptor atrophy. Early diag-nosis and treatment with hydroxycobalamin improves the survival of these patients and may improve the retinal degeneration.

C. LYSOSOMAL STORAGE DISORDERS

MUCOPOLYSACCHARIDOSIS

Most patients with **Mucopolysaccharidosis (MPS)** exhibit a **macular cherry-red spot.** MPS results from an inability to degrade glyco-saminoglycans such as dermatan sulfate, heparin sulfate, and keratan sulphate due to deficiency of various enzymes. These molecules are the degradation products of proteoglycans that normally exist in connective tissue. Once the molecules are ingested, the glycosamino-glycans are stored intracellularly in the lysosomes and accumulate, leading to cellular dysfunction. These diseases become clinically apparent not at birth but over time due to the transplacental enzyme correcting the defect *in utero.* Intracellular accumulation of metabolic products in the ganglion cells which are lacking in the fovea results in opacification during the neural disease process and hence gives rise to the cherry-red spot.

Systemic findings include skeletal abnormali-ties, coarse facial features, mental deficiency, cardiac disease, hepatosplenomegaly, ocular abnormalities, and deafness. Other ocular mani-festations include progressive corneal clouding, retinal pigmentary degeneration, optic nerve head swelling, optic atrophy, and glaucoma. Pigmentary retinopathy with abnormal ERG is found in MPS I, II, III A and B, V, VI and VII. Papilledema is a frequent finding, occurring in one-third or more of patients with certain types of MPS, such as Hunter syndrome. Optic nerve head swelling has been attributed to the hydrocephalus that results from meningeal thickening with the storage material. Collins et al. hypothesized that it could be caused by

narrowing of the scleral canal at the optic nerve head, as a result of posterior scleral thickening. Conjunctival biopsy, is a reliable screening test for patients with suspected lysosomal storage diseases. The large storage vacuoles in histiocytes, lymphocytes, or leukocytes show metachromasia. The diagnosis of MPS is based primarily on the characteristic clinical findings and on the detection of mucopolysaccharides in the urine. For definite diagnosis and for further categorization of the types and subtype of MPSs, specific enzymatic assays or gene analysis should be performed.

D. DISORDERS OF LYSOSOMAL ENZYME PHOSPHORYLATION

MUCOLIPIDOSES

The mucolipidoses have phenotypic and biochemical features of both the mucopolysaccharidoses and the sphingolipidoses without excessive urinary excretion of mucopolysaccharides. Ultrastructurally, the affected cells resemble those of the MPSs, with cytoplasmic vacuoles filled with fine fibrillogranular-material. The vacuoles also contain membranous lamellar inclusions similar to those present in the lipidoses.

Four diseases have been included in this category

i. Mucolipidosis I (MLS I) (Sialidosis Type 1; Cherry-Red Spot Myoclonus Syndrome):

There is deficiency of the enzyme sialidase that leads to a syndrome characterized by a retinal cherry-red spot and myoclonus.

ii. Mucolipidosis II (MLS II) (I-Cell Disease)

There are striking fibroblast inclusions, hence the name I-cell disease. The disease results from the absence of the enzyme that attaches a recognition phosphate group onto a mannose residue in hydrolases. There is abnormal lysosomal enzyme transport in cells of mesenchymal origin. Corneal clouding and glaucoma common. No cherry red spot or pigmentary retinopathy is seen.

iii. Mucolipidosis III (MLS III) (Pseudo-Hurler Polydystrophy):

Systemic features include joint stiffness, coarse facial features, and short stature. Carpal tunnel syndrome, aortic valve disease and mental retardation are common. Corneal clouding, mild hyperopic astigmatism and *mild retinopathy with surface-wrinkling maculo-pathy is seen.* Some patients have retinal vascular tortuosity, optic nerve head swelling, visual field defects, and abnormalities in color vision. Cultured fibroblasts have inclusion bodies. Prenatal diagnosis by means of amniocentesis is possible. There is no specific or definitive treatment.

iv. Mucolipidosis IV (MLS IV) (Berman Disease)

Deficiency of ganglioside sialidase is reported as the possible metabolic defect causing this disorder. Corneal clouding and *progressive rod-cone dystrophy is present with a subnormal or extinguished electroretinogram (ERG).* Conjunctival biopsy shows characteristic-intracellular inclusions. Prenatal diagnosis is possible.

E. DISORDERS OF GLYCOPROTEIN DEGRADATION AND STRUCTURE

1. FUCOSIDOSIS

It is caused by the deficiency of the lysosomal enzyme α-fucosidase. This results in accumulation and excretion of a variety of glycoproteins, glycolipids, and oligosaccharides containing fucoside moieties. Urine samples from individuals with fucosidosis contain excessive amounts of several fucoglycoconjugates. **Systemic features** include psychomotor retardation, coarse facies, growth retardation, dysostosis multiplex, mental retardation and angiokeratomas. The most precise way of diagnosing fucosidosis is based on enzymatic assay of α-L-fucosidase in cells of any type. The ocular features of fucosidosis are not prominent. There may be tortuosity of conjunctival vessels and a mild pigmentary retinopathy

2. SIALIDOSIS

It is caused by the deficiency of enzyme α-N-acetylneuraminidase in cultured fibroblasts.

Diagnosis is based on electron microscopy. Fibroblasts in conjunctival biopsy specimens contain small membrane-bound vacuoles containing fibrillogranular and membranous lamellar bodies detectable by electron microscopy. There is no known treatment, but prenatal diagnosis is possible. It has the following two types.

Sialidosis Type 1

The presenting symptom may be reduction in visual acuity; visual loss is progressive and often severe. *It may be associated with impaired color vision and night blindness. The macular cherry-red spot is* consistent but can be atypical. Punctate lens opacities can occur. Nystagmus, optic-atrophy, and visual field constriction have been described. An important screening test in this disorder is the examination of the urine for excessive excretion of sialic acid-containing compound using urine thin-layer chromatography. The definitive test is the demonstration of deficient sialidase in fresh cultured skin fibroblasts. As mentioned above there is no known treatment.

Sialidosis Type 2

Myoclonus, mental retarda-tion and gait ataxia is present. Grandmal seizures, deafness, and a peripheral neuropathy may occur. Skeletal abnormalities are prominent with dysostosis multiplex. Vision is retained despite the presence of a macular cherry-red spot and punctate lens opacities. Peripheral blood lymphocytes are vacuolated, and foam cells are present in the bone marrow. Sialidase is deficient in cultured fibroblasts.

F. DISORDERS OF LIPID METABOLISM

1. NIEMANN-PICK DISEASE

Niemann-Pick disease (NPD) results from impaired sphingomyelin metabolism. NPD is caused by deficient activity of acid sphingo-myelinase (ASM) that maps to 18q11–q12. It is classified in five phenotypic variants (A through E) and is based on the age of onset, the severity and type of neurologic involvement, and the

evolution of the disease. Hepatosplenomegaly and foam cells in the bone marrow are constant features in all variants.

Subtle lens opacities and corneal clouding can occur. *A cherry-red macula is present in 50% of infants in the first and second year of life.* There is deposition of fat in the ganglion cell layer of retina causing macular cherry-red spot due to absence of ganglion cells in the fovea and the choroidal vasculature shining through. There is no distinction between the appearance of the cherry-red spot in infantile NPD and in Tay-Sachs disease. Occasionally, a macular halo syndrome with a gray, granular-appearing macula is observed. Optic atrophy develops with time. ERG is abnormal. The stored lipid is localized to the ganglion and amacrine cells of the retina, most conspicuously in the parafoveal region. The other retinal layers appear unaffected. The presence of downgaze paresis is characteristic of NPD type C and has been noted in all juvenile and adult cases. Subtle slowing of vertical saccades begins in late infancy. Voluntary vertical gaze is completely paralyzed in late stages of the illness. Horizontal eye movements may be affected with a total supranuclear ophthalmoplegia. No ocular abnormalities are seen in NPD type D.

Diagnosis can be made readily by enzymatic determination of ASM activity in cells and tissues. More than 300 cases of type A and B NPD have been reported. Prenatal diagnosis has been accomplished by enzyme assays of cultured amniotic fluid cells in types A and B. Bone marrow transplantation has been successful in type B NPD. Enzyme replacement and somatic gene therapy using macrophage-targeted recombinant enzyme may be available in the future.

2. FABRY'S DISEASE

It results from a defect in glycosphingolipid catabolism due to deficient α-galactosidase A activity. Affected individuals have pain and paresthesia of the extremities around the time of puberty; vascular cutaneous lesions (angiokera-tomas) of the scalp, mucous membranes, skin, and inguinal and umbilical regions; hypohidrosis; renal failure, hypertension and cardiovascular

anomalies. The **ocular deposition** of glycosphin-golipids results in unique and diagnostic eye findings. The corneal opacities appear as whorled streaks from a central vortex and have been called cornea verticillata. Bilateral inferior granular anterior capsular or posterior subcapsular lens opacities. Conjunctival and *retinal vessel tortuosity, unilateral central retinal vascular occlusion, myelinated nerve fibers,* mild optic atrophy, papilledema, nystagmus, and internuclear ophthalmoplegia are seen. Confirmation of the **clinical diagnosis** in hemizygotes and heterozygotes requires the demonstration of deficient α-galactosidase A activity in plasma, leukocytes, or tears or increased levels of ceramide trihexaside in plasma or urinary sediment. The diagnosis in female heterozygotes can be established by linkage analysis. Prenatal diagnosis is possible by demonstration of the specific α-galactosidase A mutation in chorionic villi or cultured amniotic cells.

3. GAUCHER'S DISEASE

It is a lysosomal storage disorder caused by a recessively inherited deficiency of enzyme glucocerebrosidase (acid beta-glucosidase), which causes an accumulation of sphingolipid glucosylceramide in cells of the reticulo-endothelial systems. Three phenotypes are recognized based on the absence (type 1) or presence and severity (types 2 and 3) of primary central nervous involvement. Splenomegaly, anemia thrombocytopathic, pathologic bone fractures, bleeding episodes, and a yellow skin pigmentation are the features of the disease. **Ocular manifestations** of Gaucher's disease include infiltration of the retina, conjunctiva, and uvea, with visual loss and eye movement disorders. Brownish piguecula-like masses containing Gaucher cells are the only significant ocular feature. The classic Gaucher triad consists of trismus, strabismus, and opisthotonus. Oculomotor abnormalities often are the first manifestation of the disease, with strabismus or oculomotor apraxia. Corneal opacification is rare.

A tentative diagnosis is based on the detection of Gaucher cells (storage cells) in the bone marrow. Decreased tissue levels of gluco-cerebroside activity confirm the diagnosis.

Mutation analysis of the glucocerebrosidase gene also can be performed. Enzyme replacement treatment with intravenous recombinant glucocerebrosidase can result in dramatic improvement. Cerezyme (imiglucerase for injection), is expensive and the treatment should be continued for life. Cure theoretically is possible using bone marrow transplantation. Gene therapy may be a future step.

4. METACHROMATIC LEUKODYSTROPHY (MLD)

It is a demyelinating storage disease caused by deficiency of the lysosomal enzyme arylsulphatase A, leading to the accumulation of sulphatides in the central and peripheral nervous systems. Patients have a gait disorder characterized by flaccid paraparesis, hypotonia, and absent tendon reflexes secondary to a severe demyelinating peripheral neuropathy. Occasionally, ataxia and weakness may occur. Patients with MLD show the storage of metachromatic complex lipids in the RGCs and in the optic nerve, leading to optic atrophy. Nystagmus is present. *The cherry-red spot is similar to that in Tay-Sachs disease, but the perifoveal region is faint gray instead of white, and therefore, the cherry-red spot is much less obvious.* Electron microscopic studies of the eyes of patients with different clinical and genetic variants of MLD have revealed profound demyelination and loss of axons in the optic nerve in all cases. A variety of membrane-bound inclusions are present in the cytoplasm of glial cells; some appear whorled, homogenous, and granular, whereas others have a lamellar or prismatic configuration. Demyelination with intact axons is found in corneal and conjunctival nerves. Diagnosis relies on the demonstration of deficient arylsulfatase A or sulfatidase in leukocytes or cultured fibroblasts and demonstration of excessive excretion of sulfatide in the urine. Prenatal diagnosis has been achieved successfully using cultured amniotic fluid cells.

5. GLOBOID CELL LEUKODYSTROPHY (KRABBE'S DISEASE)

It is an autosomal recessive, rapidly progressive, invariably fatal disease in infants that begins between the ages of 3 and 6 months. There is

deficiency of the enzyme galactosyl-ceramidase or galactocerebroside-β-galactosidase which degrades galactocerebroside to ceramide and galactose. The accumulation of psychosine (galactosylsphingosine) results in the destruction of myelin-producing oligodendroglia, causing demyelination and a widespread leukodystrophy, despite a normal brain-content of galactocerebroside. Infantile and late-infantile forms are differentiated on the basis of age of onset. The gene has been mapped to chromosome 14. The clinical course is characterized by irritability, hypersensitivity, hypertonicity with hyperactive reflexes progressing to severe mental and motor deterioration, flaccidity, and hypotonicity. Optic atrophy and sluggish pupillary reactions to light are common. *Macular cherry-red spots have been reported.*

Diagnosis is based on the measurement of galactocerebroside-β-galactosidase activity in leukocytes or cultured fibroblasts. Prenatal diagnosis has been achieved using cultured amniotic fluid cells and chorionic villus samples. There is no effective therapy.

6. MULTIPLE SULPHATASE DEFICIENCY (AUSTIN DISEASE)

There is deficiency of several sulfatases, including steroid sulfatase and the various mucopolysaccharide sulfatases, with lysosomal storage of sulfatides, glycosaminoglycans, glycolipids, and sulfated steroids. Mild coarsening of the facial features, hepatosplenomegaly, joint stiffness, growth retardation, skeletal anomalies and ichthyosis. **Ophthalmologic features** include skew deviation, optic atrophy, retinal degeneration, and occasional cherry-red macula. The disease is diagnosed by demonstrating deficient activity of multiple sulfatases in fibroblasts.

7. FARBER LIPOGRANULOMATOSIS

It is characterized by tissue accumulation of ceramide caused by lack of lysosomal acid ceramidase. There are seven subtypes. **Clinical manifestations** are irritability, intermittent fever, hoarseness, failure to thrive, painful, progressively deformed swollen joints, and subcutaneous periarticular nodules near the joints. Swallowing difficulties with fever and pulmonary consolidation are common. Systolic cardiac murmurs, generalised lymphadenopathy and rarely hepatosplenomegaly are seen.

Visual function is unaffected. Granulomatous nodules have been observed in the conjunctiva. Subepithelial corneal opacities and lens changes also have been documented. Microscopic examination of conjunctival granulomas shows a histologic picture similar to that of the subcutaneous granulomas, with groups of irregular large foam cells that have a granular cytoplasm weakly positive for fat stains. Diffuse grayish opacification of the retina about the fovea is seen, producing a mild cherry-red macula with no effect on vision. The appearance of the macula in Farber disease differs from that of Tay-Sachs disease because the former has a subtle appearance and no pallor of the optic disc. It resembles the cherry-red macula of MLD. The retinal vessels are normal.

Specific **diagnosis** depends on demonstration of a deficiency of acid ceramidase in cultured fibroblasts and leukocytes. Prenatal diagnosis has been performed using cultured amniotic fluid cells. At this time, there is no specific therapy.

G. GANGLIOSIDOSIS

They are autosomal recessive neuronal lipid storage disorders characterized by progressive mental and motor deterioration due to the storage of GM1 or GM2 gangliosides in neurons.

1. GENERALIZED GANGLIOSIDOSIS (GM1 GANGLIOSIDOSIS)

GM1 is divided into infantile (type I), late-infantile or juvenile (type II), and adult or chronic (type III) types. Mental retardation, generalized spasticity, facial dysmorphism, hepatosplenomegaly, and generalized skeletal dysplasia are present. There is diffuse atrophy of the brain. It is caused by deficiency of acid β-galactosidase. Mild, diffuse corneal clouding has been reported. Conjunctival vascular tortuosity may be a feature. GM1 gangliosides accumulate in—the cytoplasm of corneal epithelium and keratocytes. *A cherry-red spot*

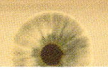

is present in a least 50% of patients and is characteristic. Nystagmus, decreased visual acuity, retinal hemorrhages, and optic atrophy may be seen.

β-galactosidase deficiency can be demonstrated in leukocytes and serum. The urine has increased keratan sulfate levels. High levels of GM1 ganglioside are found in erythrocytes, and foamy storage cells are present in the bone marrow.

2. GALACTOSIALIDOSIS

It is a lysosomal storage disease associated with combined deficiency of neuraminidase and β-galactosidase. Patients may have neonatal edema, proteinuria, coarse facies, inguinal hernias, telangiectasia, visceromegaly, psychomotor delay, and skeletal changes. *Ocular abnormalities include corneal clouding and cherry-red maculae.* Prenatal diagnosis has been established in cultured amniotic fluid cells. No specific therapy is available.

3. GM2 GANGLIOSIDOSES

They are disorders caused by excessive intra-lysosomal accumulation of ganglioside GM2 and related glycolipids. They result from the deficiency of β-hexosaminidase A (Hex Λ) [Tay-Sachs disease], β-hexosaminidase A and β-hexosaminidase B (Hex B) [Sandhoff disease] or GM2 activator deficiency which results from mutation of the GM2A gene. Patients with Tay-Sachs disease show signs of progressive CNS deterioration, such as dementia, blindness, convulsions, and early death. *Tay-Sachs disease is the most common storage disease causing macular cherry-red spots. No ganglion cells are present at the very center of the macular region, the foveola, and the central red spot simply represents the normal choroidal background color.* The ganglion cell layer surrounding the foveola is constituted of several layers of neurons. The loading of these neurons by storage products results in loss of retinal transparency and in a white parafoveal halo.

Tay-Sachs disease is diagnosed by assaying for Hex A in serum or leukocytes, cultured skin fibroblasts, cultured amniotic fluid cells obtained by amniocentesis at 16 weeks gestation, or on fresh and cultured chorionic villus cells aspirated between 8 and 11 weeks. Heterozygous carriers also can be detected by serum and leukocyte assay. Genetic counseling of carriers permits reduction in the incidence of the disease through the use of early prenatal monitoring of a pregnancy.

The clinical and neurologic features of **Sandhoff disease** and its variants are clinically indistinguishable from classic Tay-Sachs disease except for, in some cases, the presence of moderate hepatosplenomegaly and mild skeletal dysostosis. *The macular cherry-red spot in Sandhoff disease is identical to that of Tay-Sachs disease.* Blindness and optic atrophy occur. Absence of Hex A and Hex B in the serum and leukocytes confirms the diagnosis. Prenatal diagnosis has been performed successfully.

H. DISORDERS OF CARBOHYDRATE METABOLISM

GLYCOGEN STORAGE DISEASE TYPE I (VON GIERKE'S DISEASE)

It is caused by a deficiency of glucose-6-phosphatase activity in the liver, kidney, and intestinal mucosa, with excessive accumulation of glycogen in these organs. Delayed growth, feeding difficulties, massive hepatomegaly, hypoglycemia, lactic acidemia, hyperuricemia, hyperlipidemia, and upper respiratory infections are noted in infancy. The developing child has short stature and poor muscle tone. There is a low fasting blood sugar, high blood lipids, high uric acid, and increased platelet count. Death frequently is caused by ketoacidosis. Faint brown cloudy infiltration of the corneal periphery has been described. Increased bilateral subcutaneous fat in the lower eyelids and inverted eyelashes have been described recently. *Multiple yellowish discrete perimacular lesions may be present. These changes appear to correlate with the degree of hyperlipidemia.*

Definitive diagnosis requires a liver biopsy to demonstrate a deficiency of glucose-6-phosphatase activity. In the past, many patients died and prognosis was guarded. With maintenance of normal blood glucose levels

after early diagnosis and initiation of treatment, the prognosis has improved dramatically. Prenatal diagnosis has been accomplished by fetal liver biopsy.

I. LIPOPROTEIN AND LIPID DISORDERS

I. ABETALIPOPROTEINEMIA (BASSEN-KORNZWEIG SYNDROME)

It is a disorder of lipid metabolism characterized by the absence of very low-density lipoproteins (VLDLs) and LDLs from plasma due to defect in the microsomal triglyceride transfer protein. *There are five characteristic features: abetalipoproteinemia, malabsorption of fat, acanthocytosis (crenated erythrocytes with spiny excrescences), ataxic neuropathy, and retinitis pigmentosa.* Defects of transport of tocopherol in the blood result in spinocerebellar ataxia, peripheral neuropathy, ceroid myopathy, and degenerative pigmentary retinopathy.

Ophthalmoplegia due to primary aberrant regeneration of the oculomotor nerve, lens opacities, choroiditis, anisocoria, and ptosis also have been reported. *A typical retinitis pigmentosa is the most common ophthalmic abnormality in abetalipoproteinemia.* The vision and retinal appearance apparently are normal at birth and in early childhood. Retinal degeneration generally occurs between 5 and 10 years of age. By adolescence or early adulthood, most patients have decreased visual acuity, visual field defects, loss of night vision, loss of color vision, and retinal pigmentary disturbance. Major pathologic features are loss of photoreceptors and pigment epithelium in the fundus periphery. Electroretinography and dark adaptometry reveal diminished rod function.The retinal degeneration is probably secondary to absence of plasma carotenoids and low concentrations of vitamin A.

Diagnosis is made by examining peripheral blood smears for acanthocytosis. The erythrocytes apparently assume the acantholytic form because of abnormal distribution of lipids between the bilayered plasma membrane. The lipid abnormalities can be detected by electrophoretic and ultra-centrifugal studies.

2. REFSUM'S DISEASE

Inheritance of Refsum's disease is AR. The infantile and adult forms are genetically distinct. Pathogenesis includes deficiency in phytanic acid alpha-hydrolase results in accumulation of phytanic acid throughout the body. Early detection and treatment with a diet low in phytanic acid can arrest disease progression. Systemic features of infantile disease are characterized by dysmorphic facies, mental handicap, hepatomegaly and deafness. Adult disease is characterized by cerebellar ataxia, polyneuropathy, anosmia, deafness, cardiomyopathy and ichthyosis. *Fundus appearance may be similar to RP or merely show salt-and-pepper changes.* Treatment with a low-phytol and low phytanic acid diet results in the lowering of serum phytanic acid and stabilisation of retinal function. Other ocular features include cataract, prominent corneal nerves, optic atrophy, nystagmus and poorly dilating pupils.

J. MISCELLANEOUS CONDITIONS

1. MENKES DISEASE

A mutation in a copper-transporting ATP7A gene causes this disease which is characterised by low serum copper levels and low ceruloplasmin levels. The clinical features of Menkes disease are abnormal kinky hair, abnormal facies, progressive cerebral degeneration, hypopigmentation, emphysema, bone changes, arterial rupture and thrombosis, and hypothermia. Premature delivery, neonatal hypothermia, and hyperbilirubinemia are very common. *Abnormal sluggish pupillary response and retinal venous tortuosity, iris cysts, and retinal degeneration have been described. Scotopic ERG and VER are abnormal.*

The liver content of copper is diminished grossly, and duodenal or jejunal biopsy shows greatly increased copper content. No form of treatment has been proven to be truly effective. Any or all of the disturbances of copper metabolism in cultured cells can be used for prenatal diagnosis on cultured amniotic cells or cultured chorionic villus samples.

2. NEURONAL CEROID LIPOFUSCINOSES (NCLs)

It is the general name for a family of at least eight genetically separate neurodegenerative disorders that result from excessive accumulation of lipopigments (lipofuscin) in the body's tissues.

Juvenile NCL (JNCL, Batten disease) usually arises between 4 and 10 years of age; the first symptoms include considerable vision loss due to **retinitis pigmentosa (RP),** with seizures, psychological degeneration, and eventual death in the mid- to late-20s. This disease has been mapped to CLN3 gene on 16p12. *The ophthalmoscopic findings begin with a decreased foveolar reflex followed by a bulls-eye maculopathy and pigment mottling and clumping.* Progressive optic atrophy and retinal vessel attenuation occur. The ERG is non-recordable. Night blindness and color blindness also may occur.

To **diagnose** Batten's disease/NCL, the neurologist needs the patient's medical history and information from various laboratory tests. One of the tests is skin/tissue sampling under electron microscope which shows typical NCL deposits. These deposits are found in many different tissues, including the skin, muscle, conjunctiva, and others. Mostly fingerprint profiles are typically found in JNCL. Visual evoked responses and ERGs, can detect various eye problems common in childhood Batten's disease/NCLs. Enzyme assays are used that look for specific missing lysosomal enzymes for infantile and late infantile disease only. Prenatal diagnosis based on DNA testing and electron microscopic search for inclusions has been possible from chorionic villus samples.

Treatment with antioxidants such as sodium selenite and vitamin E, B_2, and B_6 has been tried with insignificant effects on the relentless clinical course of these disorders. Gene therapy and bone marrow/neural stem cell transplants is under trial for patients with Battens disease.

CONCLUSION

Early diagnosis of IMDs is important, as in most cases, dietary restriction and early treatment prevents onset of disability. Prenatal diagnosis using amniocentesis and chorionic villus sampling may help to reduce the burden due to IMDs. Carrier testing is also helpful. The role of genetic counselling is invaluable in reducing the load due to IMDs and thus helps in preventing high incidence in most cases.

A combined approach of management by an ophthalmologist, pediatrician, biochemist, and medical geneticist is warranted in most cases. Recent advances in diagnosis and treatment have significantly improved the prognosis for many infants with inborn errors of metabolism.

BIBLIOGRAPHY

1. Ashworth JL, Biswas S, Wraith E, Lloyd IC. Mucopolysaccharidoses and the eye. Surv Ophthalmol 2006;51:1–17.

2. Cogan D, Kuwabara T. The sphingolipidosis and the eye. Arch Ophthalmol 1968;79:437.

3. Collins M, Traboulsi E, Maumenee I. Optic nerve head swelling and optic atrophy in the mucopolysaccharidoses. Ophthalmology 1990; 97:1445.

4. Costa T, Scriver CR, Childs B. The effect of Mendelian disease on human health: a measurement. Am J Med Genet 1985;21:231–42.

5. Freund C, Horsford DJ, McInnes RR. Transcription factor genes and the developing eye: a genetic perspective. Hum Mol Genet 1996;5:1471–88.

6. Kivlin J, Snaborn G, Myers G. The cherry-red spot in Tay-Sachs and other storage diseases. Ann Neurol 1958;17:356.

7. Kumta NB. Inborn errors of metabolism, an Indian perspective. Indian J Pediatr 2005;72: 325–32.

8. Poll-The BT, Maillette de Buy Wenniger-Prick LJ, Barth PG, Duran M. The eye as a window to inborn errors of metabolism. J Inherit Metab Dis 2003;26:229–44.

9. Rattner A, Sun H, Nathans J. Molecular genetics of human retinal disease. Annu Rev Genet 1999;33:89–131.

10. Van Heyningen V. Developmental eye disease—a genome era paradigm. Clin Genet 1998;54: 272–82.

11. Verma IC. Burden of genetic disease in India. Indian J Pediatr 2000;67:893–8.

12. Waisbren SE, Albers S, Amato S, Ampola M, Brewster TG, Demmer L, et al. Effect of expanded newborn screening for biochemical genetic disorders on child outcome and parental stress. JAMA 2003;290:2564–72.

13. Wang T, Milan AH, Steel G, Valle D. A mouse model of gyrate atrophy of the choroid and retina: early pigment epithelium damage and progressive retinal degeneration. J Clin Invest 1996;97:2753–62.

14. Weleber RG, Kurz DE, Trzupek KM. Treatment of retinal and choroidal degenerations and dystrophies: current status and prospects for gene based therapy. Ophthalmol Clin North Am 2003;16:583–93.

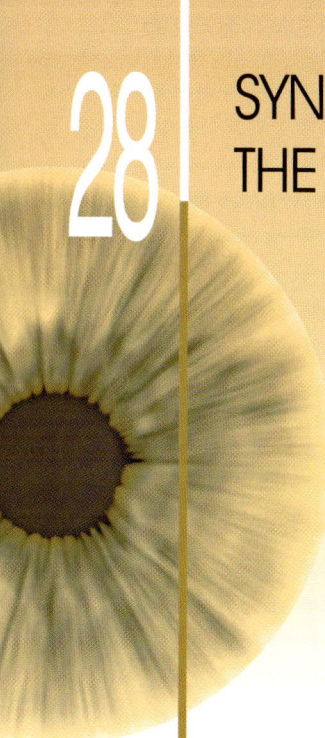

28 | SYNDROMES INVOLVING THE RETINA

Parul Chawla, Sunandan Sood

CHONDRODYSPLASIAS ASSOCIATED WITH VITREORETINAL DEGENERATION
- Stickler syndrome
- Marshall syndrome
- Kneist dysplasia
- Knobloch syndrome
- Weissenbacher-Zweymuller syndrome

SYNDROMES ASSOCIATED WITH RETINITIS PIGMENTOSA
- Usher's syndrome
- Bardet-Biedl syndrome
- Joubert syndrome
- Jeune syndrome
- Alport syndrome
- Kearns-Sayre syndrome
- Cohen syndrome
- Cockayne syndrome
- Methylmalonic aciduria
- Abetalipoproteinemia (Bassen-Kornweig disease)
- Cystinosis
- Mucopolysaccharidoses
- Refsum's disease
- Neuronal Ceroid Lipofuscinosis

CILIOPATHIES: NOVEL SYSTEMIC RETINAL DYSTROPHIES
- Bardet-Biedl syndrome
- Alström syndrome
- MORM syndrome
- Senior-Loken syndrome
- Joubert syndrome
- Jeune syndrome

PEDIATRIC SYNDROMES WITH RETINAL DEGENERATION AND FEATURES OF THE ECTODERMAL SPECTRUM (HAIR, SKIN, TEETH)
- Hypotrichosis with juvenile macular dystrophy
- Ectodermal dysplasia, ectrodactyly, macular dystrophy syndrome
- Oliver-McFarlane syndrome, trichomegaly and chorioretinopathy with pituitary dysfunction
- Refinal dystrophy and dental abnormalities: Jalili's syndrome
- RP syndrome with prominent skeletal involvement
- Spondylometaphyseal dysplasia, short stature with cone dystrophy

MISCELLANEOUS SYNDROMES INVOLVING RETINA
- Enhanced S-cone syndrome (1990) and Goldman-Favre vitreoteptoretinal degeneration (1957)
- Diffuse subretinal fibrosis syndrome
- Aicardi syndrome
- Whipple's disease
- Urbach-Wieth syndrome
- Down syndrome
- Turner syndrome
- Klinefelter syndrome
- Marfan syndrome
- Ehler-Danlos syndrome
- Paraneoplastic syndrome of CNS
- Rothmund syndrome
- McKusick-Kaufman syndrome
- Shaken baby syndrome
- Terson syndrome
- Gardner syndrome and CHPRE
- Hellp syndrome
- Reiter syndrome
- Organoid nevus syndrome
- Fat embolism syndrome

CHONDRODYSPLASIAS ASSOCIATED WITH VITREORETINAL DEGENERATION

- Stickler syndrome
- Marshall syndrome
- Kneist dysplasia
- Knobloch syndrome
- Weissenbacher-Zweymuller syndrome

Chondrodysplasias consist of number of heritable disorders characterized by abnormal proportions of limbs, trunk or skull along with vitreoretinal degeneration. It includes the following

1. *Stickler syndrome* is the most common out of all these which is often termed hereditary progressive arthro-ophthalmopathy and it has been discussed in Chapter 10 page 156.

2. *Marshall syndrome and Stickler* are both characterized by dominant inheritance, pathological myopia and liquefied vitreous. The systemic features include mid facial hypoplasia, cleft palate and hearing loss. The gene responsible for Marshall syndrome is COL11A1 whereas it is COL2A1 with Stickler.

3. *Kneist dysplasia:* It has autosomal dominant inheritance. The vitreoretinal lesions include myopia, optically empty vitreous with retrolental and peripheral vitreous membranes, lattice degeneration and retinal detachment. The systemic findings include short-trunk dwarfism with kyphoscoliosis, enlarged joints with decreased motion, flat mid face, cleft palate and hearing loss. The gene responsible for Kneist dysplasia is COL2A1.

4. *Knobloch syndrome:* It is an autosomal recessive disorder with high myopia, rhegmatogenous RD. The gene was mapped to chromosome COL18A1. The systemic features include flat nasal bridge, mid facial hypoplasia, occipital scalp defects and encephalocele.

5. *Weissenbacher-Zweymuller syndrome:* It is a rare autosomal recessive disorder with high myopia and retinal detachment. The systemic features include small size at birth, Pierre Robbin sequence (Cleft palate, micrognathia and small tongue), proximal limb shortness, metaphyseal widening of the long bone and midfacial hypoplasia. The genes responsible for Weissenbacher-Zweymuller syndrome and nonocular Stickler syndrome (type III) are all associated with mutations in chromosome COL11A2.

In all these types of chondrodysplasias electro-physiological studies are usually normal, color vision is normal and visual fields are also normal unless the patient is having retinal detachment.

The management of these hereditary disorders required multidisciplinary approach, consisting of the services of orthopedician, ENT surgeons and a vitreoretinal surgeon. Since the incidence of retinal detachment is very high with poor surgical prognosis therefore prophylactic laser therapy of all retinal breaks and all areas of lattice degeneration is recommended.

SYNDROMES ASSOCIATED WITH RETINITIS PIGMENTOSA

Retinitis pigmentosa (RP) syndromes refer to retinal degenerations associated with extraocular manifestations. Mutations of the gene or the group of genes involved in the syndrome lead to retinal degeneration associated with mani-festations in other organs as defined by the specific biologic role of the protein. Retinal degeneration in these syndromes shows the inherent biologic complex nature of the retina. The photoreceptor cell is extremely sensitive to alterations in many biologic pathways but the clinical presentation is often indistinguishable between syndromes with the classical features of retinal degeneration: night-blindness, visual field constriction, and reduced visual acuity.

In the early phases of the retinal degeneration, the fundus may appear normal although the electroretinogram (ERG) is altered. In the later stages of the disease, the fundus will show pigment mottling, pigment migration with spicules, optic disc pallor, narrowed vessels, and macular changes.

All the conditions are rare inherited diseases; the most frequent syndromes are Usher's syndrome (USH) and Bardet-Biedl syndrome (BBS).

1. USHER'S SYNDROME

Usher's syndrome (USH) is an autosomal recessive syndrome and is associated with sensorineural deafness and progressive retinal degeneration. It is the most frequently inherited syndrome with deafness and is the most common syndrome among the deaf–blind.

Types of Usher's syndrome

It is of three types: Usher's type 1 (USH1), type 2 (USH2), and type 3 (USH3). USH1 and 2 are diagnosed in early or late childhood, respectively. Vestibular dysfunction is mostly associated with USH1.

Cochlear implantation is highly beneficial for these children (especially in patients of USH1). However, no therapy is yet available for the retinal degeneration.

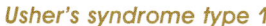

Usher's syndrome type 1

Children with USH1 are affected with congenital very severe sensorineural hearing loss associated with delayed milestones (sitting and walking) due to abnormal vestibular function. Retinal degeneration occurs early in childhood. ERG can confirm the diagnosis of retinal degeneration although the fundus appears to be normal. Five causative genes are known: MYO7A (main USH1 gene mutated in half of the cases), USH1C, CDH23, PCDH15, and USH1G.

Usher syndrome type 2

Children with this are associated with congenital mild to severe stable sensorineural hearing loss with normal vestibular function. The retinal degeneration occurs later in life than in USH1, usually during puberty. USH2 and USH3 are mostly not symptomatic in the first decade and initially have a normal fundus appearance. Many patients have a good visual acuity in spite of having constricted visual fields. The ERG may be normal in the early stages; however, ERG changes may be detected in asymptomatic young children. During the second decade, night-blindness and loss of peripheral vision are noticed. Three genes have been identified: USH2A (Usher is also seen as mutated in isolated RP cases), GPR98, and DFNB31.

Usher's syndrome type 3

The onset of retinal degeneration in USH3 is variable and is often identified after the second decade of life. Sensory hearing loss is after the child acquires language skills (as opposed to the prelingual loss in USH1 and USH2). Vestibular dysfunction of variable intensity occurs in half of the patients. The USH3A gene has been identified most commonly in Askenazi Jews and in Finns. USH3 has also been seen mutated in patients with USH1 and USH2.

Pathogenesis of usher's syndromes

They affect the inner ear stereocilia and photoreceptor cells of the retina. Alteration of the USH gene proteins lead to early dysfunction of the inner ear and of the retina simultaneously. Cochlear implantation is highly recommended for these children (especially in USH1). No therapy is yet available for the retinal degeneration.

2. BARDET-BIEDL SYNDROME (BBS)

Clinical features

The cardinal features of the BBS syndrome are early onset retinal degeneration, obesity, polydactyly, renal failure, hypogonadism, and cognitive impairment. Secondary features may include anosmia, diabetes, cardiac anomalies, hepatic fibrosis, brachydactyly, and Hirschprung's disease.

Retinal dystrophy is early in onset leading to severe visual handicap before adulthood. Profound ERG abnormalities can be detected as early as 3 years old. Legal blindness usually results before the second decade of life. Retinal dystrophies in BBS are mainly a rod-cone dystrophy or a cone-rod dystrophy, usually classified as a global retinal degeneration because both rods and cones are affected.

Obesity is the second major feature, present in 72–96% of BBS patients, usually beginning in early childhood and worsening with age. The origin of obesity is both central (the hypothalamic eating control) and peripheral (the adipose tissue). **Limb anomalies** are found in almost 95% of BBS patients, usually a postaxial polydactyly (69%). Other limb malformations such as brachydactyly or syndactyly are frequently reported for both hands and feet and have a diagnostic value. **Abnormalities of the genitalia** are common: hypogonadism in males or vaginal atresia in females. Rarely, there is hydrometrocolpos, a neonatal vaginal malformation leading to a massive abdominal tumor. Renal dysfunction can occur in late childhood and may lead to kidney failure.

Neuropsychiatric symptoms can include developmental delay, mental retardation, learning difficulties, speech deficit, and behavioral problems. Intellectual function ranges from severe mental retardation (29%) through weak intelligence and average intelligence (29%). Slow ideation and hyperemotive status are common.

Genetics and inheritance

BBS is an autosomal recessive heterogeneous condition with 16 genes identified accounting for about 85% of cases. All the genes have been

related to cilium biogenesis and/or function. BBS1 and BBS10 are the two most common, each accounting for about 20% of the cases. Implication of the other BBS genes ranges from a unique family to a few percentage of mutated families. The classical autosomal recessive inheritance model has been challenged by molecular and functional investigations with the oligogenic model and the effect of addi-tional genetic modulators on the phenotype.

3. JOUBERT SYNDROME

Joubert syndrome may be autosomal recessive or inherited as an X-linked pattern. This syndrome is a combination of cognitive impairment, ataxia, tachypnea, eye movement abnormalities with frequent retinal degeneration and kidney manifestations. Cerebellar vermis hypoplasia is a pathognomonic finding on MRI named "the molar tooth" sign. Multiple other features can be associated with this midbrain–hindbrain malformation leading to the denomination of Joubert syndrome and associated disorders (JSAD). Kidney mani-festations are cystic dysplasia, caused by multiple cysts of different sizes, or nephronophthisis (NPH). More than 30% of Joubert patients develop kidney failure. Hepatic fibrosis occurs in 10% of patients. Skeletal findings are rarer and include polydactyly and cone-shaped epiphyses. **The ocular phenotype** is broad and may include abnormal motility, nystagmus, and ocular motor apraxia (saccade initiation failure). Coloboma has been reported rarely. RP occurs in a third of patients with either very early onset (mimicking) Leber's congenital amaurosis (LCA) or later onset night-blindness. Ten genes have been identified to be mutated in JSAD: *INPP5E, AHI1, NPHP1, CEP290/ NPHP6, MKS3, RPGRIP1L, ARL13B, CC2D2A, TMEM216,* and *OFD1* (oral-facial-digital syndrome 1).

The RP phenotype varies with the mutated gene. Eighty percent of *AHI1* mutated patients present with a retinal dystrophy and NPH-related renal disorder but no hepatic defects. RP has been observed in one family out of two mutated in *ARL13B. CC2D2A* is found mutated in JSAD patients with or without RP. The same mutation in *TMEM216* was identified in eight

JSAD-related families presenting psychomotor retardation and frequent retinopathy.

4. JEUNE SYNDROME

Jeune's asphyxiating dystrophy or Jeune's syndrome is an autosomal recessive chondro-dysplasia. The phenotype is highly variable and can lead to death in early infancy because of a severely constricted thoracic cage and respiratory insufficiency. Patients present with a long narrow thorax due to short ribs, shortened long bones, and sometimes polydactyly. Kidney cysts, hepatic fibrosis, and RP may occur as early as 5 years old. The molecular basis of the syndrome has been partially elucidated indicating involvement of the IFT 80 (3q25.33), DYNC2H1 (11q22.3), WDR19 (4p14) and TTC21B (2q24.3) genes, each encoding an intraflagellar transport protein, which confirms that Jeune syndrome belongs to the ciliopathies group.

5. ALPORT SYNDROME

Clinical features

The classical Alport's syndrome is an inherited disorder characterized by progressive nephritis, sensorineural high-tone hearing loss, and ocular lesions. The clinical course is more predictable in males than in females. In males, there is often hematuria very early in childhood. Renal failure develops at the end of the first decade, the second decade, or the beginning of the third decade. Females have a more variable course. Some are as severely affected as males but others have very mild symptoms or stay asymptomatic. **Ocular lesions** are an additional feature of the Alport's syndrome. Pathognomonic features are anterior lenticonus, retinal flecks and corneal posterior polymorphous dystrophy. Anterior lenticonus is a localized, well-defined protrusion of the lens in the anterior chamber. It is bilateral and far more common in affected males than in females. An oil droplet retinoscopy reflex is an early clinical sign. Visual dysfunction and progressive myopization appear later on. The lenticonus is never present at birth but develops progressively.

There are two major types of retinal flecks: The more common macular and the rare peripheral flecks. The macular flecks appear as bilateral, faint, densely packed, whitish, dot-like lesions

in the perifoveal area. They do not cause visual dysfunction and electrophysiological and fluoroangiographic evaluations are normal. If electrophysiological abnormalities do occur, they can be explained by renal dysfunction, dialysis or renal transplantation in nearly all cases. These flecks carry a poor prognosis with respect to renal outcome: renal failure develops at early age. Most authors accept a superficial position of the macular flecks in the internal limiting membrane, but recently a dissemination in various levels of the retina has been suggested. The Miiller cells are proposed as the progenitors. The midperipheral retinal flecks are also a specific feature of the Alport's syndrome. They appear associated with the pigment epithelium and Bruch's membrane, which is confirmed by the early, mild hyperfluorescence on FFA. Other retinal changes reported in patients with Alport's syndrome are an abnormal macular reflex, pigment dispersion syndrome, a macular hole, and optic drusen. Another specific ocular feature is corneal posterior polymorphous dystrophy, which consists of endothelial vesicles and can be associated with subepithelial opacities. A fragile corneal epithelium can cause recurrent erosions and a painful eye. An arcus juvenilis, spherophakia, anterior polar, cortical and posterior capsular cataract, posterior lenticonus, and lens coloboma have been described.

Diagnosis

The ocular manifestations of Alport's sydrome consist of anterior as well as posterior segment abnormalities. The anterior segment lesions are responsible for the subjective complaints of the patient. Troubled media due to corneal and/or lenticular opacities cause visual dysfunction. Progressive myopization and refraction difficulties, as well as a higher risk of lens capsule rupture are caused by anterior lenticonus. Corneal erosions may cause a painful eye. Macular flecks do not cause visual dysfunction, but contain important information for the nephrologist, since they reflect a more severe affection of the kidneys.

Kidney biopsies can also be tested for the presence or absence of the type IV collagen alpha-3, alpha-4 and alpha-5 chains. A skin biopsy can be performed when X-linked Alport syndrome is suspected. The type IV collagen alpha-5 chain (COL4A5) is normally present in the skin and a biopsy of the skin can be tested for the presence or absence of this collagen chain. If diagnosis still remains doubtful, screening for COL4A3, COL4A4, and COL4A5 can be done.

Treatment

Since Alport syndrome is a consequence of mutations in type IV collagen genes, a cure may be effected by replacement of the defective genes or by supplying the gene product (namely type IV collagen). To date, gene therapy in models of Alport syndrome, as in other diseases, has been a disappointing failure. Stem cell transfer from amniotic fluid or bone marrow present a potential therapeutic intervention.

6. KEARNS-SAYRE SYNDROME

Kearns-Sayre syndrome is a neuromuscular disease characterised by an onset before the age of 20 years, **ophthalmoplegia, ptosis and pigmentary retinitis.** More than 200 cases have been published. The prevalence is estimated between 1 and 3/100000. The disease often starts with the hallmark ocular symptoms, followed by the progressive occurrence of several other signs, depending on the tissue distribution of the molecular anomaly. The most frequently associated symptoms include deafness, heart involvement (cardiomyopathy, cardiac conduction defect), cerebral involvement (ataxia, high cerebrospinal fluid protein content, intellectual deficit), skeletal muscle myopathy, intestinal disorders, hormonal deficit (hypoparathyroidism, diabetes), and renal failure. The disease progresses slowly, with new symptoms appearing and previous symptoms slowly worsening. Kearns-Sayre syndrome is caused by deletions of large portions of mitochondrial DNA. Deletions are heteroplasmic, i.e. a single cell can harbour both deleted and normal DNA molecules. Symptoms only appear if the proportion of abnormal DNA is high. The threshold depends on the organ; about 60% for the skeletal striated muscle. Most cases of Kearns-Sayre syndrome are sporadic. In fact, deletions of mitochondrial DNA are only

exceptionally transmitted from one generation to the next.

The diagnosis is suggested by the clinical picture and by the presence of typical morphological alterations in the skeletal muscle (fibers presenting with mitochondrial proliferation or 'Ragged Red Fibers' and cytochrome c oxydase deficient fibers). It can be confirmed by the detection of high proportion of deleted mitochondrial DNA in a clinically or morphologically affected tissue (usually in the skeletal muscle). Differential diagnosis includes conditions with an overlapping clinical picture, such as Pearson syndrome or chronic ophthalmoplegia. Treatment of the various symptoms is supportive. The prognosis essentially depends on the number of organs involved. The disease progresses slowly over decades.

7. COHEN SYNDROME

It is a rare autosomal recessive disorder common in Finish population. The gene responsible for the condition has been identified which encodes for Vps13B.

Early onset myopia and retinal dystrophy is classically seen. The onset of myopia is before 5 years of age and exceeds 7 Dioptres by the second decade. The macula may develop a "bull's eye" appearance due to cone-rod dystrophy. Myopia and night blindness are followed by reduced visual acuity, constricted visual fields and pigmentary retinopathy with bone spicules and abnormal (isoelectric) electroretinogram (ERG).

Other systemic features include mental retardation, delayed milestones, truncal obesity, stridor due to laryngomalacia, microcephaly, episodic granulocytopenia facial dysmorphism with down slanting palpebral fissures, short philtrum, heavy eyebrows, prominent nasal base. Long tapering fingers, joint laxity and prominent upper central incisors are common.

8. COCKAYNE SYNDROME

It is a DNA repair disorder due to a dysfunction of the transcription-related DNA repair genes. Mutations in two genes have been seen: CSA (group 8 excision-repair cross-complementing protein; ERCC8) and CSB (group 6 excision-repair cross-complementing protein; ERCC8).

The main characteristics of the disease are UV skin sensitivity and severe physical and mental retardation with progressive neurologic impairment, sensorineural deafness and retinal degeneration.

The fundus has "salt and pepper" pigmentation with optic disc pallor and progressive deterioration in the rod and cone ERG. The progression is usually rapid.

Congenital cataracts and poorly developed iris dilator muscle (difficult to dilate and examine). Exposure keratopathy may occur secondary to lagophthalmos as well as chronic blepharitis. Profound vision loss occurs by third decade. Early death has been seen in patients with early onset cataracts.

All the cells are hypersensitive to UV light, which is used as the basis for the diagnostic tests of cultured fibroblasts from a skin biopsy.

9. METHYLMALONIC ACIDURIA

See (p-483).

10. ABETALIPOPROTEINEMIA (BASSEN-KORNWEIG DISEASE)

See (p-489).

11. CYSTINOSIS

See (p-481).

12. MUCOPOLYSACCHARIDOSES

See (p-483).

13. REFSUM'S DISEASE

See (p-489).

14. NEURONAL CEROID LIPOFUSCINOSIS

See (p-490).

CILIOPATHIES: NOVEL SYSTEMIC RETINAL DYSTROPHIES

A single non-motile cilium ("primary cilium") is present in almost every vertebrate cell. Motile cilia are present only in specific organs such as the respiratory or the reproductive system. The primary cilium acts as the "antenna" of the cell allowing transport of sensorial information from the extracellular environment to the cell. The photoreceptor cell has a connecting cilium and hence is a ciliated cell.

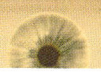

Ciliopathies are rare genetic disorders characterized by primary cilium dysfunction, frequently affecting photoreceptors and causing retinal degeneration either as an isolated condition (e.g. Leber's congenital amaurosis with CEP290 mutations) or as a ciliopathy syndrome affecting more than one organ system.

PATHOGENESIS OF THE CILIOPATHIES

The retinal degeneration in ciliopathies is related to dysfunction of the connecting cilium, a major site of transport and transit for proteins synthesized in the inner segment and necessary for phototransduction taking place in the outer segment. The ciliary-specific transport machinery is known as the intraflagellar transport (IFT) machinery and is composed of molecular motors linked to IFT protein complexes that organize anterograde and retrograde transport. Jeune's syndrome is the only ciliopathy known to be related to IFT gene mutations, namely *IFT80*, a potential regulator of IFT particles and *DYNC2H1*, a retrograde motor. To regulate cargo delivery to the cilium, two main regulatory pathways occur: vesicular sorting from the Golgi to the ciliary base and selective transport along the cilium. BBS proteins (the BBSome complex) are involved in these regulatory processes.

The extraocular manifestations are linked to specific roles of ciliary proteins involved in the development or function of many organs. As an example, the kidney epithelial cells' primary cilia are mechanosensors. Primary cilia are implicated in major developmental processes and especially in planar cell polarity, body asymmetry, or limb development.

1. BARDET–BIEDL SYNDROME

See (p-328, 494).

2. ALSTRÖM SYNDROME

Alström syndrome (ALMS) manifestations include **RP in early childhood, hearing impairment, and metabolic defect leading to hyperinsulinemia and type 2 diabetes mellitus and obesity in childhood.** Polydactyly does not occur. Dilated cardiomyopathy, often fatal, in infancy or later in life and renal dysfunction are reported in half of ALMS cases. Developmental or motor delays occur, but most children have normal intelligence.

The first manifestation of ALMS is severe early onset cone rod retinal dystrophy, sometimes mimicking Leber's congenital amaurosis (LCA) with very early visual impairment, photophobia, and nystagmus. Children usually become truncally obese during their first year. Sensorineural hearing loss presents in the first decade in up to 70%; it may progress to the moderately severe range (40–70 db) by the end of the first to second decades. Insulin resistant type 2 diabetes mellitus often presents in the second decade and is accompanied by acanthosis nigricans (pigmentation mostly in body folds). Other endocrine and metabolic abnormalities include hypothyroidism, diabetes insipidus, growth hormone deficiency, hyperuricemia, hyperlipidemia, hypothyroidism, and hypogonadotrophic hypogonadism. Hepatic and renal dysfunction can be present in the second decade. This syndrome requires a multidisciplinary follow-up to detect complications once the diagnosis is confirmed. A single gene is involved in all the cases, ALMS1. ALMS1 protein is found at the base of cilia.

3. MORM SYNDROME

MORM syndrome **(mental retardation, truncal obesity, retinal dystrophy, and micropenis)** is very rare. A congenital nonprogressive retinal dystrophy with poor night vision occurs within the first year of life with reduced visual acuity by 3 years that remains stable thereafter. The identified gene, INPP5E (inositol polyphosphate-5-phosphatase), classifies this syndrome as a ciliopathy. It is related to Joubert syndrome. It is transmitted in an autosomal recessive manner. The causative locus has been mapped to chromosome region 9q34. It shows similarities to Bardet-Biedl syndrome and Cohen syndrome, but can be distinguished by clinical features; the age of onset and nonprogressive nature of the visual impairment, the lack of characteristic facies, skin or gingival infection, microcephaly, 'mottled retina', polydactyly and small penis without testicular anomalies. However, linkage to the known Bardet-Biedl (BBS1-8) and Cohen syndrome loci has been excluded.

4. SENIOR-LOKEN SYNDROME

Senior-Loken syndrome (SLS) **combines nephrono-phthisis (NPH) and retinal degeneration.** NPH, the most common cause of inherited renal failure in childhood, is characterized by initial normal kidney size that will eventually shrink, tubulo-interstitial nephritis, and a loss of corticomedullary differentiation leading to cyst formation. The first symptoms are polyuria and polydypsia caused by a urinary concentration defect. The end-stage of the renal failure is variable – infantile, juvenile, or adolescent. The occurrence of the retinal dystrophy is higher in the juvenile form of NPH. The early retinal dystrophy usually occurs years before the kidney involvement is detected. The retinal dystrophy may be very early, mimicking isolated Lebers Congenital Amaurosis (LCA) or may have a later onset. Thus, clinical diagnosis of LCA should lead to clinical and molecular testing for LCA-SLS associated genes and, according to the results, annual kidney follow-up may be indicated.

SLS is a ciliopathy and the kidney involvement is explained by the role of the *NPHP* proteins at the level of the tubular epithelial renal cells that each carry a primary cilium in contact with the urinary flow.

Eleven genes (*NPHP1* to *NPHP11*) are known to be involved in NPH, and for all of them, except *NPHP7*, cases of SLS associated with RP have been reported. Mutations in *NPHP562* and *NPHP663* are more often linked to severe and early RP. A milder retinal phenotype is observed with mutations in other *NPHP* genes.

5. JOUBERT SYNDROME

See (p-329, 495)

6. JEUNE SYNDROME

See (p-495)

PEDIATRIC SYNDROMES WITH RETINAL DEGENERATION AND FEATURES OF THE ECTODERMAL SPECTRUM (HAIR, SKIN, TEETH)

Retinal degeneration observed in children with abnormalities related to the ectodermal dysplasia spectrum (affecting hair, skin, nails, or sweat glands or teeth) is rare.

1. HYPOTRICHOSIS WITH JUVENILE MACULAR DYSTROPHY

Congenital hypotrichosis associated with juvenile macular dystrophy is an autosomal recessive condition with early hair loss and juvenile macular degeneration in the first decade that can show phenotypic variability. **The retinal involvement becomes widespread and is a cone-rod dystrophy.** Mutations have been identifed in a P-cadherin gene, *CDH3*, that encodes an integral membrane glycoprotein responsible for calcium-dependent cell-cell desmosomal adhesion.

2. ECTODERMAL DYSPLASIA, ECTRODACTYLY, MACULAR DYSTROPHY SYNDROME

The ectodermal dysplasia, ectrodactyly, macular dystrophy (EEM) syndrome inherited as an autosomal recessive entity is a specific ectodermal entity because of the unusual associated retinal features. **The retinal involvement has a typical severe macular onset with geographic atrophy that has a peripheral progression.** The patients are characterized by hypotrichosis with sparse and short hair, eyebrows and eyelashes, partial anodontia, and limb defects with syndactyly or "lobster-claw" hands. The syndrome shares features with the hypotrichosis with juvenile macular degeneration (HJMD) syndrome and the *CHD3* gene is mutated, showing allelic variability.

Interestingly, cadherins constitute a superfamily of genes found mutated in various genetic disorders including Usher's syndrome type 1 (USH1). For the latter, there is a crucial role of transient fibrous links formed by cadherin 23 and protocadherin 15 in the cohesion of the developing hair bundle as well as the involvement of these cadherins in the formation of the tip link, a key component of the mechanoelectrical transduction machinery. This illustrates that proteins of the same superfamily may have different roles in inherited systemic retinal degenerative syndromes.

3. OLIVER-MCFARLANE SYNDROME, TRICHOMEGALY, AND CHORIORETINOPATHY WITH PITUITARY DYSFUNCTION

The Oliver-McFarlane syndrome is extremely rare, possibly autosomal recessive, and most often reported as sporadic cases with long eye

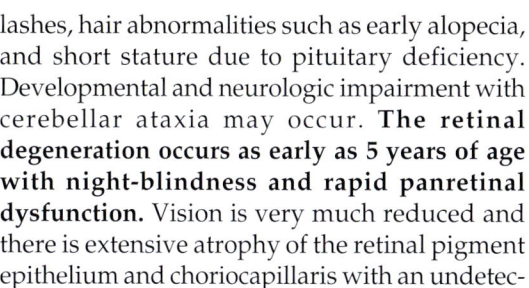

lashes, hair abnormalities such as early alopecia, and short stature due to pituitary deficiency. Developmental and neurologic impairment with cerebellar ataxia may occur. **The retinal degeneration occurs as early as 5 years of age with night-blindness and rapid panretinal dysfunction.** Vision is very much reduced and there is extensive atrophy of the retinal pigment epithelium and choriocapillaris with an undetectable ERG.

4. RETINAL DYSTROPHY AND DENTAL ABNORMALITIES: JALILI'S SYNDROME

Jalili's syndrome was first reported in 1988 by an Iraqi ophthalmologist named Ismail K. Jalili. It is a rare hereditary disorder of the teeth and eyes found primarily in the Middle East. Jalili's syndrome is characterized by the **association of amelogenesis imperfecta (AI) and cone-rod retinal dystrophy (CORD).** AI is a generic term for an inherited group of dental diseases in which the common clinical feature is an abnormality of tooth enamel. The enamel may be thin but normal, and/or hypomineralized. CORD is a rare retinal disorder that leads to an initial loss of central vision, color vision and photophobia before the age of 10 years with subsequent night blindness and visual field restriction. Jalili's syndrome is transmitted in an autosomal recessive manner. Mutations in the CNNM4 gene (2q11.2), which is implicated in metal ion transport, have been identified in several families.

Ophthalmologists and dentists together can make this diagnosis. There is no treatment for the retinal condition but dental care is required for the teeth. Lifespan is normal. Low vision aids may be useful for selected patients who have visual difficulties.

5. RP SYNDROME WITH PROMINENT SKELETAL INVOLVEMENT

Retinal degeneration may rarely be associated with inherited skeletal dysplasias. A child with spondylometaphyseal/epiphyseal dysplasia should undergo systematic ocular check-up. Genes and pathogenesis remain unknown although theories linking them to ciliopathies have been suggested.

6. SPONDYLOMETAPHYSEAL DYSPLASIA SHORT STATURE WITH CONE DYSTROPHY

This autosomal recessive condition has postnatal growth deficiency, profound short stature, platyspondyly (flattened vertebral bodies) and rhizomelic foreshortening of the limbs and early bowing of the long bones of the legs with shortening of all the tubular bones. **The retinal degeneration occurs in early childhood; it initially involves the macula with a cone-rod evolution.** A phenotypically less severe skeletal axial spondylometaphyseal dysplasia with features of retinal dystrophy has been reported.

MISCELLANEOUS SYNDROMES INVOLVING RETINA

1. ENHANCED S-CONE SYNDROME (1990) AND GOLDMANN-FAVRE VITREOTEPTORETINAL DEGENERATION (1957)

It is inherited as autosomal recessive trait. Mutation NR2E3 with locus at 15q23 lead to an absolute increase in S cones at the expense of M&L cones, decreased rod development and retinal degeneration. Severe loss of rod sensitivity is evident throughout the retina, along with characteristic enhanced S-cone electroretinogram.

Clinical feature

Goldmann-Favre syndrome was described in 1957 and is rare condition affecting retina, vitreous body and lens. **The patients have progressive loss of vision by retinoschisis both at center and periphery, cataract and clinically resembling retinitis pigmentosa.** Nyctalopia usually start early in first decade of life and pigmentary changes are in clumps rather than bone corpuscles types and an unusual enhanced S-cone electroretinogram which was demonstrated subsequently in 1990. Thus enhanced S-cone syndrome was named after the enhanced sensitivity of the S-cone syndrome system.

The most striking vitreous change is liquefaction thus converting large portion of vitreous body into an optically empty space and the **patients are at high risk of developing retinal detachment.** ERG is either markedly reduced or extinguished. As discussed earlier, the response

from the S-cone system account for waveform under both photopic and scotopic conditions.

Management

No satisfactory treatment except prophylactic laser therapy of retinal breaks if there are any.

2. DIFFUSE SUBRETINAL FIBROSIS SYNDROME (DSF)

It is a rare syndrome described by Palestine and associates in 1984. Majority of patients are young females under the age of 45 who present with multifocal choroiditis progressing to subretina fibrosis. The lesions are classically clustered at posterior pole.

Clinical features

The presentation is acute and most patients manifest with unilateral decreased vision, floaters, scotomata metamorphopsia and occasional photopsia initially. The lesion are typically clustered in the macula and few may be seen in midperiphery and these are usually at sub RPE level. Turbid fluid may accumulate around lesions which coalesce to form a yellow exudative detachment. It usually progress to subretinal fibrosis. In the meantime the second eye may also be involved with in 6 months leading to severe loss of vision. The cause is not known.

FFA in active phase of DSF demonstrate early hypo followed by late leakage in areas of the lesion and turbid subretinal fluid. There may be an evidence of choroidal neovascular membrane.

3. AICARDI SYNDROME

Aicardi syndrome is a rare congenital disorder that was first described by a French neurologist, Jean Aicardi in 1965. It is a X-linked dominant disorder and is seen almost exclusively in females. It is characterized by a **classic triad of agenesis or hypogenesis of the corpus callosum, infantile spasms and chorioretinal lacunae**. Of these three, chorioretinal lacunae is the most constant feature present. Infantile spasms typically start in early childhood. Developmental delay is generally profound involving both motor and language skills. Costovertebral malformations such as hemivertebrae, fusion of vertebrae, kyphoscoliosis,

absent or malformed ribs, and occasionally cleft lip and palate may also be associated with Aicardi syndrome. **Chorioretinal lacunae are well-defined, multifocal pale areas with minimally pigmented borders, and they are usually clustered around the optic disc.** They are peculiar punched out areas of choroidal and retinal pigment epithelium (RPE) atrophy. Other ocular abnormalities reported are optic nerve colobomas, which was seen in our case, optic nerve hypoplasia, optic disc pigmentation, microphthalmos, retrobulbar cyst, pseudoglioma, retinal detachment, macular scars, cataract, pupillary membrane remnants, iris synechiae and iris coloboma. Good visual function is seen if fovea is spared of the chorioretinal lacunae.

Dissociated burst suppression or burst suppression pattern appearing asymmetrically in either cerebral hemisphere is a characteristic EEG finding in this syndrome. ACTH, prednisolone, valproic acid and clonazepam have been used with variable success.

4. WHIPPLE'S DISEASE

Whipple's disease is a rare bacterial infection that may involve any organ system in the body. It occurs primarily in Caucasian males older than 40 years. The gastrointestinal tract is the most frequently involved organ, with manifestations such as abdominal pain, malabsorption syndrome with diarrhea, and weight loss. Other signs include low-grade fever, lymphadenopathy, skin hyperpigmentation, endocarditis, pleuritis, seronegative arthritis, uveitis, spondylodiscitis, and neurological manifestations, and these signs may occur in the absence of gastrointestinal manifestations. **Ocular symptoms of Whipple's disease are rare** (about 5% of patients) and include uveitis, vitritis, retinitis, retrobulbar neuritis, papilledema, and direct involvement of the lens epithelium. The usual patient complaints are blurred or complete loss of vision. Oculomasticatory myorhythmia (OMM) and oculofacial-skeletal myorhythmia (OSFM), are pathognomic of the disease. Supranuclear gaze palsy is also seen. In general, ocular manifestations occur in patients who also have gastrointestinal or CNS involvement. Whipple's disease of the eye without or with only minimal CNS involvement is very rare in

the absence of intestinal manifestations and, consequently, is very difficult to recognize clinically.

Due to the wide variability of manifestations, clinical **diagnosis is very difficult** and is often made only years or even decades after the initial symptoms have appeared. Trimethoprim-sulfamethoxazole for at least 1 year is usually considered adequate to eradicate the infection. The microbiological diagnosis of this insidious disease is rendered difficult by the virtual lack of culture and serodiagnostic methods. It is usually based on the demonstration of periodic acid-Schiff-positive particles in infected tissues and/or the presence of bacteria with an unusual trilaminar cell wall ultrastructure by electron microscopy. Recently, the Whipple bacteria have been characterized at the molecular level by amplification of their 16S rRNA gene(s). Phylogenetic analysis of these sequences revealed a new bacterial species related to the actinomycete branch which was named "*Tropheryma whippelli.*" Based on its unique 16S ribosomal DNA (rDNA) sequence, species-specific primers were selected for the detection of the organism in clinical specimens by PCR. This technique is currently used as one of the standard methods for establishing the diagnosis of Whipple's disease.

5. URBACH-WIETHE SYNDROME

Urbach-Wiethe syndrome (UWS) (also known as lipoid proteinosis or hyalinosis cutis et mucosae) is an autosomal recessive disorder, first described by Urbach and Wiethe in 1929. UWS has a strong tendency towards the white with no sex preponderance. It is more common among Europeans, especially the Dutch and Germans. Mutations responsible for UWS are known to occur on ECM1 gene located on 1q21. Pathophysiology of this multisystem disorder mostly includes deposition of hyaline-like material in the body.

Systemic features involve diffuse skin infiltration, thickening and hair loss, hoarseness resulting from vocal cord involvement and behavioral problems. Generally, eyelid lesions are reported in at least two-third of the cases. As mentioned before, classic presentation of such lesions is called moniliform blepharosis, which is generally believed to be one of the most pathognomonic features of UWS. This hallmark presents as tiny papules on eyelid margins just like a string of yellowish and waxy beads and is particularly known as a strong diagnostic clue. Also infiltration of glands of Zeiss, Moll, and Meibomian can consequently cause madarosis, trichiasis, and sometimes distichiasis. Trichiasis can cause corneal ulceration. **Also focal degeneration of macula and drusen formation in Bruch's membrane** have been observed in a third to a half of the examined patients. In some patients with documented histopathological evaluations, thickening of Bruch's membrane, as well as partial infiltration of vessel walls of the choroid/retina by hyaline PAS positive material are described. Other complications include uveitis, deposition of hyaline inclusions in the trabecular meshwork leading to open angle glaucoma, bilateral cataracts with bilateral lens subluxation, retinitis pigmentosa, impaired color vision and light hypersensitivity, corneal opacities as well as the deposition of hyaline on the Descemet's membrane, hyaline deposits on the iris along with corectopia, infiltration of hyaline material in conjunctiva, dry eye syndrome due to involvement of meibomian glands by the deposits, or epiphora due to punctal stenosis and calcification and thrombosis of the internal carotid artery which caused a transient blindness of the right eye.

Urbach-Wiethe disease is typically diagnosed by its clinical dermatological manifestations, particularly the beaded papules on the eyelids. The discovery of the mutations within the ECM1 gene has allowed the use of genetic testing to confirm an initial clinical diagnosis. Periodic acid-Schiff (PAS) and immunohistochemical staining may also be used for diagnosis.

Currently, there is no cure for Urbach-Wiethe disease although there are ways to individually treat many of its symptoms. The discovery of the mutations of the ECM1 gene has opened the possibility of gene therapy or a recombinant ECM1 protein for Urbach-Wiethe disease treatment, but neither of these options is currently available.

6. DOWN SYNDROME

Down syndrome (DS), first comprehensively described in 1866 by a British physician named

Langdon Down, is a genetic condition in which a person has 47 chromosomes instead of 46, with an extra copy of chromosome 21. This extra genetic material disrupts the normal developmental processes, leading to characteristic intellectual, medical, and physical abnormalities in persons with DS. DS (trisomy 21) is associated with characteristic features that include physical (short stature, small heads, flat nasal bridges, oblique palpebral fissures, prominent epicanthal folds, medical conditions such as cardiac defects, skeletal abnormalities, obesity and oculo-visual anomalies. **Ocular manifestations** include poor visual acuity, amblyopia, nystagmus, strabismus, congenital lid anomalies like prominent epicanthal folds, upward slanting of the palpebral fissures, and congenital ectropion (rare). Patients frequently have lid infections, including blepharitis, blepharoconjunctivitis, chalazion, and hordeola, meibomitis, nasolacrimal duct obstruction. Keratoconus, keratoglobus, corneal hydrops, iris brushfield spots, glaucoma and retinal detachments. Prenatal screening for Down syndrome can be done by amniocentesis and chorionic villus sampling. A multidisciplinary approach is required and medical and surgical management of ocular conditions should be done wherever required.

7. TURNER SYNDROME

Turner syndrome has been recognised since the 1930s when Otto Ullrich and Henry Turner described female subjects with the association of short stature, sexual infantilism, webbed neck, cubitus valgus, mental retardation and primary ovarian failure resulting in 'streak ovaries'. Turner syndrome is best known for the XO karyotype (45X). **Ocular features** include ametropia, amblyopia, strabismus, reduced accommodation, convergence insufficiency, ptosis, epicanthus, hypertelorism, anti-mongloid slant, red-green deficiency, nystagmus, presenile cataract, congenital glaucoma, blue sclera, keratoconus, anterior segment dysgenesis, anterior lenticonus, retinal neovascularisation, choroidal neovascular membrane and retinal detachment.

Patients with Turner syndrome require multidisciplinary care. This is normally coordinated by a pediatrician, with appropriate input from endocrinologists, cardiologists, nephrologists, psychologists, and others. Early orthoptic screening and referral to ophthalmologist may be required. General treatment strategies include hormone replacement (both growth hormone and estrogen).

8. KLINEFELTER SYNDROME

Klinefelter syndrome (KS) defines a group of chromosomal disorders in which there is at least one extra X chromosome compared with the normal 46,XY male karyotype (47, XXY). The effects on physical features and on physical and cognitive development increase with the number of extra X's, and each extra X is associated with an intelligence quotient (IQ) decrease of approximately 15–16 points, with language most affected, particularly expressive language skills. Hypospadias, small phallus or cryptorchidism, developmental delay, eunuchoid body habitus, gynecomastia and breast malignancies. **Ocular findings associated** with Klinefelter's syndrome include colobomas of the iris, choroid and optic nerve, microphthalmia, and strabismus. Cases of high myopia also have been reported in association with 49, XXXXY syndrome, a variant of Klinefelter's syndrome. Formal cytogenetic analysis is necessary to make a definite diagnosis. Prenatal diagnosis can be made by amniocentesis or chorionic villus sampling. Androgen replacement therapy should begin at puberty (around 12 years of age) and the dose should be increased so that it is sufficient to maintain age-appropriate serum concentrations of testosterone, estradiol, follicle stimulating hormone (FSH), and luteinizing hormone (LH).

9. MARFAN SYNDROME

Marfan syndrome is an inherited connective-tissue disorder transmitted as an autosomal dominant trait. Marfan syndrome is caused by mutations in FBN1 gene located on chromosome 15q21.1 and, occasionally, by mutation in TGFβR1 or TGFβR2 gene located on chromosome 9 and on chromosome 3p24.2-p25, respectively.

More than 500 fibrillin gene mutations have been identified. Almost all of these mutations are unique to an affected individual or family.

Different fibrillin mutations are responsible for genetic heterogeneity.

Clinical features

- Delayed achievement of gross and fine motor milestones secondary to ligamentous laxity of the hips, knees, ankles, arches, wrists, and fingers
- A decrescendo diastolic murmur from aortic regurgitation
- An ejection click at the apex followed by a holosystolic high-pitched murmur from mitral prolapse and regurgitation
- Dysrhythmia (a primary feature)
- Abrupt onset of thoracic pain, which occurs in more than 90% of patients with aortic dissection (Other signs include syncope, shock, pallor, pulselessness, and paresthesia or paralysis in the extremities. Onset of hypotension may indicate aortic rupture.)
- Low back pain near the tailbone, burning sensation and numbness or weakness in the legs in serious dural ectasia (Dural ectasia may cause headaches and even neurologic deficits).
- Joint pain in adult patients
- Dyspnea, severe palpitations, and substernal pain in severe pectus excavatum
- Breathlessness, often with chest pain, in spontaneous pneumothorax
- Visual problems, possibly loss of vision, from lens dislocation or retinal detachment (The most common refractory errors are myopia and amblyopia.)
- Skeletal involvement is often the first sign of the disease and can include dolichostenomelia (excessive length of extremities) large size, arachnodactyly, joint hypermobility, scoliotic deformations, acetabulum protrusion, thoracic deformity (pectus carinatum or pectus excavatum), dolichocephaly of the anteroposterior axis, micrognathism or malar hypoplasia.
- Cardiovascular findings include aortic root dilatation involving the sinuses of Valsalva, aortic dissections involving the ascending aorta, mitral valve prolapse, dilatation of proximal main pulmonary artery in the absence of peripheral pulmonic stenosis or other cause, calcification of mitral annulus (patients

< 40 years) and dilatation of abdominal or descending thoracic aorta (patients < 50 years)

Pulmonary system findings include spontaneous pneumothorax and apical blebs on chest radiography.

Skin and integumentary include striae atrophicae and recurrent or incisional hernia

Dural findings include dural ectasia which can be seen on CT and MRI

Retinal detachment is the most serious eye complication in 10–25% patients with Marfan's syndrome (Fig. 27.4). It is bilateral in 70% of patients. Ectopia lentis is there in all eyes and pupils mostly fail to dilate. The patient present with all varieties of breaks ranging from holes to giant retinal tears with or without PVR and more than 50% have multiple breaks may be >4 breaks. As regards to refractive error >50% have myopia of >6D. The result of RD surgery are good whether it is scleral buckling or parsplana vitrectomy and it is approximately 86%. Since the condition is bilatearal in vast majority therefore prophylaxis of the breaks in the other eye if there are any is justified.

Diagnosis

Marfan syndrome is currently diagnosed using criteria based on an evaluation of the family history, molecular data, and 6 organ systems. The diagnosis cannot be based on molecular analysis alone because molecular diagnosis is not generally available, mutation detection is imperfect, and not all FBN1 mutations are associated with Marfan syndrome. With the previous Berlin criteria, Marfan syndrome was diagnosed on the basis of involvement of the skeletal system and 2 other systems, with the requirement of at least one major manifestation (i.e. ectopia lentis, aortic dilatation or dissection, or dural ectasia).

Major criteria include the following:
- A first-degree relative (parent, child, or sibling) who independently meets the diagnostic criteria
- Presence of an FBN1 mutation known to cause Marfan syndrome
- Inheritance of an FBN1 haplotype known to be associated with unequivocally diagnosed Marfan syndrome in the family

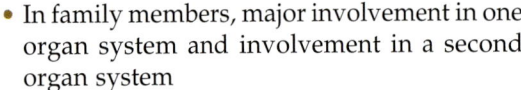

- In family members, major involvement in one organ system and involvement in a second organ system

If the family and genetic histories are not contributory, major criteria in 2 different organ systems and involvement of a third organ system are required to make the diagnosis.

Because no common mutations have been identified, genetic testing includes screening the entire FBN1 gene. Molecular studies of the fibrillin gene should be performed in patients in whom Marfan syndrome is suspected.

10. EHLER-DANLOS SYNDROME

EDS is usually transmitted as a dominant trait, although an X-linked form has been described. Blue sclera and myopia might be additional features of an uncommon recessive ophthalmological form of the EDS. The main features of the Ehlers-Danlos syndrome (EDS) are cutaneous hyperextensibility, articular laxity, and fragility of the tissues. Systemic ramifications may lead to orthopedic, cardiovascular, and gastrointestinal problems. **Various ocular abnormalities** have been observed in patients with the Ehlers-Danlos syndrome (EDS). McKusick found that epicanthal folds were the most common associated ocular abnormality. Other less frequent ocular changes occurring in this disease were strabismus, blue sclerotics, microcornea, myopia, keratoconus, ectopia lentis, hypertelorism, and intraocular hemorrhage. Bonnet described depigmentation in the preequatorial region of the fundus. Retinal detachment, retinitis proliferans and macular degeneration have been observed in the other eye. Angioid streaks have been seen in patients who were affected with pseudoxanthoma elasticum and EDS.

11. PARANEOPLASTIC SYNDROME OF CENTRAL NERVOUS SYSTEM

Cancer-associated retinopathy (CAR) is a rare paraneoplastic process in which antibodies are thought to be formed against a protein produced by the tumor that has homology to specific retinal proteins. Patients with CAR were initially found to have antibodies to a 23-kd retinal protein, later identified as recoverin. Recoverin is a retinal photoreceptor calcium-binding protein that is involved in light and dark adaptation through the regulation of rhodopsin phosphorylation. Recoverin has been identified in the tumor of a patient with small cell carcinoma of the lung, a patient with endometrial carcinoma, and in malignant mixed müllerian tumor. Anti-recoverin antibodies have been shown to induce photoreceptor apoptosis. Fifty percent of patients have retinopathy as the first manifestation of their underlying neoplasm.

The presentation of CAR typically involves a few key symptoms. First, patients report dimming of their vision occurring over days to weeks. Second, they also complain of acute-onset nyctalopia. Finally, patients often describe positive visual symptoms such as swirling and flashing lights.

On examination, patients have decreased acuity, diminished color vision, and ring scotoma visual field defects. The posterior segment of the eye can appear totally normal, but occasionally there is a mild inflammatory reaction in the vitreous and the retinal vasculature is attenuated. The electroretinogram, a test of retinal function, is markedly reduced. Serum antibody testing may confirm the diagnosis. Histopathology of the retina demonstrates loss of the photoreceptors.

Treatment for CAR involves modulation of the immune system to reduce the autoimmune response. The most widely reported therapy consists of 250 mg of intravenous methylprednisolone 4 times daily or 60 to 80 mg of oral prednisone daily, followed by a slow taper to a low maintenance dose. Other options being investigated include intravenous immunoglobulin and plasmapheresis. Most recently, Tolpa Torf preparation, a naturally occurring immunomodulator, has been shown to be effective in reducing antibody levels.

Overall, the **clinical course of CAR** is one of deterioration. Patients typically experience progressive visual loss, worsening of their visual field defects, and flattening of their electroretinogram.

12. ROTHMUND SYNDROME

Rothmund syndrome is an autosomal recessive disorder, more commonly seen in females. It is a genodermatosis presenting with a characteristic

facial rash (poikiloderma), hypogonadism, hypomenorrhea, skeletal head deformity (enlarged head with depressed nasal bridge as well as microcephaly), small stature, short or malformed distal phalanges, radial ray defects, premature ageing and a predisposition to cancer. **The ocular findings** in patients with Rothmund syndrome include sparse or absent eyebrows and hypertelorism. Bilateral cataracts are a common ocular feature of this syndrome. Isolated cases of bilateral glaucoma, retinal coloboma, and chorioretinal atrophy have also been documented in the literature.

13. MCKUSICK-KAUFMAN SYNDROME

McKusick-Kaufman syndrome (MKKS) is an autosomal recessive multiple malformation syndrome characterized by hydrometrocolpos and polydactyly and together with congenital heart disease form the distinctive triad of symptoms. Choanal atresia, pituitary dysplasia, esophageal atresia and distal tracheoesophageal fistula, Hirschsprung disease, vertebral anomalies, and hydrops fetalis have occasionally been associated with this syndrome. The disease is autosomal recessive and the causative gene, MKKS, has been mapped to 20p12. This syndrome is more frequent in females, whose parents are first-degree cousins. Most mutations in MKKS cause one of the forms of Bardet-Biedl syndrome (MKKS is also labelled BBS6), a disorder that is characterized by obesity, retinitis pigmentosa manifesting before age 10 years, polydactyly, hypogenitalism, renal malformations/insufficiency, endocrinologic dysfunctions and learning difficulties. Some of the patients diagnosed with McKusick-Kaufman syndrome at birth, later develop obesity and retinal dystrophy and in fact have Bardet-Biedl syndrome. Prenatal diagnosis of McKusick-Kaufman syndrome is possible by ultrasound visualisation of an abdominal mass combined with polydactyly. There is no therapy at present.

14. SHAKEN BABY SYNDROME

Child abuse is a major public health issue. It is well recognized that shaken baby may not show the classic stigmata of child abuse such as fractures, bruises and other visible injuries which may pose difficulty in the actual recognition of child abuse victims. Thus the ophthalmologist has an important role in diagnosing child abuse in the absence of visible marks of injury. Shaken baby syndrome is largely restricted to children <3 years of age with majority in the first year of life.

Pathogenesis

The most accepted mechanism is sudden indirect acceleration-deceleration traction stresses combined with forceful striking of the head against a soft surface, the latter may not leave behind visible marks of injury.

Ocular features

Retinal hemorrhages are found in 65 to 95% of patients. These may vary from focal hemorrhages in one layer to massive hemorrhages in all the layers of retina with extension into the vitreous. The massive hemorrhages are almost invariably associated with brain hemorrhage and with retinal detachment. In addition depending upon the quantum of injury the child may have hyphema, angle recession and cataract in the anterior segment and signs of periorbital injury.

Diagnosis

If the classical physical findings as mentioned above are present then the diagnosis is easy. However, the presence of only retinal hemorrhage make the task of diagnosis difficult. The other causes of non-accidental trauma such as coagulopathy and actual accidental injury should be explored. It should always be kept in mind that Shaken baby syndrome by and large is a diagnosis of exclusion. The diagnosis needs to be considered and vigorously explored if the facts and circumstantial evidence do not explain the nature or extent of injury.

15. TERSON SYNDROME

Terson, in 1900, described intraocular hemorrhage in association with any form of intracranial hemorrhage, this is known as Terson syndrome.

The most common cause of Terson's syndrome is acute subarachnoid hemorrhage resulting from ruptured intracranial aneurysm. Mostly it is unilateral, but bilateral involvement is common.

In acute stage one may see multiple preretinal, intraretinal and subretinal hemorrhages.

Vitreous hemorrhage is seen in about 3 to 8% patients following subarachnoid hemorrhage. The preretinal hemorrhage is characteristically boat shaped (D shaped) between the internal limiting membrane and posterior hyaloid surface. It is also known as subhyaloid hemorrhage.

Mechanism

Intracranial hemorrhage leads to acute rise of intracranial pressure which is transmitted via vaginal sheaths of optic nerve to the central retinal vein. This inturn cause rise of intraocular venous pressure, distention and rupture of capillaries resulting in retinal and vitreal hemorrhage.

Management

- The vitreous hemorrhage is treated on lines as followed in other instances (p-162). It is logical to wait for 2 months which not only facilitates PVD but will have minimal deleterious effect on the retina. If the vitreous hemorrhage does not resolve with in that period, patient is subjected to pars plana vitrectomy.
- Subhyaloid hemorrhage at the posterior pole mostly covers macula thereby diminishing the vision markedly. The vision can be restored almost instantaneously by subjecting the patient to hyaloidotomy with YAG laser at the lowest dependent part of the hemorrhage. The hemorrhage gravitates inferiorly into the vitreous which resolves spontaneously leaving behind clear macula.
- Subretinal and intraretinal hemorrhages resolves in due course of time.

16. GARDNER SYNDROME AND CHRPE

Solitary and unilateral lesions of congenital hypertrophy of retinal pigment epithelium (CHRPE) are not associated with any ocular or extraocular abnormality. However, multiple and bilateral lesions of CHRPE have been found to be associated with familial adenomatous polyposis (FAP) of large and small intenstine, hamartomas of skelton and various tumefactions of soft tissue when it is termed as Gardener Syndrome.

FAP usually appear during the third decade of life and carcinomatous change occur by 5th decade. The pigmented fundus lesions are usually identified by indirect ophthalmoscopy. Four or more such lesions in one or both eyes are thought to be a specific and sensitive marker of FAP.

Thus the detection of multiple, bilateral pigmented fundus lesions (CHRPE) (p-465) in members of families with inherited intestinal polyposis allows the ophthalmologist to make an important contribution to the early recognition of persons at risk for the development of intestinal malignancies.

17. HELLP SYNDROME

It is a syndrome associated with pregnancy induced hypertension (PIH). When PIH is severe the women may develop hepatic involvement and progress to HELLP syndrome. It consists of hemolysis (H) elevated liver enzymes (EL) and low platelet counts (LP). It is said to occur in approximately 20% patients of severe PIH. Ocular features include bilateral serous retinal detachment and yellow white subretinal opacities in addition to usual retinal signs of arteriolar attenuation, superficial flame shape hemorrhages and cotton wool spots.

Usually with timely intervention of termination of pregnancy the abovementioned signs gradually resolve and visual disturbances are restored. However, blurred central vision and central field defect have been reported in HELLP syndrome. Rarely vitreous hemorrhage unilateral CRVO and cortical blindness has also been reported in five patients with HELLP syndrome in one study.

As with severe PIH, HELLP syndrome is associated with an increased risk of adverse outcome and even fetal or maternal death.

18. REITER SYNDROME

It is characterized by classic triad of arthritis, urethiritis/cervicitis and conjunctivitis. It is rare for a patient to present with the classic triad. It has a genetic predisposition, in that 63 to 95% patients are HLA-B27 positive. The disease tends to follow an episodic and relapsing course.

The ocular features includes conjunctivitis which occur in the early part of the disease. The

more serious ocular manifestation is nongranulo-matous acute anterior uveitis (AAU) which is said to occur in 5 to 20% patients with initial attack and almost 50% of patients with long-term follow-up.

Posterior segment lesions are unusual, however, spill over vitritis and CME secondary to AAU have been described. Rarely associated panuveitis and multifocal choroiditis have been reported. The diagnosis is not difficult and steroid are the main stay of treatment.

19. ORGANOID NEVUS SYNDROME

An occuloneurocutaneous condition characterized by the sebaceous nevus of Jadassohn, cerebral atrophy, epibulbar complex choristoma and posterior scleral cartilage. The full blown syndrome is uncommon and the exact incidence is unknown. It is a sporadic condition and familial occurrence is extremely rare.

Ocular features

Two most important features are the epibulbar complex choristoma of the conjunctiva and posterior scleral cartilage which produces yellow-white discoloration of the fundus in the area of involvement. The latter is a bone density plaqaue at the level of choroid and sclera that correspond to cartilage in the posterior sclera and not bone as seen in choroidal osteoma. The clinical picture of involvement of conjunctiva, sclera along with dermatological features and CNS involvement helps in the diagnosis. CT scan orbit and ultrasonography clinch the diagnosis.

Management

There is no treatment of fundus lesion. Epibulbar choristoma and sebaceous nevus require close follow up and surgical resection is considered in case these progress.

20. FAT EMBOLISM SYNDROME (FES)

It was described in 1861 as part of clinical findings in certain patients suffering from fractures of long bones particularly thigh bones. It is clinically observed in about 50% patients of long bones fractures and may have adverse outcome in about 20% of severe cases.

The ocular findings are similar to Purtscher's retinopathy which has been reported after chest compression injury. The fundus findings include, cotton wool spots and retinal hemorr-hages and retinal whitening.

Sytemic features include petechial rash, respiratory insufficiency, radiographic changes and CNS involvement. The visual prognosis for patients of FES is generally good because of macular sparing, however, permanent visual scotamata have been reported.

BIBLIOGRAPHY

1. Al-Ani RM, Mohsin TM, Hassan ZM, Al-Dulaimy HI. Importance of ophthalmological examination in children with congenital sensorineural hearing loss. Saudi Med J 2009; 30:1197–201.
2. Albrectsen B, Svendsen IB. Hypotrichosis, syndactyly, and retinal degeneration in two siblings. Acta Derm Venereol 1956; 36:96–101.
3. Baker K, Beales PL. Making sense of cilia in disease: the human ciliopathies. Am J Med Genet C Semin Med Genet 2009; 151C:281–95.
4. Beales PL, Bland E, Tobin JL, et al. IFT80, which encodes a conserved intraflagellar transport protein, is mutated in Jeune asphyxiating thoracic dystrophy. Nat Genet 2007; 39:727–9.
5. Beales PL, Elcioglu N, Woolf AS, et al. New criteria for improved diagnosis of Bardet-Biedl syndrome: results of a population survey. J Med Genet 1999; 36:437–46.
6. Bhojwani R, Lloyd IC, Alam S, Ashworth J. Blepharokeratoconjunctivitis in Cockayne syndrome. J Pediatr Ophthalmol Strabismus 2009; 46: 184–5.
7. Bielas SL, Silhavy JL, Brancati F, et al. Mutations in INPP5E, encoding inositol polyphosphate-5-phosphatase E, link phosphatidyl inositol signaling to the ciliopathies. Nat Genet 2009; 41: 1032–6.
8. Bolz HJ, Roux AF. Clinical utility gene card for: Usher syndrome. Eur J Hum Genet 2011; 19(8).
9. Bork K, Stender E, Schmidt D, et al. Familial congenital hypotrichosis with "uncombable hair," retinal pigmentary dystrophy, juvenile cataract and brachymetacarpia: another entity of the ectodermal dysplasia group. Hautarzt 1987; 38:342–7.
10. Coene KL, Roepman R, Doherty D, et al. OFD1 is mutated in X-linked Joubert syndrome and interacts with LCA5-encoded lebercilin. Am J

Hum Genet 2009; 85:465–81.

11. Dagoneau N, Goulet M, Genevieve D, et al. DYNC2H1 mutations cause asphyxiating thoracic dystrophy and short rib-polydactyly syndrome, type III. Am J Hum Genet 2009; 84: 706–11.

12. Dollfus H, Porto F, Caussade P, et al. Ocular manifestations in the inherited DNA repair disorders. Surv Ophthalmol 2003; 48:107–22.

13. Egly JM, Coin F. A history of TFIIH: Two decades of molecular biology on a pivotal transcription/repair factor. DNA Repair (Amst) 2011; 10: 714–21.

14. Flores-Guevara R, Renault F, Loundon N, et al. Usher syndrome type 1: early detection of electroretinographic changes. Eur J Paediatr Neurol 2009; 13:505–7.

15. Fryns JP, Legius E, Devriendt K, et al. Cohen syndrome: the clinical symptoms and stigmata at a young age. Clin Genet 1996; 49:237–41.

16. Girard D, Petrovsky N. Alström syndrome: insights into the pathogenesis of metabolic disorders. Nat Rev Endocrinol 2011; 7: 77–88.

17. Hampshire DJ, Ayub M, Springell K, et al. MORM syndrome (mental retardation, truncal obesity, retinal dystrophy and micropenis), a new autosomal recessive disorder, links to 9q34. Eur J Hum Genet 2006; 14:543–8.

18. Hildebrandt F, Benzing T, Katsanis N. Ciliopathies. N Engl J Med 2011; 364:1533–43.

19. Hildebrandt F, Benzing T, Katsanis N. Ciliopathies. N Engl J Med 2011; 364:1533–43.

20. Indelman M, Eason J, Hummel M, et al. Novel CDH3 mutations in hypotrichosis with juvenile macular dystrophy. Clin Exp Dermatol 2007; 32: 191–6.

21. Indelman M, Hamel CP, Bergman R, et al. Phenotypic diversity and mutation spectrum in hypotrichosis with juvenile macular dystrophy. J Invest Dermatol 2003; 121:1217–20.

22. Keppler-Noreuil KM, Adam MP, Welch J, et al. Clinical insights gained from eight new cases and review of reported cases with Jeune syndrome (asphyxiating thoracic dystrophy). Am J Med Genet A 2011; 155A:1021–32.

23. Kimberling WJ, Hildebrand MS, Shearer AE, et al. Frequency of Usher syndrome in two pediatric populations: implications for genetic screening of deaf and hard of hearing children. Genet Med 2010; 12:512–6.

24. Kivitie-Kallio S, Norio R. Cohen syndrome: essential features, natural history, and heterogeneity. Am J Med Genet 2001; 102:125–

35.

25. Kjaer KW, Hansen L, Schwabe GC, et al. Distinct CDH3 mutations cause ectodermal dysplasia, ectrodactyly, macular dystrophy (EEM syndrome). J Med Genet 2005; 42:292–8.

26. Kolehmainen J, Black GC, Saarinen A, et al. Cohen syndrome is caused by mutations in a novel gene, COH1, encoding a transmembrane protein with a presumed role in vesicle-mediated sorting and intracellular protein transport. Am J Hum Genet 2003; 72:1359–69.

27. Lainé JP, Egly JM. When transcription and repair meet: a complex system. Trends Genet 2006; 22:430–6.

28. Leibu R, Jermans A, Hatim G, et al. Hypo-trichosis with juvenile macular dystrophy: clinical and electrophysiological assessment of visual function. Ophthalmology 2006; 113:841–7.

29. Liu XZ, Angeli SI, Rajput K, et al. Cochlear implantation in individuals with Usher type 1 syndrome. Int J Pediatr Otorhinolaryngol 2008; 72:841–7.

30. Malm E, Ponjavic V, Möller C, et al. Alteration of rod and cone function in children with Usher syndrome. Eur J Ophthalmol 2011; 21:30–8.

31. Marren P, Wilson C, Dawber RP, Walshe MM. Hereditary hypotrichosis (Marie-Unna type) and juvenile macular degeneration (Stargardt's maculopathy). Clin Exp Dermatol 1992; 17:189–91.

32. Marshall JD, Bronson RT, Collin GB, et al. New Alstrom syndrome phenotypes based on the evaluation of 182 cases. Arch Intern Med 2005; 165: 675–83.

33. Merrill A E, Merriman B, Farrington-Rock C, et al. Ciliary abnormalities due to defects in the retrograde transport protein DYNC2H1 in short rib-polydactyly syndrome. Am J Hum Genet 2009; 84: 542–9.

34. Millan JM, Aller E, Jaijo T, et al. An update on the genetics of Usher syndrome. J Ophthalmol 2011. doi:10.1155/2011/417217.

35. Mockel A, Perdomo Y, Stutzmann F, et al. Retinal dystrophy in Bardet-Biedl syndrome and related syndromic ciliopathies. Prog Retin Eye Res 2011; 30:258–74.

36. Muller J, Stoetzel C, Vincent MC, et al. Identification of 28 novel mutations in the Bardet-Biedl syndrome genes: the burden of private mutations in an extensively heterogeneous disease. Hum Genet 2010; 127: 583–93.

37. Nance MA, Berry SA. Cockayne syndrome: review of 140 cases. Am J Med Genet 1992; 42: 68–84.

38. Nikolopoulos TP, Lioumi D, Stamataki S, O'Donoghue GM. Evidence-based overview of ophthalmic disorders in deaf children: a literature update. Otol Neurotol 2006; 27:S1–24.

39. Ohdo S, Hirayama K, Terawaki T. Association of ectodermal dysplasia, ectrodactyly, and macular dystrophy: the EEM syndrome. J Med Genet 1983; 20:52–7.

40. Oliver GL, McFarlane DC. Congenital trichomegaly with associated pigmentary degeneration of the retina, dwarfism and mental retardation. Arch Ophthalmol 1965; 74:169–71.

41. Parisi MA. Clinical and molecular features of Joubert syndrome and related disorders. Am J Med Genet C Semin Med Genet 2009; 151C: 326–40.

42. Pennings RJ, Damen GW, Snik AF, et al. Audiologic performance and benefit of cochlear implantation in Usher syndrome type I. Laryngoscope 2006; 116:717–22.

43. Rapin I, Lindenbau Y, Dickson DW, et al. Cockayne syndrome and xeroderma pigmentosum. Neurology 2000; 55: 1442–9.

44. Reiners J, Nagel-Wolfrum K, Jürgens K, et al. Molecular basis of human Usher syndrome: deciphering the meshes of the Usher protein network provides insights into the pathomechanisms of the Usher disease. Exp Eye Res 2006; 83:97–119.

45. Sattar S, Gleeson JG. The ciliopathies in neuronal development: a clinical approach to investigation of Joubert syndrome and Joubert syndrome-related disorders. Dev Med Child Neurol 2011; 53:793–8.

46. Seifert W, Holder-Espinasse M, Spranger S, et al. Mutational spectrum of COH1 and clinical heterogeneity in Cohen syndrome (Letter). J Med Genet 2006; 43: e22.

47. Sprecher E, Bergman R, Richard G, et al. Hypotrichosis with juvenile macular dystrophy is caused by a mutation in CDH3, encoding P-cadherin. Nat Genet 2001; 29:134–6.

48. Tobin JL, Beales PL. Bardet-Biedl syndrome: beyond the cilium. Pediatr Nephrol 2007; 22: 926–36.

49. Traboulsi EI, De Becker I, Maumenee IH. Ocular findings in Cockayne syndrome. Am J Ophthalmol 1992; 114:579–83

50. Tuysuz B, Baris S, Aksoy F, et al. Clinical variability of asphyxiating thoracic dystrophy (Jeune) syndrome: evaluation and classification of 13 patients. Am J Med Genet 2009; 149A: 1727–33.

51. Venema J, Mullenders LHF, Natarajan AT, et al. The genetic defect in Cockayne syndrome is associated with a defect in repair of UV-induced DNA damage in transcriptionally active DNA. Proc Natl Acad Sci USA 1990; 87:4707–11.

52. Weidenheim KM, Dickson DW, Rapin I. Neuropathology of Cockayne syndrome: Evidence for impaired development, premature aging, and neurodegeneration. Mech Ageing Dev 2009; 130: 619–36.

53. Wolf MT, Hildebrandt F. Nephronophthisis. Pediatr Nephrol 2011; 26:181–94.

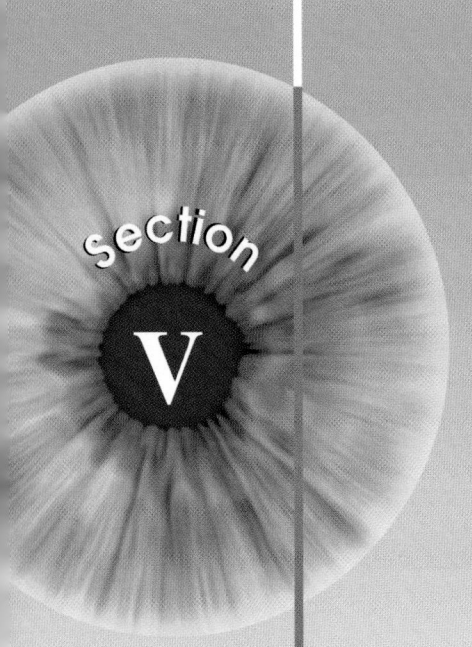

Section

V

Endophthalmitis

29. Endophthalmitis

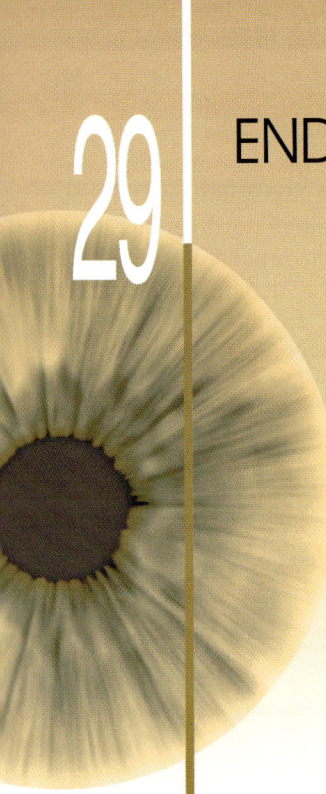

29 | ENDOPHTHALMITIS

Subina Narang and Shyna Kansal Jain

DEFINITION AND CLASSIFICATION

DEFINITION

Endophthalmitis is defined as inflammation of the anterior or posterior segment or both, with involvement of the adjacent ocular wall or as, an inflammatory reaction occurring as a result of intraocular colonization by bacteria, fungi, or rarely parasites.

CLASSIFICATION

Endophthalmitis is classified as infectious and non infectious (sterile) endophthalmitis. The infectious endophthalmitis is further classfied as endogenous and exogenous, whereas non infectious endophthalmitis has been termed as toxic anterior segment syndrome (TASS p-526).

Endogenous endophthalmitis. Endogenous is also known as metastatic endophthalmitis. It is due to hematogenous spread of micro-organisms to eye.

Exogenous endophthalmitis is due to inoculation of organism from extraneous source after surgery or trauma.

- *Postoperative endophthalmitis* incidence is 0.05–0.28%.

- *Post-traumatic endophthalmitis* accounts for 2.4–18.4% of open globe injuries.

- *Bleb relatd endophthalmitis* incidence is reported to be 0.2% to 1.3%.

ENDOGENOUS ENDOPHTHALMITIS

INCIDENCE

Endogenous or metastatic endophthalmitis is a potentially blinding complication of hematogenous spread of microorganisms to eye. It accounts for 2–17% of all cases of endophthalmitis and is misdiagnosed in more than 50% cases. It can be classified as anterior (focal

or diffuse), posterior (focal or diffuse) and panophthalmitis.

MICROBIAL SPECTRUM AND RISK FACTORS

More than 40% cases may not have any evident systemic source of infection and ocular disease may be due to transient bacteremia and fungemia. There is predisposition for diabetics, immune compromised patients, patients with malignancy, organ transplant, neutropenia, or those on intravenous hyperalimentation, intravenous or indwelling catheter, hemodialysis, contaminated intravenous infusion (Fig. 29.1). The common sites of extraocular infection are liver abscess, pneumonia, endocarditis, meningitis, soft tissue infection, gastrointestinal or urinary tract infection, renal abscess, pyonephrosis, brain abscess, etc. The bacteria responsible for endogenous endophthalmitis include *Streptococcus sp, Staphylococcus aureus, Bacillus* and *Serratia*. The common fungal isolates include *Candida* and *Aspergillus*. The

studies from Asia show *Klebsiella* liver abscess in a diabetic is the commonest cause of endogenous endophthalmitis. In India, aspergillus endophthalmitis 4–6 weeks after single intravenous fluid injection has also been reported frequently (Fig. 29.2). Schiedler et al demonstrated, in his series from the USA, fungal etiology as a common cause of endogenous endophthalmitis (62% of cases positive for *Candida albicans).*

CLINICAL FEATURES

The disease is binocular in 15% cases. The male preponderance is seen and the peak age is in 3rd decade in bacterial and less than 1 year and middle age in fungal. The right eye is twice as often prone for a focus of infection than the left, because of comparatively direct blood flow to the right carotid artery.

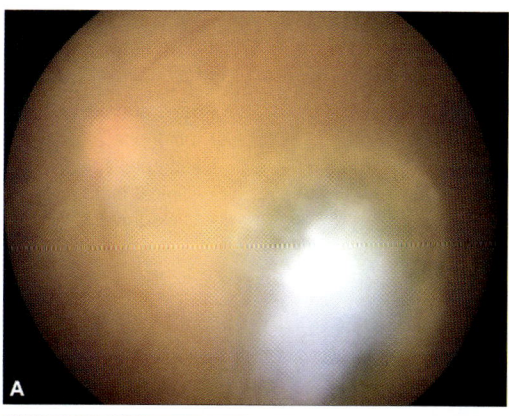

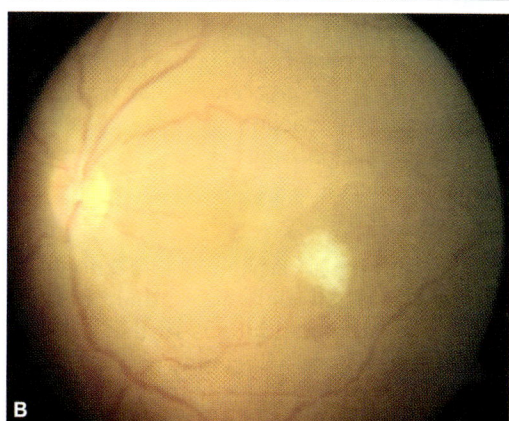

Fig. 29.2 *(A) Fundus picture of a patient with history of intravenous dextrose 3 weeks prior to decreased vision showing fluff ball exydates abd sybretubak abscess; (B) The same eye after PPV and intravitreal amphotericin B showing resolution with macular scar formation*

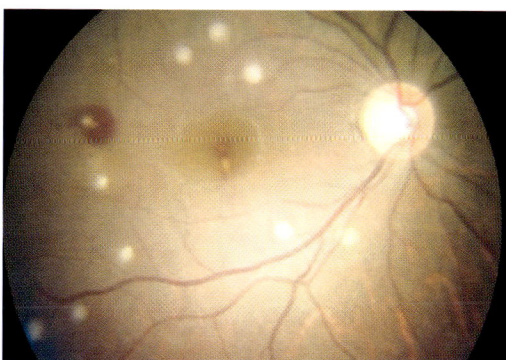

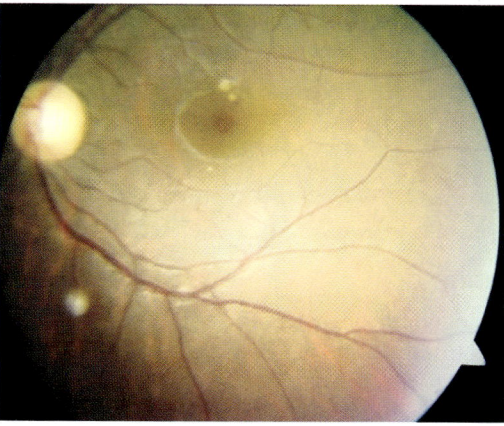

Fig. 29.1 *Fundus picture showing multiple retinal abscesses in IV drug abuser with Candida septicemia*

The patient typically presents with ocular pain, blurred vision, lid swelling, discharge, injected and chemosed conjunctiva, elevated IOP, corneal edema, anterior chamber and vitreous reaction including hypopyon, reduced red reflex, retinal cotton wool spots, Roth's spots, hemorrhages, choroidal abscess or vitreous abscess. B. cereus is the common cause of metastatic endophthalmitis in drug abusers. The patients may exhibit a ring-shaped corneal ulcer with brownish anterior chamber exudates. If brownish hypopyon occurs without corneal involvement then *Listeria monocytogenes* should be considered as diagnosis. Endophthalmitis could be grouped as anterior focal, anterior diffuse, posterior focal, posterior diffuse, pan-ophthalmitis. It is commonly misdiagnosed as granulomatous uveitis, fungal endophthalmitis, angle closure glaucoma, mucor mycosis, cavernous sinus thrombosis or orbital cellulitis.

DIAGNOSIS

B-scan ultrasonography is a useful adjunct to the clinical evaluation of infectious endophthalmitis especially in an eye with opaque media as it tells about for vitritis and retinal detachment. Vitreous exudates are seen as low to moderate intensity point like echoes in vitreous cavity. The membranous structure seen on USG is thick posterior vitreous detachment (PVD) or retinal detachment (RD). Other investigations include blood cultures which give higher positivity rate up to 94% compared to intraocular samples. It has vitreous culture positivity rate of 44–70%. It is necessary to take cultures from multiple sites and also repeated samples if suspicion of endogenous endophthalmitis is strong. For intraocular specimen for cultures, aqueous tap, vitreous sample by needle aspiration or cutter could be taken. Microbiology gram stained film of a centrifuged deposit of vitreous sample should be used for gram stain and cultures should be set up for aerobic and anaerobic bacteria and fungi. The samples should be incubated for at least a week before giving a negative report.

Polymerase chain reaction is being increasingly used nowadays for quick differentiation of bacterial from fungal endophthalmitis. PCR helps in quicker assay in small quantity samples.

TREATMENT

Thorough history taking and examination is recommended to look for the primary focus of infection once diagnosis of metastatic endophthalmitis is suspected. The primary focus of infection is the source of the ocular infection and is presumed to be **bacterial.** The empiric broad spectrum antibiotic therapy is given with vancomycin and an aminoglycoside or a third generation cephalosporin. The antibiotic therapy can later be tailored depending on the culture reports if the patient does not respond. The patients with culture-positive endogenous endophthalmitis are more likely to have fungal isolates with a predominance of Candida. In case of **fungal** endophthalmitis, antifungal of choice is intravitreal amphotericin 5–10 µg along with systemic triazoles. Systemic voriconazole and caspofungin are newer options.

Prompt treatment with intravitreal antibiotics and vitrectomy can result in improvement in ocular signs and visual acuity in majority of the patients. It has been seen that eyes that undergo pars plana vitrectomy are three times likely to retain useful vision and more than three times less likely to require enucleation or evisceration. It has also been seen that intravitreal antibiotics lowers chances of evisceration and enucleation. The definite indications for vitrectomy are:

- Worsening of signs and symptoms
- Rapid progression
- Retinal necrosis
- Extensive, subretinal abscess
- Retinal detachment.

PROGNOSIS

The poor prognosticators for endogenous endophthalmitis include delayed diagnosis and treatment (>4 days), poor initial visual acuity <20/200, presence of hypopyon and more virulent microorganisms. The visual outcomes are poor especially when it is *Klebsiella* species. *Aspergillus* has worse prognosis than *Candida*). Evisceration/enucleation is required in 25% cases. Only 5% of eyes with bacterial endogenous endophthalmitis can achieve visual acuity of 20/20 and 69% have vision worse than counting fingers.

EXOGENOUS ENDOPHTHALMITIS

POSTOPERATIVE ENDOPHTHALMITIS

INCIDENCE

The incidence of postoperative endophthalmitis decreased from 5–10% in early 20th century to 0.13–0.7% in 21st century. As over 2 million cataract surgeries are performed each year, endophthalmitis is encountered most commonly after cataract extraction. Penetrating keratoplasty has been associated with the highest incidence of postoperative endophthalmitis (0.38%).

Endophthalmitis could present as cluster infection or isolated cases. A cluster infection is described as the occurrence of two or more than two infections at a time or the occurrence of repeated postoperative infections. Patient factors are mainly responsible for isolated cases like immune compromised patient, uncontrolled diabetes mellitus, poor lid hygiene, chronic dacryocystitis, inadequate preoperative medications or prolonged use of preoperative antibiotics which alters the normal conjunctival flora. In cluster infections surgeon factors are mainly responsible for endophthalmitis. These include poor sterlization of operation room (OR) or instruments, contami-nated irrigating solution, viscoelastics agents or other consumables. Cluster infections have been reported due to contamination of IOLs, irrigating solutions, viscoelastics, ventilation system, hospital construction activity, noncompliance of OR standards as reuse of dehumidifiers. It can be acute or chronic. The acute endophthalmitis mostly present within 1–2 weeks and chronic endophthalmitis presents ≥ 6 weeks of surgery.

MICROBIAL SPECTRUM AND RISK FACTORS

The microbial spectrum of postcataract surgery endophthalmitis includes 33–77% coagulase-negative staphylococci (CNS), 0.9–21% *Staphylococcus aureus*, 9–19% ß-haemolytic streptococci (BHS), S. pneumoniae, a haemolytic, streptococci including *S. mitis* and *S. salivarius*, 6–22% gram-negative bacteria including *P. aeruginosa* (occurs rarely), up to 8–18.6% fungi (*Candida* sp., *Aspergillus* sp., *Fusarium* sp.). A study from South India, however, shows higher percentage of gram-negative and fungi accounting for 29.2% and 18.6% respectively and lesser percentage (37.2%) of CNS compared to Western data (Table 29.1).

Delayed postoperative capsule bag endophthalmitis is primarily due to *Propionibacterium acnes*, corynebacteria including *C. macginleyi*. The most common organism of Post-operative (glaucoma surgery) endophthalmitis is CNS (67%).

Factors that increase the risk of POE from cataract surgery include patient-related factors (male sex, concomitant diabetic retinopathy, same day cataract surgery combined with another intraocular surgery) and surgeon-related factors (low surgical volume, limited experience, prolonged operating time, operating on patients who are most prone to adverse events).

The multi-center randomized control trial by European Society for Cataract and Refractive Surgery Study (ESCRS) of antibiotic prophylaxis of endophthalmitis found that patients receiving the clear corneal incision were 5.88 times more likely to experience endophthalmitis than patients receiving scleral tunnel. The ESCRS study also demonstrated that patients experiencing complications at the time of surgery and the patients receiving a silicone intraocular lens had a 4.95 times and 3.13 times higher risk of infection respectively.

CLINICAL FEATURES

In microbial endophthalmitis, three phases of infection can be observed: an incubation phase, an acceleration phase and a destructive phase. A clinically inapparent incubation phase is of

Table 29.1 *Microbial spectrum of postoperative endophthalmitis*

	S. India %ge	Endophthalmitis vitrectomy study (EVS)%
S epidermidis	37.2	70
S. aureus	0.9	9.9
Staphylococcus sp.	2.7	0
Streptococcus sp.	11.5	9
Bacillus sp.	4.4	0.3
Propionibacterium sp.	2.7	0.6
Gram negative	29.2	5.9
Filamentous fungi	18.6	0

at least 16 to 18 hours duration. The incubation phase is determined mainly by the generation time of the pathogen (e.g. *Pseudomonas aeruginosa* it is up to 10 min and *Propioni-bacterium* sp. > 5 hours) and toxin production.

Intraocular bacterial inoculation above a critical level then leads to breakdown of the aqueous barrier with fibrin exudation and cellular infiltration. With *Staphylococcus epidermidis* (CNS) and Staphylococcus aureus, the greatest infiltration is observed only three days after infection. Thus acute early endophthalmitis after cataract operations commences between the first postoperative day and approximately two weeks after the operation.

Acute Postoperative Endophthalmitis

The initial symptoms of **acute postoperative endophthalmitis** are usually pain and decreased vision. The presence of unexpectedly high intraocular inflammation is pointer towards endophthalmitis. Lid edema is seen in 35% cases. Congestion is almost universal in more than 80% cases and hypopyon is seen in 75–86% cases. Media clarity decreases and there is loss of red reflex due to vitreous clouding. The poor prognosticators are poor initial visual acuity, relative afferent pupillary defect, corneal involvement and rubeosis iridis. The endophthalmitis is sometimes preceded for days or weeks by eyebrow pain, headache, blepharitis and conjunctivitis. In fungal endophthalmitis, usually long incubation period is reported, but the largest series from India on fungal endophthalmitis reports fungi even in acute cases. The typical fluff ball exudates and string of pearls appearance may be seen (Fig. 29.3A and B).

Chronic Late Endophthalmitis

Chronic late endophthalmitis after cataract operations commences only after two weeks, but may also take many months to appear. It is usually caused by *Propionibacterium acnes, S. epidermidis* (CNS), diphtheroids and fungi. The whitish plaques are seen in capsular bag in 40–89% cases of chronic endophthalmitis especially in propionibacterium endophthalmitis. Corneal edema is present in 48% cases and keratitis in 26% cases of chronic postoperative endophthalmitis (Fig. 29.4).

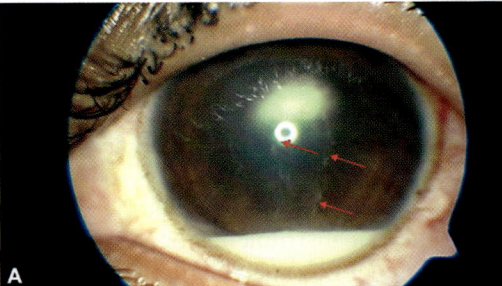

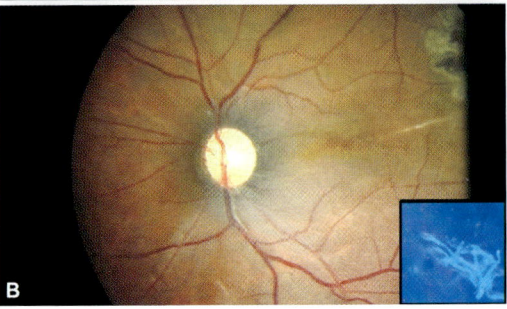

Fig. 29.3 (A) *Anterior segment picture of a case of Aspergillus fungal endophthalmitis showing convex hypopyon fluff balls and string of pearls appearance (arrow);* **(B)** *fundus picture after pars plana lensectomy and vitrectomy with antifungal agents; inset showing acutely branching hyphae from vitreous biopsy*

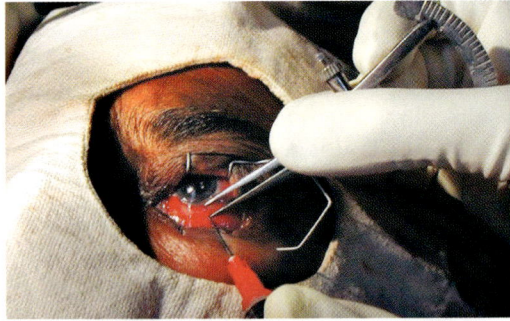

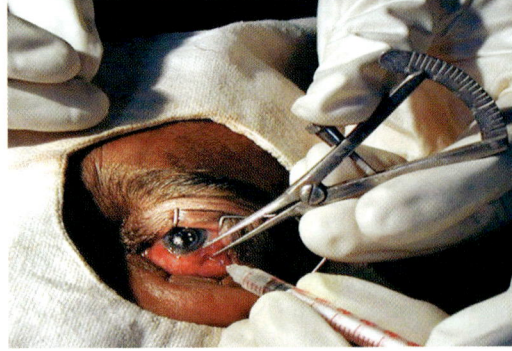

Fig. 29.4 *Showing vitreous tap and injection with 30 G needle 3 mm from limbus in pseudophakic patient*

POE needs to be differentiated from **toxic anterior segment syndrome** (TASS) is an acute inflammation of the anterior chamber of the eye. TASS may be related to any of the irrigating solutions, medications, or materials that gain access to the eye during anterior segment surgery. In addition, factors related to the cleaning and sterilisation of instruments. Some cases have been related to heat stable endotoxins from overgrowth of gram-negative bacilli in water baths of ultrasonic cleaners. TASS rarely occurs in one patient only, but usually in three or more, because most or all the patients have been exposed to the incriminating toxin during one or two operating sessions. Patients present within 12 to 48 hours of cataract surgery. The common signs include blurred vision, marked increase in anterior segment inflammation, including hypopyon formation as well as fibrin in the anterior chamber of the eye. There may be diffuse corneal edema, classically from limbus to limbus, with endothelial cell damage. It is always gram stain and culture negative. TASS responds well to intense topical corticosteroid treatment.

MANAGEMENT

Diagnosis

Apart from clinical features, microbiological results, ultrasonography guides us in treatment. In hazy media it is required to rule out retinal detachment, choroidal detachment. The presence of vitreous membranes on ultrasonography are poor prognosticators.

Prophylaxis of postoperative endophthalmitis

It has been shown in the past that 85% of endophthalmitis cases could be traced to the patient by comparing DNA profiles of vitreous isolates of bacteria with those collected from the lid and skin flora of the patient. Thus proper perioperative antisepsis significantly decreases incidence of endophthalmitis. The use of **5% povidone-iodine** 3 minutes prior to surgery decreases the incidence of postoperative endophthalmitis to 0.06% from 0.24% in the control group in which silver-protein solution was used as prophylaxis. ESCRS study has investigated if use of perioperative **topical levofloxacin,** which reaches significantly higher concentrations in the anterior chamber than ofloxacin and ciprofloxacin. To maintain an adequate level of levofloxacin in the anterior chamber it may be considered continuing to dose every two hours postoperatively on the day of surgery. The prolonged use of topical antibiotics, however, is not recommended before surgery. This is associated with replacement of normal ocular flora with resistant strains in conjunctival sac. **Intravenous antibiotic** prophylaxis is not used for conventional intra- and extra-ocular procedures and is not proven to be of benefit against postoperative endophthalmitis. The routine cataract surgery does not require oral prophylaxis unless the patient has severe atopic disease when the lid margins are more frequently colonized with *S. aureus*. ESCRS has shown periocular use **of intracameral injection of cefuroxime** at the end of surgery has lowered the incidence of endophthalmitis by five folds.

The use of topical quinolone is recommended 24 or 48 hours prior to surgery and one drop one hour prior to surgery and one drop one half-hour prior to surgery into conjunctival sac. It is recommended that after scrubbing the doctor should wear sterile gloves and patient's eyelashes should not be trimmed but covered with plastic sterile adhesive drapes.

Treatment

Endophthalmitis vitrectomy study (1990–1995) based initial management for acute post-operative endophthalmitis on the basis of presenting visual acuity. It was 3 port pars plana vitrectomy if patients present with vision worse than hand motions, but that an initial vitreous tap/biopsy with intravitreal antibiotics should generally be sufficient if presenting vision is hand motions or better (Fig. 29.5). Systemic antibiotics were not found of benefit in this study. The major limitations of this study were given as follows.

- It only included cases of acute postoperative endophthalmitis, 70% of which were due to Staph. Epidermidis. The results cannot be extrapolated to other forms of endophthalmitis and to postoperative endophthalmitis in countries where gram, negative organisms and fungal infection form a big chunk.

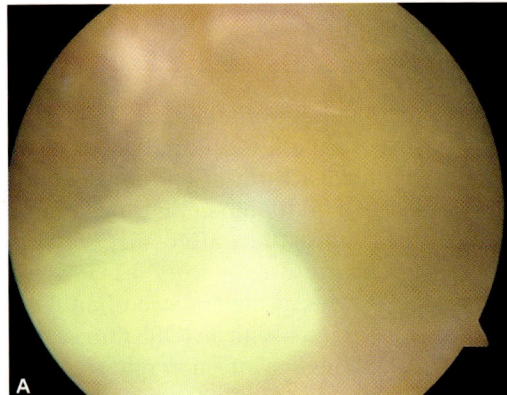

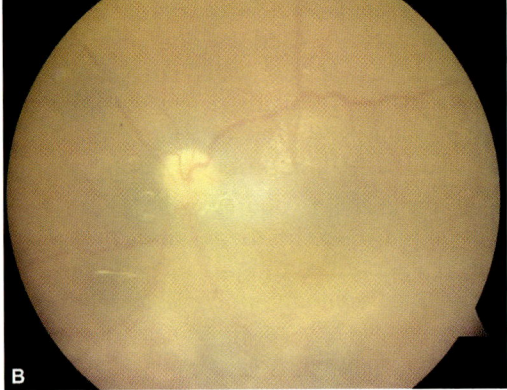

Fig. 29.5 *(A) Fundus picture of a case of chronic post operative fungal endophthalmitis showing retinal abscess; (B) Fundus picture of the same patient 6 weeks after PPV with voriconazole*

- Amikacin and ceftazidime were the only systemic antibiotics evaluated in the EVS. Although patients in the EVS derived no demonstrable benefit from these systemic antibiotics, the study made no recommendations regarding treatment with additional anti-microbial agents (e.g. systemic fluoroquino-lones) or systemic antimicrobial agents for other types of endophthalmitis (e.g. chronic, bleb related)

- Follow-up EVS analyses showed differences between diabetics and non-diabetics. Diabetics with a visual acuity of hand movements or better obtained vision of 20/40 more often (57%) by vitrectomy than after vitreous tap (40%) but the results ultimately were not statistically significant because of the low number of diabetic participants in the study.

There has been change in EVS guidelines for endophthalmitis management after report of ESCRS. In acute virulent POE there is an achievement of only one metre vision in 44–53% cases with bacterial infection and 41–70% for fungal infection. To improve the anatomical and functional outcome in endophthalmitis ESCRS gives guidelines for management of endophthalmitis. They recommend prompt action in such cases. The gold standard treatment is immediate diagnostic and therapeutic vitrectomy. If this is not possible due to the lack of a vitreoretinal surgeon and a vitreoretinal operating room then ESCRS recommends vitreous biopsy and intravitreal injection of the antibiotics. The samples for microbiology investi-gation (Gram stain, culture and PCR) should be sent at the earliest. The highest rate of pathogen identification is obtained with microscopic and microbiological processing of vitreous material, obtained using the vitrectomy cutter before switching on the irrigation. The use of a syringe and needle gives an unreliable sample that is often dry and culture-negative. The anterior chamber samples are less successful. The culture media should be inoculated directly in the operating theatre to get maximum yield. If this is not possible then samples should be carried in the same syringe plugging the needle with sterile rubber cork to the microbiology laboratory at the earliest.

The antibiotics given empirically for bacterial endophthalmitis are vancomycin 1 mg in 0.1 ml and 2.25 mg in 0.1 ml (first choice) or amikacin 400 µg in 0.1 ml and vancomycin 2 mg in 0.1 ml (second choice) in separate syringes with 30 G needle. The needle has to be directed away from macula into the mid-vitreous. This could be given in combination with intravitreal dexamethasone (400 µg in 0.1 ml) as it is the inflammation which is the basic culprit in endophthalmiti. For acute virulent endophthal-mitis, ESCRS recommends systemic therapy with the same antibiotics as those used intravitreally for 48 hours to maintain higher levels within the posterior segment of the eye. The corticosteroids should also be given orally to control inflammation (prednisolone 1 or even 2 mg/kg/day).

Vitrectomy should be also be the treatment of choice in chronic endophthalmitis, fungal endophthalmitis, deterioration of signs after initial management. The intravitreal antibiotics may be repeated at 48 hours if required.

In cases of **chronic endophthalmitis** early vitrectomy is advisable. A trial of therapy should be given with clarithromycin 250 mg twice daily which can be effective without surgery because the drug is well absorbed and concentrated 200 times into macrophages and other cells.

Special considerations in PPV

While doing pars plana vitrectomy in endophthalmitis

1. Use of 6 mm infusion cannula due thickened retinochoroid in inflamed eye.

2. AC maintainer is needed to clear AC exudates and exudative membrane to visualize posterior segment cannula before starting pars plana infusion.

3. Before starting the infusion we must collect undiluted vitreous sample from midvitreous cavity.

4. The aim is to clear only core vitreous.

5. A small posterior capsulotomy helps as it makes anterior and posterior segments one unit and proper circulation of antibiotics is there.

6. The IOL explantation is done only in cases of gross infection, plaques in the capsule, recurrent endophthalmitis

For *P acnes* **endophthalmitis** intravitreal vancomycin 1 mg/0.1 ml may be given into the capsular bag during first PPV and if it fails to respond then vitrectomy may be combined with total capsulectomy and IOL explantation.

In case of **fungal endophthalmitis**, Amphotericin B (5–7.5 µg) is the only fungicidal antibiotic available for intravitreal injection, but its spectrum does not cover all fungi; in particular *Pseudallescheria boydii* is resistant to it but sensitive to miconazole which can be used instead. Miconazole is fungistatic but can be given intravitreally. Systemic anti-fungal therapy is also required and the source of the infection needs to be identified.

POST-TRAUMATIC ENDOPHTHALMITIS

INCIDENCE

Post-traumatic endophthalmitis (PTE), along with postoperative endophthalmitis, is the second commonest form of endophthalmitis. The incidence of endophthalmitis after trauma is 100 times more than after surgery. The reported incidence ranges from 3.1–11.9% of open globe injuries in the absence of an IOFB. The incidence in cases with an IOFB ranges from 3.8–48.1%, with higher infection rates reported in eyes with retained IOFBs contaminated with organic matter from a rural setting. In a study, the occurrence of post-traumatic endophthalmitis was reported in 30% in rural districts in contrast to 11% in non-rural districts. Post-traumatic endophthalmitis comprises approximately 25–30% of all cases of infectious endophthalmitis.

The prognosis is poorer in PTE because of various reasons. The diagnosis is delayed as signs of endophthalmitis are often masked due to disrupted anatomy, polymicrobial infection is seen in 20–42% cases and more virulent organisms including *Bacillus* are cultured from 20–40% cases (Fig. 29.6).

MICROBIAL SPECTRUM AND RISK FACTORS

PTE can be categorized as culture-independent or culture positive. The former includes all clinically diagnosed cases of endophthalmitis and the latter includes only culture-positive

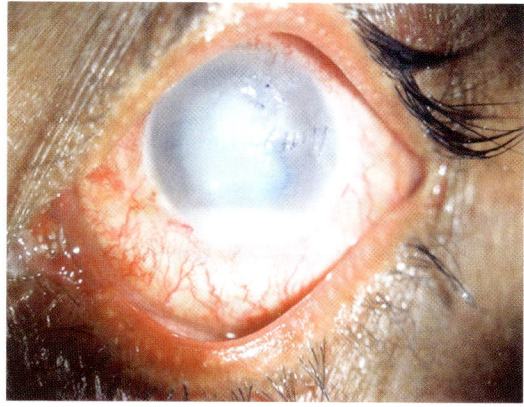

Fig. 29.6 *Anterior segment picture of a case of zone 1 injury showing corneal sutures and hypopyon*

cases. The overall incidence of culture-independent post-traumatic endophthalmitis is higher than culture positive endophthalmitis cases. It must be understood that the presence of positive cultures following open globe trauma is not synonymous with the development of post-traumatic endophthal-mitis. Ariyasu et al cultured 30 ruptured globes. Although one third of these patients had positive anterior chamber fluid cultures, no patient developed endophthal-mitis. In our experience, contamination after OGI was seen in 26% cases but only 18% developed endophthalmitis. Similar to postoperative endophthalmitis, two thirds of the bacteria in PTE are gram-positive and 10–15% are gram-negative and 15% are fungi. Culture positivity is seen in 38–60% cases of post-traumatic endophthalmitis. In contrast to postoperative endophthalmitis, virulent *Bacillus* species are the common pathogens in post-traumatic endophthalmitis. Polymicrobial infection is seen in 20–30% cases.

Microbial spectrum of PTE is depicted in Table 29.2.

Table 29.2 *Microbial spectrum of post-traumatic endophthalmitis (Kunimoto et al 2007)*

	S. India	West
S. epidermidis	21.2	8–21
S. aureus	4.4	6
Staphylococcus sp.	0.9	0
Streptococcus sp.	26.5	8–21
Bacillus sp.	17.7	17–32
Gram negative	22.1	11–18
Filamentous fungi	17.7	4–14

The major risk factors for PTE include rural setting trauma, vegetative matter associated injury, delayed repair after 24 hours, dirty wound, age greater than 50 years, female gender, large wound size, location of wound, ocular tissue prolapse, placement of primary intraocular lens (IOL), extent of injury, lens disruption. Thompson and coworkers reported endophthalmitis in 13.6% of 88 ruptured globe cases with lens disruption and in only 0.9% (1 case) of 117 cases with an intact crystalline lens. In their series, when both an IOFB and lens rupture were present, 15.6% of cases developed endophthalmitis. Delayed repair beyond 24

hours is another risk factor for PTE. The risk of PTE was 2.3% versus 15.7% if the repair was delayed by >24 hours. The sports related injuries like due to fish hook or homemade bow and arrow are at high risk of endophthalmitis. Seventy-five per cent of bow and arrow injuries in India develop endophthalmitis. The presence of IOFB leads to 2 fold increase in relative risk of PTE Wood IOFBs (18%) may be associated with a statistically higher risk of infectious endophthalmitis compared to metallic IOFBs (9%).

CLINICAL FEATURES

The start, course and symptoms of endophthal-mitis after trauma are very varied, corresponding to the causative organisms. Symptoms of extreme pain with hypopyon and vitritis indicate an infection until proven otherwise. It is present at initial presentation in 50% cases of post-traumatic endophthalmitis. The peak interval between trauma and endophthalmitis is 3–6 days. The signs and symptoms of endophthalmitis may occur days, weeks, months, and even years after the injury (Fig. 29.6). Fungi are the causative organisms in 10–15% of cases of endophthalmitis after trauma. Fungal endo-phthalmitis usually commences only weeks to months after the injury. The initial symptoms are usually pain, purulent discharge, photophobia out of proportion to the injury and visual loss increasing intraocular inflammation, hypopyon, corneal edema, loss of a red reflex, lid edema, proptosis, and vitreous clouding, periphlebitis or gas bubbles (Fig. 29.6). Inflammation that progresses slowly following primary repair may be indicative of fungal endophthalmitis. In fungal endophthalmitis string of pearls appearance or fluff ball opacities may be seen.

Metallic non-magnetic IOFBs (for example, copper) can cause non-infectious inflammation, termed **reactive endophthalmitis**, if left in the eye. A 100% **copper IOFB** can cause a rapid sterile endophthalmitis-like reaction with hypopyon. Lower per cent copper IOFBs can cause chalcosis that includes chronic uveitis-related complications such as hypotony and phthisis. Green discoloration of iris, greenish-brown discoloration of the peripheral cornea

(Kayser-Fleisher ring, due to copper deposition in Descemet's membrane), sunflower cataract, and copper. Plain radiography and computed tomography scans are then used to detect IOFBs. In order to detect small objects by computed tomography, the cut width should be less than 2 mm. B scan ultrasound may be used to help locate radiolucent foreign bodies such as glass or plastic. Extreme caution should be used if there is any suspicion of an open globe. Minimal pressure should be applied during echography, and the probe should be placed on the eyelid and not directly on the ocular surface. IOFBs containing greater than 85% copper can cause severe vision loss.

IOFBs with **free iron** content can cause siderosis; the iron ions interact with the epithelial cells causing cytotoxicity with cell degeneration and visual loss. Glass, plastic, and porcelain are inert materials that generally are well tolerated in the eye. However, all IOFBs (inert or noninert) increase the risk of endophthalmitis because they may be contaminated with infectious material.

MANAGEMENT

Diagnosis

Any inflammation in a case of trauma more than anticipated should be tabken as endophthalmitis. All PTE cases where the view of posterior segment is not possible must be subjected to a gentle ultrasound to rule out the presence of intraocular foreign body (high echnogenicity with after shadow). It also gives information regarding retina and other membranes. If not possible CT scan may also need to be done for proper localization of foreign body.

Prophylaxis

At the time of repair, the wound should be properly irrigated to clean any debris on it. Any dead or dirty looking tissue should be sent for cultures. Cultures may be obtained from the wound, anterior chamber, and/or vitreous as well as the conjunctiva, and they may be plated on blood and chocolate agar. Thioglycolate broth and heart-brain infusion are also used as a culture medium, and Gram stain of excised tissue or fluid should be performed. Fungal infection can be detected via Grocott's silver stain, periodic acid-Schiff stain, by culturing on Sabaroud's dextrose, or by potassium hydroxide (KOH) preparation The aqueous and vitreous samples can be inoculated directly into blood culture bottles.

After repair, systemic antibiotics in addition to topical with wider organism coverage should be used routinely for prophylaxis against PTE. Quinolone may be administered orally if access to the operating room is delayed and if intravenous antibiotics are not immediately available. The use **prophylactic intravitreal injections** is debatable. The decision to use at the time of initial repair depends on whether the patient is a high-risk case for endophthalmitis—provided that the injections can be given safely and reliably into the vitreous cavity. In our experience, prophylactic intravitreal antibiotics in absence of foreign body decreases the incidence of post-traumatic endophthalmitis to negligible. The use of subconjunctival steroids should be considered along with antibiotics at the time of surgical repair of a ruptured globe.

In our practice, prophylactic **intravenous quinolones** are given in trauma cases for at least 3 days. These antibiotics cross the blood-ocular barrier reasonably well and may reach therapeutic levels in the eye. Their entry into the eye is also aided by the weakening of the blood-ocular barrier that results from infection and trauma-induced inflammation. After 5 days of intravenous antibiotics, the patient (after discharge) is placed on 1 week of oral quinolones.

Treatment

The principles of management are the same for post-traumatic and acute postoperative endophthalmitis, but the visual outcome is poorer. After the diagnosis of PTE is considered early pars plana vitrectomy is recommended as soon as possible provided the corneal clarity permits. If the same is not possible at least vitreous biopsy/tap must be done and vitreous samples sent for microbiological evaluation and PCR. The antibiotics given include combination of intravitreal vancomycin (1 mg/0.1 mL and intravitreal ceftazidime (2.25 mg/0.1 mL through pars plana. The type and nature of the injury may guide the choice of antibiotics. For example, *Clostridium* should be considered if soil

contamination of the wound is present, and fungal infection should be considered if there is contamination with vegetable matter. Results of the culture, if obtained at the initial open globe repair, may also direct the choice of antibiotics. For injuries that run a high risk of contamination with *Bacillus* species (homemade bow and arrow injuries) intravitreal clindamycin (0.5 mg/0.1 mL) may also be given. Subconjunctival cefazolin (100 mg) or vancomycin (25 mg) with subconjunctival ceftazidime (100 mg) may be given after the procedure. Topical fortified cefazolin (50 mg/mL) or fortified vancomycin (50 mg/mL) every 1–2 h, alternating with fluoroquinolones (0.3%) may be used after surgery.

A related disorder is **sympathetic ophthalmia** in which injury to the eye, especially the uveal tract, can result in a harmful autoimmune T-cell mediated response. The inciting event is trauma to one eye, which is then followed by involvement of the sympathizing eye.

The causes of poor visual outcome include recurrent/chronic endophthalmitis, macular infarction, optic atrophy, epiretinal membrane, macular edema.

BLEB-RELATED ENDOPHTHALMITIS

INCIDENCE

Bleb-related endophthalmitis (BRE) is the second most frequent (16.7%) cause of postoperative endophthalmitis after acute and chronic post-cataract surgery endophthalmitis. The incidence of isolated blebitis is 2 percent with average follow-up of 2.7 years (range, 0.3 to 7.3). Early post-operative endophthalmitis following glaucoma surgery has an incidence of about 0.1 per cent. However, the majority of cases of endophthalmitis after glaucoma surgery occur after months or years; the incidence is reported to be between 0.2% to 1.3%, and is more common with the use of antiproliferative agent (up to 3%) and even higher when the bleb is placed inferiorly (up to 9.4%). With anti proliferative use, one of every 100 patients developed endophthalmitis each year and 4 percent of patients developed a bleb-related complication consisting of a bleb leak, blebitis or endophthalmitis.

MICROBIAL SPECTRUM AND RISK FACTORS

Bleb leakage has been shown to increase 26 fold the risk of bleb infection. Most believe that bleb related infections begin secondary to bleb leakage, which allows bacteria from the tear film and the periocular structures access into the eye. Early leakage is defined as leakage within the first 3 months following surgery, while late-onset leakage is defined as that occurring more than 3 months following surgery. Early leakage is most commonly caused by wound dehiscence or incomplete conjunctival closure. Late-onset leakage has been associated with the use of adjunctive anti-metabolites, which are used to prevent fibrosis and scarring of the scleral flap and bleb in order to promote long-term patency. The use of Mitomycn-C (MMC) has been associated with a 15% risk of leak at 5 years. The use of anti-metabolites such as 5-fluorouracil (5-FU) and MMC reduce the population of goblet cells, which produce mucin that serves as a protective barrier against leakage and bacteria. Their use also promotes general conjunctival thinning, reduced cellularity, and avascular blebs .

Blebitis describes an isolated bleb infection with signs of anterior segment inflammation, without vitreous involvement. It may represent a limited form or early stage of endophthalmitis. If untreated, blebitis progresses into endophthalmitis.

If inflammatory or infectious material in a blebitis extend beyond the anterior chamber, the diagnosis is bleb associated endophthalmitis. BRE can be grouped into early onset (within 6 weeks) or late onset (after 6 weeks). BRE can have a clinical presentation similar to blebitis, except that the vitreous is involved. A positive vitreous culture is pathognomonic for BRE.

Coagulase negative staphylocci (CNS) are responsible for endophthalmitis in 67% cases of early BRE. Delayed BRE is caused by Streptococci species and gram negative organisms especially Haemophilus influenza (23%).

CLINICAL FEATURES

Prodromal signs and symptoms have been identified days or weeks before the diagnosis of blebitis or endophthalmitis is made. These

include browache, headache, external eye inflammation or infection such as blepharitis or conjunctivitis. One must always maintain a high index of suspicion and pay careful attention to any of the above complaint in a patient who has undergone trabeculectomy. Blebitis must be differentiated from bleb related endophthalmitis (BRE) depending on the vitreous involvement. The patients with endophthalmitis have more rapidly progressive presentations, often with worsening pain, redness and decreasing visual acuity over a period of hours. Endophthalmitis can occur years after the initial filtering surgery. The defining feature of endophthalmitis is the presence of vitritis.

Like other forms of endophthalmitis, BRE usually presents with decreased visual acuity, redness, pain, lid swelling, diffuse conjunctival congestion, opalescent blebs (typical white on red appearance) with intense fibrin and/or hypopyon in the anterior chamber, and florid vitritis. These signs may be influenced by different variables and factors such as time to initial treatment, causative organism, wound leak (seidel's positive) and the presence of a vitreous wick.

MANAGEMENT

No clear management algorithm has been established for bleb associated endophthalmitis.

The use of fluoroquinolones alone in the initial management of isolated blebitis. These could also be used in combination with one or two other fortified antibiotics for gram negative and gram positive organisms such as an aminoglycoside, vancomycin or cephalosporin.

The use of topical corticosteroids is controversial till such time improvement of the blebitis is noted or once topical antibiotic therapy is well-established. There is no consensus regarding obtaining conjunctival cultures at initial diagnosis of blebitis.

Cases in which the vitreous is not well-visualized or in which the diagnosis of isolated blebitis is in doubt, should be treated for potential endophthalmitis. Aggressive treatment is important to prevent poor outcomes. Early PPV with intravitreal vancomycin (1mg/0.1mL) and either ceftazadime (2.25mg/0.1mL) or amikacin(0.4mg/0.1mL) with subconjunctival antibiotics is the preferred approach.

OUTCOME

Blebitis typically responds to therapy within 24 to 48 hours, both clinically and symptomatically. Most patients in one study noted a marked improvement in pain with rapidly improving anterior chamber reaction and conjunctival injection within 24 to 48 hours of the initiation of therapy.

In contrast, BRE has a poor visual prognosis even with aggressive medical and surgical treatment. Retrospective studies have shown that 94% of cases of endophthalmitis resulted in visual acuity of 20/200 or less. Busbee et al. showed that 35% of patients had no light perception, and only 10% achieved 20/40 or better. They also demonstrated that those with a positive vitreal culture had poorer outcomes, likely due to a higher bacterial load at time of diagnosis. Additionally, poorer outcomes are thought to be the result of more virulent organisms, such as gram-negative bacteria that produce exotoxins and streptococcus species. A significant number of eyes with BRE can end up being eviscerated or enucleated due to pain.

FUNGAL ENDOPHTHALMITIS

INCIDENCE

Fungal endophthalmitis results more commonly from exogenous infection and less commonly from endogenous infection. Exogenous fungal infections secondary to trauma or surgery are reported in much higher number of cases from India than West. Fungi comprise of 18.6– 21.8% of culture positive post operative cases and 17.7% of post traumatic culture positive cases in India. Endogenous fungal endophthalmitis results from intraocular dissemination of a systemic fungal infection.

MICROBIAL SPECTRUM AND RISK FACTORS

Normally, the blood-ocular barrier prevents invasion from infective organisms but if this is breached (directly through trauma or indirectly due to a change in its permeability secondary to inflammation), infection can occur.

Candida albicans is by far the most common cause of fungal endogenous endophthalmitis. They are commensal organisms that reside in the human body and are found normally in the female genital tract, the gastrointestinal tract, and the respiratory tract. When a breakdown in the host's immune system occurs, fungi may spread throughout the body. However, immunosuppression alone does not increase significantly the risk of fungi entering the bloodstream. Patients who are at risk include patients with longstanding indwelling catheters; persons who use intravenous drugs; postpartum women; premature infants; patients undergoing hyperalimentation; patients with a history of recent abdominal surgery; and patients with debilitating diseases, such as diabetes mellitus, postorgan transplantation, or malignancies.

Exogenous fungal endophthalmitis are mostly caused by filamentous fungi. *Aspergillus flavus* and *Aspergillus fumigatus* are the most common pathogenic organisms in humans. Its conidia, the asexual spores of aspergilli organisms are airborne and trauma and surgery are important routes of entry into the human body. In patients who are at risk, such as those patients with uncontrolled diabetes mellitus, chronic pulmonary diseases or those patients with orthotopic liver transplants, renal transplants, leukemia and other hematologic disorders, Goodpasture syndrome, alcoholism, prematurity, and bone marrow transplants, disseminated aspergillosis may result. Other less common causes include cryptococal endophthalmitis which is caused by inhalation of spores in pigeon droppings.

CLINICAL FEATURES

Endogenous endophthalmitis Diminished visual acuity, severe vitreous inflammation with persistent iritis, whitish puff balls and strands seen in Candida and Aspergillus infections. Choroidal neovascularization in C albicans endophthalmitis is a potential cause of late visual loss in patients who have had sepsis and endogenous chorioretinitis. It also shows macular chorioretinal abscess, subretinal hypopyon and final outcome is very poor due to frequent macular involvement.

Postoperative endophthalmitis is more localised and exhibits focal choroiditis, "string of pearls" infiltrates and puff balls in AC and vitreous. It is usually delayed presentation after surgery, however, acute cases as early as 24 hours after surgery are also reported from India. It probably depends on the load of innoculum in the eye.

Post traumatic fungal endophthalmitis is usually after trauma with vegetative matter. Classical signs of fungal endophthalmitis may not be there as anatomy of the globe is disrupted after trauma.

MANAGEMENT

DIAGNOSIS

A presumptive diagnosis of endogenous fungal endophthalmitis can be made if the fungus is isolated from anywhere in the body and the typical intraocular findings are present. Vitreous biopsy is taken and direct examination of fungi with Giemsa, Gomori-methenamine-silver (GMS), and periodic-acid Schiff (PAS) stains should be obtained. Vitrectomy samples are more sensitive for fungal cultures than vitreous needle biopsies. Vitreous biopsy by pars plana vitrectomy is important in obtaining undiluted specimens for culture and sensitivity. Vitreous samples should be concentrated either by centrifugation or by millipore filtration.

If *C neoformans* is suspected, the sample should be stained with mucicarmine and undergo membrane filtration cytology.

A useful, recently introduced diagnostic tool for fungal endophthalmitis is the polymerase chain reaction (PCR). The main advantages of PCR over conventional fungal cultures are the higher sensitivity and the rapid results obtained with PCR. Where available, DNA microarray analysis may be useful for obtaining a rapid diagnosis.

Treatment

The following drugs are used in treating of fungal endophthalmitis:
- Amphotericin B
- Fluconazole
- Ketoconazole
- Miconazole

- Flucytosine
- Itraconazole
- Caspofungin

Systemic amphotericin has been the treatment of choice because of its broad-spectrum coverage; however, the penetration of the vitreous cavity is poor. Doses of 5- to 10-mg intravitreal amphotericin have been used. Retinal toxicity has been reported in animal models at these doses thus it must be combined with intravitreal dexamethasone 400-mg to combat macular toxic effects. Fluconazole and flucytosine have good intraocular penetration, but Candida species show high resistance to flucytosine.

A new systemic treatment is voriconazole; when administered orally or intravenously, it has good intravitreal concentrations. Intravitreal administration of voriconazole also seems safe without evidence of retinal toxicity with concentrations up to 25 mg/mL. The echinocandins (caspofungin, micafungin, and anidulafungin) are newer agents that exert their antifungal activity by inhibiting D-glucan synthase, an enzyme involved in fungal cell wall synthesis. Because mammalian cells lack a cell wall, it also represents an ideal and specific target for antifungal therapy. Echinocandins exert antifungal activity against *Candida* and *Aspergillus* species.

In *endogenous fungal endophthalmitis*, it is important to initiate systemic broad spectrum antibiotics to treat the primary source of infection, but if the response to medical therapy is poor, parsplana vitrectomy along with amphotericin 5–10 µg along with systemic triazoles is instituted. Systemic Voriconazole and caspofungin are newer options. It has been seen that eyes that undergo parsplana vitrectomy are three times likely to retain useful vision and more than three times less likely to require enucleation or evisceration. It has also been seen that intravitreal antibiotics lower chances of evisceration and enucleation. For Candida endophthalmitis treatment has been recommended by Sato et al. They recommend PPV only if vitreous is involved in the form of vitreous exudates and no antibiotic response. The use of steroids is controversial and should be used with extreme caution.

In *exogenous fungal endophthalmitis*, as a general rule, moderate-to-severe vitreous involvement requires vitrectomy because most systemic antifungals have poor vitreous penetration. The advent of pars plana vitrectomy has improved the treatment results of fungal endophthalmitis. The advantages of pars plana vitrectomy are that it provides material for culture, removes viable organisms and inflammatory end products from the infected vitreous, and provides intravitreal access to antifungal agents (e.g. amphotericin B).

Given the narrow therapeutic range of amphotericin B, it should not be given in a gas-filled eye.

The prognosis following fungal endophthalmitis depends on the virulence of the organism, the extent of intraocular involvement, and the timing and mode of intervention.

TOXIC ANTERIOR SEGMENT SYNDROME

The toxic anterior segment syndrome (TASS) is an acute inflammation of the anterior chamber of the eye. TASS is an acute sterile anterior chamber inflammatory reaction that develops 12–48 hours after anterior segment surgery. TASS is a form of sterile, noninfectious endophthalmitis with or without pain.

PATHOPHYSIOLOGY

The etiology of TASS is multi-factorial. TASS may be related to any of the irrigating solutions, medications, or materials that gain access to the eye during anterior segment surgery. The causes could be inflammatory reaction to intraocular irrigating solutions with abnormal pH, osmolarity or ionic composition, denatured ophthalmic viscosurgical devices (OVD), intraocular medications (antibiotics in the irrigation solutions or intracameral antibiotics), topical ointments, inadequate sterilization of surgical instruments and tubing, inadequate flushing of instruments between cases resulting in build-up of ophthalmic viscosurgical devices (OVD), preservatives, metallic precipitate, and rarely bacterial endotoxins or particulate contamination of balanced salt solutions.

It is always Gram stain and culture negative.

CLINICAL FEATURES

It is associated with early marked decrease in vision 12–24 hours after surgery. There is diffuse corneal edema that extends limbus to limbus associated with endothelial cell damage., severe anterior chamber reaction, occasionally with hypopyon.

TASS rarely occurs in one patient only, but usually in three or more, because most or all the patients have been exposed to the incriminating toxin during one or two operating sessions. If an outbreak occurs, then the surgeon must stop operating and investigate for the source of the problem.

TREATMENT

The focus should be primary prevention. This can be done by following proper protocol during surgery. Proper balance salt solution (BSS) with the correct pH, osmolarity, and ionic composition should be used. We should avoid use of intraocular solutions, intracameral medications or irrigating solutions with preservatives. Adequate sterlization of instruments and tubing according to the manufacturer's protocol should be done.

Most patients do well with medical management using topical steroids (1% Prednisolone acetate) given hourly. In rare cases, depending on the severity there may be a need for systemic steroid treatment. The clearing may take up to 3–6 weeks which is a longer response than in mild cases. In the severe case, there may be permanent damage, persistent corneal edema, chronic persistent inflammation, fixed dilated pupil, refractory glaucoma secondary to trabecular meshwork damage and cystoid macular edema. In severe cases there may be a need for systemic steroid treatments.

The severe cases may have compromised recovery and may need cornea transplant, glaucoma surgery or both.

TREATMENT OUTCOME IN ENDOPHTHALMITIS

The treatment outcome as improved treamendously in present ear. In EVS study, visual acuity of 20/40 or better was achieved in 33%

cases of acute endophthalmitis after vitrectomy, and 20/100 or better acuity was achieved in 56% patients. In a recent review article, the visual outcome of 20/40 or better could be achieved in up to 56% of postoperative endophthalmitis patients. Significant factors associated with poor visual outcome are corneal involvement, hypopyon larger than 1.5 mm, detection of bacterial species other than a CNSP, the absence of fundus visibility, neovascularisation of iris and relative afferent papillary defect and above all the virulence of the causative organisms. Endophthalmitis due to gram-negative organisms, fungi and polymicrobial infections are associated with poor visual outcomes. Fungal infection is associated with a more unfavourable prognosis where more than 20% patients have severe visual impairment (worse than 5/200).

The visual prognosis is poorer in posttraumatic endophthalmitis than postoperative endophthalmitis. It is further poorer in geriatric and pediatric age group. The late sequelae of endophthalmitis include macular edema, disc edema, optic atrophy, epiretinal membrane, macular infarction and scarring (Fig. 29.7).

PREPARATION OF ANTIBIOTICS AND CLINICAL TRIALS

PREPARATION OF ANTIBIOTICS

The preparation of antibiotics (Adopted from ESCRS)

The antibiotics should be supplied freshly diluted by the hospital pharmacy department. However, for emergency cases, a method for diluting the drugs in the operating theatre is given below. The procedure must use sterile equipment and be undertaken on a sterile surface; ideally, the hospital makes up sterile packs with drugs, bottles for dilution and instructions in advance for this purpose. All drugs should be mixed by inverting or rolling the bottle 25 times, avoiding frothing.

Some important "Dos" and "Don'ts"

- Never return diluted drugs to the same or original vial for further dilution
- Never dilute at greater than 1 in 10

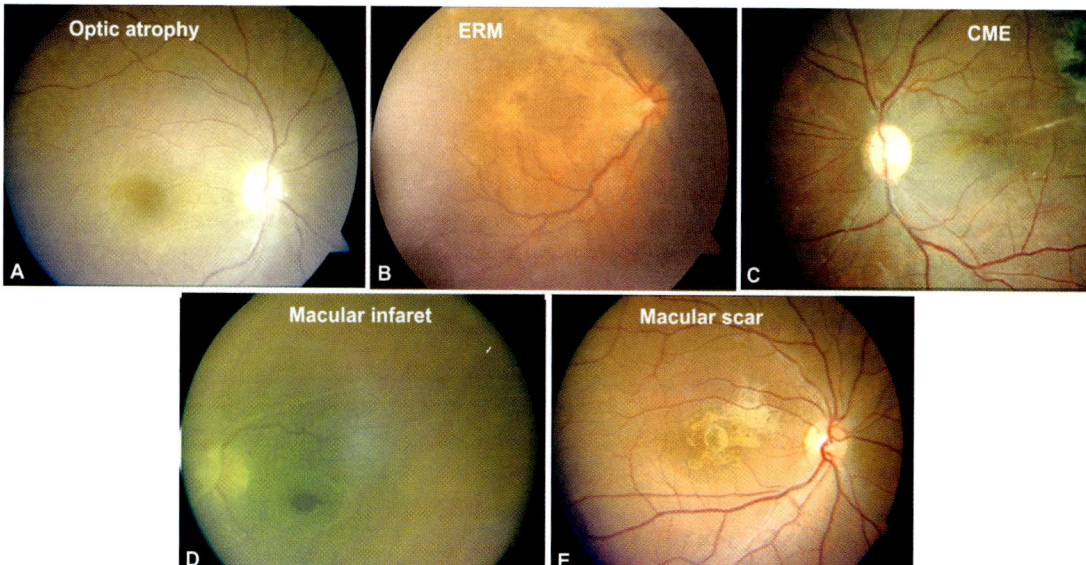

Fig. 29.7 *Fundus pictures showing sequalae of exogenous endophthalmitis **(A)** optic atrophy; **(B)** epiretinal membrane; **(C)** cystoid macular edema; **(D)** macular infarct induced by gentamycin and **(E)** macular scar*

- Do not use syringes more than once
- Do not reuse bottles
- Avoid use of drugs with preservatives if possible
- Do inject the drugs slowly over 1 to 2 minutes
  Prior to preparing the dilutions. It is mandatory to check the amount of the antibiotic in the vial as the same antibiotic may be sold in different strengths in each europlan country.

Important antibiotics

1. *Vancomycin.* Dose for use = 1000 mg. Reconstitute one vial of 250 mg and make up to 10 ml with sterile normal (0.9%) saline (SNS) in a sterile bottle with lid. Mix well. Withdraw 2 ml accurately and add to 3 ml of SNS in a sterile bottle with lid. Mix well (= 10 mg/ml). Use 0.1 ml = 1000 mg.

2. *Ceftazidime* (or other cephalosporin) Dose for use = 2000 mg. Reconstitute one vial of 500 mg and make up to 10 ml with SNS in a sterile bottle with lid. Mix well. Withdraw 2 ml accurately and add to 3 ml of SNS in a sterile bottle with lid. Mix well (= 20 mg/ml). Use 0.1 ml = 2000 mg.
   Note: the percentage of drug precipitation is less when using SNS instead of BSS.

3. *Amikacin.* Dose for use = 400 mg. Reconstitute one vial of 500 mg and make up to 10 ml with SNS or balanced salt solution (BSS) in a sterile bottle with lid. Mix well. Withdraw 0.8 ml, using a 1 ml syringe, and add to 9.2 ml of SNS or BSS in a sterile bottle with lid. Mix well (= 4.0 mg/ml). Use 0.1 ml = 400 mg.

4. *Clindamycin.* Dose for use = 1000 mg. Transfer the contents of a 2 ml ampule containing 300 mg to a sterile bottle and add 1 ml SNS or BSS, replace lid, and mix well. Withdraw 1ml, using a 1 ml syringe, and add to 9 ml of SNS or BSS in a sterile bottle with lid. Mix well (=10 mg/ml). Use 0.1 ml = 1000 mg.

5. *Amphotericin.* Dose for use = 5 mg. Reconstitute a 50 mg vial with 10 ml water for injection. Withdraw 1 ml, using a 1 ml syringe, and add to 9 ml of water in a sterile bottle with lid for injection. Mix well. Withdraw 1 ml of this dilution, using a 1 ml syringe, and add to 9 ml of dextrose in a sterile bottle with lid, to complete a dilution of 1/100. Mix well (= 50 mg/ml). Use 0.1 ml = 5 mg. (A dose of 10 mg has been used by some clinicians.)

CLINICAL TRIALS

Important trials include:
European society for Cataract and refractive surgery study, endophthalmitis vitrectomy study (EVS), and (ESCRS). These are summarized in Table 29.3

Table 29.3 *Clinical trials in endophthalmitis*

	Enrollment	Criteria	Number	Endpoint	Aim / Follow up	Intervention	Results
Endo-phthalmitis vitrectomy study (EVS)	1990–1995	Acute post cataract or sec IOL endophthal-mitis within 6 weeks of presentation Pt with clear cornea, VA < ETDRS 36 letters at 4 m, > PL and media clarity to obscure view of second order vessels	420 patients	Visual acuity and clarity of ocular media, final outcome assessment was at 9 months.	• To determine the role of initial pars plana vitrectomy in the management of postoperative bacterial endophthalmitis. • To determine the role of intravenous antibiotics in the management of vitreous tap/biopsy thalmitis. • To determine which factors, other than treatment, predict outcome in postoperative bacterial endophthalmitis	Eyes received either (1) initial pars plana vitrectomy with intra-vitreal antibiotics, followed by retap and reinjection at 36–60 hours for eyes that did poorly as defined in the study or (2) initial anterior chamber and chance of va> 20/ with injection of intravitreal antibiotics, followed by vitrectomy and reinjection at 36–60 hours in eyes doing poorly. In addition, all eyes were randomized to either treatment or no treatment with intra-venous antibiotics.	Only 11% had va LP only vision, 33% chance of 20/40 vision with ppv than without ppv (11%) and double chance of receiving 20/100 final VA eyes with better than LP, 40 in 66% vs 62% with or without with or without ppv; 20/100 in 86% vs 84% No diff in media clarity or va outcome with systemic a/b
				bacterial endoph-			
ECRS	2003–2006		16,603 patients treated at 24 clinical centres in nine European countries		• To evaluate the prophylactic effect of intracameral cefuro-xime with or without perioperative topical levofloxacin on post-operative endophthal-mitis after cataract surgery	Four treatment groups. One group received vehicle drops peri-operatively and no intracameral injection. The second group received placebo drops and an intra-cameral injection of	Injection of the antibiotic cefuroxime at the end of surgery reduced the incidence of endophthalmitis by nearly five-fold.

Contd..

Table 29.3 *Clinical trials in endophthalmitis (Contd...)*

Enrollment	Criteria	Number	Endpoint	Aim / Follow up	Intervention	Results
				• Secondary questions included finding a more reliable estimate of the true rate of endophthalmitis and identifying risk factors for the complication.	1.0 mg of cefuroxime in 0.1 ml saline at the end of surgery. The third group received levofloxacin eye drops perioperatively but no intracameral injection and the fourth group received both perioperative levofloxacin eye drops and intracameral cefuroxime. All groups received povidone iodine preoperatively and topical levofloxacin postoperatively for six days.	The use of clear corneal incisions increased the risk for the complication by nearly eight-fold and the implantation of silicone IOLs increased the risk by over three-fold. Other risk factors identified included the sex of the patient, with men being nearly three times more likely than women to develop the complication, and the occurrence of complications during surgery which increased the risk nearly five-fold.
Traumatic endophthalmitis Trial research group	Prophylaxis of traumatic endophthalmitis.	346 eyes	Occurrence of endophthalmitis within 2 weeks.	• Evaluate the efficacy of intraocular gentamicin sulfate and clindamycin in the prevention of acute post-traumatic bacterial endophthalmitis following penetrating eye injuries.	Randomized to intracameral or intravitreal injection of 40 µg of gentamicin sulfate and 45 µg of clindamycin (cases) vs balanced salt solution (controls).	

BIBLIOGRAPHY

1. Aboltins CA, Allen P, Daffy JR. Fungal endo-phthal-mitis in intravenous drug users injecting buprenorphine contaminated with oral Candida species. Med J Aust 2005; 182:427.

2. Ayyala RS, Bellows AR, Thomas JV, et al. Bleb infections: clinically different courses of "blebitis" and endophthalmitis. Ophthalmic Surg and Lasers 1997; 28:452–460.

3. Bucci FA: An in vivo study comparing the ocular absorption of levofloxacin and ciprofloxacin prior to phacoemulsification. Am J Ophthalmol 2004:137,308–12.

4. Carolee M. Cutler Peck, Jacob Brubaker, Sue Clouser, Chris Danford, Henry E. Edelhauser, Nick Mamalis Toxic anterior segment syndrome: Common causes Journal of Cataract & Refractive Surgery July 2010; Vol. 36(Issue 7): 1073–108

5. Colin J, Simonpoli S, Geldsetze K, Ropo A. Corneal penetration of levofloxacin into the human aqueous humour: a comparison with ciprofloxacin. Acta Ophthalmol Scand 81, 2003, 611–613.

6. Endophthalmitis Vitrectomy Study Group: Results of the Endophthalmitis Vitrectomy Study. A randomized trial of immediate vitrectomy and of intravenous antibiotics for the treatment of post-operative bacterial endophthalmitis. Arch Ophthalmol 1995; 113: 1479–96.

7. Engstrom RE Jr, MondinoBJ, GlasgowBJ, Pitchekian-Halabi H, Adamu SA. Immune response to *Staphylococcus aureus* endophthalmitis in a rabbit model. Invest Ophthalmol Vis Sci 1991; 32;1523–33.

8. ESCRS Endophthalmitis Study Group: Prophylaxis of post-operative endophthalmitis following cataract surgery: results of the ESCRS multicenter study and identification of risk factors. J Cataract Refract Surg 2007;33, 978–88.

9. ESCRS guidelines on prevention investigation and management of postoperative endophthal-mitis–Peter Barry, Wolgang Behrens-Baumann, Uwe Pleyer and David Seal. August 2007.

10. Holladay JT. Proper method for calculating average visual acuity. J Refract Surg 1997; 13: 388–91.

11. Keswani T, Ahuja V, Changulani M. Evaluation of outcome of various treatment methods for endogenous endophthalmitis. Indian J Med Sci 2006; 60: 454–60.

12. Kobayakawa S, Tochikubo T, Tsuji A. Penetration of levofloxacin into human aqueous humor. Ophthalmic Res 2003:35.

13. Koch HR, Kulus S C, Roessler M, Ropo A, Geldsetzer K. Corneal penetration of fluoro-quinolones: aqueous humour concentrations after topical application of levofloxacin 0.5% and ofloxacin 0.3% eye drops. J Cataract Refract Surg 2005: 31: 1377–85.

14. Kunimoto DY, Das T, Sharma S et al. Microbiologic spectrum and susceptibility of isolates: part I. Postoperative endophthalmitis. Endophthalmitis Research Group. Am J Ophthalmol. 1999 Aug; 128(2):240–2.

15. Kunimoto DY, Das T, Sharma S et al. Microbiologic spectrum and susceptibility of isolates: part II. Posttraumatic endophthalmitis. Endophthalmitis Research Group. Am J Ophthalmol. 1999 Aug; 128(2):242–4.

16. Michael S, Kresloff MD, Castellarin AA, Zarbin MA. Endophthalmitis—Major review. Surv Ophthalmol 1998; 43:193–224.

17. Mochizuki K, Jikihara S, Ando Y, et al. Incidence of delayed onset infection after trabeculectomy with adjunctive mitomycin C or 5-fluorouracil treatment. Br J Ophthalmol 1997;81:877–883.

18. Narang S, Gupta A, Gupta V et al.Fungal endophthalmitis following cataract surgery: clinical presentation, microbiological spectrum, and outcome. Am J Ophthalmol2001;132:609-617.

19. Narang S, Gupta A, Gupta V, Dogra M R, Ram J, Pandav SS, Chakrabarti A. Fungal endo-phthalmitis following cataract surgery: Clinical presentation, microbiological spectrum, and outcome. Am J Ophthalmol 2001, 132:609–17.

20. Narang S, Gupta V, Gupta A, Dogra MR, Pandav SS, Das S. Role of prophylactic intravitreal antibiotics in open globe injuries. Indian J Ophthalmol 2003;51:39–44.

21. Narang S, Gupta V, Simalandhi P, Gupta A, Raj S, Dogra MR. Pediatric open globe injuries. Visual outcome and risk factors for endophthalmitis. Indian J Ophthalmol. 2004; 52:29–34.

22. Peyman G, Lee P, Seal DV. Endophthalmitis—diagnosis and management. Taylor and Francis, London: 2004; 1–270.

23. Pflugfelder SC, Flynn HW Jr, Zwickey TA, Forster RK, Tsiligianni A, Culbertson WW, Mandelbaum S. Exogenous fungal endophthal-mitis. Ophthalmology 1988; 95:19–30.

24. PP Connell, et al. Endogenous endophthalmitis–10 year experience at a tertiary referral center. Eye 2011;25(1):66–72.

25. Schiedler V, Scott IU, Flynn Jr HW, Davis JL, Benz MS, Miller D. Culture-proven endogenous endophthalmitis: clinical features and visual acuity outcomes. Am J Ophthalmol 2004; 137: 725–31.

26. Seal D V, Barry P, Gettinby G, Lees F, Peterson M, Revie C W, Wilhelmus KR. ESCRS study of prophylaxis of postoperative endophthalmitis after cataract surgery: Case for a European multi-center study. J Cataract Refract Surg 2006; 32:396–406.

27. Seal DV, Barry P, Gettinby G, Lees F, Peterson M, Revie CW, Wilhelmus K R. ESCRS study of prophylaxis of postoperative endophthalmitis after cataract surgery: Case for a European multi-center study. J Cataract Refract Surg. 32, 2006, 396–406.

28. Seal DV, Reischl U, Behr A, Ferrer C, Alio J, Koerner R, Barry P. ESCRS Endophthalmitis Study Group: Laboratory management of endophthalmitis: comparison of microbiology and molecular biology methods in the European multi-center study and appropriate chemotherapy. Manuscript in preparation.

29. Smith RS, Kroll AJ, Lou PL, et al. endogenous bacterial and fungal endophthalmitis. Int Ophthalmol Clin 2007;47:173–183.

30. Soheilian M, Rafati N, Mohebbi M R, Yazdani S, Habibabadi H F, Feghhi M, Shahriary H A, Eslamipour J, Piri N, Peyman G A. Traumatic Endophthalmitis Trial Research Group: Prophylaxis of acute posttraumatic bacterial endophthalmitis: a multi-center, randomized clinical trial of intraocular antibiotic injection, report 2. Arch Ophthalmol 2007; 125:460–5.

31. Speaker MG and Menikoff JA. Prophylaxis of endophthalmitis with topical povidone-iodine. Ophthalmology 1991; 98, 1769–75.

32. Yan H, Chen S, Zhang JK, Yu JG, Han JD. Treatment of postoperative endophthalmitis following cataract surgery without intraocular lens removal. Zhonghua Yan Ke Za Zhi 2009; 45:684–7.

33. Yoon YH, Lee SU, Sohn JH, Lee SE. Result of early vitrectomy for endogenous Klebsiella pneumoniae endophthalmitis. Retina 2003; 23: 366–70.

34. Zhang YQ, Wang WJ. Treatment outcomes after pars plana vitrectomy for endogenous endophthalmitis. Retina 2005; 25:746–50.

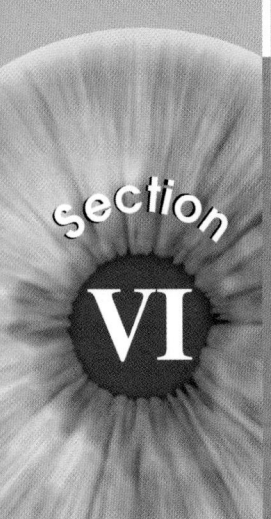

30 SCLERAL BUCKLING SURGERY

Atul Kumar

GENERAL CONSIDERATIONS

INTRODUCTION

Retinal detachment (RD) is defined as a separation of the neurosensory retina, at the level of the photoreceptor outer segments, from the retinal pigment epithelium (RPE). Rhegmatogenous retinal detachments are caused by retinal breaks. Usually resulting from vitreoretinal traction. The main goals of retinal reattachment surgery are to relieve the vitreoretinal traction and to close the retinal breaks (so that fluid from the vitreous cavity cannot gain access to the sub-retinal space). Once the retinal breaks are closed, remaining subretinal fluid will be removed by the retinal pigment epithelial "pump."

The three most important reattachment procedures are scleral buckling, pars plana vitrectomy, and pneumatic retinopexy. The choice of reattachment procedure typically depends upon the number, location, size of retinal breaks extent of proliferative vitreo-retinopathy (PVR). Additional considerations include the lens status, presence of vitreous opacities, and to some degree, the surgeon's preference.

In some instances of retinal detachment, where the vitreoretinal traction is minimal, retinal breaks can be treated with pneumatic retinopexy. At other times, severe vitreoretinal traction necessitates vitrectomy. Scleral buckling surgery accomplishes the goal of reattachment by indenting the underlying sclera, choroid, and retinal pigment epithelium with buckling elements (i.e. solid silicone tires or silicone sponges) to relieve mechanically the vitreo-retinal traction and approximate the edges of the retinal break to the underlying retinal pigment epithelium.

HISTORY OF RETINAL REATTACHMENT SURGERY

Prior to the 20th century, there were no effective treatments for rhegmatogenous RD because the pathophysiology of the disease was not understood. Jules Gonin reported in 1918 that rhegmatogenous RD was caused by retinal

breaks secondary to vitreous traction, although this was not published in the English literature for another 12 years. Gonin also pioneered the first successful reattachment procedure, ignipuncture, which involved cauterization of the retinal break(s) and external drainage of subretinal fluid. The most difficult step in this procedure was the precise localization of the retinal break(s). This localization became more predictable with the invention of the binocular indirect ophthalmoscope by Charles Schepens in 1947. Two major advances assisted the sealing of breaks to the RPE. Meyer-Schwickerath developed photocoagulation in the 1950s and Lincoff pioneered modern cryopexy in the 1960s. The three major categories of retinal reattachment surgery were developed in the second half of the 20th century. Scleral buckling was the first type of modern surgical repair. Contemporary buckling techniques date back to the 1950s and the work of Schepens, Ernst Custodis and Hermengildo Arruga. In general, Schepens advocated encircling scleral buckling (cerclage), frequently with external subretinal fluid drainage, while Custodis advocated non-drainage segmental scleral buckling. These two divergent schools of thought continue to the present day.

PATHOGENESIS OF RHEGMATOGENOUS RETINAL DETACHMENT

The pathogenesis of rhegmatogenous RD is now well understood. Around any retinal break exists a balance of forces. Some forces tend to maintain retinal apposition to the RPE, while other forces promote rhegmatogenous RD. Most retinal breaks do not cause rhegmatogenous RD. Rhegmatogenous RD develops when the forces promoting retinal detachment overwhelm the forces maintaining retinal attachment.

Forces maintaining retinal attachment

Forces maintaining retinal attachment include hydrostatic pressure, oncotic pressure, and active transport.

- *Intraocular pressure* creates a higher hydrostatic pressure within the vitreous than within the choroid.

- *Oncotic pressure.* The choroid contains more dissolved substances than the vitreous and thus has a higher oncotic pressure.

- *Active transport.* The RPE pump actively transports solutes (and fluid) from the subretinal space into the choroid.

These three forces result in a net vitreous-to-choroid fluid vector that tends to maintain retinal apposition.

Forces promoting retinal detachment

Forces promoting retinal detachment include vitreous traction, gravity, and eye movements. Active traction on the flap of a horseshoe tear accelerates the passage of liquid vitreous into the subretinal space. Gravity promotes the spread of subretinal fluid, particularly with superior breaks. Eye movements are probably the least powerful of these three mechanisms but do appear to accelerate rhegmatogenous RD formation in at least some cases.

Role of retinal breaks and vitreous traction

The two most important factors in the development of rhegmatogenous RD are retinal breaks and vitreous traction. Therefore, the two goals of retinal reattachment surgery, by any modality, are to seal all retinal breaks and to relieve all vitreous traction. In general, unsuccessful surgery is a result of failure to achieve one or both of these objectives.

There are two important exceptions to this rule. First, an untreated retinal break, if supported on a scleral buckle, does not necessarily cause surgical failure. This is in direct contrast to pars plana vitrectomy or pneumatic retinopexy, in which an untreated break usually does cause surgical failure. Second, pneumatic retinopexy does not truly relieve vitreous traction, yet it remains a highly successful procedure. The most critical factors in choosing a surgical technique are the number and location of retinal breaks. Other important factors to consider are the size of the breaks, the lens status (phakic, pseudophakic, or aphakic), the macular status (attached or detached), the surgeon's preference, and the patient's ability to comply with postoperative positioning requirements.

SCLERAL BUCKLING

Scleral buckling works through a variety of proposed mechanisms, some of which are generally agreed upon and some of which are not. Scleral buckling indirectly relieves radial vitreous traction, by supporting the retina and RPE in the area of the retinal breaks. Scleral buckling also displaces subretinal fluid away from breaks, bringing the neurosensory retina and RPE into closer proximity. Traditional teaching held that scleral buckling had two other beneficial effects. First, it was thought to displace liquid vitreous away from retinal breaks, allowing (in a nonvitrectomized eye) the breaks to become tamponaded by cortical vitreous. Second, buckles were thought to somehow offset the deleterious actions of intraocular fluid currents caused by rotational eye movements (see above). Both of these effects, however, are somewhat speculative and there are few supporting data in the modern peer-reviewed literature. Scleral buckling may be performed in several different ways. The two main decisions involve the extent of buckling and whether or not to drain subretinal fluid. Many surgeons perform encircling scleral buckling (cerclage) or placement of the buckling element(s) for 360° around the eye (Fig. 30.1). Cerclage has the advantage of more extensive support and is more likely to support breaks that were not identified. As discussed above, an untreated retinal break, if supported on the buckling element, does not necessarily lead to

surgical failure. This is, in fact, one of the distinct advantages of scleral buckling.

Buckling elements sutured to the external surface of the sclera are called *explants,* or *episcleral implants.* If the sclera is dissected, the imbedded buckling material is called a *scleral implant.* The choroid and retinal pigment epithelium (RPE) in the vicinity of all of the retinal breaks is treated with a thermal irritant (i.e., cryopexy, or laser photocoagulation) to form a permanent chorioretinal adhesion (i.e. a permanent seal) surrounding the retinal break.

However, encerclage (Fig. 30.1) is a more extensive and morbid procedure than segmental buckling. In rhegmatogenous RD with only one break or with multiple but closely spaced breaks, cerclage is not necessary to achieve reattachment. A properly placed segmental element will support the break(s) and achieve success with a less extensive procedure and a lower risk of complications. In some cases, external drainage of subretinal fluid increases the single-operation success rate and allows for quicker resolution of the rhegmatogenous RD. However, drainage is associated with several vision-threatening complications, including vitreous incarceration, retinal incarceration, suprachoroidal/subretinal hemorrhage, and potentially endophthalmitis. Drainage should be considered an intraocular step within an otherwise extraocular procedure. Typically, segmental scleral buckling is performed without drainage; cerclage may be performed either with or without drainage.

Frequently, it is necessary to drain subretinal fluid in order to close the retinal breaks. In general, this combination decreases operating time, and allows easier intraoperative readjustment of the buckle, if necessary.

An alternative scleral buckling technique may be useful in select cases with very bullous retinal detachments. Drainage, air, cryopexy, and encircling (DACE) may be thought of as a conventional scleral buckling procedure in reverse. Subretinal fluid drainage is performed as the first step, intraocular pressure is restored with an intravitreal injection of air (or other gas), and cryopexy and cerclage proceed as usual.

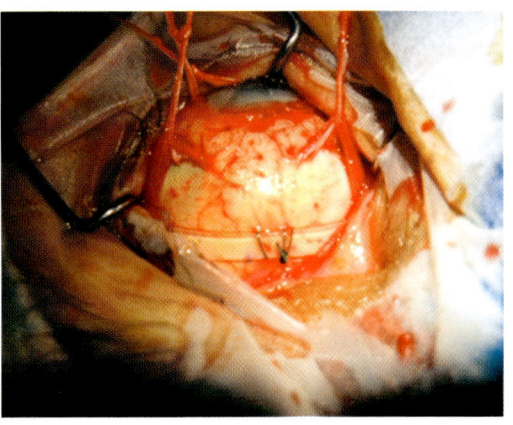

Fig. 30.1 *Encircling silicone band*

Regardless of specific technique, scleral buckling offers several advantages compared with other procedures. It is the most established procedure with the longest documented follow-up. Scleral buckling is appropriate for virtually all primary rhegmatogenous RDs (the exception would be cases with very posterior breaks and advanced PVR) and remains the best approach, with or without concomitant pars plana vitrectomy, for inferior breaks. In general, postoperative positioning is supine, which is well tolerated by most patients.

A crucial part of the procedure is identifying all of the retinal breaks, since there are frequently more than one. The detailed fundus drawing should always be available in the operating room. Fundus landmarks in the drawing (such as vortex veins, retinal vessels, and regions of lattice degeneration) can help the surgeon to locate retinal breaks if intraoperative media problems prevent adequate visualization.

PREOPERATIVE WORK UP

Thorough preoperative evaluation of the patient with retinal detachment is as important as the surgical procedure itself. The surgical strategy can be planned preoperatively after examination of the patient is completed. Specific aspects of the management strategy to be considered are a segmental or radial buckle versus an encircling scleral buckle, the necessity for drainage of subretinal fluid, the possible need for air or gas tamponade or the need for vitrectomy to mobilize fixed or star folds resulting from proliferative vitreoretinopathy. Alternative techniques for the management of retinal detachment without permanent scleral buckling such as a temporary parabulbar balloon or pneumatic retinopexy, may also be appropriate in selected cases. The preoperative evaluation should include a detailed clinical history, comprehensive ophthalmic evaluation of both anterior and posterior segments of the eye, and informed consent from the patient following detailed explanation of the planned surgical procedure.

Clinical history

The duration of symptoms resulting from vitreous opacities should be determined as accurately as possible. Often patients report symptoms such as spots, lines, cobwebs, or floaters (Fig. 30.2). A history of photopsia may also be reported. Many patients are not aware of the significance of floaters or photopsia and

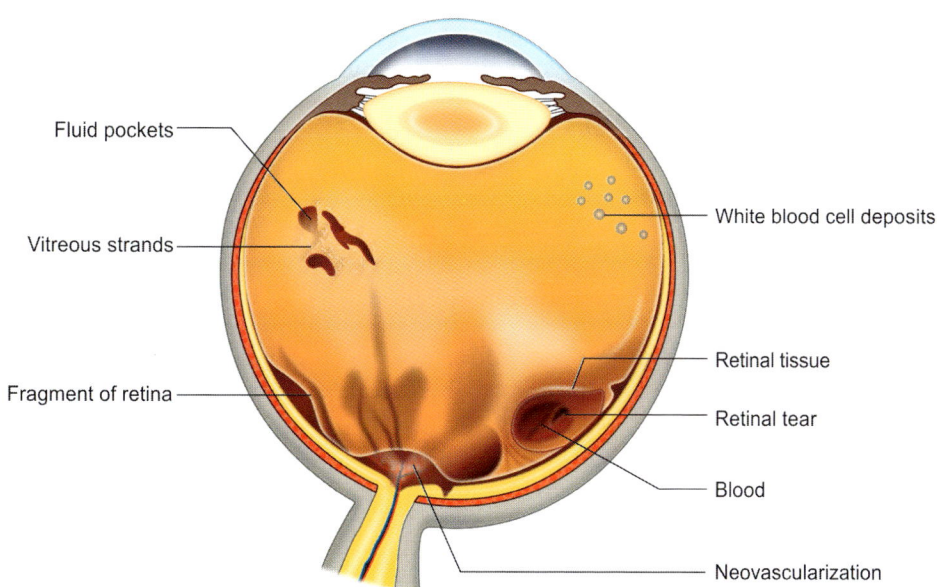

Fluid pockets

Vitreous strands

Fragment of retina

White blood cell deposits

Retinal tissue

Retinal tear

Blood

Neovascularization

Fig. 30.2 *Floaters are seen because of entoptic phenomenon due to the presence of opaque material in the transparent vitreous, casting their shadow on the retina. It shows presence of common material in the vitreous cavity close to retina responsible for variety of floaters*

do not seek attention until a peripheral field defect or central visual loss occurs secondary to macular detachment. Precise description of the symptoms may aid in localizing the retinal breaks. If the patient has had retinal detachment previously the details and results of prior surgery should be obtained if possible. Any previous history of ocular disease relevant to retinal detachment such as myopia, cataract surgery, ocular inflammation, trauma, glaucoma should be documented. A family history of retinal detachment should also be noted. There is wide variation in the ability of patients to recall their symptoms. Some patients are able to relate a very detailed history of the direction of field loss and associated symptoms, while others are unable to describe their symptoms precisely.

Patients who have had a retinal detachment previously are often more alert to symptoms that may occur in the fellow eye.

Ocular examination

The ocular examination should include a complete general eye examination as well as a detailed fundus study. The refractive error should be recorded. In eyes with a history of amblyopia, an autorefractor or retinoscopic evaluation may determine the true refractive status. The corrected visual acuity should be recorded for each eye. An afferent pupillary defect if present in the affected eye should be noted. Applanation tonometry may be used to record the intraocular pressure. In most cases the intraocular pressure is lower as a result of the retinal detachment, but the presence of hypotony should raise the possibility of accompanying choroidal detachment.

The lids and conjunctiva should be examined for blepharitis or conjunctivitis prior to pupillary dilation. Phenylephrine hydrochloride may constrict conjunctival blood vessels and mask an ocular infection. The presence of severe blepharitis or conjunctivitis should lead to a delay in surgery until the condition has been treated. Limitations in ocular motility or strabismus should be measured and noted. Patient should be informed of the increased possibility of diplopia after the retina is reattached.

Slit lamp examination

On slit lamp examination abnormalities in corneal clarity or size should he noted. The depth of the anterior chamber should be checked in patients with a narrow peripheral angle. In patients with Marfan's syndrome or a history of ocular trauma, lens subluxation or phacodonesis may also be present. If an intraocular lens implant has been inserted, the type of implant and integrity of the posterior capsule following extracapsular cataract extraction should be noted. In aphakic patients, vitreous fibrils may be displaced anteriorly through the pupil by the bullous retinal detachment. Vitreous strands to the cataract wound should be studied. The hyaloid face may be in contact with the corneal endothelium, resulting in localized corneal edema. In phakic patients with symptoms of posterior vitreous separation, it is helpful to examine the anterior vitreous with the slit lamp. The presence of pigment almost invariably indicates the presence of a retinal tear (Schaffer's sign).

Maximum pupillary dilation should be obtained prior to fundus examination. Tropicamide 1% and phenylephrine hydrochloride 2.5% (or 10% in refractory cases) can be used in combination at 20–30 minute intervals until maximum dilation occurs.

Fundus examination

The fundus examination consists two parts: (1) Indirect ophthalmoscopy with scleral depression. (2) Non-contact biomicroscopy of vitreoretinal relationships using an aspheric lens.

An indirect ophthalmoscope should be chosen that is lightweight and fits comfortably.

A small pupil attachment is helpful for poorly dilated eyes or in pseudophakic eyes with peripheral lens remnants. The room is darkened and indirect ophthalmoscopy is started when the examiner is dark adapted. The patient is placed supine on an examining chair or table. The chin is extended forward slightly. The examiner stands at the head of the patient and the fundus drawing paper is kept next to the head of the patient on the side of the examiner's writing hand. The 12:00 clock meridian of the drawing is directed toward the patient's feet and

the examiner is positioned opposite to the meridian of interest and sketches exactly what is observed. By placing the drawing upside-down, one obviates the need to transpose the inverted image of the indirect ophthalmoscope. The beginning examiner should learn to hold the lens with the non-dominant hand so that the writing hand can be used for drawing or scleral depression.

Conventional color scheme used for fundus drawing is:

- *Light blue:* Retinal detachment.
- *Dark blue:* Retinal veins, margins of retinal breaks.
- *Light red:* Attached retina.
- *Dark red:* Retinal arteries, pre-retinal or intra-retinal hemorrhages.
- *Green:* Vitreous or lens opacities.
- *Black:* Chorioretinal pigmentation/laser scars.
- *Yellow:* Intra-retinal or subretinal exudates. Subretinal bands (broken yellow lines).
- *Brown:* Choroidal detachment, nevi or melanomas.

At the beginning of the examination. The intensity of the light of the indirect ophthalmoscope is reduced to allow the patient to adjust to the brightness of the light. Initially a broad survey of the funduscopic findings is obtained without scleral depression. When the patient is more comfortable with the examining light, the illumination can be increased. The meridians delimiting the edges of the retinal detachment are first noted and the extent of detachment is sketched onto the fundus drawing on Amsler-Dubois chart, which contains three concentric circles (Fig. 30.3). The inner circle represents the equator of the fundus, the middle circle represents the ora serrata and the outer band the pars plana.

Retinal breaks visible without scleral depression are localized and drawn. Following the retinal blood vessels out to the periphery allows systematic examination of the entire fundus. Scleral depression is required for examination of the peripheral retina. The patient is more comfortable when scleral depression is started temporally. The temporal periphery is more easily visualized, and as the eye softens from scleral depression the nasal fundus can be

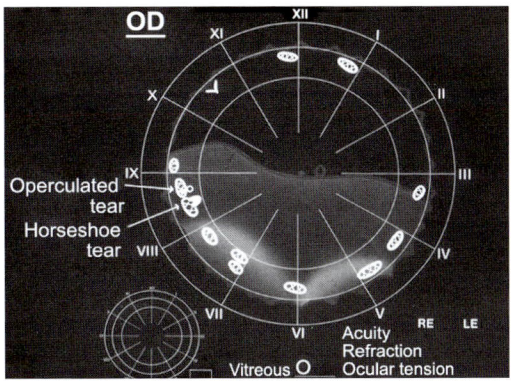

Fig. 30.3 *Amsler-Dubois chart*

more easily examined. Optimal visualization of the peripheral fundus is usually obtained when the examiner stands directly opposite to the meridian of interest. In patients with small pupils or peripheral lens opacities, visualization of retinal breaks may also be improved by turning the patient's head toward the examiner and asking the patient to look toward that meridian.

Specific features of the retinal detachment should be noted on the fundus drawing:

1. *Relationship of retinal blood vessels and vortex veins to the location of breaks* should be drawn to provide landmarks for intra-operative localization. These may be helpful during surgery if visualization decreases due to corneal edema or vitreous hemorrhage. Avulsed or bridging blood vessels over retinal tears should also be noted.

2. *The height or elevation of the retinal detachment* should be studied to determine whether drainage of sub retinal fluid is required. More bullous areas are preferable for possible drainage sites.

3. *Areas of chorioretinal pigmentation* and demarcation lines should be indicated. Demarcation lines may help to localize the region of the retinal breaks.

4. *Areas of peripheral lattice degeneration* and areas suspicious for retinal breaks should be noted.

5. *When multiple breaks are present* their antero-posterior location should be accurately depicted. As a general rule, vortex veins delineated the equator and can be helpful in the precise determination of anteroposterior

location. This information will be used to plan the size and extent of scleral buckling.

6. *Lines of circumferential traction* in the anterior retina and star or fixed folds should be indicated. By observing the mobility of the retina as the patient moves the eye, the severity of traction can be evaluated. Poor mobility [proliferative vitreorertinopathy (PVR) Table 30.1 and Fig. 30.4] indicates that the retina is stiffened by epiretinal membranes and may require vitrectomy.

The posterior pole is usually reserved for the final part of the examination with indirect ophthalmoscopy. Macular holes, cysts, or macular pucker may be present. Posterior breaks may also be present near the edge of a staphyloma or coloboma or adjacent to larger retinal blood vessels.

When the examination is completed in the supine position, the patient is examined in the sitting position this may allow folds within the retinal detachment to open revealing previously

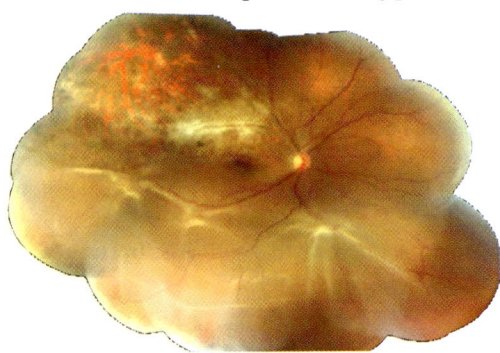

Fig. 30.4 *Grading of PVR*

unseen retinal breaks. The patient is returned to the slit lamp and undergoes biomicroscopy using the 90 diopter aspheric lens. The depth of focus permits excellent visualization of vitreoretinal interface and the macular examination.

Lincoff 's Rules of Retinal Detachment

When the funduscopic examination has been completed and the location of retinal breaks found, the examiner should consider whether the configuration of the detachment is consistent with the location of the retinal breaks. Retinal detachments accumulate subretinal fluid in a predictable manner around the retinal break of origin. These observations have been extensively described and are known as Lincoff's Rule. The shape of the retinal detachment indicates the location of the break in 96% of cases. Some concepts that may be useful in finding the break are as below (Fig. 30.5):

1. In superonasal or temporal retinal detachments, the retinal break lies within one and one-half clock hours of the highest border 98% of the time;
2. In superior detachments that cross the midline, the primary retinal break is at 12 o'clock or within a triangle the apex of which is at the ora serrata and that intersects the equator I hour to either side of 12 o'clock, this is present 93% of the time;
3. In inferior detachments, the higher side indicates to which side of the 6 o'clock meridian an inferior hole lies 95% of the time (Fig. 30.5A to C).

Table 30.1 *Retina society grading of proliferative vitreoretinopathy*	
Grade	*Characteristics*
A	Vitreous haze, pigment clumps
B	Wrinkling of the inner retinal surface. Rolled edge of retinal break, retinal stiffness, vessel tortuosity
C	Full thickness retinal folds
C1	1 quadrant
C2	2 quadrants
C3	3 quadrants
D	Fixed retinal folds in 4 quadrants
D1	Wide funnel shape
D2	Narrow funnel (optic nerve visible)
D3	Closed funnel (optic nerve not visible)

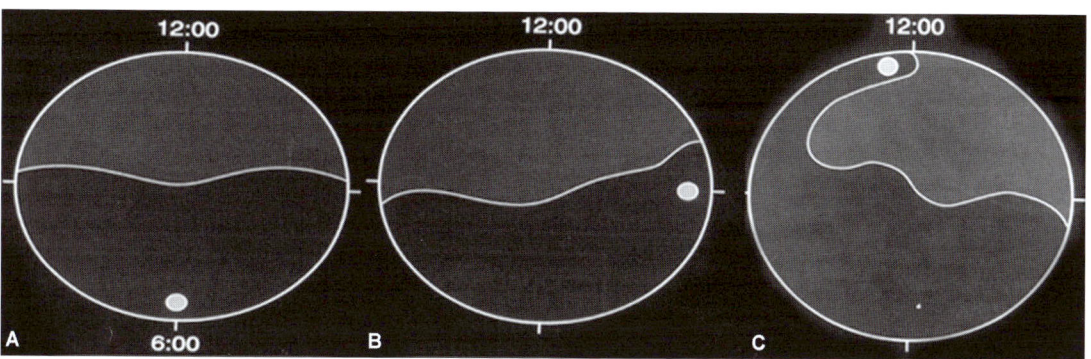

Fig. 30.5 *Schematic representation of Lincoff's rules for localisation of retinal break (for explanation see text)*

4. When an inferior retinal detachment has a bullous configuration, the primary hole lies above the horizontal meridian (Fig. 30.6).

These rules are most applicable in the absence of proliferative vitreoretinopathy since significant tractional forces can alter the distribution of subretinal fluid. If the location of the retinal breaks does not explain the retinal detachment, additional study of the retinal detachment is suggested to seek any possible missed retinal breaks.

Once the decision is made to perform scleral buckling surgery, it is important that selected cases be performed in a timely manner. "Macula-on" and recent "macula-off" (i.e. up to 5 days) retinal detachments should be operated upon as soon as possible, preferably within 48 hours. Since outer segments of the retina depend upon blood supply from the choriocapillaris. Prompt reattachment of the macula (or prevention of a macular detachment) maximizes the chance of preserving good vision. Chronic "macula-off" retinal detachments can be scheduled electively.

Patients with "macula-on" retinal detachments threatening the macula are kept at bed rest until the surgery can be performed. Reading should be discouraged since saccadic eye movements can lead to further accumulation of subretinal fluid. Watching a distant television is not a problem since this requires little, if any angular eye movements. The patient's head should be positioned so that subretinal fluid remains away from the macula. If elevated intraocular pressure is anticipated during surgery (i.e. large buckle required, little subretinal fluid to drain), patients may be treated with pressure lowering drops (i.e. beta blockers or carbonic anhydrase inhibitors) or systemic acetazolamide preoperatively. Intravenous mannitol (1 g/kg) can also be used preoperatively or intraoperatively.

The anesthesia choice in the present day practice is the peribulbar infiltration anesthesia where the combination of 2% lidocaine and 5% bupivacaine is used and is well tolerated by the patients.

SURGICAL TECHNIQUE

Positioning, scrubbing and draping

• When *positioning the patient's* head (preferably on a donut-shaped pillow or a rolled towel),

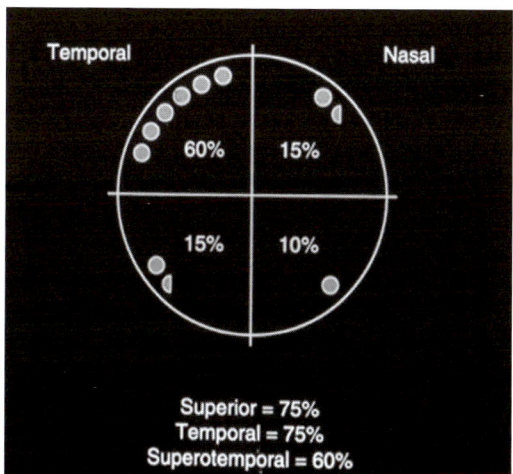

Fig. 30.6 *Quadrantic distribution of retinal breaks*

the chin should be elevated slightly, so that the brow and the lower orbital rim form a horizontal plane.

- *The lids, brow, and upper cheek are scrubbed* with a 10% povidone-iodine (Betadine) solution. Cotton tipped applicators are used to cleanse the lashes. A drop of 5% povidone-iodine is placed in the conjunctiva sac. The eye and lids are then rinsed with sterile water and the periorbital area is dried with a sterile towel.

- *A plastic adhesive drape* with iodophor on the "sticky" side can be used as a further precaution against infection. A horizontal incision is made in the drape with in the palpebral fissure unless a fenestrated drape is used. The conjunctiva (including the fornices) is then vigorously rinsed with a physiologic saline solution. Adequate exposure is usually provided with a lid speculum. The buckling is also discussed on p-425, Chapter 25.

Conjunctival peritomy

- A 360-degree limbal peritomy is usually performed and the incision made close to the limbus. A more posterior peritomy can be performed in one or more quadrants if needed.

- The conjunctiva (together with Tenon's capsule) is then undermined using blunt Wescott scissors. The conjunctiva must always be handled carefully to prevent buttonholing, especially when it is thin and atrophic (as in elderly patients). At this point it is a good idea to check pupillary dilatation and add more topical drops if needed.

- *Tenon's space in the four quadrants is then carefully opened* with blunt dissection (using blunt, tenotomy scissors) attempting to avoid damage to the vortex veins. A cotton-tipped applicator is then used to strip the intermuscular fascia from the extraocular muscles. The four recti muscles are looped and traction sutures of 3–0 silk/cotton passed beneath their tendons with fenestrated muscle hooks. It is important to isolate the entire muscle tendon during this step and not "split" the muscle. The oblique muscles are purposely avoided. Knots are tied close to the muscle and at approximately 4 inches away: this helps to

prevent tangling with buckle sutures later in the operation. The scleral surface is then examined. This is best accomplished by grasping two adjacent traction sutures and pushing Tenon's capsule and conjunctiva to the side with a small retractor (Fig. 30.4). This examination should document the occurrence of anomalous vortex veins, as well as regions of scleral thinning (scleral dehiscence) and staphyloma.

Localisation of the retinal breaks

Indirect ophthalmoscopy is used to locate the retinal breaks, usually with a 20-diopter lens. As previously mentioned, it is helpful to have the large fundus drawing available in the operating room at this time. The surgeon then performs scleral depression with a moistened, cotton-tipped applicator or instrument to localize the exact position of the retinal breaks on the corresponding external surface of the sclera. The straight (O'Conner) scleral marker is particularly helpful for posterior breaks. If the retinal break is small, just the posterior margin need be marked. If it is large the lateral margins should also be included. Large "horseshoe tears" usually require three marks to localize the posterior margin, as well as the extent of the two anterior horns. The localization should be checked; this can be readily accomplished by placing the backend of a cotton-tipped applicator on the scleral mark and depressing while viewing the fundus with the indirect ophthalmoscope. Areas of lattice degeneration usually should be marked so that bands (or buckles) can cover the regions, particularly if retinal breaks are present and areas are treated with cryopexy. After the retinal breaks are found, it is recommended that the surgeon examine the eye one final time by depressing the oraserrata 360 degrees in the hope of finding previously unrecognized retinal pathologic conditions over the retinal periphery to ensure completeness of the examination.

Cryopexy

Cryopexy should be performed to the regions surrounding each retinal break and to the areas of lattice degeneration. Contiguous freezes are

applied, usually in a V shape for horseshoe tears. Treatment is usually extended to the ora serrata for anterior or equatorial tears. For large tears, one full row of freezes is placed peripheral to the margins of the retinal break.

Treatment of bare RPE in the middle of large retinal breaks should be avoided since this serves no purpose and may cause dispersion of viable RPE cells into the vitreous cavity leading to subsequent periretinal membrane formation. If the cryoprobe is used to indent the outer eyewall, the RPE frequently can be brought into contact with the retina. In this situation, the endpoint of the treatment is the instant the first whitening appears within the retina (the foot pedal should be immediately released at this point to avoid over treatment).

If the RPE cannot be brought into close proximity to the retina, a color change (pale yellow) can be seen in the RPE itself; this represents an alternative endpoint. Freezing can take place relatively quickly in an eye with thin sclera and/or choroid (i.e. a myopic eye). Freezing also takes place rapidly in an air-filled eye (if the treated section of the retina is in contact with the air). Care must be taken always to slide the cryoprobe under the conjunctiva and rectus muscles and to direct the functioning portion of the probe against the scleral surface. The position of the opening of the protective plastic sheath covering the probe must always be checked. It is important to allow the probe to thaw completely with the help of irrigating fluid) before separating it from the scleral surface to avoid the unnecessary risk of choroidal hemorrhage of fracture of sclera.

Choice of explant

In general, the choice of explant in scleral buckling surgery is influenced by the following factors:

1. Size, number, and location of retinal breaks.
2. Amount of vitreoretinal traction.
3. Aphakia or pseudophakia.
4. Available volume for the buckle (amount of subretinal fluid that can be safely drained).
5. Distribution of the subretinal fluid.
6. Presence of proliferative vitreoretinopathy (PVR).
7. Concern for choroidal detachment.

Although the choice of the buckling element is always based upon the previous experience of the individual surgeon, it is beneficial for the retinal surgeon to be as open-minded as possible to other surgical techniques which are alternative to buckling procedure. This flexibility will allow for optimal results, particularly in challenging cases. The buckling element can either be circumferential (parallel to the limbus) or radial (perpendicular to the limbus). The two most widely used materials are solid silicone and silicone sponge. The solid silicone "tyres" are usually grooved to accommodate an overlying band. A wide variety of solid silicone bands, strips.tires, and accessories are available; although the most commonly used are silicone bands of 240 and silicone tyre 276 (asymmetrical tire). Band no. 41 is used as a isolated enciraling element. Silicone sponges that can used are 505G (grooved sponge), 510 (half sponge), 505T (tunnel sponge).

Encirclement (i.e. with either a band or a 360-degree circumferential buckle) is specifically recommended in the following circumstances:
- Treatment of aphakic and pseudophakic retinal detachment.
- Multiple retinal breaks and/or large tears.
- No retinal break found.
- Preretinal membrane formation, star folds, vitreous membranes PVR.
- High myopia.
- Extensive drainage of subretinal fluid.
- Extensive lattice degeneration.
- Desire to create a permanent buckling effect.

It is frequently not necessary to drain subretinal fluid, it is however, necessary to close the retinal breaks.
Buckle sutures can be temporarily tied to check for closure of retinal breaks without drainage. In general, situations that tend to favor drainage include:
- Long-standing retinal detachment (with viscous subretinal fluid that may require long periods of time for resorption).
- Highly elevated retinal detachment (particularly with elevated retinal breaks).
- Inferior retinal breaks.
- Presence of PVR.

- Absence of a recognized retinal break.
- Elderly patients (with poorly functioning RPE "pumps").
- Eyes that cannot tolerate intraocular pressure elevations (i.e. recent intraocular surgery, severe glaucoma).

Radially oriented buckles are most effective for treating single, large. posterior horseshoe tears. This can prevent the posterior gaping of retinal tears ("fish-mouthing") that can result with circumferential buckles. In addition to free standing radial sponges, radial accessories may be placed beneath circumferential buckles to prevent the fish-mouthing.

Segmental circumferential buckles (usually of silicone sponge) can be used to treat straight forward anterior breaks when the pathologic condition is limited to discrete regions (i.e. clock hours) and buckle height is not crucial. It also can be helpful if limited buckling volume is available. As a general rule, solid silicone explants produce broader buckles and sponge explants produce higher indentation. For this reason, subretinal fluid need not be drained in a higher proportion of cases in which sponges are used.

When planning a circumferential solid silicone buckle, the following recommendations should be considered:

- Bands may be used to support small retinal breaks, as well as areas of lattice degeneration.
- Extend the explant at least one clock hour beyond the margins of the retinal break.
- When possible, position the posterior margin of the retinal break near the middle of the tyre width (summit of the buckle indent).
- Attempt to extend the buckle anteriorly to cover the ora serrata to prevent anterior leakage (an anterior "gutter"). Suture placement at the line of muscle insertion will accomplish this goal. If the posterior extent of the planned tyre is inadequate, an accessory can provide adequate posterior coverage, yet allow the anterior buckle suture to be placed near the muscle insertion line. The posterior suture should be placed at least 3 mm posterior to the posterior margin of the actual break.

The following recommendations pertain to the use of radial sponges:

- The diameter of the radial explant should be at least twice the width of the retinal break (i.e. if the retinal break is 2.5 mm across, a sponge at least 5 mm in diameter should be used).
- Posterior coverage is crucial: start posterior radial sutures at the posterior margin of the retinal break and continue 2–3 mm posteriorly. If exposure is a problem, both suture bites may be made in the same anterior to posterior direction.
- Tie buckle sutures slowly (using temporary ties) to avoid excessive intraocular pressure elevation; watch the optic nerve head for arterial closure. (Paracentesis can be used to lower intraocular pressure; it is safest in phakic eyes or pseudophakic eyes with an intact posterior capsule.)
- Trim radial sponges at the line of muscle insertion.

If a retinal break cannot be identified, it is a good idea to encircle the eye, supporting the vitreous base since small, unrecognized breaks are most likely to be present in this location. Suspicious areas in the vicinity of the vitreous base are treated with cryopexy. Many surgeons prefer to drain subretinal fluid in this situation.

Once the buckle configuration has been chosen, the appropriate explant material should be soaked in an antibiotic solution.

Intrascleral suture placement

For circumferential buckles one to two buckle sutures are usually placed in each quadrant, preferably directly over the retinal breaks. In general explant segments should be secured by at least two buckle sutures. Suture material should be of the permanent variety. Usually nylon 5–0 or ethibond 5–0 is used. Suture needles should be of the spatula type. The sclera is engaged with the tip of the needle to approximately half depth and the needle is then passed along the same plane for a total length of 2–3 mm. Bluish-appearing areas of sclera represent thin regions and should be avoided. Sutures are placed in a mattress fashion, according to the orientation of the buckling

element. The free ends of the suture are held together with a Serrefine clamp until the sutures are tied. The distance between the anterior and posterior bites for silicone tires should be approximately 2 mm larger than the actual width of the explant. If a sponge explant is used the distance between the suture bites should be 1.5 times the diameter of the sponge.

If the suture is placed too deeply (penetrating the sclera, choroid, pigment epithelium, and possibly retina) and/or fluid is noted to leak from the needle tract, the tract should usually be marked and the suture removed and placed more posteriorly. The underlying retina is then examined with indirect ophthalmoscopy, and if a retinal break is noted, it is treated accordingly. Band sutures are placed in a very shallow fashion, to avoid unnecessary risk of scleral perforation.

The anterior and posterior bites are placed approximately 3 mm apart for a 2 mm band. One band suture is placed in each quadrant that does not already contain at least one buckle suture. When all sutures have been placed, buckling elements are positioned appropriately beneath the sutures and the recti muscles. Grooved, circumferential explants with the overlying bands are grasped together by a small, curved hemostat that has been placed beneath the buckle sutures and muscles.

Drainage of subretinal fluid

In general, it is desirable to drain subretinal fluid:
- Away from the retinal breaks (particularly largebreaks) to prevent drainage of liquid vitreous through the retinal breaks.
- Beneath the areas of maximal retinal elevation.
- Beneath retinal star folds (since these areas of the retina tend to remain elevated until other areas of the retina flatten).
- In the bed of the buckle (under preplaced buckle sutures).

Areas adjacent to the medial rectus muscle are the most desirable because of the easy accessibility. It is important to avoid areas adjacent to vortex veins (i.e. mid-quadrant), because of the higher risk of choroidal bleeding. Anterior drainage sites are preferable, again. To limit the risk of choroidal bleeding, it is prudent

to recheck the configuration of the subretinal fluid immediately before drainage. Since the subretinal fluid may shift when the eye position is altered and buckling elements are positioned.

The drainage site is prepared by radially oriented cuts in the sclera with Beaver blade. Diathermy to the scleral lips (using a conical tip) can be used to open the scleral wound by lateral tissue contraction. The endpoint of the scleral dissection (3–4 mm in length) is the herniation of a small, dark knuckle of choroid into the lips of the sclera wound. A preplaced suture (of nylon) is placed in the lips of the sclera incision if the drainage site is not in the bed of the buckle. The scleral lips are then held open with a fine-toothed forceps (0.12 mm) and all traction is released on the globe. If the intraocular pressure is still elevated, some of the preplaced buckling material must be temporarily removed to normalize the intraocular pressure prior to drainage, diathermy to the choroidal bed as a precaution against choroidal bleeding, prior to penetration of the choroid and pigment epithelium with a sharp suture needle, 30-gauge needle (with a 90-degree bend) can be used. Penetration is promptly stopped and the needle withdrawn when fluid leakage is first noted. We use modified needle drainage technique where a sclerotomy is not required. A paracentesis needle is used with a 90 degree bend and transcleral drainage is performed. After choroidal penetration, fluid can be gently expressed using cotton-tipped applicators. The cotton-tipped applicators are placed adjacent to the globe to take up volume temporarily and prevent hypotony. It is desirable to place the drainage site in a gravitationally dependent position. Endpoints of drainage include stoppage of fluid flow, or appearance of pigment. If stoppage of flow is followed by a sudden gush of fluid, retinal incarceration and perforation in the drainage site must be suspected. The overlying buckle sutures (or intrascleral mattress sutures if the drain is not in the bed of the buckle) are then tied temporarily with slip knots and the retina examined with indirect ophthalmoscopy. One observes the amount of remaining subretinal fluid and its proximity to the drainage site, and

looks carefully for possible complications, such as subretinal hemorrhage, retinal breaks at the drainage site, and retinal incarceration and they are managed appropriately.

When the drainage is completed, buckle sutures are pulled up and tied permanently. If a band is used, the ends may be joined with a permanent suture 'clove hitch' or a Watzke sleeve. The ends of the encircling sponges (or tyres) may be joined directly (end-to-end), using a permanent mattress suture. While tying the buckle sutures, the intraocular pressure should be checked periodically. If it is elevated the perfusion of the retinal arterioles (i.e. arterial pulsation near the optic nerve head) must be checked; the arterioles should be open at least 50% of the time. A paracentesis can be performed if the intraocular pressure is excessively high. This manoeuvre is safer in phakic eyes or pseudophakic eyes with an intact posterior capsule. A 30-gauge paracentesis needle is introduced over the peripheral iris (to avoid risking damage to the lens). If pressure elevation is anticipated, temporary ties can be used and the tension loosened appropriately. Slow intermittent tying of the buckle sutures is frequently an effective technique for dealing with elevated intraocular pressure. As previously mentioned, mannitol may be administered intravenously (1 g/kg) for marked intraocular pressure elevation.

The fundus is then re-examined to check the position of retinal breaks on the buckle. Although the margins of the retinal breaks need not be flat on the buckle, the buckle element must entirely underlie the retinal break.

The buckling elements and the subconjunctival space are irrigated with an antibiotic solution.

Closure of Tenon's capsule and conjunctiva

Tenon's capsule should be attached to the anterior muscle insertion or episclera with 7–0 Vicryl sutures in quadrant-where sponge material has been used (especially radially oriented sponges). This special two-layer closure helps to prevent sponge extrusion and infection. The conjunctiva is closed with sutures of 7–0 Vicryl, incorporating episcleral tissue. Relaxing incisions and other dehiscences in the conjunctiva should be meticulously repaired to prevent buckle exposure, infection, and extrusion.

I prefer to inject subconjunctival antibiotic with atropine and a peribulbar depot preparation of depo medrol 0.5 cc at the conclusion of the procedure. A combination antibiotic/steroid drops are used, along with a cycloplegic eye drops to relieve postoperative pain and discomfort.

BIBLIOGRAPHY

1. Arruga H. Certain considerations of the surgical treatment of retinal detachment. Trans Am Acad Ophthalmol Otolaryngol 1952;56:535–42.
2. Chang S. Low viscosity liquid fluorochemicals in vitreous surgery. Am J Ophthalmol 1987;103: 38–43.
3. Cibis PA, Becker B, Okun E, Canaan S: The use of liquid silicone in retinal detachment surgery. Arch Ophthalmol 1962;68:590–9.
4. Custodis E. Treatment of retinal detachment by circumscribed diathermal coagulation and by scleral depression in the area of tear caused by imbedding of a plastic implant. Klin Monatsbl Augenheilkd 1956;129:476–95.
5. Foulds WS. The vitreous in retinal detachment. Trans Ophthalmol Soc UK 1975;95:412–6.
6. Gilbert C, McLeod D. D-ACE surgical sequence for selected bullous retinal detachments. Br J Ophthalmol 1985;69:733–6.
7. Gonin J. The treatment of detached retina by sealing the retinal tears. Arch Ophthalmol 1930; 4:621.
8. Hilton GF, Grizzard WS. Pneumatic retinopexy. A two-step outpatient operation without conjunctival incision. Ophthalmology 1986;93: 626–41.
9. Lincoff HA, Kreissig I, Hahn YS. A temporary balloon buckle for the treatment of small retinal detachments. Ophthalmology 1979;86:586–96.
10. Lincoff HA, McLean JM, Nano H. Cryosurgical Treatment of Retinal Detachment. Trans Am Acad Ophthalmol Otolaryngol 1964;68:412–32.
11. Machemer R, Buettner H, Norton EW, Parel JM. Vitrectomy: a pars plana approach. Trans Am Acad Ophthalmol Otolaryngol 1971;75:813–20.
12. McPherson AR, Schwartz SG, Kuhl DP. Principles of retinal reattachment surgery, in Boyd BF, Boyd S (eds): Retinal and Vitreoretinal Surgery. Mastering the Latest Techniques. Panama, Highlights of Ophthalmology, 2001, 355–91.

13. Michels RG. Scleral buckling methods for rhegmatogenous retinal detachment. Retina 1986:6.

14. Peyman GA, Dodich NA. Experimental vitrectomy. Instrumentation and surgical technique. Arch Ophthalmol 1971;86:548–51.

15. Rosengren B, Osterlin S. Hydrodynamic events in the vitreous space accompanying eye movements. Significance for the pathogenesis of retinal detachment. Ophthalmologica 1976; 173:513–24.

16. Schepens CL, Okamura ID, Brockhurst RJ: The scleral buckling procedures. I. Surgical techniques and management. Arch Ophthalmol 1957; 58:797–811.

17. Schepens CL: A new ophthalmoscope demonstration. Trans Am Acad Ophthalmol Otolaryngol 1947;51:298.

18. Schwartz SG, Kuhl DP, McPherson AR, et al: Twenty-year follow-up for scleral buckling. Arch Ophthalmol 2002;120:325–9.

19. Thompson JT: The effects and action of scleral buckles in the treatment of retinal detachment, in Ryan SJ (ed): Retina. St. Louis: Mosby, 2001, ed 3, pp 1994–2009

20. Williams GA. Aaberg TM. Techniques of scleral buckling. In: Ryan SJ. et al., ells. Retina. 2011 ed. St. Louis: Mosby, 1994:1979–2017.

31

PARS PLANA VITRECTOMY, VITREOUS SUBSTITUTES AND MANAGEMENT OF GIANT RETINAL TEARS

Atul Kumar

PARS PLANA VITRECTOMY

GENERAL CONSIDERATIONS

INTRODUCTION

Pars plana vitrectomy represented an entirely new approach to the treatment of rhegmatogenous RD. It was first reported by Robert Machemer in 1971, who developed the 17-gauge one-port vitrectomy system using a full-function vitreous cutter including infusion cannula. O'Malley and Heinz then developed the three-port vitrectomy system in 1972, which is essentially the same system we are currently using now. There are other instruments that

have made a breakthrough, including the laser system, fluid-air exchange (Steven Charles in 1977), long-acting gas, silicone oil (Paul Cibis in 1962), and heavy liquid. Recently, the 25-gauge vitrectomy system was developed by Fujii, de Juan and colleagues, followed by the similar innovation of the 23-gauge system developed by Eckardt.

Another breakthrough is the bright illumination system with a Xenon light source that can provide bright illumination through narrow light pipe (available in 23 and 25 gauge) and as also in the chandelier system, it allows the surgeon to carry out vitrectomy with the 25-gauge system and to use truly bi-manual techniques.

ADVANTAGE OVER THE CONVENTIONAL SCLERAL BUCKLING

Regardless of tamponade agent, pars plana vitrectomy has three distinct advantages over scleral buckling or pneumatic retinopexy. First, pars plana vitrectomy is the only procedure that directly removes vitreous traction by lysing the vitreous strands adherent to the flap of the horseshoe tear. Scleral buckling only indirectly relieves vitreous traction, and pneumatic retinopexy does not relieve traction at all.

Second, pars plana vitrectomy directly removes vitreous hemorrhage and pigment, clearing the visual axis. It therefore makes cases with proliferative vitreoretinopathy and combined (tractional+rhegmatogenous retinal detachments) operable. In cases with significant vitreous opacity, this allows for better intra-operative visualization and the potential for faster postoperative visual recovery.

Third, pars plana vitrectomy is the only procedure that can reliably achieve complete, intra-operative retinal reattachment. This is attained either by internal drainage of subretinal fluid or by use of perfluorocarbon liquids to displace the subretinal fluid and relieve all the traction because of proliferative vitreoretinopathy. In contrast, scleral buckling with subretinal fluid drainage typically achieves only partial reattachment, while scleral buckling without drainage and pneumatic retinopexy never achieves immediate reattachment. Immediate intraoperative retinal reattachment has improved the prognosis for giant retinal tears, although its importance for uncomplicated primary rhegmatogenous RD is much less significant. Anatomic success rates generally are about 90%. While this may appear to be nearly that of scleral buckling, the outcome is dependent upon case selection. In pseudophakic patients without proliferative vitreoretinopathy, the success rate is approximately 90% with a single operation.

BASIC INSTRUMENTATION FOR PARS PLANA VITRECTOMY

Pars plana vitrectomy requires the most specialized equipment and support staff, and is by far the most expensive of all reattachment procedures.

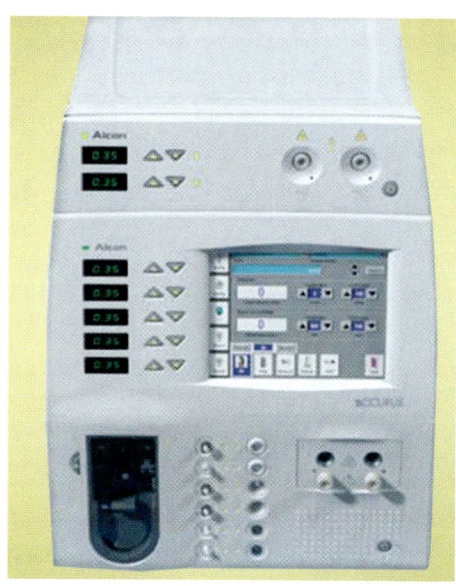

Fig. 31.1 *Vitrectomy systems with inbuilt xenon illumination system*

Essential features of modern vitrectomy system are:

- Vitrectomy systems with VGFI (vented gas fluid infusion system), have inbuilt xenon illumination system (Fig. 31.1).
- Vitrectomy systems now can provide with high speed cutting (2500) and some machines can provide up to 5000 cuts/minute.
- They have a builtin intraocular pressure sensors for smooth infusion flow rate and to keep unwanted fluctuation in intraocular pressure. The VGFI system is used to achieve a pre-set IOP at a push of a button to achieve hemostasis/fluid air exchange.
- For making the port a 20 gauge MVR is used, in case of 23 and 25 gauge system trochar and cannula system are available.

VITRECTOMY CUTTER

There are two different kinds of vitreous cutter, the pneumatic cutter driven by air pressure and the motor-driven cutter (Fig. 31.2). Each has its advantages and disadvantages. The pneumatic cutter driven by air-pressure is light and has minimal vibration, while the motor-driven one has more precise control of the blade motions. Recently developed cutters have a maximum cutting speed limit of as fast as 2,500–5000 rpm

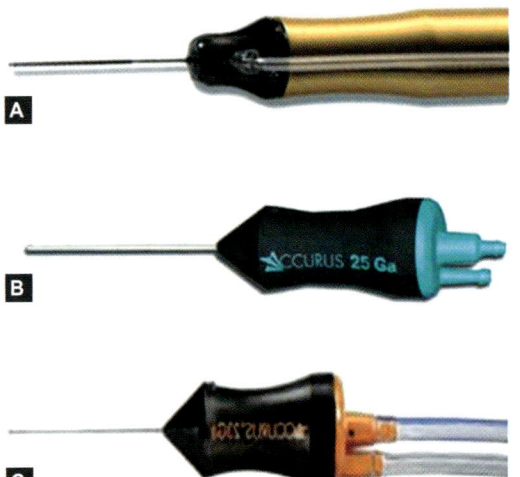

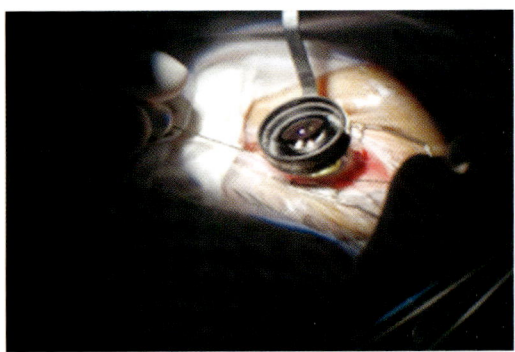

Fig. 31.3 *Volk wide angle contact viewing system*

Fig. 31.2 *Vitrectomy cutters (both electric and pneumatic)*

as in the 20-gauge system. Because of the narrow aperture of the 23-gauge vitreous cutter, the aspiration rate is smaller than that of the 20-gauge cutter. Therefore, the aspiration vacuum is usually set to 500–600 mmHg instead of 200 mmHg to achieve enough aspiration flow.

VIEWING SYSTEM

The viewing system can be classified into two:

1. The contact viewing systems

- Plano-concave irrigating contact lenses: better stereoscopic vision along with higher magnification and smaller field of view).
- Wide angle viewing system e.g. PWL,Volk (Fig. 31.3) and AVI system of lenses provide wide field of view even in small pupil, negates corneal astigmatisms, but the view is minified.

2. The non-contact viewing systems

- BIOM (binocular indirect ophthalmo-microscope) (Fig. 31.4).
- EIBOS (erect indirect binocular ophthalmo-microscope).

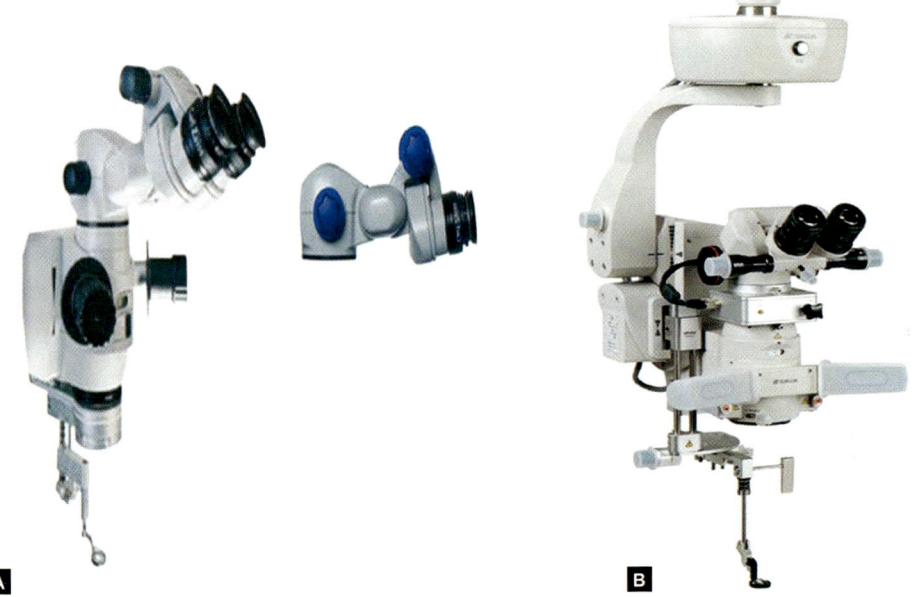

Fig. 31.4 *Non-contact viewing system (BIOM and OFFISS)*

- OFFISS (optical fiber-free intravitreal surgery system) is a new wide-angle viewing system combined with a surgical microscope (Fig. 31.4).

ILLUMINATION SYSTEMS

Recently, a bright illumination system using a xenon light source was developed (Fig. 31.5).

The xenon light source can shine a brighter light than the regular halogen light source and a spherical reflector plays an important role in introducing the bright light to the light fiber. It has a complex design with expensive optics; however, it can introduce uniform illumination without a dark spot in the center of the output pattern, as in the illumination system with a parabolic reflector.

PARS PLANA VITRECTOMY SURGERY

Vitrectomy techniques and intraoperative endolaser photocoagulation allow visual rehabilitation in many eyes that are otherwise untreatable. Discerning the indications and timing for Vitrectomy is increasingly important as the treatment of complications of retinal pathology continues to undergo modification and redefinition.

INDICATIONS OF PARS PLANA VITRECTOMY

Most common indications of PPV include:
- Rhegmatogenous retinal detachment (simple or complicated by PVR).

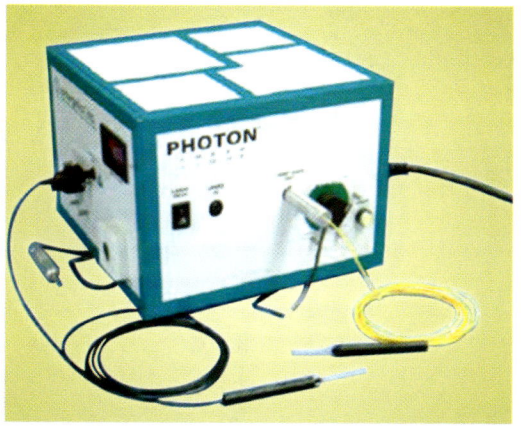

Fig. 31.5 *Illumination system (endoilluminator light probe and chandeliers)*

- Severe non-clearing vitreous hemorrhage (of various etiologies).
- Traction retinal detachment involving the macula; (diabetic patients mainly with or without associated vitreous hemorrhage).
- Combined traction and rhegmatogenous detachment.
- Progressive fibrovascular proliferation.
- Macular hole and ERM.
- Endopthalmitis.
- Posteriorly dislocated IOL/nucleus fragments.
- Retained intraocular foreign body.

Other less common indications in selected cases include dense premacular hemorrhage, ghost cell glaucoma, macular edema with premacular traction, anterior hyaloidal fibrovascular proliferation, and fibrinoid syndrome with retinal detachment, severe vitreous floaters/vitreous membranes secondary to pars planitis.

PPV in diabetic retinopathy. Vitreous surgery addresses several problems of advanced diabetic retinopathy. Media opacities can be removed and elevated retina reattached. More-over, removal of the vitreous has a stabilizing effect on the subsequent development of the proliferative process. In a vitrectomized eye there is no anatomical scaffold which could be used as a matrix for in growth of fibro-vascular tissue into the eye. Relief of traction on retinal vessels may also improve blood flow within these vessels and reduce leakage. In addition, unrestricted circulation of fluid in the vitreous cavity after vitrectomy seems to improve the oxygen supply to the inner retina and prevents accumulation of vasoactive cytokines in the retina. A serious complication of vitrectomy for diabetic retinopathy is the progression of iris rubeosis and the development of neovascular glaucoma. Pathophysiologically two mechanisms are involved in the development of this complication. In eyes with active preretinal neovascularisation these new vessels contribute to the supply of oxygen and nutrients to the inner retina. Surgical removal of these new vessels will aggravate retinal ischemia and stimulate the production of growth factors. It is therefore important to extensively treat the ischemic retina with endolaser, especially in eyes where active preretinal neovascularisations

are surgically removed. If the retina is edematous, laser effects may be difficult to apply. Here, it is helpful to inject perfluorcarbon liquids into the eye. Under perfluorocarbons the application of effective laser treatment to an edematous retina is much easier.

CONVENTIONAL 20 GAUGE OR SMALLER GAUGE?

Classically the surgical system of choice for operating is the conventional 20-gauge vitrectomy system (still considered gold standard by most vitreo retina surgeons), which has come a long way since its inception to the present day pneumatic cutter (light weight and ergonomically designed, capable of cutting at high speed 5000 rpm) all the instruments used for the posterior segment surgery were initially developed as 20-gauge instrumentation and has come a long way now. The armamentarium of 20-gauge is complete and the surgeon feels more secure as it is time tested. The ports are made with 20-gauge micro vitreo retina blades (MVR), for light source an endoillumination fiberoptic light probes are used, for fluid air exchange flute needles are used, silicone tips are very helpful in fluid-air exchange as they cause minimal trauma to the retina and complete fluid air exchange. And the retinopexy is achieved with endophotocoagulation probes which are powered by solid state laser (either diode or Nd:YAG). For the visualisation of the retina during surgery, various lens systems can be used. The most commonly used in teaching institution is the contact wide angle viewing system (Volk lenses) but the disadvantage is that it is to be held by an assistant or it can be placed on a presewn limbal ring, and it has to be coupled with a SDI (stereo diagonal inverter).

Basic steps of pars plana vitrectomy

- Conjunctival peritomy required in 20 g, although it is transconjunctival in smaller gauge surgery.
- There ports are made with MVR blade at a distance from the limbus of 3.0 mm in aphakia, 3.5 mm in pseudophakia and 4.0 mm in phakic patients (after the first port the infusion cannula is connected and checked weather its is indeed in the vitreous cavity).

- This is followed by core vitrectomy with a cut rate of 1500 to 1800 and suction of 150 mmhg.
- An active posterior hyaloid separation can be induced with suction alone up to 150 mmhg with 20 g and higher suction rates required in 23 and 25 g.
- This is followed by peripheral vitrectomy using higher cut rates (2500 to 5000) and low suction 100 mmHg or lesser.
- Any traction/proliferation taken care of and removed by using the cutter and PFCL as an surgical adjuvant.
- After peripheral vitrectomy fluid air exchange is done followed by laser photocoagulation.

Complications

The most important disadvantage of pars plana vitrectomy is its relatively high morbidity for other intraocular structures. This includes trauma to the lens, retina, and optic nerve. Intraocular gas or silicone oil may cause cataract formation in a phakic eye; for this reason, many surgeons are hesitant to use pars plana vitrectomy in phakic detachments. Furthermore, an untreated retinal break will typically cause pars plana vitrectomy to fail. Postoperative positioning requirements are stricter than for scleral buckling and depend on the location of the breaks.

SMALLER GAUGE VITRECTOMY

In the 1980s, Visitec introduced the first 23-gauge cutter for vitreous biopsy and in 1993, Chang presented his own 23-gauge system for vitrectomy. However, the 23-gauge system was not adopted by the surgeons at that time and it was not until the introduction of transconjunctival sutureless entry that such microincisional techniques became popular, first through the work of Eugene De Juan in 2001 with his 25-gauge system and then Claus Eckhardt with his 23-gauge system in 2005.

The limitations that most surgeons faced when the smaller gauge vitrectomy systems surfaced were lower intensity of the endoilluminators, instruments that were flexible and hence posed problems while operating complex conditions like anterior hyaloid trimming, membrane dissections and peeling, and enbloc dissections, as most of the instrumentation was available

only in 20 gauge. Also the surgical time was prolonged due to the port area of the cutter was smaller than the conventional 20-gauge instrument and the duty cycle was poorer, leading to prolonged vitrectomy time. Postoperative hypotony and endophthalmitis were other problems faced due to leaky ports.

Recent developments in the transconjunctival sutureless vitrectomy (TSV) systems have considerably transformed patient management outlook in the field of vitreous surgery. In fact, based on the several reported advantages, TSV is becoming increasingly popular. The vitrectomy incision construction using the trocar and cannula method in the TSV systems differs from the conventional 20-gauge (20-G) vitrectomy incisions in several important aspects; either pre- or intra- or postoperative. It facilitates easy entry, with minimal trauma to the conjunctiva, sclera and the pars plana. *Through-out the surgery, all instrument shafts pass through the sleeve of the cannula.* This minimizes tissue manipulation and micro-trauma due to repeated insertion and removal of instruments. Transconjunctival sutureless vitrectomy has been shown to significantly *decrease the overall operating time compared with conventional 20-G vitrectomy. Reduction in the convalescence period* and the postoperative

inflammatory response has been reported. The concept of port based flow limitation has been hypothesized to increase the safety margin of this procedure. It decreases vitreous manipulation during the procedure and lowers the risk of drag on the peripheral retina, as compared with a larger port of 20-G system (Fig. 31.6).

Original 23-gauge system developed by Claus Eckhardt MD required two separate steps for incision creation and micro-cannula insertion. Recently developed 23-gauge vitrectomy system (Alcon) that provides simplified one-step incision and entry. It has a trocar-cannula design similar to the Alcon 25-gauge system, with a sharp and solid trocar blade. Alcon's new 23-gauge system also has machined disposable titanium cannulas which reduce friction against the metal instrument shafts. The smoother movement provides a higher level of control when working close to the retina surface, Moreover, the system's vitreous cutter includes many innovative features which enable more precise control and easier manipulation of the probe in vitrectomy procedures. *The 23-gauge vitrectomy probe is an outstanding probe, with a cut rate of 5000 cuts per minute.* The probe is stiffer and less flexible and the port is closer to the tip. I have found the cutting performance to be better than that of the 20-gauge.

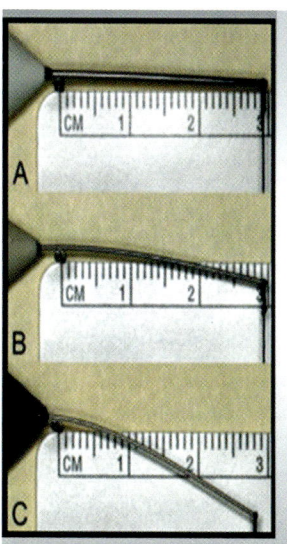

Vitrector flexibility

The extreme flexibility of 25-G cutters compared to 20 and 23-G cutters is demonstrated a syringe filled with 20 ml of water was suspended from the cutter port via a 6-0 silk suture on each of a

A : 20-gauge,
B : 23-g and
C : 25-g cutter held
    horizontally

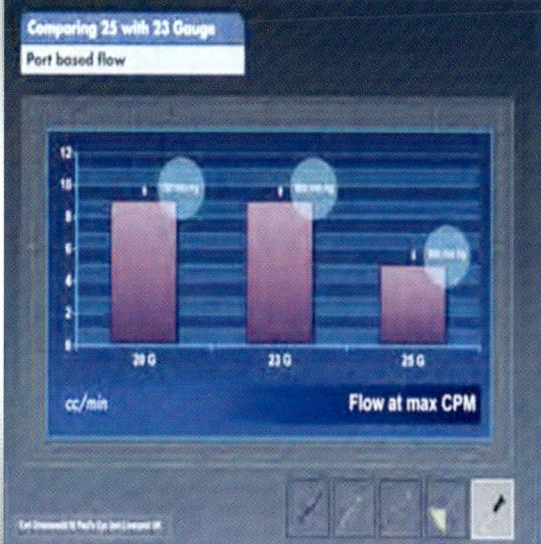

Fig. 31.6 *Vitrector flexibility and port based flow parameters of various gauge cutters*

It has been noted that the *greater proximity of the probe's port to its tip* makes it easier to shave tissue close to the surface of the retina and the smaller tip enables access into smaller spaces than is possible with 20-gauge. Furthermore, the high speed cutting reduces the traction on the retina as it is being cut and can reduce the need for scissors in the eye. In addition, the 23-gauge light probe is designed to be stiffer and provide greater illumination. It couples a 20-gauge fiber with a 23-gauge light fiber in the handle. The 23-gauge endo laser probe is also stiffer than the 25-gauge instrument (Fig. 31.7). Other additions include the disposable scissors and forceps. The ILM forceps are the same platform as the 25-gauge variety but with a stiffer shaft. There are also 23-gauge and 25-gauge needles, multi-gauge viscous fluid injection, re-usable handheld instruments, a wide angle endoilluminator, to complement the system.

Tips for 23–25 G TSV

- Displacement of conjunctiva helpful (misalign conjunctival and scleral wounds).
- Try not to rotate trocars will damage pars plana epithelium and vitreous base.

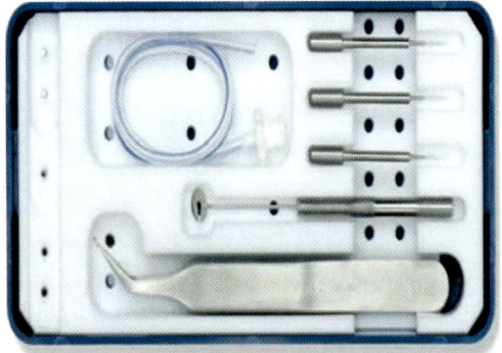

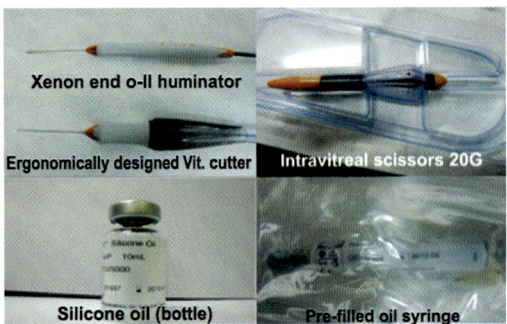

Xenon end o-II huminator

Ergonomically designed Vit. cutter   Intravitreal scissors 20G

Silicone oil (bottle)   Pre-filled oil syringe

Fig. 31.7 *Instrumentation used in 23-gauge vitrectomy*

- Avoid subconjunctival antibiotics near open sclerotomies.
- Conjunctival massaging may be avoided at end of surgery; creates more incidence of vitreous incarceration and leak.
- Use of chandelier light (e.g. Xenon source) useful to increase illumination.

Vitrectomy in advanced diabetic eye disease, rhegmatogenous retinal detachment with severe proliferative vitreoretinopathy are certainly more complex than simple vitreous hemorrhage, as there are tractional bands and tractional retinal detachment, fibrovascular membranes, adherent hyaloid, macular edema that is secondary to vitreomacular traction and may require 20-gauge instrumentation, however with the improving 'learning curve' of the surgeons there is a gradual shift to MIVS.

Using the 23- and 25-gauge microincision vitrectomy surgery most of these complex cases can be operated with success comparable to the conventional 20-gauge system. The clearing of the hemorrhage, the dissection, peeling and trimming of the fibrovascular membranes can be achieved by the cutter and the available 23-gauge disposable instrumentation. Another important aspect of treating complex retinal condition while performing vitreous surgery is endophotocoagulation, and this has also seen some innovations in the form of directional probes to easily reach the area of interest and the solid state laser with pulse modes are also available now.

The wide range of disposable Grieshaber Revolution DSP MIVS line, we have been able to peel tractional membranes, diabetic membranes, PVR membranes and ILMs with as much ease as we did with 20-gauge reusable instruments (Fig. 31.8).

A few years ago, 25 G surgery was often associated with significant hypotony and wound leak; recent surgical modifications and instrument design enhancements, however, have resulted in a very low incidence of both hypotony and wound suturing. More recently, Dr Rizzo has developed an oblique incision which is made parallel instead of perpendicular to the sclera fibers. It therefore avoids cutting

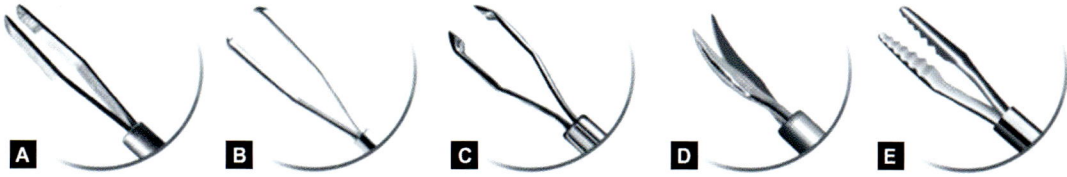

Fig. 31.8 *Newer instrumentation in vitrectomy: (A) end gripping; (B) ILM peeling forceps; (C) asymmetric forceps; (D) intra vitreal scissors; and (E) end opening forceps*

the scleral fibers, which in turn allows the wound to close more efficiently (Fig. 31.9).

Until recently, 25 G instruments were used only to perform macular surgery. It was found that the vitrectors were less efficient than the larger gauge instruments; thus, vitreous removal, although possible, was a time-consuming process. With the new 25 G+ vitrectors, however, it is now possible to gain the same, if not better, aspiration and cutting rates than those achieved with bigger calibre instruments, and the improved duty cycle makes it possible to achieve exceptional performance in retinal pathologies where proximity to the retina is required, a small vitrector is in fact favourable. For example, in fibrovascular proliferations, it is possible to use

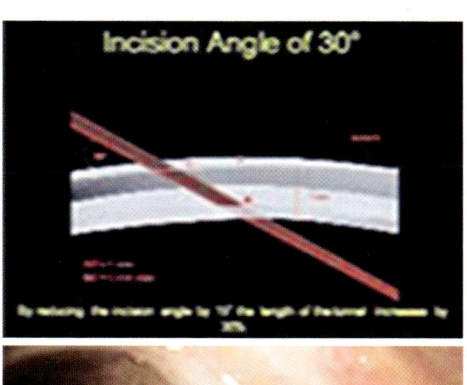

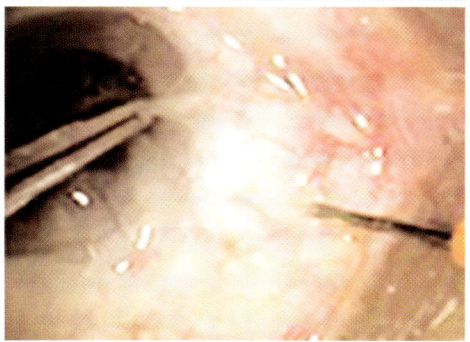

Fig. 31.9 *Art of wound construction for 23-gauge vitrectomy*

25 G instruments successfully to remove epiretinal membrane tissue without the need for either numerous instrument changes or difficult bimanual maneuvres.

The biggest inconvenience that was encountered with 25 G instruments is, without a doubt, the tool flexure, which made working in the periphery of the vitreous chamber very difficult, and for several years caused 25 G surgery to be restricted to uncomplicated cases of vitreous and macular surgery. Thankfully, however, with today's stiffer and more durable instruments, the number of conditions that can be treated with this minimally invasive approach is growing. In fact, results from the American Society of Retina. Specialists Preferences and Trends (ASRS PAT) annual survey show that the minimally invasive technique is gaining favour rapidly in the US. In 2007, the survey revealed that 70% of vitreoretinal surgeons use 25 G technology occasionally and 25% used it in more than 75% of their cases.

NEWER DEVELOPMENTS IN SMALL GAUGE VITRECTOMY

Y. Oshima et al developed a prototype pneumatic 27-gauge cutter in collaboration with DORC, the port area of the cutter is wider than that of commercially available 25-gauge cutters. A shorter shaft provides rigidity similar to a conventional 25-gauge. He further claims that 27-gauge system offers several advantages over the currently widely used 23- and 25-gauge systems. Using the 27-gauge system removes concerns about complications related to wound-sealing. In a pilot study approved by the institutional review board, they have performed 27-gauge vitrectomy in 28 eyes of 28 patients for a variety of vitreo-retinal diseases, including epiretinal membrane proliferation, idiopathic

macular hole, diabetic vitreous hemorrhage with fibrovascular membrane proliferation, and nonclearing vitreous opacity. The settings for 27-gauge vitrectomy were similar to that for 23- and 25-gauge instrumentations.

CONCLUSION

The current microincision vitrectomy surgery (MIVS) with 25- or 23-gauge instrumentation has simplified the vitrectomy procedure and offers numerous potential advantages over traditional 20-gauge surgery including shorter operating time, reduced corneal astigmatism, diminished conjunctival scaring, less postoperative inflammation, improved patient comfort, and earlier visual recovery, compared to the conventional 20-gauge vitrectomy.

VITREOUS SUBSTITUTES

VITREOUS HUMOR AND RETINAL DETACHMENT

VITREOUS HUMOR

In order to better understand the role of vitreous substitutes, it is important to first understand the basic properties of the vitreous.

The vitreous body is the clear substance present in the posterior portion of the eye, behind the lens. It is approximately 99% water by weight and is a paucicellular natural hydrogel that is made up primarily of unbranched Type II collagen fibrils and hyaluronic acid. Within the vitreous body, the non-crosslinked collagen forms a semi-random polymer network that runs from one end of the vitreous cavity to the other. Hyaluronic acid is interspersed within the collagen polymer network and is also present in regions of liquefied vitreous. Hyaluronic acid is a glycosaminoglycan, made up of two alternating monosaccharides (N-acetylglucosamine and glucuronic acid, linked by glycoside bonds), and forms a 1,000–10,000 MW unbranched, coiled polyanion that has a high hydrated specific volume (2,000–3,000 cc/g). The concentration of hyaluronic acid varies from 0.03 to 0.10% in human vitreous.

The vitreous is non-uniform in density. Cloquet's canal, the central portion of the vitreous that is present anterior to the optic nerve, frequently contains thin, multilayered, fenestrated sheaths of basal lamina tissue. In addition, there is a 100–200 µm-thick layer of solid cortical gel adjacent to the retina, ciliary body, and lens. The vitreous is firmly attached to the anterior retina at the vitreous base, where collagen fibers penetrate the retina and attach to the basement membrane of the ciliary epithelium and peripheral retinal pigment epithelium (RPE). The retina is otherwise in contact with the vitreous along its inner surface, at the internal limiting membrane.

ROLE OF THE VITREOUS IN RHEGMATOGENOUS RETINAL DETACHMENTS

As a person ages, the vitreous body normally undergoes a non-uniform transition from a gel like substance in a young child to a more fluid-like substance in an older adult. Associated with this transition is a number of vision threatening phenomena such as macular holes, retinal tears, retinal detachments, and vitreous hemorrhage. The mechanism for these phenomena is thought to involve traction of the liquefying vitreous gel on the retina and retinal vessels when convective currents are created in the vitreous by eye movements. During the acute phase of this separation (known as a posterior vitreous detachment or PVD), the vitreous may be abnormally attached to the retina at some focal point. The vitreous will naturally move within the eye during normal eye movement and in the process can create a tear or hole in the retina at the point of adhesion. This retinal tear should be repaired promptly, using laser or cryopexy, as it can lead to retinal detachment with the risk of blindness. Treatment of a retinal detachment involves relieving the traction and blocking egress of fluid through the hole by re-approximation of the retina to the underlying tissues. An increasingly common technique to achieve successful re-attachment of the retina is vitrectomy surgery.

VITRECTOMY AND VITREOUS SUBSTITUTES AND ADJUVANTS

When a patient undergoes a vitrectomy, much of the vitreous is removed by using aspiration

and cutting techniques to relieve the traction on the retina. The eye is then typically filled with air or a perfluorinated hydrocarbon, and the retina is re-attached to the back of the eye by surface tension. Thermal laser photo-coagulation is then applied around any retinal tears or holes to create an inflammatory scar. Finally, a vitreous substitute is injected into the eye to maintain the retina in position. Vitreous substitutes in common use include sulfur hexafluoride gas (SF6), n-perfluorpropane gas (C3F8), air, and polydimethylsiloxane (silicone oil). The role of each substance shall be discussed in detail.

GASES

Frequently a gas (air, sulfur hexafluoride, or n-perfluoropropane) is introduced into the eye to hold the retina against the back of the eye (the RPE) until a scar is formed around the retinal tear, between the retina and the underlying tissue. This process can take weeks, and during this time, the installed compound must remain in contact with the retinal hole. For this reason, patients who have received intraocular gas are usually positioned for a week or more in a facedown position that many find difficult to maintain. Obviously, holes located in the inferior retina are not easily amenable to closure by intraocular gas.

THE PHYSICS OF INTRAOCULAR GAS AND PERFLUORINATED SMALL-MOLECULE LIQUIDS

A rigorous evaluation of the behavior of intra-ocular gas has recently been conducted and the primary findings are summarized here. Although it might seem natural to consider buoyancy forces when gas bubbles are immersed in liquids, this concept is applicable only in systems where the bubble is much smaller than the area of detached retina. For larger injected gas volumes, as is typically used in retinal re-attachment procedures, the re-adhesion force actually arises from the gas-liquid surface tension of a thin fluid film wetting the detached flap. Consider the typical case of a large gas bubble that envelops the entire tear. "Since the pressure inside the gas phase is uniform, the gas exerts equal pressures on both sides of the retinal flap. Because the gas bubble has risen to

the posterior of the inverted eye, there is no longer a buoyant force on the flap, which simply hangs inside a pocket of gas. However, a re-adhesion force arises from the surface tension of the wedge-shaped liquid film covering retina-RPE juncture at the base of the detached flap."

The situation might be better visualized if you consider an eye containing a large amount of injected gas as simply a vessel with gas in the upper portion and liquid in the lower portion of the vessel. A retinal flap tear at the top of the vessel hangs into the gas phase and clearly experiences no buoyancy force. On the other hand, re-approximating the retina to the top of the vessel allows the gas within the vessel to assume a more spherical shape, and thus, reduce the energy of the system (energy = surface tension time surface area). *In summary,* although the gas bubble clearly must be in contact with the hole or tear in order to seal it, surface tension is responsible for keeping the retina re-approximated to the back of the eye. The gas only provides a gas-liquid interface and the related surface tension that seals the hole or tears in the retina. If we take into account the facts that, because of the hydrogen bonding of water molecules, the surface tension at the air-gas interface is one of the highest in nature (72 mN/m) and that gases absorb into the circulation, leaving minimal residue, it will be difficult to find a better compound to repair simple, superior retinal detachments. This is particularly true in patients who can appropriately position themselves.

In order to improve on intraocular gases, compounds must reduce the incidence of post-operative cataract formation, re-detachment of the retina from PVR, transient ocular hypertension, or the need for extensive face-down positioning.

Physical characteristics of gases

Physical characteristics of gases are summarized in Table 31.1.

SILICONE OILS

Paul Cibis, of St. Louis, was responsible for the early popularity of intraocular silicone oil. John

Table 31.1 *Physical characteristics of gases*

Gas	Purity	Expansion	Longevity (days)	Non expansile concentration
C3F8	99.7	3.3	30–35	14%
SF6	99.9	2.0	10–14	18%
Air	—	0	5–7	
Xe	99.995	0	1	—

Scott used silicone oil as an instrument to separate membranes and push the retina back, without vitrectomy. It was Haut who first combined use of silicone oil as internal tamponade after vitrectomy. Zivojnovic popularized this technique and contributed immensely to its successful usage by defining its role clearly. The observations of Reidel et. al defined the complications of intravitreal silicone oil and aided in the purification of the material and production of a silicone oil with more homogeneous chain length, thereby reducing emulsification significantly.

PROPERTIES OF SILICONE OILS

Silicone oils are polymers of a number of molecular weights of polydimethylsiloxane. Differences among silicone oils are determined by the length of the polymer, which affects the viscocity and the hydrocarbon radicals, which constitute the side groups of the polymer. It is not miscible with water. Silicone oil is transparent and has a refractive index of 1.40, which is higher than that of vitreous. Hence, the optics of silicone oil filled eye changes. In the phakic eye, if the silicone globule is in contact with the lens and the anterior surface of the globule is thus concave, a hyperopic change to about +6 D is induced. Since the front of the silicone globule is convex in an aphakic eye, the refractive power of the eye is increased such that the hyperopia is reduced. The convex anterior surface of the silicone oil can be altered by the position of the head, thus making it difficult to correct an aphakic silicone oil filled eye by utilizing a spectacle lens or contact lens.

The viscocity of silicone oil is designated in centistokes. The viscocity of a specific silicone oil is determined most importantly by the average molecular weight and the entanglement of individual strands. High-viscosity silicone oils have been speculated, less likely, to undergo emulsification. A 1000 centistokes silicone oil with an average molecular weight of 30,000 daltons has 403 such repeating units. Silicone oil of 5000 Centistokes has a molecular weight of 50,000 daltons and 673 repeating units. Most clinical studies have been performed with 1000 and 5000 Centistoke silicone oils. Although higher Centistoke silicone oil may reduce the risk of emulsification, they are more difficult to insert and remove from the eye.

The main purpose of silicone oil is to permit long-term tamponade of the retina. Its surface tension is significantly less than a gas-water interface. Because it has a specific gravity of approximately 0.971 (less than that of water), it produces a buoyant force within the eye. This buoyant force is only one-third of that of the pressure produced by a gas bubble, which may provide a helpful force in maintaining reattachment of the superior retina if it is free of traction but is insufficient to resist radially directed tractional forces on the retina. There are other mechanisms by which intravitreal silicone oil can deter redetachment. The presence of silicone globule in close proximity to the surface of the retina may impose a redirection of tractional forces, so that they are realigned parallel to the retina (tangential) and are correspondingly less effective than radially transmitted traction. When a large silicone globule occupies the vitreous cavity, the posterior retinal surface is covered by only a thin layer of aqueous. Perhaps under these conditions, intraocular fluid currents are not sufficient to redetach the retina unless the traction is significant.

Long-term tamponade force is produced primarily by interfascial surface tension. It is important to avoid blood and surgical debris within the eye, in order to maintain the highest possible surface tension. The silicone oil bubble has the ability to produce a tamponade effect as well as to compartmentalize the eye. The interfascial tension of the silicone oil with water forms a bubble that does not easily migrate through open holes. The blockage of open retinal holes prevents passage of fluid into the

subretinal space and may allow the retinal pigment epithelium to pump out any residual fluid. Because it is impossible to completely fill the eye with silicone oil, there is always an inferior space filled with vitreous fluid, having restricted movement. Occasionally, inferior open holes close spontaneously because the pigment epithelium can remove fluid with enough rapidity to overcome the diminished fluid currents, thereby resulting in spontaneous retinal reattachment. This restricted fluid space can also harbour the potential for perisilicone proliferation. The small remaining fluid cavity gradually concentrates proteins and other factors that may stimulate tissue proliferation, thereby explaining the propensity for reproliferation in oil-filled eyes treated for retinal detachments.

SURGICAL TECHNIQUE

A standard three port vitrectomy is done with the goal of removing all formed vitreous. It is of extreme importance that all retinal traction be released and the retina be completely reattached before the use of silicone oil. The PFCLs can be useful in producing traction in the posterior pole and stabilizing the anterior retina, to facilitate dissection of membranes. PFCLs may be removed before the gas exchange or during fluid-air exchange. An inferior iridectomy (Ando's PI) is performed in aphakic eyes, which may also be beneficial in eyes with a posterior chamber intraocular lens if zonular rupture is suspected. Extremely high buckles prevent the silicone oil from forming a proper tamponade in areas posterior to the buckle, and therefore should be avoided. Pre-existing very high buckles may need to be removed. Following reattachment of the retina by the fluid-air exchange and endolaser photocoagulation, the silicone oil is infused into the eye through 20 gauge thin walled cannula attached to the silicone pump. Fluid silicone oil exchange also can be done. In eyes where PFCL is used, direct PFCL silicone oil exchange is done. The interface between the two liquids is well made out, and this avoids the unnecessary step of PFCL air exchange. This also eliminates the miosis, corneal descemet's folds and other visualisation problems that go with an air filled eye. The eye should be left normotensive or slightly soft at the end of the procedure. The eye must be relatively soft before this maneuver to avoid migration of BSS posteriorly.

SILICONE OIL REMOVAL

The technique of oil removal is relatively simple. A formal three port vitrectomy is favourable as any residual or recurrent preretinal membranes or other media opacities can be removed. Balanced salt solution is infused through the pars plana using the infusion cannula. In aphakic patients, where additional surgery is not required, a small corneal incision made by the MVR blade is sufficient to allow the egress of the oil. An 18 or 19 gauge thin-walled needle inserted through the pars plana and attached by a small piece of tubing to a 60 ml syringe allows generation of sufficient suction force to evacuate oil in phakic or pseudophakic eyes. Mechanised viscous fluid extractors can also be used. Silicone oil tends to be trapped in the vitreous base and under the iris and in membranes. Flute needle wash out of small bubbles of silicone oil may need to be done for a long time. However, total removal of all oil traces is never possible. The minimal time after which silicone oil can be removed is considered to be 3 weeks. In general, it is preferred that the silicone oil be removed by 3 to 6 months postoperatively and even earlier. There are, however, several cases in which silicone liquid has remained in eyes for several years.

INDICATIONS FOR SILICONE OIL USE

1. Proliferative vitreoretinopathy (PVR)

Rhegmatogenous retinal detachments complicated by PVR constitute the major group of eyes in which silicone oil could be of some benefit. These eyes exhibit a propensity for reproliferation that has resulted in the anatomical success rate of only 40 to 70%. In general, perfluoropropane is indicated in most patients as a primary procedure for severe PVR. The use of C3F8 helps avoid a second surgery for oil removal and results in similar or slightly better results in eyes untreated with previous vitrectomy. Silicone oil should be considered in patients if previous vitrectomy has not achieved

retinal reattachment. One- eyed patients can regain mobility faster with silicone oil. It may be preferable in patients who are not able to position themselves. In eyes with an intraocular pressure less than 5 mmHg and recurrent severe retinal detachment, silicone oil may be preferred. Despite the potential benefits, because of its buoyancy it rises to the superior pole of the vitreous cavity and is thus most effective when a retinal tear detachment is located superiorly and is less effective for inferior lesions. Consequently, the inferior quadrants in which PVR also tends to be most severe, are usually the locus of persistent or recurrent detachments following silicone oil injection. Redetachment has obvious consequences for visual function and may also secondarily precipitate lens and corneal complications by forcing the intravitreally placed silicone globule anteriorly. Buckling of an inferior tear, in conjunction with intravitreally placed silicone oil, is advocated so that the silicone globule, deformed by the buckle, will contact the retinal tear.

The 20% incidence of retinal detachment with oil removal is similar to the ultimate retinal detachment rate in eyes with oil retention. Silicone oil removal may, however, help in avoiding long-term corneal and retinal complications and often results in immediate improvement in visual acuity. The oil removal operation can be combined with further surgery to peel off any residual or reproliferated membranes. Silicone oil removal should not be considered a simple procedure. A thorough evaluation of the retina pre- and intraoperatively is needed to look for (1) recurrent preretinal fibrosis, (2) areas of shallow detachments especially in the periphery that can be easily missed, (3) open retinal breaks that may not cause retinal detachment in the presence of silicone oil but may produce the same following its removal. Careful removal of reformed membranes, and treatment of identified retinal breaks helps to reduce incidence of recurrent retinal detachment following silicone oil removal. The thoroughness of initial vitrectomy, (especially peripheral traction relief), very often dictates the type of recurrence that occur under silicone oil. In the presence of significant

recurrence, further surgery is done under silicone oil to remove the traction and reattach the retina. In this case a silicone oil filled syringe is connected to the infusion cannula to top up the eye whenever needed. The silicone oil study was a multicenter, randomized clinical trial supported by the National Eye Institute, Bethesda, Maryland.

The outcome of the study has been published as several reports. Silicone oil tamponade has been found to be superior to sulfur hexafluoride, but when compared to perfluoro propane gas (C3F8), silicone oil had similar anatomic and functional results. Abnormalities in intraocular pressure postoperatively were noted both in silicone oil and C3F8 groups. In eyes needing relaxing retinotomy also, C3F8 was found to be as effective as silicone oil. Removal of silicone oil was found to lead to increased likelihood of improved vision as well as recurrent retinal detachment. Oil removed eyes in general showed a trend towards reduced incidence of complications. Corneal abnormalities were noted in both gas and oil filled eyes.

2. Proliferative diabetic retinopathy

Vitrectomy used with aggressive sectioning and removal of fibrovascular membranes, endophotocoagulation and improved case selection result in 70 to 80% anatomical success rate in eyes with proliferative diabetic retinopathy, vitreous hemorrhage or localized retinal detachment. The ability of silicone oil to compartmentalize the eye and prevent or at least attenuate the passage of angiogenic factors into the anterior segment can produce regression of the anterior neovascularization in many eyes. There is evidence that it acts as a diffusion-convection barrier to oxygen, an effect that is postulated to alter the stimulus for neovascularization. Stabilization or regression of rubeosis iridis can occur in up to 80% cases. Nevertheless, an effect on the anterior segment neovascularization has not always been observed and may be dependent on factors such as the degree of filling. However, the improvement in the anterior segment frequently does not correlate with posterior segment changes and often there is reproliferation of fibrovascular tissue behind the silicone oil. To

avoid reproliferation, all bleeding sites must be sealed. Hemorrhage behind silicone oil will usually result in reproliferation leading to recurrent hole formation. Silicone oil has been found to be useful in eyes with attached retinas in which all proliferative tissue has been removed but continued hemorrhage is a consequence of rubeosis iridis. These eyes may respond to oil injection and often have the potential for useful vision, although silicone oil cannot be removed because rubeosis will recur. Silicone oil is also useful in the management of severe tractional retinal detachment secondary to anterior hyaloid proliferation. Extensive retinotomies may be required necessitating the use of silicone oil.

3. Giant Retinal tears

Cibis described the use of silicone oil to unfold the posterior edge of a giant tear. Silicone oil was found to work well as an intraocular device to unfold the retina and a success rate of approximately 85% were reported. A fluid silicone exchange was done, allowing manipulation of the posterior flap under the oil as it entered the eye, subretinal fluid was drained through retinotomies or by a flute needle from under the retinal flap. The introduction of PFCL obviates the need to use silicone oil for the purpose of reattaching the retina intraoperatively, although it still is useful for the long-term tamponade postoperatively.

4. Trauma

Acutely injured eyes with unstable scleral wounds, hemorrhagic choroidal and retinal detachment, vitreous hemorrhage and incarcerated retina having propensity for intraocular fibrous proliferation may benefit from silicone oil injection. Silicone oil placed in the vitreous cavity stabilizes the ocular wound and helps in avoiding extension of the hemorrhagic choroidal detachments. It may also be useful in cases of ocular injuries resulting in massive choroidal and ciliary body detach-ment and hypotony. It stabilizes the intraocular pressure and avoids postoperative hypotony that may eventually lead to phthisis bulbi. Severely traumatised eyes with traumatic PVR and retinal detachment often need extensive relaxing retinotomies and hence benefit by long-term tamponade with silicone oil.

5. Retinal detachment in acquired immunodeficiency syndrome (AIDS)

The use of silicone oil in detachments, associated with cytomegalo virus (CMV) retinitis, has been shown to be effective for anatomical correction and in many cases can preserve some degree of functional vision. The surgical technique is essentially same, however, the type of complications encountered may require some deviations. A pars plana vitrectomy is done. Relatively younger patients do not have posterior vitreous detachments. Cortical vitreous is removed utilizing silicone-tipped flute cannula. In areas of necrotic retina, it may be safer to circumcise the adherent cortical vitreous. Internal drainage is done either utilizing a preexisting hole or by making a retinotomy in detached retina. The retina is reattached utilizing fluid-air exchange. Endophotocoagulation may be done to surround retinal breaks, retinotomy and areas of severely necrotic retina. Subsequently, air-silicone exchange is done. Despite anatomical success, optic atrophy may occur and result in severe visual loss. It is most likely due to viral infection, although the possibility that silicone oil may play some role has not been conclusively excluded.

6. Retinal detachments due to coloboma choroids

Retinal detachment caused by coloboma of the choroid are attributable to breaks located in the diaphanous retinal tissue located in the colobomatous area. These are difficult to directly close because of the lack of retinal pigment epithelium and choroid. Retinopexy is not effective and buckling is very difficult. Hence, vitrectomy with silicone oil tamponade and endolaser along the colobomatous margin serve to isolate the colobomatous area from the rest of the retina.

COMPLICATIONS OF SILICONE OIL

1. *Emulsification:* Emulsification probably occurs because of the shearing effect created by the difference between the velocity of movement

of the silicone bubble and that of the eye and the fluid meniscus around the silicone bubble. The protein concentrated in the vitreous fluid may contribute to the shearing effect. It occurs in variably in all cases.

2. *Keratopathy:* Band keratopathy or stromal opacification may occur in 30% cases. Band keratopathy responds well to debridement of the cornea with diluted disodium ethylene-diaminetetraacetic acid (EDTA), with application of a bandage lens postoperatively. Stromal opacification is treated by corneal transplant, in eyes with visual potential. Corneal transplant is usually carried out at the time of silicone oil removal.

3. *Cataract:* All phakic eyes containing intravitreal silicone oil develop cataracts. This is related to contact between the silicone globule and the posterior lens capsule and the resulting mechanical obstruction to diffusion of nutrients. The incidence of cataract is most pronounced between 6 and 18 months after surgery and opacification can develop or progress even after silicone withdrawal.

4. *Pupillary block:* The inferior iridectomy by Ando has reduced the incidence of pupillary block, however, the inferior iridectomies close in the postoperative period from iris retraction and recurrent proliferation of tissue at the vitreous base. Postoperative closure of peripheral iridectomy is highly correlated with forward oil migration and occurs most frequently in eyes with proliferative diabetic retinopathy. Silicone oil can migrate into the anterior chamber even in phakic eyes. This occurs through unsuspected zonular dehiscences. If small, this can be ignored and be removed along with the main bubble later. Removal of the bubble from the anterior chamber alone usually is followed by the migration of oil into anterior chamber from the main bubble.

5. *Glaucoma:* Glaucoma occurs in 3 : 5% cases. Since the advent of purified oil, its incidence has decreased. When used in eyes that have had previous procedures, there is presumably some destruction of the ciliary body which reduces the production of intraocular fluid.

6. *Perisilicone proliferation and macular pucker:* Macular pucker has been reported to occur in approximately 30% cases. Membranes should be removed at the time of oil removal.

SILICONE OIL AS INTRAOPERATIVE TOOL

Silicone oil has been used during pars plana vitrectomy to reposition retina, to stabilize the retina during the removal of epiretinal membranes, and to unroll the flaps of retinal tears. As a liquid having a density lower than water (specific gravity of 0.97), it lacks the physical properties that, with the patient in supine position, would provide a downward force to flatten the retina and collapse the subretinal space or unroll the retinal tear in a posterior to anterior direction. Fluorosilicone, because of its high specific gravity of 1.28, has been advocated as an alternative intraoperative tool. Perfluorocarbon liquids have replaced fluorosilicone liquids as intraoperative tools because of their favourable physical properties.

PERFLUOROCARBON LIQUIDS (PFCL)

Low viscosity liquid perfluorocarbons are optically clear compounds, having a specific gravity higher than saline, which make them a useful surgical tool for flattening a detached retina, intraoperatively. Since their initial use in vitreous surgery as a surgical tamponade in 1987, they have been found to be useful in the management of complex vitreoretinal conditions.

PROPERTIES

Several low viscosity PFCLs have been studied for their potential intraoperative use. These include, perfluoro-tributylamine (C12F27N), perfluoro-decalin (C10F18), perfluoro-phenanthrene (C14F24), perfluoro-ethylcyclo-hexamine (C8F16), for alkyl AC-6, perfluoro-octylbromide and perfluoro-n-octane (C8F18). Perfluoro-n-octane, perfluoro-tributylamine, perfluoro-decalin and perfluorophenanthrene are the liquid perfluorocarbons currently in use. They are optically clear with indices of refraction similar to that of water. Hence, no optical aberrations occur when working through PFCLs. An interface can be visualized between

the PFCL and saline, since they are immiscible. Visualizing the interface is important as it facilitates the complete removal of PFCL and reduces the incidence of residual droplets in the vitreous cavity. The specific gravity of PFCL is nearly twice that of water. Thus, the tamponade force exerted by PFCL against retina is considerably greater than that exerted by equivalent volume of fluoro-silicone oil. This characteristic makes it possible for the PFCL to flatten the retina intraoperatively. The inter-fascial tension of PFCL with water is roughly equivalent to that of silicone oil and the material tends to be cohesive, so that liquid remains in one large bubble. The surface tension though not as pronounced as long acting gas still provides some deterrence to passage of PFCL through a break. The low viscosity of PFCL (0.8 to 8 Centistokes at 25°C vs 1000 to 5000 Centistokes at 25° C of silicone oil) facilitates easy introduction and removal with small gauge instruments and allows them to demonstrate areas of residual traction. PFCLs have variable vapour pressures. A higher vapour pressure is desirable because a residual layer of PFCL, on the surface of retina, will evaporate during fluid-air exchange, thus reducing the incidence of residual droplets. The boiling point of PFCL exceeds that of saline and this allows safe endophotocoagulation without causing vaporization.

Perfluoro-n-octane is the preferred PFCL. It is obtained as a highly purified compound. It does not contain protonated impurities (NMR spectroscopy analysis). The major impurities that could be present in PFCLs are hydrogen containing and would result from the incomplete fluorination of the hydrocarbon precursor; hydrogen-containing impurities are suspected to cause tissue reactivity. In addition to being free of detectable impurities, it can also be manufactured with a uniformity of 99.9%. It has a relatively lower boiling point and higher vapour pressure than do other PFCLs.

The high stability of the carbon-fluorine bond in a PFCL can render the liquid virtually inert. Experience with PFCLs as artificial blood replacements also suggests that they are biologically inert. Various studies, evaluating short-term tolerance of different PFCLs have not shown electro-physiologic or morphologic evidences of retinal toxicity for as long as 48 hours. Electron microscopic studies of intravitreal PFCLs have not shown any toxicity in pig eyes for a period up to 3 hours. Perfluoro-phenanthrene has shown reduced incidence of dispersion into small droplets during long-term tamponade and appears to be well tolerated intravitreally up to 1 week and perhaps longer.

Experimental extended vitreous replacement with perfluoro-n-octane, in rabbit eyes, elicited a macrophage response with epiretinal membrane formation on the surface of retina. Narrowing of the outer plexiform layer and thinning of the outer nuclear layer, in the inferior retina, was observed as the PFCL remained longer in the eye. These changes suggest the mechanical effect of PFCL. Similar changes, due to pressure-induced mechanism, have been observed in the superior retina of rabbit eyes filled with silicone oil. Small droplets of perfluoro-n-octane injected into the vitreous cavity of rabbit elicited mild macrophage response but no retinal alterations at 6 months. Clinically, no observable inflammatory effects have been seen after 6 months, in patients with residual PFCL droplets. Nevertheless, whether these small droplets can induce intraocular proliferation is unknown and the long-term effects of residual PFCLs are uncertain.

In general, PFCLs are used as intraoperative tools and not as postoperative tamponade agents, in view of the propensity for emulsi-fication, although perfluorophenanthrene has been used as a short-term tamponading agent.

INDICATIONS FOR USE OF PFCL

1. Proliferative vitreoretinopathy (PVR)

The use of PFCLs in the management of retinal detachment complicated by severe degrees of PVR was first described by Chang. Subsequent studies found a reattachment rate of 78% and 96.5% with the use of PFCL. These results compare favourably with the silicone study group. The surgical technique in most of these cases includes removal of the crystalline lens to allow anterior dissection. Intraocular lenses are left in place. A scleral buckle or encircling band is used to support the vitreous base. In eyes with

anterior PVR, PFCLs open peripheral folds by pulling the peripheral retina posteriorly. This action allows better visualization of the membranes and therefore their complete removal. The anterior proliferations in the vitreous base are better defined when the posterior retina is immobilized by PFCL. The use of PFCLs permit initial dissection of posterior PVR. Posterior membrane dissection is begun at the optic nerve and 0.5–1.0 ml PFCL is injected over the optic nerve. This opens the funnel and flattens the posterior retina, exposing residual membranes and creating counter-traction to allow anterior dissection. PFCL interface is kept posterior to areas of epiretinal membranes and their removal continues in a posteroanterior direction. As the retina becomes more mobile further PFCL is added. The level of PFCL is kept posterior to the retinal breaks and to the scleral buckle area. Once the retina is completely flattened, PFCL-air or a PFCL-silicone oil exchange is done.

There are numerous advantages of PFCLs. A posterior retinotomy is not necessary for drainage of subretinal fluid because it is displaced and aspirated through peripheral breaks. This reduces injury to the retina and the risk of reproliferation from the retinotomy site. Areas of retinal traction can be readily visualized and it can be determined if all traction has been relieved or when subretinal membrane removal or retinotomies are needed. The size of relaxing retinotomies can be precisely moni-tored because PFCLs flatten the retina as it is cut. Even 360° retinotomies can be easily handled by PFCLs without need for agents such as retinal tacks. Besides flattening and immobilizing the posterior retina, it acts as a barrier, protecting the posterior retina from cells and biochemically active substances produced during surgery which may contribute to reproliferation. Finally, PFCLs in contrast to air do not cause pupillary miosis when injected into the eye to flatten the retina.

2. Proliferative diabetic retinopathy

PFCLs can be useful in the management of patients with severe proliferative diabetic retinopathy. PFCLs make it possible to flatten the retina in cases of combined traction-rhegmatogenous detachments to facilitate the removal of fibrovascular proliferation and to allow endophotocoagulation to be applied intraoperatively. Care should be taken in cases where there is significant bleeding, since droplets may be hidden under blood clots, making their removal difficult. Anatomic re-attachment, using PFCLs, has been reported in eyes with diabetic traction detachments complicated by a rhegmatogenous component.

3. Giant retinal tears

Liquid perfluorocarbons offer the greatest advantage in the management of giant retinal tears. Previously described techniques involved use of silicone oil, fluorosilicone, prone fluid-gas exchange, sodium hyaluronate, and the expanding bubble method. Chang et al initially described the use of PFCLs for giant retinal tears. Subsequent reports showed a reattach-ment rate of 100 and 90% in giant retinal tear cases complicated with PVR.

Vitrectomy is necessary when the flap of the tear is inverted and immobile. Lensectomy is done if better visualization is required. A central and anterior vitrectomy is done and epiretinal membranes, if present, are removed. The flap of the tear is bimanually unfolded and a small amount of PFCL is introduced over the disc. More PFCL is added to flatten the retina up to the edge of the tear. Membranes on the edge of the tear are removed and the vitreous base is trimmed. After all the traction has been removed, the level of PFCL is raised over the edge of the tear. A fluid-air exchange or a fluid-silicone exchange is done, removing all the fluid anterior to the PFCL. The PFCL is then aspirated anteroposteriorly. If slippage occurs in the air-filled eye, a small amount of saline is injected into the vitreous and the patient is rotated postoperatively to steamroll the retina.

The choice of tamponade depends on the extent of tear and presence of PVR. If giant tear is around 90° to 180° with no PVR, gas tamponade with perfluoro propane gas may be preferred. Silicone oil is preferred in most other situations. *When silicone oil is used, it is preferable to do direct PFCL silicone oil exchange.* The retinal edge is manipulated hydraulically, thus avoiding trauma by mechanical manipulation.

In cases without PVR, a scleral buckle can be avoided.

4. Trauma

Traumatic retinal detachments are often complicated by vitreous hemorrhage, subretinal or choroidal hemorrhage, lens injury, foreign bodies and severe proliferation. PFCLs have been used in the management of penetrating ocular trauma. In cases with extensive vitreous hemorrhage and retinal detachment, PFCLs can stabilize the retina, drain subretinal fluid anteriorly and permit safe removal of blood from the vitreous base with a posteriorly flattened retina. Injected into subhyaloid space PFCL can induce posterior vitreous separation and make vitrectomy simpler. If subretinal hemorrhage is present, the PFCL displaces it anteriorly so that it can be aspirated through a peripheral break. The higher specific gravity of PFCL allows stabilisation of eye, preventing collapse and reducing risk of intraocular hemorrhage. Traumatic retinal detachments complicated by epiretinal or subretinal membrane or large breaks and dialyses are managed in the same manner as PVR. PFCLs may assist in the management of traumatic retinal incarceration to stabilize the retina during manipulations and retinectomies. Intraocular wood or plastic foreign bodies can be floated on the surface of PFCL and removed. Metallic foreign bodies can be held in place by covering them with PFCL and removing them through PFCL thus minimizing the potential for retinal damage.

5. Posteriorly dislocated crystalline lens and intraocular lens

PFCLs facilitate the safe removal of a posteriorly dislocated crystalline lens, nucleus, and nuclear fragments. The PFCL allows the crystalline lens to float off the retinal surface into the anterior vitreous cavity. In the presence of retinal tear, PFCL prevents the retina from detaching. Prior to aspiration, lens fragments may be produced intentionally. The crushed material may remain on the surface of the bubble, avoiding damage to the retina from posteriorly falling particles. Retrieval, removal, repositioning or exchange of a posteriorly dislocated IOL by using PFCL,

eliminates the risk of injuring the posterior retina. While elevating the IOL, the high density vitreous substitute can flatten an associated retinal detachment without the need for a posterior drainage retinotomy and an air-fluid exchange. It also supports the eye from collapsing, thus allowing a safer IOL exchange or fixation. PFCLs have been used in the management of retinal detachments associated with dislocated crystalline or intraocular lenses. PFCLs, while elevating the lens, displace subretinal fluid through an anterior break, successfully flattening the retina.

6. Surgical excision of subretinal membrane

PFCLs have been used during the surgical excision of subfoveal membranes. Following removal of the subretinal membrane, PFCL is injected to tamponade any bleeding from subretinal space.

7. Retinal incarceration

Retinal incarcerations may be repaired by injecting PFCLs. PFCL applies counter traction which helps to pull the incarcerated retina back into the vitreous cavity. Unrelieved incarcerations may be managed by relaxing retinotomy.

8. Endophthalmitis

PFCL to cover posterior pole during vitrectomy for endophthalmitis, which prevents contact of the antibiotic with macula, avoiding possible macular toxicity has been described. However, this application of PFCL is not very popular with most surgeons.

9. Retinal detachments secondary to macular holes

Retinal detachments secondary to macular holes can be managed by injecting a small amount of PFCL to flatten and stabilise the retina so that internal limiting membrane can be peeled without causing extension of the macular hole. In cases where there is doubt whether there is a peripheral break in addition to macular hole, PFCL can be injected to flatten the retina. If a peripheral break is present, the fluid will drain through it flattening the retina peripherally, this phenomenon is called schleren.

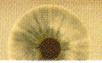

10. Massive subretinal hemorrhage

Cases of massive subretinal hemorrhage are managed by creating retinotomy through which a fibrinolytic agent is injected to dissolve the clotted blood. PFCL can be injected into the eye to express the liquefied blood through the retinotomy.

11. Retinopathy of prematurity

PFCLs can also be used in the management of open-funnel or closed-funnel retinal detachments of advanced retinopathy of prematurity.

12. Retinal detachments associated with choroidal coloboma

Perfluoroperhydrophenanthrene, in the area of retinal detachment associated with an inferior coloboma provides prolonged inferior tamponade.

13. Retinal detachments associated with posterior retinal breaks

PFCL has been injected into eyes with complicated retinal detachments with posterior breaks without complications to help anterior dissection and endophotocoagulation. It was thought initially that PFCL could not be used in situations where posterior-posterior breaks were present since the liquid would migrate subretinally.

15. Suprachoroidal hemorrhage

The use of perfluorophenanthrene in the management of non-expulsive suprachoroidal hemorrhage. The PFCL was inserted into the vitreous cavity with simultaneous drainage of blood from anterior sclerotomies.

COMPLICATIONS OF PFCL

1. *Retinal break.* A retinal break can occur from forceful injection of PFCL into the vitreous cavity. This complication can be avoided by slow injection of the fluid and by directing stream at the optic disc.

2. *Subretinal migration of PFCL.* PFCL can migrate subretinally during surgery. It can either be aspirated by an extrusion needle or displaced anteriorly and evacuated through a peripheral break by filling the vitreous cavity with more PFCL.

3. *Dispersion of PFCL.* Dispersion of PFCL into multiple bubbles can occur if the level of PFCL goes above the infusion cannula or if injection is not done into the PFCL bubble.

4. *Residual PFCL.* Large amount of PFCL can damage the corneal endothelium in aphakic and pseudophakic eyes, and should be removed. Patients with residual droplets of PFCL in the subretinal space and vitreous cavity have been followed without any evident inflammatory problems. These small droplets tend to decrease in size over time and eventually disappear.

COMBINATION OF SILICONE OIL AND PFCL

The combined use of silicone oil and a non-toxic PFCL may be useful in the treatment of complex retinal detachments. Such a combination supports both superior and inferior areas of the pathology, because, silicone oil apposes the superior retina and PFCL apposes the inferior retina. As both substances are immiscible, the meniscus delineating them is visible during fundus examination. Based on experimental studies, it has been concluded that a 2:1 ratio of silicone and PFCL would take advantage of the greater ability of PFCLs compared with silicone oil to resist traction retinal detachment while ensuring that the interface between the two liquids did not involve the visual axis. Silicone oil, because of its greater viscocity, is less likely to enter the anterior chamber in aphakic eyes than are PFCLs and may resist the movement of PFCL into the anterior chamber. Silicone oil tends to delay the emulsification of PFCLs when both are used together. Clinical studies have demonstrated good tolerance of the combination of silicone oil and perfluoroperhydrophenanthrene in human eye intraoperatively and as a short term tamponade.

HEAVIER THAN WATER SILICONE OILS

In order to achieve more effective tamponading of the posterior pole, Jonas and Jäger used a heavier-than-water endotamponade, perfluorohexyloctane(F6H8), which is a semifluorinated alkane, in the treatment of recurrent macular hole. They achieved good anatomical and functional results, but the incidence of complications (emulsification, epiretinal membrane formation) was significant.

HSO (Oxane HD) as a heavier-than water endotamponade in the treatment of persistent macular holes was found to be effective, after failure of vitrectomy, ILM peeling, long-acting gas endotamponade, and prone positioning. HSO, due to its specific gravity, achieved effective endotamponade of the foveal region in the upright position, allowing a good anatomic and functional recovery.

VISCOELASTIC FLUIDS

Viscous fluids used in vitreoretinal surgery include sodium hyaluronate, chondroitin sulphate and hydroxypropyl methylcellulose. These are polymers with molecular weights ranging from approximately 30,000 to 4 million daltons. It is the viscoelastic properties of these materials that make them most useful for intraocular surgery. Shearing occurs when fluid is made to flow. At zero shear rate (steady state) they exhibit high viscosity whereas at high shear rates their viscocity decreases. This behaviour allows the material to be injected through small gauge cannula and yet ensures that the material will regain its shape.

Sodium hyaluronate (1%; Healon) has the most favorable viscoelastic properties. Its molecular weight is nearly 4 million daltons and has a viscocity greater than 400,000 Centistokes at near zero shear. At high shear, the viscosity decreases to 110 Centistokes. The viscoelastic properties of sodium hyaluronate can be helpful in the separation of epiretinal membranes. The term *viscodissection* describes the hydraulic elevation of epiretinal membranes as the fluid is injected into the plane between the retina and proliferative tissue. The membranes are separated from the retinal surface with less trauma and the remaining attachments can be dissected more easily. *In proliferative diabetic retinopathy blood can be displaced* so that the planes between membranes and retina can be seen more easily. This approach should be used cautiously when the retina is atrophic because iatrogenic retinal breaks may develop if too much injection force is used. Sodium hyaluronate has also been used to unfold the retina during repair of giant retinal tears and to manage hemorrhage. Postoperative elevation of intraocular pressure can result if large volumes

are left in the vitreous cavity after surgery. *Sodium hyaluronate has been used in surgery for Stage V retinopathy of prematurity,* as a volume maintainer. Being a viscous substance, it does not leak out rapidly and enables bimanual dissection through 2 ports although infusion is absent.

During fluid air exchange, in aphakic and pseudophakic eyes, problem in visualisation can occur sometimes. In aphakic eyes, especially wherein the epithelium has been removed, or wherein the cornea has been cut and sutured (as in combined cataract surgery and pars plana procedure), descemet's folds form or get exaggerated during fluid air exchange. This substantially interferes with visualisation. The situation can be countered by coating the posterior corneal surface with viscoelastic substances. In pseudophakic eyes with a posterior capsulotomy, the exposed portion of the IOL tends to become dry during fluid air exchange leading to break down of fluid film into fine droplets. This again can interfere with visualisation and can be countered by coating this surface with sodium hyaluronate or methyl cellulose.

MANAGEMENT OF GIANT RETINAL TEARS

FEATURES AND PATHOGENESIS

FEATURES OF GIANT RETINAL TEAR

A giant retinal tear (GRT) is a full-thickness retinal break that extends circumferentially around the retina for three or more clock hours/ 90 degrees or more (Fig. 31.10), in the presence of a posteriorly detached vitreous, the vitreous gel is attached essentially to the anterior flap thereby allowing independent mobility of the posterior edge of tear.

One of the differential diagnosis for GRT is a giant retinal dialyses which is retinal disinsertion from the ora serrata with 90 degrees or more of circumferential extent. These conditions differ markedly in their vitreoretinal relationships and prognosis. In dialysis, vitreous bridges the dialysis gap and is attached to the posterior margin of the dialysis and posterior vitreous detachment is absent thus preventing it from

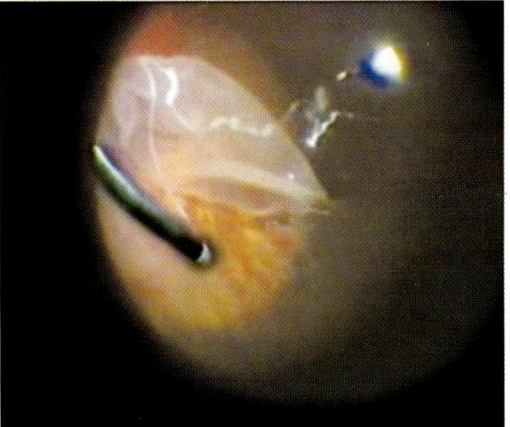

Fig. 31.10 *Giant tear with no flap inversion*

inversion. Conversely, in giant tear vitreous remains strongly attached to the anterior margin of the tear and the posterior flap, without any vitreous adhesion is free to move and inverts towards disc due to gravity (Fig. 31.11). Dialysis is generally amenable to buckling whereas giant tear requires highly specialized techniques especially for unfolding the inverted retinal flap. Schepens described three types of giant retinal tears: Idiopathic seen in 70%, traumatic in 20% and in 10% at the posterior edge of chorioretinal degeneration.

Giant retinal tears (idiopathic or traumatic) occur more frequently in males. Myopia was a frequent finding, with approximately 40% of eyes in this series having more than 8 diopters of myopia.

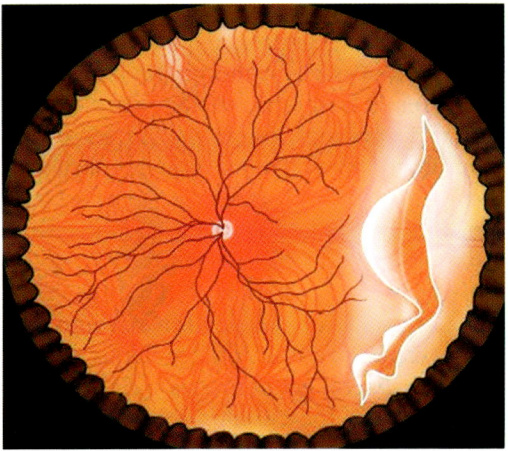

Fig. 31.11 *GRT with inverted flap*

Vitreous anomalies may be associated like in Stickler syndrome and Marfan syndrome (Fig. 31.12). Subluxation of the crystalline lens and cataract may also be present.

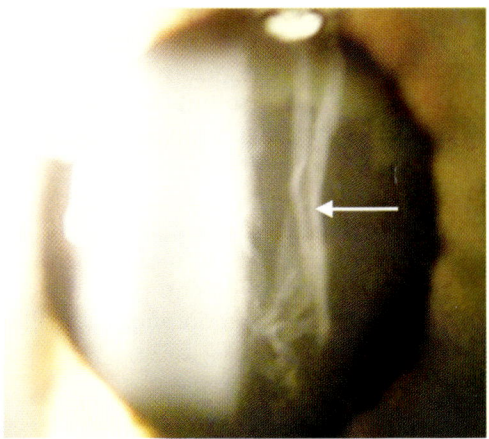

Fig. 31.12 *Vitreous anomaly as in stickler*

Fellow eyes of patients with giant tear are at considerable risk of retinal breaks, giant tears and retinal detachment. In a study of 226 patients with giant tears, 51% developed retinal tears in the fellow eye including 13% who developed giant tears.

PATHOGENESIS

The pathogenesis of idiopathic GRT is a liquefying process of the central gel forming a cavity while there is relentlessly progressive shrinkage of the remaining gel in the vitreous base exerting traction on the base and the peripheral retina causing GRT. Posterior flap folds because it is not sustained by intact vitreous face. Radial extensions may occur generally at either end of the tear and if large in size may present difficulties in surgical repair.

Giant retinal tears resulting from blunt trauma occurs along the posterior border of vitreous base and may be associated with avulsion of vitreous base. Giant tears also occur along the posterior edge of large areas of chorioretinal scarring especially in eyes with acute retinal necrosis. Giant retinal tears have been known to occur frequently in Sticklers syndromes, Marfan's syndrome and Ehler-Danlos syndrome.

GRT have also been noted as a complication of attempted removal of intravitreal nuclear

fragment during cataract surgery by the anterior segment surgeon using the limbal approach while performing open sky blind deep anterior vitrectomy. These have also been described as a complication of pars plana vitreous surgery. This could be due to detachment of the residual peripheral vitreous after surgery combined with pre-existing or surgically induced retinal pathology, the use of blunt instrumentation and invariable traction force exerted during pars plana vitreous surgery.

It is an uncommon retinal condition with a guarded prognosis, as it can cause significant visual morbidity from retinal detachment. Recurrent retinal detachment, predominantly due to proliferative vitreoretinopathy (PVR), occurs in up to 49% of GRT cases.

PREOPERATIVE CONSIDERATIONS

PREOPERATIVE EVALUATION

Careful indirect ophthalmoscopy of both eyes should be done and the size of the tear, mobility of the posterior flap, radial extension if any, amount of vitreous liquefaction, abnormal areas of vitreous condensation and the extent of proliferative vitreoretinopathy (PVR) should be noted. Preoperatively, extension of a giant tear, possibly with creation of radial extensions may occur with violent head movement, and patients should not be subjected to extensive manipulation or physical activity.

GRT A COMPLEX CONDITION TO OPERATE

Giant retinal tear by definition have a large tear. Large area of bare choroid causing pigment release in the pre-, intra- and postoperative phase causing intraocular inflammation and proliferative vitreoretinopathy.

Large areas of bare choroid opens up alternative aqueous drainage pathways and severe hypotony causing choroidal detachment. The flap of the GRT as described is inverted both due to vitreous attachment and PVR, which makes it difficult to unfold as there is risk of retinal damage while unfolding the flap.

Hypotony increases the risk of placement of subretinal infusion cannula and damage to the crystalline lens.

SURGICAL MANAGEMENT

Since the advent of pars plana vitreous surgery giant tears have stimulated the development of many innovative approaches to unroll the flap of the tear and the results of surgery for GRT have steadily improved. All the vitreous traction can be relieved under direct visualisation during pars plana vitrectomy.

The introduction of perfluorocarbon liquids (PFCL) by Chang et al supplanted all of the previous techniques (retinal sutures, tacks, prone fluid air exchange) for unrolling and repositioning inverted giant retinal tears. PCFLs have a higher specific gravity than water with relatively low viscosity and assume a liquid form at room temperature.

The retinal flattening forces exerted by these compounds are significantly higher than those exerted by either air or silicone oil. PFCLs allow for precise, controlled and accurate rare positioning of the retina with minimal manipulation. The surgical principles involved in the management include complete vitrectomy, unfolding of the retinal flap, sealing the tear with chorioretinal adhesion and providing long-term intraocular tamponade.

SURGICAL MANEUVERS

Various surgical maneuvers involved in the management of giant retinal tear are described as follows:

VITRECTOMY

Good results in the management of giant retinal tears greatly depend on removal of as much vitreous as possible. A thorough vitrectomy of the vitreous base around its entire circumference, extending close to the surface of pars plana and peripheral retina, is mandatory in the management of a giant tear. It is important to remove the condensed vitreous gel attached to the anterior edge of giant tear, otherwise this might be pushed posteriorly by air infusion and cause slippage of the posterior retinal flap after it has been unfolded. Meticulous removal of the peripheral gel permits a more complete replacement of the vitreous volume by gas or silicon oil, decreases the likelihood of new breaks along the posterior insertion of the

vitreous base, and diminishes the occurrence of anterior PVR. Optimal visualization of the vitreous base is vital for its dissection. This is aided by maximal pupillary dilatation pharmacologically, or with help of iris retractors, scleral indentation with cotton tipped applicator by the assistant or by using wide angle viewing system (panoramic viewing). Wide-angle viewing allows the surgeon to assess the overall, panfundoscopic vitreoretinal relationship and enhances visualization of mid peripheral and anterior vitreoretinal pathology. Thus it is an ideal surgical viewing system in cases of giant retinal tears.

MANAGEMENT OF THE LENS

The main indications for lens removal in giant tears are cataract, lens subluxation and the presence of proliferative vitreoretinopathy. Controversy remains as for need for clear lens extraction in fresh giant tears. The advantages of lens removal are visualization of the edge of the tear during fluid-air exchange, and improved access to the region of the vitreous base. The use of wide angle viewing systems for giant tear surgery improves the ability to see the peripheral retina under air in phakic and pseudophakic eyes. Thus, lensectomy to increase fundus visualization is not necessary. Many eyes with giant tears are highly myopic have large axial length and have broader pars

plana region. This anatomic variation allows adequate shaving of the vitreous base with less risk of lens touch. The clears lens should be removed when it impedes adequate peripheral vitreous dissection. It appears reasonable to conclude that the surgeon should not compromise the initial surgery for giant tear by diminishing other surgical goals to preserve the lens. Some surgeons recommend phacoemulsification and intraocular lens implantation because it makes possible optimal visualization for thorough debulking of the vitreous base and provides excellent visualization intraoperatively for vitrectomy and photocoagulation and avoids subsequent cataract surgery.

COMPLETE TRACTION REMOVAL

After vitrectomy attention should be turned to the epiretinal membranes and proliferative tissue especially near the posterior edge of the giant tear.

ROLE OF PFCL

Once the retina is mobilized by membrane peeling, the inverted retinal flap is unfolded to expose the optic disc and posterior pole and liquid perfluoro-octane is slowly injected over the optic disc (Fig. 31.13). Care is taken to prevent the injection of multiple bubbles by ensuring that the tip of injection needle is always within the PFCL bubble and the size of the

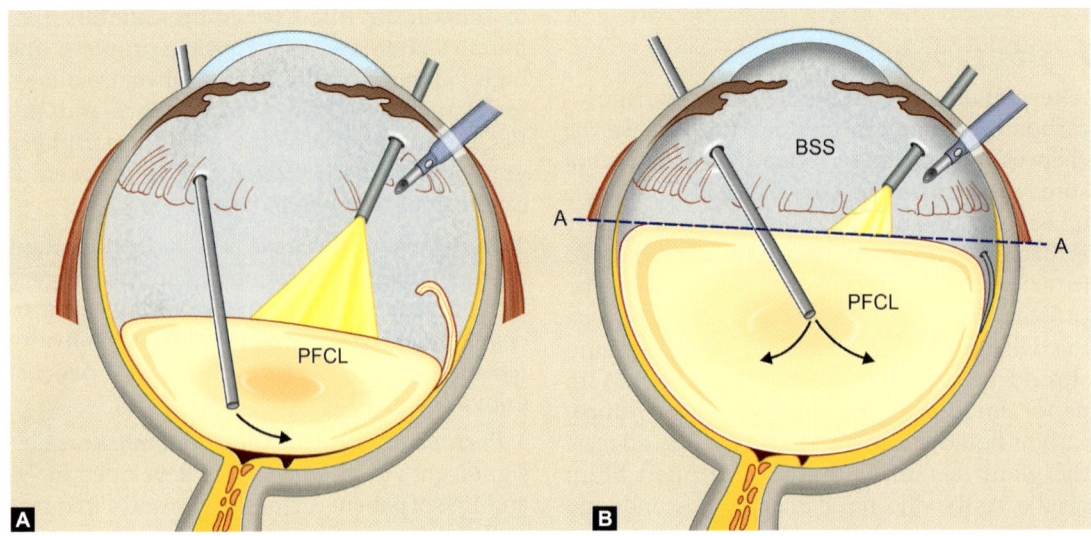

Fig. 31.13 *PFCL assisted unfolding of the inverted flap of GRT:* **(A and B)**

bubble is gradually increased as subretinal and vitreous cavity fluid is displaced anteriorly and out of the eye.

ROLE OF ENDOPHOTOCOAGULATION

With the retina fully attached under PFCL eight to ten rows of endophotocoagulation of 200–500 micron spot size are applied to the posterior edge and anterior retinal flap and at least five rows are placed in the fundus periphery not involved in giant tear.

GAS-FLUID EXCHANGE

The perfluorocarbon liquids can then be directly exchanged with gas or silicone oil. If the surgeon is sure of total vitreous base removal, and drying of free retinal edges, air-PFCL exchange followed by gas/silicon oil exchange may also be done. A flute needle with a soft silicone tip is positioned at the edge of the giant break as air-enters the vitreous cavity. The anterior retina is flattened as the bubble descends towards the perfluorocarbon meniscus. Fluid should be aspirated at the edge of the break, at the air/perfluorocarbon interface, to prevent posterior slippage of retina. Slippage may occur when persistent subretinal fluid is trapped posteriorly by descending air bubble causing the retina to slide. It is important to maintain adequate intraocular pressure during PFCL air exchange to prevent posterior slippage of retina.

PFCL-OIL EXCHANGE

Alternatively, a direct silicone oil perfluorocarbon exchange can be done to decrease the chances of slippage of retina if surgeon is not sure of tear edges being dry. Since PFCL silicone oil have relatively similar surface tension, there is preferential attraction between the two interfaces. This characteristic reduces the problem of having an aqueous layer between the two interfaces. A silicone oil infusion pump should be used during the exchange. With panoramic viewing, aspiration of perfluorocarbon liquid should be started at the edge of the giant tear using a silicone tipped blunt needle. As the silicone oil interface descends and covers the edge of the tear, the liquid overcomes any residual intrinsic elastic forces that may

result in posterior slippage. The aspirating tip is then placed just below the anterior surface of the PFCL as the oil continues to fill the vitreous cavity.

COMPLICATIONS

1. *Posterior slippage of a giant tear* after successful reapproximation indicates residual fluid at the margin of the tear and it requires a repeat PFCL exchange with careful anterior drainage. Incidence of intraoperative slippage was noted in 10.7 to 49% of cases in two trials. Postoperative slippage may also occur and was noted in 1.5% of cases. This can be managed by careful implementation of head positioning and by additional posterior coverage with postoperative laser.

2. *Retention of PFCL bubble in vitreous* cavity: Experimental studies have shown damaging retinal changes after 1 week with retention of perfluoro N-octane.

• *Retinal damage,* especially macular damage, may occur within 1–3 days of retention of a PFCL bubble. Hence, its almost total removal is prudent. Supine position in a patient with leftover PFCL bubble should be prohibited for fear of macular damage and also prone position need to be avoided in aphakia for fear of corneal damage. Removal of liquid PF-Octane from vitreous cavity is simplified by allowing the eye to remain air filled for approximately five minutes after removal of visible droplets. The high vapour pressure of this substance allows for evaporation from retinal surface and any PFCL entrapped elsewhere in the periphery gravitates to the posterior pole from where it can be easily removed.

3. *Recurrent detachment.* The most important postoperative complication in giant tear surgery is recurrent detachment principally due to development of proliferative vitreo retinopathy reported to occur in 49.4 and 31.5% of patients in two separate studies.

4. *Postoperative epimacular membranes* causing significant visual impairment developed in 7.4 and 15% of patients in these series and a frequent cause of reoperation after otherwise successful repair of giant tear.

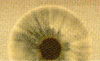

ROLE OF SCLERAL BUCKLING

Scleral buckling in the era of modern pars plana vitreous surgery and PFCL surgical techniques in cases of giant retinal tears without PVR is controversial. There is a general consensus in favor of buckling in giant tear cases with PVR. Scleral buckling along with vitreous surgery has traditionally been done to reduce the chances of redetachment. The proposed mechanisms are: it reduces early and late traction ensuring GRT will remain closed and will not extend, supports areas where unrecognized retinal breaks develop after surgery away from GRT, counteracts later traction on peripheral retina from contracture of residual vitreous gel by epiretinal membrane.

Buckling can complicate the closure of GRT by causing a gaping of retinal tissue, redundant retinal folds, fishmouthing and increased tendency of slippage of retina posteriorly. In a prospective randomized controlled trial conducted at RP Centre, we used 360 degree 9 mm silicone band in 10 cases and none in cases of GRT without PVR, the success of primary surgery was 100% in scleral buckle group (SB) as compared to 37.5% in no scleral buckle group (NSB). Resurgeries were required in 8 out of 11 cases in NSB group whereas only one required re-surgery in SB group. The final visual acuity regained in SB group was better than NSB group as the re-surgeries done were less in this group. Buckle sutures and buckle should be placed at the beginning of the surgery but not tied. They should be tied after the PFCL-air exchange to reduce the chances of slippage of retina and ensure proper fill of silicone oil. The height of the buckle should be relatively low and broad to reduce the formation of radial folds as the circumferential dimension of the globe is shortened.

The current technique used by us now is a 3.5 mm encircling band along with the final tie placed at the diagonally opposite to the GRT, we recommend a PFCL-silicone oil exchange in all cases of GRT.

SCLERAL BUCKLING IN GIANT TEARS WITHOUT AN INVERTED FLAP

These can be managed by conventional buckling surgery with cryotherapy, low broad scleral buckle throughout the length of the retinal break and drainage beneath the elevated flap. Zone of cryotherapy should extend beyond the edges of the tear to prevent recurrent detach-ment due to fluid passing posteriorly from beneath the anterior edge of the tear. Low buckling is preferred to decrease the antero- posterior opening of the break and for the same reason buckling effect should extend well posterior to the original posterior edge of the tear.

PROPHYLACTIC SCLERAL BUCKLING IN FELLOW EYE

- Idiopathic giant retinal tears have high incidence of retinal pathology in the fellow eye. Freeman noted several high-risk characteristics in his study on fellow eyes of giant retinal tears: high myopia (> −10 diopters), increasing white with pressure, and increasing condensation of the vitreous base. The studies of fellow eyes indicate that increasing condensation of vitreous base and subsequent traction plays a major role in the pathogenesis of giant retinal tears.
- The main objective in management of high-risk fellow eyes is to relieve this vitreous traction. It is recommended that all the high risk fellow eyes should have prophylactic scleral buckle. A prophylactic scleral buckle in phakic eye with an attached retina is challenging and not without complication. 360 degree retinopexy, either in the form of cryopexy or laser photocoagulation may be considered.

How the prophylactic encircling works

It is believed that GRT would occur in areas of abnormal vitreoretinal adhesion and traction, often at the vitreous base, especially when there are already pre-existing vitreoretinal degenerations that could predispose to the development of retinal breaks (Freeman 1978; Schepens 1962; Scott 1976). A 360-degree encircling buckle would reduce the internal circumference of the eye at the site it is placed, thus reducing the amount of peripheral vitreoretinal traction. Cryotherapy and laser photocoagulation would result in an increased neurosensory retina-retinal pigment epithelium adhesion (scar) over 360 degrees and would

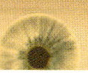

likely reduce the risk of neurosensory retinal detachment from the retinal pigment epithelium and/or limit its extension if it were to occur.

BIBLIOGRAPHY

Pars Plana Vitrectomy

1. 2007 American Society of Retina Specialists Patterns and Trends Survey. Poster presented at 2007 Annual ASRS meeting; 1–5 December 2007; Palm Springs, California, USA
2. Abrams GW, Edelhauser HF, Aaberg TM, et al. Dynamics of intravitreal sulfur hexa-fluoride gas. Invest Ophthalmol 1974;13:863–868.
3. Ando F, Sasano K, Suzuki, et al. Indocyanine green-assisted ILM peeling in macular hole surgery revisited. Am J Ophthalmol1 2004;38:886–7.
4. Asami T, Terasaki H, Kachi S, et al. Ultrastructure of internal limiting membrane removed during plasmin-assisted vitrectomy from eyes with diabetic macular edema. Ophthalmology 2004;111:231–7.
5. Brooks-HL (1995) ILM peeling in full thickness macular hole surgery. Vitreoretinal Surg Technol 7:2.
6. Burk SE, Da Mata AP, Snyder ME, et al. Indocyanine green-assisted peeling of the retinal internal limiting membrane. Ophthalmology 2000;107:2010–14.
7. Chang S. Low viscosity liquid fluoro-chemicals in vitreous surgery. Am J Ophthalmol. 1987;103:38–43.
8. Charles S. Fluid-gas exchange in the vitreous cavity. Ocutome/Fragmatome News-letter 1977; 2:1
9. Coll GE, Change S, Sun J, et al. Perfluorocarbon liquid in the management of retinal detachment with proliferative vitreo-retinopathy. Ophthalmology 1995;102:630–638.
10. Da Mata AP, Burk SE, Foster RE, et al. Long term follow-up of indocyanine green-assisted peeling of the retinal internal limiting membrane during vitrectomy surgery for idiopathic macular hole repair. Ophthalmology 2004;111:2246–53.
11. Diabetic Retinopathy Vitrectomy Study Group Early Vitrectomy for severe vitreous hemorrhage in diabetic retinopathy. Four-year results of a randomized trial: Diabetic Retinopathy Vitrectomy Study Report 5. Arch Ophthalmol 1990;108:958–964

12. Eckardt C. Transconjunctival sutureless 23-gauge vitrectomy. Retina 2005;25:208–211.
13. Engelbrecht NE, Freeman J, Sternberg P Jr, et al. Retinal pigment epithelial changes after macular hole surgery with indocyanine green-assisted internal limiting membrane peeling. Am J Ophthalmol 2002;133:89–94.
14. Feron EJ, Veckeneer M, Parys-Van Ginderdeuren R, et al. Trypan blue staining of epiretinal membranes in proliferative vitreoretinopathy. Arch Ophthalmol 2002;120:141–4.
15. Fleischman JA, Schwartz M, Dixon JA. Argon laser photocoagulation. An intraoperative trans-pars plana technique. Arch Ophthalmol 1981;99:1610–12.
16. Fujii GY, De Juan E Jr, Humayun MS et al. Anew 25-gauge instrument system for trans-conjunctival sutureless vitrectomy surgery. Ophthalmology. 2002;109:1807–12.
17. Fujii GY, de Juan E, Humayun MS, et al. A new 25-gauge instrument system for trans-conjunctival sutureless vitrectomy surgery. Ophthalmology 2002;109:1807–13.
18. Fujii GY, de Juan E, Humayun MS, et al. Initial experience using the transconjunctival sutureless vitrectomy system for vitreoretinal surgery. Ophthalmology 2002;109:1814–20.
19. GandorferA, Kampik A. Pars plana Vitrectomy in diabetic retinopathy. From pathogenetic principle to surgical strategy. Ophthalmologe 2000;97:325–30.
20. Gandorfer A, Messmer EM, Ulbig MW, Kampik A. Resolution of diabetic macular edema after surgical removal of the posteriorhyaloid and the inner limiting membrane. Retina 2000;20:126–33.
21. Haritoglou C, Gandorfer A, Gass CA, et al. Indocyanine green-assisted peeling of the internal limiting membrane in macular hole surgery affects visual outcome: a clinicopathologic correlation. Am J Ophthalmol 2002;134:836–41.
22. Helbig H, Kellner U, Bornfeld N, Foerster MH. Rubeosis iridis after Vitrectomy for diabetic retinopathy. Graefes Arch Clin Exp Ophthalmol 1998;236:730–3.
23. Horiguchi M, Kojima Y, Shima Y. Removal of lens material dropped into the vitreous cavity during cataract surgery using an optical fiber-free intravitreal surgery system. J Cataract RefractSurg 2003;29:1256–9.
24. Kadonosono K, Itoh N, Uchio E, Nakamura S, Ohno S. Staining of internal limiting membrane in macular hole surgery. Arch Ophthalmol 2000;118:1116–8.

25. Kanda S, Uemura A, Yamashita T, et al. Visual field defects after intravitreous administration of indocyanine green in macular hole surgery. Arch Ophthalmol 2004;122:1447–51.
26. Kimura H, KurodaS, Nagata M. Triamcinolone acetonide-assisted peeling of the internal limiting membrane. Am J Ophthalmol 2004;137: 172–3.
27. Kirchhof B,Wong D, Van Meurs J, et al. Use of perfluorohexyloctane as a long-term internal tamponade agent in complicated retinal detach-ment surgery. Am J Ophthalmol 2002;133:95–101.
28. Kwok AK, Lai TY, Man-ChanW, Woo DC. Indocyanine green assisted retinal internal limiting membrane removal in stage 3 or 4 macularhole surgery. Br J Ophthalmol 2003;87: 71–74.

Vitreous Substitutes

1. Abrams GW, Williams GA, Neuwirth J, et al. Clinical results of titanium retinal tacks with pneumatic insertion. Am J Ophthalmol 1986; 102:13.
2. Alexandribes E. Silicone oil tamponade in management of severe hemorrhagic detachment of the choroid and ciliary body after surgical trauma. Ophthalmology 1990;200:189.
3. Alfaro DV, Liggett PF. Perfluorocarbon liquids in the management of tarumatic retinal detach-ment. Vitreoretinal Surg Technol 1993;15:1.
4. Ando F, Miyake Y, Oshima K, et al. Temporary use of intraocular silicone in the treatment of complicated retinal detachment. Graefe's Arch Clin Exp Ophthalmol 1984;224:32.
5. Ando F. Intraocular hypertension resulting from pupillary block by silicone oil. Am J Ophthalmol 1985;99:87.
6. Ando, Kondo J. A plastic tack for the treatment of retinal detachment with giant tear (Letter). Am J Ophthalmol 1983;95:260.
7. Benson WE, Brown GC, Tasman W, et al. Complications of vitrectomy for non-clearing vitreous hemorrhage in diabetic patients. Ophth Surg 1988;19:862.
8. Berrocal MH, Chang S. Perfluorocarbon liquids in vitreous surgery. OphthalmolClin North America 1994;7:67.
9. Blinder KJ, Peyman GA, Desai UR, et al. Vitreon, a short-term vitreoretinal tamponade. Br J Ophthalmol 1992;76:240.
10. Bothner H, Wik O. Rheology of intraocular solutions. In: Rosen ES, Ed. Vision and Visual Health Care, Vol. 2. Viscoelastic materials. New York, Pergamon Press 1986.
11. Brod RD, Flynn HW Jr, Clarkson JG, et al. Management options for retinal detachment in the peresence of a posteriorly dislocated intraocular lens. Retina 1990;10:50.
12. Brourman ND, Blumenkranz MS, Cox MS, et al. Silicone oil for treatment of severe proliferative diabetic retinopathy. Ophthalmology 1989; 96:759.
13. Brown GC, Benson WE. Use of sodium hyaluronate for the repair of giant retinal tears. Arch Ophthalmol 1989;107:1246.
14. Chan C, Okun E. The question of ocular tolerance to intravitreal liquid silicone oil. Ophthalmology 1986;93:651.
15. Chang S, Lincoff H, Zimmerman NJ, et al. Giant retinal tears. Surgical techniques and results using perfluorocarbon liquids. Arch Ophthalmol 1989;107:761.
16. Chang S, Ozmert E, Zimmerman NJ, et al. Intraoperative perfluorocarbon liquids in the management of proliferative vitreoretinopathy Am J Ophthalmol 1988;106:668.
17. Chang S, Repucci V, Zimmerman NJ, et al. Perfluorocarbon liquids in the management of traumatic retinal detachments. Ophthalmology 1989;96:785.
18. Chang S, Sparrow JR, Iwamoto T, et al. Experimental studies of tolerance to intravitreal perfluoro-n-octane liquid. Retina 1991;11:367.
19. Chang S, Wieland M, Zimmerman NJ. Results and complications of perfluorocarbon liquids in proliferative vitreoretinopathy. Presented at the 17th meeting of Club Jules Gonin, Lausanne, September 1990;2–6.
20. Chang S, Zimmerman NJ, Iwamoto T, et al. Experimental vitreous replacement with perfluoro-tributyline. Am J Ophthalmol 1987; 103:29.
21. Chang S. Low viscosity liquid fluorochemicals in vitreous surgery. Am J Ophthalmol 1987; 103:38.
22. Chang TS, Pelzek CD, Nguyen RL, Purohit SS, Scott GR, Hay D. Inverted pneumatic retinopexy: a method of treating retinal detachments associated with inferior retinal breaks. Ophthalmology 2003; 110: 589–94.
23. Chung H, Acosta J, Refojo MJ, et al. Use of high-density fluorosilicone oil in open sky vitrectomy. Retina 1987;7:180.
24. Cibis PA, Becker B, Okun E, et al. The use of liquid silicone in retinal detachment surgery. Arch Ophthalmol 1962;68:590.
25. Claes C, Zivojnovic R. The use of perfluoro-carbon liquids in vitreous surgery. Bulletin De La SocieteBelge D Ophthalmologie 1990; 238:145.

26. Clark LJ, Gollan F. Survival of mammals breathing organic liquids equilibrated with oxygen at atmospheric pressure. Science 1966; 152:1755.

27. Clark LJ. Whole animal perfusion with fluorocarbon dispersions. Fed Proc 1970;29:1695.

28. Corcostegui B. Use of perfluorocarbon liquid in vitrectomy for diabetic rhegmatogenous retinal detachment. J Retina 1992;1:30.

29. Cox MS, Trese MT, Murphy PL. Silicone oil after advanced proliferative vitreoretinopathy. Ophthalmology 1986;93:636.

30. Crisp A, dejuan E Jr, Tiedeman J. Effect of silicone oil viscocity on emulsification. Arch Ophthalmol 1987;105:546.

31. De Juan E Jr, McCuen BW II, Machemer R. The use of retinal tacks in the repair of complicated retinal detachments. Am J Ophthalmol 1986; 102:20.

32. De Juan E, Hardy M, Hatchell DL, et al. The effect of intraocular silicone oil on anterior chamber oxygen pressure in cats. Arch Ophthalmol 1986;104:1063.

33. deBustros S, Michels RG. Surgical treatment of retinal detachment complicated by proliferative vitreoretinopathy. Am J Ophthalmol 1984; 98:694.

34. DeCorral LR, Peyman GA. Pars plana vitrectomy and intravitreal silicone oil injection in eyes with rubeosisirides. Can J Ophthalmol 1986;21: 10.

35. DeMarchis J, Chang S, Ortiz R, et al. Electrophysiologic evaluation of short-term vitreous replacement by perfluorocarbon liquids. Invest Ophthalmol Vis Sci. 30 (suppl) 1989;102.

Management of Giant Retinal Tears

1. Aaberg TM Jr, Rubsamen PE, Flynn HW Jr, et al. Giant retinal tear as a complication of attempted removal of intravitreal lens fragments. Am J Ophthalmol 1997; 124: 222–6.

2. Ahmed H. Giant retinal tears after pars plana vitrectomy. Eye 1997;11:325–7.

3. Aylward GW, Cooling RJ, Leaver RK. Trauma induced retinal detachment associated with giant retinal tears. Retina 1993;13:136–41.

4. Billington BM, Leaver PK, McLeod D. Management of retinal detachment in the Wagener Stickler Syndrome. Trans Ophthalmol Soc 1985; 104:875.

5. Chang S, Lincoff H, Zimmermann NJ, Fuchs W. Giant retinal tears: Surgical techniques and results using perfluorocarbon liquids. Arch Ophthalmol 1989;l07:761–6.

6. Freeman HM. Discussion of Lewis H, Kamei M, Masdia SH. Treatment with and without scleral buckles for uncomplicated giant retinal tears: randomized clinical trial.

7. Freeman HM. Fellow eyes of giant retinal breaks. Trans Am Ophthalmol Soc 1978; 76: 343–82.

8. Freeman HM. Giant retinal tears: 207 cases from the perfluorom study (Abstract). Am Acad Ophthalmol Vitreoretinal up data 1997; 168–71.

9. Kertes Pl, Wafapoor H, Peyman GA et al. The management of giant retinal tears using perfluorophenanthrene: A multicenter Case Series. Ophthalmol 1997;104:1159–65.

10. Schepens LL, Dobbie JG, McMeel JW. Retinal detachments with giant retinal breaks: preliminary report. Trans Am Acad Ophthalmol Otolarynogol 1962;66:471–68.

11. Sharma YR, Reddy PR, Azad RV, et al. 360 degree scleral buckling in vitreous surgery for giant retinal tears without proliferative vitreoretinopathy changes presented at American Academy of Ophthalmology, Dulles 2000.

12. Topilon HW, Nussbaum JJ, Freeman HM, et al. Bilateral acute retinal necrosis. Clinical and ultrastructural study. Arch Ophthalmol 1982; 00: 1901.

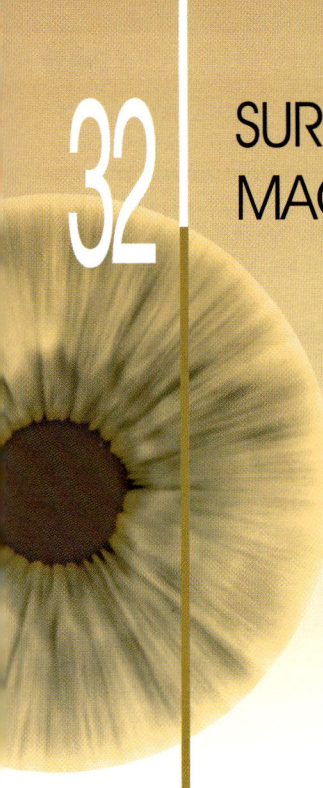

32 SURGICAL MANAGEMENT OF MACULAR HOLE

Atul Kumar

GENERAL CONSIDERATIONS

INTRODUCTION

The rationale for the surgical management of idiopathic macular holes, originally described by Kelly and Wendel in 1991, is to relieve vitreofoveal traction and to flatten and reappose the macular hole edges by intraocular tamponade. This is achieved by three-port pars plana vitrectomy with meticulous removal of posterior cortical vitreous and of any epiretinal membranes at the macula and adequate peeling of the internal limiting membrane of the retina (modification to the originally described technique) so as to completely relieve the tangential traction. A peripheral vitrectomy is completed and the retinal periphery inspected for iatrogenic retinal breaks. An air-fluid exchange is performed and the intraocular air is usually exchanged for long-acting gas like C3F8 or SF6 or very rarely silicone oil for internal tamponade. Patients may be advised to posture in a face-down position for up to 3 to 5 days postoperatively.

TRIALS IN MACULAR HOLE SURGERY

In eyes with full-thickness macular holes, vitrectomy with intraocular gas tamponade significantly improves the rate of both anatomical closure and visual function. Outcomes are particularly favourable for stage 2 holes and holes of less than 6 months' duration. In their original series, Kelly and Wendel reported an anatomical closure rate of 58%, and visual improvement in 73% of eyes in which holes were closed. The vitrectomy for macular hole study (VMHS) was a multicenter trial that included 171 eyes followed for 12 months postoperatively and the Moorfields macular hole study (MMHS) was a single surgeon trial that followed 185 eyes over 2 years. In the MMHS the overall anatomic closure rate for stage 2, 3, and 4 macular holes was 81% at 24 months following surgery compared with 11% in the observation group, and surgery was associated with a significant reduction in macular hole dimensions. Operated eyes improved in median Snellen acuity from 6/36 to 6/18, compared with deterioration from

6/36 to 6/60 in the observation group. Median near acuity improved even more dramatically in the operated group from N10 to N5, compared with deterioration from N10 to N14 over 24 months in the observation group. The number of eyes with Snellen acuity of 6/12 or better increased from 0% at baseline to 44% at 24 months in the operated group in contrast to the number in the observation group, which increased from 0% at baseline to 7% over the same period. The VMHS demonstrated a clear benefit of surgical management in reducing the rate of progression of stage 2 to stage 3 or 4 macular holes. While this study did not demonstrate statistically significant effect on ETDRS visual acuity at 6 or 12 months, it was not statistically powered to detect modest differences and the study design precluded surgery for cataract that may have masked an improvement in potential visual acuity in eyes randomized to surgery. Indeed, operated eyes in this study did perform significantly better than un-operated eyes at word reading and on potential acuity meter testing, a measure less influenced by cataract development than ETDRS acuity.

In the MMHS, 96% of treated stage 2 holes were closed at 24 months compared with 21% in the observation group that closed spontaneously. Surgery was associated with a mean difference of 2 Snellen lines of acuity.

Both the VMHS and the MMHS demonstrated a clear benefit of surgical management of stage 3 and stage 4 macular holes on the rate of anatomical closure and on final visual acuity. In the VMHS, after 6 months follow-up of 129 eyes with stage 3 and stage 4 macular holes, anatomical closure was achieved in 69% of eyes randomized to surgery compared with only 4% of eyes randomized to observation alone. The surgically treated eyes had significantly better visual acuity at 6 months as measured ETDRS visual acuity (mean acuity was 20/115 in operated eyes versus 20/166 in observed eyes, p < 0.01) and higher word reading scores. In the MMHS, anatomical closure was achieved in 77% of eyes with stage 3 and 4 holes randomized to surgery, compared with only 6% of eyes in the observation group associated with a mean difference of 2 Snellen lines of acuity between

the treatment groups. The surgical techniques and results have improved since these two trials began and many case series now report primary anatomical closure following conventional surgery in approximately 80–90% of eyes with full thickness macular holes.

SURGICAL TECHNIQUES FOR MACULAR HOLE

CONVENTIONAL SURGERY OF MACULAR HOLE

A three port pars plana core vitrectomy is performed. A complete posterior vitreous detachment is induced; the posterior hyaloid face at the optic disc is elevated by active aspiration using the vitreous cutter or passively using a flute needle. Separation of the hyaloid from the retina is evident from the appearance of a Weiss ring and by an advancing wave-like demarcation line between attached and detached posterior hyaloid. Posterior cortical vitreous and any epiretinal membranes are meticulously removed using a pic and membrane forceps. A peripheral vitrectomy is completed and the retinal periphery is searched for iatrogenic breaks. An air-fluid exchange is performed and usually a long-acting gas (SF6 or C3F8) is infused. Patients may be advised to posture face-down for up to 5 days postoperatively.

CURRENT SURGICAL TECHNIQUES

Peeling of the inner limiting membrane (ILM) from the macula is a technique advocated in an attempt to further improve anatomical and visual outcomes of surgery for macular holes. The rationale for peeling the ILM is to relieve tangential traction from the edges of the hole and to promote closure by stimulation of wound healing. Peeling the ILM ensures thorough removal of any tangential tractional components implicated in the development of macular holes. The removal of a potential scaffold for re-proliferation of myofibroblasts may reduce the possibility of late reopening of surgically closed holes. Furthermore, peeling of the ILM is also believed to stimulate wound healing at the macula, possibly by inducing local expression

of undefined growth factors that promote glial repair. A number of nonrandomized comparative series suggest that ILM peeling results in a higher rate of hole closure and that this is associated with improved visual outcomes. In one study of 160 eyes ILM peeling was associated with 100% hole closure rate and no re-openings, compared with 82% closure with 25% re-openings in the non-ILM peeled group. Further the development of ergonomically designed forceps and better microscopes the surgical experience is less tiring now.

VITAL STAINS USED IN MACULAR HOLE SURGERY

Many vital stains have been used. Indo-cyanine green (ICG) dye selectively stains the ILM (Table 32.1). The improved contrast between the green ICG-stained ILM and the unstained underlying retina facilitates initiation of the peel and enables precise monitoring of its extent (Fig. 32.1). Furthermore, the application of ICG is believed to create a cleavage plane that facilitates removal of the ILM. Indocyanine green-assisted ILM peeling is associated with high rates of macular hole closure. In a nonrandomized comparative trial of 68 eyes, macular hole surgery with ICG-assisted ILM peel (5 mg/ml) resulted in 91.2% primary closure rate and 82% improvement in visual acuity above baseline, versus 73.5% primary closure rate and 53% improvement in vision following ILM peeling without ICG (p=0.056). The best staining properties are seen with indocyanine green but it has photoreceptor toxicity and is unpopular with current day

Table 32.1 *Dyes for ILM staining*
• Indocyanine green (0.5%)
• Infracyanine green
• Brilliant Blue G (2.5%)
• Trypan blue
– Retiblue: 0.1%
– Membrane blue (DORC): 0.20%
• Triamcinolone
• Rhodamine 6G
• Bromophenol blue 0.2%
• Patent blue 0.48%

macular surgeons. ICG-assisted ILM peeling resulted in anatomical closure in 97.1% versus 97.7% without ICG. Postoperative visual acuity, however, was 20/50 or better in only 51.4% of eyes following ICG use versus 70.4% without ICG, trypan blue has no such toxicity but has poor staining properties. The dye used most commonly in todays practice is brilliant blue G, this dye can be used after PVD induction for staining and peeling ILM under fluid itself.

LONG-TERM TAMPONADE

Intraocular tamponade following vitrectomy for macular holes is believed to facilitate re-apposition of the rim of a detached neuro-sensory retina and to provide an interface with the vitreous fluid component that serves as a template for glial migration across the macular hole.

Consistently favourable anatomic and visual outcomes can be achieved by long-acting gas tamponade with strict face-down posturing

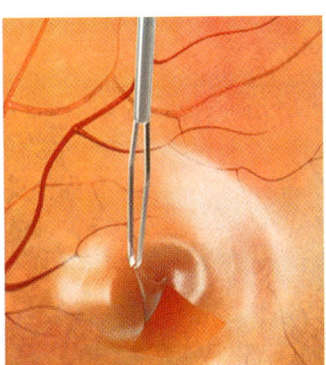
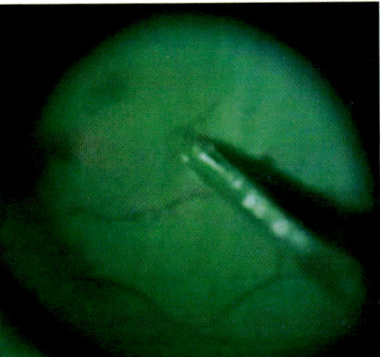
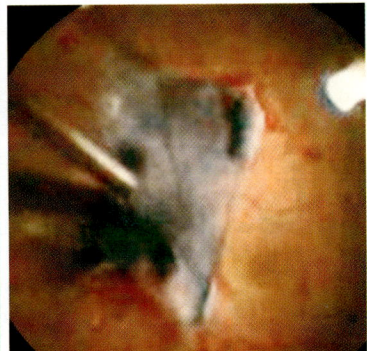

Fig. 32.1 *Picture showing ILM peeling unstained and using a vital stain*

originally advocated. In a comparative study of 52 eyes, use of 16% perfluoropropane gas resulted in anatomical closure in 97% and improvement in visual acuity by a mean of 3.1 lines whereas use of air resulted in closure in only 53.3% and improved mean acuity by only 1.3 lines. In another comparative series of 149 eyes, tamponade by 16% per fluoropropane and face-down posturing for 2 weeks resulted in an anatomical closure rate of 94%, compared with 65% following tamponade by lower concentrations of perfluoropropane and shorter durations of posturing; visual outcomes paralleled the rates of macular hole closure. Prolonged face-down posturing is a task that presents a formidable challenge for many patients, and for some may be an unrealistic expectation. A number of studies have suggested that the use of shorter acting gases or shorter durations of face-down posturing can result in anatomical and visual outcomes comparable to those of longer tamponade with a more rapid recovery of visual acuity post-operatively (Fig. 32.2).

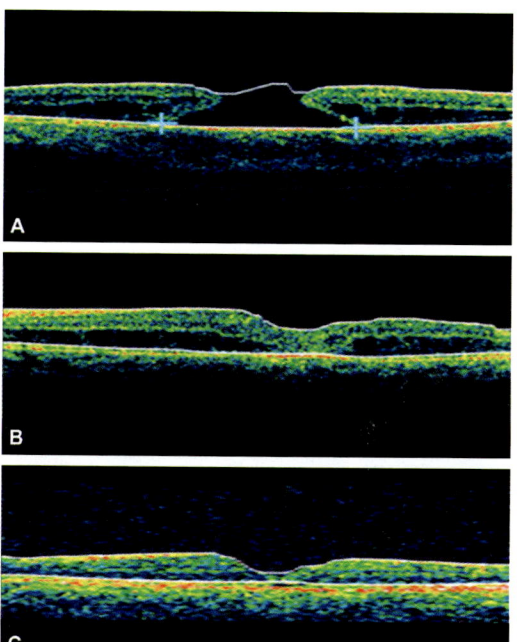

Fig. 32.2 OCT pictures of macular hole: **(A)** Preoperative, **(B)** postoperative 1 week, and **(C)** postoperative 12 weeks

COMPLICATIONS AND PROGNOSIS

COMPLICATIONS OF MACULAR HOLE SURGERY

1. *Iatrogenic retinal tears.* Peeling of the posterior vitreous cortex from the retinal surface can result in iatrogenic retinal tears. In the MMHS, retinal tears occurred in 3.2% of eyes and were effectively treated intraoperatively by retinopexy.

2. *Retinal detachments* occurred in 5.6% of eyes in the MMHS and in 11% of eyes in the VMHS. Retinal detachments generally occur within the first 6–8 weeks postoperatively and have a high success rate of anatomic reattach-ment following further surgery. Although retinal detachment does not preclude improved final visual acuity, involvement of the macula and the development of proliferative vitreo-retinopathy indicate poorer prognosis.

3. *Transient elevation of intraocular pressure* is very common postoperatively and intraocular pressures of greater than 30 mmHg have been reported in over 50% of patients following tamponade by 14% perfluoropropane gas. Transient elevation of intraocular pressure generally can be controlled by appropriate topical medication.

4. *Postoperative peripheral visual field defects,* consistent with damage to the retinal nerve fiber layer, have been described in up to 17% of cases. These visual field defects are believed to result from damage to the nerve fiber layer by the infusion of dry air under high pressure; the incidence of the field defects is dependent on the air pressure and its position is consistently located contralateral to the site of the infusion cannula, whether placed temporally or nasally. The development of field defects can be almost eliminated by limiting the air infusion pressure to 30 mmHg.

5. *Cataract development* is almost inevitable following macular hole surgery. Lens opacity has been reported in 46% of eyes at 3 months postoperatively, and in greater than 80% by 2 years. Since the development of cataract is predictable, combined cataract and vitrectomy surgery for macular hole has been advocated in order to obviate the requirement for subsequent

cataract surgery. Combined surgery has the added advantages afforded by excellent visibility of the retina per-operatively and a large fill of intraocular gas for optimal tamponade.

6. *Alterations in the retinal pigment epithelium* have been reported in as many as 33% of eyes following macular hole surgery. Retinal pigment epitheliopathy, which has been attributed to surgical trauma or phototoxicity, may limit visual outcome and predispose to the development of choroidal neo-vascularization.

7. *Cystoid macular edema (1%) and post-operative endophthalmitis (1%).* Rare complications of macular hole surgery.

PROGNOSIS FOLLOWING MACULAR HOLE SURGERY

Visual recovery following surgical closure of macular holes may be gradual. Although substantial improvement in visual acuity occurs soon after cataract extraction as cataract is known to commonly occur following macular hole surgery, further improvement may be observed for up to 2 years.

Factors affecting prognosis of macular surgery

- *OCT based visual outcomes dependent* on IS/OS line continuity and ELM line presence as an uninterrupted line has been emphasized in recent reports (Fig. 32.3).

- Visual recovery is also inversely correlated with vision in the fellow eye, tending to be greater where vision in the fellow eye is subnormal. Bilateral visual function improves in a significant proportion of patients after macular hole surgery, particularly where vision in the fellow eye is subnormal.

- Successful closure improves stereo acuity and has a beneficial effect on patients' subjective perception of visual function, but the effect of macular hole surgery on patients quality of life has yet to be fully evaluated.

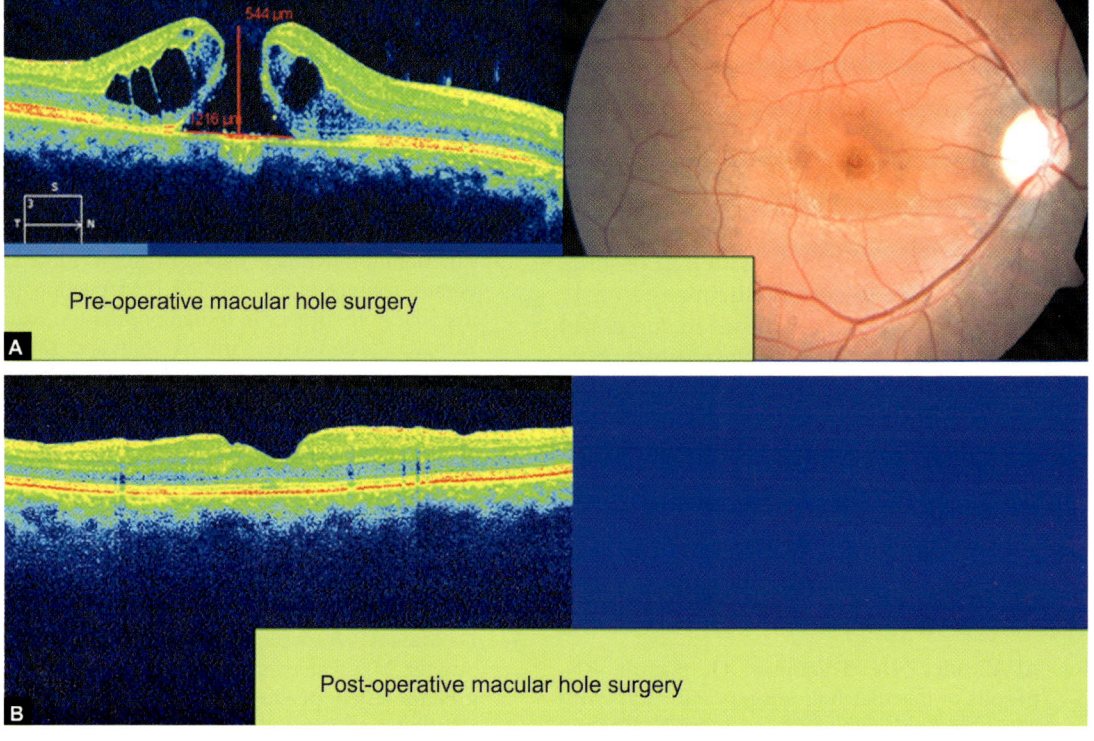

Pre-operative macular hole surgery

A

Post-operative macular hole surgery

B

Fig. 32.3 *(A) Macular hole index >0.5, improves hole closure rates and (B) discontinuous IS/OS line and ELM affects visual acuity outcome*

- The outcome of macular hole surgery is dependent on the *stage of the hole* and the duration of symptoms, but is not dependent on the age of the patient. Anatomic and visual outcomes are inversely correlated to the stage of the hole and are greatest following surgery for small stage 2 holes.

- *The closure rate in* patients undergoing surgery within 1 year of onset is 94.0%, and in those waiting 1 year or more it is 47.4%. However in our study we found even chronic macular holes improved vision after surgery with a closure rate of upto 94%. Although the best functional results are obtained if surgery is performed within 6 months of the onset of symptoms, visual improvement may be achieved in patients who have been symptomatic for much longer.

- Surgery for macular holes secondary to trauma can result in closure rates comparable to those of idiopathic holes, but high myopia or the presence of a localized macular detachment are associated with a relatively poor prognosis.

- Following failure of primary surgery to close macular holes, further surgery involving rigorous dissection of epiretinal membranes, with or without ILM peeling, and long-acting gas tamponade can result in anatomical closure and improvement in visual acuity.

- Alternatively, in eyes with unclosed macular holes following vitrectomy with ILM peeling, additional gas injection during the early postoperative period can result in successful closure. In the MMHS, eyes in which hole closure was achieved after a second procedure attained slightly poorer Log-MAR and Snellen acuities than eyes in which closure had been achieved after a single procedure, but achieved similar near acuities.

BIBLIOGRAPHY

1. Al-Abdulla NA, Thompson JT, Sjaarda RN. Results of macular hole surgery with and without epiretinal dissection or internal limiting membrane removal. Ophthalmology 2004; 111(1):142–9.

2. Ando F, Sasano K, Ohba N, Hirose H, Yasui O. Anatomic and visual outcomes after indocyanine green-assisted peeling of the retinal internal limiting membrane in idiopathic macular hole surgery. Am J Ophthalmol 2004; 137(4): 609–14.

3. Ando F, Sasano K, Suzuki F, Ohba N. Indocyanine green-assisted ILM peeling in macular hole surgery revisited. Am J Ophthalmol 2004; 138(5):886–7.

4. Apostolopoulos MN, Koutsandrea CN, Moschos MN, Alonistiotis DA, Papaspyrou AE, Mallias JA, et al. Evaluation of successful macular hole surgery by optical coherence tomography and multifocal electroretinography. Am J Ophthalmol. 2002;134(5):667–74.

5. Banker AS, Freeman WR, Azen SP, Lai MY. A multi-centered clinical study of serum as adjuvant therapy for surgical treatment of macular holes. Vitrectomy for Macular Hole Study Group. Arch Ophthalmol 1999; 117(11):1499–1502.

6. Banker AS, Freeman WR, Kim JW, Munguia D, Azen SP. Vision-threatening complications of surgery for full-thickness macular holes. Vitrectomy for Macular Hole Study Group. Ophthalmology 1997; 104(9):1442–52; discussion 1452–53.

7. Brooks HL Jr. Macular hole surgery with and without internal limiting membrane peeling. Ophthalmology 2000; 107(10):1939–48; discussion 48–49.

8. Chen CJ. Glaucoma after macular hole surgery. Ophthalmology. 1998; 105(1):94–9; discussion 99–100.

9. Comparative evaluation of anatomical and functional outcomes using brilliant blue G versus triamcinolone assisted ILM peeling in macular hole surgery in Indian population Atul Kumar, Varun Gogia, Vinit M. Shah and Tapas C. Nag. Graefe's Archive for Clinical and Exp Ophthalmology. 2011; Vol 1, 1854, Vol 249; 452–60.

10. Da Mata AP, Burk SE, Foster RE, Riemann CD, Petersen MR, Nehemy MB, et al. Long-term follow-up of indocyanine green-assisted peeling of the retinal internal limiting membrane during vitrectomy surgery for idiopathic macular hole repair. Ophthalmology 2004; 111(12):2246–53.

11. Da Mata AP, Burk SE, Riemann CD, Rosa RHJr, Snyder ME, Petersen MR, et al. Indocyanine green-assisted peeling of the retinal internal limiting membrane during vitrectomy surgery for macular hole repair. Ophthalmology 2001; 108(7):1187–92.

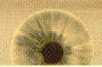

12. Engelbrecht NE, Freeman J, Sternberg P Jr, Aaberg TM Sr, Aaberg TM Jr, Martin DF, et al. Retinal pigment epithelial changes after macular hole surgery with indocyanine green-assisted internal limiting membrane peeling. Am J Ophthalmol 2002; 133(1):89–94.

13. Ezra E, Aylward WG, Gregor ZJ. Membranectomy and autologous serum for the retreatment of full-thickness macular holes. Arch Ophthalmol 1997;115(10):1276–80.

14. Ezra E, Gregor ZJ. Surgery for idiopathic full thickness macular hole: two-year results of a randomized clinical trial comparing natural history, vitrectomy, and vitrectomy plus autologous serum: Moorfields Macular Hole Study Group Report no. 1. Arch Ophthalmol 2004;122(2):224–36

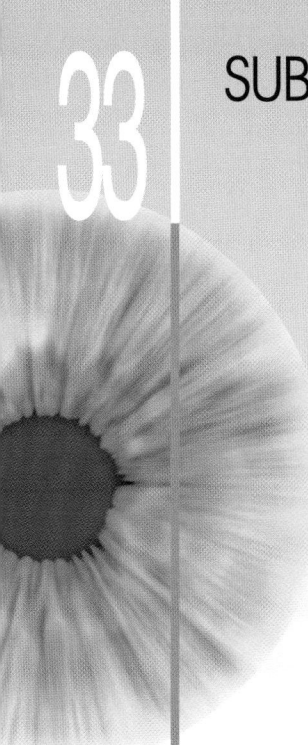

SUBMACULAR SURGERY

Atul Kumar

SUBMACULAR SURGERY: HISTORICAL BACKGROUD AND PREOPERATIVE CONSIDERATIONS

HISTORY OF SUBMACULAR SURGERY

In the late 1980s, initial attempts at surgical removal of choroidal neovasacular membranes (CNVMs) were reported. De Juan and Machemer pioneered a technique that involved performing a vitrectomy followed by a large retinotomy around the macula. A retinal flap was reflected, the membrane was removed, the retina was repositioned, and endophoto-coagulation was used to create adhesions to hold the retina in place. Unfortunately, poor visual results and the development of proliferative vitreoretinopathy with retinal detachment occurred. In an attempt to limit this complication, Blinder et al performed scatter photocoagulation outside the vascular arcades prior to surgery. Vitrectomy was followed by endodiathermy to the retina just inside the arcades. Again a large flap retinotomy was created, the retina was folded

back, the membrane was removed, the retina was once again repositioned, endophoto-coagulation was applied to the retinotomy, and silicone oil was injected for prolonged tamponade. Oil removal was performed later, without the development of retinal detachments. These eyes had extensive macular pathology with poor preoperative vision, and visual results remained poor despite the lack of retinal detachments.

CLINICAL RELEVANCE

Vitrectomy techniques may be an appropriate management option for some patients with choroidal neovascularization (CNV). Available techniques allowed safe extraction of most subretinal membranes regardless of etiology but not all patients respond favourably to such an approach. Certain clinical and angiographic characteristics as well as underlying disease processes may allow favorable outcomes.

Laser photocoagulation and photodynamic therapy had both been shown to be advantageous over observation in the management of

some eyes with AMD-associated subfoveal CNV. Although the macular photocoagulation study (MPS) demonstrated effective laser treatment for some choroidal neovascular membranes (CNVM) in AMD, years after treatment the visual outcome was poor, ranging from 20/100 to 20/400. The rate of persistent or recurrent CNV ranged from 50 to 70%. Additionally, MPS guidelines excluded many patients from laser treatment. These limitations along with no available safer options like anti-VEGF had stimulated the search for other therapies.

Surgical excision of subretinal membranes was an alternative to laser treatment, and techniques for surgical removal have become quite safe. Currently available data of the prospective randomized submacular surgery clinical trial (SST) and the advent of effective pan anti VEGF inhibitors the submacular surgery at present is the least viable option for a patient with CNVs.

PATIENT PROFILE FOR SUBMACULAR SURGERY

The best surgical candidates are those patients with type 2 CNV [membranes between the retinal pigment epithelium (RPE) and neurosensory retina] and with extrafoveal in growth sites. Clinically, the appearance of well-defined borders, a thin layer of blood between the membrane and the RPE, pigmented edges, patient age less than 50, and absence of biomicroscopic and stereoscopic fluorescein evidence of elevation of the RPE beyond a well-defined CNVM all suggest that the CNVM is between the RPE and retina. An anterior location can be determined by finding a rim of blocked fluorescence and absent late staining of surrounding tissues with fluorescein angiography. In addition, ocular coherence tomography can help reveal the position of the CNVM and thus help predict which eyes will do well with surgery.

Excision of CNVM may be accompanied by loss of underlying RPE. Angiography is often useful in predicting the size of this postoperative defect. This defect is generally greater for patients with AMD than those with multifocal choroidopathies or idiopathic CNVM. In AMD, the area of the CNVM and the hyperfluorescent halo seen in the latephase of the angiogram before surgery is approximately 80% the size of the postoperative defect.

In many non-AMD eyes, the initial site of presumed ingrowth by the choroidal vessels can be detected preoperatively. The best surgical outcomes were seen with eccentric ingrowth sites. Eyes with an unidentifiable ingrowth site probably have more diffuse RPE involvement and may have worse outcome following surgery. A light colored spot noted during fundus examination may indicate the ingrowth site. Fluorescein angiography may reveal a stalk in the earliest frames or a focal area of hyperfluorescence from which the membrane arises. Such characteristics may allow a preoperative indication for better postoperative outcomes.

GOALS OF THE PROCEDURE

The goal of subretinal membrane removal is to remove the pathological tissue and leave as much RPE and choroid as possible. Prevention of retinal detachment and hemorrhage is also important. Careful selection of the retinotomy site, gentle dissection of the membrane from overlying retina and underlying RPE, and control of intraocular pressure are essential to achieving these goals.

SUBMACULAR SURGERY: OPERATIVE AND POST OPERATIVE CONSIDERATIONS

OPERATIVE TECHNIQUE

The technique is as follows: complete vitrectomy is followed by removal of the posterior hyaloid, and a 36-gauge pick is used to pierce the neurosensory retina (Fig. 33.1). A localized retinal detachment over the CNVM is created by infusing balanced salt solution through the retinotomy using a 33-gauge angled cannula (Fig. 33.2). The subretinal pick is then reinserted through the retinotomy to separate the neovascular complex from overlying retina and surrounding tissues. Subretinal forceps are then passed through the retinotomy, and the membrane is grasped and removed very slowly, to minimize RPE loss and to allow the retinotomy to stretch around the CNVM (Figs. 33.3 and 33.4).

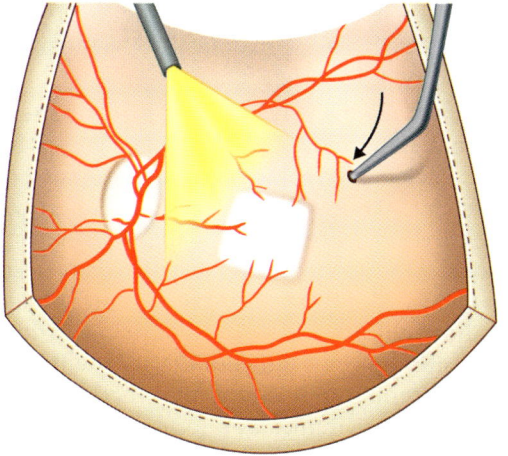

Fig. 33.1 *Creating a RD by infusing BSS with a 33 G infusion needle*

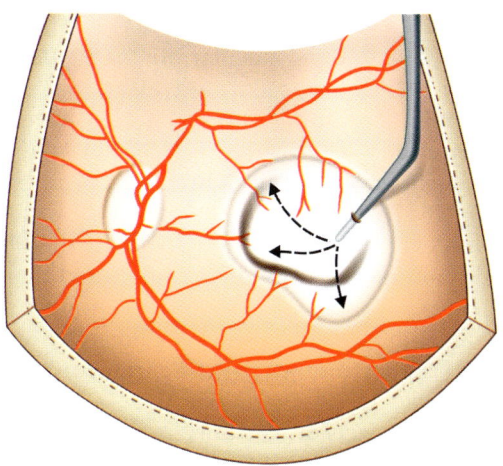

Fig. 33.2 *Perforating retinotomy using 36 G pointed subretinal pick*

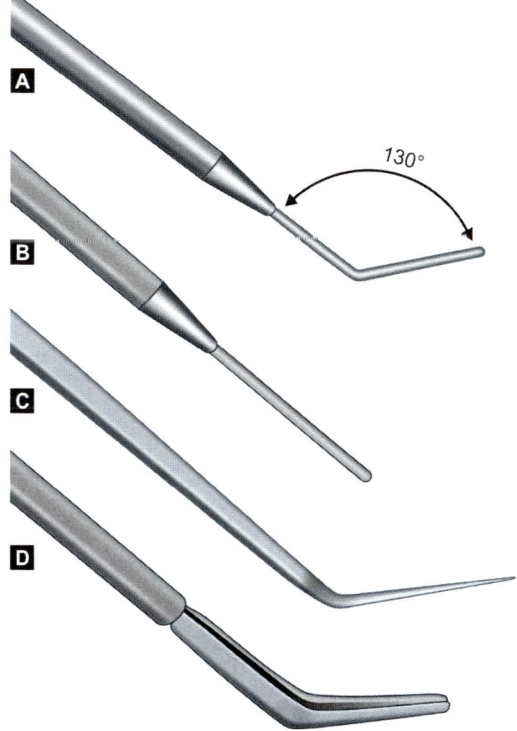

Fig. 33.3 *Instruments used in submacular surgery: (A) 33G subretinal infusion needle; (B) 33G straight cannula; (C) Sharpened subretinal picks; and (D) horizontal subretinal forceps*

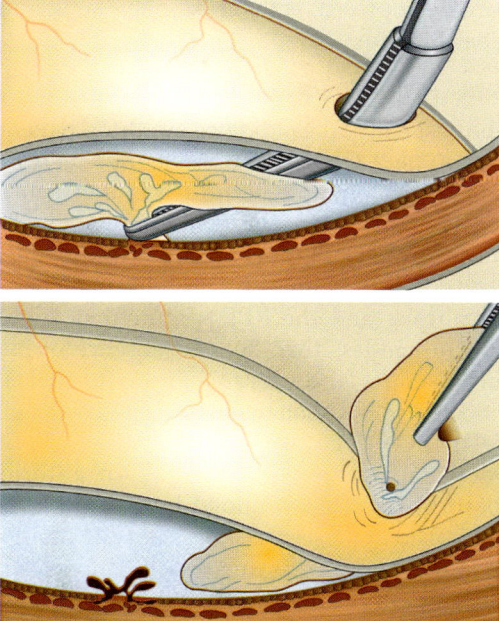

Fig. 33.4 *Showing removal of the CNV membrane*

Great care is taken to achieve hemostasis by elevating the intraocular pressure before the membrane is disconnected from the choroid. A gradual return to normal pressure while directly visualizing the excision site allows for immediate recognition of any subretinal bleeding. If any bleeding is seen, the pressure is promptly raised until hemostasis is verified.

Once hemostasis is achieved and the intraocular pressure has been returned to

normal, the membrane can be removed from the eye.

The intraocular fluid is exchanged for air and residual fluid is removed from the retinotomy site by aspirating just anterior to the retinotomy with a 33-gauge extrusion needle. If the retinotomy has not enlarged, fluid is infused until a 10–15% air bubble is left. Face-down postoperative positioning facilitates air tamponade of the retinotomy and prevents cataract formation. These techniques result in a low rate of complications.

OUTCOMES OF THE SURGERIES

Many studies have examined the role of submacular surgery in patients suffering from AMD-related CNVMs. The results are mixed and may reflect the aspect of visual function that is measured. For example, after subretinal membrane removal, patients with AMD may occasionally have residual retinal function in the surgical site when tested with the scanning laser ophthalmoscope. Additionally, a recent retrospective case series of surgical removal of subfoveal membranes from patients suffering from AMD demonstrated vision improvement (gained three lines) in 30% or stabilized vision in 42% of surgically treated eyes. Unfortunately, 28% of patients also lost three or more lines of vision. The authors concluded that vision improved or stabilized in the majority of patients. While 72% of patients improved or remained stable, one could also argue that 70% of these patients remained stable or worsened. Previous reports suggest that most patients with AMD do not improve in visual function following surgery. Additionally, one recent report demonstrates possible worsening of visual acuity following surgery and the authors recommend not operating on AMD-associated subfoveal CNVMs. *Patients with AMD generally do not achieve good vision after surgical excision of subretinal membranes* because of the widespread nature of the disease. Another cause for visual decline following surgical treatment may be the loss of perfusion to the underlying choriocapillaris. Preserved perfusion of the choriocapillaris is associated with better postoperative results. Unfortunately, the choriocapillaris may continue to

atrophy after surgery in patients with macular degeneration. This progressive atrophy may be due to the RPE loss that usually accompanies surgery for subretinal membranes in AMD.

Many patients with CNVM present with **subretinal hemorrhage.** Subretinal blood in patients with macular degeneration is often associated with decreased vision if left untreated.

Numerous studies have documented either stabilization or improvement of vision after surgical removal of subretinal hemorrhage. In addition, evacuation of this blood may result in a smaller scotoma for patients with AMD.

However, the best candidates for removal of subretinal blood are those who are young and have thick hemorrhages due to causes other than AMD. Most of the previously mentioned studies are small series or retrospective reviews.

The submacular surgery trials (SST) are a prospective randomized series of studies that are currently enrolling patients and seek to illuminate the potential role this surgical approach may play in managing patients with CNV. The SST pilot study number 1 enrolled 70 patients who had previously received extrafoveal laser photocoagulation for an AMD associated CNV and then developed subfoveal recurrent neovascularization. This trial was created to test methods and attain an estimate of the number of patients necessary for the larger multicenter trial. The published results from this pilot study suggest no reason to prefer surgery over photocoagulation for eyes with recurrent subfoveal CNV associated with AMD. There were few perioperative complications and the size of the surgically affected area was not significantly larger 2 years following surgery than the area of the neovascular lesion at baseline. The SST pilot study number 2 examined quality-of-life outcomes following surgery and laser treatment of recurrent subfoveal CNVM associated with AMD. Of the 70 patients in SST pilot study number 1, 54 were interviewed with the 36-item short form health survey prior to randomization. At the conclusion of the study, there were no significant differences in quality-of-life outcome scores between the two treatment arms.

Further at the conclusion of the trial the SST group has concluded that submacular surgery,

as performed in the trial, did not improve or preserve VA for 24 months in more eyes than observation and is not recommended for patients with similar lesions.

SUBMACULAR SURGERY IN OTHER DISEASE

Surgical treatment of CNVM is most successful in patients with focal abnormalities of the RPE. Patients with presumed ocular histoplasmosis syndrome (POHS), punctate inner choroido-pathy, and CNVM formation following focal laser treatment presumably have only focal disturbances of the RPE. Those with myopia and angioid streaks have more diffuse disease, while those with AMD are thought to have widespread RPE disease. Surgery for CNVM in these disorders has variable reported success rates. CNV from idiopathic juxtafoveolar retinal telangiectasis probably should not be approached with our current surgical techniques. The membranes seen in this disease probably arise within the neurosensory retina and only secondarily do they connect to the choroid. Attempted removal has resulted in retinal defects and poor outcomes.

Large pocket of subretinal blood can be treated with intravitreal tissue plasminogen activator followed by removal with variable success.

COMPLICATIONS

Complications can occur both during and after surgery.

A. *Intraoperative complications* include those potentially associated with any pars plana vitrectomy, such as retinal tears or detachment, and bleeding. Intraoperative complications unique to this surgery include enlarged retino-tomy sites with persistent subretial fluid or detachment, extensive subretinal hemorrhage, and large RPE defects.

B. *Delayed postoperative complications* may include cataract formation, retinal detachment, and recurrent membrane formation.

C. *Recurrence of CNV* after surgical removal of subretinal membranes has been reported to occur in 23–52% of cases. Melberg et al. found that when CNV recurred following surgery, the best visual outcomes were achieved for patients who underwent laser treatment for an extrafoveal recurrence. Benson et al have noted that repeat surgery was not associated with worse visual outcome. Photodynamic therapy may also play a role in controlling recurrences. Recurrent membranes should be treated with laser if extrafoveal and with either laser photo-coagulation or repeat surgery if juxtafoveal and with either repeat surgery, photodynamic therapy, or observation if the regrowth is central, however, the treatment protocol has significantly been changed in the present day practice.

FUTURE OF SUBMACULAR SURGERY

- With the conclusion of the submacular surgery trial, it has been established that the visual gain with submacular surgery in patients with AMD with classical CNV was not favourable.
- Surgery for hemorrhagic choroidal neo-vascular lesions of age-related macular degeneration did not increase the chance of stable or improved VA (the primary outcome of interest) and was associated with a high risk of rhegmatogenous RD, but did reduce the risk of severe VA loss in comparison with observation.
- Further with the availability and the favourable results (improvement of visual acuity and not just stabilisation) with anti-VEGF drugs and considering the invasive nature of the subretinal surgery, it has been used lesser and lesser in the present day practice.

BIBLIOGRAPHY

1. Adelberg DA, Del Priore LV, Kaplan HJ. Surgery for subfoveal membranes in myopia, angioid streaks and other disorders. Retina 1995; 15:198–205.

2. Akduman L, Del Priore LV, Desai VN, Olk RJ, Kaplan HJ. Perfusion of the subfoveal chorio-capillaris affects visual recovery after submacular surgery in presumed ocular histoplasmosis syndrome. Am J Ophthalmol 1997; 123(1):90–6.

3. Atebara NH, Thomas MA, Holekamp NM, Mandell BA, Del Priore LV. Surgical removal of extensive peripapillary choroidal neo-vasculari-zation associated with presumed ocular histo-plasmosis syndrome. Ophthalmology 1998; 105(6): 1598–605.

4. Avery RL, Fekrat S, Hawkins BS, Bressler NM. Natural history of subfoveal hemorrhage in age-related macular degeneration. Retina 1996; 16:183–9.

5. Bennett SR, Folk JC, Blodi CF, Klugman M. Factors prognostic of visual outcome in patients with subretinal hemorrhage. Am J Ophthalmol 1990; 109:33–7.

6. Benson MT, Callear A, Tsaloumas M, Chhina J, Beatty S. Surgical excision of subfoveal neovascular membranes. Eye 1998; 12:768–74.

7. Berger AS, Conway M, Del Priore LV, Walker RS, Pollack JS, Kaplan HJ. Submacular surgery for subfoveal choroidal neovascular membranes in patients with presumed ocular histo-plasmosis. Arch Ophthalmol 1997; 115:991–6.

8. Berger AS, Kaplan HJ. Clinical experience with the surgical removal of subfoveal neovascular membranes. Ophthalmology 1992; 99:969–76.

9. Berger AS, McCuen BW, Brown GC, Brownlow RL. Surgical removal of subfoveal neo-vascularization in idiopathic juxtafoveolar retinal telangiectasis. Retina 1997; 17(2): 94–8.

10. Berrocal MH, Lewis ML, Flynn HW. Variations in the clinical course of submacular hemorrhage. Am J Ophthalmol 1996; 122:486–93.

11. Blinder KJ, Peyman GA, Paris CL, Gremillion CM. Submacular scar excision in age-related macular degeneration. Int Ophthalmol 1991; 15:215–22.

12. Bottoni F, Perego E, Airaghi P, Cigada M, Ortolina S, Carlevaro G, et al. Surgical removal of subfoveal choroidal neovascular membranes in high myopia. Graefes Arch Clin Exp Ophthalmol 1999; 237(7):573–82.

13. Bressler NM, Bressler SB, Childs AL, Haller JA, Hawkins BS, Lewis H, MacCumber MW, Marsh MJ, Redford M, Sternberg P Jr, Thomas MA, Williams GA; Submacular Surgery Trials (SST) Research Group. Ophthalmology. 2004 Nov.; 111(11):1993–2006.

14. Castellarin AA, Nasir M, Sugino IK, Zarbin MA. Progressive presumed choriocapillaris atrophy after surgery for age-related macular degeneration. Retina 1998; 18(2):143–9.

15. Chen CJ, Urban LL, Nelson NC, Fratkin JD. Surgical removal of subfoveal iatrogenic choroidal neovascular membranes. Ophthalmology 1998; 105(9):1606–11.

16. De Juan E, Machemer R. Vitreous surgery for hemorrhagic and fibrous complications of age-related macular degeneration. Am J Ophthalmol 1988; 105:25–9.

17. Freund KB, Yannuzzi LA, Sorenson JA. Age-related macular degeneration and choroidal neovascularization. Am J Ophthalmol 1993; 115:786–91.

18. Gass JD. Biomicroscopic and histopathologic considerations regarding the feasibility of surgical excision of subfoveal neovascular membranes. Am J Ophthalmol 1994; 118:285–98.

19. Giovannini A, Amato GP, Mariotti C, Scassellati-Sforzolini B. OCT Imaging of choroidal neovascularization and its role in the determination of patients' eligibility for surgery. Br J Ophthalmol 1999; 83:438–42.

20. Giovannini A, Mariotti C, Scassellati-Sforzolini B, D'Altobrando E. Usefulness of fluorescein angiography in predicting the size of the atrophic area after surgical excision of choroidal neovascularization. Ophthalmologica 1999; 213:139–44.

21. Green WR, Enger C. Age-related macular degeneration histopathologic studies: the 1992 Lorenz E. Zimmerman Lecture. Ophthalmology 1993; 100:1519–35.

22. Grossniklaus HE, Gass JD. Clinicopathologic correlations of surgically excised type 1 and 2 type submacular choroidal neovascular membranes. Am J Ophthalmol 1998; 126 (1):59–69.

23. Hochman MA, Seery CM, Zarbin MA. Patho-physiology and management of subretinal hemorrhage. Surv Ophthalmol 1997; 42:195–213.

24. Holekamp NM, Thomas MA, Dickinson JD, Valluri S. Surgical removal of subfoveal choroidal neovascularization in presumed ocular histoplasmosis: stability of early visual results. Ophthalmology 1997; 104:22–6.

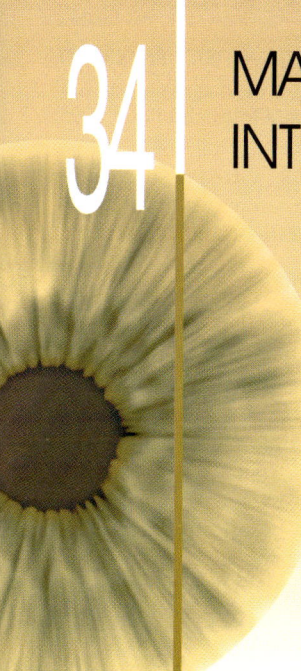

34 MANAGEMENT OF RETAINED INTRAOCULAR FOREIGN BODY

Atul Kumar

GENERAL CONSIDERATIONS

INTRODUCTION

Open-globe injuries with a retained intraocular foreign body (IOFB) may cause severe vision loss, either due to the trauma or due to secondary events related to IOFB. Currently use of commercially available pars plana vitrectomy and microsurgical techniques can maximize favorable outcomes. The combination of a standard 3-port pars plana vitrectomy with a wide-field viewing system, xenon illumination, and IOFB forceps, rare earth endomagnets allows the surgeon to efficiently and safely remove an IOFB, thus reducing the rate of complications. Furthermore, the addition of newer generation broad-spectrum systemic antibiotics has led to reduced rates of post-traumatic endophthalmitis.

HISTORICAL PERSPECTIVE

Historically, intraocular foreign body (magnetic) were removed through the pars plana using an external magnet, after a thorough and meticulous localisation with a limbal ring as a reference plane and radiograms taken in anteroposterior, and lateral views in various gazes. However, external magnetic extraction of metallic IOFB was associated with a high incidence of intraocular damage. With the development of the pars plana vitrectomy (PPV) and the addition of vitrectomy instrumentation and IOFB forceps both magnetic and non-magnetic IOFBs could be removed from the vitreous cavity with minimum collateral damage.

Intraocular foreign body removal was originally localized using scout films of the orbit. This technique has long been replaced by improvements in ultrasonography and computed tomography (CT) technology. The advances in CT have enabled better pre-operative planning by using improved resolution to determine the exact location and size of an IOFB.

Williams et al published the first large series of visual outcomes using PPV microsurgical

techniques, with 60% retaining better than 20/40 best-corrected visual acuity. Chow and colleagues found no difference in visual acuity when comparing an external magnet versus an internal PPV approach for IOFB removal. Over the last 10 years, numerous authors have published their experiences with IOFB removal using a PPV approach. Current IOFB removal techniques incorporate the most recent advances in PPV microsurgical instrumentation and technology.

METHODICAL STEPWISE APPROACH FOR OPEN-GLOBE INJURY WITH POSSIBLE IOFB

Open-globe injury with a possible IOFB should start with an extensive methodical stepwise approach. The first step is the IOFB preoperative planning and testing. An open-globe injury with a suspected retained IOFB needs a systemic evaluation to rule out any life threatening emergency if necessary (not needed in a chisel hammer type of injury but mandatory in blast victims). After ruling out any concomitant injury that may require more emergent attention, an extensive history should be obtained in the patient who is conscious and able to communicate. The surgeon should document the etiology of the injury; the type of material that may have entered the eye such as metallic (magnetic/nonmagnetic), nonorganic (stone), organic (plant/wood), or autologous (bone, cilia); time of injury; last meal; and allergy to penicillin.

A complete ophthalmic examination should include an initial visual acuity, pupillary examination to rule out an afferent pupillary defect, a slit lamp examination to rule out endophthalmitis, and a dilated fundus examination to possibly visualize the IOFB and rule out a retinal detachment. Intraocular pressure and B-scan ultrasonography may be deferred until the primary globe repair is completed to evaluate the retina and the choroid.

The surgeon should immediately order broad-spectrum antiobiotics. Today's top choices for IOFB endophthalmitis prophylaxis include

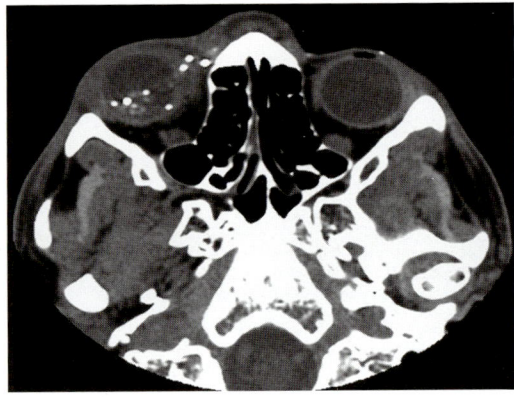

Fig. 34.1 *Axial CT scan of the orbit multiple foreign bodies*

moxifloxacin 400 mg intravenously/orally once per day or levofloxacin 500 mg intravenously/orally once per day. The minimum inhibitory concentration needed to inhibit the growth of 90% of organisms (MIC90) of these 2 antibiotics penetrating into the vitreous will cover most bacterial causes of post-traumatic endophthalmitis except *Pseudomonas aeruginosa* and *Bacillus cereus*.

The patient should have an urgent CT helical scan of the orbits and the brain (Fig. 34.1). The surgeon should rule out any intracranial foreign bodies or roof fractures that may need neurosurgical consultation. Depending on the etiology of the injury, orbital fractures may need otolaryngology consultation as well. The newer generation helical CT scans can reformat IOFB images in axial, coronal, and sagittal views. The high-resolution CT scan generate images as thin as 0.625 mm. The patient with a suspected open-globe injury without a foreign body on the CT scan, can then proceed to the operating room for primary globe repair.

Although CT scan is very sensitive in picking up RIOFB **ultrasonography** (Fig. 34.2) gives valuable information regarding site of impaction of foreign body status of posterior vitreous detachment, any associated retinal detachment, presence of concurrent vitreous hemorrhage or endophthalmitis.

PRIMARY REPAIR VERSUS TWO-STAGE OPERATION

The timing and type of surgery are the next major decisions in the management of an IOFB. The surgeon can either primarily close the open-

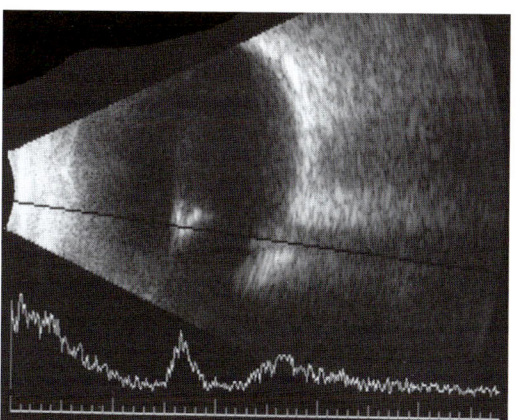

Fig. 34.2 *USG showing a hyperechoic RIOFB in the vitreous cavity with post-acoustic shadowing*

23/25-gauge PPV. Very small IOFBs less than 0.5 mm can be removed through the cannulas without enlarging the sclerotomy wounds. And in case of larger foreign bodies a hybrid 23 (two ports) and a 20 gauge port at the surgeons active hand may be used.

CONVENTIONAL 20 GAUGE VERSUS SMALL PORT VITRECTOMY

• *The 20-gauge PPV uses a microvitreoretinal blade* to create an incision in the sclera and can be enlarged if needed to remove the IOFB. The 20-gauge sutured sclerotomy PPV is better suited for most IOFB injuries, unlike the insertion of a 23-/25-gauge trocar, the intraocular pressure does not increase.

• *Trocar insertion in IOFB cases* may exacerbate a traumatic optic neuropathy, worsen corneal edema, and cause wound leakage from a recent primary globe closure (all these complications are often pre-existing in cases with RIOFB).

• *Suprachoroidal hemorrhage* has been documented in 6% of IOFB cases. Visual outcomes after a suprachoroidal hemorrhage are extremely poor, with high rates of no light perception visual acuity, chronic post-operative hypotony, and non-repairable retinal detachment.

• *At the beginning of the PPV, a vitreous sample* can be obtained and sent for immediate Gram stain and culture. Intraocular foreign body removal will start with a pars plana lensectomy, if associated with a traumatic cataract. The anterior capsule not damaged by the IOFB should remain intact for possible future intraocular lens (IOLs).

The most conservative approach is to leave the eye surgically aphakic and return for secondary IOL implantation 3 to 6 months after IOFB removal. The other option in the case of a RIOFB without any evidence of endophthalmitis is a preparatory phacoemulsification which can be done with IOL, provided the foreign body is less than 5 mm × 5 mm × 5 mm.

• *IOL implantation at the time of IOFB* has many pitfalls. The IOL may be subluxated postoperative by the gas tamponade used for retinal detachment repair. The IOL may develop synechiae to the iris during the immediate

globe and secondarily remove the IOFB or combine both surgeries at the same time. An open-globe injury with a retained IOFB must be stable for extended surgery if both a globe repair and IOFB are planned together. An open-globe repair, IOFB removal, and intravitreal antibiotics are necessary with a post-traumatic endophthalmitis.

A very important factor is the availability of trained operating room personnel who are skilled in assisting during very complicated and lengthy primary open-globe closure and IOFB removal cases. Operating with unskilled personnel after hours may not be the safest setting for an IOFB removal; therefore, primary globe closure with secondary IOFB removal may be a safer option in certain circumstances. Corneal clarity is also a very important consideration when determining primary globe closure with or without IOFB removal. Corneal edema and stromal haze improve dramatically from 7 to 10 days after primary globe repair.

Once the surgeon decides to remove an IOFB, the operating room planning must include the necessary equipment and supplies needed for the surgical case. The first step is to decide whether the IOFB is isolated in the anterior segment and can be safely removed through a limbal incision and intralenticular IOFBs can be removed after a lens aspiration.

Retained IOFBs in the posterior segment will require a PPV. The vitreoretinal surgeon may choose from a 20-gauge PPV or a small gauge

postoperative period, with permanent changes in the pupil. The artificial IOL implant may lead to a higher risk of delayed endophthalmitis, considering the fact that a contaminated foreign body was removed from the eye at the time of IOL implantation.

• *Once core vitrectomy is performed,* it is important to achieve a complete posterior hyaloid separation from the posterior pole and also from the foreign body site so as to prevent iatrogenic breaks while foreign body retrieval. The methods of posterior hyaloids separation are beyond the scope of this chapter.

• *The size of the IOFB* is the most important factor in determining the instrumentation for IOFB removal. A magnetic metallic IOFB less than 1 × 1 × 1 mm in dimension is most easily removed using a positive action IOFB endomagnet (Grieshaber). This instrument uses the magnet to capture the small IOFB and retracts the IOFB into a sleeve before removal from the sclerotomy site. This prevents the IOFB from catching on the edge of sclerotomy and falling back into the eye. Intraocular foreign body ranging in size from 1 to 3 mm regardless of composition is best removed with a Grieshaber Pannarale basket forceps (Fig. 34.3). The Grieshaber Machemer diamond-coated foreign body forceps (Fig. 34.4) are very commonly used in our set up and they are useful for grabbing an IOFB that is 3 to 5 mm in smallest dimension and are necessary when removing large pieces of glass off the macula. The diamond coating prevents slippage of smooth foreign bodies during retrieval.

• *Sclerotomy incisions* larger than 5 mm tend to leak fluid faster than infusion through a 20-gauge infusion line. Globe collapse prevents

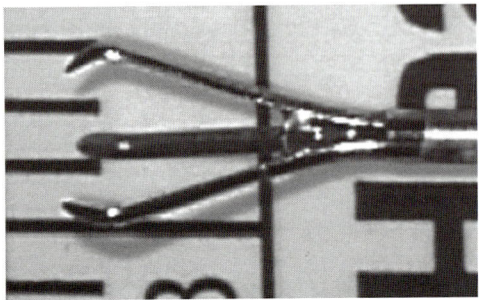

Fig. 34.3 *Pannarale basket foreign body retrieval forceps*

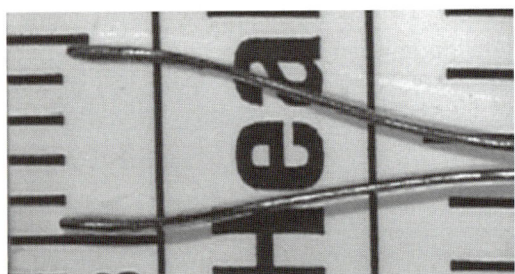

Fig. 34.4 *Diamond dusted Machemer foreign body forceps*

observation and safe removal of an IOFB. IOFBs requiring larger than 5 mm sclerotomy should be retrieved through a sclera tunnel/limbal incision.

• *Corneal clarity* is the most important aspect of intraocular foreign body removal. Injured corneas become more edematous as IOFB cases progress. Particular attention to intraocular pressure is imperative to reduce progression of corneal edema.

• *The illumination of the retina during PPV* has significantly improved visualization of IOFBs and retinal tears.

– *The newer generation xenon light* sources enable the surgeon to see past an edematous cornea and safely retrieve IOFBs. Xenon-illuminated laser probes enable the management of retinal tears and detachments especially when used in conjunction with perfluoro-n-octane.

– *Chandelier light sources* are also commercially available to perform bimanual removal of large IOFBs.

– *Preservative-free intraoperative triamcinolone* is extremely useful in identifying residual cortical vitreous through an edematous cornea.

• *Without signs of retinal injury, the globe can be left with balanced salt solution,* and the sclerotomies closed with Vicryl 7-0. Air may be used as a tamponade after laser retinopexy for retinal tears.

• *After IOFB removal, retinal detachments* may be repaired in the standard fashion with or without an encircling band. Intraocular foreign body related retinal detachments can be repaired with sulfur hexafluoride (SF6), perfluoropropane (C3F8), or silicone oil (1000 or 5000 centistoke) depending on the severity of

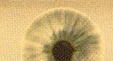

the injury. The most severe IOFB-related retinal detachments and perforating injuries need silicone oil for long-term tamponade to prevent the effects of proliferative vitreoretinopathy.

SCHEMATIC OUTLINE OF FOREIGN BODY

Figure 34.1 summarizes the schematic outline of foreign body removal.

Open globe injury with possible IOFB

Initiate broad-spectrum antibiotics, (e.g. moxifloxacin and gatifloxacin)

History and ophthalmic examination, without IOP or B-scan ultrasound

CT orbits without contrast, is an IOFB visulized on CT? Size? Location? → No IOFB → Primary globe repair

+ IOFB

1. Is patient stable for extended surgery?
2. Does the eye have an active infection?
3. Is operating room personnel equipped to safely remove IOFB?

Yes → Primary closure with IOFB removal

No → Consider primary closure with delayed IOFB removal

Perform complete vitrectomy to safely free IOFB from vitreous base/adhesions, +/− cataract extraction if poor view

*Stat gram stain/Cx, intravitreal vancomycin/ceftazidime unless fungal/atypical organisms found

IOFB removal strategies: size?, material?

<1.0 mm, magnetic → Magnet

1–3 mm, stone → Basket forceps

3–5 mm, glass → IOFB diamond-coated forceps

IOFB removal site: is IOFB > 4 × 4 × 4 mm?
Yes → Scleral tunnel
No → Sclerotomy

IOL: is there adequate capsule for an intraocular lens implant?
Yes → Implant intraocular lens
No → Leave aphakia

Temponade: is there a retinal tear, RD, or choroidal?
RT → Laser, air
No → Balanced salt solution

RT/RD → RD repair, SF$_6$, C$_3$F$_3$

RD/choroidal → RD repair, silicone oil

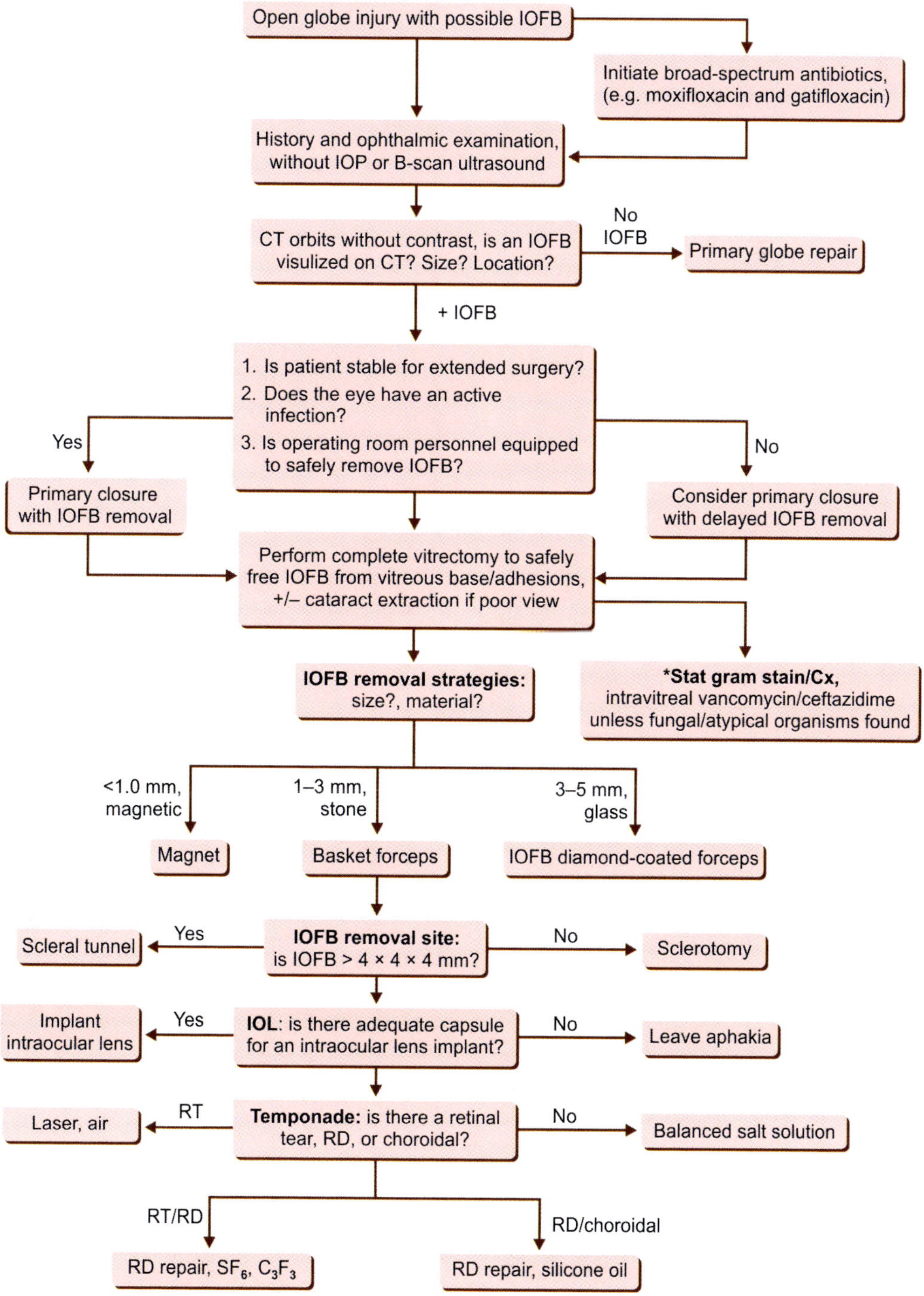

Fig. 34.1: *Schematic outline of foreign body removal*

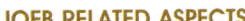

IOFB RELATED ASPECTS

Visual outcomes after IOFB injury

Visual outcomes after IOFB injury can vary depending on other concomitant globe injuries. Preoperative visual acuity is usually reduced by traumatic cataract or vitreous hemorrhage. These 2 media opacities are removed during IOFB removal. The major contributing factors for long term poor visual acuity are traumatic optic neuropathy, corneal scarring, residual effects of post-traumatic endophthalmitis, and suprachoroidal hemorrhage as well as proliferative vitreoretinopathy (PVR) causing irreparable chronic retinal detachment.

Most common type of IOFB injury

Most common type of IOFB injury involves a small corneal laceration with traumatic cataract and vitreous hemorrhage in more than 50% of these cases. These IOFB injuries have excellent visual recovery, with most obtaining best-corrected visual acuity 20/40.

Corneal scarring and astigmatism

Corneal scarring and astigmatism are significant factors for vision loss after an IOFB injury. Anterior segment reconstruction for a traumatic iridodialysis is commonly repaired using a double-armed McCannell suture to repair a sectoral iris defect. Aniridia IOL can be used to manage traumatic aniridia with symptomatic photophobia. Traumatic optic neuropathy can be followed using visual field or multifocal visual evoked potential testing.

The rate of preoperative retinal detachment

The rate of preoperative retinal detachment associated with an IOFB has been reported at 31%. Intraocular foreign body removal associated with a retinal detachment can be extremely complicated, especially with subretinal IOFBs located away from the entry site of the IOFB. Its been found that an IOFB left in the subretinal space after PPV is a nidus for PVR formation regardless of IOFB composition and recommend removing a subretinal IOFB through the existing retinal hole or another retinotomy site. Postoperative IOFB-related retinal detachment can also contribute to poor visual outcome, with large IOFB and endophthalmitis as the strongest predictive factors.

Late rhegmatogenous retinal detachments

Late rhegmatogenous retinal detachments have been documented after posterior segment IOFB removal. Proliferative vitreoretinopathy is another major risk factor for vision loss after an IOFB injury. Cardillo and colleagues reported an 11% rate of PVR after IOFB, with vitreous hemorrhage as a major risk factor. PVR can lead to chronic non-repairable total retinal detachment, with resulting phthisis bulbi and enucleation. Increased depth of IOFB penetration and more extensive, intraocular injuries are associated with higher rates of PVR. Intraocular foreign body injuries, which penetrate through the retina, develop PVR in up to 75% of the cases. On the contrary, an IOFB, that penetrates into the vitreous cavity or ricochets off the retina surface, only carries roughly a 5% rate of PVR formation.

Post-traumatic endophthalmitis

Post-traumatic endophthalmitis has historically averaged 4 to 8% of all IOFB injuries, with up to 30% in rural settings. Bacteria such as *B. cereus*, *Staphylococcus aureus*, *Streptococcus pneumonia*, and *Pseudomonas aeruginosa* can lead to extremely poor visual results. Reported risks factors for post-traumatic endophthalmitis include delay in primary closure, delay in IOFB removal, disruption of the crystalline lens, and sustaining ocular trauma in a rural setting.

Clinical features associated with favorable visual acuity outcomes

Clinical features associated with favorable visual acuity outcomes in post-traumatic endophthalmitis include better presenting visual acuity, culture of a non-virulent organism, lack of a retinal detachment, absence of clinical endophthalmitis, and shorter wound length.

Broad-spectrum systemic antiobiotics

Broad-spectrum systemic antiobiotics with third- or fourth-generation fluoroquinolones have been increasingly used by ophthalmologists after open-globe injuries. The levels of orally administered fluoroquinolones in the

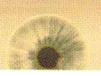

aqueous and vitreous have been shown to exceed the MIC90 of the major organisms causing post-traumatic endophthalmitis.

Meta-analysis of all published post-traumatic endophthalmitis

Meta-analysis of all published post-traumatic endophthalmitis cases reported an average rate of 8.7% in open-globe injuries. Recent published studies have suggested a reduction in this rate of post-traumatic endophthalmitis of 1 to 2% over the last 10 years.

Non-reactive or encapsulated and fixed intraocular foreign bodies

Ocassionally there might be some delayed presentation of retained intraocular foreign body in which the foreign body although metallic but with well-formed encapsulation, or totally inert foreign bodies like large graphite foreign bodies (pencil leads) rubber pellets which are fixed in the vitreous or a few foreign bodies which have pierced in the optic nerve head which carry a huge risk of torrential hemorrhage with attempted removal, these kind of foreign bodies can be safely left alone and the patient can be monitored with clinical examination and electrophysiological test like electroretinogram (ERG) and VER (visually evoked potentials). Intervention can be planned if there is a risk of retinal detachment/endophthalmitis.

CONCLUSION

Current IOFB removal techniques have advanced with improving imaging using ultrasound and helical CT scan for localisation and preoperative planning and improved PPV technology and instrumentation combined with newer broad-spectrum antibiotics. All these put together have improved visual outcome and mitigated complications from IOFB injuries.

BIBLIOGRAPHY

1. Al-Omran AM, Abboud EB, Abu El-Asrar AM. Microbiologic spectrum and visual outcome of post-traumatic endophthalmitis. Retina 2007; 27(2): 236–42.

2. Boldt HC, Pulido JS, Blodi CF, et al. Rural endophthalmitis. Ophthalmology 1989; 96(12): 1722–26.

3. Chow DR, Garretson BR, Kuczynski B, et al. External versus internal approach to the removal of metallic intraocular foreign bodies. Retina. 2000;20(4):364–9.

4. Coleman DJ, Lucas BC, Rondeau MJ, et al. Management of intraocular foreign bodies. Ophthalmology 1987; 94(12): 1647–53.

5. Colyer MH, Weber ED, Weichel ED, et al. Delayed intraocular foreign body removal without endophthalmitis during Operations Iraqi Freedom and Enduring Freedom. Ophthalmology 2007; 114(8):1439–47.

6. de Smet MD, Mura M. Minimally invasive surgery vs endoscopic retinal detachment repair in patients with media opacities. Eye 2008; 22(5):662–5.

7. De Souza S, Howcroft MJ. Management of posterior segment intraocular foreign bodies: 14 years' experience. Can J Ophthalmol 1999; 34(1):23–9.

8. El-Asrar AM, Al-Amro SA, Khan NM, et al. Retinal detachment after posterior segment intraocular foreign body injuries. Int Ophthalmol 1998; 22(6): 369–75.

9. El-Asrar AM, Al-Amro SA, Khan NM, et al. Visual outcome and prognostic factors after vitrectomy for posterior segment foreign bodies. Eur J Ophthalmol 2000; 10(4):304–11.

10. Ersanli D, Sonmez M, Unal M, et al. Management of retinal detachment due to closed globe injury by pars plana vitrectomy with and without scleral buckling. Retina 2006; 26(1): 32–6.

11. Fison PN, Chignell AH. Diplopia after retinal detachment surgery. Br J Ophthalmol 1987; 71(7): 521–5.

12. Gallemore RP, Bokosky JE. Penetrating keratoplasty with vitreoretinal surgery using the Eckardt temporary keratoprosthesis: modified technique allowing use of larger corneal grafts. Cornea 1995; 14(1): 33–38.

13. Gelender H, Vaiser A, Snyder WB, et al. Temporary keratoprosthesis for combined penetrating keratoplasty, pars plana vitrectomy, and repair of retinal detachment. Ophthalmology 1988; 95(7): 897–901.

14. Greven CM, Engelbrecht NE, Slusher MM, et al. Intraocular foreign bodies: management, prognostic factors, and visual outcomes. Ophthalmology 2000; 107(3): 608–12.

15. Hariprasad SM, Shah GK, Mieler WF, et al. Vitreous and aqueous penetration of orally administered moxifloxacin in humans. Arch Ophthalmol 2006; 124(2):178–182.

16. Imrie FR, Cox A, Foot B, et al. Surveillance of intraocular foreign bodies in the UK. Eye. May 25, 2007.

17. Irvine AR. Old and new techniques combined in the management of intraocular foreign bodies. Ann Ophthalmol 1981; 13(1):41–7.

18. Jonas JB, Budde WM. Early versus late removal of retained intraocular foreign bodies. Retina 1999; 19(3): 193–7.

19. Jonas JB, Knorr HL, Budde WM. Prognostic factors inocular injuries caused by intraocular or retrobulbar foreignbodies. Ophthalmology 2000; 107(5):823–8.

20. Klistorner A, Fraser C, Garrick R, et al. Correlation between full-field and multifocal VEPs in optic neuritis. Doc Ophthalmol 2008; 116(1): 19–27.

21. Kramer M, Kramer MR, Blau H, et al. Intravitreal Voriconazole for the treatment of endogenous Aspergillus endophthalmitis. Ophthalmology 2006; 113(7): 1184–86.

22. Kuhn F, Morris R. Posterior segment intraocular foreign bodies: management in the vitrectomy era. Ophthalmology 2000; 107(5): 821–2.

23. Kwong JS, Munk PL, Lin DT, et al. Real-time Sonography in ocular trauma. AJR Am J Roentgenol 1992; 158(1) 179–182.

24. Lakits A, Prokesch R, Scholda C, et al. Multiplanar imaging in the preoperative assessment of metallic intraocular foreign bodies. Helical computed tomography versus conventional computed tomography. Ophthalmology 1998; 105(9): 1679–85.

25. Lieb DF, Scott IU, Flynn HW Jr, et al. Open globe injurieswith positive intraocular cultures: factors influencing final visual acuity outcomes. Ophthalmology 2003; 110(8): 1560–66.

26. Machemer R. A new concept for vitreous surgery; Surgical technique and complications. Am J Ophthalmol 1972; 74(6): 1022–33.

27. Pavlovic S. Primary intraocular lens implantation duringpars plana vitrectomy and intraretinal foreign body removal. Retina 1999; 19(5): 430–6.

Index

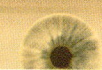

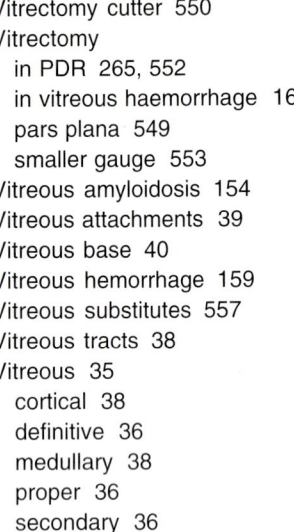